ELECTROENCEPHALOGRAPHY AND CLINICAL NEUROPHYSIOLOGY

Volume 27 (1969)

"THE EEG JOURNAL"

ELECTROENCEPHALOGRAPHY and CLINICAL NEUROPHYSIOLOGY

Official Organ of the International Federation of Societies for Electroencephalography and Clinical Neurophysiology

This Journal was founded in 1947 by an International Committee of EEG Societies. Publication began in 1949, with H. H. Jasper as first Editor, and in the same year the Journal became the official organ of the International Federation of Societies for Electroencephalography and Clinical Neurophysiology, then set up by the above Committee.

Although the electrical activity of the brain is the central theme of this Journal, studies of the spinal and peripheral nervous systems are welcomed, particularly those concerned with the clinical and experimental electrophysiology of muscle and nerve.

To reach the largest proportion of readers, communications must be submitted in English. In special circumstances manuscripts in French will be considered for publication. Each manuscript must be accompanied by a summary in English and may also have summaries in French, German or Spanish if the author wishes. Proceedings of EEG Societies must be submitted in English and will be published exclusively in that language.

SUBMISSION OF PAPERS:
Manuscripts from the Americas and the Far East should be sent to:
Dr. Peter Kellaway, Editor, The EEG Journal,
Baylor College of Medicine, Houston, Texas 77025, U.S.A.

Manuscripts from Europe, the Middle East and Africa should be sent to:
Dr. W. A. Cobb, Editor, The EEG Journal,
The National Hospital, Queen Square, London W.C.1, England.

BOOKS FOR REVIEW should be sent to the *Consulting Editors for Book Reviews;*
from Europe, the Middle East and Africa to:
Dr. H. Petsche
Neurologisches Institut der Universität, Schwarzspanierstrasse 17, Wien IX, Österreich
and from the Americas and the Far East to:
Dr. J. R. Hughes
Northwestern University Medical Center, Ward Memorial Building, 303 E. Chicago Avenue, Chicago, Illinois 60611, U.S.A.

SUBSCRIPTION: The subscription rate is Dfl. 41.40 per volume (plus Dfl. 3.60 postage and handling). Additional charges for copies by air mail are available on request. Two volumes appear per year in monthly issues. Subscriptions, advertisements, payments and all business correspondence should be addressed to:
Elsevier Publishing Company, P.O. Box 211, Amsterdam, The Netherlands.

"INSTRUCTIONS TO AUTHORS" SHOULD BE READ BEFORE SUBMITTING ANY MANUSCRIPT FOR PUBLICATION (1964, 16: 318–320. Reprints available from either regional Editor on request). Failure to comply with them may result in the return of the manuscript. The Editors will consider manuscripts only if two complete copies of text and figures are submitted.

ELECTROENCEPHALOGRAPHY

AND

CLINICAL NEUROPHYSIOLOGY

JOURNAL OF THE INTERNATIONAL FEDERATION OF SOCIETIES FOR ELECTROENCEPHALOGRAPHY AND CLINICAL NEUROPHYSIOLOGY

VOL. 27 1969

ELSEVIER PUBLISHING COMPANY
AMSTERDAM

ELSEVIER PUBLISHING COMPANY, AMSTERDAM

PRINTED IN THE NETHERLANDS

TABLE OF CONTENTS

VOLUME 27, 1969

Page

EDITORIAL 1

PROCEEDINGS OF THE 7TH INTERNATIONAL CONGRESS 641

MAIN ARTICLES

Electroencephalographic activity after prolonged sleep loss
by P. NAITOH, A. KALES, E. J. KOLLAR, J. C. SMITH and A. JACOBSON (San Diego and Los Angeles, Calif., U.S.A.) 2

Changes of the EEG, intracranial pressure and other variables during sleep in patients with intracranial lesions
by R. COOPER and A. HULME (Bristol, Great Britain) 12

The average visual response in patients with cerebrovascular disease
by H. J. G. H. OOSTERHUIS, L. PONSEN, E. J. JONKMAN and O. MAGNUS (Wassenaar, The Netherlands) 23

Variability of the human visual evoked potential: normative data
by L. CIGÁNEK (Bratislava, Czechoslovakia) 35

Rhythmic mid-temporal discharges. An electro-clinical study
by I. J. LIPMAN and J. R. HUGHES (Chicago, Ill., U.S.A.) 43

Étude des effets électrophysiologiques de la psilocybine chez un cercopithecinae, *Papio papio*
par F. BERMOND et J. BERT (Dakar, Sénégal) 48

Frequency analysis of EEG during milk drinking
by N. W. GRANDSTAFF (Stanford, Calif., U.S.A.) 57

Frequency control of motor unit action potentials
by J. H. PETAJAN and B. A. PHILIP (College, Alaska, U.S.A.) 66

Relationship of slow potential changes to response speed and motivation in man
by M. WASZAK and W. D. OBRIST (Durham, N.C., U.S.A.). 113

Acoustic evoked responses in newborn infants: the influence of pitch and complexity of the stimulus
by H. G. LENARD, H. VON BERNUTH and S. J. HUTT (Groningen, The Netherlands) 121

EEG sleep patterns in mental retardation
by I. FEINBERG, M. BRAUN and E. SHULMAN (Brooklyn, N.Y., U.S.A.) 128

Averaged visual evoked potentials in humans: mechanism of dichoptic interaction studied in a subject with a split chiasma
by D. LEHMANN and D. H. FENDER (San Francisco and Pasadena, Calif., U.S.A.) . . 142

Comparison of evoked gross and unit responses in association cortex of waking cat
by R. F. THOMPSON, L. A. BETTINGER, H. BIRCH and P. M. GROVES (Irvine, Calif., U.S.A.) 146

TABLE OF CONTENTS VOLUME 27, 1969

MAIN ARTICLES

Page

Slow potential changes in cat brain during classical appetitive and aversive conditioning of jaw movement
by C. S. REBERT and D. A. IRWIN (Iowa City, Iowa, U.S.A.) 152

The influence of intra-hippocampal gamma-aminobutyric acid on the orienting reflex
by R. ROGOZEA, J. UNGHER and V. FLOREA-CIOCOIU (Bucharest, Rumania) 162

Variations in human physiological finger tremor, with particular reference to changes with age
by C. D. MARSDEN, J. C. MEADOWS, G. W. LANGE and R. S. WATSON (London and Teddington, Great Britain) 169

The relation between physiological tremor of the two hands in healthy subjects
by C. D. MARSDEN, J. C. MEADOWS, G. W. LANGE and R. S. WATSON (London and Teddington, Great Britain) 179

EEG response to photic stimulation as a function of cognitive style
by W. VOGEL, D. M. BROVERMAN, E. L. KLAIBER and K. J. KUN (Worcester, Mass., U.S.A.) 186

Aspects dynamiques de l'électroencéphalogramme humain.
Premiers résultats d'une étude radio-télémétrique
par G. ARFEL, C. CASANOVA et M. COULMANCE (Suresnes, France) 225

Selective suppression of cerebral evoked potentials to patterned light in amblyopia ex anopsia
by C. T. LOMBROSO, H. F. DUFFY and R. M. ROBB (Boston, Mass., U.S.A.) . . . 238

Changes induced in stabilized image visibility by experimental alteration of the ongoing EEG
by U. T. KEESEY and D. J. NICHOLS (Madison, Wisc., U.S.A.) 248

Modifications des activités évoquées corticales et thalamiques au cours d'un conditionnement sensoriel. I. Localisation des réponses et variations avec la vigilance
par G. LELORD et C. MAHO (Paris, France) 258

Modifications des activités évoquées corticales et thalamiques au cours d'un conditionnement sensoriel. II. Évolution des réponses avec les stades du conditionnement
par G. LELORD et C. MAHO (Paris, France) 270

Long-term EEG changes during direct cortical stimulation
by M. J. O'CONNOR, M. ROSENTHAL and F. F. JÖBSIS (Durham, N.C., U.S.A.) . . 280

Functional changes of somato-sensory system during deep sleep
by C. CASATI, N. DAGNINO, E. FAVALE, M. MANFREDI, A. SEITUN and A. TARTAGLIONE (Genoa and Sassari, Italy) 289

Action of drugs on the electrical activity of the red nucleus
by G. GOGOLÁK, G. LIEBESWAR and CH. STUMPF (Vienna, Austria) 296

Electroencephalographic findings in experimentally induced intracranial hypertension
by S. L. H. NOTERMANS and S. BOONSTRA (Groningen, The Netherlands) 337

Human vigilance and auditory evoked responses
by H. FRUHSTORFER and R. M. BERGSTRÖM (Helsinki, Finland) 346

Effect of LSD on visually evoked responses to color in visualizer and non-visualizer subjects
by B. B. BROWN (Sepulveda and Orange, Calif., U.S.A.) 356

TABLE OF CONTENTS VOLUME 27, 1969

MAIN ARTICLES Page

The visual evoked response: a comparison of bright and dull children
by L. E. Rhodes, R. E. Dustman and E. C. Beck (Salt Lake City, Utah, U.S.A.) 364

Evoked visual, somato-sensory and retinal potentials in photosensitive epilepsy
by R. Broughton, K.-H. Meier-Ewert and M. Ebe (Montreal, Canada) 373

EEG spikes and the averaged evoked response to clicks and flashes
by E. M. Ornitz, E. R. Ritvo, P. E. Tanguay and R. D. Walter (Los Angeles, Calif., U.S.A.) 387

An analysis of the effect of 1,2-dihydroxybenzene on transmission through the dorsal column sensory pathway
by A. Angel (London, Great Britain) 392

Effect of brain-stem lesions on Metrazol-induced seizures in cats
by D. Jinnai, H. Mogami, J. Mukawa, Y. Iwata and K. Kobayashi (Osaka, Japan) 404

Thalamo-cortical recruiting responses during sleep characterized by a low voltage fast EEG
by I. Lehtinen and P. Valleala (Turku, Finland) 412

Alterations of the human electroencephalogram induced by stressful verbal activity
by J. Berkhout, D. O. Walter and W. R. Adey (Los Angeles, Calif., U.S.A.) . . 457

EEG changes during performance of various tasks under open- and closed-eyed conditions
by H. Legewie, O. Simonova and O. D. Creutzfeldt (Munich, West Germany) . 470

EEG average frequency and intelligence
by D. Giannitrapani (Chicago, Ill., U.S.A.) 480

Electrophysiological and behavioural changes owing to splitting of the brain-stem in cats
by M. Mancia (Milan, Italy) 487

Discrimination of behavioral state in the cat utilizing long-term EEG frequency analysis
by M. D. Fairchild, D. J. Jenden and M. R. Mickey (Long Beach and Los Angeles, Calif., U.S.A.) 503

Reticular multiple unit activity during a progression of states induced by CNS excitants. III
by W. D. Winters, K. Mori, M. B. Wallach, R. J. Marcus and C. E. Spooner (Los Angeles, Calif., U.S.A.) 514

EEG changes in Wilson's disease
by P. Hansotia, R. Harris and J. Kennedy (London, Great Britain) 523

The effect of non-paralytic doses of D-tubocurarine on individual motor end-plates in man, studied with a new electrophysiological method
by J. Ekstedt and E. Stålberg (Uppsala, Sweden) 557

A correlation of EEG, reticular multiple unit activity and gross behavior following various antidepressant agents in the cat. IV
by M. B. Wallach, W. D. Winters, A. J. Mandell and C. E. Spooner (Los Angeles, Calif., U.S.A.) 563

Effects of antidepressant drugs on wakefulness and sleep in the cat
by M. B. Wallach, W. D. Winters, A. J. Mandell and C. E. Spooner (Los Angeles, Calif., U.S.A.) 574

TABLE OF CONTENTS VOLUME 27, 1969

MAIN ARTICLES Page

Effects of lowered body temperature on hyperoxic seizures
by M. L. GIRETTI, F. S. RUCCI and M. LA ROCCA (Sassari, Sardinia, Italy) 581

Primary auditory evoked potentials after section of brachium of the inferior colliculus
by J. MAJKOWSKI and P. P. MORGADES (New York, N. Y., U.S.A.). 587

A test of an "efferent model" of the function of inferotemporal cortex in visual discrimination
by P. A. SCHWARTZKROIN, A. COWEY and C. G. GROSS (Cambridge, Mass., U.S.A.) . 594

CLINICAL AND LABORATORY NOTES

Bereitschaftspotential enhancement with increased level of motivation
by D. W. MCADAM and D. M. SEALES (Rochester, N.Y., U.S.A.) 73

Digital computer classifications of EEG sleep stages
by T. M. ITIL, D. M. SHAPIRO, M. FINK and D. KASSEBAUM (St. Louis, Mo., U.S.A.) 76

Modified pupillary diameter and evoked potential component variation in waking cats
by D. E. FLEMING (Phoenix, Ariz., U.S.A.) 84

EEG patterns in juvenile cerebral lipidosis
by R. J. ELLINGSON and R. J. SCHAIN (Omaha, Neb., U.S.A.). 191

The auditory evoked response in babies during REM sleep
by E. M. ORNITZ, E. R. RITVO, Y. H. LEE, L. M. PANMAN, R. D. WALTER and A. MASON (Los Angeles, Calif., U.S.A.). 195

The influence of end-tidal carbon dioxide tension on EEG changes during routine hyperventilation in different age groups
by C. D. BINNIE, P. A. COLES and J. H. MARGERISON (London, Great Britain) . . 304

Behavioural and EEG arousal induced by stimulation of unspecific projection systems in a patient with post-traumatic apallic syndrome
by R. HASSLER, G. DALLE ORE, G. DIECKMANN, A. BRICOLO and G. DOLCE (Verona, Italy and Frankfurt/M., W. Germany) 306

Spontaneous sleep in healthy subjects in long-term serial electroencephalographic recordings
by P. F. PRIOR and P. A. DEACON (Sittingbourne, Kent, Great Britain) 422

Cortical evoked potentials in hepatolenticular degeneration
by H. LÜDERS, M. KATO and Y. KUROIWA (Fukuoka, Japan). 425

Effects of intravenous diazepam (Valium) upon evoked potentials of photosensitive epileptic and normal subjects
by M. EBE, K.-H. MEIER-EWERT and R. BROUGHTON (Montreal, Canada) 429

Effects of *para*-chlorophenylalanine on sleep in man
by R. J. WYATT, K. ENGELMAN, D. J. KUPFER, J. SCOTT, A. SJOERDSMA and F. SNYDER (Bethesda, Md., U.S.A.). 529

The Kleine-Levin syndrome with intermittent abnormality in the EEG
by M. ELIAN and B. BORNSTEIN (Petah Tikva, Israel) 601

The EEG in a case of periodic hypersomnia
by V. R. THACORE, M. AHMED and I. OSWALD (Lucknow, India, and Edinburgh, Great Britain) 605

Abnormal connections between skeletal muscle fibers
by J. EKSTEDT and E. STÅLBERG (Uppsala, Sweden) 607

TABLE OF CONTENTS VOLUME 27, 1969

TECHNICAL CONTRIBUTIONS

Page

A novel method for preparing and implanting brain electrode assemblies in rats
by A. SAYERS and G. STILLE (Berne, Switzerland) 87

Behavioral experimental epilepsy in monkeys. II. Video-tape control gate for the detection and recording of motor seizures
by R. I. BARENSTEN and J. S. LOCKARD (Seattle, Wash., U.S.A.). 89

Specular reflectance photometric detection of cortical displacement
by C. TEAGUE, J. ELFERT, G. TIMM and W. BRADLEY (Minneapolis, Minn., U.S.A.). . 92

Z-axis modulation in neural spike display
by C. J. CONWAY and W. E. BRADLEY (Minneapolis, Minn., U.S.A.) 199

Multi-barreled coaxial micro-pipettes with independent control of the central recording barrel
by R. SPEHLMANN (Chicago, Ill., U.S.A.) 201

A technique for the chronic implantation of multiple movable micro-electrodes
by E. R. JOHN and P. P. MORGADES (New York, N.Y.). 205

A printed circuit swivel for recording from freely moving animals
by A. EDELSON and T. L. HOLDSTOCK (Johannesburg, S. Africa). 209

Discriminant analysis in average evoked response studies: the study of single trial data
by E. DONCHIN (Moffett Field, Calif., U.S.A.) 311

Étude du bruit résiduel des potentiels évoqués moyens
par D. ARNAL et P. GERIN (Lyon, France) 315

A method for detecting change in a time series applied to newborn EEG
by R. H. JONES, D. H. CROWELL and L. E. KAPUNIAI (Honolulu, Hawaii, U.S.A.) 436

An electrode for the study of lingual sensitivity
by D. A. MAJEAU and A. K. PLEASONTON (New Orleans, La., U.S.A.) 440

Implantation of sterile electrodes in chronic animals
by V. MILSTEIN (Portland, Ore., U.S.A.) 442

On-line analysis of EEG with a small computer (period–amplitude analysis)
by H. LEGEWIE and W. PROBST (Munich, West Germany) 533

Oscilloscopic recording of muscle fiber action potentials. The window trigger and the delay unit
by J. CZEKAJEWSKI, J. EKSTEDT and E. STÅLBERG (Uppsala, Sweden) 536

The construction of needle multi-electrodes for single fiber electromyography
by J. EKSTEDT, P. HÄGGQVIST and E. STÅLBERG (Uppsala, Sweden) 540

Micro-electrode tip position marking in nervous tissue: a new dye method
by B. B. LEE, G. MANDL and J. P. B. STEAN (London, Great Britain) 610

A stereotaxic frame assembly for investigating the cat auditory system
by C. W. DUNLOP (Sydney, N.S.W., Australia). 614

BOOK REVIEWS

Structure and function of the limbic system
edited by W. R. ADEY and T. TOKIZANE 110

BOOK REVIEWS Page

The brain stem of the cat
by A. L. BERMAN 111

Neurologie des Neugeborenen
by G. JOPPICH and F. J. SCHULTE. 112

Physiological basis of the alpha rhythm
by P. ANDERSEN and S. A. ANDERSSON 222

An atlas of pathological pneumoencephalographic anatomy
by G. DI CHIRO, M. M. SCHECTER and I. WICKBOM 223

Hypothalamus und Thalamus. Experimental-Dokumente
by W. R. HESS 224

Neurophysiological basis of normal and abnormal motor activities
edited by M. D. YAHR and D. P. PURPURA. 336

Klinische Elektroenzephalographie. Lehrbuch und Atlas
by W. CHRISTIAN 453

Elektricheskie reakcii mozga na tormoznye signaly [Electrical reactions of the brain to inhibitory signals]
by J. G. KRATIN. 453

Cerebral circulation
edited by W. LUYENDIJK 454

Hepatocerebral circulation
by H. ASAO and K. OJI 456

Atlas des Mittel- und Zwischenhirns des Kaninchens. Atlas of the mes- and diencephalon of the rabbit
by L. GERHARD 555

Chemische, physikalische und radiologische Probleme in der Neurochirurgie (Beiträge zur Neurochirurgie, Heft 13)
edited by G. MERREM 555

Membranes, ions, and impulses
by K. S. COLE. 556

The dizzy patient
by J. C. ELIA 640

SOCIETY PROCEEDINGS (for details see *Index of Subjects*) . . .96, 211, 322, 444, 544, 617, 641

ANNOUNCEMENTS (for details see *Index of Subjects*). 224, 421, 435

INDEX OF AUTHORS VOLUME 27, 1969. 737

INDEX OF SUBJECTS VOLUME 27, 1969. 747

ERRATA 754

INDEX TO CURRENT LITERATURE Nos. 11 and 12 were enclosed with the August and November numbers, respectively

EDITORIAL

It is with great regret that we have to announce the retirement of Dr. Cosimo Ajmone Marsan from the post of Editor for the Western Hemisphere and the Far East. Dr. Marsan was appointed at the beginning of 1961, an important moment in the history of the Journal, marking the end of the "amateur" (but highly proficient) regime of Dr. H.H. Jasper and the beginning of professional publication by Elsevier. During these eight and a half years the Journal has grown by nearly fifty percent but the volume of material submitted has increased even faster. With a new paper arriving on his desk almost every working day (each accepted paper to be read at least twice, often three or four times, before publication) it would have been small wonder if Dr. Marsan had lowered his initial high standards but his editing remains now as careful and meticulous of detail as when he began. The Journal has been very fortunate in its "American" editors and it is fitting that both will have prominent roles to play in the 7th International Congress in September, and satisfying that Dr. Marsan will continue to serve the interests of the Federation and the Journal.

The task of finding a new editor seemed likely to be long and difficult: though some might have the right qualities of mind and experience few would have the willingness to accept the heavy demands which the Journal makes on time and effort. We were fortunate indeed that our search was quickly rewarded. Dr. Peter Kellaway of Houston, who takes over from Dr. Marsan on July 1, is too well known in the United States, and throughout the world, to need any introduction. He has an "international" background which will be valuable to our Journal and we hope that his tenure of the office will be as long and successful as were those of his predecessors

An important feature of the editorial policy of the Journal is that every paper should be read by at least two reviewers in addition to the Editor. For this to be possible each Editor has to make heavy inroads on the time and goodwill of numerous colleagues whose services cannot be given adequate recognition. The moment is opportune to thank them all and to hope that those who have served Dr. Marsan so well will continue to give their help to Dr. Kellaway.

London, June 1969

W. A. Cobb
Managing Editor

Electroencephalography and Clinical Neurophysiology
Elsevier Publishing Company, Amsterdam – Printed in The Netherlands

ELECTROENCEPHALOGRAPHIC ACTIVITY AFTER PROLONGED SLEEP LOSS[1]

P. NAITOH, A. KALES, E. J. KOLLAR, J. C. SMITH AND A. JACOBSON

Navy Medical Neuropsychiatric Research Unit, San Diego, Calif. 92152, and Departments of Psychiatry and Anatomy, University of California, Los Angeles, Calif. (U.S.A.)

(Accepted for publication: October 1, 1968)

Blake and Gerard (1937) were the first to report the EEG change of a progressive reduction of alpha activity as hours of sleep loss accumulated, a finding subsequently confirmed by others (see Mirsky and Cardon 1962, Kollar *et al.* 1966 and others in Discussion). Beyond 100 h of sleep loss, no systematic study of the EEG is available until 264 h of sleep loss in one subject (Johnson *et al.* 1965; Ross 1965; Gulevitch *et al.* 1966). West *et al.* (1962) suggested that there is a critical period around 120 h of sleep loss; the production of adenosine triphosphate (ATP), a critical energy substance, becomes minimal at 96 h of sleep deprivation (Luby *et al.* 1960).

The major purposes of this EEG study were: (a) to fill in the gap between the reported effects of 100 h of sleep loss and the effects of 264 h of sleep; (b) to compare the relation of behavioral, autonomic, and biochemical changes to the reduction of alpha activity with sleep loss; and (c) to resolve the conflicting interpretation of this reduction.

MATERIALS AND METHOD

Four healthy young adult males (21–23 years old) were continuously observed for 15 days in the research ward of the U.C.L.A. Neuropsychiatric Institute. After 3 baseline days, sleep deprivation was started at 6 a.m. (September 22) and continued for 8 nights and 9 days until about 7 p.m. (September 30), a total sleep deprivation of 205 h. There were 3 recovery days: the subjects were awakened after 12 h sleep on the first night, and after 8 h of sleep on recovery nights 2 and 3. Follow-up EEG records were obtained 1 month later for three of the subjects and 2 months later for the remaining one subject. Monetary rewards were: \$100 for 6 nights of sleep loss, \$250 for 7 nights, or \$400 if they completed 205 h of sleep deprivation. All subjects completed 205 h.

A light breakfast was served at 6 a.m. and the other meals at noon, 6 p.m., and midnight. Caffeine and other stimulants were prohibited. The first subject was started on his EEG recordings promptly at 9 a.m., 3 p.m., 9 p.m. and 3 a.m. The last subject started his EEG recording session 1.5–2 h after the first. The EEG reported in this paper, therefore, represented the EEG of early morning, late morning, late afternoon, and late evening.

An Offner 8-channel type R Dynograph was used to record the EEGs (P_3–O_1; P_4–O_2), the EKG, respiration, skin resistance, EMG of the neck muscle, and stimulus marks. The EEG was also recorded on magnetic tape with a Sanborn-Hewlett-Packard model 3907. All records were taken from the standing subjects.

The percent alpha time (*i.e.*, the duration in mm of all waves at 8–13 c/sec of >20 μV) was scored visually from 3 samples of 20 sec each, using a paper speed of 10 mm/sec during an eyes-open relaxed state just prior to the command "close eyes", during the eyes-closed period, and during the eyes-open relaxed period immediately following the 1 min eyes-closed period. The observed alpha duration was divided by the total length of 200 mm to derive the % alpha time (or alpha index).

[1] Presented in part at the 24th Western EEG Society annual meeting in Park City, Utah. This study was partly supported by research grant MH08441 from the National Institute of Mental Health.

Forty sec of the same eyes-closed EEG periods used in the visual analysis of alpha index were spectro-analyzed, using a Space Biology Laboratory computer program (French *et al.* 1966). Spectral intensity was expressed by an arbitary unit of squared digitizer counts which had constant linear relation to squared microvolt unit. A scheme of Walter (1963) was modified to describe the EEG auto-spectral intensities: delta (2–3 c/sec), theta (4–7 c/sec), alpha (8–13 c/sec), and beta (14–20 c/sec).

To supplement the auto-spectral analysis, the entire P_4–O_2 EEG records were analyzed with electronic filters (Krohn-Hite model 33OAR). In addition, the filtered alpha and delta outputs were full-wave rectified, and integrated with a Beckman resetting integrator coupler. Both integrators were set to reset (*i.e.*, dump their contents) whenever they reached the integrator value corresponding to 5 mm of pen deflection.

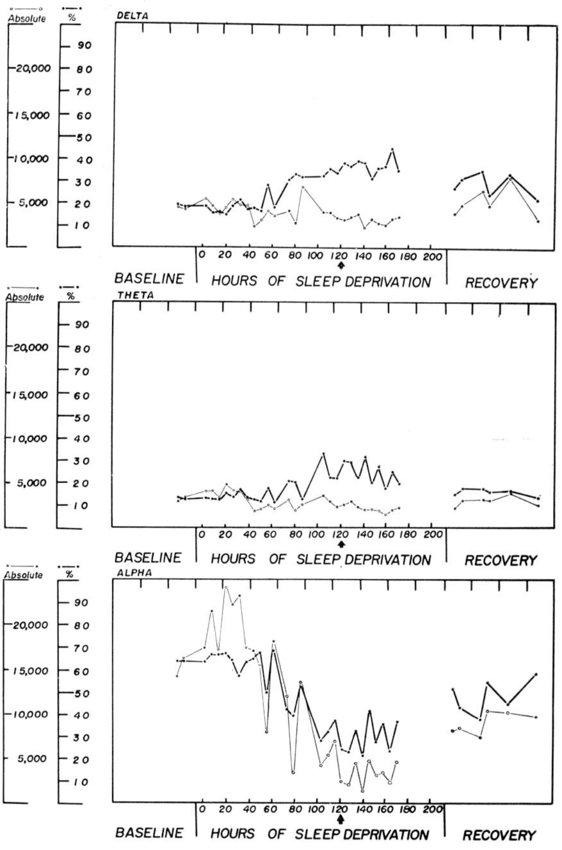

Fig. 1

The time course of average auto-spectral intensity of four subjects at delta, theta or alpha activity (a thin line). A heavy line shows the percentages of these EEG band activities in terms of the total EEG output. The arrow indicates the time of "fifth day turning point" suggested by West *et al.* (1962).

Tracking data were obtained from the standing subject who viewed a 5 in. CRO screen in which a 2 mm spot of light was driven vertically over a 6 cm course by a sinusoidal signal (*i.e.*, the tracking signal) from a low frequency function generator. The subject tried to keep this spot of light within a 1 cm circle in the center of the screen by moving a thumbwheel (*i.e.*, the tracking response). The difference between the tracking signal and the thumbwheel movement generated a score of time-*off*-target (TOT) (Malmo and Surwillo 1960; Kelley 1967). After each session, the subject indicated the effort expended in the tracking task. The phrases "considerable" amount of extra effort and "normal" amount of effort appeared at opposite ends of a 20 cm scale. To indicate the degree of fatigue, the subject marked on a 20 cm scale on which 5 phrases, "very tired", "tired", "as usual", "fresh", and "very fresh" were evenly spaced. Scores were based on the distance of the subject's mark from "normal" and "very fresh". These scales were adapted from Malmo and Surwillo (1960).

Oral temperature, respiration and pulse rates, arterial pressure, and blood samples (for 17-hydroxycorticosteroids—17-OHCS) were obtained at 6 a.m., noon, 6 p.m., and midnight.

RESULTS

I. *EEG activity and sleep loss*

Fig. 1 shows the changes in delta, theta, and alpha EEG activity expressed both in percentage of the total EEG output for a given sample and in absolute intensity of squared digitizer count unit. There was a marked decrease in both percentage and absolute alpha intensity with sleep loss. Although there was an increase in delta and theta percentage with respect to the total EEG output, the absolute intensities did not increase: absolute delta remained unchanged, and absolute theta decreased slightly. Lubin's (1961) rank order test showed no significant[1]

[1] "Significant" ordinarily refers to the 0.05 level or better. *K* is the average Spearman correlation with the *a priori* rank order.

increase in the absolute delta intensity during sleep loss ($K= +0.25$). Similarly, absolute beta intensity failed to show a significant increase during sleep loss ($K= +0.30$). The absolute alpha and theta intensities decreased significantly during sleep loss (for alpha, $K= +0.79$; for theta, $K= +0.43$).

In all four subjects, the alpha index decreased up to 120 h of sleep loss (Fig. 1–3). Before sleep loss, the eyes-closure always generated alpha activity (Fig. 2, *A*), but not much after 117 h of sleep loss. Beyond 120 h (see arrow in Fig. 3), the subjects regained some of the lost alpha activity. In spite of marked individual difference and time of day effects on alpha reduction (Fig. 3), statistical analysis showed definite alpha reduction due to sleep loss, particularly when the analysis was performed separately on the alpha indices of "3 a.m.", "9 a.m.", "3 p.m.", and "9 p.m.". By fitting a curve using a BMD program of the U.C.L.A. Health Sciences Computing Facility, it was found that alpha index decreased linearly over the hours of sleep loss.

Rank order correlations between the alpha index and auto-spectral intensity for the alpha range within four subjects indicated a high degree of agreement (+0.85, +0.86, +0.89, and +0.91). Thus, alpha abundance data appear to be measured adequately by a relatively simple visual analysis.

II. *Circadian rhythmicity of alpha*

Fig. 3 shows a regular appearance of peaks and troughs in alpha output for all subjects. The method of Frank *et al.* (1966) was used to study circadian rhythmicity of alpha activity. The sleep loss period of 177 h was divided into 6 overlapping epochs of 30 h each and with a 6 h

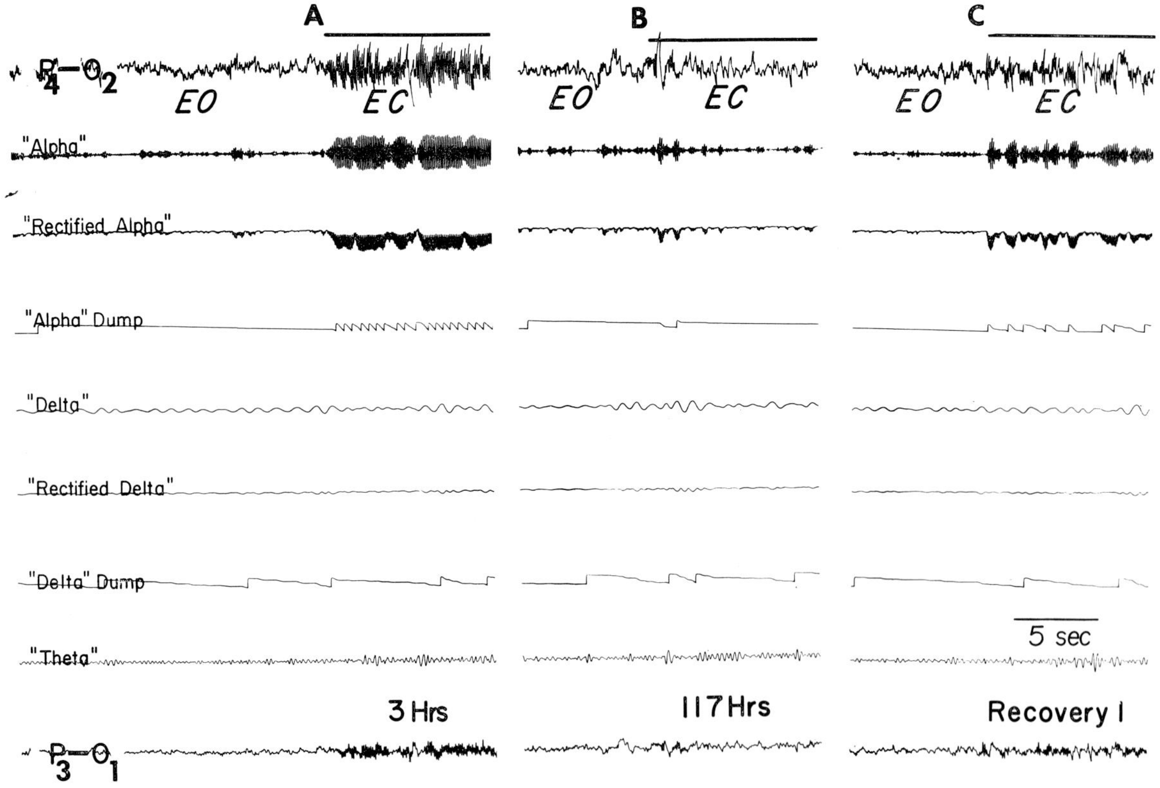

Fig. 2

Filter analysis of the P_4–O_2 of one subject, J. L., showing the effects of 3 h (*A*), 117 h of staying awake (*B*), and after the night of 12 h first recovery sleep (*C*). The P_4–O_2 derivation was subjected to additional amplification for the filter analysis. This figure shows only a part of the EEG which was used for visual and auto-spectral analyses. EC = eyes closed; EO = eyes open.

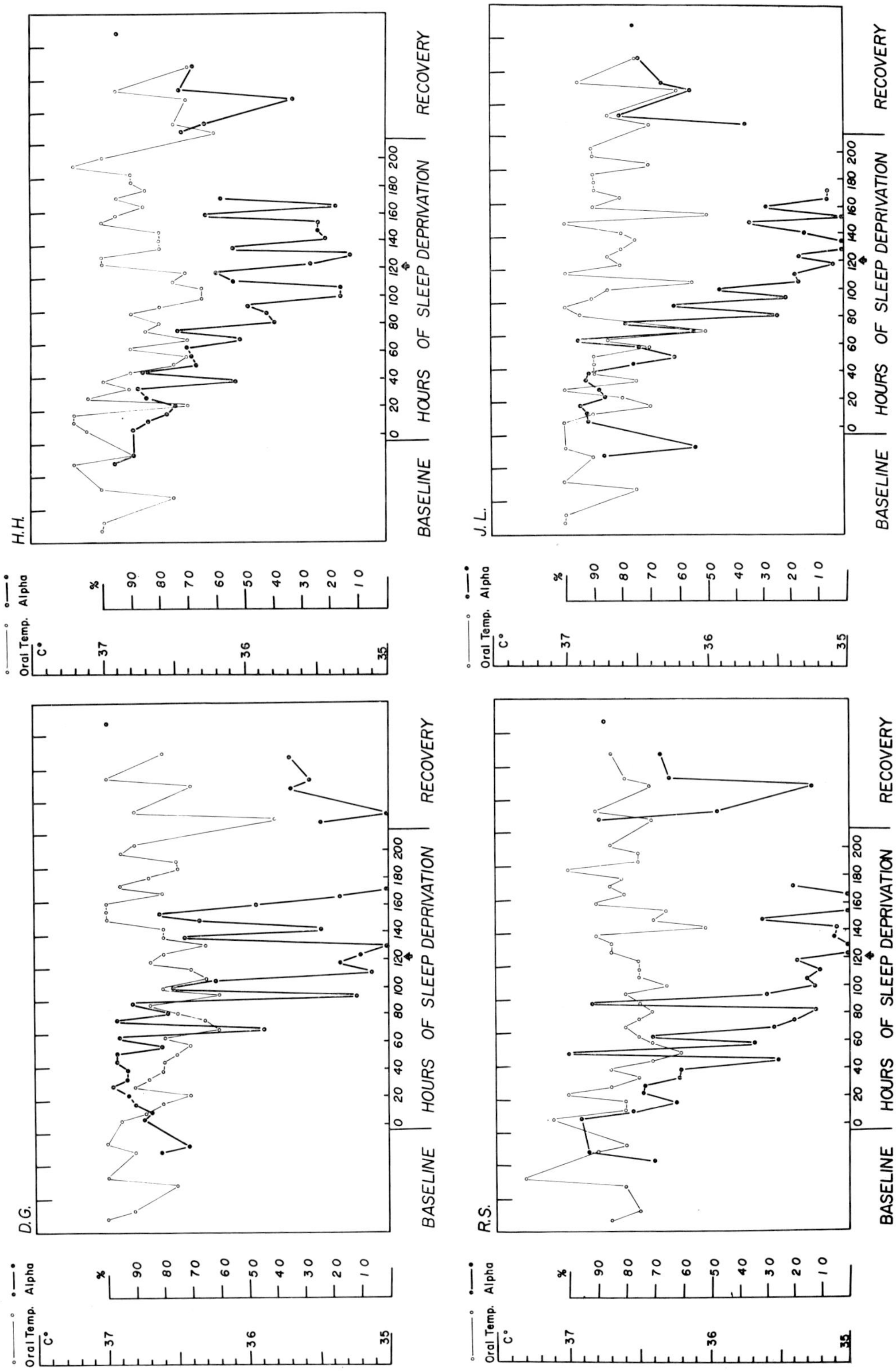

Fig. 3

Individual plot of the percent alpha of the P_4–O_2. The initials of four subjects appear on the top left corner of each graph. The dot seen in the extreme right represents the alpha index obtained from the follow-up examination. Notice that the lowest oral temperature in all four subjects was not observed near the end of sleep deprivation, but much earlier.

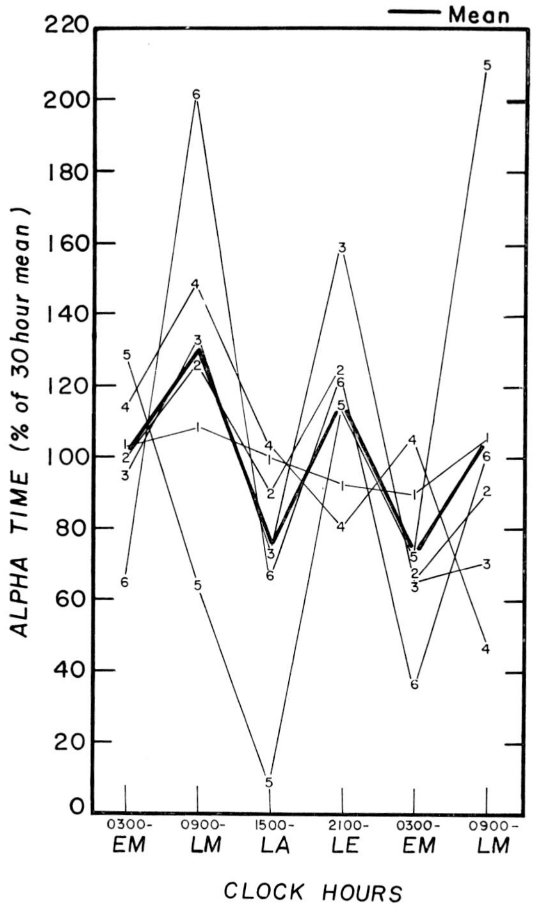

Fig. 4
Circadian rhythmicity of alpha activity during sleep deprivation. See text for explanation. E = early; L = late; M = morning; A = afternoon; E = evening.

overlap. Numerals 1–6 were assigned to epochs: the numeral 1 to the 30 h epoch, 27–57 h of sleep loss (3 a.m. to 3 a.m.). The numeral 2 was given to the epoch of 51–81 h of sleep loss, etc. The average alpha index was computed for each 30 h epoch. Then, the alpha time as shown in Fig. 4 was calculated by dividing the alpha index observed at the given clock hour by the 30 h mean alpha index, and then multiplying by 100. These results are shown in Fig. 4. Line 1, which represents the first 30 h, shows little change with time. However, the amplitude of the circadian rhythm increased during the 2nd, 3rd, and 4th epochs. There was a disruption of rhythm in the 5th epoch, coinciding with minimum alpha output, followed by a return of rhythmicity coinciding with the somewhat higher alpha activity in the 6th epoch (lines 5 and 6).

III. *Concomitants of alpha reduction during sleep loss*

The time course of the averages of oral temperature, heart rate, 17-OHCS, TOT, "feeling" and "effort" is shown in Fig. 5.

Table I summarizes rank order correlations between these variables. To evaluate statistical significance of the observed correlation, Fisher's Z transformation was used and these transformed scores were subjected to the zero-mu t test (Winer 1962). Table I shows that higher alpha index is significantly correlated with lower level of 17-OHCS, smaller tracking error, less "effort", and better "feeling". More exertion of "effort" was correlated significantly with elevated oral temperature, higher 17-OHCS level, greater tracking error and smaller alpha index. Other intercorrelations were not significant.

Table II shows the averages of EEG (P_4–O_2), autonomic and behavioral variables before, during and after 205 h sleep loss.

Beyond 130 h of sleep loss there was a slight improvement in the subject's psychological ratings. Resting oral temperature and 17-OHCS followed the same course as the alpha index: a decrease until about 100 h of sleep deprivation, and then an increase—a partial recovery (see Fig. 3 for oral temperature in relation to alpha index). Heart rate did not show any systematic change.

The maximal effects of sleep loss were observed not during the terminal hours of the 153–171 h, but earlier (see Table II). For absolute alpha intensity, the minimal alpha occurred during 141–153 h (the average time when minimal alpha occurred was 144 h $\pm$ 2.5 h). The maximal oral temperature drop occurred during 87–141 h (the average of 108 h $\pm$ 11.6 h). During 111–141 h, the heart rate was minimal (122.3 $\pm$ 6.6 h). The subjective ratings showed the maximal sleep loss effects during 99–111 h for "feeling" (102 $\pm$ 3 h), and for "effort" at 110 $\pm$ 6.5 h. The 17-OHCS reached its minimum at 72.8 $\pm$ 19.2 h.

The increase in the alpha index after 120 h of sleep loss was, then, either anticipated or accompanied by partial recuperation and im-

TABLE I

Average rank correlations during sleep deprivation

	Oral temp. (higher)	17-OHCS (higher)	TOT (more)	Effort (more)	Feeling (tired)
Alpha index (higher)	0.05	−0.22**	−0.65**	−0.58*	−0.52*
Oral temperature (higher)		0.27*	0.14	0.28**	0.14
17-OHCS (higher)			0.38	0.23*	0.05
Time-*off*-target (more)				0.56*	0.44*
Effort (more)					0.76**

* $P = 0.05$. ** $P = 0.01$. Number of subjects = 4, except for TOT ($N = 3$). A larger rank order correlation may be less significant than a smaller one, depending on inter-subject variability. See Fig. 5 for the plots of these averages.

TABLE II

Averages of EEG (P_4–O_2), autonomic and behavioral variables

Variables	Baseline (Sept. 21)	Sleep deprivation hours		Recovery days			Follow-up*
		3–21	123–171	1	2	3	
EEG							
Alpha index (%)	80	84	23	65	41	61	60
Alpha intensity**	15,221	19,957	3,317	8,269	8,961	10,197	9,873
Theta intensity	3,019	4,017	2,170	2,653	3,131	3,960	2,481
Delta intensity	4,379	4,351	3,096	4,345	5,559	7,833	3,186
*Behavior****							
Feeling	7.4	6.5	12.7	8.2	6.4	4.4	
Effort	4.1	1.2	11.1	6.9	1.7	1.8	
Time-*off*-target	—	1.1	63.4	24.8	2.2	22.7	
Autonomic							
Oral temperature (°C)	36.9	36.8	36.7	36.4	36.4	36.6	
Heart rate (/min)	88	84	88	89	79	90	
Systolic blood pressure (mm Hg)	119	121	124	121	121	128	
Respiration rate (/min)	20	21	21	21	21	20	
Biochemical							
17-OHCS (μg%)	26	15.6	23.7	22.4	14.2	24.7	

* Taken 30 or 60 days after the recovery day 3.
** Expressed as squared digitizer count.
*** Figures indicate distance in mm; see Method.

proved clinical status in oral temperature, 17-OHCS, and subjective ratings. Fig. 5 shows, however, an exception to this "recuperation"—continued deterioration of tracking throughout the hours of sleep loss.

IV. *Effects of recovery sleep*

After 205 h of sleep deprivation, the subjects were permitted to sleep for 12 h, then they continued the daily testing schedule.

The alpha index of the first recovery day was significantly smaller than that of the first 3–21 h of sleep loss. On the second recovery night, the subjects slept 8 h. The average alpha indices then returned to pre-deprivation levels. Only one subject, D.G., failed to show an increase of the

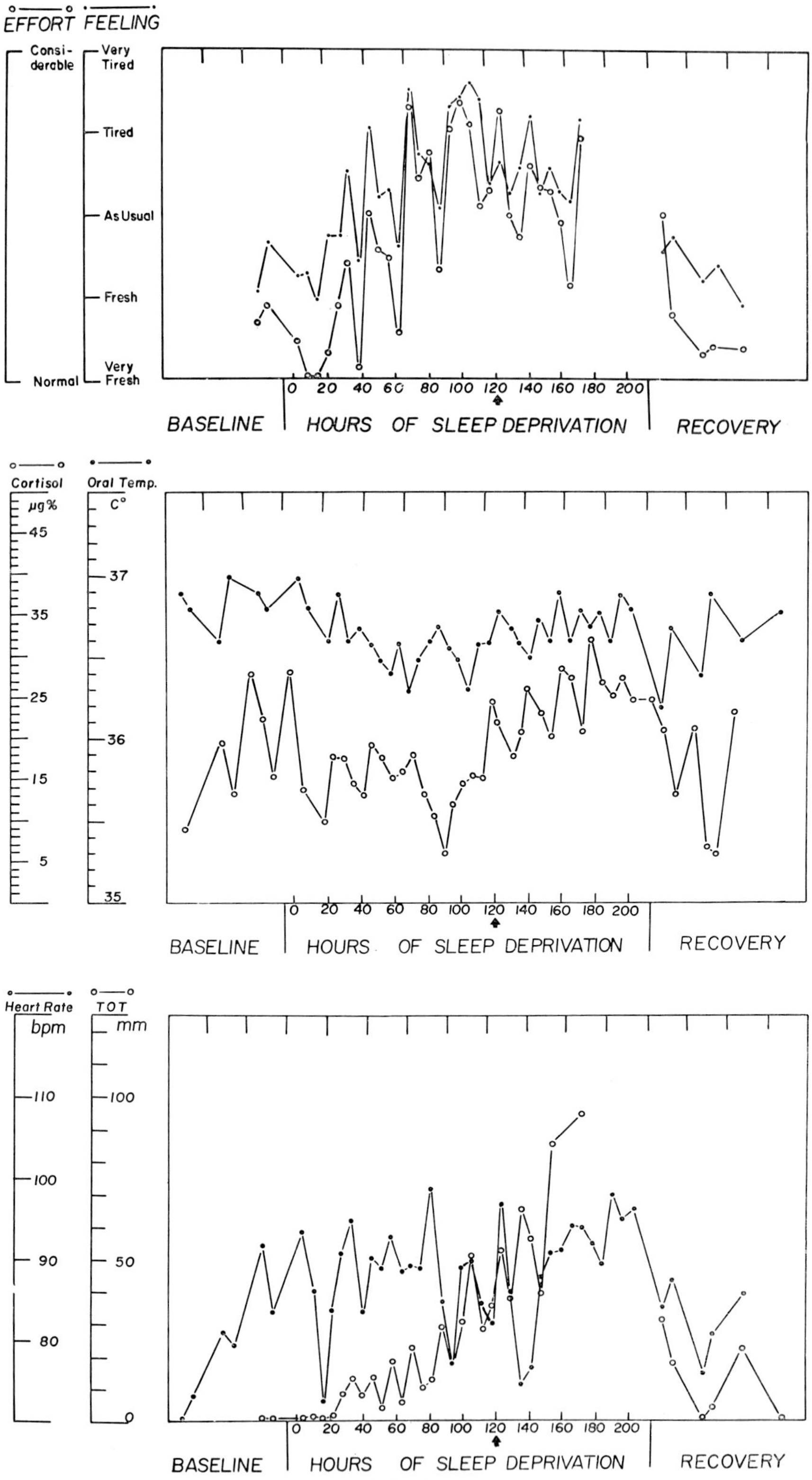

Fig. 5

The time course of subjective rating of fatigue and effort, TOT, 17-OHCS levels, heart rate, and oral temperature.

absolute alpha intensity to pre-deprivation level even after all 3 nights of recovery sleep. However, the average alpha index returned to pre-deprivation level.

Similar carry-over effects were observed in other variables. Tracking response recovered only after 2 nights of recovery sleep.

DISCUSSION

Our findings of a decreased alpha activity during the first 120 h of sleep loss corroborates previous studies (Tyler *et al.* 1947; Armington and Mitnick 1959; Williams *et al.* 1959; Rodin *et al.* 1962; Johnson *et al.* 1965), some of which utilized only visual EEG analysis. In our study the results from simple visual analysis of the alpha index were consistent with those from auto-spectral analysis. The latter, however, clarified the effects of sleep loss on other EEG bands (delta and theta) in agreement with the findings of Tyler *et al.* (1947) and Johnson *et al.* (1965).

We agree with Frank *et al.* (1966) that sleep loss of less than 50 h enhances the periodicity of alpha activity. This enhancement of diurnal variation in alpha activity was accompanied by marked diurnal variations in the subjective sense of sleepiness, which was most intense and impelling during early morning when the alpha intensity was also lowest.

Tyler *et al.* (1947) and Malmo and Surwillo (1960) concluded that the low voltage characteristics of sleep deprivation EEG is the result of increased central nervous system activation secondary to the sleep-deprived subjects' efforts to remain awake. However, Armington and Mitnick (1959), Williams *et al.* (1962) and Johnson *et al.* (1965) concluded that the decrease in alpha activity is an EEG concomitant of drowsiness (see Bjerner 1949), or the sleep stage 1 of Dement-Kleitman classification (1957). Wilkinson (1965) suggested that if the subject was successful in his efforts to stay awake, this was reflected in a reduction of the alpha activity. If he failed, the EEG showed the low voltage non-alpha pattern of the sleep stage 1. During the early period of sleep loss in our study, the EEG showed a pattern in which alpha bursts punctuated an otherwise flat low voltage record. This could be interpreted in terms of Wilkinson's schema. However, such an interpretation does not seem to be adequate to explain many of the observations of later stages of sleep deprivation in which the EEG does not show frequent alpha bursts, although the subjects remain in good contact and are able to mobilize themselves to logically and correctly deal with short intellectual tasks. Wilkinson's concept is unable to account for such things as performance lapses (Williams *et al.* 1959) and hypnagogic illusions (Pasnau *et al.* 1968) during later periods of prolonged sleep loss. Unlike Bjerner's study (1949), examination of the eyes-closed EEG of our subjects did not show K complexes, or 12–14 c/sec sigma spindles. This difference may have been due to a fact that Bjerner's subject was in bed, whereas our subjects remained standing.

A partial recovery of alpha activity at about 120–130 h of sleep deprivation was observed rather unexpectedly in all subjects. Perhaps the recovery reflects shifts in coping mechanisms manifested by the "second wind" phenomenon, or the "fifth day turning point". Performance on tracking task continued to deteriorate with sleep loss, and there was no performance recovery after 120–130 h. Thus, psychomotor performance, unlike other psychological modalities, showed no compensating mechanisms to counteract the effects of prolonged sleep loss.

SUMMARY

The P_4–O_2 EEG of four subjects was measured by visual inspection and by auto-spectral analysis before, during and after 205 h of total sleep deprivation. A marked reduction of alpha activity which overrode circadian variations and individual differences was observed.

Alpha reduction was paralleled by deterioration of subjective ratings on feeling and effort, by deterioration of tracking performance, and by reports of hypnagogic illusions. These findings are not unlike those made during the sleep stage 1.

After 120 h of sleep loss, there was a slight increase of alpha activity which was accompanied or "anticipated" by partial returns of oral temperature, subjective ratings, and 17-hydroxycorticosteroids to pre-sleep deprivation levels. The increase of alpha activity and other changes are postulated to reflect shifts in basic coping mechanisms.

After 2 nights of recovery sleep (12 h and 8 h), the return to the pre-deprivation levels was complete for all variables, except the absolute alpha activity of one subject. The follow-up study conducted 1 month or 2 months later showed that all subjects had a complete recovery.

Alpha activity can be reasonably estimated by alpha index and, as such, it will be sufficient to indicate a gross sleep debt. In those who lack dominant alpha activity, the simple subjective ratings associated with standardized tasks may be used for detection of sleep debt. The poor indicators of sleep loss were 17-hydroxycorticosteroids, oral temperature, and time-*off*-target. Respiration rate, heart rate, and arterial pressure were useless in detecting even a gross sleep starvation.

RÉSUMÉ

ACTIVITÉ ÉLECTROENCÉPHALOGRAPHIQUE APRÈS PERTE PROLONGÉE DE SOMMEIL

L'EEG pariéto-occipital de quatre sujets a été mesuré au moyen de l'inspection visuelle et l'analyse autospectrale avant, pendant et après 205 h de déprivation totale de sommeil. Une nette réduction de l'activité alpha, qui dépasse les variations circadiennes et les différences individuelles, est observée.

Parallèlement à la réduction de l'alpha, on note une détérioration de l'évaluation subjective du sens et de l'effort, une détérioration des performances de précision et des récits d'illusions hypnagogiques. Ces données ne sont pas différentes de celles qui ont été observées au cours du stade I de sommeil.

Après 120 h de perte de sommeil, on note une légère augmentation de l'activité alpha qui s'accompagne de, ou précède, un retour partiel de la température orale, des mesures subjectives et des 17-hydroxycorticostéroïdes à des niveaux pré-déprivation de sommeil. L'augmentation de l'activité alpha et les autres modifications paraissent refléter des variations dans les mécanismes d'adaptation de base.

Après 2 nuits de récupération de sommeil (12 h et 8 h), le retour au niveau pré-déprivation est complet pour toutes les variables, exceptée l'activité alpha chez un sujet. L'étude évolutive poursuivie un ou deux mois après a montré que tous les sujets avaient une récupération complète.

L'activité alpha peut être raisonnablement évaluée par un index qui, comme tel, est suffisant pour indiquer une dette importante de sommeil. Chez ceux qui manquent d'activité alpha dominante, des mesures subjectives simples associées à des tâches standardisées peuvent être utilisées pour détecter une dette de sommeil. Le niveau des 17-hydroxycorticostéroïdes, la température orale, et le "time-*off*-target" sont de mauvais indicateurs de perte de sommeil. La vitesse respiratoire, la vitesse cardiaque et la pression artérielle se sont révélées inutiles dans la détection d'une déprivation de sommeil même massive.

Digital computer analyses of the brain waves were made possible through D. O. Walter of the Space Biology Laboratory, J. Mason of the Data Processing Laboratory, and the UCLA Health Sciences Computing Facility. Bibliographical work was assisted by the UCLA Brain Information Service. Technical supports of S. Sugent, B. Ray, E. Truttner, and N. Willis are deeply appreciated. The editorial assistance of L. C. Johnson and A. Lubin is gratefully acknowledged.

REFERENCES

ARMINGTON, J. C. and MITNICK, L. L. Electroencephalogram and sleep deprivation. *J. appl. Physiol.*, **1959**, *14*: 247–250.

BJERNER, B. Alpha depression and lowered pulse rate during delayed actions in a serial reaction test: a study in sleep deprivation. *Acta physiol. scand.*, **1949**, *19*, *Suppl. 65*, 93 p.

BLAKE, H. and GERARD, R. W. Brain potentials during sleep. *Amer. J. Physiol.*, **1937**, *119*: 692–703.

DEMENT, W. C. and KLEITMAN, N. Cyclic variations of EEG during sleep and their relation to eye movements, bodily motility, and dreaming. *Electroenceph. clin. Neurophysiol.*, **1957**, *9*: 673–690.

FRANK, G., HALBERG, F., HARNER, R., MATTHEWS, J., JOHNSON, E., GRAVEM, H. and ANDRUN, V. Circadian periodicity, adrenal corticosteroids, and the EEG of normal man. *J. psychiat. Res.*, **1966**, *4*: 63–86.

FRENCH, J. D., ADEY, W. R. and WALTER, D. O. *Computer analysis of EEG data for a normative library.* Final Report to NASA, NAS 9–1970. Brain Research Institute, UCLA, April 15, **1966**, 187 p.

GULEVITCH, G., DEMENT, W. C. and JOHNSON, L. C. Psychiatric and EEG observations in a case of prolonged (264 hours) wakefulness. *Arch. gen. Psychiat.*, **1966**, *15*: 29–35.

JOHNSON, L. C., SLYE, E. S. and DEMENT, W. C. Electroencephalographic and autonomic activity during and after prolonged sleep deprivation. *Psychosom. Med.*, **1965**, *27*: 415–423.

KELLEY, C. R. *The measurement of tracking proficiency.* Final Report on Contract Nonr-4986(00), Office of Naval Research, Dunlap, Santa Monica, Calif., **1967**, 43 p.

KOLLAR, E. J., SLATER, G. R., PALMER, J. O., DOCTER, R. F and MANDELL, A. L. Stress in subjects undergoing sleep deprivation. *Psychosom. Med.*, **1966**, *28*: 101–113.

LUBIN, A. L'utilisation des corrélations par rang pour éprouver une tendance dans un ensemble de moyennes. *Bull. Centre Étude Rech. psychotechn.*, **1961**, *10*: 433–444.

LUBY, E. D., FROHMAN, C. E., GRISELL, J. L., LENZO, J. E. and GOTTLIEB, J. S. Sleep deprivation: Effects on behavior, thinking, motor performance, and biological energy transfer systems. *Psychosom. Med.*, **1960**, *22*: 182–192.

MALMO, R. B. and SURWILLO, W. W. Sleep deprivation: Change in performances and physiological indicants of activation. *Psychol. Monogr.*, **1960**, *74*, No. 15 (Whole No. 502), 24 p.

MIRSKY, A. F. and CARDON, P. V. A comparison of the behavioral and physiological changes accompanying sleep deprivation and chlorpromazine administration in man. *Electroenceph. clin. Neurophysiol.*, **1962**, *14*: 1–10.

PASNAU, R. O., NAITOH, P., STIER, S. and KOLLAR, E. J. The psychological effects of 205 hours of sleep deprivation. *Arch. gen. Psychiat.*, **1968**, *18*: 496–505.

RODIN, E. A., LUBY, E. D. and GOTTLIEB, J. S. The electroencephalogram during prolonged experimental sleep deprivation. *Electroenceph. clin. Neurophysiol.*, **1962**, *14*: 544–551.

ROSS, J. J. Neurological findings after prolonged sleep deprivation. *Arch. Neurol. (Chic.)*, **1965**, *12*: 399–403.

TYLER, D. B., GOODMAN, J. and ROTHMAN, T. The effect of experimental insomnia on the rate of potential changes in the brain. *Amer. J. Physiol.*, **1947**, *149*: 185–193.

WALTER, W. G. Technique-interpretation. In D. HILL and G. PARR (Eds.), *Electroencephalography: A symposium on its various aspects.* Macmillan, New York, **1963**, 86 p.

WEST, L. J., JANZEN, H. H., LESTER, B. K. and CORNELISOON JR., F. S. The psychosis of sleep deprivation. *Ann. N. Y. Acad. Sci.*, **1962**, *96*: 66–70.

WILKINSON, R. T. Sleep deprivation. In O. G. EDHOLM and A. L. BACHARACH (Eds.), *The physiology of human survival.* Academic Press, New York, **1965**: 399–430.

WILLIAMS, H. L., GRANADA, A. M., JONES, R. C., LUBIN, A. and ARMINGTON, J. C. EEG frequency and finger pulse volume as predictors of reaction time during sleep loss. *Electroenceph. clin. Neurophysiol.*, **1962**, *14*: 64–70.

WILLIAMS, H. L., LUBIN, A. and GOODNOW, J. J. Impaired performance with acute sleep loss. *Psychol. Monogr.*, **1959**, *73*, No. 14 (Whole No. 484), 26 p.

WINER, B. J. *Statistical principles in experimental design.* McGraw-Hill, New York, **1962**, 672 p.

Reference: NAITOH, P., KALES, A., KOLLAR, E. J., SMITH, J. C. and JACOBSON, A. Electroencephalographic activity after prolonged sleep loss. *Electroenceph. clin. Neurophysiol.*, **1969**, *27*: 2–11.

Electroencephalography and Clinical Neurophysiology
Elsevier Publishing Company, Amsterdam – Printed in The Netherlands

CHANGES OF THE EEG, INTRACRANIAL PRESSURE AND OTHER VARIABLES DURING SLEEP IN PATIENTS WITH INTRACRANIAL LESIONS

RAY COOPER AND A. HULME

Burden Neurological Institute, Stapleton, Bristol, and Frenchay Hospital, Bristol (Great Britain)

(Accepted for publication: September 27, 1968)

Although high levels of intracranial pressure can cause partial or even total stoppage of the cerebral blood flow the effect on the EEG is not well defined. Several workers, for example Walter (1937), Cobb (1945), Cavazzuti (1959) and Bagchi *et al.* (1961), have suggested that the bilateral or paroxysmal EEG abnormalities recorded from patients with tumours or hydrocephalus are not due to the associated raised intracranial pressure but due more directly to the disorder itself. Mani and Townsend (1964) reported a preponderance of "generalized bursts of activity" (delta and theta waves) in cases of benign intracranial hypertension and to a lesser degree in cases of obstructive hydrocephalus and suggested that they may be related to the rise in intracranial pressure. However Wilson *et al.* (1965) showed that no EEG abnormalities occurred when the intracranial pressure was artificially raised to levels approaching that of the diastolic blood pressure (approximately 1000 mm of water) for periods of 2–5 min. This work clearly demonstrates that acute rises of intracranial pressure *per se* do not give rise to EEG abnormalities. Langfitt *et al.* (1966), using supratentorial balloons in monkeys, also showed that EEG abnormalities did not occur during intracranial hypertension if adequate perfusion was maintained. These authors also demonstrated that the rate of rise of intracranial pressure was important. With continuous recording of ventricular fluid pressure Ingvar and Lundberg (1961) showed that during periods of high pressure the EEG changes were "strikingly small, often only of a subtle nature".

In a previous paper we showed that, in patients with intracranial hypertension, large increases of intracranial pressure occurred during the so-called "paradoxical" or rapid eye movement (REM) stage of sleep (Cooper and Hulme 1966). During this state there is a reduction of EEG activity and it was suggested that this reduction might be associated with a high cerebral metabolic rate, producing cerebral vasodilatation and raised intracranial pressure. In the present paper changes of the EEG in stage II of sleep are shown to be correlated with changes of intracranial pressure and other variables.

METHODS

Most of the techniques used in these investigations have been described in detail in other publications. The intracranial pressure (ICP) was measured by using a pressure transducer in contact with the cortex (Hulme and Cooper 1966). Gold electrodes (4 mm long, 150 μ diameter) and thermistors were placed in the subdural space when the pressure transducer was implanted. One or more of the electrodes was used to measure oxygen availability by a polarographic method (Clark *et al.* 1958; Meyer and Portnoy 1959; Cooper 1963). In the present study the bare electrodes were polarized with a 0.9 V negative potential with respect to a silver/silver chloride electrode on the scalp. The mean current flowing through each electrode was "backed off" and the changes of oxygen availability (O_2a) were displayed on the recorder.

The electrical impedance (electroplethysmograph) of two electrodes in the subdural space is primarily determined by the thickness of the layer of cerebrospinal fluid, which is of low impedance compared with blood and other tissue (Porte. *et al.* 1964; Robinson and Tompkins 1964). The impedance rises if brain volume increases, as in generalized cerebral vasodilatation (Moskalenko *et al.* 1964). In these studies the impedance was measured at 1 kc/sec or 20 kc/sec.

The temperature of the subdural thermistor beads was raised about 1.5°C above blood temperature by direct current and the change of temperature, as measured by the resistance, was used to indicate blood flow.

Silver/silver chloride electrodes and time constants of 1 sec were used for the recording of the EEG and lateral eye movements. Heart rate was determined by expressing the beat to beat (ECG) interval as an equivalent heart rate and displayed as a deviation from a chosen norm. A variable resistance carbon microphone strapped to the chest was used to indicate respiration. In some patients respiratory CO_2 was measured, using an infra-red analyser with air samples obtained via a catheter in a nostril. An 8- or 16-channel Beckman/Offner EEG machine was used and selected variables were preserved on tape, using a Precision Instruments 8-channel tape recorder. Whenever possible the classification of Dement and Kleitman (1957) was used to describe the state of sleep. Most of the recordings were made with the patient in a side room of the neurosurgical ward.

Twenty patients suffering from a variety of intracranial abnormalities were studied on one or more nights by some or all of these techniques. There were fifteen cases of intracranial tumour (11 supratentorial, 3 infratentorial and one in the third ventricle), four cases of hydrocephalus and one case of intracranial haematoma.

RESULTS

As might be expected most of the patients did not fall asleep easily and many of them were restless for much of the night, with frequent awakenings. These deviations from the normal sleep pattern were probably due to natural anxiety about their illness as well as to the disturbance caused by the recording. The identification of the Dement and Kleitman stages of sleep in such circumstances was difficult. Only a few patients went through stage IV sleep (continuous delta activity) before awakening.

Groups of generalized slow waves in the EEG, closely correlated with changes of the intracranial variables, were recorded from fifteen patients. This delta activity occurred in a phase of sleep similar to stage II of the normal pattern. It was not found in the waking state or during other stages of sleep. Fig. 1, *a* is a slow speed polygraphic record, with two samples of EEG from vertex/frontal scalp electrodes displayed on a faster time scale (but still slow compared with normal EEG practice). The intracranial pressure fluctuated periodically from 400 to 900 mm of water at about 1 min intervals. The cortical impedance showed similar rhythmic activity with the impedance rising and falling with the pressure. There were reductions of available oxygen and blood flow when the pressure was high. The respiration and respiratory CO_2 showed marked periodicity (Cheyne-Stokes) correlated with the change of pressure, the sudden increase of tidal volume occurring at about the peak of the pressure wave (see later). Increases of heart rate also occurred at this time. At about the peak of each pressure wave there was a group of slow waves in the EEG lasting about 20 sec.

This record is in marked contrast to that shown in Fig. 1, *b* taken 30 min later when the patient was in stage IV sleep. During this recording there were no marked rhythmic changes of intracranial pressure, although there was a long slow rise and fall in the first half of the figure.

We found that the association of intracranial variations and the EEG with disturbance of respiration was very common during stage II sleep, although it was not often as clear as in Fig. 1, *a*. Usually the sequence of events leading to the collapse of a pressure wave appeared to be started by a deep breath and the occurrence of the EEG slow waves, as shown at the end of the record in Fig. 2. The decrease of the pressure at A (Fig. 2) which was associated with changes of the EEG, heart rate, oxygen availability and blood flow was one of the few occasions when there was no obvious change of respiration. In the first half of this figure the K complexes are associated with small increases of intracranial

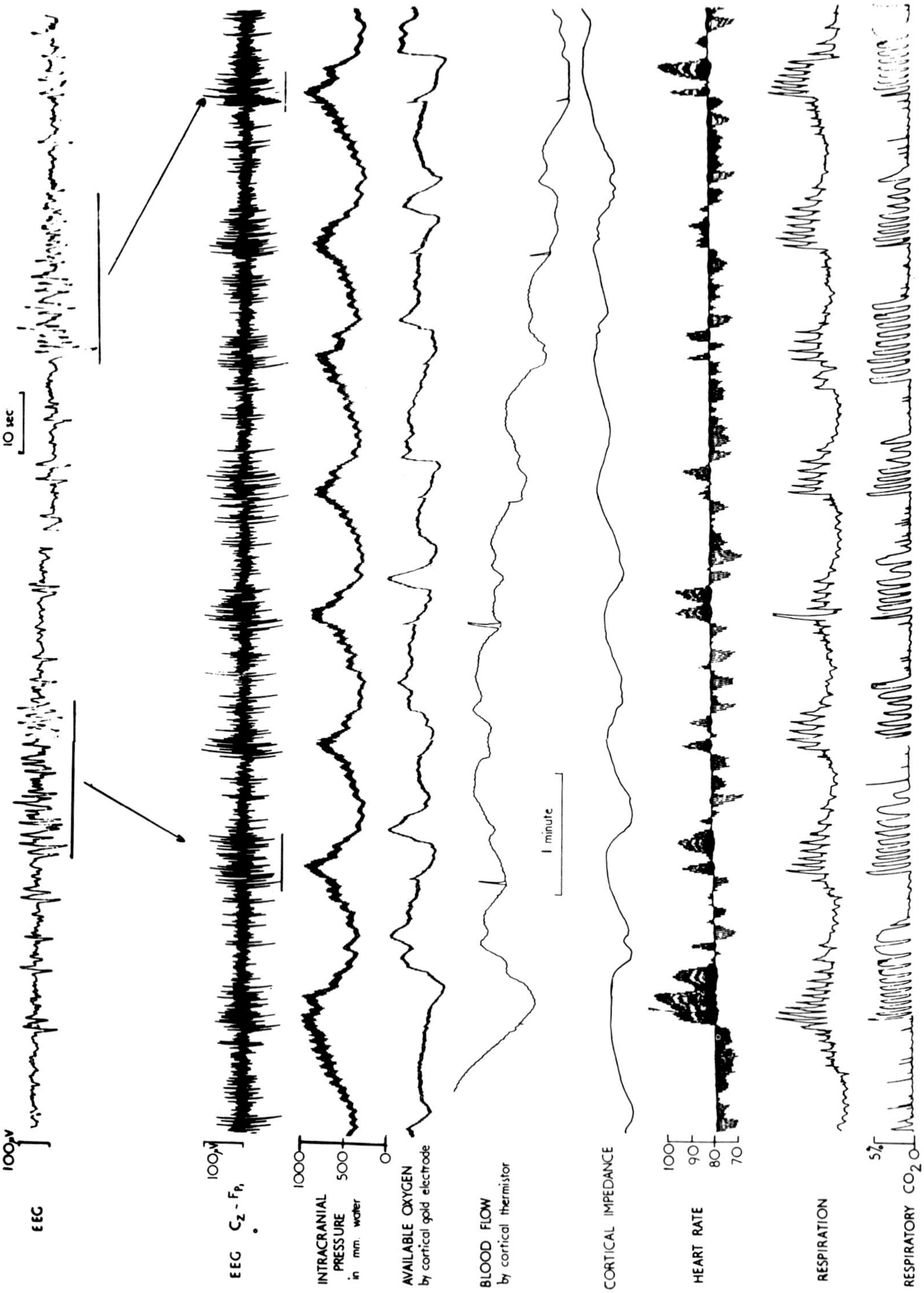
EEG
100μV
EEG C_z - Fp_1
100μV
INTRACRANIAL PRESSURE in mm. water
1000
500
0
AVAILABLE OXYGEN by cortical gold electrode
BLOOD FLOW by cortical thermistor
CORTICAL IMPEDANCE
HEART RATE
100
90
80
70
RESPIRATION
RESPIRATORY CO_2
5%
0
10 sec
1 minute

(a)

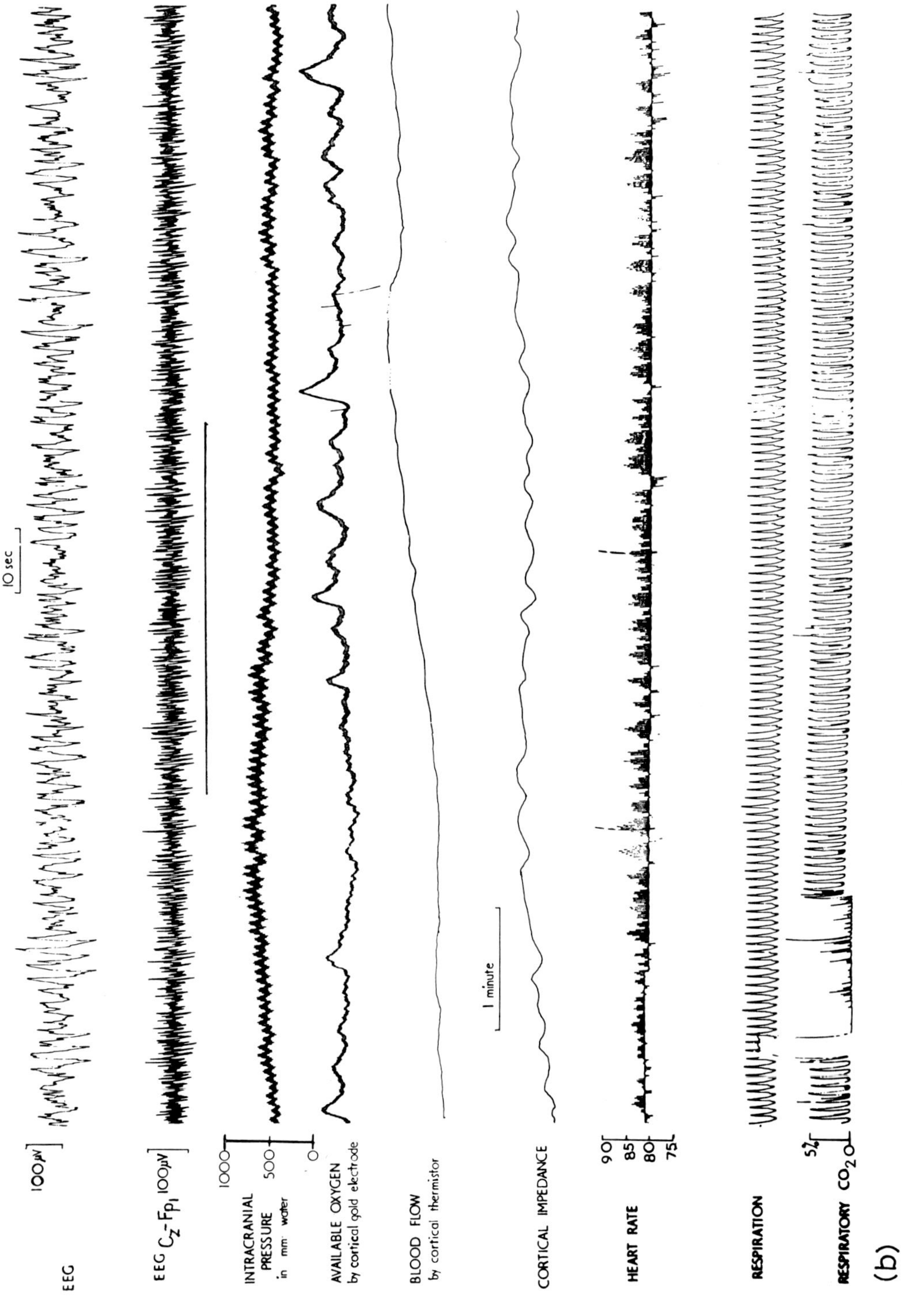

Fig. 1

Polygraphic record from patient with communicating hydrocephalus. Upper traces are EEG at faster paper speed. Record taken: (*a*) during stage II sleep, and (*b*) during stage IV sleep. In all figures an upward pen deflection is an increase in value of the variable displayed.

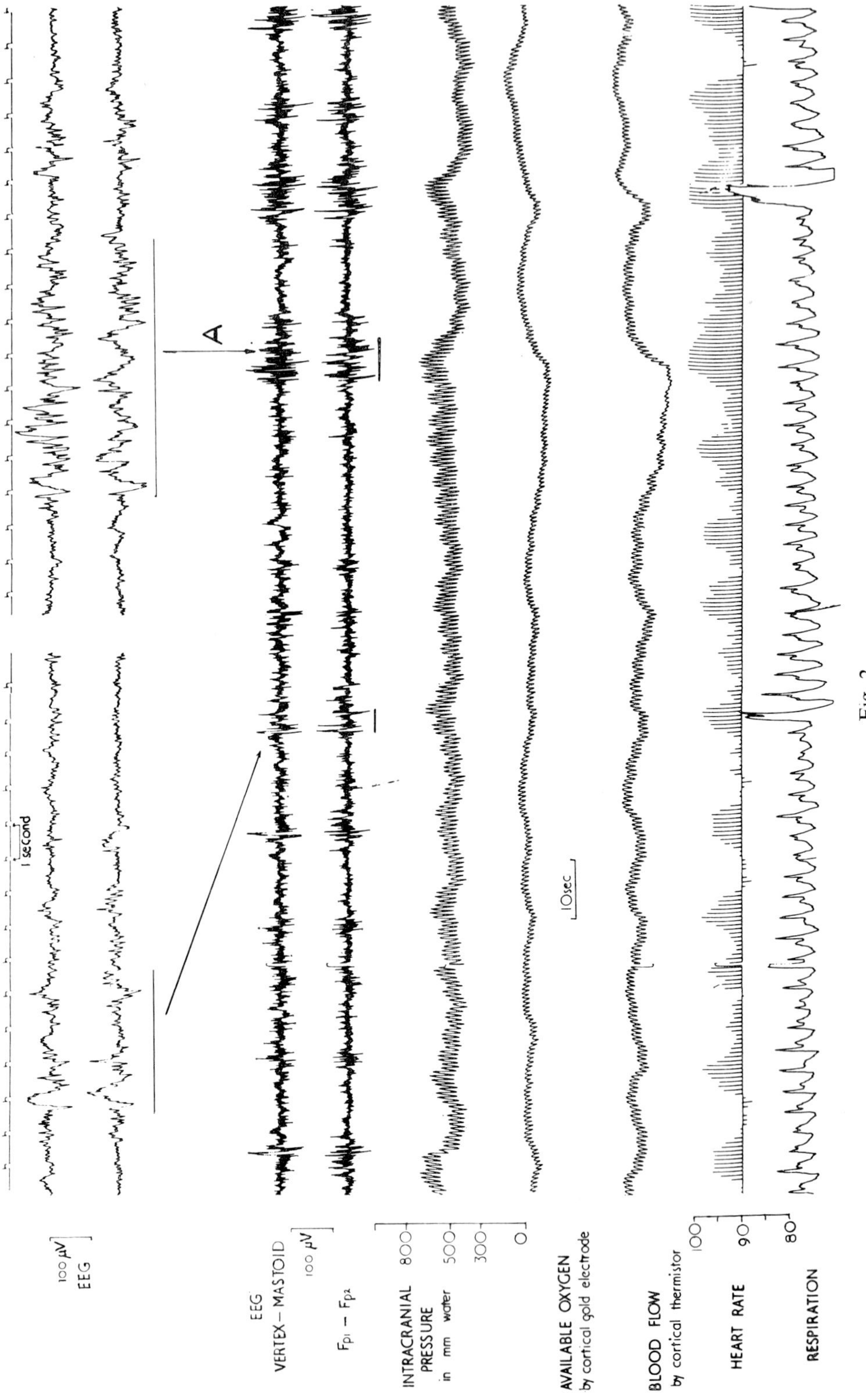

Fig. 2

Record showing small changes of intracranial pressure and other variables associated with K complexes. Towards end of the section shown (A) there was a marked change of intracranial pressure and other variables without an obvious change of respiration.

pressure, available oxygen, blood flow and heart rate.

Cerebral CO_2 is an important factor in the intracranial vascular system and information about the cortical pCO_2 would be very valuable in our studies. Unfortunately this is difficult to measure in man and we were able only to determine the respiratory CO_2, the alveolar sample of which corresponded to the arterial tension. However these records showed that during the increase of intracranial pressure there was usually no significant rise of respiratory CO_2 (Fig. 3). There was a slight but definite reduction (approx. 0.2%) during the time when the intracranial pressure was falling. The mean level of the respiratory CO_2 in this stage II of sleep was not significantly different from that during stage IV.

The association of EEG slow waves and changes of intracranial pressure during sleep is not a phenomenon confined to patients with high intracranial pressure as we found similar, but smaller, changes in a patient whose intracranial pressure was only a little above normal. In this patient there were no obvious changes of heart rate and respiration associated with the changes of intracranial pressure and EEG (Fig. 4).

The temporal relationships of some of the variables of Fig. 1 are shown in detail in Fig. 5. This record shows that the onset of the slow waves coincided with the hyperpnoea and tachycardia. The pressure began to fall 15 sec after the beginning of the delta waves and only after it had fallen considerably did the available oxygen and blood flow increase.

In Fig. 6 the increase in flow, as recorded by the thermistor, was earlier than in Fig. 5 and coincided with the tachycardia. The available oxygen in this record rose only when the pressure fell.

The results presented are representative of the features seen in the records of fifteen patients (12 cases of intracranial tumour and 3 cases of hydrocephalus due to non-neoplastic causes). Five patients who did not show these effects were three cases of intracranial tumour (2 supratentorial, 1 in the third ventricle), one case of hydrocephalus and the case of intracranial

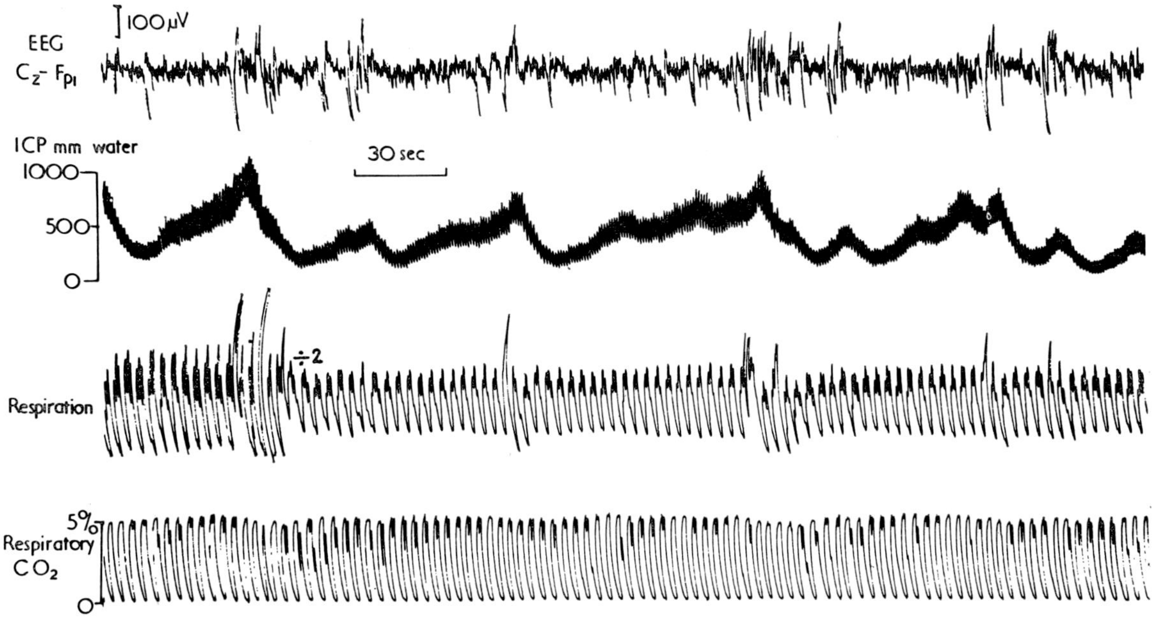

Fig. 3
Record showing changes of respiratory CO_2 during pressure waves. There was a small transient reduction of CO_2 following the increase in respiration which occurred at the time of the collapse of the pressure wave. There was no significant increase of CO_2 during the increase of intracranial pressure.

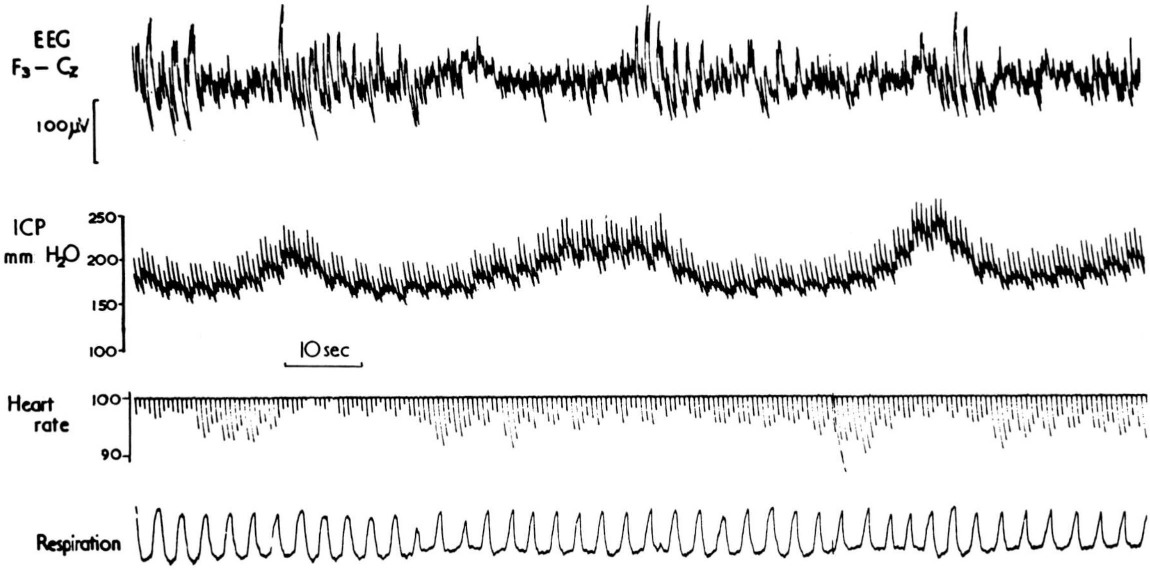

Fig. 4
Polygraphic record from patient with low intracranial pressure (communicating hydrocephalus). The changes are similar in type, but less in amplitude, to those seen in patients with high intracranial pressure.

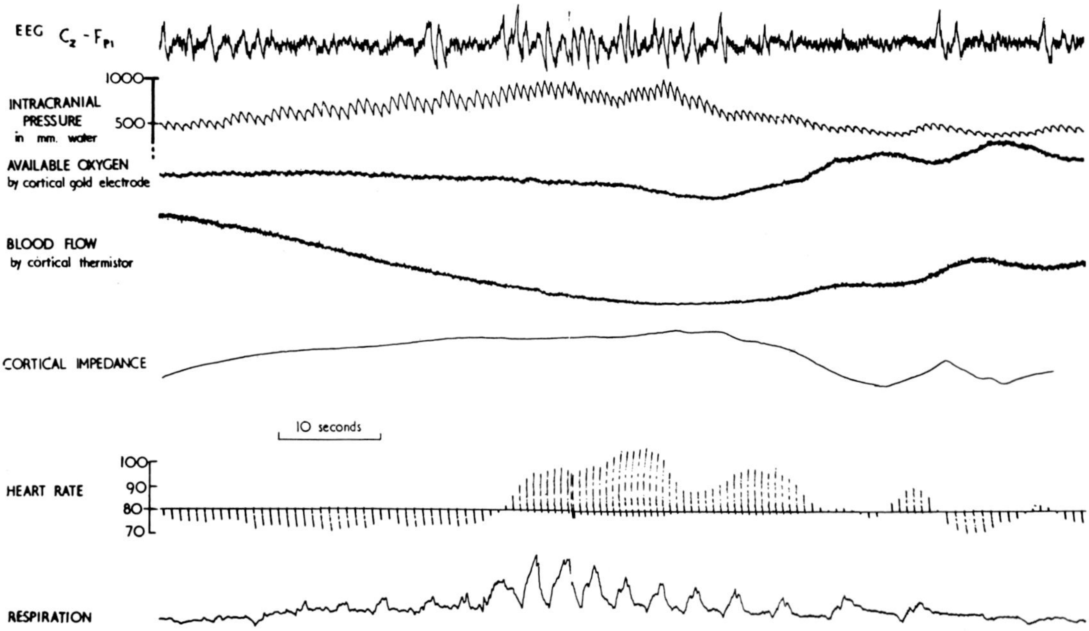

Fig. 5
Record showing the considerable delay between the increase of respiration and the change of pressure, O_2a, blood flow and cortical impedance. Same patient as in Fig. 1.

haematoma. The long lasting groups of slow waves in the EEG, with which the changes of pressure and other variables were clearly associated, were not seen in the sleep records of these five patients. Papilloedema was present in twelve of the fifteen patients showing the effects and in one of the five others. We could not find any relationship between the presence

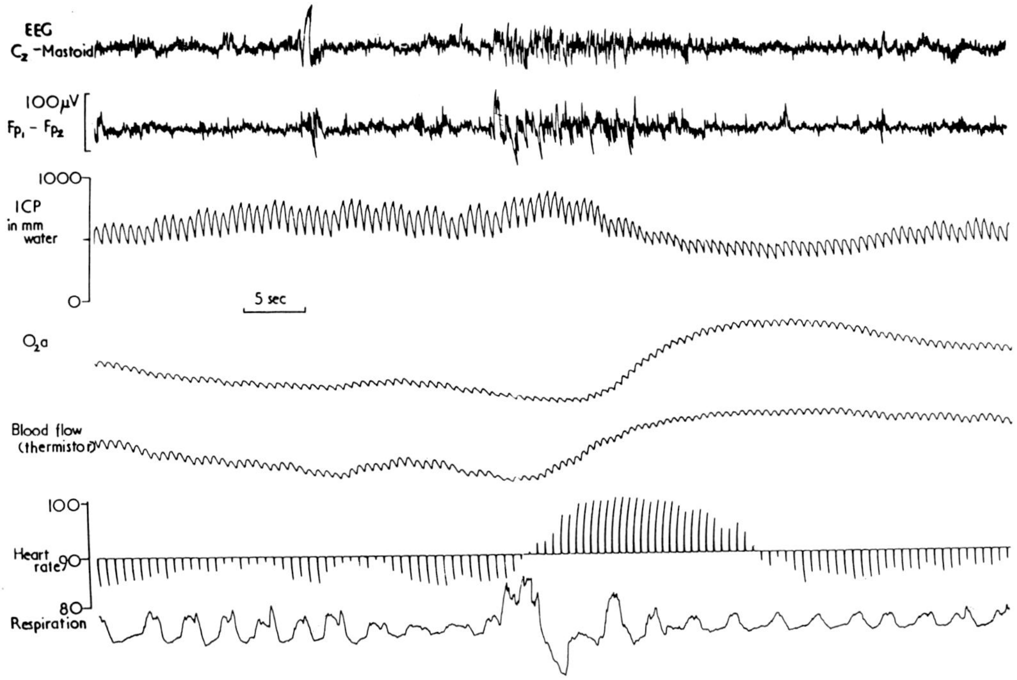

Fig. 6
In this patient (same as in Fig. 2) the increase of blood flow occurred at the same time as the tachycardia although the pressure continued high for several seconds.

or absence of these effects and the mental state, ventricular dilatation or midline shifts. Nor was their occurrence dependent upon a high mean intracranial pressure as they were observed in a case of communicating hydrocephalus in which the pressure was only a little above normal (200 mm H_2O, Fig. 4).

DISCUSSION

The results shown here were not evoked by artificial increases of intracranial pressure but occurred during natural sleep. Thus comparison with animal experiments, often performed under anaesthesia, in which changes are procured by inflating balloons, intracranial injections etc., is difficult. A comparable investigation, that of Ingvar and Lundberg (1961) showed very little change in EEG pattern during pressure waves, although their report did not include normal sleep.

Our records demonstrate clearly that during certain stages of sleep diffuse EEG activity can occur which is associated with changes of the intracranial dynamics. The rhythmical fluctuations of intracranial pressure and other variables appear to depend upon the occurrence of groups of slow waves in the EEG. If they do not occur, as in REM sleep, then the pressure builds up over a much longer period (several minutes) before collapsing (Cooper and Hulme 1966). In our records the biggest change of intracranial variables occurred when the groups of slow waves were of long duration (20 sec or more) and when the mean intracranial pressure was high. The delta activity observed in these patients is not a feature of the sleep records of normal people, although the K complexes in Fig. 2, which were associated with small fluctuations of intracranial pressure, were within the normal range. Whether the abnormalities were due to the intracranial pathology or to their great anxiety and restlessness is not known. We recorded these slow waves from patients with tumours and with hydrocephalus, when the intracranial pressure was very high (greater than 500 mm water) and just above normal (200 mm water). The frequent awakenings of these patients and their inability to fall asleep easily could be considered an exaggerated form of the "first night effect" observed in normal people acting as subjects for sleep studies (Agnew *et al.* 1966; Mendels and Hawkins 1967).

In previous publications (Lundberg 1960; Cooper and Hulme 1966) transient increases of intracranial pressure (plateau waves) were attributed to cerebral vasodilatation, although the evidence was indirect. Recently Cronquist and Lundberg (1968) reported that angiograms taken at the peaks and troughs of such waves showed that the cerebral vessels were dilated at the height of the pressure waves. Although the pressure fluctuations we have seen in sleep are not always typical plateau waves it is reasonable to assume that they are due also to fluctuations of vascular diameter. This assumption is supported by the increases of cortical impedance, indicating increases of brain volume (Moskalenko *et al.* 1964), and by the loss of the spontaneous fluctuations of cortical oxygen availability which occurs during vasodilatation (Clark *et al.* 1958; Cooper *et al.* 1966 and others). The paradoxical fall of cortical flow and oxygen availability seen in our records during this vasodilatation is most probably due to an increase of cerebral vascular resistance by the compression of the thin-walled venules by the raised intracranial pressure (Cronquist and Lundberg 1968).

Although cerebral vasodilatation and constriction may account for the changes observed in our records we do not know why the tone of the vessels should change at these times. It is generally accepted that the calibre of the cerebral vessels is determined largely by pH and pCO_2 in the region of the arterioles. This chemical environment can be altered systemically by changing the contents of the arterial blood or locally by changes in the metabolism of the tissue or accumulation of metabolites. Another factor affecting the tone of the vessels is cerebral oxygen tension which, when low, causes vasodilatation. There is also a possibility that the cerebral vessels, which are known to be innervated, might be under significant neurogenic control by the brain-stem (Scheinberg 1968). Yet another intrinsic mechanism of vascular control is the differential pressure across the walls of the cerebral vessels. As the differential pressure decreases, for example by decrease of blood pressure or increase of intracranial pressure, the vessels relax.

Nearly all of the intracranial pressure changes reported here were associated with changes of respiratory pattern. The Cheyne-Stokes type of respiration shown in Fig. 1, *a* and 5 would cause a rise of arterial, and therefore cerebral, pCO_2 during the apnoeic periods, thus causing an increase of intracranial pressure etc. The time relations of events leading to the fall of pressure in this case are interesting (Fig. 5). The increase of heart rate and depth of respiration and the start of the group of EEG slow waves occur practically simultaneously, whereas the changes of pressure, impedance (brain volume), blood flow and oxygen availability are delayed by 8–15 sec.

In Fig. 6, in which there is a deep breath associated with the collapse of the pressure wave, the increase of blood flow, as shown by the cortical thermistor, occurs at the same time as the heart rate increases.

From our observations it is not possible to determine with any degree of certainty which of the various mechanisms of altering cerebral vascular tone are in operation during these stages of sleep. It is possible that more than one are involved, interacting in a complex manner. The hypoxia or more probably the hypercarbia associated with the reduction of flow could stimulate the brain-stem, causing a respiratory gasp, increase in heart rate and EEG changes. When the intracranial pressure was high this increase in heart rate could lead to a significant increase in average blood flow (since the flow is partly pulsatile, Fig. 6), a reduction of cortical pCO_2 and vasoconstriction. As the intracranial pressure fell the blood flow would continue to increase because of the decreased cerebral vascular resistance, thus reducing the cerebral pCO_2 to a normal value. If this sequence of events overcompensated and reduced the pCO_2 to a subnormal value there would then be an apnoeic pause, as in Cheyne-Stokes respiration. In this explanation there need be no functional significance attached to the changes of the EEG, which could be a result of the brain-stem stimulation.

It is possible, however, that the cerebral

metabolic rate may be reduced during the time of diffuse delta activity, just as it is in deep sleep as compared with the activated REM stage, although the evidence for this is indirect (Brebbia and Altshuler 1965; Evarts 1962, 1964; Reivich *et al.* 1968). The reduced cerebral metabolic rate would reduce the cerebral pCO_2, cause vasoconstriction etc. and act as a protective mechanism. It would also reduce utilization of oxygen during adverse circumstances.

Although it is well known that the pial blood vessels are innervated there is only a little direct evidence (Mchedlishvili and Nikolaishvili 1967) that these nerves provide a control mechanism for cerebral blood flow. It is possible that the EEG slow waves described in this paper are the electrical control signals acting directly on the cortical blood vessels causing constriction.

Which, if any, of these hypotheses is correct must await further investigation.

SUMMARY

Indwelling pressure transducers, thermistors and gold electrodes have been used to measure intracranial pressure and other variables in neurosurgical patients. During stage II sleep diffuse scalp EEG activity is associated with changes of intracranial pressure and other variables. Possible mechanisms are discussed and it is suggested that, as in animals, cerebral metabolism is increased when the amplitude of the EEG is small (desynchronized) and decreased during periods of large amplitude slow waves.

RÉSUMÉ

MODIFICATIONS DE L'EEG, DE LA PRESSION INTRACRÂNIENNE ET D'AUTRES VARIABLES AU COURS DU SOMMEIL CHEZ DES MALADES PORTEURS DE LÉSIONS INTRACRÂNIENNES

Chez des malades neuro-chirurgicaux des capteurs de pression, des thermistors et des électrodes en or implantés ont été utilisés pour mesurer la pression intracranienne et d'autres variables. Au cours du stade II l'activité EEG diffuse de sommeil recueillie au niveau du scalp s'associe à des modifications de la pression intracranienne et des autres variables. Les mécanismes possibles de ces changements sont discutés; les auteurs suggèrent que, comme chez l'animal, le métabolisme cérébral augmente lorsque l'amplitude de l'EEG est faible (désynchronisée) et qu'il diminue pendant les périodes d'ondes lentes de grande amplitude.

It is a pleasure to acknowledge the help of our colleagues, especially Mr. W. J. Warren, who made this work possible. The Medical Research Council, W. Clement and Jessie V. Stone Foundation and Mr. M. S. Leslie-Rowe provided financial assistance.

REFERENCES

AGNEW, H. W., WEBB, W. B. and WILLIAMS, R. L. The first night effect: an EEG study of sleep. *Psychophysiology*, **1966**, *2*: 263–266.

BAGCHI, B. K., KOOI, K. A., SELVING, B. T. and CALHOUN, H. D. Subtentorial tumours and other lesions; an electroencephalographic study of 121 cases. *Electroenceph. clin. Neurophysiol.*, **1961**, *13*: 180–192.

BREBBIA, D. R. and ALTSHULER, K. Z. Oxygen consumption rate and electroencephalographic stage of sleep. *Science*, **1965**, *150*: 1621–1623.

CAVAZZUTI, G. B. EEG findings in infantile hydrocephalus. *Electroenceph. clin. Neurophysiol.*, **1959**, *11*: 383P.

CLARK, L. C., MISRAHY, G. A. and FOX, R. P. Chronically implanted polarograph electrodes. *J. appl. Physiol.*, **1958**, *13*: 85–91.

COBB, W. A. Rhythmic slow discharges in the electroencephalogram. *J. Neurol. Neurosurg. Psychiat.*, **1945**, *8*: 65–78.

COOPER, R. Local changes of intracerebral blood flow and oxygen in humans. *Med. Electron. biol. Engng.*, **1963**, *1*: 529–536.

COOPER, R., CROW, H. J., WALTER, W. G. and WINTER, A. L. Regional control of cerebral vascular reactivity and oxygen supply in man. *Brain Res.*, **1966**, *3*: 174–191.

COOPER, R. and HULME, A. Intracranial pressure and related phenomena during sleep. *J. Neurol. Neurosurg. Psychiat.*, **1966**, *29*: 564–570.

CRONQUIST, S. and LUNDBERG, N. Regional cerebral blood flow in intracranial tumours with special regard to cases with intracranial hypertension. *Scand. J. clin. Lab. Invest.*, **1968**, *Suppl. 102*: XV: A.

DEMENT, W. and KLEITMAN, N. Cyclic variations in EEG during sleep and their relation to eye movements, body motility and dreaming. *Electroenceph. clin. Neurophysiol.*, **1957**, *9*: 673–690.

EVARTS, E. V. Activity of neurons in visual cortex of the cat during sleep with low voltage fast EEG activity. *J. Neurophysiol.*, **1962**, *25*: 812–816.

EVARTS, E. V. Temporal patterns of discharge of pyramidal tract neurons during sleep and waking in the monkey. *J. Neurophysiol.*, **1964**, *27*: 152–171.

HULME, A. and COOPER, R. A technique for the investigation of intracranial pressure in man. *J. Neurol. Neurosurg. Psychiat.*, **1966,** *29*: 154–156.

INGVAR, D. H. and LUNDBERG, N. Paroxysmal symptoms in intracranial hypertension, studied with ventricular fluid pressure recording and electroencephalography. *Brain*, **1961,** *84*: 446–459.

LANGFITT, T. W., TANNANBAUM, H. M., KASSELL, N. F. and ZAREN, H. Acute intracranial hypertension, cerebral blood flow and the EEG. *Electroenceph. clin. Neurophysiol.*, **1966,** *20*: 139–148.

LUNDBERG, N. Continuous recording and control of ventricular fluid pressure in neurosurgical practice. *Acta psychiat. scand.*, **1960,** *Suppl. 149*: 36.

MANI, K. S. and TOWNSEND, H. R. A. The EEG in benign intracranial hypertension. *Electroenceph. clin. Neurophysiol.*, **1964,** *16*: 604–610.

MCHEDLISHVILI, G. I. und NIKOLAISHVILI, L. S. Zum nervosen Mechanismus der funktionellen Dilatation der Piaarterien. *Pflügers Arch. ges. Physiol.*, **1967,** *296*: 14–20.

MENDELS, J. and HAWKINS, D. R. Sleep laboratory adaption in normal subjects and depressed patients ("first night effect"). *Eejctroenceph. clin. Neurophysiol.*, **1967,** *22*: 556–558.

MEYER, J. S. and PORTNOY, H. D. Post-epileptic paralysis. *Brain*, **1959,** *82*: 162–185.

MOSKALENKO, YU. E., COOPER, R., CROW, H. J. and WALTER, W. G. Variations in blood volume and oxygen availability in the human brain. *Nature (Lond.)*, **1964,** *202*: 159–161.

PORTER, R., ADEY, W. R. and KADO, R. T. Measurement of electrical impedance in the human brain. *Neurology (Minneap.)*, **1964,** *14*: 1002–1012.

REIVICH, M., ISAACS, G., EVARTS, E. and KETY, S. The effect of slow wave sleep and REM sleep on regional cerebral blood flow in cats. *J. Neurochem.*, **1968,** *15*: 301–306.

ROBINSON, B. W. and TOMPKINS, H. E. Impedance method for localizing brain structures. *Arch. Neurol. (Chic.)*, **1964,** *10*: 563–574.

SCHEINBERG, P. Evidence for a brain-stem center regulating CBF. *Scand. J. clin. Lab. Invest.*, **1968,** *Suppl. 102*: VI: C.

WALTER, W. G. The electroencephalogram in cases of cerebral tumour. *Proc. roy. Soc. Med.*, **1937,** *30*: 579–598.

WILSON, W. P., TINDALL, G. T. and GREENFIELD JR., J. C. Effects of an acute rise of intracranial pressure upon the electroencephalogram. *Electroenceph. clin. Neurophysiol.*, **1965,** *19*: 184–186.

Reference: COOPER, R. and HULME, A. Changes of the EEG, intracranial pressure and other variables during sleep in patients with intracranial lesions. *Electroenceph. clin. Neurophysiol.*, **1969,** *27*: 12–22.

Electroencephalography and Clinical Neurophysiology
Elsevier Publishing Company, Amsterdam – Printed in The Netherlands

THE AVERAGE VISUAL RESPONSE IN PATIENTS WITH CEREBROVASCULAR DISEASE[1]

H. J. G. H. OOSTERHUIS[2], L. PONSEN, E. J. JONKMAN AND O. MAGNUS

The Neurological and Neurosurgical Hospital "St. Ursula Kliniek", Wassenaar (The Netherlands)

(Accepted for publication: October 24, 1968)

The significance of the average visual response (AVR) for the diagnosis of brain disease has been mainly investigated in patients with visual field defects (Cohn 1963; Gastaut *et al.* 1963; Vaughan *et al.* 1963; Vaughan and Katzman 1964; Kooi *et al.* 1965; Crighel and Botez 1966). In patients with homonymous defects in the visual fields abnormalities were found in the so-called primary response (waves I and II according to Cigánek's nomenclature). In patients with brain lesions without visual field defects wave II appeared to have a longer latency on the side of the lesion, but the difference between the latencies on the normal and the abnormal sides was much less than in patients with a hemianopia (Vaughan *et al.* 1963). A smaller amplitude of wave V appeared to be associated with a reduced amplitude of the alpha rhythm (Kooi *et al.* 1965).

It is still not clear whether this method of investigation, employed complementary to the "routine" EEG, is useful for the diagnosis or the localization of a cerebral lesion. Moreover, the specificity of an abnormal AVR has not been sufficiently investigated.

In addition to the investigations of one of our team (Jonkman 1967), we decided to initiate an exploratory investigation on the AVR in patients with a lesion in one cerebral hemisphere. Patients with a cerebrovascular accident seemed to be well suited for this purpose, as the unaffected hemisphere could serve as a control.

Jonkman (1967) compared the AVR in 115 patients with various brain disorders with those of sixteen normal young adults and ten older normal controls. The AVR was asymmetrical in twenty-one out of twenty-two patients with a homonymous visual field defect. However, asymmetrical responses were frequently found in the presence of unilateral lesions without homonymous hemianopia. Out of fourteen patients with cerebrovascular lesions with an asymmetrical AVR eight had a homonymous hemianopia and in six the visual fields were normal. Asymmetry of the secondary response was always associated with asymmetry of the primary response. The secondary response was asymmetrical only when the lesion affected the occipital or parieto-occipital area or in the presence of a unilateral lesion of the visual pathways.

METHODS

Patients

AVRs have been recorded in a group of thirty patients varying in age between 35 and 80 years (35–39: 5; 40–49: 1; 50–59: 10; 60–69: 11; 70 and older: 3); seventeen were male and thirteen female. All patients were admitted to the St. Ursula Kliniek. Diagnosis of a cerebrovascular lesion was made on the combined data of a history of acute onset, clinical examination which usually included arteriography, and a follow-up. The lesion was on the left side in seventeen patients, on the right in eleven, bilateral in two patients. Six patients had a hemianopia. Twenty-three patients were examined once, five twice and two patients 3 times. The data obtained in such repeated examinations were treated as

[1] These investigations have been carried out with support from the Netherlands Research Organisation T.N.O.

[2] Present address: Neurological Clinic, Wilhelmina Gasthuis, University of Amsterdam, The Netherlands.

TABLE I

Average visual responses in thirty patients with cerebrovascular lesions

Cerebral pathology	Ischaemic lesion in area of: middle cerebral a.	basilar a.	Intra-cerebral haematoma	Total
Moderate	5	5 (3)	1	11 (3)
Severe	12	2 (2)	5 (1)	19 (3)
Total	17	7 (5)	6 (1)	30 (6)

( ), patients with visual field defects.

new data, as they were obtained after a material change of the clinical picture. According to the severity of the disturbance but without taking into account the EEG findings the cases were divided into two groups. A moderate cerebrovascular disturbance was considered to be present when there was a partial (motor or sensory) hemisyndrome, or a hemianopia with sparing of central vision, or an incomplete aphasia. There was considered to be a severe disturbance when there was a complete hemisyndrome, or a complete aphasia, or a complete homonymous hemianopia, or a combination of various partial disturbances. The distribution according to the location of the lesion and according to the severity of the cerebral pathology is seen in Table I.

Controls

Obviously it was necessary to study the AVR in normal controls from the same age group. Fourteen control subjects were examined with the same method as the patients. The ages varied between 46 and 74 years, eight were male and six female. Six were admitted because of low back pain, one because of a disorder of the spinal cord and the others had no illness or complaints. The routine EEGs were unremarkable in ten, one had a low voltage fast EEG, one an alpha rhythm at 8 c/sec, one a dominant rhythm in the posterior regions at 14–16 c/sec and one had sporadic slow waves in the temporal regions. These findings were not considered to be pathological for the age.

Stimulation and recording

The method has been described in detail by Jonkman (1967). Orange-red flashes with a duration of 4.8 msec and a light intensity of 2 lux/sec at the level of the eyelids were presented at a frequency of 1/1.5 sec. The lamp was placed at a distance of 15 cm from the closed eyes. The patient was urged to stay awake.

Prior to the recording of the AVR a routine EEG was made in all patients and controls. The EEG was also recorded simultaneously with the AVR in order to monitor the level of vigilance. A 16-channel van Gogh electroencephalograph, type EST 16B, was used.

The electrodes were applied with collodion at the positions of the 10–20 system with additional electrodes bilaterally in the suboccipital regions at the same inter-electrode distance. Occasionally one midline electrode on the inion was used. Bipolar serial derivations from the frontal poles to the suboccipital electrodes over the convexity and derivations over the central, parietal and occipital regions were used. A derivation between one occipital electrode and the ipsilateral ear was included routinely. In the last third of the experiments no recording was made from the anterior region of the scalp as it had become evident that the response, recorded by this method, did not extend significantly into this area.

The electrical activity recorded during presentation of 500 or 250 flashes was stored in an FR 1300 Ampex tape recorder, which had 13 FM channels and 1 AM channel, in order to record from 13 channels simultaneously, so that the potential distribution could be determined with 2 series of flashes. Afterwards the visual response recorded in each channel was summated by the Computer of Average Transients (Mnemotron type 400 B) for 2 or 3 analysis periods (usually 125 and 500 msec). The resulting averages were plotted with a Moseley X–Y plotter (Autograf model 135). In this way at least 50 curves were obtained for each subject per experiment. The pupils were not dilated artificially and their diameter was not measured. This did not appear to be essential for our purpose. It was ascertained that the media of the eyes were clear. The various data obtained in the present investigations were submitted to statistical analysis with the χ^2 test.

Evaluation of the AVR

In accordance with the publications of Cigánek (1961a and b) the AVR was divided into a primary response during the period of 0–100 msec after the stimulus, a secondary response between 100 and 300 msec and a rhythmic response. A detailed analysis was made of the AVR in the parieto-occipital and occipital-to-ear derivations on both sides. The potential distribution was evaluated in the same way as is done for the interpretation of an ordinary EEG. For this purpose composite antero-posterior and transverse derivations were used such as are used routinely in electroencephalography. On the basis of the findings of Vaughan *et al.* (1963) and those obtained in normal controls by Jonkman (1967) in our hospital and the additional controls investigated for comparison with the present series of patients, the following criteria for the limits of normal values were fixed. The primary response was considered to be normal in configuration when there was at least one peak in the period between 60 and 100 msec after the flash (wave III) and the symmetry was considered to be within normal limits when the difference between the peak latencies on both sides did not exceed 5 msec and the difference in amplitude was not more than 50% of the smaller of the values on each side. When the earliest components (wave I or wave II) were present the same criteria were applied as regards the symmetry.

The secondary response was considered to be normal and symmetrical when, in the period between 100 and 300 msec after the flash, a bi- or polyphasic curve was obtained which appeared to be reasonably symmetrical in shape, with a difference of peak latency not exceeding 25 msec and a difference of amplitude not greater than 50%. Similar criteria were applied for the rhythmic response.

Evaluation of the EEG

The EEGs were described and interpreted by two of the authors independently, without knowledge of any data of the case or of the AVR. They were classified in 3 groups. Group 1: the EEGs were normal or showed slight or questionable abnormalities such as some asymmetry of the background activity, a low voltage fast pattern, sporadic slow waves in temporal regions. Such patterns usually have no pathological significance for the age group of the present series. Group 2: EEGs with definite local abnormalities, usually consisting in depression of normal background activity or local or unilateral slow waves. Group 3: EEGs with severe diffuse disturbances.

As could be expected there was a good correlation between the degree of abnormality of the EEG and the severity of the cerebral lesion ($P < 0.001$).

RESULTS

In these investigations it was evident that there were considerable differences in the AVR as recorded in different subjects and that the configuration and peak latency of the AVR varied markedly with the level of consciousness. This was of considerable importance as patients with vascular lesions are often drowsy and in some cases there was a continuous impairment

TABLE II

AVR waves I and II (occipital-to-ear derivation)

AVR	Controls	Cerebral pathology	
		Moderate	Severe
Symmetrical	9	6	7
Absent	3	5 (2)	5 (3)
Asymmetrical	2	6 (4)	10 (3)
Smaller on abnormal side		4 (3)	7 (3)
Larger on abnormal side		2 (1)	3

Figures represent number of records. ( ), records of patients with visual field defects.

TABLE III

AVR peak latency and amplitude of wave II (occipital-to-ear derivation)

	Patients		Controls	
	Affected hemisphere	Unaffected hemisphere	Left	Right
Records with recognizable wave II	23	26	8	7
Mean peak latency (msec)	51.5	51.2	53	56
Standard deviation	8.7	7.9	8.7	8.8
Variation	41–72	40–73	42–68	42–68
Mean amplitude (μV)	2.2	2.1	2.3	1.6
Standard deviation	1.2	1.6	—	—
Variation	0.8–5.0	0.5–6.5	0.5–5.0	1.0–3.0

TABLE IV

Peak latencies and amplitudes of wave III (occipital-to-ear derivation)

	Patients		Controls	
	Affected hemisphere	Unaffected hemisphere	Left	Right
Experiments	34	35	14	14
Mean peak latency (msec)	83	83	82	83
Standard deviation	10	10	11	12
Variation	67–110	60–117	70–106	70–106
R–L difference > 5 msec	6 ×		0 ×	
Mean amplitude (μV)	8.4	8.6	6.6	6.6
Standard deviation	5.3	4.9	3.5	3.5
Variation	2–26	1–19	2–16	2–15
R–L difference > 50%	4 ×		0 ×	

of consciousness. However, this did not affect the degree of symmetry substantially.

A. *The primary response*

1. Waves I and II (Cigánek 1961a and b). Some data concerning waves I and II in controls and patients are summarized in Tables II and III. From these tables it can be seen that bilateral absence of waves I and II as recorded by this method is not to be considered a sign of pathology and that it was not correlated with the presence of a disturbance in the visual pathways. Asymmetrical responses were found more frequently in patients than in controls, but there was no correlation with the degree of cerebral pathology. Waves I and II could, when present, practically be recorded only at the occipital electrodes.

It is remarkable that no difference was found, in average peak latencies and amplitudes of the early waves, between the affected and the unaffected hemispheres, or between the patients and controls.

2. Wave III. This component was present in all control subjects and it was only absent in three patients, two of whom had severe cerebral pathology. Some data concerning wave III are summarized in Table IV.

A difference of peak latency of more than

5 msec between the two sides, or a difference of amplitude of more than 50% between the right and left sides (the test criteria for abnormality!) was present in six patients, two of whom had a visual field defect. Of the other four patients three had a severe, and one a moderate, cerebral disturbance.

Wave III, or at least a distinct peak with the same latency of approximately 80 msec, was not infrequently found to be surface positive in the occipital region, but sometimes it was surface negative. The polarity showed no correlation with the severity of the cerebral pathology, the duration of the affection, the occurrence of patterns of sleep or drowsiness in the EEG or with the amplitude of the alpha rhythm. There was, however, a correlation with the age of the subject. As stated by Jonkman (1967), wave III was relatively more often positive in older subjects than in younger ones. This was particularly evident when younger control subjects from the previous study by Jonkman were included in the present series (Table V). The amplitude of wave

TABLE V

Polarity of wave III in relation to age

	20–29		30–49		50–59		60–69		70–	
	+	–	+	–	+	–	+	–	+	–
Patients	0	0	1	5	7	3	7	3	3	0
Controls	0	10	0	2	2	3	2	1	2	0
Total	0	10	1	7	9	6	9	4	5	0

III in the patients was not correlated with the amplitude of the alpha rhythm, the severity of the cerebral abnormalities or the degree of abnormality of the AVR as a whole. Wave III was generally recorded over the entire posterior part of the scalp, with a maximum in the occipital region.

3. The primary response in relation to the cerebral pathology. The degree of abnormality of the primary response *as a whole*, as judged according to the standards established above, was determined both in the parieto-occipital and in the occipital-to-ear derivations. In the parieto-occipital derivation there was significantly more often an abnormal primary response in patients with severe cerebral pathology than in those with moderate pathology ($P < 0.05$); in the occipital-to-ear derivation such a correlation could not be established. In the presence of disturbances of the visual system the primary response as a whole was more often abnormal, independent of the degree of cerebral pathology.

B. *The secondary response*

The AVR usually had its greatest amplitude in the secondary response; it varied between 2 and 40 μV in patients and between 7 and 20 μV in controls. The amplitude of the secondary response was more often greater than 20 μV in patients than in controls ($P < 0.05$). It showed no correlation with the amplitude of the alpha rhythm. Differences in amplitude of more than 50% between the left and right sides were seen 5 times (in 4 patients), in all instances in patients with a disturbance of the visual system; in these cases there was also a pathological asymmetry of the primary response.

In the parieto-occipital derivation an abnormal secondary response was more often found in patients with severe than in those with moderate cerebral pathology ($P < 0.1$); in the occipital-to-ear derivation there was no such correlation. In the fourteen control subjects the secondary response showed no abnormalities.

C. *The rhythmic response (R.R.)*

The amplitude of this part of the AVR was correlated with the amplitude of the alpha rhythm ($P < 0.05$). In the parieto-occipital derivation the R.R. was normal in 21 records, abnormal in 12 and absent in 6; in recording from the occipital-to-ear derivation these figures were 18, 15 and 6. When there was a difference in amplitude of more than 50%, the R.R. was usually smaller on the pathological side (8 ×), but in 2 instances it was larger on this side; in the latter cases the alpha rhythm was also greater on this side. In the parieto-occipital derivation the R.R. was abnormal or absent significantly more often in patients with severe cerebral pathology than in those with moderate pathology ($P < 0.05$). In the group of fourteen controls the rhythmic response was always normal in the parieto-occipital and occipital-to-ear derivations.

TABLE VI

Score of the AVR and degree of cerebral pathology (parieto-occipital derivation)

Cerebral pathology	Scores				Total
	0	1	2	3	
Moderate	11 (2–1)	2	2 (2–2)	2 (2–1)	17 (6–3)
Severe	5 (1–1)	5	4 (2–1)	8 (3–2)	22 (6–3)
Total	16 (3–2)	7	6 (4–3)	10 (5–3)	39 (12–6)

In parentheses: the first figure represents the number of records of patients with visual field defects, while the second one gives the number of patients with such defects.

D. *The evaluation of the AVR as a whole*

A "score" of the AVR as a whole was made up of the separate scores of the primary, secondary and rhythmic responses (0 = normal, 1 = abnormal). In this way the score of the AVR ranged from 0 (normal) to 3 (most abnormal). The correlation of the score of the AVR with the degree of cerebral pathology, the duration since the occurrence of the cerebral vascular accident and the severity of the EEG abnormalities was investigated (Tables VI and VII). It appears from Table VI that the AVR in the parieto-occipital derivation was less abnormal in patients with a moderate lesion than in patients with a severe lesion. However, the difference is not significant ($0.1 < P < 0.2$). The same holds true for the records (patients) with a disturbance of the visual system.

As regards the AVR from the occipital-to-ear derivation there was no difference between the two categories of cerebral pathology. No correlation was found between the time elapsed since the cerebrovascular accident and the score of the AVR. The degree of EEG disturbance was only partially correlated with the abnormality of the AVR. Only in the occipito-parietal derivation did it appear that patients with an abnormal EEG had an abnormal AVR more often than patients with an EEG within normal limits for the age ($P < 0.05$; Table VII). In the occipital-to-ear derivation there was no such correlation. In the group of controls ten subjects had a normal AVR (score 0), four subjects had a primary response which, according to our criteria, had to be classified as "abnormal" (score 1). The difference between the AVR in the patients and in the control group is highly significant ($P < 0.005$).

TABLE VII

Correlation between the AVR and the EEG

Score of AVR in P–O lead	EEG		Total
	Normal	Abnormal	
0	12 (3)	4	16 (3)
1	2	5	7
2 + 3	7 (4)	9 (5)	16 (9)
Total	21 (7)	18 (5)	39 (12)

( ), records of patients with visual field defects.

ILLUSTRATIVE CASE HISTORY

Patient A, male, 25 years of age, when watching a football match suddenly fell ill with headache and vomiting; he noticed a disturbance of his left visual field. On admission he was found to have a left hemianopia and nuchal rigidity. The CSF contained blood. The EEG showed a smaller amplitude of the alpha rhythm and local delta activity in the right temporo-occipital region. Angiography of the carotid and vertebral arteries showed no abnormalities. A diagnosis of intracerebral and subarachnoid haemorrhage was made. Since the first week after the onset of his illness he noticed that he could not recognize faces (prosopagnosia).

After 1 month, when the AVR was recorded, the visual fields (Fig. 1) showed no defects for gross movements, but when determined with small test objects there appeared to be a ribbon-shaped homonymous defect reaching the midline; there was a disturbance of the left visual field for colours and for the recognition of

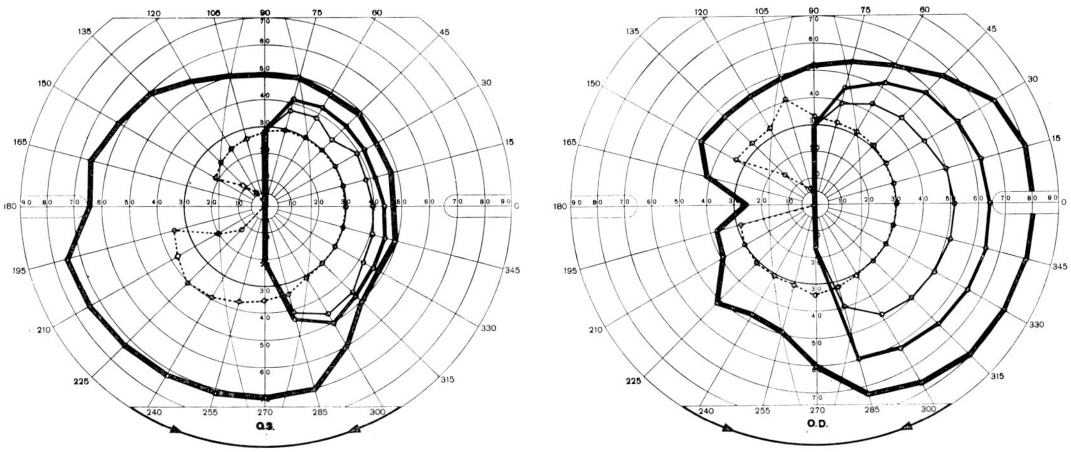

Fig. 1

Visual fields of patient A, 7 weeks after cerebrovascular accident. Solid lines, in decreasing order of thickness = white, blue and red respectively, with a 16 mm² object and relative intensity 1; broken line = white, 1 mm² object, relative intensity 1.

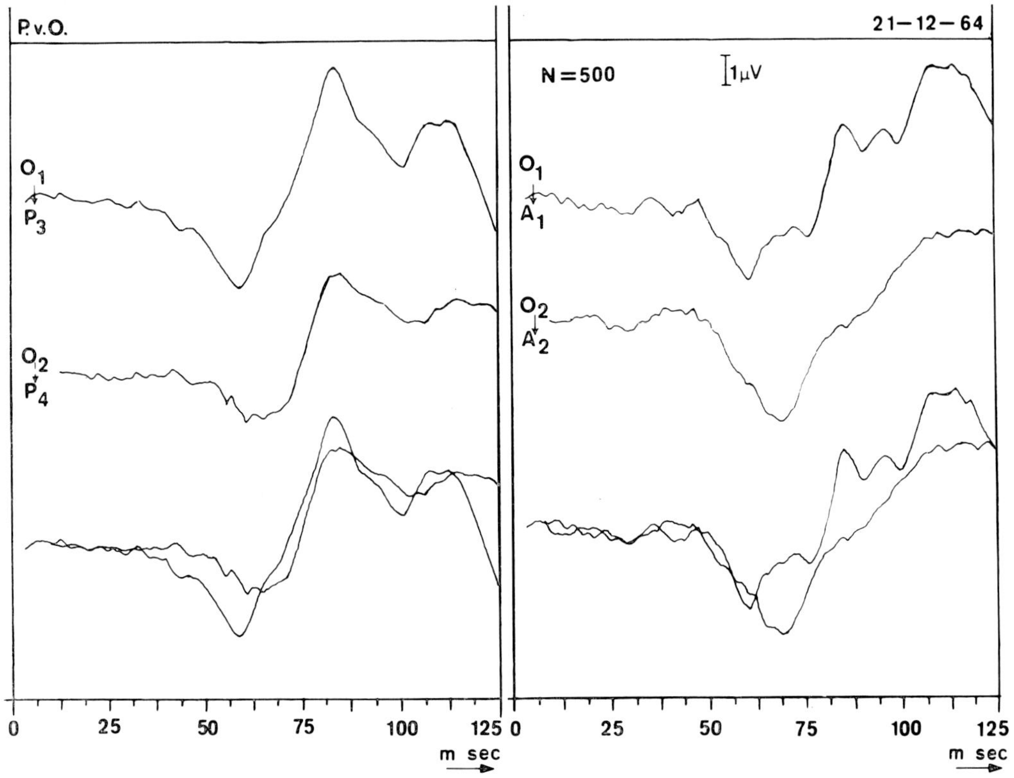

Fig. 2

Responses of patient A, 1 month after the cerebrovascular accident. *Top*: left side; *centre*: right side; *bottom*: the above superimposed.

objects. No other neurological or psychiatric abnormalities were found. The patient had no disturbance of consciousness or vigilance and was very cooperative. Optokinetic nystagmus and localization on imagination were normal. Faces looked strange and could only be recognized with difficulty.

During the second recording, 3 months after the onset, he still had a prosopagnosia; now the visual fields were normal for movement and colours; however, recognition of objects was still impaired in the left visual field. The picture had not changed 10 and 16 months after the cerebrovascular accident. The EEG at the time of the second AVR had not changed.

The AVR (Fig. 2) always showed abnormal differences between the right and left sides, in shape as well as in latency and amplitude. The abnormalities were maximal in the occipital-to-ear derivation. The AVRs recorded in subsequent investigations differed considerably from each other in this case (Fig. 3). The differences between the left and the right sides also proved to be present during sleep.

DISCUSSION

Particularly in older persons the average visual response appears to show considerable individual variations. On comparison with the results obtained by other investigators (Ciganek 1961a and b; Kooi and Bagchi 1964; Kooi *et al.* 1965; Vaughan *et al.* 1963; Vaughan and Katzman 1964; Gastaut 1966) there appear to be considerable differences, particularly as regards

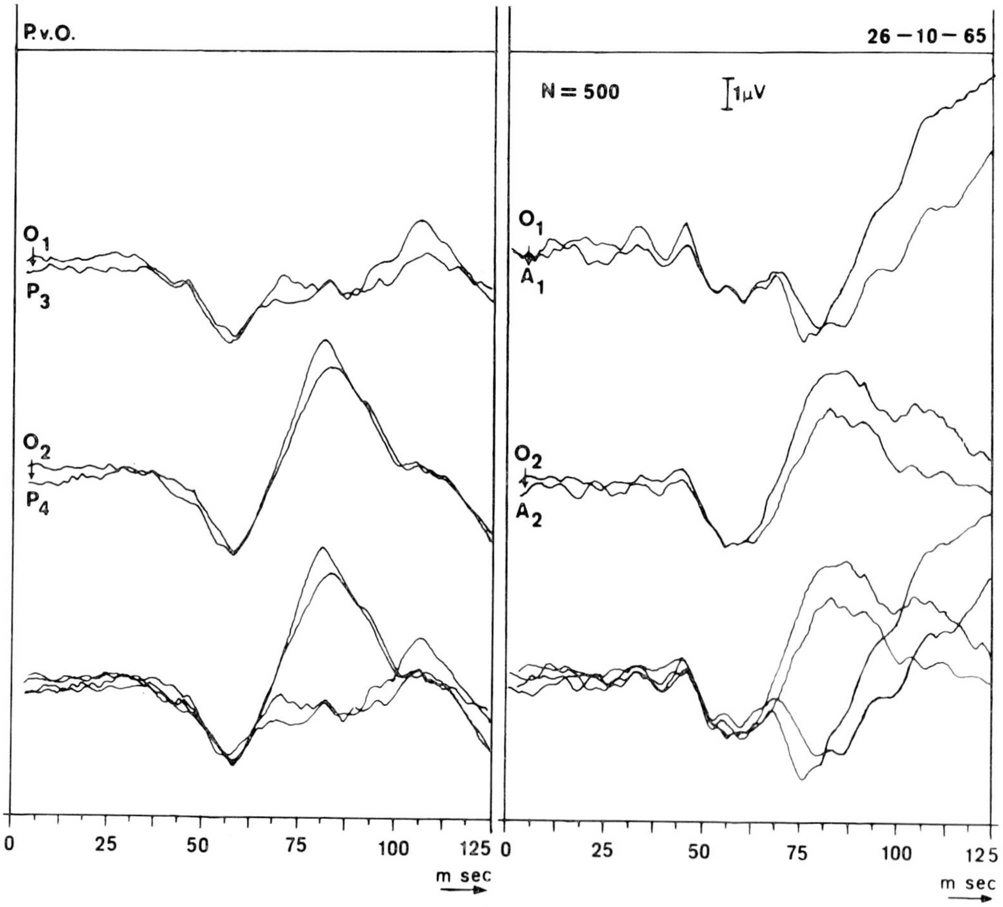

Fig. 3
Responses of patient A, 11 months after the cerebrovascular accident. *Top*: left side; *centre*: right side; *bottom*: the above superimposed. Each trace shows two AVRs superimposed.

the presence or absence and the latencies of the components of the primary response.

Notwithstanding that 500 flashes were presented waves I and II were both absent in 10 out of 30 records of patients and in three out of fourteen control subjects; *i.e.*, in about one out of four of all AVR recorded. Wave I was absent in 65% of the patients. One of the control subjects had an asymmetric primary response according to our criteria. In Cigánek's (1961a) group of normal controls wave I was absent only in 15%, in one-third of the series of normals and patients with cerebral lesions of Vaughan *et al.* (1963). Wave II was absent in six out of fourteen of our older controls; in this respect our findings also differ from those of Cigánek (1961a), who apparently mainly investigated younger control subjects. Vaughan *et al.* (1963) and Vaughan and Katzman (1964) considered the absence, or a marked asymmetry, of this second component more or less characteristic of a lesion of the visual pathways. On the other hand Gastaut (1966) found all components of the AVR only in 20% of his group of control subjects. The differences between the results of various authors could be due to differences in technique, particularly in colour and intensity of the flashes, but also at least partly to differences of age. Jonkman's results in young and older adults, obtained with the same technique, seem to point in this direction.

Apparently the absence of the first and second component of the primary response is not *per se* pathological with our technique and for the age group of our patients. Absence or a marked asymmetry of wave III (approximately 80 msec after the flash) does appear to indicate pathology: this component was only absent in two patients (3 recordings) with visual field defects associated with other signs of the presence of severe cerebral pathology. It appears that there is not infrequently a distinct surface positive wave with the same latency as Cigánek's wave III. It is likewise fairly diffuse over the posterior part of the head with a maximum in the occipital region. We have considered this wave as a "positive wave III" though such an interpretation may not be generally acceptable. This wave is also apparent in the illustrations of the AVR of a few patients in the series of Vaughan *et al.* (1963). The present observations confirm the previous findings from our laboratory (Jonkman 1967). From our group of subjects it appears that the percentage of cases in which wave III is surface positive increases steadily with age; this holds true for patients as well as for controls. The correlation is highly significant ($P < 0.01$).

When the AVR was considered as a whole and a score was given for the degree of abnormality the score for the AVR in the occipito-parietal derivation showed some correlation with the severity of cerebral pathology, the presence of visual field defects and the degree of abnormality of the EEG; such a correlation was not found in the occipital-to-ear derivations. Patients with lesions of the visual pathways did not always have the most marked abnormalities of the AVR. In two patients with a homonymous hemianopia with only a small central sparing the response was entirely normal. In one of these patients this was confirmed by a second recording. In two patients with a homonymous hemianopia reaching to the fixation point the AVRs were abnormal (score 2 and 3, later confirmed in one patient). Particularly interesting were the findings in patient A with prosopagnosia. This patient's AVR remained very abnormal after his visual fields had become normal apart from a slight defect for the recognition of small geometric figures. This tends to indicate that the primary response does not depend only on the primary occipital projection area (area 17) as Cigánek supposed (1961a). With the patients of the present series the disturbance of the entire AVR was generally more marked as the cerebral lesion was more extensive, even without there being an impairment of the visual fields.

It must be concluded that the characteristic features of the AVR, even of the primary response, are not determined only by the visual pathways and the visual projection areas in the cerebral cortex. This is in itself not as surprising as it seems: for we know from electroencephalography that areas with abnormal spontaneous electrical activity may still function normally. It will need further investigations to ascertain which type and location of lesion give rise to specific changes in the AVR. The conclusion of one of us (Jonkman 1967) that the secondary response is only abnormal when there is a lesion of the visual pathways or the occipital cortex was confirmed in this series. This was also true for the finding that an abnormal asymmetry of the secondary response was always associated with an abnormal primary response.

The use of a 13-channel FM tape recorder made it possible to record routinely in patients the AVR for different analysis times and enabled us to study the potential distribution of the main components of the AVR in a similar way to reading an ordinary EEG. It has been confirmed that only wave III and the later components extend (with decreasing amplitudes) to parietal, posterior temporal and sometimes also to the central regions. It must be stressed that this only holds true for the visual response averaged after a great number of stimuli. This probably explains the practically complete absence of a response in the vertex area, where it is sometimes seen in the ordinary EEG and where it can often be obtained by averaging responses to a small series of flashes.

The parieto-occipital derivation appears to provide a more satisfactory curve than the occipital-to-ear derivation as the abnormality of the AVR in the latter tended to correlate with the severity of the cerebral disorder and with the degree of EEG abnormality, whereas the occipital-to-ear AVR did not show such a correlation. The earliest components were sometimes only seen in parieto-occipital derivations, but there were cases in which they were only obtained in occipital-to-ear derivations. Therefore it is recommended to record between the occipital electrode and a distant reference such as the ear or the vertex in addition to the parieto-occipital derivation. The absence or asymmetry of waves I and II is not in itself abnormal; an asymmetry of these components occurred much less frequently in controls than in patients, but there was no correlation with the degree of cerebral pathology. In order to obtain these early components with our method it is necessary to use 500 stimuli. The later components can nearly always be obtained with 200 flashes and often even with 50–100 flashes. As the application of a great number of stimuli is time-consuming and very tiring, particularly for patients with brain lesions, it is probably in most cases sufficient to use 200 flashes.

Our investigations have indicated that the AVR is often modified by hemisphere lesions, even when they do not interfere with the visual pathways. It is usually only by comparison with the response from the other side (if this is not or much less affected) that criteria of abnormality can be established. The variation of the AVR in normals is such that only in rare cases can an AVR be considered to be abnormal as such.

So far the determination of the AVR in patients with a cerebrovascular accident has not revealed specific features which would make it of value for clinical diagnosis. The expensive and complicated equipment, the fact that the recording must be made by a highly qualified investigator and the time-consuming nature of each investigation are so far additional important limitations to the usefulness of this method for clinical diagnosis. Further studies may eventually lead to a simplification of the method and to specific indications for its application. Before that time it will be necessary to continue research in order to gain a better insight into the origin of the different components of the AVR and the factors determining changes in the parameters of its various components.

SUMMARY

The average visual response (AVR) was recorded in thirty patients after a cerebrovascular accident and in fourteen control subjects from the same age group. The AVR was obtained with the aid of a 16-channel EEG machine, a Computer of Average Transients and a tape recorder with 13 FM channels. This made it possible to study different periods after the stimuli and to study the potential distribution of the various components.

Primary and secondary parts of the response and the rhythmic response were considered separately and the AVR was also considered as a whole. There were large inter-individual differences in both the patients and the controls. Therefore no general criteria of abnormality of the AVR could be established from the control subjects; criteria of abnormality of the degree of asymmetry between the AVR from the affected and unaffected sides were defined. The absence of waves I or II could not be considered pathological. In our series wave III (peak latency approximately 80 msec) was not infrequently surface positive in the occipital region. The presence of such a positive wave III correlated with the age of the subject both in the patient group and in the group of controls.

The primary and secondary responses and the AVR as a whole, recorded from the parieto-occipital derivation, were more frequently abnormal in patients with severe cerebral pathology than in those with moderate pathology. Such a correlation could not be found for the AVR recorded from the occipital-to-ear derivation. Similar findings were obtained, independent of the degree of cerebral pathology, for the patients with a disturbance of the visual system. An abnormal asymmetry of the amplitude of the secondary response only occurred in patients with disturbance of the visual system. The amplitude of the rhythmic response was correlated with the amplitude of the alpha rhythm; such a correlation could not be demonstrated for the other components of the AVR.

A normal AVR was found more often in controls and in patients with a normal EEG than in patients with moderate or severe EEG disturbances. Determination of the potential field of the AVR with the aid of multi-channel recording did not appear to furnish significantly more information for diagnostic purposes than recording from both parieto-occipital areas. The AVR from the parieto-occipital derivation appeared to provide a better picture of the disturbances of cerebral function than did the occipital-to-ear derivation.

RÉSUMÉ

LA RÉPONSE VISUELLE MOYENNE CHEZ DES MALADES ATTEINTS D'UNE AFFECTION CÉRÉBROVASCULAIRE

Les réponses visuelles moyennes (RVM) ont été enregistreés chez trente malades atteints d'affection cérébrovasculaire et chez quatorze sujets de contrôle d'age comparable. Les RVM ont été obtenues à l'aide d'un appareil d'EEG à 16 plumes et un "Computer of Average Transients (C.A.T.)". L'enregistrement sur bande magnétique à 13 canaux M.F. nous a permi à étudier des périodes différentes suivant les stimuli ainsi que les champs de potentiel des composants de la RVM.

Les réponses dites primaires, secondaires et rythmiques ont été envisagées et en plus la RVM a été étudiée dans sa totalité. De grandes différences inter-individuelles ont été constatées aussi bien chez les malades que chez les sujets normaux. Pour cette raison il était impossible d'établir des critères de normalité de la RVM; par contre des critères d'anomalie du degré d'asymétrie ont été définis entre la RVM du côté atteint en comparaison avec le côté sain. L'absence des ondes I et II (suivant la définition de Cigánek) ne pouvait être considerée comme pathologique. Dans notre série une onde III (ou bien une onde avec la même latence d'environ 80 msec) avec un signe positif dans la région occipital a été assez souvent enregistré. Une corrélation a été établie entre la présence d'une telle onde positive et l'âge des malades aussi bien que des sujets normaux.

La RVM enregistrée dans la dérivation parieto-occipitale était plus souvent anormale chez les malades atteints d'une affection cérébrale grave que chez ceux avec une affection moderée. Une telle corrélation n'a pu être établie en ce qui concerne la RVM enregistrée dans la dérivation occipito-auriculaire. Des résultats similaires ont été obtenus des malades atteints de troubles du système visuel, indépendant du degré de la pathologie cérébrale. Une asymétrie anormale de l'amplitude de la réponse secondaire se trouvait seulement chez des malades souffrant d'une atteinte du système visuel. Il y avait une corrélation entre l'amplitude de la réponse rythmique et l'amplitude du rythme alpha; une telle corrélation n'a pas été constatée pour les autres composants de la RVM.

Une RVM normale a été enrégistrée plus fréquemment chez les sujets de contrôle et chez les malades avec un EEG normal que chez les malades souffrants des affections cérébrovasculaires modérées et graves. L'analyse du champs de potentiel de la RVM en utilisant une bande magnétique à 13 canaux ne nous a pas fourni d'une façon significative plus de données diagnostiques que l'enregistrement des deux aires parieto-occipitales. La dérivation parieto-occipitale nous a paru plus utile que la dérivation occipito-auriculaire.

Electroenceph. clin. Neurophysiol., **1969**, *27*: 23–34

REFERENCES

CIGÁNEK, L. *Die elektroencephalographische Lichtreizantwort der menslichen Hirnrinde.* Vydavatel'stvo Slovenskej Akadémie Vied, Bratislava, **1961**a, 151 p.

CIGÁNEK, L. The EEG response (evoked potential) to light stimulus in man. *Electroenceph. clin. Neurophysiol.*, **1961**b, *13*: 165–172.

CRIGHEL, E. and BOTEZ, M. I. Photic evoked potentials in man in lesions of the occipital lobes. *Brain*, **1966,** *89*: 311–316.

COHN, R. Evoked visual cortical responses in homonymous hemianopic defects in man. *Electroenceph. clin. Neurophysiol.*, **1963,** *15*: 922P.

GASTAUT, H. New developments in clinical electroencephalography. In W. S. FIELDS (Ed.), *Neurological diagnostic techniques.* Thomas, Springfield, **1966,** 147 p.

GASTAUT, H., FRANCK, G., KROLIKOWSKA, W., NAQUET, R., RÉGIS, H. et ROGER, J. Études des potentiels évoqués visuels chez les hémianopsiques présentant des crises épileptiques visuelles dans leur champ aveugle. *Rev. neurol.*, **1963,** *108*: 316–322.

JONKMAN, E. J. *The average cortical response to photic stimulation.* Thesis, Amsterdam, **1967,** 160 p.

KOOI, K. A. and BAGCHI, B. K. Visual evoked responses in man, normative data. *Ann. N.Y. Acad. Sci.*, **1964**, *112*: 254–269.

KOOI, K. A., GUVENER, A. M. and BAGCHI, B. K. Visually evoked responses in lesions of the higher optic pathways. *Neurology (Minneap.)*, **1965,** *15*: 841–854.

VAUGHAN, H. G. and KATZMAN, R. Evoked response in visual disorders. *Ann. N.Y. Acad. Sci.*, **1964,** *112*: 305–312.

VAUGHAN, H. G., KATZMAN, R. and TAYLOR, J. Alterations of visual evoked response in the presence of homonymous visual defects. *Electroenceph. clin. Neurophysiol.*, **1963,** *15*: 737–746.

Reference: OOSTERHUIS, H. J. G. H., PONSEN, L., JONKMAN, E. J. and MAGNUS, O. The average visual response in patients with cerebrovascular disease. *Electroenceph. clin. Neurophysiol.*, **1969,** *27*: 23–34.

Electroencephalography and Clinical Neurophysiology
Elsevier Publishing Company, Amsterdam – Printed in The Netherlands

VARIABILITY OF THE HUMAN VISUAL EVOKED POTENTIAL: NORMATIVE DATA

L. CIGÁNEK

Institute of Normal and Pathological Physiology, Slovak Academy of Sciences, Bratislava (Czechoslovakia)

(Accepted for publication: October 9, 1968)

In the present period of very detailed quantitative studies of the human evoked potentials, an exact knowledge of their variability becomes increasingly important. Great inter-individual and intra-individual variability of the averaged responses is widely admitted and emphasized, but their systematic study has rarely been undertaken (Kooi and Bagchi 1964; Jonkman 1967). The computers of average transients, generally used in these studies, do not preserve any information about the variability of the single samples (responses) constituting the averaged responses, so that very little is known about this kind of variability (Townsend 1967; Zerlin and Davis 1967). One of the computers designed by Barlow (1959) permits computing of the variance of single evoked potentials, which he himself commented on in one of his recent studies (Barlow 1966). Most recently, automatic computation of standard deviations was introduced by Brazier (1967).

The aim of the present study was to obtain information mainly about the variability of the single responses constituting the visual average response in normal human subjects.

METHODS AND MATERIAL

In order to obtain applicable normative data, the same stimulation and recording techniques were used as in previous studies (Cigánek 1959, 1961a and b, 1964, 1965, 1966, 1967, in press). The responses were evoked by bluish-white flashes of the "Vareclat-ALVAR" stroboscope with its reflector placed immediately in front of the subject's closed eyes. The flashes lasted 50 μsec and their energy was 0.3 J/flash. Bipolar derivation O_z–P_z (Jasper 1958) was used in such a way that the relative negativity of the electrode O_z resulted in an upward deflection of the record. The stimuli were given at random with intervals ranging from 3 to 6 sec. The frequency response of the amplifiers was flat from 1.4 to 8.0 c/sec and its value decreased by half at 0.22 and 45 c/sec. The record during the time interval of 300 msec after the flash was used for further analysis. The responses to each flash were photographed separately (not superimposed) from the screen of the cathode ray oscilloscope and projected on an 8 times enlarged scale; ordinates each 5 msec were measured separately for each response and used for further mathematical analysis by means of a universal digital computer (Zeiss ZRA-1).

Twenty normal subjects were examined in this study and in each of them 50 single, not superimposed, responses were recorded. For further study the material was grouped in three logical subgroups: (1) 20 sets of 50 single responses, one set from each subject; (2) one set of 20 individual average responses, each averaged from the 50 single responses for each subject; (3) one set of 1000 single responses, 50 from each of the twenty subjects. The average of these 1000 single responses represented the average response of the whole group (average group response).

RESULTS

1. *Amplitude variability*

As expected, the amplitude variability was very high. The minimal standard deviation (S.D.) found in the subject with the smallest variability was 1.33 μV (mean amplitude: $-5.20\,\mu$V); the maximal, in another subject with the greatest variability, was 10.33 μV (mean amplitude: 1.20 μV.

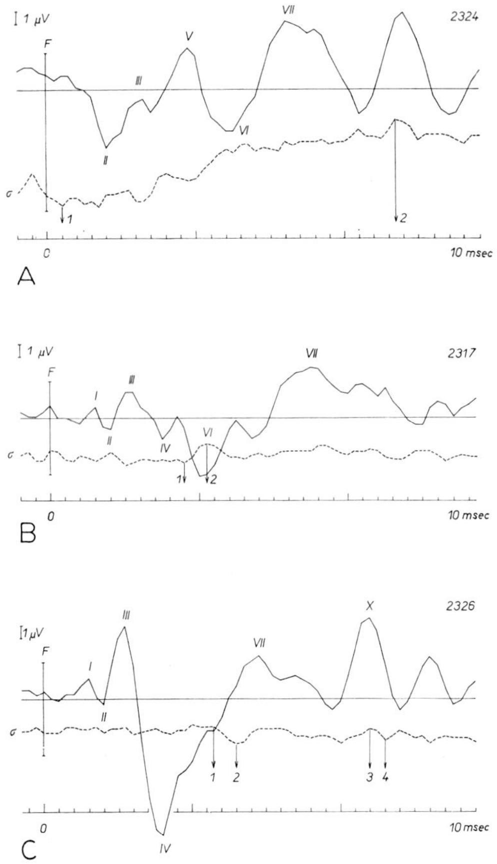

Fig. 1

Individual average human evoked response to a flash, marked by vertical line (F), in three different subjects. The probability with which individual waves (Roman numerals) can be due to insufficiently averaged background activity (noise) alone is:
A: II, $P < 0.01\%$; V, $P < 0.3\%$; VI, $P < 0.01\%$; VII, $P \ll 0.01\%$.
B: I, $P < 10\%$; II, $P < 5\%$; III, $P < 0.01\%$; IV, $P < 0.1\%$; VI, $P \ll 0.01\%$; VII, $P \ll 0.01\%$.
C: I, $P < 0.01\%$; II, $P < 30\%$; III, $P \ll 0.01\%$; IV, $P \ll 0.01\%$; VII, $P \ll 0.01\%$; X (wave of the rhythmic after-discharge), $P \ll 0.01\%$.
Dashed line: standard deviations for single responses, constituting the individual average response. Significance levels (*F* test) of some differences between these values (the compared values are marked by arrows and labelled by Arabic numerals) are: *A*: 1–2, $P \ll 0.5\%$; *B*: 1–2, $P < 0.5\%$; *C*: 1–2, $P < 0.5\%$; 3–4, $P < 5\%$. For details see text. Calibration intervals = 10 msec.

This was the mean amplitude 10 msec after the stimulus). The minimal range of S.D. in one subject (the difference between the maximal and minimal S.D. in this subject) was 1.50, the maximal 7.67 μV. The corresponding range of mean amplitudes was 2.63 and 5.00 μV, respectively.

In slightly more than half of the subjects there was a more or less pronounced decrease of the S.D. beginning, on average, 81.35 msec (measured from the digital data) after the flash and lasting till the end of the analysed 300 msec period (Fig. 1, *A*, dashed line). This decrease could be significant at different, sometimes very

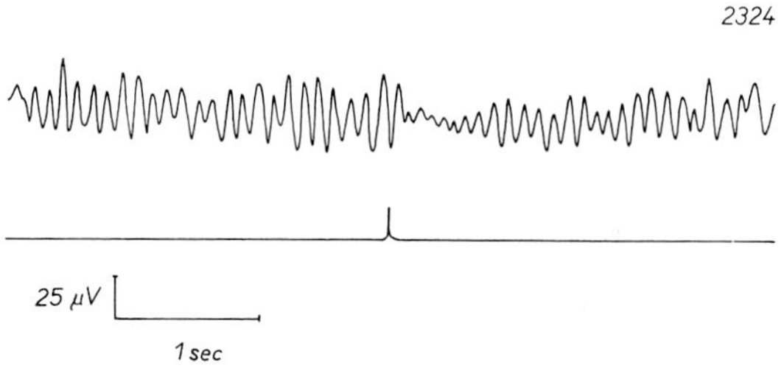

Fig. 2

Routine EEG of one of the single responses averaged in Fig. 1, *A*. Notice the prominent alpha blocking after the flash.

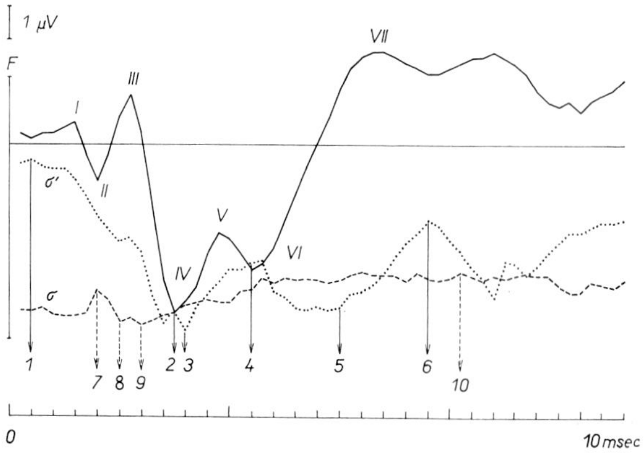

Fig. 3

Average group response (of 1000 single responses, 50 in each of the 20 subjects) to a flash marked by vertical line (F). The probability with which the single waves (Roman numerals) can be due to insufficiently averaged background activity (noise) only, is: waves I, II, III: $P < 0.01\%$; waves IV, VI, VII: $P \ll 0.01\%$.
Dashed line: standard deviations for the 1000 single responses. Dotted line: standard deviations for the 20 individual average responses. In both S.D. curves significance levels (*F* test) of some differences (at points indicated by arrows and labelled by Arabic numerals) are: dotted line: 1–3, $P < 0.5\%$; 2–3, $P > 5\%$; 3–4, $P < 1\%$; 5–6, $P < 0.5\%$; dashed line: 7–8, $P < 1\%$; 9–10, $P < 0.5\%$. For details see text. Calibration intervals = 10 msec.

high, levels. In cases where it was very prominent a clear-cut blocking of the background EEG activity after the flash could be seen in the routine EEG record (Fig. 2). In spite of the fact that the described S.D. decrease was present only in slightly more than half of the subjects, it was clearly visible and highly significant also in the average group response, across the whole group of subjects (Fig. 3, dashed line) with a latency of 75 msec. Thus, this decrease, when present, appeared about 40 msec after the end of the latent period. There was no systematic change of the S.D. correlating with the appearance of the evoked potential. On the other hand, very often there were short oscillations of the S.D. values, sometimes significant in comparison with the immediately preceding and following parts of the S.D. curve (Fig. 1, *B* and *C*). These oscillations were frequently—though not in all cases —time-linked to some of the evoked potential waves (Fig. 1, *B*). No similar significant oscillations were present in the S.D. curve of the average group response (Fig. 3, dashed line), evidently because they were not exactly time correlated with the stimulus in all subjects.

Fig. 3 represents the average response across the whole group (average group response) and shows all standard components described in previous studies (Cigánek 1961a,b). Average

TABLE I

Latency of the whole response, peak latencies of separate waves, and their amplitudes, with corresponding standard deviations of the average group response. σ represents the standard deviation of all 1000 single responses, σ' is the standard deviation of the 20 individual average responses. For details see text and Fig. 3. The amplitude of wave V is given as the distance between its peak and the zero line in μV

	Peak latency msec	σ	Amplitude μV	σ	σ'
Whole response	20–25	—	—	—	—
Wave I	30	9.25	−0.67	5.22	1.10
II	40	5.33	+1.17	4.83	2.18
III	55	6.75	−1.50	5.33	2.85
IV	75	7.35	+5.17	5.15	4.78
V	95	8.89	+2.67	4.17	4.22
VI	110	10.98	+3.83	4.38	3.67
VII	160	20.20	−2.68	4.00	4.32

amplitudes and latencies of separate waves are given in Table I. The dotted line in Fig. 3 represents the S.D. values computed for the individual average amplitudes at each of the 5 msec intervals, indicating the dispersion of the 20 individual average responses, while the dashed line shows the dispersion of all 1000 single responses. These S.D. values for the individual average responses present a significant increase shortly after the end of the latent period with a maximum at the time of the peak latency of wave IV. Partly significant oscillations are visible in correlation with waves III, IV, VI and after wave VII. Comparing this average response of the whole group with the individual average responses we could find some of the latter which were very similar to (Fig. 1, *C*), and others rather different from, the average group response, as well as many intermediate types (Fig. 1, *A* and *B*). As usual the same waves as in the average group response could be identified also in the individual average responses but sometimes some of them were absent.

According to Tassy (1966), it is possible to compute the probability of noise making a deflection at a given point of an averaged response equal to or higher than the maximal amplitude of the signal or, *vice versa*, the probability that the given deflection is due to the averaged signal and not to the insufficiently averaged noise. For the average group response (Fig. 3) the probability that the separate waves were due only to noise was $<0.01\%$ for waves I, II, III and $\ll 0.01\%$ for waves IV, VI and VII. Thus all waves were certainly signals linked to the stimulus. There were technical difficulties in computing the same probability for wave V. In individual average responses the probability that waves were due to noise was in some waves higher than in the average group response, mainly if the wave was small, because of the 20 times smaller number of averaged single responses, but in the majority it was also less than 0.01% (see Fig. 1, *A*–*C*).

As the majority of computations have assumed that the distribution of the reported samples was of a Gaussian character (Tassy 1966), we computed the distribution curve of the 1000 amplitudes in the whole group, separately for each wave peak of the average group response,

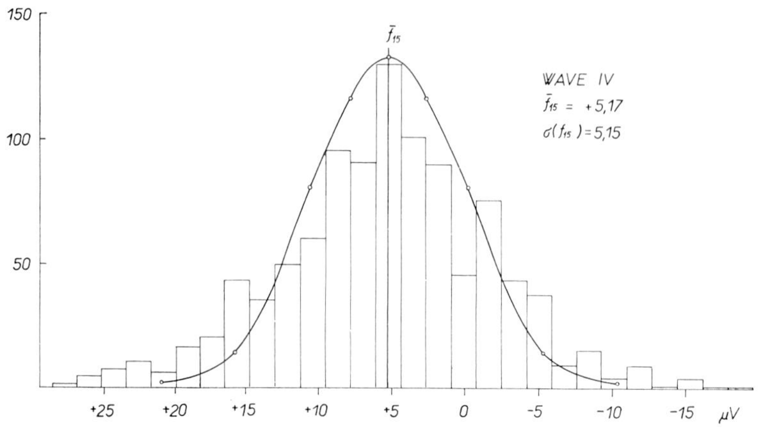

Fig. 4
Distribution of 1000 amplitudes measured at the peak of wave IV of the average group response (Fig. 3). The line with circles represents the theoretical normal distribution for the computed statistical parameters (top right). It is in good accord with the experimentally obtained distribution shown by the columns. The amplitude scale is given in μV but for technical reasons the digital amplitudes were measured and also plotted in relative units, where 1 rel. unit = 1.667 μV.

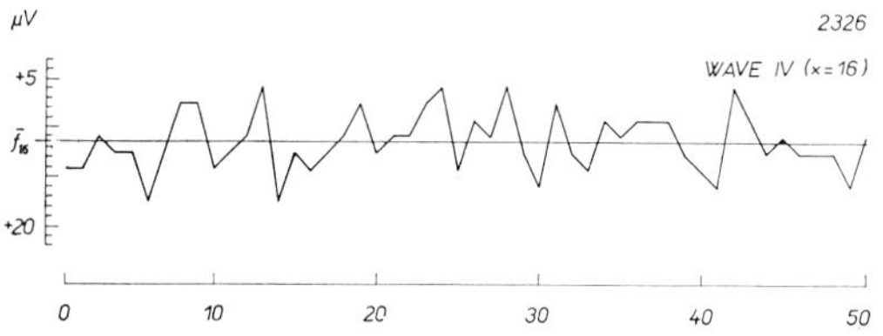

Fig. 5
Amplitudes of 50 single responses measured at the peak latency of wave IV of the individual average response (see Fig. 1, *C*) in the same subject. The amplitudes are ranged from 1 to 50 in the same order as they were evoked. The amplitude mean is marked by a horizontal line. The variability of the amplitudes about the mean does not seem to change in any systematic way during the period of averaging.

as well as at one point at the time of the stimulus. The distribution was very similar to a Gaussian distribution, as illustrated in Fig. 4. An orienting study of the stationariness, in the wide sense, of the amplitudes was made by simple inspection of curves (Fig. 5), each of which consisted of 50 single response amplitudes measured at the time of a definite peak latency in the individual average response. The single response amplitudes were ranged in the same order as they had been evoked. The study was made for 37 well pronounced individual average waves in nine subjects. The distribution of the 50 amplitudes about the mean did not change in any systematic way during averaging of one individual response, lasting from 200 to 250 sec (Fig. 5).

2. *Latency variability*

The duration of each wave was usually determined from both marginal zero crossing points in the averaged curves. In the study of individual average responses in all these time intervals the peak latency of the highest (positive or negative, according to the wave polarity in the average curve) amplitude in each of the 50 single responses was determined and thus the arithmetic means and standard deviations could be computed separately for each average wave latency. The computed arithmetic means were in all cases identical with or very near to the latencies of peaks computed by previous amplitude averaging, proving in this way that the measured single response latencies were due predominantly to the signal rather than to the noise waves. The latency variability for the average group response was computed analogically, using the peak latencies of corresponding waves of the 20 individual average responses. The results are shown in Tables I and II. Only well pronounced and defined waves were used for this analysis. The tables show the lowest dispersion in waves II and III. As usual

TABLE II

Peak latencies (PL) with corresponding standard deviations (σ) in selected, clearly measurable waves in some individual average responses. The waves are labelled by Roman numerals

Response	I		II		III		IV		V		VI		VII		After discharge	
Subj. No.	PL	σ	PL	σ	PL	σ	PL	σ	PL	σ	PL	σ	PL	σ	PL	σ
1884			39.45	5.68	64.50	3.18	86.15	6.39	105.00	5.42	122.05	6.74	198.80	18.95		
R					64.45	5.35	88.80	4.02					159.60	6.20	274.45	11.15
2301			45.70	10.90	83.60	7.20	127.15	10.35					228.20	11.25		
2310					48.25	7.10	76.85	8.10							205.20	8.45
2019					37.60	10.75	79.50	8.50					143.75	8.18	215.25	7.83
2316			38.30	4.02	53.50	3.35	76.60	3.74					155.85	8.12		
2320			36.90	3.76	56.00	4.26	77.45	5.43	91.90	5.80	129.45	7.40	180.70	11.35		
2326	28.00	3.85	38.60	2.53	53.95	2.10	78.10	2.69					144.10	8.89	218.80	6.15

the dispersion increased with later waves, but the first waves I and II often presented greater dispersion than the subsequent waves III and IV.

DISCUSSION

The mathematical model of the EEG response $f(t)$ after a sensory stimulus (light flash in our case) assumes a linear sum of the more or less stable evoked potential $s(t)$, which is time-locked to the stimulus, and of the background EEG activity, often considered in this connection as noise $n(t)$:

$$f(t)=s(t)+n(t) \qquad (1)$$

As follows from our method, the analogue form of the curve $f(t)$ was digitalized, *i.e.*, transformed into a series of ordinates f_x, in which $x=1, 2, 3, \ldots k$ denoted the numerical rank of ordinates measured every 5 msec after the stimulus. In this form the arithmetic mean of each of the ordinates f_x after averaging repeated evoked single responses is

$$\bar{f_x}=\bar{s_x}+\bar{n_x} \qquad (2)$$

After averaging 50 single responses for instance, $\bar{f_x}$ represents any of the amplitudes of the individual average response. The mean of the noise (background activity) $\bar{n_x}$, which is not time-locked to the stimulus, is assumed to be near to zero, so that

$$\bar{f_x}\approx\bar{s_x} \qquad (3)$$

this representing the main axiom of the averaging technique. The analogy with the average group response is evident. The variance (second power of S.D.) of the response ordinates f_x is:

$$\sigma^2(f_x)= \sigma^2(s_x)+ \sigma^2(n_x) \qquad (4)$$

i.e. the sum of the variances of the evoked potential and the noise (background activity) ordinates. Therefore also

$$\sigma(f_x)=\sqrt{\sigma^2(s_x)+ \sigma^2(n_x)}. \qquad (5)$$

We have shown, as can be seen in Fig. 3 and 1, *B* and *C*, that there was no systematic change of the S.D. in correlation with the appearance of the evoked potential, *i.e.*, between the S.D. before the stimulus or during the latent period (both representing the pure S.D. of the noise, without the evoked potential, *i.e.*, $\sigma(n_x)$) and the S.D. during the manifestation of the evoked potential $\sigma(f_x)$, before the reported occasional long latency S.D. decrease, which will be discussed later. Mathematically expressed this experimental result means that

$$\sigma(f_x) \approx (n_x) \quad (6)$$

which supposes, according to the equation (5) that the S.D. of the evoked potential $\sigma(s_x)$ is negligible in comparison with the S.D. of the noise $\sigma(n_x)$.

The decrease of S.D. seen in about half of the subjects (Fig. 1, *A*), and in the average group response (Fig. 3), does not seem to be due to the evoked potential since the latency of the former was much longer than that of the evoked potential. It can be considered rather to be a quantitative expression of the background activity blocking to the flash. The blocking can be seen in the routine records (Fig. 2) and the latencies of the reported S.D. decrease, 81.35 and 75 msec respectively, correspond to the expected blocking latency to a flash of the characteristics used. Our findings are in accordance with those of Barlow (1959, 1966).

The short S.D. oscillations (Fig. 1, *B* and *C*) are not easy to interpret. One, and perhaps the most probable, explanation is that they are due to sudden increase or decrease of the evoked potential S.D. $\sigma(s_x)$ correlated with a definite component of the evoked potential, though such a correlation was not quite convincing in our material. This conclusion is supported by our preliminary findings (Cigánek, in press) that such small oscillations sometimes appear at the same time after the stimulus when the responses are repeatedly evoked. It is less probable that these oscillations are due to the amplitude variability of insufficiently averaged background waves (Barlow 1966). It is well known that a very regular and highly auto-correlated background (mainly alpha) rhythm is present in the average curve even with a large number of averaged samples.

The average group response (Fig. 3) yields the same components as group responses repeatedly obtained by less exact methods (Cigánek 1959, 1961a and b, 1964, 1965, 1966, 1967). At variance with the opinion of Rietveld (1963) and of Werre and Smith (1964) we believe that, in spite of the enormous inter-individual variability, there actually is a standard visual evoked response in man. As we have shown above, the probability that the waves of the average group response are due to the noise is less or much less than 0.01%. The inter-individual variability is expressed by the S.D. of the 20 individual average responses about the average group response (Fig. 3, dotted line). When compared with the values during the latent period, it rises slightly but progressively for waves I, II and III and is very high for the rest of the response. This is in accordance with our previous findings (Cigánek 1959, 1961a and b) and we cannot confirm the conclusion of Jonkman (1967) that there is no distinct difference in amplitude variability in peaks II and III on the one hand and IV on the other. Nevertheless, we have to admit that the amplitude variability measured in our way can be influenced by different peak latencies in separate subjects, since the compared time points are related to the stimulus rather than to the peaks of separate waves.

The probability that the waves of the individual average responses are due to the noise was determined from the table according to Tassy (1966) by finding the value coordinated with the coefficient:

$$\frac{\bar{f_x}\sqrt{N}}{\sigma(n_x)}$$

As has been shown above, the S.D. of the evoked potential is negligible in comparison with the S.D. of the noise so that, according to the expression (6), $\sigma(f_x)$ could be used instead of $\sigma(n_x)$ though the latter is also available in the period before the appearance of the evoked potential. The higher the value of the reported coefficient, the lower the probability that the wave is due to noise only. On the other hand, it follows from the coefficient that this probability rises with increasing $\sigma(n_x)$, decreasing number N of averaged responses, and decreasing amplitude of the averaged evoked potential $\bar{f}_x$. The last situation appears with the small initial waves of the evoked potential (see waves I and II in Fig. 1, *B* and wave II in Fig. 1, *C*). This can be one explanation of the common experience (many personal communications) that wave I and even II is rarely seen with the averaging technique (there is for instance no distinct wave I in Fig. 1, *A*). Dawson's superimposition technique (Dawson 1947) sometimes seems to be more advantageous in this respect as it gives mode rather than mean, the former being less influenced by large noise deflections than the latter. Another cause of the absence of waves I and II in averaged curves can be the insufficient vertical discrimination of the device used (Danthine *et al.* 1966). In our method, the single responses could be measured in steps of 1.667 μV. The probability of wave III and later waves being due to noise was always less than 0.01%.

It follows from the method that the latency S.D. is composed of the S.D. of the evoked potential itself and of the S.D. of the background activity. The contribution of the former seems to be more substantial as the computed latency means are very near to, or identical with, the peak latencies of the amplitude means. The slightly higher variability of the very short latency waves is probably due to the rising relative contribution of the background activity to the variability as the evoked potential waves become too small. On the other hand the high variability of the late waves is probably their inherent characteristic.

SUMMARY

1. Visual evoked responses of twenty normal subjects (50 from each of them) were recorded, graphically digitalized and studied by means of digital computer techniques, mainly for their variability.

2. The amplitude variability of the individual average responses—averaged from the 50 single responses of each subject— is due mainly to the background activity, the variability of the evoked potential being mostly negligible. In about one half of the subjects there is a significant decrease of variability about 80 msec after the stimulus, due to blocking of background activity. Other significant short oscillations in variability of less clear origin are described and discussed.

3. The average group response (across the whole group of subjects) supports the existence of a standard, though inter-individually very variable, human visual evoked potential. The dispersion of the amplitudes of the individual average responses about the average group responses rises with the wave latency.

4. With the method used it is possible to compute the probability with which a particular wave of the average response is due to the evoked potential or to noise (background activity). Examples are given mainly in connection with the problem of reliability of low voltage, short latency waves of the EEG response.

5. The latency variability is greater with long than with short latency waves. There is also a slight increase in variability in the initial short latency waves (I and II) but this is probably due to the background constituent as these evoked potential waves are of low voltage.

RÉSUMÉ

VARIABILITÉ DU POTENTIEL ÉVOQUÉ VISUEL CHEZ L'HOMME: DONNÉES NORMATIVES

1. Les réponses évoquées visuelles de vingt sujets normaux (50 réponses pour chacun d'entre eux) ont été enregistrées, mesurées à la main et étudiées au moyen d'un calculateur digital surtout en ce qui concerne leur variabilité.

2. La variabilité d'amplitude des réponses moyennes individuelles—moyenne des 50 réponses isolées d'un individu—est due essentiellement à l'activité de fond, la variabilité du potentiel évoqué étant tout à fait négligeable. Dans près de la moitié des cas on note une diminution significative de la variabilité 80 msec environ après le stimulus, due au blocage de l'activité de fond. D'autres brèves mais significatives fluctuations de variabilité d'une origine moins évidente sont décrites et discutées.

3. La réponse moyenne pour l'ensemble du groupe (tenant compte du groupe total) montre l'existence d'un potential évoqué visuel humain standard bien que très variable d'un individu à l'autre. La dispersion des amplitudes de la réponse moyenne individuelle par rapport à la réponse moyenne du groupe s'augmente avec la latence des ondes.

4. Avec la méthode utilisée, il est possible de calculer la probabilité avec laquelle une onde particulière de la réponse moyenne est due au potentiel évoqué ou au bruit (activité de fond). L'auteur donne des exemples, surtout en rapport

avec le problème de l'authenticité des ondes de bas voltage et de courte latence de la réponse EEG.

5. La variabilité de latence est plus grande pour les ondes de latence longue que pour les ondes de latence courte. Il existe également une légère augmentation de la variabilité des ondes initiales de latence courte (I et II) mais ceci est dû probablement à l'activité de fond, étant donné que ces potentiels évoqués sont de bas voltage.

The author wishes to express his appreciation to Mrs. V. Cigánková for her excellent assistance, to Ing. I. Plander and his collaborators, mainly Ing. T. Ferenczy, Miss M. Postulková and Mrs. M. Kasmanová, from the Institute of Technical Cybernetics for computing the results and to Ing. J. Mravec for his consultation on mathematical problems.

REFERENCES

Barlow, J. S. A small electronic analogue averager and variance computer for evoked potentials of the brain. *Med. Electron.*, **1959**: 113–119.

Barlow, J. S. Electronic simulation as an aid in evaluating computer-analyzed data. *Electroenceph. clin. Neurophysiol.*, **1966,** *22*: 109–117.

Brazier, M. A. B. Varieties of computer analysis of electrophysiological potentials. *Electroenceph. clin. Neurophysiol.*, **1967,** *Suppl. 26*: 1–8.

Cigánek, L. The effect of Largactil on the electroencephalographic response (evoked potential) to light stimulus in man. *Electroenceph. clin. Neurophysiol.*, **1959,** *11*: 65–71.

Cigánek, L. *Die elektroencephalographische Lichtreizantwort der menschlichen Hirnrinde.* Vydavatel'stvo Slovenskej Akadémie Vied, Bratislava, **1961**a, 151 p.

Cigánek, L. The EEG response (evoked potential) to light stimulus in man. *Electroenceph. clin. Neurophysiol.*, **1961**b, *13*: 165–172.

Cigánek, L. Excitability cycle of the visual cortex in man. *Ann. N.Y. Acad. Sci.*, **1964,** *112*: 241–253.

Cigánek, L. A comparative study of visual and auditory EEG responses in man. *Electroenceph. clin. Neurophysiol.*, **1965,** *18*: 625–629.

Cigánek, L. Evoked potentials in man: interaction of sound and light. *Electroenceph. clin. Neurophysiol.*, **1966,** *21*: 28–33.

Cigánek, L. The effects of attention and distraction on the visual evoked potential in man: a preliminary report. *Electroenceph. clin. Neurophysiol.*, **1967,** *Suppl. 26*: 70–73.

Cigánek, L. Visually evoked potential correlates of attention and distraction in man. *Neurol. Psychiat. (Basel)*, in press.

Danthine, A. A. S., Deliège, M. et Faidherbe, J. Performances et limitations du computer of average transients (C.A.T.) pour l'extraction des potentiels évoqués électroencéphalographiques. *Bull. Soc. roy. Sci. (Liège)*, **1966,** *35*: 250–266.

Dawson, G. D. Central responses to electrical stimulation of peripheral nerve in man. *J. Neurol. Neurosurg. Psychiat.*, **1947,** *10*: 137–140.

Jasper, H. The ten–twenty electrode system of the International Federation. *Electroenceph. clin. Neurophysiol.*, **1958,** *10*: 371–375.

Jonkman, E. J. *The average cortical response to photic stimulation. A study in normal subjects and neurological patients.* Thesis, Amsterdam, **1967,** 160 p.

Kooi, K. A. and Bagchi, B. K. Visual evoked responses in man: normative data. *Ann. N.Y. Acad. Sci.*, **1964,** *112*: 254–269.

Rietveld, W. J. The occipito-cortical response to light flashes in man. *Acta physiol. pharmacol. neerl.*, **1963,** *12*: 373–407.

Tassy, A.-F. *Utilisation de la méthode de sommation en électrophysiologie et électrodiagnostic ophtalmologique.* Leydet, Marseille, **1966,** 101 p.

Townsend, H. R. A. A technique for studying the time course of small evoked potentials. *Electroenceph. clin. Neurophysiol.*, **1967,** *23*: 397.

Werre, P. F. and Smith, C. J. Variability of response evoked by flashes in man. *Electroenceph. clin. Neurophysiol.*, **1964,** *17*: 644–652.

Zerlin, S. and Davis, H. The variability of single evoked vertex potentials in man. *Electroenceph. clin. Neurophysiol.*, **1967,** *23*: 468–472.

Reference: Cigánek, L. Variability of the human visual evoked potential: normative data. *Electroenceph. clin. Neurophysiol.*, **1969,** *27*: 35–42.

Electroencephalography and Clinical Neurophysiology
Elsevier Publishing Company, Amsterdam – Printed in The Netherlands

RHYTHMIC MID-TEMPORAL DISCHARGES. AN ELECTRO-CLINICAL STUDY[1]

IVAN J. LIPMAN[2] AND JOHN R. HUGHES

Division of Laboratory Sciences, Department of Neurology and Psychiatry, Northwestern University Medical Center, Chicago, Ill. 60611 (U.S.A.)

(Accepted for publication: October 22, 1968)

INTRODUCTION

Gibbs *et al.* (1937) described rhythmic waves of 4–7/sec recorded during an ictal automatism. The same pattern, which was later found during the inter-ictal period in patients with psychomotor seizures (Gibbs *et al.* 1938), was termed "psychomotor variant" by Gibbs and Gibbs (1952). Very few studies have thoroughly investigated the clinical correlates of this EEG pattern, and disagreement exists in the literature concerning the clinical significance of this entity (Gibbs *et al.* 1948, 1963; Garvin 1953, 1968; Gastaut 1953; Gibbs and Gibbs 1964; Small *et al.* 1968). This study was designed to determine the spectrum of clinical symptomatology in patients with this EEG abnormality and to assess the significance of these findings, as compared to appropriate control populations.

METHODS

This study was based on the analysis of 16,800 EEGs recorded during a 51 month period in the EEG laboratories of Chicago Wesley Memorial Hospital, Passavant Memorial Hospital, Evanston Hospital Association and the Northwestern University Medical School.

All records showing bursts of rhythmic mid-temporal discharges (RMTD) at a theta frequency were included in the study and comprise the experimental group. Most of these bursts occurred at 6/sec. Usually, the harmonic frequency of 12/sec was clearly seen, and only rarely did the frequencies vary significantly from 6 and 12/sec (see Fig. 1). The bursts lasted 1–8 sec and occasionally up to 1 min. This pattern was most often seen during drowsiness or light sleep and never during the waking state exclusively. The RMTD was often deceptively blunt in configuration, especially when seen at the basic frequency of 6/sec without a clear 12/sec harmonic, but always co-existed with isolated sharp waves on the temporal region(s).

Three control groups were utilized. EEGs and clinical records were reviewed for each control group as for the group under study. Each control population consisted of patients individually matched for age and sex with the experimental group. The controls were as follows: Control Group A included tracings showing temporal lobe sharp waves, seen as isolated events, but never in rhythmic bursts. Control Group B included completely normal EEGs, but this group was not truly representative of the "normal" population, since it contained a high percentage of psychiatric cases, as well as patients with various neurological complaints. Control Group C included charts selected from the medical records library of Chicago Wesley Memorial Hospital, which provided the majority (67%) of the cases in the group under study. These controls were age and sex matched, but were otherwise selected in a totally random fashion, so as to represent a "typical" hospital in-patient population. EEGs could not be obtained on these patients.

EEGs were done using the 10–20 international system of electrode placement (collodion or bentonite) with 8-channel Grass Model 6 or

[1] This study was supported, in part, by Grants NB 5049 and NB 05377 from the National Institute of Neurological Diseases and Blindness (U.S. Public Health Service).

[2] Present address: Division of Neurology, Medical College of Virginia, Richmond, Va.

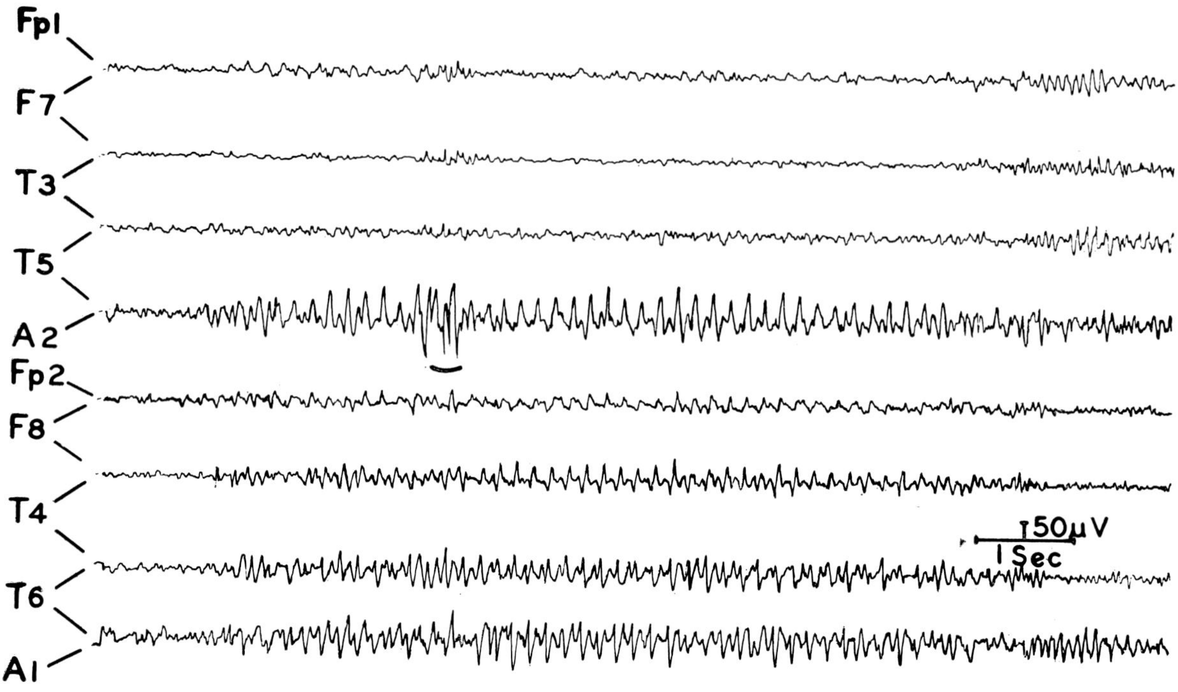

Fig. 1

Rhythmic mid-temporal discharges seen during sleep. Note the 5.5–6/sec frequency, seen well on A_2 (Channel 4) and T_4 (Channels 6 and 7), and the harmonic frequency of 11–12/sec. Note also a short burst of positive spikes (underlined on Channel 4), which are seen in some patients with RMTD.

Offner Type T EEG equipment. All patients had a 20 min waking record, with photic stimulation and with 5 min of hyperventilation. A sleep record was also obtained in every case, usually with the aid of chloral hydrate. Both referential and bipolar montages were employed.

RESULTS

Fifty-five of 16,800 consecutive EEGs (0.3 %) showed RMTD. The sexes were represented almost equally, with twenty-nine females (53 %) and twenty-six males (47 %). The age distribution of patients with RMTD is shown in Table I. The mean age was 34.1 years, the median was 36 and the range was 7–82 years.

RMTDs were unilateral in fifteen cases (27 %) and bilateral in forty (73 %). The bilateral bursts could appear independently on the two sides or simultaneously with various degrees of symmetry. Eight of the unilateral bursts occurred on the right and 7 on the left; of the bilateral bursts 18 were approximately equal on the two sides, 11 were more prominent on the right and 11 on the left.

These discharges were maximal on the mid-temporal area (T_3 or T_4 electrodes) in fifty-three out of fifty-five cases. They appeared to predominate on the anterior temporal area (F_7 or F_8 electrodes) in one instance and on the posterior temporal (T_5 or T_6 electrodes) area in another.

Presumed etiologic factors for this abnormality included post-natal head trauma in thirteen

TABLE I

Age distribution of patients with RMTD

Age (years)	Number of patients	%
1–10	2	3.6
11–20	11	20.0
21–30	12	21.8
31–40	11	20.0
41–50	8	14.5
51–60	7	12.7
Over 60	4	7.3

cases ("serious" in 9), infection in five and birth trauma, cerebrovascular disease and multiple sclerosis each in two cases. No etiology was apparent in 32 cases (58 %).

Slow wave abnormalities were found in twenty-five cases (45 %). In seventeen (31 %) of these the slowing occurred on one or both temporal areas. When present, temporal slowing was almost always (95 %) found on the same side as the RMTD.

Positive spikes at 6–7 and 14/sec were seen in eleven cases of RMTD (20 %). The patients with positive spikes had an age of 12–40 years, with a mean of 24.4 years and a median of 25 years. Of these eleven patients, seven (64 %) were females and four (36 %) were males. Thus, positive spikes occurred in 24% of all females in this series and in 33% of all females below 40 years of age with RMTD.

The occurrence of clinical manifestations in the group under study and in the control groups is shown in Table II. The total incidence of all types of ictal episodes was significantly greater in patients with single temporal lobe sharp waves (Control Group A) than in those with RMTD ($P<0.018$). This difference was even greater when major motor seizures were considered alone ($P<0.005$), but no significant difference was found in the incidence of psychomotor attacks between these two groups. The incidence of seizures in patients with normal EEGs (Group B) and in the "typical" hospital in-patient population (Group C) was significantly less than in those with RMTD ($P<0.003$ for Group B). The difference in incidence of vegetative disorders between the RMTD group and Control Group A was significant ($P<0.049$); this difference was greater when headache was considered alone ($P<0.002$). Psychiatric disturbances also were significantly more common in the RMTD group than in Control Group A ($P<0.03$). The most frequent psychiatric diagnoses were neuroses, character disorders and behavior problems.

DISCUSSION

The above data suggest that the RMTD should be considered as a distinct electrographic entity, with definable clinical correlations. The 0.3 % incidence in this study agrees closely with the values of 0.5 % reported by Gibbs *et al.* (1963) and 0.28 % by Garvin (1968). The RMTD occurs chiefly in adolescents and young adults, and shows little sex preference. Other authors also have found similar distributions of RMTD (Gibbs *et al.* 1948; Gibbs and Gibbs 1964; Small *et al.* 1968). Gibbs and Gibbs (1964) reported a history of trauma in 24 % and no apparent etiology in 56 %, similar to the incidences of 24 % and 58 %, respectively, in the present study.

RMTDs occur with equal frequency on the right and left sides, in contrast to isolated temporal lobe sharp waves, which often show a prefer-

TABLE II

Symptomatology in fifty-five patients with RMTD and in three control groups

	RMTD	Group A	Group B	Group C
All seizures	20 (36 %)	31	7	1
Major motor seizures	9	25	3	1
Psychomotor attacks*	16	14	5	0
Vegetative disorders**	33 (60 %)	24	23	5
Headache***	24	10	19	3
Dizzy spells (or vertigo)	11	7	6	0
Syncope (or fainting or blackouts)	11	9	6	2
Gastrointestinal	4	3	1	0
Psychiatric disorders	26 (47 %)	16	34	4

* "Psychomotor attacks" were considered to include the following: trances, vague states, staring spells, automatisms, episodic bizarre behavior, micropsia, macropsia, psychic manifestations such as déjà-vu, jamais-vu and paroxysmal fears or terrors, and paroxysmal olfactory, gustatory and auditory phenomena.

** "Paroxysmal vegetative disorders" included headache, syncope (also "fainting" and "blackouts"), spells of dizziness or vertigo and gastrointestinal symptoms of clearly paroxysmal nature.

*** Headaches that were the major presenting complaint were included, as were all that were significant by virtue of their severity, chronicity or periodicity. Mild, brief or infrequent headaches were excluded.

ence for the left side (Ajmone Marsan and Ralston 1957; Hughes and Schlagenhauff 1961). The mid-temporal location of RMTD may be significant in view of the observations of Hughes and Schlagenhauff (1961) that temporal discharges occurred most often anteriorly in temporal lobe epileptics with generalized seizures or ictal automatisms. Mid-temporal discharges, on the other hand, were more commonly seen in patients with a preponderance of "vegetative" and psychiatric disorders, and with fewer convulsive attacks than in the anterior temporal group. Patients with RMTD more closely resemble their mid-temporal group.

Using the electrocorticogram in temporal lobe epileptics, Chatrian (1953) recorded "local theta" on the infero-mesial temporal lobe (rhinencephalic structures). He viewed this activity as an incomplete ("frustre") temporal discharge, representing involvement of deep structures projecting onto the temporal lobe, rather than as a primary superficial cortical discharge. The RMTD is likely the same pattern as these rhythmical discharges described by Chatrian.

Although the RMTD group showed a significantly lower incidence of major motor seizures compared to patients with single temporal lobe discharges, the former group had a nearly equal incidence of psychomotor attacks and a higher incidence of paroxysmal vegetative symptoms. The RMTD is therefore viewed as an epileptiform type of activity on the basis of both its clinical correlates and electrographic characteristics. It is possible that the differences in the clinical symptomatology between patients with RMTD and those with single temporal discharges are related to differences in the locus of the discharge or in the excitability cycles of the involved neuronal populations.

The picture thus emerges of a clinical spectrum similar to that of the 6/sec spike and wave phenomenon in its correlation with seizures, "vegetative" symptoms or psychiatric disorders[1] (Table III). Patients with 6/sec spike and wave complexes have a higher incidence of these 3 types of symptoms. Previous authors (Gibbs *et al.* 1948; Gastaut 1953; Penfield and Jasper 1954; Gibbs and Gibbs 1964) have also found psychiatric or behavioral disorders to be frequent in patients with RMTD. The paucity of frank psychoses in RMTD patients in the present study was also noted in patients with 6/sec spike and wave complexes (Small 1968). The absence of psychomotor attacks in patients with 6/sec spike and wave complexes is the major clinical difference between these patients and those with RMTD. In the general hospital population (Group C), seizures, vegetative symptoms and psychiatric disorders were uncommon, and an even lower incidence would be expected in a group of non-hospitalized "healthy" persons.

[1] A similar clinical profile has been found by some investigators in patients with the positive spike phenomenon (Gibbs *et al.* 1963; Hughes 1965).

TABLE III

Comparative symptomatology in patients with RMTD and 6/sec spike and wave

	RMTD	6/sec S & W*
All seizures	36%	62%
Major motor seizures	16%	50%
Vegetative disorders	60%	72%
Headache	44%	50%
Psychiatric disorders	46%	78%

* Hughes *et al.* 1965.

The high incidence of headaches and psychiatric disorders in the normal EEG population (Control Group B) represents the previously mentioned clinical bias of that group.

Follow-up observations were not possible in this study. Investigation of the clinical and EEG evolution of these patients, both with and without anticonvulsant therapy, will be the object of future study.

The term, "psychomotor variant", would seem unacceptable, since the use of clinical terminology in describing EEG phenomena has been discouraged (Storm van Leeuwen *et al.* 1966). Also, the strong or exclusive association with psychomotor attacks implied by this term was not found in the present study. Therefore, the name "Rhythmic Mid-Temporal Discharges" (RMTD) is suggested. This term describes the entity strictly on EEG grounds, with no clinical inferences. It draws attention to the three most striking characteristics of the pattern: its rhythmicity, mid-temporal origin and discharging nature.

SUMMARY

This study is concerned with a rare EEG abnormality, the rhythmic bursts of 6 and 12/sec temporal lobe sharp waves, previously known as "psychomotor variant". This discharge is seen mainly on the mid-temporal area, and appears most often in adolescents and young adults.

Seizures (36%), major motor and psychomotor in type, vegetative complaints (60%), especially headache, and psychiatric disorders (46%) were the most common symptoms seen in these patients. Compared to a group with single temporal lobe sharp waves, these patients showed fewer major motor seizures but an equal incidence of psychomotor attacks. The semiological similarity of this disorder to the 6/sec spike and wave pattern was noted. The term "Rhythmic Mid-Temporal Discharges" (RMTD) is suggested for this EEG abnormality.

RÉSUMÉ

DÉCHARGES RYTHMIQUES MÉDIO-TEMPORALES. ÉTUDE ÉLECTRO-CLINIQUE

Cette étude se rapporte à une anomalie EEG rare, les bouffées rythmiques temporales d'ondes pointues de 6 et 12 c/sec, connues précédemment comme "pattern psychomoteur variant". Ces décharges s'observent essentiellement au niveau de la région médio-temporale et apparaissent le plus souvent chez les adolescents et les adultes jeunes.

Les crises (36%), de type grand mal et psychomoteur, les troubles végétatifs (60%), spécialement les migraines, et les perturbations psychiatriques (46%), sont les symptômes les plus habituels observés chez ces malades. Si on les compare à un groupe de malades présentant des ondes pointues temporales isolées, ces malades montrent moins de crises motrices majeures, mais une proportion égale de crises psychomotrices. La similarité sémiologique de ce trouble et du pattern pointe-onde à 6/sec est soulignée. Le terme "décharge rythmique médio-temporale" est proposé pour définir cette anomalie EEG.

REFERENCES

AJMONE MARSAN, C. and RALSTON, B. *The epileptic seizure*. Thomas, Springfield, Ill., **1957**, 228 p.

CHATRIAN, M. G. E. Étude électroencéphalographique et électrocorticographique du rythme thêta local dans les épilepsies temporales. *Rev. neurol.*, **1953**, *88*: 384–386.

GARVIN, J. S. Psychomotor epilepsy: a clinicoencephalographic syndrome. *J. nerv. ment. Dis.*, **1953**, *117*: 1–8.

GARVIN, J. S. Psychomotor variant pattern. *Dis. nerv. Syst.*, **1968**, *29*: 307–309.

GASTAUT, H. So-called "psychomotor" and "temporal" epilepsy. *Epilepsia (Amst.)*, **1953**, *2*: 59–76.

GIBBS, E. L., GIBBS, F. A. and FUSTER, B. Psychomotor epilepsy. *Arch. Neurol. Psychiat. (Chic.)*, **1948**, *60*: 331–339.

GIBBS, F. A. and GIBBS, E. L. *Atlas of electroencephalography. Vol. 2*. Addison-Wesley, Cambridge, Mass., **1952**: 356–374.

GIBBS, F. A. and GIBBS, E. L. *Atlas of electroencephalography. Vol. 3*. Addison-Wesley, Reading, Mass., **1964**: 60–61.

GIBBS, F. A., GIBBS, E. L. and LENNOX, W. G. Epilepsy: a paroxysmal cerebral dysrhythmia. *Brain*, **1937**, *60*: 377–388.

GIBBS, F. A., GIBBS, E. L. and LENNOX, W. G. Cerebral dysrhythmias of epilepsy. *Arch. Neurol. Psychiat. (Chic.)*, **1938**, *39*: 298–314.

GIBBS, F. A., RICH, C. L. and GIBBS, E. L. Psychomotor variant type of seizure discharge. *Neurology (Minneap.)*, **1963**, *13*: 991–998.

HUGHES, J. R. A review of the positive spike phenomenon. In W. P. WILSON (Ed.), *Applications of electroencephalography in psychiatry*. Duke Univ. Press, Durham, N.C., **1965**: 54–101.

HUGHES, J. R. and SCHLAGENHAUFF, R. E. Electroclinical correlation in temporal lobe epilepsy with emphasis on inter-areal analysis of the temporal lobe. *Electroenceph. clin. Neurophysiol.*, **1961**, *13*: 333–339.

HUGHES, J. R., SCHLAGENHAUFF, R. E. and MAGOSS, M. Electro-clinical correlations in the six per second spike and wave complex. *Electroenceph. clin. Neurophysiol.*, **1965**, *18*: 71–77.

PENFIELD, W. and JASPER, H. *Epilepsy and the functional anatomy of the human brain*. Little, Brown, Boston, Mass., **1954**: 634.

SMALL, J. G. The six per second spike and wave—a psychiatric population study. *Electroenceph. clin. Neurophysiol.*, **1968**, *24*: 561–568.

SMALL, J. G., SHARPLEY, P. and SMALL, I. F. Positive spikes, spike-wave phantoms and psychomotor variants. *Arch. gen. Psychiat.*, **1968**, *18*: 232–238.

STORM VAN LEEUWEN *et al.* Proposal for an EEG terminology by the Terminology Committee of the International Federation for Electroencephalography and Clinical Neurophysiology. *Electroenceph. clin. Neurophysiol.*, **1966**, *20*: 293–320.

Reference: LIPMAN, I. J. and HUGHES, J. R. Rhythmic mid-temporal discharges. An electro-clinical study. *Electroenceph. clin. Neurophysiol.*, **1969**, *27*: 43–47.

Electroencephalography and Clinical Neurophysiology
Elsevier Publishing Company, Amsterdam – Printed in The Netherlands

ÉTUDE DES EFFETS ÉLECTROPHYSIOLOGIQUES DE LA PSILOCYBINE CHEZ UN CERCOPITHECINAE, *PAPIO PAPIO*

F. Bermond et J. Bert

Laboratoire de Neurobiologie, Faculté de Médecine, Dakar (Sénégal)

(Accepted for publication: September 26, 1968)

La psilocybine est un des principes actifs des champignons hallucinogènes du Mexique, extraite par Hofmann *et al.* (1958). Il existe une parenté particulière entre la psilocybine et la diéthylamide de l'acide lysergique (LSD25): ce sont deux dérivés indoliques dont le système indolique est substitué en position 4. Bien qu'à des doses différentes, ces deux composés présentent une activité psychodysleptique chez l'homme. Isbell (1959) a souligné la similitude entre les réactions induites par ces deux drogues dont l'aspect le plus spectaculaire est représenté par des hallucinations visuelles. De multiples travaux ont déjà été réalisés concernant l'action de la psilocybine et d'autres drogues psychotropes sur l'EEG et les potentiels évoqués, avec des résultats variables. Ce travail a été entrepris dans le but de définir de façon claire les effets de la psilocybine sur certaines activités du système nerveux d'un singe; celui-ci constituant un modèle suffisamment proche du système nerveux humain pour permettre une certaine identification.

MATÉRIEL ET MÉTHODE

Les animaux utilisés sont de babouins *Papio papio* femelles adultes. Quarante-et-un animaux ont été utilisés pour cette expérimentation.

Huit électrodes corticales sont implantées chirurgicalement au contact de la dure-mère sur les aires occipitale et somesthésique et sur la ligne médiane. Un autre type d'implantation est utilisé pour l'étude topographique: trente électrodes sont implantées en lignes parallèles en avant et en arrière du sulcus lunatus. Une électrode bipolaire concentrique est introduite de façon stéréotaxique dans le corps genouillé latéral (CGL). Les mouvements oculaires sont enregistrés entre deux électrodes sous cutanées placées verticalement à un demi-centimètre de l'angle externe de chaque oeil. Pour l'enregistrement de l'électrorétinogramme, l'électrode active est un verre de contact qui maintient sur la cornée une mèche de coton imbibée de sérum physiologique.

L'animal non anesthésié est placé sur une chaise de contention, ses pupilles sont dilatées par un collyre mydriatique et il est soumis à une stimulation lumineuse, sonore ou électrique, à un rythme de 1/sec, pendant une heure au cours de laquelle les différentes dérivations sont enregistrées sur bandes magnétiques (Ampex/SB 1300), l'ERG étant photographié directement à l'oscillographe chaque minute. L'animal reçoit alors une injection i.v. de 3 mg de psilocybine (Laboratoire Sandoz = Indocybin cy 39)[1] et l'expérience se poursuit pendant une heure.

Les potentiels évoqués seront étudiés à l'aide d'un calculateur de moyennes Enhancetron 1024. L'action de la drogue est étudiée statistiquement en utilisant le test du *t*.

Les relations avec l'histologie du cortex ont été étudiées chez trois animaux: avant de sacrifier l'animal, la position des électrodes est repérée sur le cortex, l'animal est formolé et l'étude histologique est faite au niveau des différentes électrodes.

RÉSULTATS

1. *Électroencéphalogramme*

L'EEG du *Papio papio* en contention a été étudié par Bert et Collomb (1963, 1964, 1965).

[1] Nous remercions les Laboratoires Sandoz (Bâle) qui ont bien voulu nous fournir les produits d'expérimentation.

L'action de la psilocybine sur l'EEG a été étudiée au cours de 18 expériences réalisées sur neuf animaux. La psilocybine ne provoque que de brèves modifications des rythmes. Pendant les 5 min qui suivent l'injection, il y a une diminution de la durée des phases de synchronisation; la comparaison par rapport à une même période sans drogue montre une différence hautement significative au seuil de 0,001 (t = 5,3). Cette action est de courte durée puisqu'à partir de la 5ème minute la différence n'est plus statistiquement significative (t = 1,7 pour la période comprise entre la 5ème et la 10ème minute).

Si l'on compare les durées des périodes synchronisées avant et après l'injection de psilocybine pendant une heure, aucune différence statistiquement significative n'apparaît (t = 0,84).

2. *Réponses évoquées visuelles*

Électrorétinogramme (ERG). Les caractéristiques de l'ERG du babouin *Papio papio*, recueillies dans les mêmes conditions expérimentales, ont été décrites par Bermond *et al.* (1967).

L'action de la psilocybine est étudiée sur les ondes a et b de l'ERG au cours de 17 expériences réalisées sur neuf animaux. L'analyse statistique des résultats montre que la drogue ne provoque aucune modification, sur la latence de l'ERG, sur les culminances et les durées des ondes a et b. Dans la plupart des expériences, les amplitudes des deux ondes ne varient pas de façon statistiquement significative. Cependant, une augmentation statistiquement significative de l'onde a, a été observée lors de 4 expériences (augmentation comprise entre 1,6 et 35 μV), de l'onde b, lors d'une seule expérience (augmentation comprise entre 9 et 30 μV).

Mouvements oculaires. Les mouvements oculaires ont été étudiés sur neuf animaux au cours de 20 expériences. Dès l'injection, les mouvements oculaires augmentent d'amplitude et de fréquence. Cette augmentation de fréquence est hautement significative au seuil 0,001 pendant les 10 premières minutes (t = 8,35 sous les 5 premières minutes; t = 4,69 de la 5ème à la 10ème minute). La durée de cet effet est variable; chez certains singes, dès la 10ème minute, l'oculogramme est redevenu identique au tracé de contrôle, chez d'autres, l'effet diminue progressivement. Vers la 40ème minute, avec la dose utilisée, l'effet de la psilocybine sur les mouvements oculaires est terminé chez tous les animaux (t = 0,77 de la 35ème minute à la 40ème minute: variation non significative). Cet effet est sans relation avec l'augmentation passagère des périodes de désynchronisation, celle-ci ne durant que 5 min.

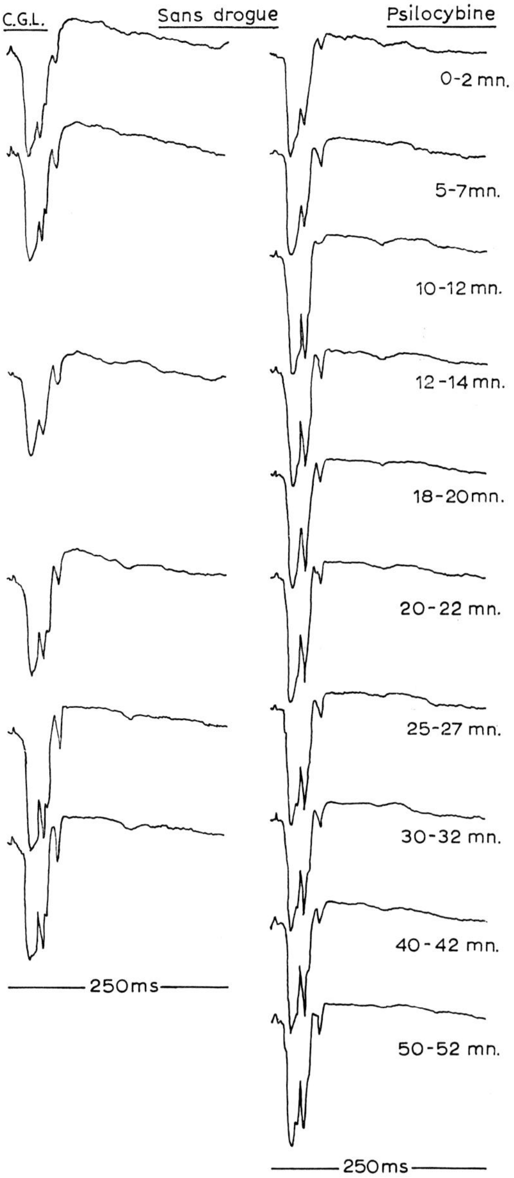

Fig. 1
Action de la psilocybine sur les potentiels évoqués au niveau du CGL. Potentiels recueillis pendant une heure avant et après l'injection. Aucun effet de la drogue n'est observé.

Corps genouillé latéral. Chez le cynocéphale *Papio papio*, le potentiel a été étudié à partir de 12 expériences réalisées sur six animaux: recueilli par l'intermédiaire d'une électrode bipolaire concentrique, le potentiel évoqué par un éclair présente 2 ondes de polarité opposée (Rovetta 1956); tout le décours du potentiel est surchargé par de nombreux potentiels peu amples et très rapides. Les caractéristiques de ce potentiel sont: une latence de 13,15 msec (s = 2,7 msec); une première onde, toujours bien marquée, de durée de 51,7 msec (s = 21,7 msec); une deuxième onde beaucoup moins ample, plus large et de forme variable suivant les animaux.

La psilocybine ne provoque aucune modification statistiquement significative des latences, durées et amplitude générale du potentiel (comparaison des amplitudes moyennes des potentiels évoqués pendant une heure avec et sans drogue: t = 0,02) (Fig. 1). Les potentiels peu amples et rapides qui surchargent la courbe demeurent inchangés. Il faut cependant noter que dans la moitié des expériences, les potentiels présentent une légère diminution d'amplitude pendant les quelques minutes suivant l'injection.

TABLEAU I

PEV: latence en msec des différentes ondes. Moyennes établies à partir de 31 expériences réalisées sur dix-sept animaux

	I	II	III	IV
m = moyennes	45	112	153	192
s = écart type	8,6	14,1	19,2	56,3

TABLEAU II

Étude statistique des effets de la psilocybine sur le PEV (réalisée à partir de 32 expériences)

	Latence en msec				Amplitude en unité arbitraire		
	I	II	III	IV	I	II	III
d	1,28	0,4	1,26	12,9	7,8	46,13	54,89
sd	2,46	3,33	4,87	6,63	5,48	7,62	8,83
t	0,52	0,12	0,25	1,94	1,47	6,05	6,21
	ns	ns	ns	ns	ns	hs	hs

d = différence entre les moyennes avec et sans drogue.
sd = écart type estimé de la différence.

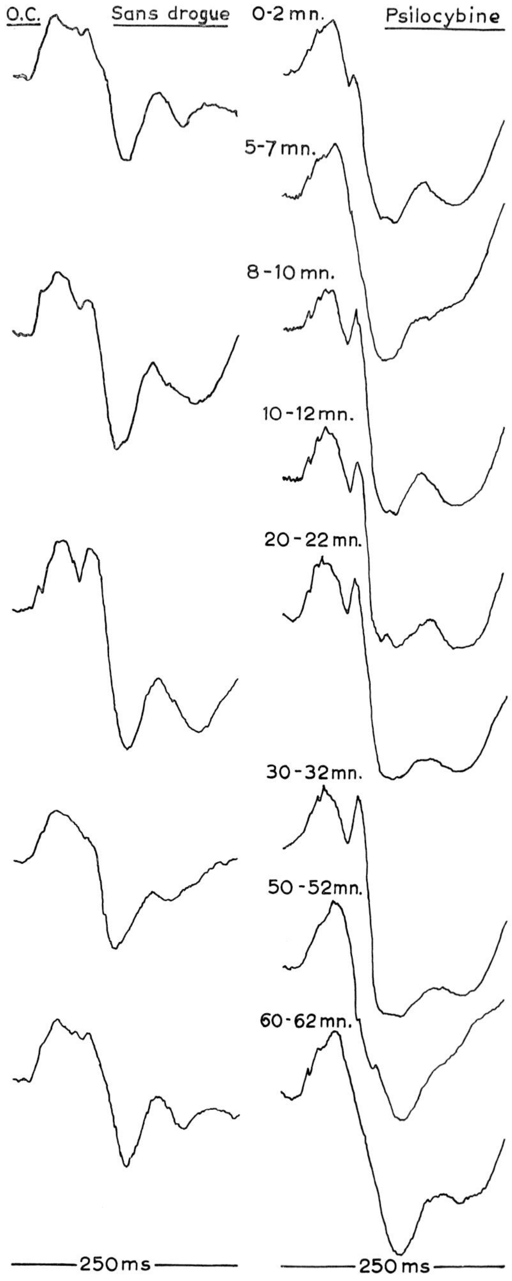

Fig. 2

Action de la psilocybine sur le PEV recueilli au niveau du cortex primaire. Potentiels étudiés pendant une heure avant et après l'injection; on note un effet immédiat de la drogue, un début de retour à la normale vers 60 min.

Cortex visuel: (a) *effets de la psilocybine sur la morphologie du PEV recueilli sur le cortex visuel primaire.* L'étude en dérivation bipolaire comme en monopolaire montre une succession d'ondes de polarité opposée débutant par une onde négative (Tableau I); la forme du PEV a été étudiée par Bermond *et al.* (1966). La psilocybine provoque une modification importante, constante et durable du PEV (Tableau II). La drogue n'a aucun effet sur les latences des ondes quand celles-ci subsistent; son action porte essentiellement sur l'amplitude des ondes II et III: l'onde positive II est considérablement augmentée, la différence des amplitudes avec et sans drogue est hautement significative au seuil 0,001 et comprise avec un risque de 5 % entre 70 % et 150 % de la valeur moyenne de l'amplitude de l'onde sans drogue; l'onde négative III subit également une modification hautement significative au seuil de 0,001; elle est profondément déprimée ou même complètement supprimée. La psilocybine provoque une modification profonde du PEV se traduisant par l'apparition d'une très grande positivité après la première onde négative (Fig. 2). Cette action se manifeste immédiatement après l'injection et persiste pendant 1 h–1 h 30.

(b) *Étude topographique de l'action de la drogue*. En arrière du sulcus lunatus, l'action de la drogue est identique en importance et en durée. En avant du sulcus lunatus, les effets de la psilocybine sont plus variables, plus discrets et plus brefs, les effets sont d'autant moins visibles que l'électrode est placée plus en avant du sulcus lunatus (Fig. 3). Cette action discrète n'excède jamais 20 min et les potentiels sont redevenus normaux alors que l'action en arrière du sulcus lunatus est encore maximum. Or l'étude histologique du cortex montre que l'aire striée

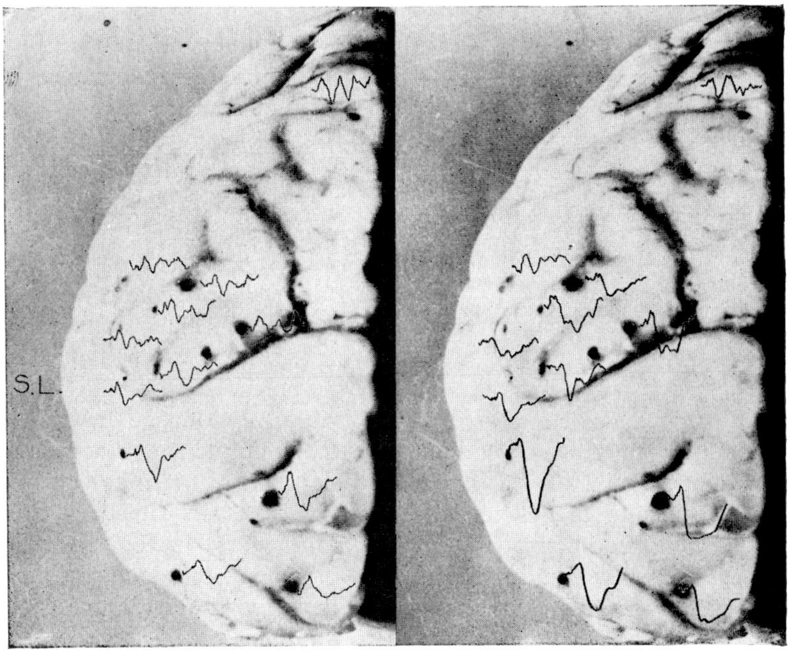

Fig. 3

Étude topographique de l'action de la psilocybine sur le cortex visuel primaire et péristrié. (Vue arrière du cerveau.) S.L. = sulcus lunatus.

À gauche: potentiels évoqués sans drogue; à droite: potentiels évoqués pendant le premier quart d'heure suivant l'injection. Une action importante de la drogue s'observe uniquement sur le cortex visuel primaire.

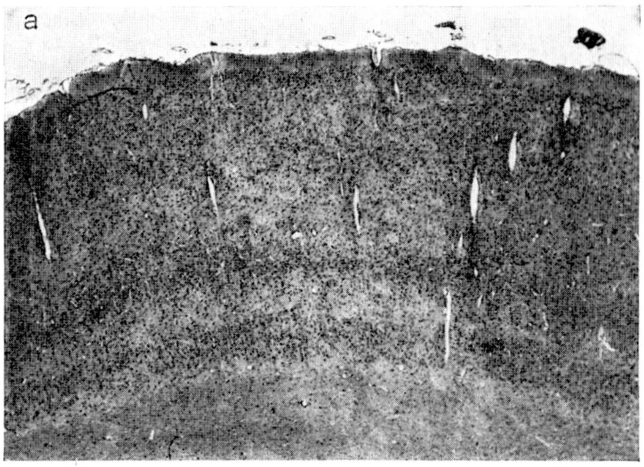

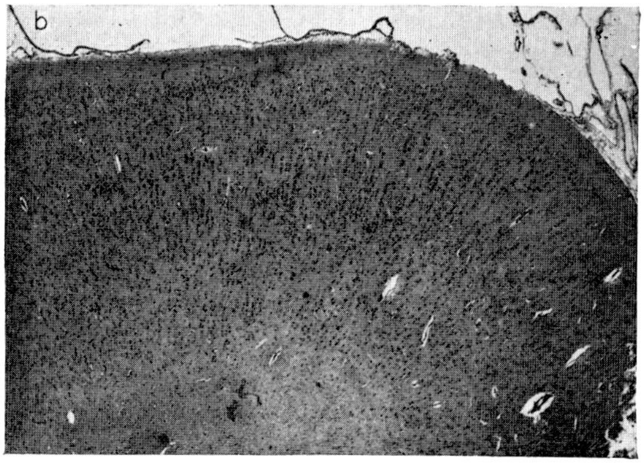

Fig. 4
a: Coupe du cortex en arrière du sulcus lunatus; à ce niveau une action importante de la drogue a été enregistrée.
b: Coupe en avant du sulcus lunatus; l'action de la drogue est ici faible et inconstante.
Seule la coupe *a* montre une structure de koniocortex; la division de la couche IV par une bande claire (strie de Gennari) permet de reconnaître facilement l'aire striée 17 sur la coupe *a*.

(aire 17), facilement reconnaissable à la division frappante de la couche IV par l'apparition d'une bande claire horizontale au milieu de la couche (strie de Gennari), occupe toute l'étendue du cortex en arrière du sulcus lunatus; cette structure ne se retrouve pas en avant de sulcus lunatus (Fig. 4) où se localisent les aires 18 et 19. Sur les berges du sulcus lunatus, l'action de la drogue est variable; on observe un effet comparable soit à celui observé au niveau de l'aire 17, soit à celui observé plus antérieurement; or, l'étude histologique des berges montre soit une structure de cortex primaire, soit une structure parastriée.

3. *Potentiels évoqués somesthésiques* (*PES*)

L'action de la psilocybine sur le PES en réponse à une stimulation du nerf médian contralatéral a été étudiée au cours de 17 expériences réalisées sur douze animaux. Caractéristiques du PES: une latence très précoce: 12,18 msec (s = 1,8 msec); une onde positive très brève culminant à 20,47 msec (s = 4,1 msec). Cette onde précoce est suivie par: une onde négative culminant à 36 msec (s = 7,4 msec); cette onde pouvant être dédoublée, présentant alors une première culminance à 36 msec, une deuxième à 53 msec; une onde positive culminant à 74,8 msec (s = 14 msec).

Cette partie initiale du potentiel est très stable d'un animal à l'autre, les ondes plus tardives présentant une plus grande variabilité ne seront pas considérées.

Ainsi que le constatent Allison *et al.* (1963) chez le macaque, on ne retrouve pas la première onde négative du PES de l'homme. Les 3 ondes suivantes ont des latences voisines de celles décrites chez l'homme (Giblin 1964).

La psilocybine ne modifie ni la forme ni les latences des différentes ondes. Dans 15 expériences, l'amplitude générale du potentiel subit une légère diminution; au cours de 2 expériences, une légère augmentation.

4. *Potentiels évoqués au niveau de la ligne médiane*

Ces potentiels évoqués, soit par stimulation lumineuse, soit par stimulation sonore, présentent une succession d'ondes de polarité opposée, identique dans les deux cas; la première onde étant de polarité négative. Les ondes I (se décomposant en deux pointes a et c) et II constituent la partie précoce du potentiel (latence inférieure à 100 msec), les ondes III, IV, V, la partie tardive du potentiel; ces dernières ondes sont moins stables dans leur chronologie que les composantes précoces. Les latences des différentes ondes sont indiquées dans le Tableau III.

La psilocybine n'a aucun effet sur les latences. L'amplitude des ondes précoces I–II ne subit aucune variation statistiquement significative (stimulation lumineuse: t = 1,68; stimulation sonore: t = 1,25). L'amplitude des ondes tardives III–IV subit une diminution légère mais statistiquement significative au seuil 0,05. Donc une dépression significative mais discrète s'observe

TABLEAU III

Potentiels évoqués au niveau de la ligne médiane—latences des différentes ondes en msec

		I		II	III	IV	V
		a	c				
Stimulation	m	29,2	48,9	79,9	131,1	169,4	200,2
lumineuse	s	5,2	8,4	12,9	21,2	22	13,9
Stimulation	m	25	46,6	81,5	140,6	178	213,75
sonore	s	3	5	3,6	18,1	18,5	4,8

Moyennes établies: à partir de 20 expériences réalisées sur dix-sept animaux pour la stimulation lumineuse; à partir de 9 expériences réalisées sur neuf animaux pour la stimulation sonore.

sur les ondes tardives des potentiels évoqués au niveau de la ligne médiane.

5. *Étude comparative des effets du LSD*

Réalisée sur trois animaux au cours de 8 expériences. Une dose de 0,1 mg i.v. de LSD est utilisée. L'effet sur l'EEG est immédiat; dès la première minute suivant l'injection s'installe un rythme rapide (30–35 c/sec), plus important dans les régions fronto-pariétales, moins sensible au niveau du lobe occipital.

L'effet sur le PEV est identique à celui observé sous psilocybine mais dure plus longtemps.

DISCUSSION

Sous l'action du LSD de très nombreux auteurs ont observé chez de nombreuses espèces animales et chez l'homme une modification de l'EEG: désynchronisation du tracé avec diminution d'amplitude et accélération du rythme. Chez le babouin, le LSD produit également une modification de l'EEG.

Par contre, les effets de la psilocybine sur l'EEG sont plus variables. Chez le lapin curarisé (Cerletti 1958), une injection i.v. de 1–2 mg/kg de psilocybine provoque un rythme régulier de bas voltage, 4–5 c/sec, avec disparition pratiquement complète des ondes lentes et des fuseaux. Cependant Longo (1967) obtient chez le lapin une désynchronisation immédiate du tracé sous l'action de 1 mg/kg de psilocybine, mais passagère, car dès la 5ème minute le tracé reprend un aspect synchronisé. Une désynchronisation de l'EEG sous l'action de 0,16 mg/kg de psilocybine est décrite chez le chat (Da Fonseca *et al.* 1965a,b) dans la plupart des cas et chez l'homme (Kolarik *et al.* 1966).

Chez le babouin, on observe seulement une désynchronisation partielle et passagère, n'excédant jamais 5 min.

Il est possible de faire appel, pour expliquer cette faible variation de l'EEG, aux caractéristiques fonctionnelles particulières au système nerveux du babouin: le comportement et l'EEG du babouin immobilisé sur une chaise de contention sont notablement différents du comportement et de l'EEG des autres cercopithecinae africains (*Patas—Cercopithecus aethiops*) et asiatiques (*Macacus rhésus*).

Étant donné l'importance des manifestations visuelles provoquées par les drogues hallucinogènes, la voie spécifique visuelle a été particulièrement étudiée.

Au niveau du CGL, Evarts *et al.* (1955) montrent une diminution d'amplitude de 80 % de la réponse post-synaptique à une excitation du nerf optique chez le chat anesthésié (pentobarbital) sous l'action de 30 μg/kg de LSD en injection intracarotidienne. Une dose de 160 μg/kg est nécessaire en injection i.v. pour provoquer une diminution de 60 % de la réponse post-synaptique au niveau du CGL et une dose 5 fois plus grande chez l'animal non anesthésié. Bishop *et al.* (1958) constatent également un blocage de la transmission synaptique au niveau du CGL pour de fortes doses de LSD chez le chat anesthésié.

Or les expériences réalisées sous anesthésie associent plusieurs actions pharmacologiques et une interprétation est particulièrement difficile. Purpura (1956) obtient des résultats différents suivant qu'il utilise des chats immobilisés par succinylcholine, chez lesquels il observe un effet facilitant du LSD sur les réponses évoquées visuelles, ou des chats anesthésiés (pentobarbital), chez lesquels cet effet facilitant ne s'observe jamais.

Or, pour obtenir les mêmes effets au niveau du CGL chez l'animal non anesthésié, Evarts utilise des doses très élevées (pour le singe, 0,5–1 mg/kg) provoquant une cécité temporaire aussi bien chez le chat que chez le singe (Evarts 1956, 1957).

Par contre, Killam et Killam (1956) chez le chat non anesthésié, montrent l'inefficacité de 100 μg/kg de LSD sur l'amplitude de la réponse évoquée au niveau du thalamus par stimulation électrique d'un nerf périphérique. Si l'on considère exclusivement les résultats obtenus pour des doses inférieures à 100 μg/kg utilisées sur des préparations chroniques, le LSD n'a aucun effet sur la transmission thalamique. Ceci est en accord avec les résultats obtenus chez le babouin *Papio papio* en expérience chronique avec des doses de psilocybine comparables à celles provoquant des troubles visuels chez l'homme: la réponse évoquée au niveau du CGL par stimulation lumineuse demeure inchangée.

Au niveau cortical, des résultats variables sont observés: une légère augmentation du PEV est notée chez l'homme par Rinkel *et al.* (1952), Gastaut *et al.* (1953), Bradley et Elkes (1957) sous l'action du LSD; Bacchini *et al.* (1965) observent une multiplication des ondes, en particulier des premières, et une augmentation d'amplitude des dernières composantes du PEV chez l'homme sous l'action de 1–1,5 μg/kg i.m. Cette multiplication des ondes du PEV en réponse à une stimulation isolée est également retrouvée chez le singe (Domino 1960) avec des doses de 1–25 μg/kg i.v. de LSD. Par contre, Chapman et Walter (1965) et Rodin *et al.* (1966) montrent une diminution d'amplitude de la principale onde positive du PEV chez l'homme (1 μg/kg i.v. de LSD).

Ces variations de l'action de la drogue sur le PEV chez l'homme sont également constatées avec la psilocybine par Da Fonseca *et al.* (1965a,b): 0,15 mg/kg administrée oralement provoque une augmentation d'amplitude chez huit sujets, une diminution d'amplitude chez deux sujets, et aucune modification chez un sujet.

Donc des résultats assez discordants, aussi bien sous l'action du LSD que de la psilocybine, sont obtenus chez l'homme. A cette variabilité, s'opposent l'importance et la constance des effets observés chez le babouin: les potentiels évoqués recueillis au niveau du cortex visuel primaire (aire 17) subissent une modification profonde et durable, identique chez tous les animaux, apparaissant immédiatement après injection soit de psilocybine, soit de LSD.

Cependant, au niveau des aires 18 et 19, l'action des deux drogues est beaucoup moins évidente, moins stable, et souvent très fugace. Ainsi peuvent être expliqués les résultats variables obtenus par différents auteurs chez l'homme, puisque l'étude des PEV ne peut être faite qu'au niveau des aires 18 et 19, seules accessibles lors de l'enregistrement humain.

Une autre explication pourrait être avancée pour expliquer ces divergences; Killam *et al.* (1967) ont montré que le babouin *Papio papio* (du Sénégal) est un animal particulièrement photosensible. L'effet différent de la drogue chez l'homme et le *Papio papio* pourrait provenir non seulement d'une répartition différente des aires corticales visuelles mais également de cette particularité. Cette hypothèse devrait être vérifiée en étudiant l'effet de la psilocybine sur des sujets humains particulièrement photosensibles.

Si nous récapitulons les effets électrophysiologiques de la psilocybine chez les babouins, en regard de cette importante action sur le PEV: aucune modification constante de l'ERG; aucun effet sur les potentiels évoqués au niveau du CGL ne sont observés; l'action sur les potentiels évoqués somesthésiques est variable d'un animal à l'autre, faible, se traduisant le plus souvent par une légère diminution d'amplitude; sur les potentiels évoqués au niveau de la ligne médiane, on constate seulement une légère diminution des ondes tardives; enfin, la psilocybine ne provoque aucune modification durable de l'EEG. On peut donc dire que la psilocybine a une action importante et spécifique sur le cortex visuel.

Or, Delay *et al.* (1959) notent que c'est dans la sphère visuelle que les phénomènes psychosensoriels sont le plus remarquables, la coloration des objets se modifie, les sujets insistant sur le caractère inaccoutumé de leur perception, les hallucinations visuelles sont fréquentes, apparaissant surtout les yeux fermés. L'action spécifique de la psilocybine sur le cortex visuel primaire pourrait donc constituer le support de ces manifestations observées chez l'homme. Les faibles modifications du PES sont à rapprocher de la rareté des manifestations dans la sphère somesthésique chez l'homme. De plus, cette interprétation semble pouvoir être généralisée aux autres hallucinogènes puisque les mêmes modifications au niveau du cortex visuel primaire s'observent sous l'action du LSD.

RÉSUMÉ

Les effets électrophysiologiques de la psilocybine ont été étudiés chez le cercopithecinae *Papio papio*.

1. Les réponses visuelles (électrorétinogramme, potentiels évoqués au niveau du corps genouillé latéral et du cortex visuel) ont été étudiées: seuls les potentiels évoqués au niveau du cortex visuel primaire subissent une modification importante, constante et durable.

2. L'action sur les potentiels évoqués somesthésiques est variable d'un animal à l'autre, faible, se traduisant le plus souvent par une légère diminution d'amplitude.

3. La psilocybine n'a aucun effet durable sur l'EEG.

Une action spécifique de la psilocybine sur le cortex visuel primaire peut être considérée comme le support des manifestations hallucinatoires provoquées par la drogue chez l'homme.

SUMMARY

ELECTROPHYSIOLOGICAL EFFECTS OF PSILOCYBIN IN A CERCOPITHECINAE, *Papio papio*

The electrophysiological effects of psilocybin have been studied in baboons (*Papio papio*).

1. The visual response has been studied by ERG and by lateral geniculate body and visual cortex evoked potentials. The primary visual cortex evoked potentials are the only ones to show significant constant and long lasting modifications.

2. The effects on somaesthetic evoked potentials are weak, inconsistent and most often characterized by a slight decrease in amplitude.

3. Psilocybin has no durable effect on the EEG.

A specific activity of psilocybin on the visual primary cortex may be considered as the basis of hallucinatory phenomena induced in man by this drug.

Les auteurs remercient: Docteur Lemercier pour l'interprétation histologique, Monsieur Vezard pour son assistance technique.

RÉFÉRENCES

ALLISON, T., GOFF, W. R., ABRAHAMIAN, H. A. and ROSNER, B. S. The effects of barbiturate anesthesia upon human somatosensory evoked responses. *Electroenceph. clin. Neurophysiol.*, **1963**, *Suppl. 24*: 68–75.

BACCHINI, O., VILLAR, J. I., PRIETO, S. and GARCIA AUSTT, E. Effects of psychodrugs upon sensory inflow. Changes provoked by LSD.25 on the averaged visual evoked responses in man. *Acta neurol. lat.-amer.*, **1965**, *11*: 383–390.

BERMOND, F., BERT, J. et AYATS, H. Action de la psilocybine sur les potentiels évoqués visuels chez un cercopithecinae *Papio papio*. *C.R. Soc. Biol. (Paris)*, **1966**, *160*: 2405–2409.

BERMOND, F., BERT, J. et AYATS, H. Effet de la psilocybine sur les mouvements oculaires et l'ERG chez un cercopithecinae *Papio papio*. *C.R. Soc. Biol. (Paris)*, **1967**, *161*: 1763–1767.

BERT, J. et COLLOMB, H. Sur l'EEG du babouin *Papio papio*. *C.R. Soc. Biol. (Paris)*, **1963**, *157*: 609–611.

BERT, J. et COLLOMB, H. Diversité de l'EEG des primates cynomorphes. *Electroenceph. clin. Neurophysiol.*, **1964**, *17*: 545–556.

BERT, J. et COLLOMB, H. Effet de l'immobilisation sur l'EEG du babouin. Comparaison avec les résultats obtenus par télémétrie chez l'animal en liberté. *C.R. Soc. Biol. (Paris)*, **1965**, *159*: 1202–1204.

BISHOP, P. O., FIELD, G., HENNESSY, B. L. and SMITH, J. R. Action of LSD on lateral geniculate synapses. *J. Neurophysiol.*, **1958**, *21*: 529–549.

BRADLEY, P. B. and ELKES, J. The effect of some drugs on the electrical activity of the brain. *Brain*, **1957**, *80*: 77–117.

CERLETTI, A. Pharmacology of psilocybin. *First Int. Meeting of Neuro-psycho-pharmacol.*, Rome, **1958**: 8–13.

CHAPMAN, L. F. and WALTER, R. D. Actions of LSD on averaged human cortical evoked responses to light flash. *Recent Advan. Biol. Psychiat.*, **1965**, *4*: 23–25.

DA FONSECA, J. S., FIALHO, M. L. and GRIL, T. Evoked potentials and visual information processing under the action of psilocybin in the cat. *Neuropsychopharmacology*, **1965**a, *4*: 309–315.

DA FONSECA, J. S., CARDOSO, C., SALGUIERO, E. and FIALHO, M. L. Neurophysiological and psychological study of psilocybin. Induced modifications of visual information in man. *Neuropsychopharmacology*, **1965**b, *4*: 315–319.

DELAY, J., PICHOT, P. et LEMPERIÈRE, T. La psilocybine. *Presse méd.*, **1959**, *47*: 1731–1733; *ibid.*, **1959**, *49*: 1811–1813.

DOMINO, E. Effect of LSD 25 on photic driving in monkeys with chronically implanted electrodes. *Electroenceph. clin. Neurophysiol.*, **1960,** *12*: 264P.

EVARTS, E. V. Some effects of bufotenine and LSD on the monkey. *Arch. Neurol. Psychiat. (Chic.)*, **1956,** *75*: 49–53.

EVARTS, E. V. Review of neurophysiological effects of LSD. *Ann. N.Y. Acad. Sci.*, **1957,** *66*: 479–495.

EVARTS, E. V., LANDAU, W., FREYGANG, W. and MARSHALL, W. H. Some effect of LSD and bufotenine on electrical activity in the cat's visual system. *Amer. J. Physiol.*, **1955,** *182*: 594–598.

GASTAUT, H., FERRER, S. et CASTELLS, C. Action de la diethylamide de l'acide D-lysergique (LSD 25) sur les fonctions psychiques et l'électroencéphalogramme. *Confin. neurol. (Basel)*, **1953,** *13*: 102–120.

GIBLIN, D. R. Somatosensory evoked potentials in healthy subjects and in patients with lesions of the nervous system. *Ann. N.Y. Acad. Sci.*, **1964,** *112*: 93–142.

HOFMANN, A., FREY, A., OTT, H., PETRZILKA, T. und TROXLER, F. Konstitutionsaufklärung und Synthese von Psilocybin. *Experientia (Basel)*, **1958,** *14*: 397.

ISBELL, H. Comparison of the reactions induced by psilocybin and LSD 25 in man. *Psychopharmacologia*, **1959,** *1*: 29–38.

KILLAM, K. F. and KILLAM, E. K. Action of LSD on central afferent and limbic pathway in the cat. *J. Pharmacol. exp. Ther.*, **1956,** *116*: 35–36.

KILLAM, K. F., KILLAM, E. K. and NAQUET, R. An animal model of light sensitive epilepsy. *Electroenceph. clin. Neurophysiol.*, **1967,** *22*: 497–513.

KOLARIK, J., SEVCIK, M., DUBANSKY, B. and VYHANANKOVA, M. Comparison of EEG desynchronisation and the optical hallucinogenic effect after psilocybin in organic brain lesions. *Activ. nerv. sup. (Praha)*, **1966,** *8*: 350.

LONGO, V. G. Contribution à l'étude des effets centraux des médicaments hallucinogènes et psychomimétiques. *Actualités neurophysiol.*, **1967,** *7*: 203–216.

PURPURA, P. P. Electrophysiological analysis of psychotogenic drug action. *Arch. Neurol. Psychiat. (Chic.)*, **1956,** *75*: 122–131.

RINKEL, M., DE SHON, H., HYDE, R. W. and SOLOMON, H. C. Experimental schizophrenia-like symptoms. *Amer. J. Psychiat.*, **1952,** *108*: 572–578.

RODIN, E., LUBY, E. and DETROIT, M. D. Effects of LSD on the EEG an photic evoked responses. *Arch. gen. Psychiat.*, **1966,** *14*: 435–441.

ROVETTA, P. Effect of mescaline and LSD on evoked responses especially of the optic system of the cat. *Electroenceph. clin. Neurophysiol.*, **1956,** *8*: 15–24.

Référence: BERMOND, F. et BERT, J. Étude des effets électrophysiologiques de la psilocybine chez un cercopithecinae, *Papio papio*. *Electroenceph. clin. Neurophysiol.*, **1969,** *27*: 48–56.

Electroencephalography and Clinical Neurophysiology
Elsevier Publishing Company, Amsterdam – Printed in The Netherlands

FREQUENCY ANALYSIS OF EEG DURING MILK DRINKING[1]

NETTA W. GRANDSTAFF, PH.D.

Neuropsychology Laboratories, Department of Psychiatry, Stanford University School of Medicine, Stanford, Calif. 94305 (U.S.A.)

(Accepted for publication: September 25, 1968)

INTRODUCTION

The appearance of a 4–12 c/sec synchronized electrocortical activity localized in the striate cortex (posterior lateral gyrus) of cats has been reported to be associated with post-reinforcement during conditioning (Clemente *et al.* 1964; Sheer *et al.* 1966). Although the primary emphasis has been centered on this relationship, it has also been shown that conditioning was not a prerequisite for its elicitation, as the same type of activity was recorded from the striate cortex of a naive, hungry animal with the attainment of food. The slow wave synchronized EEG has also been reported to be present in the parietal cortex with an appetitive response (Clemente *et al.* 1964). This electrical response appears to be limited to a small portion of the cat brain, as recordings made from numerous other loci in both cortical and subcortical areas in approximately thirty cats during a period of several years have failed to show a similar rhythm when the cat was drinking milk (Grandstaff, unpublished data).

The present investigation was undertaken to further elucidate the details of the relationship of the 7.5 c/sec EEG activity in the striate cortex with the behavioral response of drinking milk. The question of primary interest was: Does the 4–12 c/sec activity in the visual cortex associated with drinking milk reflect in some way a change in the afferent visual input as such, or is it independent of vision and therefore affected by non-visual activating and/or inhibitory inputs to the striate cortex?

To test this question experimentally, the problem of blocking all visual input to the striate cortex without disrupting the non-visual inputs had to be met. The visually split-brain animal afforded such a possibility. By sectioning the optic chiasm plus the midline structures down to the brain-stem and visually occluding one eye with an opaque contact lens, the ipsilateral hemisphere had visual input blocked, while non-visual inputs were still supposedly intact. With the contact lens removed, the animal served as his own control; *i.e.*, the same recording loci in the striate cortex could be compared in the presence and in the absence of visual input. Such an approach should at least give some indication as to the role of visual/non-visual input relationships in striate cortex during food intake.

METHODS

Subjects and surgical procedures

A series of cats, four split-brain animals and two controls, were surgically prepared under aseptic conditions with chronically implanted bilateral, bipolar electrodes in the following loci: striate cortex (posterior lateral gyrus), auditory cortex (mid-ectosylvian gyrus) and mid-suprasylvian gyri, making a total of 12 electrode placements. All electrode placements were determined by the stereotaxic atlas (Jasper and Ajmone Marsan 1954). All electrodes were made of 300 μ insulated nichrome wire with approximately 1 mm separating the 0.5 mm exposed tips. They were placed both intracortically and

[1] This research was supported by U.S. Public Health Service Post-doctoral Fellowship F2-MH-23, 198-02, Grant N.I.H. MH-08304-05 and Grant MH-12970.

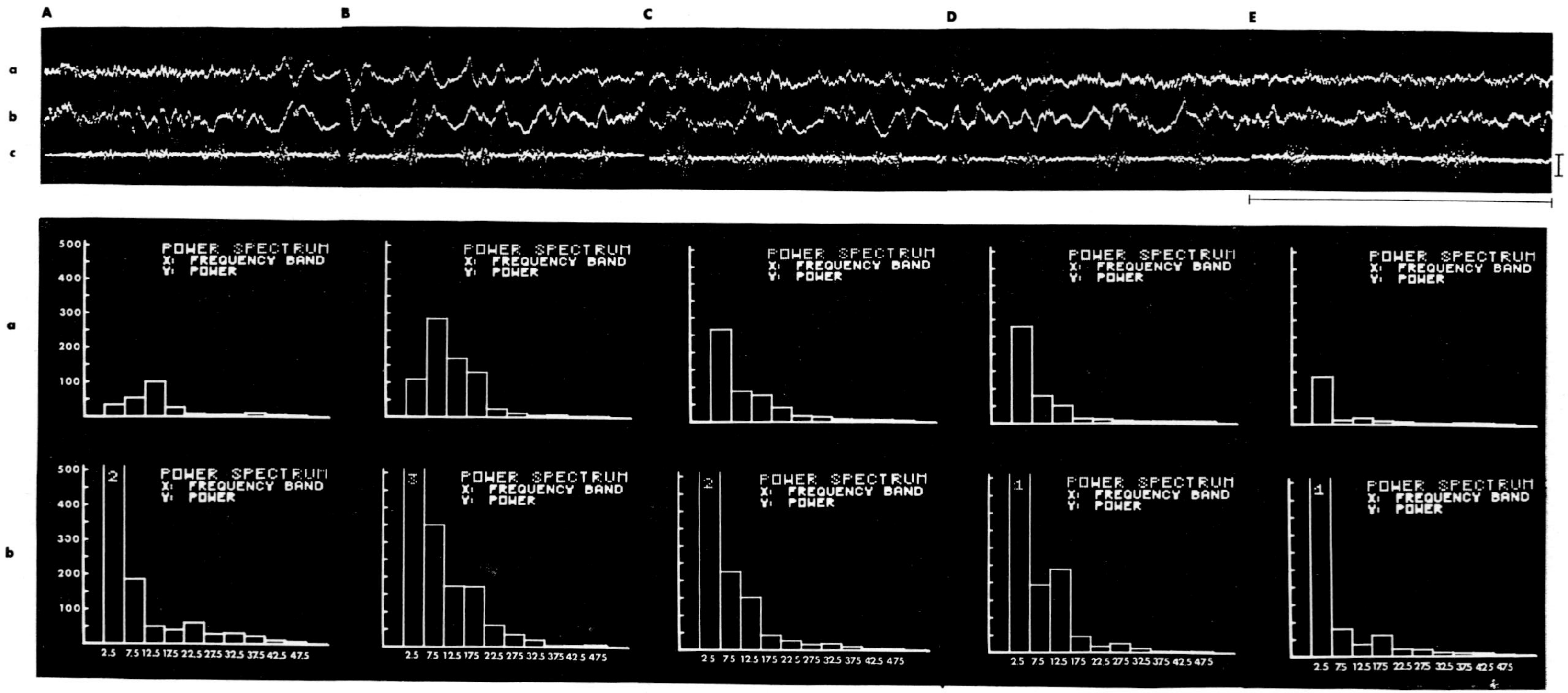

Fig. 1

EEG trace of normal cat and corresponding spectral analysis for 5 sec (*A*, *B*, *C*, *D*, *E*, respectively) of consecutive record from two different loci on the posterior lateral gyrus, showing a difference in output of the striate cortex during lapping as a function of electrode placement and time. Traces *a* and *b*: posterior lateral gyrus; trace *c*: written record of lap response. Note: an open column with a number in it indicates that the value exceeds the maximum value shown in the graph by 1, 2 or 3 times. (Calibrations: 1 sec and 50 μV).

epidurally, the latter electrodes having small balled tips. Electrode leads were crimped to a miniature Microdot plug and cemented to the skull with dental acrylic. All subjects were allowed a minimum recovery period of 2 weeks prior to testing.

Transection of the brain in the split-brain animals included the following midline structures: optic chiasm, corpus callosum, anterior and posterior commisures, fornix, massa intermedia, and superior colliculi. Surgery was done in two separate operations several weeks prior to electrode implantation. The first operation was the sectioning of the optic chiasm through a transbuccal approach. After a 2 week recovery period, the animal underwent transection of the midline structures accomplished from a dorsal approach.

Data acquisition and analysis

All data were stored on a 7-channel magnetic tape system (Ampex, Model SR-300) for later analysis on a small general purpose digital computer (PDP-8). Six channels recorded analog EEG and the seventh was used to record event data, both the milk presentation and the lapping response made by the animal.

Data analysis was on the PDP-8 computer. In the analog to digital conversion the signal was sampled at a rate of 1000 points/sec for a period of 5 sec and stored on digital tape for further processing. A special Digital Spectral Analysis program, which was adapted for the PDP-8 computer from an original program developed by the Stanford Electronics Laboratories[1] was used for the spectral analysis. The print-out gave the power in each narrow band (5 cycles) with the center frequencies of each band given in the graphed record (see samples in Fig. 1). Only frequencies up to 50 c/sec were graphed.

Apparatus and testing procedure

The feeder system was constructed entirely of plastic and was designed to eliminate the possibility of artifacts. Actuation of a solenoid valve by a short manually controlled electrical pulse allowed a small amount of milk to be delivered into the plastic feeder. A phono-cartridge placed beneath the spring-mounted plastic feeder cup picked up the lapping movements made by the cat. The spring tension was sensitive enough to allow the cup to move with the pressure produced by the tongue touching the shallow cup thereby producing a recordable signal.

The testing session for each animal consisted of putting the animal in a sound-insulated experimental box, which had a constant background noise (80 dB) and dim illumination. Milk was presented to the animal on a random schedule for approximately 10 trials under each of the following conditions: (1) visually non-occluded, and (2) visually occluded with an opaque contact lens in one eye of each of the split-brain cats. Control trials were run with the animal eating solid cat food, and with milk lapped from a bowl.

Verification of the split-brain

Histological verification of electrode placements and surgical transection of the brain in the split-brain cats is not possible at the present time as the animals are still being tested in other studies. However, electrophysiological verification by testing for the presence of evoked potentials in the occluded hemisphere during flash stimulation was carried out. There was no evidence of an evoked potential in the visually occluded hemisphere of any animal from a total of six bipolar electrodes in each hemisphere of each animal during the flash stimulation.

RESULTS

Digitized EEG for samples of milk lapping data, with the corresponding spectral analysis for each sample, are shown in Fig. 1 and 2. Records from the striate cortex showed the peak power in the 7.5 c/sec band during lapping, whereas the data from the auditory cortex for the same period of time were variable but often had a dominant power output in the 2.5 c/sec band (Fig. 2). The EEG records from the striate cortex indicated that after the burst of 7.5 c/sec activity with lapping, there was a shift to much higher frequencies as lapping became more sporadic, and subsequently all synchrony dropped out of the record.

Lapping at a fast and highly repetitive rate

[1] National Heart Institute Grant PHS HE 10202.

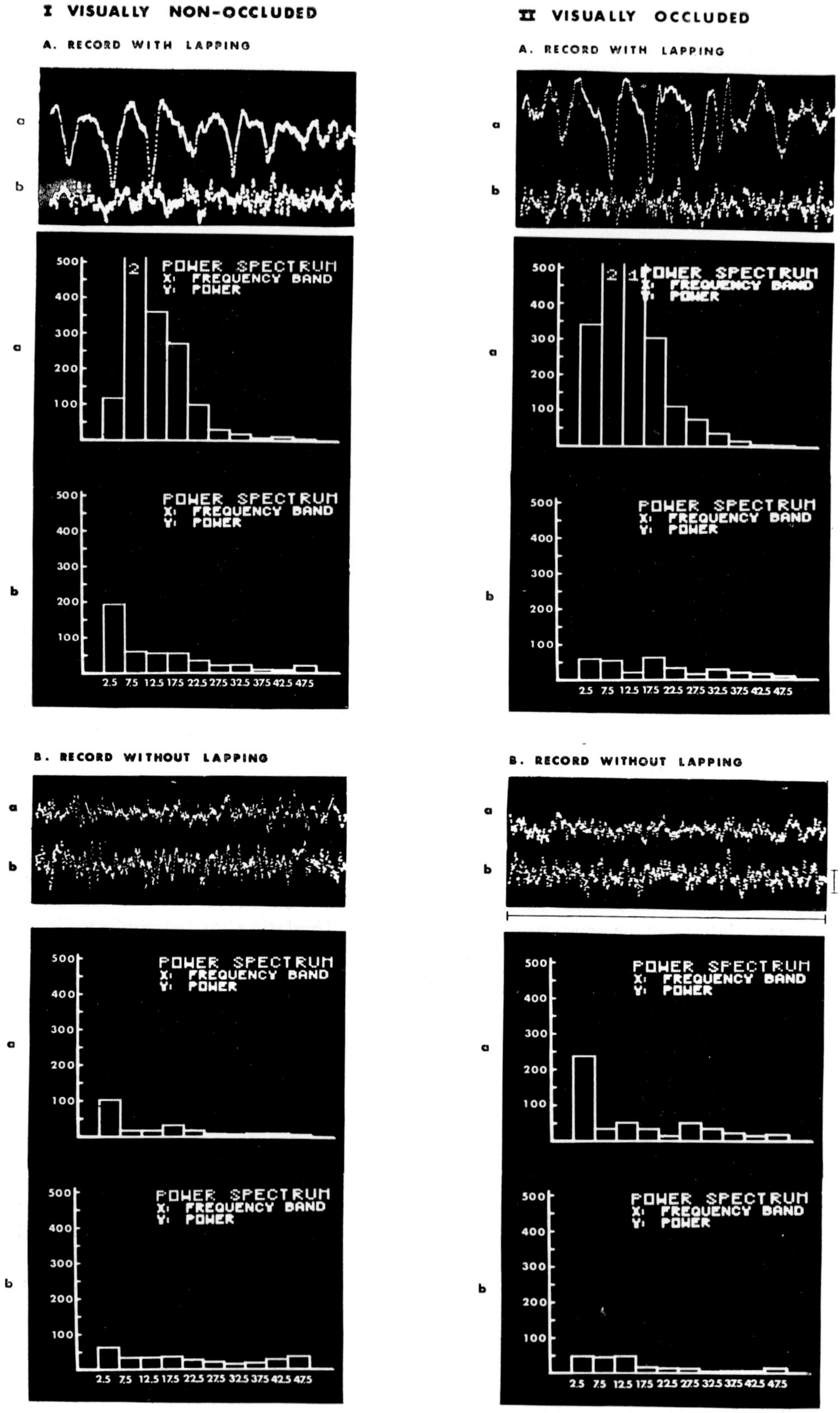

Fig. 2

Corresponding EEG trace and digital spectral analysis of split-brain cat with and without visual occlusion during lapping and not lapping. Traces *IAa*, *IBa*, *IIAa* and *IIBa* are from the same striate cortex lead and *IAb*, *IBb*, *IIAb* and *IIB* are concomitant records from the auditory cortex. Note: an open column with a number in it indicates that the value exceeds the maximum value shown in the graph by 1, 2 or 3 times. (Calibrations: 1 sec and 50 μV).

appeared to be a prerequisite for the initiation of the 7.5 c/sec activity. The EEG slow wave activity occurred approximately 300–500 msec after the onset of lapping, and then only if lapping was very repetitive; sporadic lapping simply did not produce the synchronous response. At the onset, the lapping rate was often 5 or 6 laps/sec, but after a few seconds the rate decreased and the synchronous EEG rhythm in the striate cortex evidenced a concomitant decrease. An example of the lapping response and its relationship to the EEG rhythm is shown in Fig. 1. Visual inspection of the animal during lapping, while monitoring the signal output of the phono-cartridge system designed to pick-up the tongue movements, indicated that the system produced a relatively reliable record of the lapping response.

All striate leads in all animals did not show the same proportion of synchronous EEG activity with lapping; this activity, however, was present in both epidural and intra-cortical recording sites in all animals. Electrodes having the response did so with high reliability.

An example of digitized EEG data from two striate electrodes in the same animal exhibiting different responses with lapping is shown in Fig. 1. At onset of lapping, striate electrode *b* showed a typical record of 7.5 c/sec which perseverated for several seconds. By contrast, electrode *a*, also in the posterior lateral gyrus, showed a much shorter period of oscillatory activity.

During periods when the animal was not lapping, there was a consistent shift to a more variable distribution of energy in all frequencies with a loss of all synchronous oscillatory activity in the striate cortex (Fig. 2). Auditory records taken during the same period did not exhibit a power frequency distribution that was reliably different from the records taken during lapping. The major peak of energy was often in the lowest frequency band, 2.5 c/sec, but this was not consistent from trial to trial.

A comparison of EEG data from split-brain animals with the normal cats during lapping showed that the 7.5 c/sec oscillatory activity was essentially the same in both groups of animals (Fig. 1 and 2). The major portion of energy was definitely centered in the 7.5 c/sec band.

When split-brain animals were visually occluded in one eye with an opaque contact lens and tested in the same milk lapping situation, the recordings from the ipsilateral visual cortex indicated that the peak power was distributed over the measured frequency bands in approximately the same manner as that of the non-occluded split-brain animals (Fig. 2) and the normal control animals. The same 7.5 c/sec band contained the major portion of energy. The electrical activity in the auditory cortex did not appear to vary in any systematic way from that of the normal controls or the non-occluded split-brain cats under the same behavioral conditions. Samples of analyzed records with visual occlusion of split-brain animals during periods when the animals were not lap-

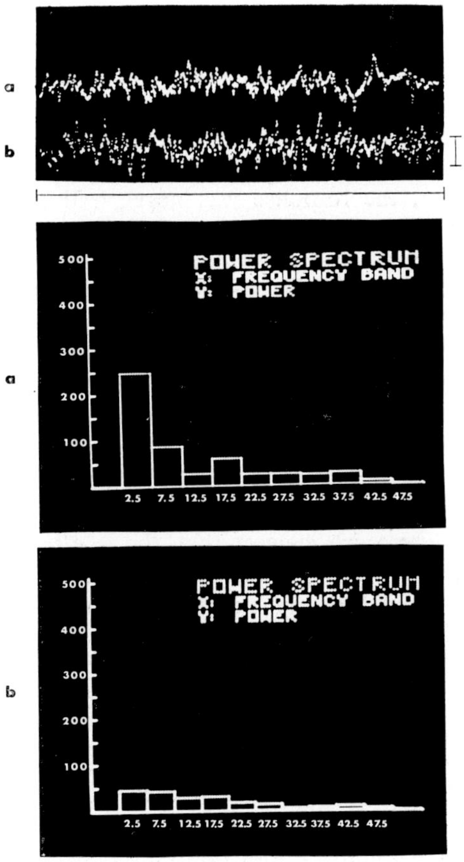

Fig. 3
EEG trace and corresponding digital spectral analysis during eating of solid cat food. Trace *a*: posterior lateral gyrus; trace *b*: mid-ectosylvian gyrus. (Calibrations: time: 1 sec and 50 μV).

ping, did not show any consistent changes when compared to similar records without occlusion (Fig. 2).

Control trials were run with the animals drinking milk from a bowl, and the frequency analysis indicated that the results were essentially the same as those with milk lapping from the feeder cup. This evidence ruled out the possibility that artifact from the feeder system somehow contaminated or was responsible for the results.

In order to ascertain whether the 7.5 c/sec oscillations were related to food intake *per se*, records were also taken with the animal eating canned cat food. Chewing and ingestion of solid food did not elicit the same electrophysiological response in the striate cortex (Fig. 3). There was no evidence of the synchronized oscillations. The major portion of power was often at 2.5 c/sec with a wider distribution over all frequencies which was continuously variable. EEG monitoring and gross observation of the animal during grooming behavior indicated that when the animal licked himself there was some evidence of a shift in the EEG to slower frequencies, however, the response was never well defined and obvious as in milk lapping. The rhythmic oscillations simply never developed.

DISCUSSION

Although previous investigations have associated the slow wave oscillatory activity in visual cortex with post-reinforcement or simply with the ingestion of food during drinking (Clemente *et al.* 1964) the results from the present research suggest that the 7 c/sec synchrony has a high correlation with the specific and highly repetitive tongue movement which occurs with lapping, and that the changes effected in the electrophysiological activity of the visual cortex seem to be a direct consequence of this complex repetitive movement.

In correlating the behavioral lapping response with the synchronized EEG response, there did not appear to be a one-to-one correspondence of the 7 c/sec activity with the motor response as such—the lapping must have been ongoing for a period of time prior to the onset of the synchronous activity occurring in the striate cortex. The latency of onset of the rhythm was quite variable. Its initiation occurred somewhere in a range of 300–500 msec or longer after the onset of vigorous lapping. The synchronous EEG activity was not invariably associated with lapping, but appeared in the record only when the animal lapped in a highly repetitive manner. If the animal lapped sporadically, the synchronous oscillatory electrical activity did not occur. Therefore, the 7 c/sec oscillatory activity does not represent a specific glossokinetic potential as such, but an electrophysiological state which is initiated and maintained as a consequence of repetitive tongue movement. If the 7 c/sec activity were a tongue potential, the potential would occur with each lick, and this certainly was not the case.

The possibility of artifactually induced electrophysiological responses should always be given serious consideration. Although artifact generated by eye movement could conceivably contribute to the 7 c/sec activity, this appears highly unlikely, as Hughes (1964) showed these potentials to be so small in the striate cortex that they were negligible when using ordinary recording techniques. If the 7 c/sec oscillations were equivalent to lambda activity in visual cortex they should disappear with visual occlusion (and they did not), as it has been shown that lambda waves disappear without patterned visual input (Hughes 1964).

The failure of previous researchers (Clemente *et al.* 1964) to elicit the same activity when a food deprived animal was given water can possibly be explained by the difference in the behavioral response; cats do not generally lap water for any prolonged period of time (and the results of Clemente *et al.* verified this), therefore the initiation of the synchronous electrical activity in the visual cortex never occurred.

Sadowski and Longo (1962) have reported "masticatory" waves in the EEG from the rabbit anterior sensori-motor cortex during eating, which were synchronized with the chewing movements. Although these researchers indicated that the "masticatory" waves spread to other cortical areas, they did not designate which areas were involved. One can only speculate that the striate cortex was one of these sites.

That the EEG synchrony in striate cortex is related to the rather global term "post-reinforcement" appears fairly obvious but hardly seems descriptively adequate and is somewhat misleading. For example, when the animal is eating solid cat food, the post-reinforcement waves do not appear. To infer a causal relationship between the initiation of the synchronized EEG and a "post reinforcement" state is indeed misleading. Unfortunately, the cat does not chew in a very rhythmic manner, therefore chewing movements do not elicit a synchronous EEG pattern.

That the 7 c/sec activity can become associated with, and elicited by the conditioned stimulus during classical conditioning (Clemente *et al.* 1964) seems plausible. If indeed the repetitive tongue movement does initiate the 7 c/sec rhythm, the "intended" tongue movements which become established with conditioning in "anticipation" of the unconditioned stimulus (milk) should also initiate the 7 c/sec activity. There could be a "sub-lapping" movement which the animal makes prior to actually lapping (similar to sub-vocal movements in speech). This question can possibly be answered by recording the EMG of the tongue during a conditioning situation.

The question of why this synchronous slow EEG activity is not present in the auditory cortex is a puzzling one and does not appear solvable at the moment. However, a possible explanation might entail a consideration of the types of non-auditorys timuli which affect activity in single cells in the primary auditory cortex, and the ratio of such units to "pure acoustic units" as well as their inhibitory/activation relationship; *i.e.*, whether these non-auditory responding units are basically inhibited and/or activated. Should these relationships appear drastically different from those present in striate cortex, the distribution and coupling of activated and inhibited units present during lapping, for example, would be reflected by EEG activity which would in turn be different in terms of c/sec, amplitude, phase, etc.

In the present experiment, the split-brain visually occluded cats afforded an excellent opportunity to evaluate the relative contribution of visual input to the 7 c/sec synchrony in striate cortex. In comparing the data from the split-brain animals, both with and without visual occlusion, there did not appear to be a reliable or significant difference in the slow wave EEG synchrony in the striate cortex with visual occlusion of the ipsilateral eye during milk lapping. The conclusion seems inevitable: even though the rhythmic 7 c/sec activity was recorded in striate cortex, it was not affected by a total blocking of visual input; therefore it could not have been visually mediated.

That the striate cortex is directly involved in activity other than processing visual inputs has been amply demonstrated by the single cell research which reports unit responses to a variety of non-visual stimuli. Jung *et al.* (1963) were among the first investigators to report multisensory convergence occurring in single units of the primary visual cortex. Recent research (in our laboratory) has illustrated that unit activity exhibiting multisensory activation is probably not simply related to just a non-specific or general arousal effect, but that single cells in striate cortex of cat have a highly specific response pattern; *i.e.*, responses to tone, when frequency is varied throughout the auditory range, produce a specific pattern in individual cells (Spinelli *et al.* 1968). However, more relevant to the present study is evidence that a large percentage of single cells in striate cortex are inhibited when the animal makes a specific movement (Skrebitsky and Gapich 1967). Thus the single unit data stand as excellent corroborative evidence that the electrical activity in striate cortex need not be visually mediated.

Although it is obvious that there are numerous non-visual inputs present in such a complex act as lapping and ingesting milk, the predominant input would still most likely be that initiated by a highly repetitive movement such as lapping. The neuronal mechanisms which seem most tenable in effecting such a dramatic and well-defined electrophysiological response as the the 7 c/sec synchrony in striate cortex may be a massive inhibition of cellular activity produced by these inputs. The distribution and coupling of inputs produced by the ratio of visual/non-visual cells activated and inhibited by such a highly specific response could conceivably initiate a reliably consistent output of highly synchronous and relatively frequency specific waves in a neuronal network such as that in the striate cortex.

SUMMARY

1. When cats were presented a small amount of milk in a plastic feeder cup, their tongue movements made during lapping were recorded concomitantly with EEG records from posterior lateral gyri, suprasylvian gyri, and mid-ectosylvian gyri. Frequency analysis of the records revealed that a 7.5 c/sec activity was present only in the posterior lateral gyri during the lapping (7.5 was one of the center frequencies of the total ten 5-cycle bands of frequencies analyzed). The 7.5 c/sec activity was of relatively large amplitude and occurred only with repetitive lapping. Its initiation was approximately 300 msec or longer after the onset of lapping.

2. The synchronous oscillatory EEG activity did not occur with ingestion of solid cat food by the animals. Therefore, the fact that the slow wave EEG occurred due to the reinforcing properties of the milk hardly seems tenable. Solid cat food should be as reinforcing as milk.

3. The 7.5 c/sec synchronous rhythm occurred in both normal and split-brain animals. With visual occlusion of the split-brain cat with an opaque contact lens over one eye, and recording from the ipsilateral striate cortex, there was no reliable difference in the EEG record when compared with a record from the same animal and electrode without visual occlusion. Therefore, the 7.5 c/sec synchrony in striate cortex associated with lapping was definitely not visually mediated.

4. It is proposed that the synchronous slow wave EEG is initiated by a massive inhibition of cells in the striate cortex effected by the non-visual inputs associated with lapping. Microelectrode data showing inhibition in single cells correlated with movement and non-visual stimuli are cited as ancillary evidence for such an interpretation.

RÉSUMÉ

ANALYSE DE FRÉQUENCE DE L'EEG PENDANT L'ABSORPTION DE LAIT

1. On présente à des chats une petite quantité de lait dans une cupule de plastique; les mouvements de la langue effectués pendant le lappage sont enregistrés, concomitament aux tracés EEG des gyri postérieurs latéraux, suprasylviens et ectosylviens médians. L'analyse de fréquence de ces tracés révèle qu'une activité à 7,5 c/sec s'observe pendant le lappage, mais seulement au niveau des gyri latéraux postérieurs (7,5 est l'une des fréquences centrales des 10 bandes totales de fréquences analysées). L'activité à 7,5 c/sec est d'une amplitude relativement grande et ne survient qu'avec le lappage répétitif. Elle commence approximativement 300 msec après le début du lappage, ou même plus tardivement.

2. Cette activité EEG rythmique synchrone ne survient pas avec l'ingestion de nourriture solide par les animaux. Toutefois, que ces ondes lentes EEG surviennent à cause de propriétés de renforcement particulières au lait paraît difficilement soutenable. La nourriture solide pour chats devrait avoir les mêmes propriétés de renforcement que le lait.

3. Le rythme synchrone à 7,5 c/sec survient chez des animaux normaux aussi bien que chez des animaux à cerveau divisé (split-brain). Si chez le chat à cerveau divisé on fait une occlusion visuelle au moyen d'un verre de contact opaque sur un oeil, et que l'on enregistre le cortex strié ipsilatéral, on ne note pas de différence significative du tracé EEG d'avec le tracé du même animal et de la même électrode sans occlusion visuelle. Ainsi, il apparaît certain que la synchronie à 7,5 c/sec du cortex strié associée au lappage n'est pas médiatisée par la vue.

4. L'auteur suggère que les ondes lentes EEG synchrones sont initiées par une inhibition massive des cellules du cortex strié due aux afférences non visuelles associées au lappage. Des données micro-physiologiques montrant une inhibition au niveau de cellules isolées en corrélation avec des mouvements et des stimuli non visuels sont citées comme arguments auxiliaires d'une telle interprétation.

The author gratefully acknowledges the able laboratory assistance of Miss J. Bonham and Mr. B. Bridgeman. In particular, she expresses her sincere thanks and appreciation to Dr. K. H. Pribram for his encouragement and support in making this work possible.

REFERENCES

CLEMENTE, C. C., STERMAN, M. B. and WYRWICKA, W. Post-reinforcement EEG synchronization during alimentary behavior. *Electroenceph. clin. Neurophysiol.*, **1964**, *16*: 355–365.

HUGHES, J. R. Response from the visual cortex of unanesthetized monkeys. *Int. Rev. Neurobiol.*, **1964**, *7*: 99–152.

JASPER, H. H. and AJMONE MARSAN, C. *A stereotaxic atlas of the diencephalon of the cat.* University of Toronto Press, Toronto, **1954.**

JUNG, R., KORNHUBER, H. H. and DA FONSECA, J. S. Multi-sensory convergence on cortical neurons. In G. MORRUZI *et al.* (Eds.), *Progress in brain research.* Elsevier, Amsterdam, **1963,** *1*: 207–240.

SADOWSKI, B. and LONGO, V. C. Electroencephalographic and behavioral correlates of an instrumental reward conditioned response in rabbits. *Electroenceph. clin. Neurophysio l.*,**1962,** *14*: 465–476.

SHEER, D. E., GRANDSTAFF, N. W. and BENIGNUS, V. A. 40-c/sec electrical activity in the brain of the cat: V. Pattern relations between visual cortex and the behavioral response in learning. Paper presented at the *4th World Congress of Psychiatry, Madrid, 1966.*

SKREBITSKY, V. G. and GAPICH, L. I. Microelectrode investigation of extinction of neuronal responses in visual cortex of waking rabbits to acoustic stimulation. *Fiziol. Zh. (Leningrad)*, **1967**, *53*: 906–914, in *Neuroscience Translations*, 1967–68.

SPINELLI, D. N., STARR, A. and BARRET, T. Auditory specificity in unit recordings from cat's visual cortex. *J. exp. Neurol.*, **1968,** *22*: 75–84.

Reference: GRANDSTAFF, N. W. Frequency analysis of EEG during milk drinking. *Electroenceph. clin. Neurophysiol.*, **1969,** *27*: 57–65.

Electroencephalography and Clinical Neurophysiology
Elsevier Publishing Company, Amsterdam – Printed in The Netherlands

FREQUENCY CONTROL OF MOTOR UNIT ACTION POTENTIALS

JACK H. PETAJAN, M.D., PH.D. AND BETTY ANNE PHILIP, PH.D.

Physiology Section, Arctic Health Research Laboratory, College, Alaska 99701 (U.S.A.)

(Accepted for publication: October 8, 1968)

INTRODUCTION

Changes in the amplitude, duration, or configuration of the motor unit action potential (MUAP), recorded by a needle electrode inserted into the muscle, may indicate diseases in the motor unit. The MUAP also provides a "window" into the central nervous system since during ordinary effort, a one to one relationship exists between the discharge of the alpha motoneuron and the MUAP. The force required of the whole muscle determines the number of active motor units and their frequency of firing. The effectiveness of control is measured by the difference between the force required and the force actually exerted. In the normal individual, the latter reflects the subjective level of effort.

Since the force delivered by the single muscle or motor unit cannot be conveniently measured, the frequency of firing of the MUAP is commonly selected for study. When the MUAP is firing at minimal effort at its lowest, most stable frequency, both the average force contribution of the single unit and the total number of motor units active in the muscles are minimal. The inter-spike interval (ΔT) of a single MUAP at this minimum level of effort is defined here as the *onset interval* and represents a lower limit of control. As effort is gradually increased, a second unit in the same territory as the first is recruited. The inter-spike interval of the first unit at the point of recruitment of the second unit is defined as the *recruitment interval.* Between the onset interval and the recruitment interval, a level of effort prevails where control is maintained by change in ΔT alone. The frequency change from onset to recruitment relative to the recruitment frequency of the single motor unit is defined as the *range of control:*

$$\frac{f_r - f_o}{f_r} = \frac{\Delta T_o - \Delta T_r}{\Delta T_o}$$

where f_r = recruitment frequency, f_o = onset frequency, ΔT_o = onset interval, and ΔT_r = recruitment interval.

METHODS

MUAPs were studied using an intramuscular coaxial needle electrode (TECA) in forty-two young adults. Muscles (Table I) were selected so that proximal and distal locations, as well as flexor and extensor actions, could be compared. Subjects were supine or prone and completely relaxed. Slight manual resistance prevented movement during minimal effort. Most often no resistance was required and no movement occurred. The MUAPs, displayed on the oscilloscope, were in full view of the subject. Units were also heard through a loudspeaker after amplification with a Grass AM-5 audio-amplifier. Thus, the MUAP became an "artificial" effector under the subjects' control while movement *per se* was not a determinant of control (Smith 1934; Harrison and Mortensen 1962; Basmajian 1963).

Data were recorded on electromagnetic tape with a Model 1028 2-channel Magnecord tape recorder (one channel being utilized for subject and muscle identification, as well as for constant recording of instructions to the subject). The subjects were instructed to familiarize themselves with the relation between conscious muscle activation and motor unit discharge. Once a MUAP was defined, the subject was instructed to try to activate it and then to keep it firing regularly but as slowly as possible. He was then told to gradually increase the rate of firing until a second MUAP appeared, and to sustain that level of effort.

TABLE I

Onset and recruitment intervals

Muscle**	Mean and standard deviation* of onset intervals (msec)	Mean and standard deviation of recruitment intervals (msec)	Number of units analyzed	Number of onset intervals	Number of recruitment intervals
Frontalis	102 ± 29	46 ± 16	72	316	78
Orbicularis oris	70 ± 19	34 ± 10	58	299	69
All facial muscles	86 ± 29	40 ± 16	130	615	147
Deltoid	116 ± 23	84 ± 16	53	353	94
Biceps	124 ± 21	86 ± 14	56	376	111
Triceps	132 ± 36	84 ± 17	49	332	80
Brachioradialis	116 ± 22	78 ± 18	36	247	42
Pronator teres	132 ± 38	88 ± 19	35	132	46
First dorsal interosseous	142 ± 39	98 ± 21	51	318	122
Multifidus	152 ± 33	102 ± 20	39	240	41
Vastus lateralis	126 ± 30	88 ± 18	80	520	143
Gluteus maximus	128 ± 30	88 ± 16	48	323	56
Tibialis anterior	124 ± 26	90 ± 13	85	594	149
Biceps femoris	132 ± 29	92 ± 16	64	411	61
Medial gastrocnemius	156 ± 29	110 ± 23	54	326	76
Extensor digitorum brevis	138 ± 29	98 ± 13	43	260	77
All muscles	132 ± 32	90 ± 19	693	4,608	1,137

* Standard deviations are calculated from the numbers of onset and recruitment intervals recorded.
** Muscles are listed in descending order on the neuraxis.

Once a unit was found during minimal effort, the examiner positioned the electrode manually to obtain and maintain the maximum amplitude and minimum duration of the MUAP. After recruitment of the second unit, subject effort was decreased and the first unit was recorded alone to verify that the electrode position had been retained. By systematic exploration of the muscle, four to five motor units were examined in a single muscle to avoid duplicate sampling of motor unit territories.

System of data analysis

The taped results were utilized as the input to a "threshold" detector, a diode rectifier, which was adjusted to select motor units preferentially by amplitude and to convert the polyphasic MUAP into a single monophasic spike. The monophasic spike then became the input for the "dot pattern analyzer" (Hind *et al.* 1960). This analyzer consists of an unblanking circuit, in combination with a sawtooth signal generator, which displays the interval between two dots on the oscilloscope screen. Intervals were read accurately to within 5 msec. Each successive interval, displayed as the distance between two dots, was then photographed on 35 mm film using a Grass C-4 oscilloscope camera. The succession of dots representing intervals between spikes from initiation of single MUAP activity to recruitment of a second MUAP was examined and the longest stable inter-spike interval, the *onset interval*, was then determined. Recruitment was signaled as an abrupt decrease in interval. The interval immediately preceding the decrease caused by recruitment of a second unit was measured as the *recruitment interval.* Selected intervals were recorded on data cards which were subsequently analyzed using an IBM-360 computer.

RESULTS

Activation of a single MUAP

Most subjects were able to activate single MUAPs with little difficulty after brief experience with the method. Characteristically, the unit was initially activated in an on-and-off manner which

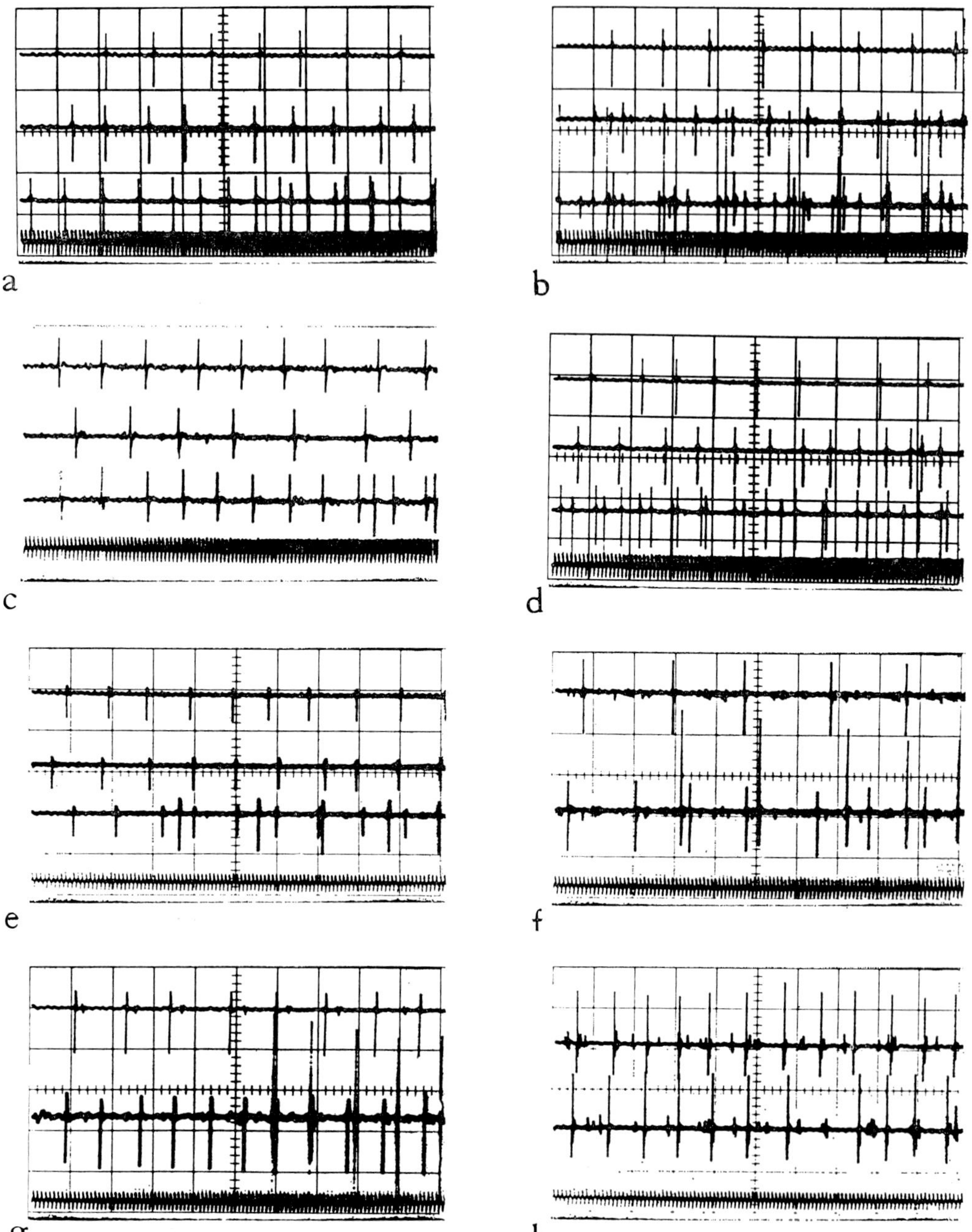

Fig. 1

Motor unit action potentials from deltoid (*a*), first dorsal interosseous (*b*), pronator teres (*c*), triceps (*d*), gluteus maximus (*e*), paraspinal (multifidus) (*f*), and vastus lateralis (*g*) muscles are shown depicting stable onset and recuitment intervals. Traces are to be read from left to right and from top to bottom since they represent single traces stored in sequence. Onset intervals are present in the uppermost trace. The recruited MUAP can be differentiated by amplitude and wave form. In (*h*) is shown the on-and-off characteristic of firing rate in first dorsal interosseous as the subject reduces effort below that essential for firing and then increases it to re-establish firing, seen as a lengthening of interval after the seventh MUAP in the second trace. Calibration signal is a 100 μV, 100 c/sec pulse. Sweep speed is 100 msec/cm for all traces.

resulted in considerable irregularity in the intervals. When a unit was finally turned on and its activity sustained, it fired regularly at a rate which could not be reproduced by intermittent conscious activation. A lapse of attention was signaled by an abrupt increase in interval, which was several times that which had been regularly sustained and which could be several seconds long. The stable intervals between such lapses were measured as the *onset interval*, since the subject was unable to reduce the firing rate by reducing effort without causing the unit to stop firing (Fig. 1).

Table I shows the mean and standard deviation of onset intervals for various muscles. The results from all units were averaged for any given muscle. Distributions were slightly skewed with essentially no values below 80 msec. Standard deviations were calculated as for normal distributions. Onset intervals tended to be greater in distal muscles and the muscles of the upper extremity. An exception was multifidus which had a long onset interval. Significant differences ($P < 0.001$) existed between muscles in different locations such as deltoid and first dorsal interosseous, and between gluteus maximus and medial gastrocnemius (see Table I). Mean onset interval for all muscles and for the facial muscles alone are also shown in Table I.

Recruitment intervals

A MUAP was considered recruited only if its amplitude was sufficient to consider the recording electrode to be within its territory. The subject was unable to activate the recruited unit alone without simultaneous activation of the first unit. After recruitment occurred, a stabilization in firing rate of the first unit was observed which was maintained until gross increases in force caused an increase in frequency.

Values for recruitment intervals are found in Table I for all subjects. Excluding facial muscles, intervals were slightly skewed to the right with a minimum interval of 60 msec and an over-all mean recruitment interval of 90 ± 19 msec. Recruitment intervals varied less than onset intervals; and where the onset interval was short, only a small decrease in interval occurred between onset and recruitment. In proximal muscles, in some instances, it was impossible to discern a difference between onset and recruitment intervals; *i.e.*, it was impossible to isolate a single MUAP.

TABLE II

Range of control $[(f_r - f_o)/f_r]$

Muscle	Mean	S.D.	*N*
Frontalis	0.52	0.16	66
Orbicularis oris	0.50	0.17	55
Triceps	0.40	0.13	41
Pronator teres	0.36	0.15	28
First dorsal interosseous	0.35	0.13	47
Deltoid	0.33	0.13	40
Biceps	0.33	0.13	43
Brachioradialis	0.33	0.13	26
Multifidus	0.32	0.12	36
Gluteus maximus	0.31	0.12	38
Vastus lateralis	0.31	0.12	71
Extensor digitorum brevis	0.31	0.14	33
Tibialis anterior	0.30	0.12	74
Medial gastrocnemius	0.29	0.11	42
Biceps femoris	0.29	0.11	44

Recruitment intervals for orbicularis oris and frontalis muscles (Table I) were approximately half the value for limb and girdle muscles.

Range of control

The variation in the range of control $[(f_r - f_o)/f_r]$ with muscle location is indicated in Table II, where the range of control is seen to be highest in facial muscles and progressively lower in more caudal muscles with significant differences ($P < 0.001$) existing between facial and upper and lower extremity regions. The values for triceps were significantly higher than those for biceps, but no significant difference was found between flexor and extensor muscles in the lower extremity. Although multifidus has a long onset interval, its range of control, 0.32, is low.

DISCUSSION

The study of single MUAP activation in a subject who is constantly aware of its activity utilizes a level of effort far less than that of ordinary movement. The method used here investigates an artificial control system in that the peripheral sensory input usually acting in normal movement is supplemented by visual and auditory cues.

During minimal effort, many motoneurons to a muscle may be active. In this study, the subject was not consciously able to activate segments of a muscle, but he could control the level of effort and thus alter the frequency of firing of single units. A further increase in the level of effort resulted in an increase in the number of units (recruitment). The awareness of the level of effort thus appeared to be critical in controlling motoneuron activation.

It is unknown whether or not the motoneurons activated at minimal effort differ in any way from those MUAPs which are recruited. As many as nine motor units may overlap in a territory within the muscle (Buchthal *et al.* 1955). Minimal effort is effective in activating a certain population of motoneurons which fire at a relatively constant rate. Reduction in effort results in abrupt cessation of firing. It is this characteristic—the on-and-off nature of firing at minimal effort—which permits establishment of onset interval values for individual muscles.

Studies of spinal motoneurons in the cat have shown higher activation thresholds for large than for small motoneurons (Henneman *et al.* 1965). The relationship between the size of the motoneuron soma and the number of muscle fibers in the motor unit has not been established in man. Further, it is unknown whether motor units which become active at minimal effort differ in size from those active at higher levels of effort.

In the baboon, "motoneurons of distal muscle groups have narrower colonies (of corticomotor neurons) commanding larger monosynaptic excitations, motoneurons of proximal groups have wider colonies commanding smaller monosynaptic excitations" (Phillips 1967). The "narrower colonies" in control of distal muscles and the greater monosynaptic excitation imply a greater degree of control. If this is accomplished by smaller force increments, then the greater monosynaptic excitation and "narrow colonies" in the motor cortex may be associated with longer onset intervals. The greater range of control, present in facial and upper extremity muscles, indicates a greater ability to vary effort by changing the frequency of firing rather than by recruitment. Thus, the number of active units might be kept at a minimum. In general, finer increments in force might be expected to be produced by small increases in frequency rather than by recruitment. This is supported by the observation that the first unit stabilizes in frequency at the moment of recruitment and that at onset, the second unit fires at a rate similar to that of the first unit. Further refinement of the control system would be anticipated when the number of muscle fibers in a motor unit is small and onset and recruitment intervals are short as is the case with facial muscles since the relative change in force with changing frequency would be smaller.

Tokizane and Shimazu (1964) and others have also studied the control of frequency of single MUAPs. They define two kinds of motor units: "tonic" units have a low variability, and intervals increase less with decreasing effort than do "kinetic" units which have highly variable intervals. Such variability exceeds many times the small variation in interval accepted here as representing a stable onset interval. In our study such instability of interval was taken to indicate that the level of effort was insufficient to keep the unit firing. Tokizane and Shimazu do not indicate how either the level or constancy of effort were controlled in their studies.

The recruited MUAP is the first of many recruited at higher levels of effort, but one which is probably contiguous in the muscle with the first MUAP being recorded. If the recruited MUAP is obtained only at higher levels of effort, if it cannot be (or is not) activated singly, and if its activation bears a constant relation to the frequency of firing of the first MUAP, then the motoneuron firing at minimal effort may participate in the activation of the motoneuron firing at higher levels of effort through the action of collateral connections. Conscious awareness of movement, or the level of effort important for initial activation of motoneurons at minimal effort, may be supplemented at higher levels of effort by the action of Renshaw cells which facilitate motoneurons through the release of inhibitory background discharge (Wilson *et al.* 1960; Wilson and Burgess 1962). Through such mechanisms, a system of control may operate so that facilitation of recruited motoneurons is related to the frequency of firing of motoneurons already firing.

The stabilization of interval at the time of

recruitment and the narrow distribution of recruitment intervals indicate that there may be a preferred or optimum frequency of discharge. This concept is compatible with the finding of a relative constancy of frequency of discharge over a wide range of effort (25–85% of maximum) with a sudden increase in frequency as effort is increased from 80 to 100% (Kaiser and Petersén 1965). The second unit is recruited when the unit appearing at minimal effort fires at an interval just below the optimum. At maximal effort Bracchi *et al.* (1966) have found a progressive increase from lower limbs to head in the firing rate of single motor units. Also firing rate was found to be quite stable. A higher frequency of firing was found associated with less recurrent inhibition. The greater relative frequency change (range of control) between onset and recruitment in more cephalad muscles is associated then with less recurrent inhibition. The observation that recruitment interval is relatively constant (excluding facial muscles) and that stabilization of firing rate occurs at the time of recruitment suggests that in more cephalad muscles greater frequency change can occur in a single unit after a second unit has been recruited. Therefore, in these muscles the range of frequency would be greater and control more dependent upon varying frequency in single units before and after recruitment has occurred. It is important to recognize that stabilization in frequency was noted at low levels of effort but effort sufficient to recruit a second unit with gross increases in effort required to increase frequency. Comparison of recruitment intervals with intervals at maximal effort from Bracchi *et al.* reveals good correspondence for lower extremity muscles (gastrocnemius, 110 msec *vs.* 100 msec; biceps femoris, 92 msec *vs.* 90 msec, respectively) but higher intervals for recruitment in upper extremities (deltoid and triceps, 84 msec *vs.* 58 msec; biceps, 86 msec *vs.* 56 msec, respectively). Therefore, considering the MUAP that fires first at minimal effort in lower extremity muscles recruitment occurs at approximately maximal frequency while in upper extremity additional frequency increase can occur after recruitment. However, all muscles could not be compared.

Facial muscles which have onset and recruitment intervals significantly below those of other muscles, nevertheless, exhibit a range of control and maximum frequency of discharge which are consistent with the observation of a cephalo-caudad gradient of frequency. This suggests that the recurrent inhibition mechanism may explain both maximum frequency and range of control but that other factors such as the size of the motoneuron and other influences upon threshold may determine onset and recruitment intervals.

Inhibitory influences may be greater on smaller motoneurons which have relatively long onset intervals. One must then explain how it is that facial motor units have such short onset intervals. One explanation would be that in facial muscles a very large motoneuron innervates a small number of muscle fibers. Recurrent inhibition may be less in motor units with a small number of muscle fibers. Further, a relationship may exist between the degree of recurrent inhibition and the threshold of recruited motoneurons.

Since changes in the force contribution of the single motor unit or the number of motor units that are active can be expected to alter the frequency of MUAP firing, measurement of the latter may prove useful in the investigation of physiological or pathological factors which affect the motor unit.

SUMMARY

The onset interval of the single motor unit action potential (MUAP), defined as the longest regular interval of firing at minimal effort, was determined for various skeletal muscles. Intervals found were 132±32 msec, mean for all limb and girdle muscles, and 86±29 msec, mean for all facial muscles studied. Distal muscles in the upper extremities had significantly longer onset intervals than did proximal shoulder girdle and lower extremity muscles. In studying single units, awareness of the level of effort seemed more critical to the control of firing rate than did movement. The recruitment interval was less variable than onset interval, with a mean of 90±19 msec for limb and girdle muscles and 40±16 msec for facial muscles.

The range of control, expressed as the difference in frequency of a MUAP between onset and recruitment relative to the recruitment frequency, decreased with cephalo-caudal location of the muscle from 0.55 for the frontalis muscle to 0.29 for the biceps femoris muscle.

RÉSUMÉ

CONTRÔLE DE FRÉQUENCE DES POTENTIELS D'ACTION MOTEURS UNITAIRES

L'intervalle de départ d'un potentiel d'action moteur unitaire isolé, défini comme l'intervalle régulier de décharge le plus long sous l'action d'un effort minime, est déterminé pour plusieurs muscles striés. La valeur moyenne des intervalles trouvés est de 132 ± 32 msec pour tous les muscles des membres et de leur attache, et de 86 ± 29 msec pour tous les muscles de la face étudiés. Les muscles distaux des extrêmités supérieures ont des intervalles de départ nettement plus longs que les muscles proximaux de la ceinture scapulaire et des extrêmités inférieures. Dans l'étude des unités isolées, la prise en considération du niveau d'effort apparaît plus importante que le mouvement pour le contrôle du taux de décharge. L'intervalle de recrutement est moins variable que l'intervalle de départ, avec une moyenne de 90 ± 19 msec pour les muscles des membres et de leur ceinture et 40 ± 16 msec pour les muscles faciaux.

La gamme de contrôle, exprimée par le rapport de la différence de fréquence d'un potentiel d'action moteur unitaire entre le début et le recrutement, par la fréquence du recrutement diminue avec la localisation céphalo-caudale du muscle de 0.55 pour le muscle frontal à 0.29 pour le muscle biceps fémoral.

The authors would like to express their appreciation to all of the subjects who volunteered for this study as well as to Mrs. S. K. Loder, who assisted in the analysis of the data.

REFERENCES

BASMAJIAN, J. V. Control and training of individual motor units. *Science*, **1963**, *141*: 440–441.

BRACCHI, F., DECANDIA, M. and GUALTIEROTTI, T. Frequency stabilization in the motor centers of spinal cord and caudal brain stem. *Amer. J. Physiol.*, **1966**, *210*: 1170–1177.

BUCHTHAL, F., GULD, C. and ROSENFALCK, P. Innervation zone and propagation velocity in human muscle. *Acta physiol. scand.*, **1955**, *35*: 174–190.

HARRISON, V. F. and MORTENSEN, O. A. Identification and voluntary control of single motor unit activity in the tibialis anterior muscle. *Anat. Rec.*, **1962**, *144*: 109–116.

HENNEMAN, E., SOMJEN, G. and CARPENTER, D. O. Excitability and inhibitibility of motoneurons of different sizes. *J. Neurophysiol.*, **1965**, *28*: 599–620.

HIND, J. E., ROSE, J. E., DAVIES, P. W., WOOLSEY, D. N., BENJAMIN, R. M., WELLER, W. I. and THOMPSON, R. F. Unit activity in the auditory cortex. In G. L. RASMUSSEN and W. F. WINDLE (Eds.), *Neural mechanisms of the auditory and vestibular system*. Thomas, Springfield, Ill., **1960**: 201–216.

KAISER, E. I. and PETERSÉN, I. Muscle action potentials studied by frequency analysis and duration measurement. *Acta neurol. scand.*, **1965**, *41*, *Suppl. 13*: 213–236.

PHILLIPS, C. G. Corticomotoneuronal organization: Projection from the arm area of the baboon's motor cortex. *Arch. Neurol. (Chic.)*, **1967**, *17*: 188–195.

SMITH, O. C. Action potentials from single motor units in voluntary contraction. *Amer. J. Physiol.*, **1934**, *108*: 629–638.

TOKIZANE, T. and SHIMAZU, H. *Functional differentiation of human skeletal muscle*. Thomas, Springfield, Ill., **1964**: 21–28.

WILSON, V. J. and BURGESS, P. R. Disinhibition in the cat spinal cord. *J. Neurophysiol.*, **1962**, *25*: 392–404.

WILSON, V. J., DIECKE, F. P. J. and TALBOT, W. H. Action of tetanus toxin on conditioning of spinal motoneurons. *J. Neurophysiol.*, **1960**, *23*: 659–666.

Reference: PETAJAN, J. H. and PHILIP, B. A. Frequency control of motor unit action potentials. *Electroenceph. clin. Neurophysiol.*, **1969**, *27*: 66–72.

CLINICAL AND LABORATORY NOTES

BEREITSCHAFTSPOTENTIAL ENHANCEMENT WITH INCREASED LEVEL OF MOTIVATION[1]

DALE W. MCADAM AND DAVID M. SEALES[2]

Departments of Psychology and Neurology, University of Rochester, Rochester, N.Y. 14627 (U.S.A.)

(Accepted for publication: October 14, 1968)

Kornhüber and Deecke (1965) were the first to describe a time-locked cerebral slow negative potential shift, the Bereitschaftspotential (BSP), occurring maximally over contralateral Rolandic cortex before a voluntary movement. Gilden *et al.* (1966), and Vaughan *et al.* (1968), have explored movement-related potentials further and have described what they call the "motor potential" (MP). The MP consists of four components: (1) N_1, a slow, small amplitude negative shift arising up to 1 sec before the movement, (2) P_1, a rapid, small amplitude positive wave, (3) N_2, a rapid, large amplitude negative wave and (4) P_2, a rapid, large amplitude positive wave. Component N_1 is the same as the BSP of Kornhüber and Deecke, and is considered by Vaughan *et al.* "to represent a physiological correlate of preparatory motor set".

The BSP phenomenon is strikingly similar to the Contingent Negative Variation (CNV) first described by Walter *et al.* (1964), as a large, slow, vertex-negative potential shift arising after the warning signal in a fixed foreperiod reaction time setting. The CNV has been shown to be linked to the motivational significance of the warning signal preceding it (Irwin *et al.* 1966; Rebert *et al.* 1967); CNV amplitude increased with increases in motivation.

Whereas Kornhüber and Deecke noted that the BSP was enhanced with "intentional engagement" on the part of the subject, the relationship between BSP and level of motivation has not been subjected to controlled experimentation. The purpose of the present study was to examine the BSP under conditions of differing motivation, and to evaluate the findings in the light of similar knowledge of the CNV.

[1] This research was supported in part under a contract with the U.S. Office of Naval Research. Such support does not imply endorsement of the content of the publication by the Navy.

[2] Mr. Seales received support as an NSF Undergraduate Summer Research Fellow.

METHODS

Eleven women between the ages of 18 and 25 served as subjects. None had prior information about the phenomenon being studied.

Silver–silver chloride recording electrodes were placed over both hemispheres in those regions presumably overlying hand motor areas. Active electrodes were placed at C_3 and C_4 (international system), reference electrodes were placed at the respective mastoids, and a ground electrode was placed either on the forehead or earlobe. Signals were amplified by a Grass 7P1 low level DC pre-amplifier and its associated 7DA driver amplifier.

The time needed for magnetic tape to pass from the record head to the reproduce head on a Precision Instrument 6208 tape recorder (about 1.26 sec) was used to obtain "on-line" analyses of brain activity preceding an overt response. Signals were taken from the polygraph to the input of the tape recorder. The output of the tape recorder was led to a Nuclear Chicago Data Retrieval Computer (DRC). The 2 sec sweep of the averager was triggered by the subject's response. Each sweep thus analyzed signals beginning 1.26 sec before the response and continuing for 0.74 sec after its occurrence. Following each experimental session, a voltage calibration was placed in the averager to allow scoring of the brain responses in μV. Averages were read out onto a Houston Model HR-80 T–Y plotter.

Subjects were seated in a cushioned chair located within a darkened sound dampened room. The experiment consisted of two conditions, *reward* and non-reward (*baseline*). Under *baseline* condition, subjects received instructions to close their eyes, relax, remain quiet, and to press a button switch, held in the right hand, once "every few seconds". Counting and "clocking" were discouraged on the basis that they might tend to mask the effects of the variable being studied. Subjects heard a brief tone with each button press. Forty trials were averaged.

Under *reward* condition subjects received identical information and instructions and, in addition, were told that for each "correct" button press they would receive 10 cents. Subjects heard the tone only after a "correct" response and heard nothing after an "incorrect" response. These instructions were kept vague and subjects were allowed to form their own hypotheses about what might be a "correct" response so that no external stimuli, which might be inimical to recording the BSP, would intrude. Reward over 40 trials was randomly determined by the experimenter such that each subject received approximately 50% rewarded responses.

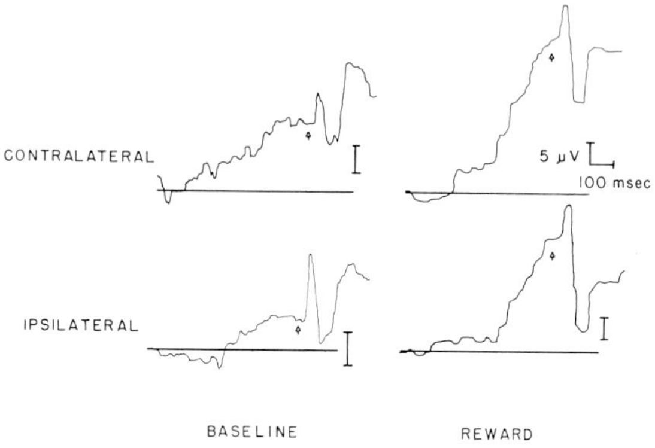

Fig. 1

Sample BSPs obtained from one subject. Negativity at the active electrode is represented by an upward deflection. Arrow indicates occurrence of response.

RESULTS

All of the records showed a measurable BSP (N_1). In addition most showed N_2 and P_2 components. Component P_1 was seen rarely, but this was probably due to the small number of responses averaged here (40 *vs.* 400 for Vaughan *et al.* 1968) and to its small size (2 μV). The BSP was measured as the amplitude above baseline at the onset of P_1 or N_2 or, if neither was identifiable, at the time of the response. The baseline was defined as the average amplitude of the response for the first 50 msec recorded. Comparison of BSP amplitudes in mm with a known calibration signal allowed their expression in μV. Fig. 1 shows tracings of one subject's responses obtained from ipsilateral and contralateral sites under the *baseline* and *reward* conditions.

Fig. 2 presents the mean BSP amplitudes for all eleven subjects. An analysis of variance on all of these data showed no interaction effect between conditions and electrode placement ($F = 0.59$, $df = 1/10$, $p > 0.20$). BSP amplitudes were larger under the *reward* condition than under the *baseline* condition for both ipsilateral and contralateral placements ($t_{ipsi} = 2.268$, $df = 10$, $p < 0.025$; $t_{contra} = 2.215$, $df = 10$, $p < 0.05$). BSP amplitudes were larger for contralateral placements than for ipsilateral placements under both conditions ($t_{baseline} = 1.928$, $df = 10$, $p < 0.05$; $t_{reward} = 3.370$, $df = 10$, $p < 0.005$).

DISCUSSION

A comparison of the results of this study of the BSP with those of Irwin *et al.* (1966) and Rebert *et al.* (1967) on the CNV show that both of these phenomena reflect motivational increases in the same manner; *i.e.*, through an increase in amplitude. The broad range of manipulations used in these studies (intensity of noxious shock, forced attention by presentation of near threshold stimuli, effort required to respond and monetary reward) points up the general nature of the psychological variable which attends these DC shifts. This perhaps implicates a general activating system as a neural substrate for these observed changes, possibly the midbrain reticular formation. Certainly, both the BSP and the CNV share some psychological and physiological substrates; both reflect preparation to respond, and both are linked to the significance of the response for the subject.

The lack of an interaction between motivation and electrode location demonstrates that BSP amplitude increases were of the same magnitude for both ipsilateral and contralateral sites. It is interesting that a laterality effect has not been reported for the CNV. In the majority of the studies on the CNV, the absence of a reported laterality effect proceeds quite simply from the fact that it was not sought; most of the studies employed only midline placements. Nonetheless, Low *et al.* (1966), report that the CNV is symmetrically distributed in the coronal plane with peak amplitude at the vertex. It is not entirely clear, however, that all of the subjects who generated that curve made their responses with the same hand. In addition, stimuli were presented bilaterally to the subject; *e.g.*, flashes of light and trains of clicks. This

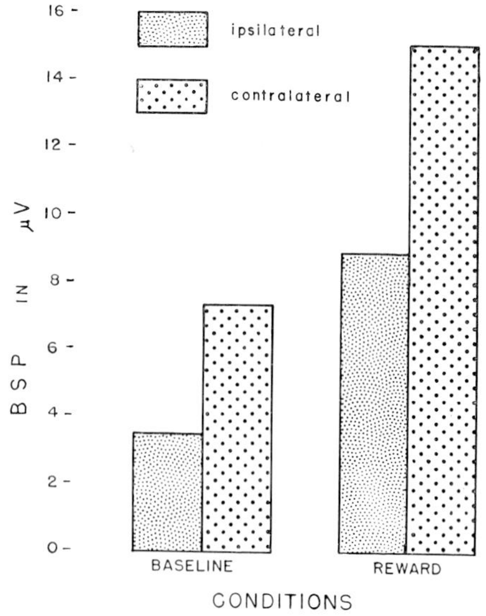

Fig. 2

Group means of BSP amplitudes for ipsilateral and contralateral locations under *baseline* and *reward* conditions.

along with the increased complexity of the CNV situation as compared to that for recording the BSP, may have masked any laterality effects. Firm answers to the question of laterality of the CNV must await appropriate experimental investigation.

SUMMARY

Bereitschaftspotentials (BSPs) were taken from scalp electrodes overlying the left and right Rolandic areas of eleven human subjects under two conditions, *baseline* (where responses resulted in no reward) and *reward* (where "correct" responses resulted in monetary reward). BSP amplitudes were significantly larger under *reward* than under *baseline* condition, and were significantly larger over the hemisphere contralateral to the responding hand for both conditions. No interaction between conditions and locations was found. These results are taken as evidence showing some common neural and behavioral substrates for the BSP and the DC shift known as the Contingent Negative Variation.

RÉSUMÉ

AUGMENTATION DE L'ONDE D'ATTENTE (BEREITSCHAFTSPOTENTIAL) PARALLÈLEMENT À UNE AUGMENTATION DU NIVEAU DE MOTIVATION

Les ondes d'attente (BSPs) ont été enregistrées à partir d'électrodes situées sur le scalp au niveau des aires rolandiques droite et gauche chez onze sujets dans deux conditions, *condition de base* (dans laquelle les réponses n'aboutissaient à aucune gratification), et *condition de gratification* (dans laquelle les réponses "correctes" aboutissaient à un paiement en argent). Les auteurs montrent que les amplitudes de ces potentiels étaient significativement plus grandes dans la *condition de gratification* que dans la *condition de base*, et qu'elles étaient, dans les deux conditions, nettement plus grandes sur l'hémisphère contralatéral à la main qui répondait. Aucune interaction n'a été observée entre les conditions d'expérience et la localisation. Ces résultats constituent la preuve qu'il existe un substrat neuronique et comportemental commun à l'onde d'attente (BSP) et à la déflexion en courant continu connue sous le terme de Variation Contingente Négative.

REFERENCES

GILDEN, L., VAUGHAN JR., H. G. and COSTA, L. D. Summated human EEG potentials with voluntary movement. *Electroenceph. clin. Neurophysiol.*, **1966,** *20*: 433–438.

IRWIN, D. A., KNOTT, J. R., MCADAM, D. W. and REBERT, C. S. Motivational determinants of the "contingent negative variation". *Electroenceph. clin. Neurophysiol.*, **1966,** *21*: 538–543.

KORNHÜBER, H. H. und DEECKE, L. Hirnpotential Änderungen bei Willkürbewegungen und passiven Bewegungen des Menschen: Bereitschaftspotential und reafferente Potentiale. *Pflügers Arch. ges. Physiol.*, **1965,** *284*: 1–17.

LOW, M. D., BORDA, A. B., FROST JR., J. D. and KELLAWAY, P. Surface-negative, slow-potential shift associated with conditioning in man. *Neurology (Minneap.)*, **1966,** *16*: 771–782.

REBERT, C. S., MCADAM, D. W., KNOTT, J. R. and IRWIN, D. A. A slow potential change in human brain related to level of motivation. *J. comp. physiol. Psychol.*, **1967,** *63*: 20–23.

VAUGHAN JR., H. G., COSTA, L. D. and RITTER, W. Topography of the human motor potential. *Electroenceph. clin. Neurophysiol.*, **1968,** *25*: 1–10.

WALTER, W. G., COOPER, R., ALDRIDGE, V. J., MCCALLUM, W. C. and WINTER, A. L. Contingent negative variation: An electric sign of sensori-motor association and expectancy in the human brain. *Nature (Lond.)*, **1964,** *203*: 380–384.

Reference: MCADAM, D. W. and SEALES, D. M. Bereitschaftspotential enhancement with increased level of motivation. *Electroenceph. clin. Neurophysiol.*, **1969,** *27*: 73–75.

Electroencephalography and Clinical Neurophysiology
Elsevier Publishing Company, Amsterdam – Printed in The Netherlands

DIGITAL COMPUTER CLASSIFICATIONS OF EEG SLEEP STAGES[1]

T. M. ITIL, M.D., D. M. SHAPIRO, D.Sc.[2], MAX FINK, M.D.[2] AND D. KASSEBAUM, B.A.

Department of Psychiatry of the University of Missouri School of Medicine, Missouri Institute of Psychiatry, St. Louis, Mo. 63139 (U.S.A.)

(Accepted for publication: October 14, 1968)

Various electronic analysis techniques have been used for quantitative analysis of the EEG during sleep, but due to the lack of reliability and the expense such procedures entail, they have not achieved general use (Knott *et al.* 1942; Kaiser *et al.* 1964; Hord *et al.* 1965; Maulsby *et al.* 1966; Agnew *et al.* 1967). The application of digital computer procedures to the analysis of the sleep EEG, including power spectrum analysis, baseline cross analysis, phase detection, and averaging techniques, shows promise of greater reliability (Bickford 1959; Brazier 1961, 1965; Adey and Walter 1963; Burch *et al.* 1964; Fink and Shapiro 1965; Johnson *et al.* 1967; Walter *et al.* 1967).

We have successfully used on-line digital computer analyses for the identification and classification of EEG changes induced by psychotropic drugs (Fink *et al.* 1967, 1968; Itil 1968a; Itil *et al.* 1968a,b). Of the methods employed, analysis of the baseline cross of the primary EEG wave and its first derivative proved to be the most useful (Burch 1959; Burch and Fink 1964; Shapiro and Fink 1966); consequently, this technique has been used to objectively classify the EEG stages in all-night sleep recordings. This report summarizes our recent investigations and suggests pragmatic solutions to the problem of rapid and consistent analysis of EEG sleep stages.

MATERIAL AND METHOD

Ten normal volunteers (22–38 years of age) were used for this study. Up to 6 consecutive nights of sleep were recorded for a full duration of 7–8.5 h in each subject. In addition to the EEG, vertical and horizontal eye movements, EMG, respiration and heart rate were recorded simultaneously on paper and on analog tape. The Fz to O2 combination was analyzed on-line using both an IBM 1710 digital computer system and an analog frequency analyzer. The computer configuration, logic of programs and statistics have been detailed elsewhere (Shapiro and Fink 1966). Baseline cross analyses of 1 min epochs at a sampling rate of 320/sec were used for the various classifications, the principles of which were detailed by Burch (1959) and Burch *et al.* (1964). Primary wave and first derivative baseline cross spectra were each divided into 7 frequency bands. In addition, an average frequency and its variability and an average absolute amplitude and its deviation were measured. A total of 20 measures provided the characteristics for the classification of each epoch (Table I).

RESULTS

These various measures were used to classify stages of sleep by one of four methods.

1. The first classification scheme was based on four subsets of these measures — the seven baseline cross frequency measures, the seven first derivative frequency measures, the average amplitude and the baseline cross frequency deviation. For each subset, the range of limiting values, divided into five levels (A,B,C,D,E), was determined for consecutive 1 min sleep EEG samples, visually classified as classic stages according to Loomis *et al.* (1937), with the addition of four intermediary sleep stages (A–B, B–C, C–D and D–E) (Itil and Shapiro 1968). For each of the four measures, a five-letter scheme (A to E) was developed representing the progression from slower to the faster frequencies (primary wave and first derivative), small to large for amplitude, and rhythmic to highly variable for the frequency spread.

To classify the samples a minimal distance function approach[3] was used to determine the most appropriate class for each subset. We first used this method to differentiate slow wave spindle (SWS) sleep, low voltage fast

---

[1] Supported, in part, by U.S. Public Health Service Grants MH-11380, 11381 and 13003; and by the Psychiatric Research Foundation of Missouri. Presented, in part, at the APSS Meeting, April 6–9, 1967, Santa Monica, Calif.

[2] Now at the Department of Psychiatry, New York Medical College, 5 East 102nd Street, New York, N.Y. 10029.

[3] The term "distance function" is used in the following sense: X_i^j, $i = 1, N_1$ is a set of N_1 variable values defining the jth classificatory group (sleep stage or letter for a particular subset). For each successive EEG epoch, the subset variable values are determined, for example, y_i, $i = 1, N_1$. The distance between the values of this EEG epoch and the jth class is defined by:

$$D_j^2 = \sum_{i=1}^{N1} (y_i - X_i^j)^2$$

That value of j for which D_j^2 is smallest is used to classify the epoch.

TABLE I

EEG period analysis measures

Measures		Description
Baseline cross		
1.	Average frequency:	Each occasion the EEG crosses the baseline (zero volt potential) the time elapsed from the last baseline crossing can be converted to a frequency. Over a given length (epoch) of EEG, there were many crossings and a mean time between crossings is calculated and converted to the average frequency.
2.	Frequency deviation: (variability)	A measure of the variance of the frequency distribution of EEG waves.
	Fractional time in band:	
3.		0–3 c/sec
4.		3–5 c/sec
5.		5–8 c/sec
6.		8–12 c/sec
7.		12–16 c/sec
8.		16–26 c/sec
9.		Over 26 c/sec
First derivative		
10.	Average frequency:	Analogous to the primary wave average wave form but of the first derivative of the EEG waves (or the wave form of the instantaneous slope of the raw EEG).
11.	Frequency deviation:	A measure of the variance of the frequency distribution of the first derivative of the raw EEG wave form.
	Fractional time in band:	
12.		0–7 c/sec
13.		7–10 c/sec
14.		10–13 c/sec
15.		13–16 c/sec
16.		16–22 c/sec
17.		22–40 c/sec
18.		Over 40 c/sec
Amplitude		
19.	Average amplitude:	The digitized absolute values for each point are averaged every second (or 320 points). The amplitude is the average of these numbers over as many seconds as there are in the epoch.
20.	Amplitude deviation:	Standard deviation for as many samples (seconds) in the epoch.

(LVF) sleep and the waking resting state. For samples of SWS sleep visually classified as B–C, C, C–D, D, D–E or E, the computer program demonstrated 19 combinations of the 4 EEG subsets from the 625 possible combinations (Table II). In more than 75% of the samples that were visually classified as stages B–C or C, the BBAB combination was produced. In sleep stages C–D, D, D–E or E, more than 75% of the samples were classified as the AABA combination. LVF sleep patterns, which were visually classified as stage B with or without rapid eye movement (REM), were placed in the BCAB combination in more than 75% of the samples. In more than 75% of the resting record samples, the DCAC combination was defined.

In this method, LVF could be differentiated from SWS sleep (particularly from stages C–D, D, D–E and E) by acceleration of the baseline cross frequency pattern, acceleration of the first derivative frequency pattern, decrease of amplitude and increase of baseline cross frequency variability. SWS sleep stages C and D as well as LVF sleep stages B with and without REM could also be differentiated from the resting record, but not in all samples.

2. As a derivative of the first method, a program was written to provide an on-line computer classification according to conventional visual classification procedures. In this method, samples of a single night's sleep EEG were visually classified into 1 to 9 sleep stages. The mean values of the period analysis variables of the visually identified samples were computed for one subject's all-night recording.

Table III represents an initial set of guidelines based on 25–100 epochs of 1 min duration for each sleep stage. In this classification, a successive increase in slow waves

TABLE II

Automatic classification of EEG of all night sleep stages

	Visual classification (according to modified Loomis *et al.* 1937)	Computer classification Subset* 1	2	3	4	
Slow wave-spindle sleep (SWS)	B–C	B	B	A	B	(>75%)
	C	B	C	A	B	
		A	B	B	B	
		B	B	A	C	
		A	A	B	B	
		A	A	B	A	
		A	B	B	A	
		A	B	A	B	
		B	B	B	D	
		B	C	A	C	
		C	B	A	C	
		A	A	A	B	
	C–D	A	A	B	A	(>75%)
	D	A	A	B	B	
	D–E	B	B	A	B	
	E	A	B	B	B	
		A	B	B	A	
		B	A	A	B	
		B	B	B	B	
Low voltage fast sleep (LVF)	B	B	C	A	B	(>75%)
	B (with REM)	B	C	A	C	
		C	C	A	C	
		B	B	A	B	
		C	C	A	B	
		D	B	B	C	
Neither	Awake	D	C	A	C	(>75%)
	A	D	B	A	D	
	A–B	D	D	A	D	
		E	D	A	D	
		D	C	A	B	
		C	C	A	C	
		C	B	A	B	
		B	B	A	C	

* Computer classification is four letters with following scheme:
Subset 1, baseline cross frequency pattern (A–E) (slow–fast).
Subset 2, first derivative frequency pattern (A–E) (slow–fast).
Subset 3, amplitude (A–E) (small–large).
Subset 4, baseline cross frequency spread (A–E) (rhythmic–highly variable).

(0–3 c/sec) from stage A to E is observed. The other frequency bands also show a continuous decrease of their mean values in the same sleep stage order except for the 3–5 c/sec band. In the first derivative analysis, no frequency bands other than 7–10 c/sec and 22–40 c/sec show systematic changes in mean values. Mean values of the amplitude show a continuous increase from stage A to stage E.

In consecutive night sleep studies in the same subject, the distance function approach was applied to classify each 1 min sample, using the mean values of the baseline cross frequency pattern of the previous sleep EEG experiment (Fig. 1, *A*).

The computer classification of the same EEG classified visually demonstrated almost identical sleep stages and the same characteristic temporal shape of the total sleep activity (Fig. 1, *B*).

In a comparison of the computer-derived and visually determined classes in 2658 sleep EEG samples, the agreement varied from 55 to 74% (average 64.6%) for the

TABLE III

Mean values of period analysis variables of visually identified EEG samples of all-night sleep stages

Stages	Frequencies																Amplitude
	Baseline cross								First derivative								
	0–3	3–5	5–8	8–12	12–16	16–26	>26	Average	0–7	7–10	10–13	13–16	16–22	22–40	>40	Average	
A	0.049	0.067	0.226	0.318	0.063	0.115	0.160	18.07	0.00005	0.0022	0.021	0.0054	0.130	0.076	0.766	52.81	83.6
A–B	0.060	0.130	0.222	0.267	0.047	0.123	0.175	18.57	0.00085	0.0015	0.013	0.0036	0.114	0.073	0.743	53.39	81.1
B with and without REM	0.166	0.209	0.205	0.138	0.026	0.087	0.165	16.45	0.00072	0.0009	0.007	0.0011	0.07	0.055	0.865	55.48	89.9
B–C	0.265	0.235	0.177	0.126	0.030	0.057	0.107	12.37	0.00352	0.0056	0.030	0.0035	0.111	0.039	0.807	53.36	133.6
C	0.333	0.229	0.157	0.112	0.028	0.048	0.089	10.92	0.00551	0.0075	0.037	0.0038	0.120	0.036	0.790	52.70	153.7
C–D	0.418	0.207	0.132	0.095	0.023	0.040	0.078	9.73	0.00524	0.0079	0.037	0.0035	0.117	0.036	0.793	53.25	171.7
D	0.559	0.163	0.089	0.072	0.015	0.028	0.060	7.69	0.00461	0.0085	0.036	0.0018	0.108	0.029	0.812	53.63	203.2
D–E	0.605	0.147	0.072	0.065	0.015	0.025	0.054	7.04	0.00682	0.0097	0.037	0.0019	0.109	0.028	0.807	53.35	219.7
E	0.642	0.132	0.067	0.060	0.014	0.023	0.046	6.45	0.0085	0.0134	0.045	0.0017	0.112	0.026	0.793	52.64	234.9

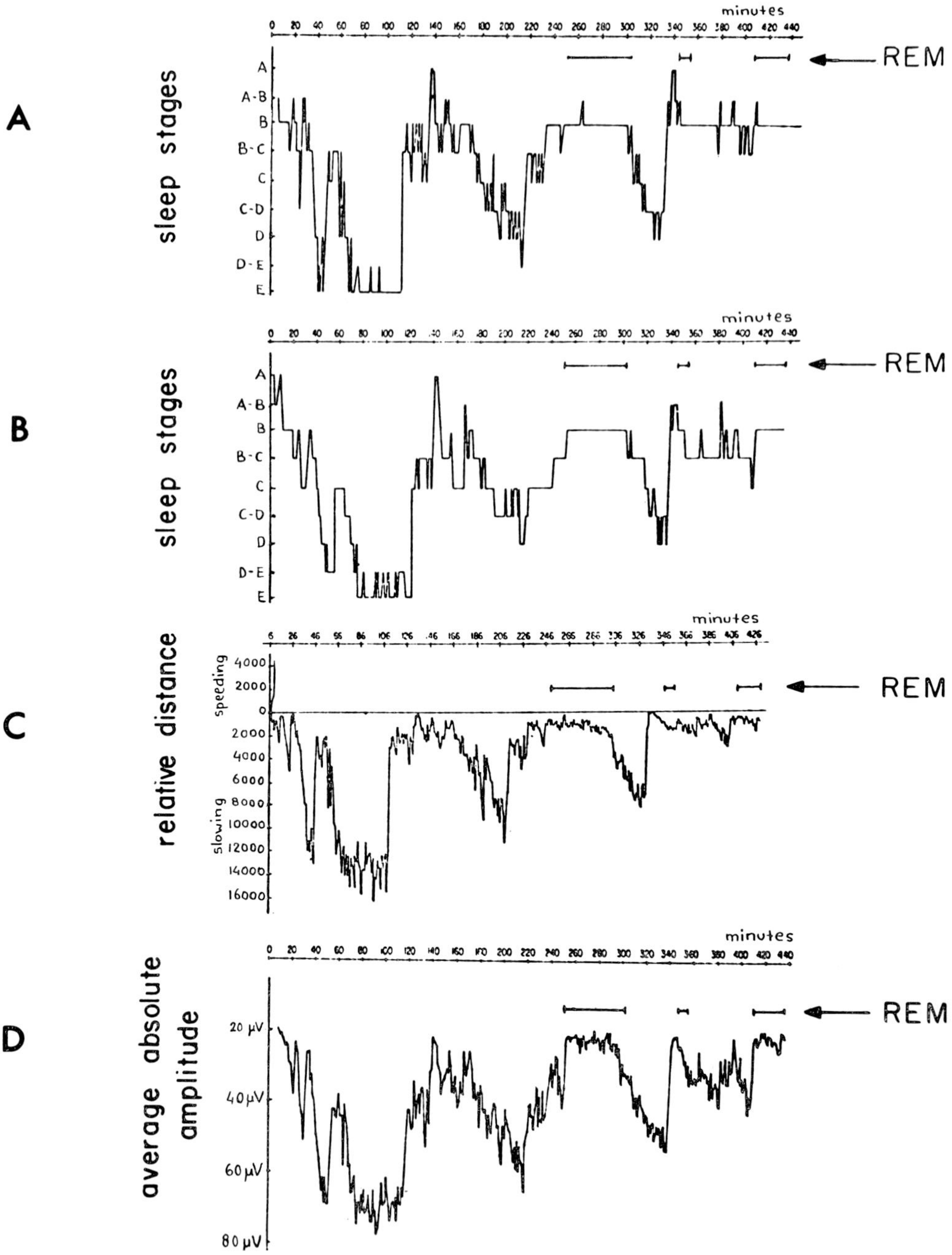

Fig. 1

Comparison between visual classification and classifications based on different computer methods. *A*: Computer classification of the all-night sleep EEG based on "sleep print" method. Every 1 min sample was classified based on the distance function of the 7 frequency bands of the primary wave of the period analysis. In the ordinate, 9 sleep stage classification. Rapid eye movement (REM) periods are hand plotted.

B: Visual classification of the same all-night sleep EEG as *A*: Every 1 min sample was classified visually based on 9 sleep stage classification. The samples were not classified continuously from 0–440 min, but all time periods were randomly selected.

C: Computer analysis of the same all-night sleep EEG based on the baseline cross frequency pattern distance function approach. The relative distance from the resting record in terms of resting record variability was scored for every 1 min sample.

D: Average absolute amplitude of the same night's sleep based on the EEG period analysis. The amplitude of every 1 min sample was averaged and scored in terms of microvolts.

TABLE IV

Percent agreement of computer and visual classifications of all-night sleep EEG samples (N: 2658) Frequency distance function

Five-stage classification		Nine-stage classification	
Stage	% of agreement	Stage	% of agreement
A (W)	74	A	77
		A–B	33
B (1)	73	B	73
		B–C	35
C (2)	55	C	29
		C–D	42
D (3)	62	D	45
		D–E	17
E (4)	59	E	55
Average = 64.6%		Average = 45.1%	

Note: If a one-stage difference is allowed, then the average % agreement is 96% for the 5-stage and 85% for the 9-stage.

five-stage classification; and from 17 to 77% (average 45.1%) for the nine-stage classification (Table IV). When one allows for a one-stage classification difference, the average agreement for all stages increases to 96% of the samples for the five-stage classification and to 85% for the nine-stage classification.

We consider the disagreement, particularly for the nine-stage classification, to be related to our use of the measures of a single subject who showed a predominant alpha waking record, and the fact that only 7 of the 20 EEG variables were used as the standard. The standard may be improved by three strategies — determining more precise limits for the variables in each sleep stage from a larger number and variety of sleep EEG records; developing different sleep classification standards for different resting (waking) records, with the computer then selecting automatically the best standards for each subject[1]; and increasing the number of EEG variables used in the classification. Our initial experiences with the first two strategies indicate that a greater agreement in the classification by visual and computer methods can indeed be achieved.

In this classification method, based exclusively on EEG criteria, no distinction between stage B-REM and stage B-without REM was made. In another study in which samples were defined as paradoxical sleep using the criteria of eye movement as well as EEG characteristics, we observed differences in the frequency spectra which may allow this distinction to be made in future analyses (Itil 1968b).

This method of sleep classification is rapid, accurate and reliable, and can be made either on-line or from FM tape at speeds faster than real-time. The programs provide rapid calculations of the usual periods of interest, such as the amount of time for each stage of sleep either for the total recording or for each hour during the night, and numeric or graphic displays of the changes in sleep pattern during a night. The "EEG sleep profile" for each night is another useful portrayal of the pattern of sleep change, and since these seem characteristic for each subject, we have called them "sleep prints" (Fig. 2) (Itil and Shapiro 1968; Itil *et al.* 1968b).

3. Seeking a different approach not dependent on predetermined sleep EEG criteria, a third method to define sleep stages was developed using the variability of the baseline cross frequency pattern during the resting record. Each epoch of the sleep record is classified by its "distance"[2] from the resting (awake) record in terms of the resting (waking) variability measure. This method gives a temporal profile similar to the visual classification (Fig. 1, *C*).

4. The utility of amplitude measures to define changes with drug and sleep stages (Agnew *et al.* 1967) led to a similar trial. This fourth method utilizes the average amplitude measure from the period analysis program and is a close approximation of the usual amplitude integration methods of Drohocki (1948). The temporal profile resembles the sleep profiles of the visual classification in one subject (Fig. 1, *D*). In a comparison of the visual and the amplitude classifications of 2504 sleep samples, the agreement varied from 18 to 52% (average 39%) for the five-stage classification and 6 to 56% (average 21%) for the nine-stage classification (Table V).

DISCUSSION

The classification of sleep stages by digital computer methods will vary according to the needs of individual projects. Both our first methods, which depended on arbitrary classes of EEG measures, and the distance approach, dependent on the variability of the resting EEG (method 3), provided reasonable classifications of sleep stages, but did not satisfy our needs. In the first method, agreement between the computer classes and the visual classes became progressively poorer as we increased the number of stages in the classification. Even for the three-stage classification, all visual sleep stages (B, C, D and E) included computer classes BBAB, BCAC, and BCAB.

We were dissatisfied with the distance approach based on variability of the resting EEG because we are particu-

[1] The type and configuration of sleep stages are determined, in part, by the type and distribution of the characteristics of the waking EEG. In schizophrenic patients who exhibit greater degrees of low voltage fast activity in the waking record, we obseı ved fewer deep sleep stages.

[2] Distance is defined by

$$D^2 = \sum_{j=1}^{N} \left(\frac{x_j - \mu_j}{\sigma_j}\right)^2$$

when $N = 7$ and μ and σ are the mean and standard deviation over time of the jth variable during the resting record.

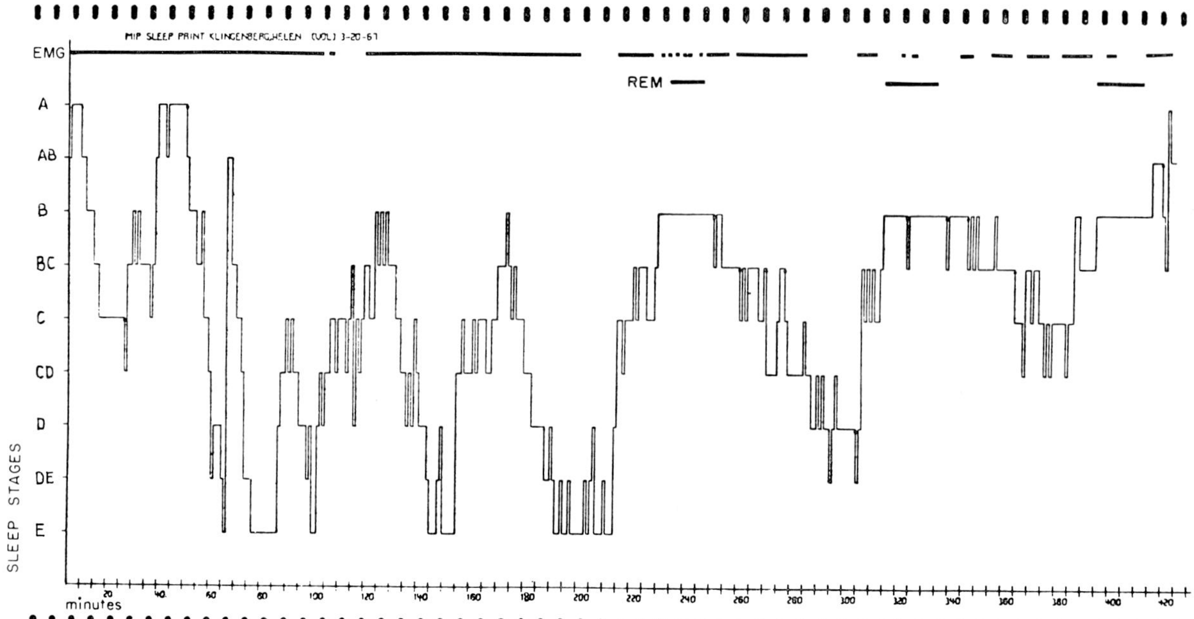

Fig. 2
Digital computer "sleep print". Automatically plotted classifications derived from baseline cross frequency pattern of the primary wave. Time in minutes in the abscissa and the sleep stages (9 stage classification) in the ordinate. EMG and REM activity were hand plotted.

TABLE V

Percent agreement of computer and visual classifications of all-night sleep EEG samples
(*N*: 2504)
Amplitude measure

Five-stage classification		Nine-stage classification	
Stage	% of agreement	Stage	% of agreement
A (W)	50	A	6
		A–B	38
B (1)	26	B	26
		B–C	28
C (2)	49	C	9
		C–D	11
D (3)	18	D	7
		D–E	8
E (4)	52	E	56
Average = 39%		Average = 21%	

larly interested in the changes in sleep from night to night as they relate to drug effects. Since these changes occur in the resting EEG also, the dependence on this measure obscures the sleep record changes of interest to us. However, this method may be particularly useful in studies of changes in vigilance, since it is independent of preconceived criteria. Applications of the "sleep print" method in human psychopharmacology also suggests that this method may readily reflect the effects of drugs on the sleep EEG (Itil 1968a).

Whereas the amplitude measure alone is inexpensive, commonly available and frequently used, we have found significantly poorer agreement with visual classifications, both five- and nine-stage, than with the frequency dependent measures ($P < 0.01$, Wilcoxon matched pairs signed-ranks).

The agreements between visual and computer methods reported here are similar to those which depend on spectral density estimates (Johnson *et al.* 1967). Their over-all agreement, based on 63 epochs, was 60.5%, varying from 91% to 0% for six EEG stages. A step-wise multiple regression procedure using power estimates and five bands was the technique used to discriminate stages. Also, the linear change between stages of vigilance occurred in all but one of the primary wave frequency bands using the period analysis method, while the power spectral results indicate a linear change for only the delta band.

In view of the similarity of these experiences, the ease which the period analytic method and distance function allow for classification and experimentation, as well as the large differences in cost, encourage us to continue the use of our methods to extend the classifications of sleep EEG stages by computer methods.

SUMMARY

Four programs have been developed to classify all-night sleep EEGs using digital computer techniques.

Method one classified sleep stages according to the baseline cross primary wave and first derivative frequency patterns, amplitude, and primary wave frequency variability. Method two (sleep print) applies the distance function approach to classify sleep stages using as a standard the mean values of the primary wave baseline cross frequency measures of EEG samples first classified visually. Method three utilizes the distance function approach to classify the sleep pattern in comparison to the pre-sleep resting record. Method four is based on the average amplitude.

The best agreement between visual and computer classification was attained with the "sleep print" method. The effect of psychotropic drugs could also be best demonstrated with this method.

The similarities of computer period analysis classification and visually classified samples, the reliability of the sampling, its rapidity and ease of statistical and visual portrayal, and its relative cost make such analyses useful and practical.

REFERENCES

ADEY, W. R. and WALTER, D. O. Application of phase detection and averaging techniques in computer analysis of EEG records in the cat. *Exp. Neurol.*, **1963,** *7*: 186–209.

AGNEW, H. W., PARKER, J. C., WEBB, W. B. and WILLIAMS, R. L. Amplitude measurement of the sleep electroencephalogram. *Electroenceph. clin. Neurophysiol.*, **1967,** *22*: 84–86.

BICKFORD, R. O. An automatic recognition system for spike-and-wave with simultaneous testing of motor response. *Electroenceph. clin. Neurophysiol.*, **1959,** *11*: 397–398.

BRAZIER, M. A. B. (Ed.). *Computer techniques in EEG analysis. Electroenceph. clin. Neurophysiol.*, **1961,** *Suppl. 20*: 1–99.

BRAZIER, M. A. B. The application of computers to electroencephalography. In R. W. STACY and B. D. WAXMAN (Eds.), *Computers in biomedical research.* Academic Press, New York, **1965,** *1*: 295–315.

BURCH, N. R. Automatic analysis of the electroencephalogram: a review and classification of systems. *Electroenceph. clin. Neurophysiol.*, **1959,** *11*: 827–843.

BURCH, N. R. and FINK, M. Comparative study of period analysis and frequency analysis of the electroencephalogram. *Electroenceph. clin. Neurophysiol.*, **1964,** *17*: 454–455.

BURCH, N. R., NETTLETON, W. J., SWEENEY, J. and EDWARDS, R. J. Period analysis of the electroencephalogram on a general purpose digital computer. *Ann. N. Y. Acad. Sci.*, **1964,** *115*: 827–843.

DROHOCKI, Z. L'intégrateur de l'électroproduction cérébrale pour l'électroencéphalographie quantitative. *Rev. neurol.*, **1948,** *80*: 619–624.

FINK, M., ITIL, T. and SHAPIRO, D. Digital computer analysis of the human EEG in psychiatric research. *Comprehens. Psychiat.*, **1967,** *8*: 521–538.

FINK, M. and SHAPIRO, D. *Computer analytic classification of EEG sleep stages.* Psychiat. Res. Found. Missouri, St. Louis, Publication No. 65-10, **1965.**

FINK, M., SHAPIRO, D. M., HICKMAN, C. and ITIL, T. Digital computer EEG analyses in psychopharmacology. In N. KLINE and E. LASKA (Eds.), *Computers and electronic devices in psychiatry.* Grune and Stratton, New York, **1968:** 109–123.

HORD, H. J., JOHNSON, L. C., LUBIN, A. and AUSTIN, M. T. Resolution and stability of tranquilizers in the autospectra of EEG. *Electroenceph. clin. Neurophysiol.*, **1965,** *19*: 305–308.

ITIL, T. M. Electroencephalography and pharmacopsychiatry. In F. A. FREYHAN *et al.* (Eds.), *Clinical psychopharmacology, modern problems in pharmacopsychiatry.* Karger, Basel, **1968**a, *1*: 163–194.

ITIL, T. M. Digital computer analysis of the dream state. *Psychophysiology*, **1968**b, *5*: 214–215.

ITIL, T. M. and SHAPIRO, D. Computer classification of all-night sleep EEG (sleep prints). *Proc. XIXth European Congr. EEG*, Bologna, **1968:** 30–40.

ITIL, T. M., SHAPIRO, D. and FINK, M. Differentiation of psychotropic drugs by quantitative EEG analysis. *Agressologie*, **1968**a, *9*: 276–280.

ITIL, T. M., SHAPIRO, D., FINK, M., HICKMAN, C., KIREMITCI, N. and HOLDEN, J. M. C. On-line computer classification of electroencephalographic sleep stages. *Psychophysiology*, **1968**b, *4*: 366.

JOHNSON, L. C., NUTE, C., AUSTIN, M. T. and LUBIN, A. Spectral analysis of the EEG during waking and sleeping. *Electroenceph. clin. Neurophysiol.*, **1967,** *23*: 80.

KAISER, E., PETERSÉN, I., SELLDÉN, U. and KAGAWA, N. EEG data representation in broad-band frequency analysis. *Electroenceph. clin. Neurophysiol.*, **1964,** *17*: 76–80.

KNOTT, J. R., GIBBS, F. A. and HENRY, C. E. Fourier transforms of the electroencephalogram during sleep. *J. exp. Psychol.*, **1942,** *31*: 465–477.

LOOMIS, A., HARVEY, F. and HOBART, G. Cerebral states during sleep as studied by human brain potentials. *J. exp. Psychol.*, **1937,** *21*: 127–144.

MAULSBY, R. L., FROST JR., J. D. and GRAHAM, M. H. A simple electronic method for graphing EEG sleep patterns. *Electroenceph. clin. Neurophysiol.*, **1966,** *21*: 501–503.

SHAPIRO, D. M. and FINK, M. *Quantitative analysis of the electroencephalogram by digital computer methods.* Psychiat. Res. Found. Missouri, St. Louis, Publication No. 66-1, **1966.**

WALTER, D. O., RHODES, J. M. and ADEY, W. R. Discriminating among states of consciousness by EEG measurements. A study of four subjects. *Electroenceph. clin. Neurophysiol.*, **1967,** *22*: 22–29.

Reference: ITIL, T. M., SHAPIRO, D. M., FINK, M. and KASSEBAUM, D. Digital computer classifications of EEG sleep stages. *Electroenceph. clin. Neurophysiol.*, **1969,** *27*: 76–83.

Electroencephalography and Clinical Neurophysiology
Elsevier Publishing Company, Amsterdam – Printed in The Netherlands

MODIFIED PUPILLARY DIAMETER AND EVOKED POTENTIAL COMPONENT VARIATION IN WAKING CATS

DONOVAN E. FLEMING

Veterans Administration Hospital, Phoenix, Ariz. 85012 (U.S.A.)

(Accepted for publication: October 23, 1968)

INTRODUCTION

It has been demonstrated that amplitude of ERG and optic chiasm responses to light pulses was clearly changed as pupillary diameter was modified. On the other hand, variations in amplitude of visual cortical potentials appeared to be the result of changes in background electrocortical activity (Naquet *et al.* 1959; Fernández-Guardiola *et al.* 1964). Whereas mydriasis produced by reticular formation stimulation resulted in an increase, miosis produced by stimulation of the Edinger-Westphal nucleus resulted in a decrease in the amplitude of ERG and chiasmatic responses. Stimulation of either locus resulted in a desynchronized cortical EEG pattern and concomitantly cortical evoked response amplitude was depressed (Fernández-Guardiola *et al.* 1964).

The question remains, however, whether or not changes in amplitude of some components of evoked cortical potentials can be shown to accompany changes in pupillary diameter when a photic stimulus is presented only during a period of desynchronized electrocortical activity in waking animal preparations. In the present investigation the relationships between pupillary size and evoked potential amplitude were examined with specific attention being directed to three regularly appearing wave components of the evoked potential complex.

METHOD

Experiments have been performed on ten[1] adult cats with indwelling electrodes (placed under direct visual control and with electrophysiological monitoring) over the left primary visual cortex. For all experimental procedures, a cylindrically shaped white reflector, 33 cm in diameter, 56.5 cm in height, encompassed (250°) the cat's head and shoulders. A Grass photo-stimulator lamp was mounted approximately 68 cm behind and slightly above the center of the cylinder. Light flashes diffused evenly over the surface of the cylinder and stimulated the cat irrespective of head position. The latter was also monitored, thus stimuli were delivered only when the head was maintained in a specified position. With the intensity setting of the photo-stimulator held constant (setting "4" on 1–16 range—the calculated illuminance of the reflector was approximately 6.7 ft.candles) three pupillary conditions were studied in each animal: (1) mydriasis (with 1% atropine sulfate); (2) miosis (with 1% pilocarpine hydrochloride); and (3) unfixed (mobile). The experiment was carried out with light adapted animals. The ambient illumination was approximately 0.16 ft.-candles. During each condition 50 light pulses, each at about 2–3 sec interval, were presented to the animal. Brain responses were amplified conventionally and were recorded on magnetic tape, fed into a Computer of Average Transients (CAT) and the summated evoked potentials were plotted with an X–Y plotter.

The EEG was monitored continuously during each experimental run. Light pulses were presented only when the animal was displaying a low voltage fast EEG pattern.

The following data were taken from each evoked potential plot: (1) latency to the initial deflection of the first primary wave component; (2) latency to peak of each component; and (3) peak-to-peak amplitude for regularly appearing wave components of the evoked potential complex. The data were analyzed statistically with analysis of variance techniques.

[1] Data on miosis were only collected from nine cats (one animal expired before the completion of the experiment).

RESULTS

The horizontal diameter of mobile pupils varied between 4 and 8 mm with ambient illumination. Mydriatic pupils were 8–10 mm and miotic pupils were approximately 1 mm in diameter.

The effects of modified pupil diameter on evoked cortical responses are summarized in Tables I and II. Although the wave components varied in form and in number from cat to cat, it was found that three positive-negative wave complexes, arbitrarily numbered in terms of polarity and order of appearance, could be consistently identified for each of the three pupil conditions (Fig. 1).

An analysis of the responses indicated that the latency to the initial deflection of the first primary wave (P_1) was reliably lengthened for miotic, when compared with mydriatic and mobile pupils. The latencies for the latter two conditions did not differ significantly. While the peak delays for individual wave components were generally longer for miotic pupils, when compared with the other two pupillary conditions, only the peak delays for the P_1

TABLE I

Mean latency and peak delay values of evoked potential components for three pupillary conditions (in msec)

	Mydriasis		Miosis		Mobile	
	Mean	S.E.*	Mean	S.E.	Mean	S.E.
Latency to initial deflection	9.6	0.3	12.7***	1.0	10.1	0.5
Peak delay						
P_1	16.8	0.7	20.3**	2.0	17.0	0.9
N_1	22.0	1.3	24.5	1.5	22.4	1.3
P_2	28.1	2.5	30.7	2.6	27.9	1.7
N_2	40.2	4.7	46.8**	6.2	40.6	4.8
P_3	78.2	7.6	81.8	9.3	76.3	7.9
N_3	114.4	14.3	113.8	13.6	114.4	14.0

* Standard error of the mean.
** Mean reliably different from mydriatic and mobile pupil conditions $P < 0.05$.
*** Mean reliably different from mydriatic and mobile pupil conditions $P < 0.01$.

TABLE II

Peak-to-peak amplitude values of evoked potential components for three pupillary conditions (in μV)

	Mydriasis		Miosis		Mobile	
	Mean	S.E.*	Mean	S.E.	Mean	S.E.
Baseline–P_1	50.5	8.2	37.9**	9.4	47.8	6.6
P_1N_1	41.9	7.4	31.1	8.4	43.5	6.8
P_2N_2	61.3	9.1	66.4	13.3	66.8	12.3
P_3N_3	57.4	8.9	48.2	14.9	61.4	11.9

* Standard error of the mean.
** Mean reliably different from mydriatic and mobile pupil conditions $P < 0.05$.

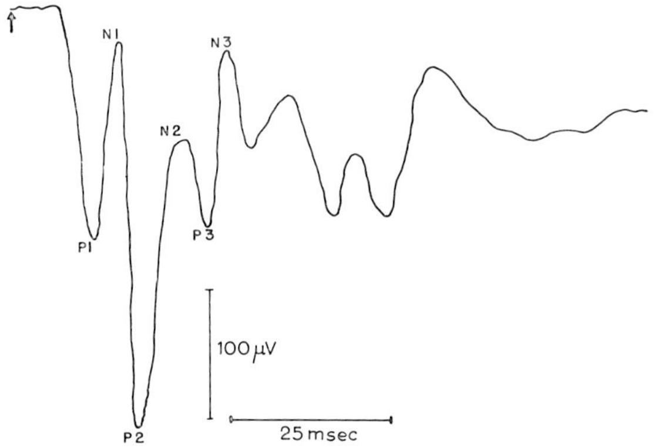

Fig. 1
Example of summed evoked potential indicating wave components examined in this study. Positivity is indicated by a downward deflection.

and N_2 components were significantly longer. Peak delay values for responses obtained under mydriatic and mobile pupil conditions did not differ reliably for any wave component.

When peak-to-peak amplitudes to responses obtained under the three conditions were compared, only the amplitude value measured from the point of the initial deflection to the peak of P_1 was reliably affected by pupillary diameter; responses obtained with miotic pupils being significantly lower. The P_1N_1 amplitude differences for the three conditions approached significance, miosis yielding lower values.

DISCUSSION

Under the conditions of the present investigation, it appears that the effects of modified pupillary diameter are restricted to the early components of the evoked potential. The latency to the initial deflection and the peak delay of P_1 were reliably lengthened by miosis and P_1 amplitude was reliably smaller with miotic pupils than with either mobile or mydriatic pupils. Bergamini *et al.* (1966) reported similar findings with human subjects. These results are consistent with the implication that the early positive component reflects a greater dependence on primary visual pathway discharges than do the other components (Wicke *et al.* 1964; Rose and Lindsley 1965). The results also are in general agreement with those of Fernández-Guardiola *et al.* (1964) and Naquet *et al.*

(1959) in spite of the difference in analytical techniques. There is no apparent explanation for the observation that N_2 peak delay was reliably longer during the miotic than during the mobile or mydriatic pupillary condition.

Response components obtained with mobile and mydriatic pupils were highly similar temporally. With the relatively low level of ambient illumination used in this study, pupil diameter values during the mobile condition were close to those of mydriatic pupils. Bartley (1951) reported that the constriction latency of the pupil was 250 msec; that constriction progresses very rapidly for the next 350 msec; and that irregular oscillations occur after 930 msec. Since less than a 250 msec epoch of the evoked potential was analyzed in the present study, pupil constriction would be of minor consequence, and on these grounds values obtained with mobile pupils would not be excepted to be different from values obtained with mydriatic pupils.

The role of pupillary motility in the habituation of visual cortical evoked potentials to iterative photic stimulation has received considerable experimental attention (Thompson 1967). Little or no satisfactory evidence has been published which demonstrates that pupillary fluctuations correlate with the amplitude lability of evoked potential complexes. The findings of the present investigation indicate that the amplitude of the initial positive component does vary with modified pupillary diameter. However, those components succeeding the initial positive deflection which were examined in the present study, those presumed to be behaviorally labile and thus sensitive to habituation procedures, are relatively unaffected by modified pupil size.

SUMMARY

Peak delay and amplitude variations of three regularly appearing components of photically evoked cortical potentials were investigated in waking cats during conditions of experimentally modified pupillary diameter. It was observed that the parameters of an early component were most sensitive to modifications in pupillary diameter. When compared with mydriatic and mobile pupil values, the values for both the latency to the initial deflection and peak delay of the first appearing component were reliably longer during miosis. The amplitude of this component was also smaller during the miotic condition than during conditions of mydriatic and mobile pupils. Component values obtained during mobile and mydriatic conditions did not differ reliably.

RÉSUMÉ

MODIFICATION DU DIAMÈTRE PUPILLAIRE ET VARIATION DES COMPOSANTES DES POTENTIELS ÉVOQUÉS CHEZ DES CHATS ÉVEILLÉS

Les variations de délai et d'amplitude du pic de trois composantes constantes des potentiels évoqués corticaux à la lumière ont été explorées chez des chats éveillés pendant des conditions de modification expérimentale du diamètre pupillaire. On observe que les paramètres d'une composante précoce sont les plus sensibles aux modifications du diamètre pupillaire. Quand on compare les valeurs en mydriase et les valeurs en pupille mobile, les valeurs de la latence de la déflexion initiale et du délai du pic de la première composante sont nettement plus longues pendant le myosis. L'amplitude de cette composante est également moindre en condition de myosis qu'en condition de mydriase ou de pupille mobile. Les valeurs des composantes obtenues en conditions de mydriase et de pupille mobile ne diffèrent pas notablement.

The technical assistance of D. Shearer and E. Watts is gratefully acknowledged.

REFERENCES

Bartley, S. H. The psychophysiology of vision. In S. S. Stevens (Ed.), *Handbook of experimental psychology*. Wiley, New York, **1951**: 921–984.

Bergamini, L., Bergamasco, B. et Mombelli, A. M. Variations du potentiel évoqué chez l'homme provoquées par les modifications du diamètre pupillaire et de l'état d'activation corticale, avec référence particulière aux phénomènes d'habituation, d'attention et de distraction. *J. Physiol. (Paris)*, **1966,** *58*: 671–685.

Fernández-Guardiola, A., Harmony, T. and Roldán, E. Modulations of visual input by pupillary mechanisms. *Electroenceph. clin. Neurophysiol.*, **1964,** *16*: 259–268.

Naquet, R., Regis, H., Fischer-Williams, M. et Fernández-Guardiola, A. Variations des réponses évoquées par la lumière de long de la voie spécifique. *C.R. Soc. Biol. (Paris)*, **1959,** *153*: 809–812.

Rose, G. H. and Lindsley, D. B. Visually evoked electro-cortical responses in kittens: Development of specific and nonspecific system. *Science*, **1965,** *148*: 1244–1246.

Thompson, R. F. *Foundations of physiological psychology*. Harper, New York, **1967,** 688 p.

Wicke, J. D., Donchin, E. and Lindsley, D. B. Visual evoked potentials as a function of flash luminance and duration. *Science*, **1964,** *146*: 83–85.

Reference: Fleming, D. E. Modified pupillary diameter and evoked potential component variation in waking cats. *Electroenceph. clin. Neurophysiol.*, **1969,** *27*: 84–86.

Electroencephalography and Clinical Neurophysiology
Elsevier Publishing Company, Amsterdam – Printed in The Netherlands

TECHNICAL CONTRIBUTIONS

A NOVEL METHOD FOR PREPARING AND IMPLANTING BRAIN ELECTRODE ASSEMBLIES IN RATS

A. SAYERS AND G. STILLE

Research Institute, Dr. A. Wander S.A., Berne (Switzerland)

(Accepted for publication: October 14, 1968)

In most methods described for implanting electrodes chronically in rats, each electrode is inserted separately by using a stereotaxic instrument, fastened in position with dental or acrylic cement and then soldered to a connector which is fixed to the skull. This method is time consuming and has the inherent danger of brain damage due to heat conduction, even if a low melting point solder is used.

The following method, developed and tried in our laboratories over the past 3 years, uses a technique suitable for preparing large numbers of animals while avoiding the possibility of brain damage due to soldering. At the same time the method permits intracerebral injections to be made on freely moving animals with simultaneous EEG recording.

A. *Preparation of the electrode complex*

1. A skull is prepared from a rat of the same sex, weight, and strain as the animals to be implanted, filled with plaster of Paris and, when this is hard, mounted in the stereotaxic instrument[1].

2. The ordinates of the brain structures in which it is intended to implant electrodes are ascertained from a brain atlas. Holes are then drilled at these points through the skull and into the plaster of Paris to the required depth to accept the electrodes and guide needles (0.4 mm diameter for depth electrodes and 0.9 mm diameter for cortical electrodes and guide needles). A further hole of 1 mm diameter is drilled to a depth of 5–6 mm at the bregma to accept a guide rod (Fig. 1, *A*).

3. A piece of cellotape is moulded over the skull in order to facilitate removal of the finished assembly. The electrodes (silver wire of 0.8 mm diameter, rounded at the end, and platinum needles of 0.3 mm diameter, insulated to within 1 mm of the tip) and guide needles (if intracerebral injections are required) are inserted through the cellotape into their respective holes (Fig. 1, *B*).

4. A Winchester subminiature connector[2] is cut and filed to shape, the number of contacts depending on the required programme. The electrodes are wired up to the socket using fine silver wire, where necessary insulated with polyethylene tubing. Soldering is accomplished with a micro-miniature soldering pencil[3]. One wire from the connector is left free to be soldered later to the indifferent electrode in situ (Fig. 1, *C*).

5. The guide rod is inserted and the whole assembly is walled in with a metal strip which is sealed to the skull with plasticine (Fig. 1, *D*). The mould thus formed is filled with Beracryl[4]. After hardening, the guide rod is withdrawn (Fig. 1, *E*) and the electrode complex is removed from the skull. The under surface is roughened with emery cloth and the guide hole slightly enlarged.

6. A dust-cap is prepared as follows: two shortened Winchester male contacts are inserted through cellotape into the connector. A mould is formed by wrapping a strip of cellotape or paper around the connector, and then filling it with Beracryl. After hardening, the cap is withdrawn from the connector and the cellotape removed.

7. Guide needles, if present, are plugged with shortened household pins to prevent the entry of foreign matter. The pins are lightly vaselined to facilitate withdrawal.

Further electrode assemblies can be made as required, the cellotape covering the skull being replaced as necessary. Assemblies can be produced for any programme by means of this technique and can be used several times if care is taken to avoid damage during removal from the animal's head.

B. *Implantation technique*

A female rat of 220–230 g is anaesthetized with sodium pentobarbital (33–35 mg/kg i.p.) and, after shaving the scalp, is fixed in the stereotaxic instrument. 1 % procaine solution (containing 4 mg% epinephrine) is injected subcutaneously at the site of operation. The skull is exposed, bleeding controlled and the surface dried. Holes are bored at the same ordinates as before (omitting that at the bregma), taking care not to damage the dura. An

[1] C. H. Stoelting Company, 424 N. Homan Ave., Chicago 24, Ill., U.S.A.

[2] Winchester Electronics, Main St. and Hillside Ave., Oakville, Conn., U.S.A.

[3] Oryx Electrical Laboratories Ltd., Meadow Road, Worthing, Sx., England.

[4] Prothoplast AG., Rothrist, Switzerland.

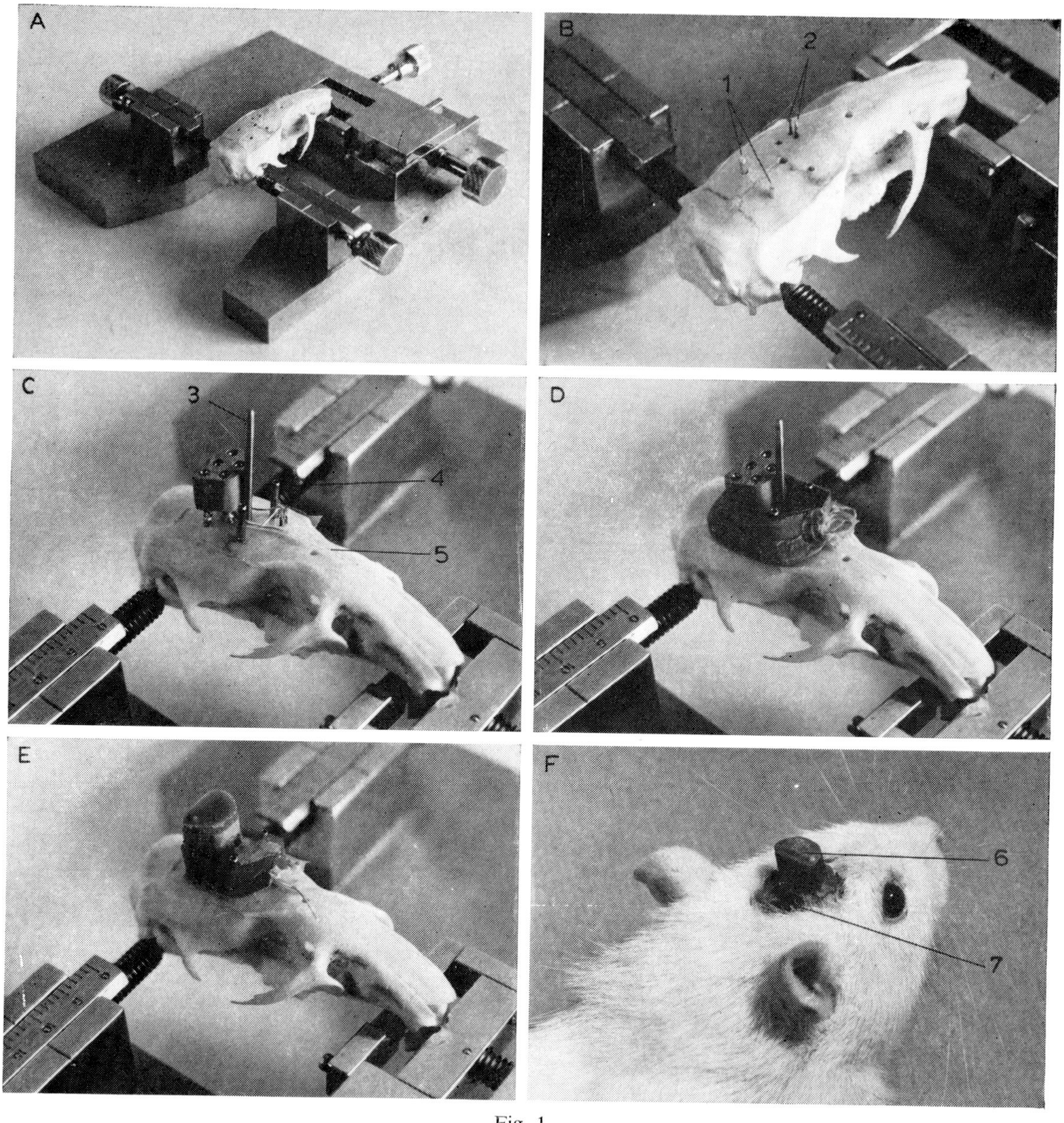

Fig. 1
Stages in the preparation of the electrode assembly. *A*: Prepared skull mounted in the holder of the stereotaxic instrument. The holes for the electrodes and guide needles have been drilled. *B*: Electrodes in position. *C*: The connector has been wired to the electrodes and the guide needles for intracerebral injections are in place. *D*: The mould ready for pouring. *E*: Finished electrode assembly, including dust cap. *F*: Animal with complete assembly. (This complex includes provision for application of substances to the dura.) Photo approx. 3 months following operation. Key: 1, cortical electrodes; 2, depth electrodes; 3, guide rod; 4, guide needle (without plug); 5, lead for the indifferent electrode; 6, dust cap; 7, area with exposed dura (cap removed).

additional hole (0.5 mm diameter) is bored in the frontal bone 10 mm anterior to the bregma and one or two similar holes are bored peripheral to the site of the electrode complex. Silver-plated watchmakers screws are threaded into these holes. The skull and the under surface of the electrode complex are thinly coated with dental cement, and the complex is lowered onto the skull by means of the guide rod mounted in the stereotaxic instrument and positioned over the bregma. The free-lying wire is soldered to the screw in the frontal bone, and the whole assembly, including the anchor screws, is coated with dental cement, leaving the Winchester connector exposed. Granulation tissue rapidly closes the wound around the electrode assembly. The rat is treated with penicillin/streptomycin following operation and at least 3 days are allowed to elapse before using the animal for experiments. We have also used this technique on animals for repeated observations on spreading cortical depression. For this purpose the mould on the skull was extended posteriorly to wall in an extra area of about 3 × 8 mm, leaving the surface of the skull exposed. After implantation of the finished assembly, openings (approx. 2 × 3 mm) were cut in the skull within the enclosed area on each side of the midline to expose the dura. Between experiments a Beracryl cap was placed over the cavity to prevent contamination with foreign matter, and was held in place with adhesive tape. Such animals have been used over a period of months without signs of infection (Fig. 1, *F*).

Histological controls have consistently shown accurate placement of the electrodes.

SUMMARY

A novel method is described for preparing and implanting brain electrode assemblies in rats. A distinct advantage over older methods is the ease with which large series of animals can be prepared, without the risk of brain damage during soldering. The technique, which is adaptable to any electrode pattern and is also suitable for intracerebral injections in unrestricted animals, has been successfully used over a number of years.

RÉSUMÉ

UNE NOUVELLE MÉTHODE POUR PRÉPARER ET IMPLANTER DES ENSEMBLES D'ÉLÉCTRODES CÉRÉBRALES CHEZ DES RATS

Une nouvelle méthode est décrite en vue de préparer et d'implanter des ensembles d'éléctrodes cérébrales chez des rats. Un avantage remarquable, comparé aux anciennes méthodes, c'est la facilité avec laquelle il est possible de préparer un grand nombre d'animaux, sans qu'il y ait un risque de léser le cerveau pendant la soudure. La technique, qui s'adapte à chaque système d'éléctrode et qui peut aussi servir pour des injections intracérébrales chez des animaux en situation libre, a été utilisée avec succès pendant plusieurs années.

Reference: SAYERS, A. and STILLE, G. A novel method for preparing and implanting brain electrode assemblies in rats. *Electroenceph. clin. Neurophysiol.*, **1969**, *27*: 87–89.

BEHAVIORAL EXPERIMENTAL EPILEPSY IN MONKEYS. II. VIDEO-TAPE CONTROL GATE FOR THE DETECTION AND RECORDING OF MOTOR SEIZURES[1]

RONALD I. BARENSTEN, E. E. AND JOAN S. LOCKARD, PH.D.

Department of Neurological Surgery, University of Washington School of Medicine, Seattle, Wash. 98105 (U.S.A.)

(Accepted for publication: November 18, 1968)

INTRODUCTION

A recording technique has been recently developed (Lockard and Barensten 1967) which permits the monitoring of gross motor seizure activity in monkeys over extensive periods of time. The technique involves the detection and video-tape verification of the seizure signature imbedded among normal motor activity of the monkey. This paper is concerned with the development, perfection and circuitry of the detection device. The main consideration has been to maximize the number of epileptic monkeys which could be monitored simultaneously (via the closed-circuit TV system) while minimizing the daily video-tape review time required. The optimal compromise from both the equipment cost and the investigator's time has been a 60 min video tape. The detection accuracy of the present device allows 24 h coverage of every motor seizure of at least four monkeys simultaneously in this tape length time. As many as 35 motor seizures have been repeatedly taped in a single night and reviewed in an hour or less the following day.

In the recording of motor seizures (Lockard and Barensten 1967) experimental epileptic monkeys are housed in primate chairs instrumented with strain gage transducers for continuous polygraph readout of gross motor activity. (To assure the welfare of the animals, periodic surveillance and maintenance are provided by trained technicians.)

In detecting the motor seizures, the video-tape control gate is operated by the electrical readout of monkey

[1] This research was supported by National Institutes of Health Grant NB-04053.

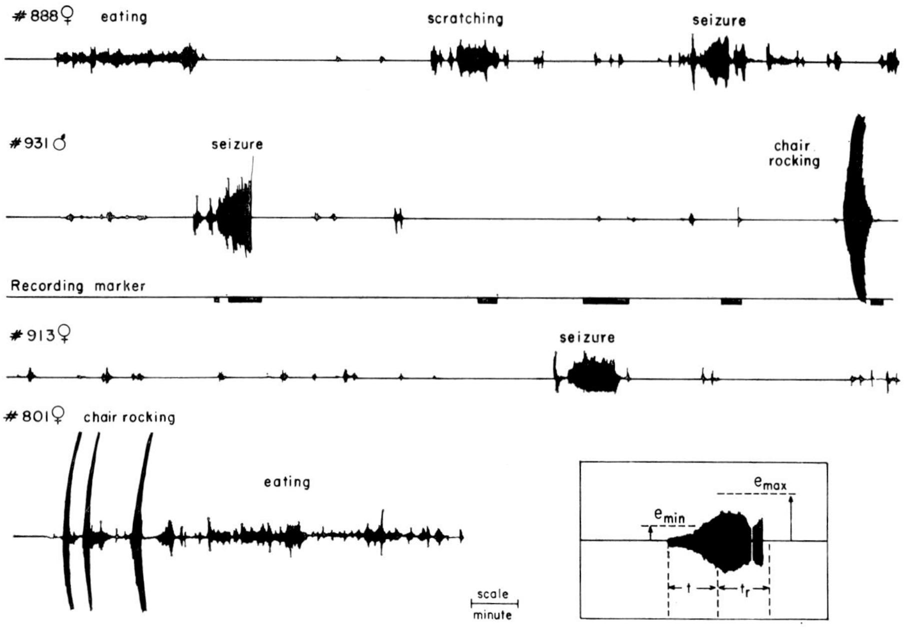

Fig. 1
Condensed polygraph records of epileptic monkey activity.

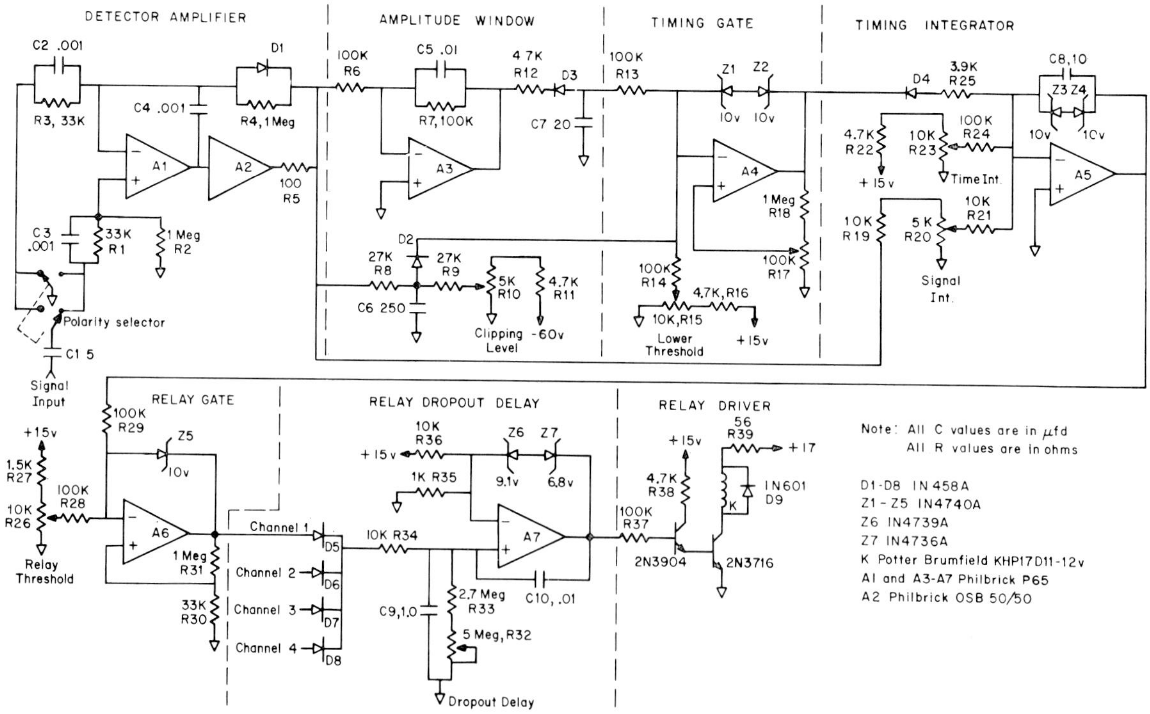

Fig. 2
Circuit diagram of video-tape control gate.

activity from the polygraph. A condensed polygraph record of typical activity is shown in Fig. 1. Empirically, the most reliable parameters of the seizure signature are its contiguous duration and an amplitude range between very high contiguous activity (*e.g.*, chair rocking) and very low contiguous activity (*e.g.*, eating). The levels of these parameters vary among monkeys but are relatively constant for individual monkeys. Therefore, what is needed is a device supplying a recording gate which turns on after time "t" when the amplitude lies between two pre-set values, e_{min} and e_{max} (Fig. 1, insert). To conserve tape, "t" should be of sufficient length to assure that the record period "t_r" includes only the last identifying segment of a particular behavior of the monkey. Moreover, "t_r" must span transitory decreases in monkey activity.

CIRCUITRY

Following is a description of the control gate circuit. The circuit diagram is shown in Fig. 2. A1 through A7 are Philbrick[1] operational amplifiers.

The I.R.I.G. output available from the power amplifier of the Grass Model 7 polygraph is amplified by A1–A2 and rectified by D1 providing a positive 0–50 V full-scale signal. The booster, A2, extends the output voltage range of A1 from 11 V to 50 V which decreases rectification errors of small signals. R5, C4, C3 and C2 provide stabilization to prevent oscillations. The Polarity Selector switch selects either the positive or negative half of the signal for processing.

The Timing Gate, a regenerative amplifier, in the absence of a signal current through R13 is held at a negative output (defined as the "off" state) by the current through R14 set by R15. The signal current through R13—derived from the unity gain inverting amplifier A3 and peak detector R12, D3, and C7—is opposite in polarity to the current in R14. When the current through R13 exceeds the current through R14, the Timing Gate switches to a positive output voltage (defined as the "on" state) regeneratively aided by the positive feedback connected to the plus input. The positive feedback voltage developed across the potentiometer R17 provides an adjustable hysteresis which allows separation of the on and off trip levels. The hysteresis prevents frequent operation of the Timing Gate on varying levels close to the trip level. The peak detector has a fast charging time constant (R12 is chosen just large enough to prevent overload of A3) and a slow discharge time constant. The latter filters the signal and prevents Timing Gate turn off on momentarily small signals.

If the signal exceeds the Clipping level set by potentiometer R10, D2 will conduct—providing a current opposite and greater than that through R13—causing the Timing Gate to turn off. C6 filters the signal and delays the turn off on brief, large amplitude signals. The signal currents through D2 and R13 form an amplitude window allowing the Timing Gate to turn on only when the signal level exists between adjustable lower and upper thresholds.

When the Timing Gate is off, its output is negative and the current through D4 will hold the Timing Integrator output reset at a positive output level. The level is determined by the zener voltage of Z4 plus the forward conductance voltage of Z3. (The zener diodes, Z1 through Z7 prevent the amplifiers from saturating which would cause undesirable delays.) R25 limits the current to prevent overload of A4. When the Timing Gate is on, its output is positive and D4 stops conducting, allowing the currents through R21 and R24 to charge C8 as a linear function of time and/or signal, set respectively by R23 and R20. The output voltage is limited to the zener voltage of Z3 plus the forward conductance voltage of Z4.

The output of the Relay Gate, a regenerative amplifier, switches to +10 V when the Timing Integrators output is within 0.25 V of maximum. This threshold is set by R26. Fixed hysteresis established by R30 and R31 insures good snap action.

The Relay Gate output, one of four channels, is connected to a four input OR gate. The OR gate output triggers the Relay Dropout Delay which behaves as a monostable multi-vibrator with a direct coupled trigger input. R35 and R36 establish a slightly positive bias at the minus input of A7.

The stable state occurs when no positive inputs are present at the OR gate and C9 has discharged through R33 and R32. This condition holds the plus input of A7 negative with respect to its minus input, driving the output negative and placing a reverse bias at the input of the Darlington connected Relay Driver. The Relay Driver will thus be at cut-off and the record relay K will not be energized.

The unstable state occurs when one or more of the OR gate inputs are positive, causing C9 to be charged through R34 and through any of the diodes D5–D8 which are forward biased by a positive input. The plus input of A7 will now be positive with respect to its minus input, driving the output positive and forward biasing the input of the Relay Driver. The Relay Driver switches to a saturated conducting condition which energizes the record relay. This state will be maintained while one or more inputs of the OR gate are positive. When the positive inputs to the OR gate are no longer present, diodes D5–D8 will be reverse biased and C9 will discharge through R33 and R32. The unstable state terminates when the voltage across C9 has decreased sufficiently to bias the plus input of A7 negative with respect to its minus input. The time constant of C9, and R33 plus R32 is adjusted by R32 to provide a 5 sec delay. The delay assures contiguous video-tape recording during transitory monkey inactivity. C10 speeds up the transition between states. R34 prevents overload of A6. (The 10 msec time constant formed by R34 and C9 is negligible.) A second set of contacts on the record relay is used to operate the polygraph marker channel. Adjustment of the circuit is normally performed with the aid of a 1 c/sec sine wave generator connected

[1] Philbrick Researches Inc. *Applications manual for computing amplifiers*. Nimrod Press, Boston, 1966.

to the polygraph pre-amplifier input. (Adjustment and maintenance are facilitated by bringing the output of each stage to front panel jacks.)

SUMMARY

An electronic control gate has been constructed which recognizes the signature of gross motor seizures of chronic experimental epileptic monkeys. This device activates a video-tape recorder which gives unattended 24 h clinical verification of the seizures.

RÉSUMÉ

ÉPILEPSIE COMPORTEMENTALE EXPÉRIMENTALE CHEZ LE SINGE. II. PORTE DE CONTRÔLE DES ENREGISTREMENTS MAGNÉTIQUES VIDEO ET ENREGISTREMENT DE CRISES MOTRICES

Une porte de contrôle électronique a été construite de telle sorte qu'elle reconnait la survenue de grandes crises motrices chez des singes avec épilepsie expérimentale chronique. Ce système met en jeu un enregistreur magnétique video qui fournit une vérification clinique automatique des crises 24 h sur 24.

The authors wish to express their appreciation to Mr. C. Beverstock and Mr. C. Dreyer for their construction contribution.

REFERENCE

LOCKARD, J. S. and BARENSTEN, R. I. Behavioral experimental epilepsy in monkeys. I. Clinical seizure recording apparatus and initial data. *Electroenceph. clin. Neurophysiol.*, **1967**, *22*: 482–486.

Reference: BARENSTEN, R. I. and LOCKARD, J. S. Behavioral experimental epilepsy in monkeys. II. Video-tape control gate for the detection and recording of motor seizures. *Electroenceph. clin. Neurophysiol.*, **1969**, *27*: 89–92.

SPECULAR REFLECTANCE PHOTOMETRIC DETECTION OF CORTICAL DISPLACEMENT

C. TEAGUE, J. ELFERT, G. TIMM AND W. BRADLEY

Departments of Neurology and Neurosurgery, University of Minnesota Medical Center, Minneapolis, Minn. 55455 (U.S.A.)

(Accepted for publication: October 30, 1968)

Cortical movement during experimental electronic recording of normal and abnormal neural events is an undefined problem. Surface cortical displacement has been observed during spreading depression (Marshall 1959). This displacement was estimated qualitatively by a spring mounted modified pore electrode mechanically coupled to a force displacement strain gauge. A probeless inertialess photometric recording system (Deferrari and Andrews 1966; Young 1967; Timm 1969; Timm *et al.* 1969), has been developed for quantitation of cortical pulsation and displacement.

DESCRIPTION OF INSTRUMENT

The photometric displacement detector consisted of a light source and a light detector. The light source was a Tungsol[1] No. 1816 incandescent bulb connected to a 12 V storage battery. The light source was mounted in an aluminum block such that light traveled through a 1.5 mm diameter, 4 cm long hole coated with flat black paint. The light detector was a Clairex[2] No. CL-604L photoconductive cell connected in series with a 1.4 V dry cell battery and a 96 Ω resistor. These were mounted in an aluminum block similar to that of the source. Both aluminum blocks were mounted opposing each other at an angle of 60° from the vertical on an aluminum bar connected to a micro-manipulator (Fig. 1, *A*). A Hewlett-Packard[3] 8875A D.C. pre-amplifier was arranged to amplify the voltage across the 96 Ω resistor. The output of the 8875A was monitored on a Tektronix 564[4] oscilloscope with a 2A63 plug in unit and recorded on an FM tape deck[5] (Fig. 1, *B*).

The principle of operation of the displacement detector is the detection of specular reflection of an essentially parallel light beam from a reflective surface. A vertical displacement of the reflective surface at the point of incidence induces a proportional displacement of the

[1] Wagner Electric Corp., Tung-Sol Division, Newark, N.J.

[2] Clairex Electronics, Inc., New York, N.Y.

[3] Hewlett-Packard Co., Palo Alto, Calif.

[4] Tektronix Inc., Beaverton, Ore.

[5] Technical Measurements Corporation, North Haven, Conn.

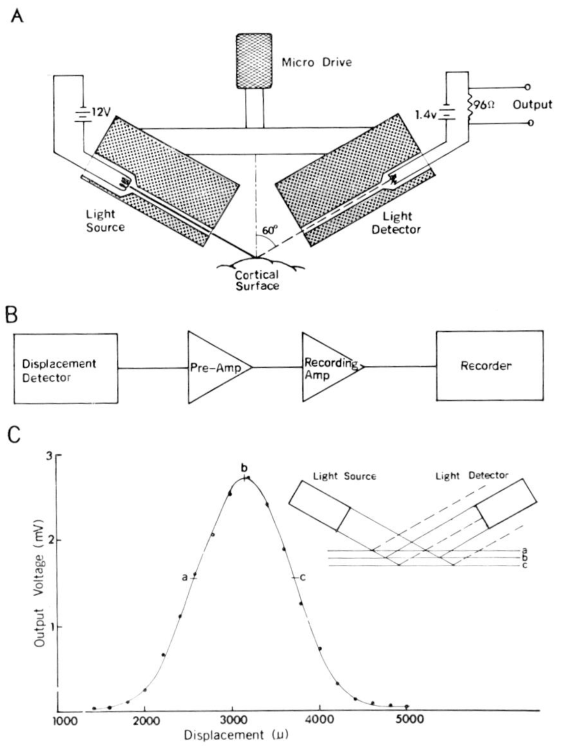

Fig. 1

A: The specular reflectance photometric displacement detector. *B*: Block diagram of the displacement detector system. *C*: The response of the displacement detector to displacement of a layer of silicone oil on water.

reflected beam. This displacement is perpendicular to the beam in the plane defined by the center of the light source aperture, the center of the detector aperture and the point of incidence. The portion of the reflected beam detected by the photocell will vary from a maximum when the entire reflected beam enters the detector aperture. Therefore, a vertical displacement of the reflective surface will result in a proportional change in the amount of the parallel beam detected by the photocell. Since the resistance of the photocell decreases with increasing light intensity a voltage proportional to the light intensity incident on the photocell can be measured across the series resistor (Fig. 1, *C*).

The cat was surgically exposed for pyramidotomy and recording of evoked response in the sensori-motor cortex as previously described (Conway *et al.* 1969). Pneumothorax was performed and bilateral chest tubes were inserted. Blood pressure was measured via a catheter in the femoral artery. A thin layer of silicone oil (Dow Corning[1] 200 fluid) was applied to the cortical surface to prevent drying and enhance surface reflection. The detector was positioned such that the axis of the micromanipulator drive was perpendicular to the cortical surface. The incident field of 7 sq.mm was selected in an area free of large blood vessels. The output voltage was then adjusted such that movement of the cortex towards the detector increased and movement of the cortex away from the detector decreased the output voltage. The former was interpreted as a positive deflection and the latter as a negative deflection. The detector was then calibrated in 50 µ steps on both sides of the center point C (Fig. 1, *C*). Calibration eliminated the need to consider the effects of surface curvature, linearity of the photoconductive cell, reflection from the oil–brain interface and change in optical path length. Two other possible sources of error, change in surface curvature with displacement and change in absorption of refracted light, were determined as negligible after comparison with concurrent mechanical displacement detection using a Model ST-2 linear motion transducer[2].

RESULTS

Two categories of cortical movement were detectable by specular reflectance. These categories differ in origin, amplitude and time course. The first movement is small in amplitude, closely related in time course to systolic and diastolic alterations in femoral artery pressure and may represent pulsation of the pial circulation (Fig. 2, *A*). The second category of movements, cortical displacements, are of larger amplitude, longer time course and may be related to overall changes in circulating blood volume (Fig. 3, *A*). Both movements were detectable in all areas of the cerebral cortex. The movements may occur spontaneously, in response to neural input and appear after administration of anesthetic agents and convulsants.

Cortical pulsations respond differentially to blood

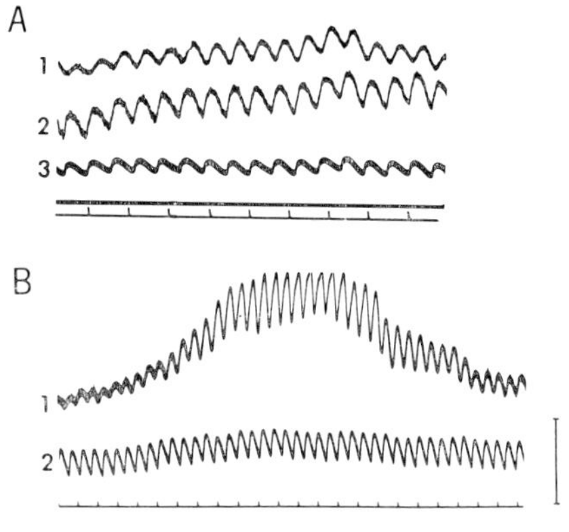

Fig. 2

A: Cortical pulsation detectable by (1) photometric and (2) mechanical displacement detectors. Trace 3 is a plot of femoral arterial blood pressure. *B*: Increase in amplitude of cortical pulsation measured by the photometric detector (1). Trace 2 shows a concurrent rise in arterial blood pressure. Amplitude marker is 20 µ and 150 mm Hg for *A*, and 40 µ and 75 mm Hg for *B*. All time marks are 1 sec.

[1] Dow Corning Co., Midland, Mich.

[2] Phipps and Bird, Richmond, Va.

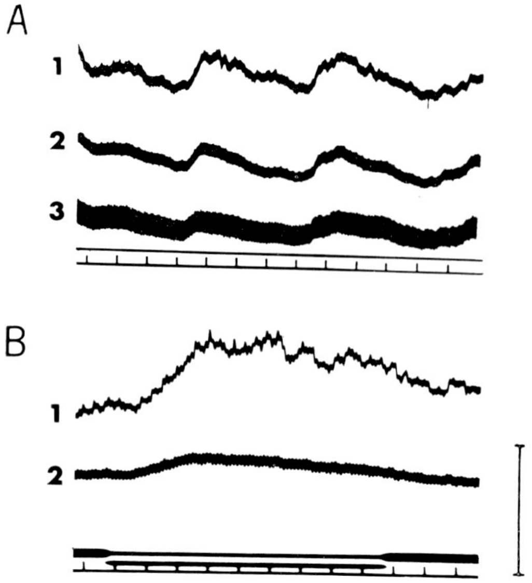

Fig. 3
A: Photometric (1) and mechanical (2) displacement detector responses to cortical displacement evoked by (3) spontaneous blood pressure alterations. *B*: Photometric displacement detector (1) and blood pressure response (2) to pyramidal tract stimulation indicated by the broken trace. Amplitude marker is 200 μ for *A* and 80 μ for *B*. Time mark is 20 sec for *A* and 5 sec for *B*.

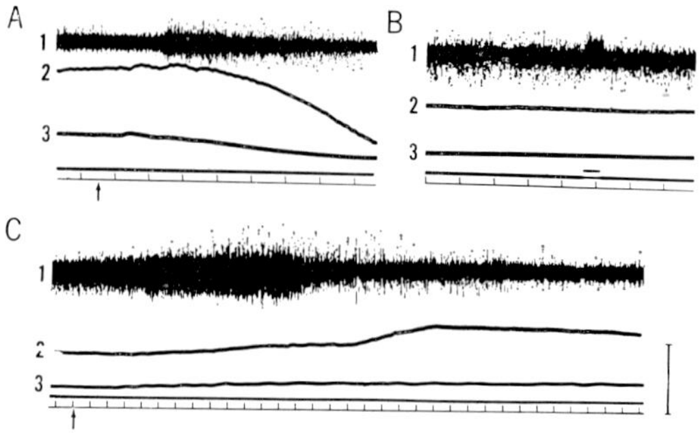

Fig. 4
A: EEG (1), photometric displacement detector (2) and blood pressure (3) responses to barbiturate administration at the time indicated by the arrow. *B*: Absence of displacement measured by the photometric detector (2) and blood pressure response (3) elicited by pyramidal stimulation 10 min after barbiturate administration; (1) EEG. *C*: EEG (1), photometric displacement detector (2), and blood pressure (3) responses to Metrazol administration at the time indicated by the arrow. Amplitude marker is 800 μ for *A* and *C*, 400 μ for *B* and 150 mm Hg for *A* and *B*, 300 mm Hg for *C*. All time marks are 20 sec.

pressure alterations (Fig. 2, *B*). With a spontaneous rise in femoral artery pressure with no alteration in systolic and diastolic excursion, cortical pulsations show an increase in amplitude in addition to cortical displacement.

Displacements were distributed over the cortical surface and were not altered in magnitude or distribution after cortical drainage. A 10 mm Hg spontaneous fluctuation in systolic blood pressure was associated with approximately a 50 μ displacement of the cortical surface. This displacement was positive and had a similar time course to the blood pressure variation.

Pyramidal tract stimulation resulted in blood pressure increases of 10–20 mm Hg which were associated with a positive cortical displacement of 50–100 μ (Fig. 3, *B*). Cortical displacements were not observed in the absence of concurrent blood pressure change.

Administration of sodium pentobarbital (25–35 mg/kg i.v.) resulted in a negative cortical displacement of greater than 750 μ, commencing 40–60 sec after injection and coinciding with a decrease in blood pressure. After 2–3 min an equilibrium was attained and large spontaneous blood pressure fluctuations and cortical movements were not evident (Fig. 4, *A*). Pyramidal tract stimulation did not elicit a blood pressure rise or cortical displacement after barbiturate administration (Fig. 4, *B*).

Administration of i.v. pentylenetetrazol in sufficient amounts to induce epileptiform EEG activity resulted in positive cortical displacements and blood pressure rise (Fig. 4, *C*).

DISCUSSION

Some of the problems involved in instrumentation included the following:

1. Since the intensity of the reflected light is small compared to the total incident light, alterations in diffuse reflection of the refracted light may be considered as a possible source of artifact. The intensity of light reflected from a transparent medium (I) in air can be calculated if the index of refraction (n) of the medium and the angle of incidence (i) is known.

$$I = \frac{I_0}{2}\left[\frac{\sin^2(i-r)}{\sin^2(i+r)} + \frac{\tan^2(i-r)}{\tan^2(i+r)}\right]$$

I_0 = intensity of the incident light; r = angle of refraction; $\sin r = (\sin i)/n$.

Given that the refractive index of silicone oil is 1.4 and that the incident angle is 60°, I is 6.75% of I_0. The other 93.25% is refracted into the oil layer and diffused by the cortical surface. Therefore the intensity of reflected light is considerably less than the intensity of the refracted light. However, the diffusional reflectance from the cortical surface is a constant for any given displacement and is taken into account by the calibration procedure.

2. If there is an alteration in systemic blood pressure there is also corresponding alteration in cortical blood flow (Brewington and Stecher 1967). Since the photocell used was sensitive to red light wavelengths vascular dilatation would increase the intensity of red light incident on the photocell. The result would appear to be a surface displacement if the alteration in spectral composition of diffuse reflected light from the cortical surface was significant in proportion to the specular reflected light. However, since simultaneous measurements with both photometric and mechanical detectors indicated the same

amount of displacement, alteration in the spectral composition of diffuse reflection from the cortical surface can be neglected.

3. Alteration of the cortical vascularity could produce a change in cortical surface curvature. Comparison with a mechanical transducer showed that there was no change in cortical curvature, at least not in the field of view of the light detector.

4. The surface of the cortex is curved and light reflected from a curved surface will be dispersed. For a constant curvature and a small field of view the error due to curvature can be eliminated by calibration of the photometric detector on the surface since the dispersion by the surface will be small and constant for a given displacement.

A photopotentiometric technique dependent upon conductivity changes of a photocell has previously been reported. However, this requires the attachment of a mechanically activated probe to vary the light intensity incident upon the photocell (McIntosh *et al.* 1965).

SUMMARY

A non-contacting photometric displacement detector was described and used to measure cortical surface displacements. The variation in the proportion of a specular reflected parallel light beam incident on a photoconductive cell with vertical displacement of the reflective surface provides an accurate method of measuring small displacements of the cortical surface. Cortical surface displacements are always associated with alterations in systemic blood pressure. Pyramidal tract stimulation, barbiturate administration and Metrazol administration alter systemic blood pressure and cause concurrent cortical surface displacement. The problems caused by surface curvature, alteration in surface curvature, diffuse reflection and alteration in the spectral composition of diffuse reflected light by absorption are discussed. Advantages include probeless and inertialess operation, precise measurement of displacement of a discrete surface area and ease of calibration.

RÉSUMÉ

DÉTECTION PHOTOMÉTRIQUE PAR RÉFLEXION DANS UN MIROIR DU DÉPLACEMENT CORTICAL

Un détecteur photométrique de déplacement à distance est décrit et utilisé pour mesurer les déplacements corticaux de surface. La variation de proportion d'un rayon lumineux parallèle réfléchi en miroir sur une cellule photo-électrique, avec déplacement vertical de la surface réfléchissante, fournit une méthode précise de mesure des petits déplacements de surface corticale. Les déplacements de surface corticale sont toujours associés à des altérations de la pression sanguine systémique. La stimulation du faisceau pyramidal, l'administration de barbituriques, et l'administration de Métrazol altèrent la pression sanguine systémique et provoquent en conséquence un déplacement de surface corticale. Les problèmes dus à la courbe de surface, l'altération de cette courbe de surface, la réflexion diffuse, et l'altération de la composition spectrale de la lumière diffuse réfléchie par absorption sont discutés. Parmi les avantages de cette méthode, il faut noter l'absence de sonde et d'inertie, la précision de mesure des déplacements d'une discrète aire de surface et la facilité de calibration.

REFERENCES

BREWINGTON, H. H. and STECHER, K. An improved technique for obtaining cortical photoelectric plethysmograms. *J. appl. Physiol.*, **1967**, *22*: 187–188.

CONWAY, C. J., WRIGHT, F. S. and BRADLEY, W. E. Electrophysiological maturation of the pyramidal tract in the post-natal rabbit. *Electroenceph. clin. Neurophysiol.*, **1969**, *26*: 565–577.

DEFERRARI, H. A. and ANDREWS, F. A. Laser interferometric technique for measuring small order vibration displacements. *J. acoustic Soc. Amer.*, **1966**, *39*: 779–780.

MARSHALL, W. H. Spreading cortical depression of Leão. *Physiol. Rev.*, **1959**, *39*: 239–279.

MCINTOSH, M., DUGGAN, P. E., WATT, D. D. and GOODSON, L. H. A photopotentiometric transducer for detecting in vitro muscle contraction. *J. appl. Physiol.*, **1965**, *20*: 349–350.

TIMM, G. W. Probeless displacement transducer. *I.E.E.E. Trans. bio-med. Engng.*, **1969** (in press).

TIMM, G., BRADLEY, W. and ELFERT, J. Photometric method of measurement of spread of excitation within the detrusor muscle. *Invest. Urol.*, **1969** (in press).

YOUNG, R. D. Ultrasensitive measurement of short distances. *Instr. Control Systems*, **1967**, *40*: 91–92.

Reference: TEAGUE, C., ELFERT, J., TIMM, G. and BRADLEY, W. Specular reflectance photometric detection of cortical displacement. *Electroenceph. clin. Neurophysiol.*, **1969**, *27*: 92–95.

Electroencephalography and Clinical Neurophysiology
Elsevier Publishing Company, Amsterdam – Printed in The Netherlands

SOCIETY PROCEEDINGS

SOCIETÀ ITALIANA DI ELETTROENCEFALOGRAFIA E NEUROFISIOLOGIA

Turin, May 25–26, 1968

Secretary: Dr. E. Lugaresi

Clinica Neurologica dell'Università di Bologna (Italy)

1. Spontaneous rhythmic cerebral electrical activity at a frequency higher than 14 c/sec seen in the waking state. — F. Rinaldi, F. Bravaccio and L. Vacca (Naples).

A series of 2000 EEGs, taken from a variety of subjects, irrespective of age and sex, was reviewed. The only selection was the exclusion of patients under drug therapy. From these records those showing sinusoidal fast activity of a frequency above 14 c/sec were considered, provided the amplitude of this activity was above 25 μV. A tentative classification of the different types of rhythmic fast activity (frequency, amplitude, continuity and regional distribution) is presented, together with a discussion of possible relationships with clinical conditions.

2. The electroencephalogram in post-convulsive coma: a study of the correlogram and power spectrum. — F. M. Puca, C. Rivano, G. Rosadini, I. Rosadini and G. F. Rossi (Genoa).

An analysis by means of the correlogram and power spectrum was made of the cerebral electrical activity of 9 patients treated with electroshock therapy before, during and after the comatose state following the seizure. (1) Immediately after the seizure, when the depth of coma is at maximum and the EEG is flat, no rhythmic activity is revealed by the correlogram and power spectrum. (2) When coma is still deep but some slow waves are present in the EEG, the correlogram and the spectrum show the presence of rhythmic activity in the delta band. (3) Two rhythmic activities are recorded when the first signs of vigilance reappear and large amplitude slow waves, with some faster activity, are present in the EEG. They are located in the delta and theta bands. (4) When the level of consciousness and the EEG return to normal there is a reduction of the two rhythms mentioned in (3) and the appearance of an alpha rhythm.

3. Results of attempts to produce certain types of epileptic seizures of conditioned reflex origin in man. — R. Zappoli (Florence).

Brief reference is made to cases of confirmed epilepsy of the conditioned reflex type described in the literature and the experimental investigations aimed at bringing about true epileptic manifestations of a conditioned reflex nature in animals. The author reports the results of attempts to produce, in humans, a temporary epileptogenic capacity with stimuli normally accommodated but associated variously with sensory stimulation capable of inducing reflex epileptic seizures. Nineteen cases of reflex epilepsy were examined. Sixteen were photosensitive epilepsy, 2 subjects had audiogenic epilepsy and 1 presented typical sensory motor reflex attacks in response to painful stimulation of the right zygomatic region.

Under normal conditions (while basic anticonvulsant therapy was maintained unchanged), using our combinations of conditioning and deconditioning stimuli, it was not possible in any of the 19 patients to obtain a true conditioning of the epileptic seizures, together with the motor manifestations that accompany them. Instead, in many cases a perfect conditioning was noted, including both the phenomenon of the alpha blocking reaction and some peripheral vegetative responses (modifications of skin resistance, vasomotor tone and of cardiac and respiratory rhythms). These reactions consistently followed the classical laws of conditioned reflexes: extinction from failure to reinforce, delay, differentiation and re-elaboration. Thus a particular phenomenon of disassociation is established in comparison with the conditioning of effects normally produced by the unconditioned stimuli: that is, between the conditionable alpha blocking reaction and peripheral vegetative responses on the one hand and epileptic seizures and their concomitant motor manifestations not influenced by the conditioning stimuli on the other.

In 9 subjects (8 affected by photosensitive epilepsy and 1 with acoustico-motor attacks) the conditioning sessions were repeated, associating stimulation with administration of progressive doses of Bemegride. With this method it was possible to reach a certain level of activation and obtain conditioning, not only of the peripheral vegetative responses but also of the polyspike-waves with myoclonic jerks, in 5 subjects with photosensitive myoclonus and absences. On some occasions when there were "conditioned" epileptic seizures it was even possible to reach a true extinction from the failure to reinforce, differentiation and re-elaboration. In 4 cases, including one with audio-motor attacks, the administration of Bemegride failed to facilitate to any important degree the conditioning of the epileptic seizures of reflex origin.

4. A case of epileptic seizures occurring spontaneously and induced by movements. — G. Gandiglio and D. Gambi (Rome).

A subject who had suffered from epilepsy since infancy noticed that abrupt movements of extension of the forearm sometimes provoked epileptic seizures completely similar to those occurring spontaneously (adversive towards the right, generally without loss of consciousness). (1) In order to demonstrate that the epileptic seizures were caused by muscle afferences strictly limited to one segment, passive movement of the right forearm was used, as well as the application of electrical stimuli over the appropriate nerves before, during and after anaesthetic block of the brachial plexus by infiltration with procaine. (2) The symptomatology of the induced seizures and their relationship with physiological night sleep in its various phases were also studied. The present case can be added to those described by Lishman *et al.*, Falconer *et al.* and other authors, describing epilepsy induced by movements. Hypotheses concerning the mechanisms of these convulsive episodes may be made.

5. Audio-motor epilepsy with atypical EEG correlates. — R. Di Perri, G. Dello Ioio and V. Supino (Naples and Messina).

A patient is described who had typical tonic fits induced by sudden auditory stimuli (startle epilepsy). Although the clinical attacks were always of the same kind, their EEG correlates could be of two different types: (a) at times a diffuse depression of cerebral electrical activity was followed by focal convulsive discharges in the left temporal region, subsequently extending to all cortical areas; (b) at other times the attacks were accompanied by synchronous, generalized, high voltage potentials beginning either simultaneously with the tonic fit or after an interval of generalized depression of the electrical activity.

This variety of EEG seizure pattern in contrast to the uniformity of the motor phenomena is discussed in the light of the current pathogenetic interpretation of audiomotor epilepsy.

6. Electro-clinical correlations in the treatment of infantile epilepsy (without hypsarrhythmia) with ACTH. — F. Bertamino, L. Luciano and M. de Negri (Genoa).

This report concerns 52 subjects aged 6 months to 6 years who suffered from a severe epileptic syndrome and were treated with ACTH; 16 of these patients with particular features have been followed up. All had certain electroclinical characteristics (akinetic, myoclonic and mixed attacks, diffuse EEG changes of "centrencephalic" type, an intellectual level which excluded serious mental damage) which enabled a more exact evaluation of the hormone therapy, both from the electro-clinical and the mental aspects. These cases have been compared with a similar group of patients who did not have hormone therapy and the findings suggest that the mental deterioration is related to the persistence of the attacks rather than to the persistence of EEG abnormalities. ACTH treatment of childhood epilepsy without hypsarrhythmia is discussed.

7. Effects of labyrinthine caloric stimulation and drugs micro-iontophoretically applied to brain-stem neurones. — G. L. Avanzini, E. A. Pallestrini, F. Carta and R. Ermirio (Genoa).

The existence of connections between the vestibular system, reticular formation and other brain-stem structures is known. The aim of this research was to study the relation between responses of brain-stem neurones to labyrinthine caloric stimulation and to various drugs with supposed transmitter action (structures below the rhomboid fossa and mainly on the nuclei reticulares gigantocellularis and pontis caudalis). Unanaesthetized, Flaxedil paralysed guinea pigs were used. In these animals the cerebellum was removed by suction. Stimulation of the labyrinth was carried out by irrigating one epitympanic recess with warm saline solution at 45–48° C or a cold solution at 10–12° C. Multi-barrelled micro-electrodes, which allow single neurone discharges to be recorded as well as the iontophoretic application of up to 4 different drugs, were introduced through the rhomboid fossa.

Many of the cells studied responded to at least one of the caloric stimuli and they were scattered in practically all the area examined. Both warm and cold stimulation could provoke either excitation or inhibition. However, in the brain-stem ipsilateral to the stimulated labyrinth both warm and cold stimulation provoked mainly excitatory effects and in the contralateral part mainly inhibitory effects. As for the drugs applied micro-iontophoretically, acetylcholine, noradrenaline and 5-hydroxytryptamine provoked both excitation and inhibition while L-glutamate produced excitation. The relationships between neuronal responses to caloric stimulation and their sensitivity to drugs, as well as the effects of the various drugs on the neuronal responses to labyrinthine stimulation, were studied.

8. Experimental study of the reliability of the visual evoked response recorded from the scalp. — J. Zattoni, F. Giunta and C. Siani (Genoa).

An experimental study of visual evoked responses has been carried out on 20 cats (acute as well as chronic preparations) using pairs of electrodes placed on the scalp and on the dura overlying the visual cortical area. The responses evoked by single visual stimuli were simultaneously recorded on multi-channel magnetic tape and electronically summated in groups of 50–150; both bipolar and unipolar (reference electrode on the mandibular bone) records were made. (a) During relaxed wakefulness the responses recorded bipolarly from the scalp and the dura might have a different appearance although the responses recorded unipolarly were quite similar. (b) The amplitude of the responses recorded bipolarly from the scalp was 19% of that recorded from the dura, but 28% and 40% when recorded unipolarly. (c) Changes in the general state of the animal (natural or pharmacological sleep) or in the intensity of the photic stimulation produced variations in the amplitude of the scalp and dural responses which were not necessarily related, especially in the bipolar recordings.

9. The auditory evoked response in the normal subject. — A. Cordone, A. Gentilomo, E. Mora and C. Rivano (Genoa).

The optimal technical conditions for the scalp recording of the cerebral response evoked by single auditory stimuli are as follows: (1) stimulus: pure tone of a duration of 0.5 msec, intensity of 80 dB, repeated every second, with bilateral earphones; (2) recording electrodes: one placed on the scalp overlying the region of the acoustic area, the other on the ipsilateral ear lobe; (3) averaging (electronic summation) of at least 100 responses.

In these conditions the auditory evoked response of normal subjects is a complex polyphasic potential formed by six main positive-negative oscillations. Some of these oscillations are present in all subjects (peak latency above 40 msec: mean peak latencies: P2: 45.09 msec; N2: 72.96 msec; P3: 142.51 msec; N3: 211.01 msec), others in some subjects only (peak latency below 40 msec: mean peak latencies: P1: 22.55 msec; N1: 31.79 msec).

The possibility of the presence of myogenic components in the evoked response has been examined by taking records in curarized patients and in patients with bipolar electrodes implanted in the temporal lobe. These show patterns similar to the usual scalp records.

10. A statistical method for automatic analysis of EEG data. — F. Ferro-Milone, P. Viviani, A. Lorizio and and F. Denoth (Pisa).

This research was carried out in order to obtain an automatic EEG analysis for both clinical and neurophysiological applications. The clinical application is concerned with a more precise and detailed subdivision of routine records. The neurophysiological studies aim at a detailed analysis of the electrical activity of the brain. Amplitude histograms were obtained from the EEG in digital form according to the usual parameters: variance, 3rd moment mode, mean square value, form factor. Statistical analysis was performed with an IBM/7090 computer. Second order conditional amplitude distribution and some new related functions were calculated for every K interval. The numerical parameters and their discriminant functions allow a differential picture to be obtained, *e.g.*, between alpha-rich and alpha-poor EEGs and between delta waves with spikes and delta waves devoid of spikes. These parameters and the related discriminant functions were inserted during the learning phase on a digital tape through the use of a fixed length scheme.

The first results are reported to show the possibilities of these new methods. In the recognition phase the programme automatically compares the parameters of an unknown case with those of the table on the digital tape.

11. Analysis of the various components of evoked muscular responses in some peripheral nerve lesions. — D. Passerini, E. Sala and G. Valli (Milan).

It is common knowledge that nerve lesions of compressive type are correlated with some scatter of evoked muscle potentials, making it difficult to distinguish the original wave form of the individual components. This makes analysis practicable only in the presence of few surviving motor units. In this case, however, two wave forms superimposable upon each other may be the final effect of manifold neural activation procedures, namely: direct excitation of motor nerve fibres at the site of the stimulus (M wave), antidromic (F wave) or monosynaptic activation (H wave) of the motoneurone and finally "straggling" of the discharge in regenerated nerve branches (axon reflex). Such possibilities must be borne in mind whenever a correct EMG screening is required in order to avoid obvious mistakes.

12. Electrophysiological findings concerning the involvement of the ulnar nerve at the elbow in a case of bilateral Mouchet's syndrome. — C. Messina (Messina).

Electrophysiological studies have been carried out in a patient with bilateral Mouchet's syndrome. The results concerning the involvement of the ulnar nerve motor fibres were as follows: (a) EMG findings of partial denervation of the hypothenar and interossei muscles bilaterally; (b) maximal nerve conduction velocity was normal above the region of the elbow, very slow through this region and relatively normal below it; (c) minimal nerve conduction velocity was normal above the elbow, very slow through the elbow region and a little slower below it; (d) different muscle potential parameters were present when stimulating above or below the elbow; (e) a normal electrical threshold was found above and below the elbow but it was higher in the elbow region. The importance of these findings is discussed in relation to a correct diagnosis and surgical therapy (which has given good results).

13. Posterior tibial nerve conduction velocity in patients with polyneuropathy. — L. Fra, F. Brignolio and M. Delsedime (Turin).

Motor and afferent conduction velocity studies of the posterior tibial nerve were carried out in 16 patients with polyneuropathy and also in 10 normal subjects. For comparative purposes patients with peripheral involvement were subdivided into four groups according to the clinical diagnosis: 6 patients with alcoholic polyneuropathy, 6 with diabetic polyneuropathy, 3 with infective polyneuritis and 3 with uraemic polyneuropathy.

In most patients maximal motor conduction velocities were below the range of normal values, but more information was obtained by determining single motor fibre conduction velocity, using threshold stimulation and bipolar needle electrodes. Conduction changes in the different types of polyneuropathy showed similar patterns and seemed to occur in both fast and slow conducting motor fibres. Sensory nerve action potentials elicited at the ankle following stimulation of the digital nerves (second and third toes) were not recorded in any patient. Mixed nerve action potentials evoked at the level of the knee by stimulation of the nerve trunk at the ankle were recorded only in some patients and were always of very small amplitude. Slight differences in motor and afferent conduction velocities between the various types of polyneuropathy were observed.

14. Somato-motor effects of isolated and simultaneous stimulation of the hypothalamus and the caudate nucleus in cats with permanent implanted electrodes. — S. Giammanco, V. La Grutta, M. T. Zagami and R. D'Anna (Palermo).

The somato-motor effects following isolated or simultaneous stimulation of the hypothalamic perifornical area and of the body of the caudate nucleus were studied in cats with permanent intracerebral electrodes, free to move in a behavioural cage.

The results may be summarized as follows: (1) isolated stimulation of the hypothalamic perifornical area produced an attack and escape reaction, or a simple escape reaction, and a rapid half-turn towards the same side as the structure stimulated; (2) isolated stimulation of the body of the caudate nucleus was characterized by: (a) no somato-motor effects (22%); (b) a slow and uniform contraversive rotation of the head and neck (32%), which may be followed by marked curving of the body (8%) or by a slow and gliding circling movement (38%); (3) simultaneous stimulation of the hypothalamic perifornical area and of the caudate nucleus was always followed by fast circling movements towards the side opposite to the caudate nucleus stimulated. The number of such movements was proportional to the intensity of the stimulus (in volts) to the caudate nucleus and to the hypothalamic perifornical area.

15. Hypersomnia with periodic apnoea: problems of classification. — E. Lugaresi, G. Coccagna, G. Berti Ceroni, M. Mantovani and P. Pazzaglia (Bologna).

Two cases of hypersomnia, apparently of essential type, showed periodic respiration beginning when the patient became drowsy and persisting throughout sleep. In the first case the apnoeic periods were of purely central type but in the second case they were often complicated by some obstruction. In both cases spirography, arterial gas measurements and lung function tests indicated the absence of a chronic condition with alveolar hypoventilation.

These observations demonstrate that hypersomnia and periodic respiration may occur even in the absence of all the other symptoms which are characteristic of either the Pickwick syndrome or the central alveolar hypoventilation syndrome (Ondine's curse). From a classification point of view these cases represent a transition between narcolepsies and hypersomnia syndromes accompanied by alveolar hypoventilation (Pickwick syndrome and central alveolar hypoventilation).

From a physiopathological point of view it is possible to suggest hypothetically that the hypersomnia syndromes accompanied by central alveolar hypoventilation are the expression of a primitive depression of the reticular activating system. Drowsiness, hypoexcitability of the respiratory centre, muscular hypotonia and possibly also the tendency to obesity, which seem to be characteristic features of these syndromes, may in fact be explained by hypoexcitability of the reticular activating substance. Chronic alveolar hypoventilation, with all its possible consequences (central hypoexcitability to CO_2, polycythaemia, pulmonary hypertension, cardiomegaly and cardiac failure) may well be the result of the severe and persistent respiratory disturbance.

16. Nocturnal EEG patterns of patients following complete or partial hemispherectomy. — S. Mingrino, A. Semerano, C. Ravenna and A. Benedetti (Padua).

Complete hemispherectomy was carried out in 4 patients and partial hemispherectomy in 3 patients because of infantile spastic hemiplegia with epilepsy. Following surgery nocturnal EEG records were carried out in order to study the organization of sleep cycles and any residual epileptic activity. The results can be summarized as follows: (1) Partial hemispherectomy did not induce significant alterations of EEG patterns during nocturnal sleep. Tracings of patients with complete hemispherectomy were characterized by absence of phase IV sleep and a reduced percentage and late appearance of REM sleep. The other three phases of slow sleep were prolonged and the cycles of sleep were reduced in number. (2) Epileptic activity was absent in the 4 completely hemispherectomized patients. Patients with partial hemispherectomy, although free from clinical attacks after surgery, showed epileptic activity in the EEG. This, however, was reduced in amount compared with the pre-operative tracing, and appeared only during the slow phase of sleep. This activity was usually localized to the cortical areas adjacent to those removed, or contralaterally over the intact hemisphere.

17. Structural aspects of sleep in depressed patients. — A. Muratorio and C. Maggini (Pisa).

In previous work we have reported the main polygraphic features of sleep in depressed patients, the relationship with the severity of depressive symptoms, and the evolution of the sleep patterns with therapy. We have suggested that the main characteristic is the appearance of awakenings during the night. Therefore, we have supposed that the awakenings had a pathogenetic role in determining some structural alterations of sleep in depressed patients. We have studied the structural features of all-night records of our depressed patients (the change from one stage to another and their relation with the awakenings) and compared them with those of normal subjects. The results are as follows: (1) The patient may awake from any sleep stage, especially from stages I, II and REM sleep. (2) The patient shows some modalities of shift which are not found in a normal subject. (3) The decrease in REM sleep seems to be due to the appearance of the awakenings. (4) The reduction of stage IV sleep seems to be due to an alteration of the mechanisms regulating sleep, as well as to the presence of awakenings.

18. Electromyographic study of the extrinsic ocular muscles in a familial ocular myopathy. — G. Amabile, G. Bernardi, C. Morocutti and P. A. Rizzo (Siena).

Three subjects out of 5 in a family affected by ocular

myopathy have had EMG studies of the extrinsic ocular muscles. The results obtained confirm the importance of EMG examination in the diagnosis of the ocular myopathies with characteristic features, namely, the disintegration of the motor units even in the ocular muscles.

The authors stress the importance of studying the motor unit as the finding of polyphasic potentials even in small numbers is an indication of muscular damage because of the limited innervation of these muscles, which does not allow spatial dispersion of the motor units. In some cases in fact indirect criteria, such as discrepancy between the clinical motor deficit and the persistence of a large amount of electrical activity during movements, with absence of EMG signs typical of neurogenic alterations (pathological activity at rest and lack of an interference pattern) are present. These may be difficult to appreciate because the muscular lesions, leading to functional loss, mask the more characteristic neurogenic features. The authors also point out the early involvement of orbicularis oculi in chronic progressive ophthalmoplegia.

19. Oculo-pharyngeal muscular dystrophy. — F. Simone and F. M. Ferro (Rome).

A syndrome characterized by ptosis and extrinsic eye-muscle weakness was observed in two patients, brother and sister. In addition, atrophy with corresponding diminution in strength of upper arm and shoulder girdle muscles was present and the brother also had dysphagia. Myopathic alterations in the upper arm were revealed by EMG and histological findings. The EMG findings excluded ocular myasthenia and neurogenic ophthalmoplegia. Radiological examination showed hypertrophy of the thymus in the brother and to a lesser extent in the sister. The immunoglobulin G (IgG) was normal in both patients. Oral glucose tolerance tests and plasma insulin responses to orally administered glucose were slightly abnormal. The relationship with myotonic dystrophy is discussed but it is nevertheless clear that this syndrome can be regarded as an oculo-pharyngeal muscular dystrophy and may be accepted as a distinctive clinical entity.

20. Preliminary study of the EEG modifications induced by a new anaesthetic drug derived from phencyclidine, Cl 581. — S. Bram and G. Marullo-Reedtz (Turin).

The EEG changes following i.v. injection of Cl 581 (1.5 mg/kg) have been studied in 10 cases. The interest of the work is due to the fact that the drug has already been considered by other authors as a dissociative anaesthetic, as it causes disturbances of consciousness such as dreaming, hallucinations, emotional lability and uncoordinated motor activity.

The EEG following the injection of the drug showed quite a different electrical picture from that obtained after injecting short acting barbiturates. In fact, with this drug, the patterns of deep sleep with delta waves were never obtained but a synchronized pattern was seen with medium voltage theta activity, lasting about 15 min with the dose used, and this was followed by a marked and prolonged period of desynchronization. The authors consider that the drug has an action on the adrenergic systems of the reticular formation. They support their hypothesis on the action of Cl 581 by comparing this effect with that of chlorpromazine.

21. EEG changes induced by high dosages of benzodiazepines. — A. Cocchi and G. Invernizzi (Milan).

The use of psychotropic drugs in attempted suicide is common. Amongst 1000 attempted suicides, the authors have studied the EEGs of about 130 patients intoxicated with benzodiazepines. (Psychiatric Emergency Ward of the "Ospedale Policlinico" of Milan). Serial EEG recordings were carried out on these patients, the number varying according to the severity of the toxic state and the symptomatology. The changes in the cerebral activity (chiefly fast rhythms of medium voltage from all the areas of the brain) are not strictly related to the quantity of the drug ingested. The results of this investigation are discussed in relation to the literature both on animals and man.

22. Frequency analysis in clinical electromyography: a preliminary report. — V. Cosi and G. L. Mazzella (Pavia).

Preliminary results of a study of frequency analysis of the EMG in 10 normal subjects are reported. The tibialis anterior muscle of each subject was tested by means of both bipolar surface leads and bipolar coaxial needle electrodes; with the latter the muscle was examined at 10 different points at various depths during an isometric contraction of weak, medium and maximal effort. A frequency analyser (Medelec FA 3) connected with an electromyograph (Medelec MS3R) was employed. The frequency range of this analyser is 150–1500 c/sec in 12 steps of nominal frequencies (logarithmic distribution).

The frequency spectrum of voluntary effort using the needle lead varies in the same muscle from one point to another and also at the same point, depending upon the degree of effort. The frequency spectrum from the surface lead is quite different from that obtained from the same muscle by means of a needle lead and changes very little with contractions of different effort. The comparison of 300 spectra from needle leads and of 50 spectra from surface leads shows the following: (1) the peak frequency is the most steady parameter (185–228 c/sec in 78–87% of cases); (2) the frequency of respectively 1/2, 1/3 and 1/10 peak value varies within broader limits (1/2: 64–70% at 347–428 c/sec; 1/3: 69–70% at 428–527 c/sec; 1/10: 73–81% at 656–989 c/sec; (3) the frequency spectra from surface leads are concentrated in the lower frequency bands. The authors emphasize the importance of examining at least 3–5 points of each muscle with needle electrodes.

23. A system for automatic processing of neuro-myoelectric data. — F. Denoth, G. Musolino, P. Antognetti and F. Ferro Milone (Pisa).

A quantitative and uniform analysis of neuro-myoelectric information can be usefully performed with the techniques of automatic computation. In order to be able to use this technique the information must be presented in numerical form. Besides, the continuing development of analysis techniques makes it necessary for information to be recorded without any decrease in the original information content so as to allow maximum flexibility in the processing.

With this in mind, a system has been worked out for processing on a digital computer the neuro-myoelectric information, formerly recorded on analogue magnetic tape. The system consists of an analogue-processing unit, an analogue-digital conversion unit and a timing unit. The analogue unit performs linear and non-linear amplification and the bandpass filtering of the signal. The conversion unit periodically samples the resulting signal and codes each sample into words of six bits. The timing unit is employed to measure the time interval between given events such as reaching some peak amplitude or crossing a predetermined threshold. The time interval is coded into words of twelve bits.

The output units are a tape puncher which punches at a rate of 110/sec, a magnetic digital tape unit, a plotter with a digital control and a CRT. The tape puncher and the magnetic digital tape unit are used for the output of digital data. The plotter and CRT are used either for displaying the results of processing or for monitoring the conversion process.

The system now described is currently utilized for analysing EEG, EMG and other data.

24. 24-hour sleep cycles and sleep stages in cats. — F. Angeleri, A. Quattrini and G. Zucconi (Perugia).

Continuous 24 h polygraphic recordings have been carried out on 27 adult cats with chronically implanted dural or bony electrodes for EEG, depth electrodes in the hippocampus, electrodes to monitor ocular movements and insulated stainless steel wires in the neck muscles for EMG studies. During the whole period of recording the animal remained in a cage which reproduced exactly, in form and dimension, the cage where the animal had previously spent some time (30–60 days). The animals were not isolated acoustically or visually but additional stimuli were avoided. Eight cats in the group had a second 24 h record during which stimuli were used to arouse their interest. A statistical study of the recurrence of waking, light and deep sleep polygraphic patterns has allowed us to compare the differences between the average percentages calculated for the entire 24 h day and for periods of 4 h. A similar comparison has also been made between the average percentages calculated on tracings recorded in the undisturbed 24 h and those recorded during the stimulated 24 h.

25. Unusual EEG findings during intermittent photic stimulation in a patient with hemiparkinsonism. — G. Dello Ioio and A. Amati (Naples).

In a female subject, affected by left hemiparkinsonism, intermittent photic stimulation was carried out. In all EEG leads synchronous and symmetrical responses appeared which had a constant time relationship with each flash (beginning from 1/sec). Myoclonic responses appeared at 20 flashes/sec but neither epileptic seizures nor disturbances of consciousness were observed. It was noticed that these EEG findings appeared to be related to the evolution of the neurological disease because the EEG responses to intermittent photic stimulation were maximal and most regular when the extrapyramidal clinical features were more evident.

26. Power spectrum analysis of the effect of aescine on the EEG activity in intracranial hypertension. — F. Ferrillo, P. Lavarello, C. Rivano and G. Rosadini (Genoa).

A power spectrum analysis has been made of the EEG of patients suffering from intracranial hypertension of different kinds and recorded before, during and after treatment with aescine. (1) In the EEG recorded before treatment there was a poverty of organized alpha activity. Both rhythmic and non-rhythmic slow (delta) EEG activities were present, the latter being recorded from the region of cerebral anatomical damage, the former at a distance. (2) Following treatment with aescine a marked reduction or disappearance of the rhythmic slow activity occurred; the non-rhythmic slow activity did not change and even increased. Moreover, the alpha rhythm increased or appeared in the cases in which it was not previously present.

27. Automatic analysis of the discharge rate of motor units during voluntary contraction. — F. Ferro-Milone, A. Starita, C. C. Perfetti and F. Denoth (Pisa).

The voluntary activity of single motor units was recorded in the extensor digitorum communis with a bipolar needle (DISA 9013K0131) in 20 normal subjects aged 20–25 years. Each patient maintained a steady muscular contraction for about 15 min under proprioceptive, auditory or visual control of the motor unit discharge rate; afterwards the rate of discharge was voluntarily modified by means of the same auditory control signal. About 8000 spikes were recorded from each motor unit on magnetic analogue tape; the time interval between peaks was measured and converted into numerical binary data and recorded on digital tape. Such data were then computed, using an IBM/7090, and (a) means, (b) variances, (c) interval histograms and (d) conditional probabilities were calculated under different experimental conditions.

28. Exhaustion of neuromuscular transmission in a case of atypical paramyotonia with hypertrophy of the thymus. — D. Gambi and P. Tonali (Rome).

A 39-year-old female patient has suffered since infancy from a myotonic syndrome with special features. Clinically, on relaxation, the myotonic phenomenon (after contraction) is obvious in the orbicularis oculi muscles. EMG studies show typical myotonic features even at the level of the limb muscles. Percussion myotonia is not present. Voluntary contraction is initially effective but the strength diminishes with the prolongation of the exertion during the first contraction; the strength returns progressively to normal with repeated contractions.

Supramaximal stimulation of the motor nerves at a frequency greater than 5/sec elicits at rest a decrease in the amplitude of the muscle action potential. The rate of decrease is greater and earlier, the higher the frequency of stimulation. The i.v. injection of 10 mg of Tensilon does not prevent such a decrease in the muscle action potential. This decrease does not occur if stimulation is performed in the phase of complete recovery of the energy of voluntary contraction after the initial exhaustion (instead of being applied at rest). This phenomenon of exhaustion is not observed in the orbicularis oculi muscles. Change of temperature, particularly cold, does not modify either the muscular performance or the intensity of the myotonic phenomenon. The histological findings (biopsy of quadriceps) are normal. Radiologically hypertrophy of the thymus was observed.

The clinical data and the EMG findings are discussed in connection with myotonia congenita, dystrophia myotonica, paramyotonia congenita and myasthenia with myotonic features.

29. Automatic multi-exponential analysis of adaptive autonomic regulation (cardiorhythmogram). — S. Gandini, F. Denoth and E. Gandini-Collodel (Pisa).

The analysis of homeostatic regulation of the autonomic nervous system in man was studied through the variations of heart rhythm. For this purpose the EKG was recorded on analogue magnetic tape and then converted into numerical data by means of suitable apparatus. Besides the parameters arising from the examination by conventional techniques (mean heart rate in both upright and horizontal positions, their differential value, and the modifications during movement), we have taken into account other parameters which will be used for a comparative evaluation and classification of clinical patterns. From the function of the interval between two successive heart beats (the cardiorhythmogram) it has been possible to extract and isolate by automatic analysis damped oscillatory responses (Selbach's relaxation oscillations). This pattern is a reliable index of the adaptive behaviour of the autonomic system to an external stimulus.

The programme was developed in three successive steps. The first consisted in recording the heart rhythm on analogue magnetic tape. The second involved the conversion of the intervals between successive heart beats into numerical data suitable for the computer. The last was an averaging process between three successive "orthoclinostatic" cycles in order to reduce accidental fluctuations. The following multi-exponential "fitting" gave seven parameters used for classifying both physiological and pathological patterns of heart rhythm.

30. Effects of ablation of the olfactory bulbs in very young rats. — S. Giammanco, V. La Grutta, V. Tessitore and C. Di Bernardo (Palermo).

Very young male and female rats with complete ablation of the olfactory bulbs were kept under observation for 3 months after the ablation and compared with control animals of the same age. The following changes were noted: (1) a decrease of daily food intake, of body weight and body length (from the occiput to the insertion of the tail) especially in male rats; (2) a delayed development of the uterus and the uterine horns, which were about half the normal; (3) no appreciable alteration of the volume and weight of the testicles and the seminal vesicles; (4) a marked atrophy of the thyroid gland, but no volume changes in the other glands tested (hypophysis, adrenal glands and gonads); (5) decreased aggression and reaction in relation to nociceptive stimuli.

31. Influence of temporal paroxysmal EEG discharges and epileptogenic lesions on conditioned responses obtainable in man by auditory stimuli. — R. Zappoli (Florence).

The development of first order conditioned responses has been studied in a group of 21 carefully selected subjects with unilateral temporal lobe epileptogenic lesions, well localized and confirmed by EEG (frequent focal discharges with little tendency to spread) and neuroradiological examinations.

It has been noted that temporal lobe epileptic discharges of brief duration do not in any way influence the conditioned responses obtained with combined sound-nociceptive stimulation either in their central (alpha blocking reaction) or peripheral (somato-vegetative) components. When, instead, the discharge produced by an epileptogenic lesion localized in the auditory cortical analyser tends to be prolonged, becoming pseudo-rhythmic, (even if it is apparently subclinical and strictly limited) it sometimes causes the temporary suppression or disorganization of the conditioned responses. In general this occurs without modifying the effects of the nociceptive stimuli. This "deconditioning" effect of the temporal epileptic discharges appears more noticeable and constant if the conditioned responses are evoked by the presentation of auditory stimuli to the sensory organ with primary projection to the cortical area involved in the prolonged paroxysmal activity (ear on the opposite side of the temporal epileptogenic focus). This temporary inhibition produced by the discharges (even when strictly unilateral) is not always rapidly reversible and this phenomenon sometimes tends to persist for some seconds.

The second problem concerns the negative influence shown by certain epileptogenic lesions on these kinds of conditioned responses when the lesion is localized in a primary cortical area for conditioning of auditory stimuli, especially when the stimulation is presented to the ear opposite the lesion. What is most impaired in these cases is the power to discriminate between positive conditioning stimuli (constantly reinforced) and negative stimuli (unreinforced differential stimuli).

As we have observed, the validity of the results obtained by Morrell with monkeys has been demonstrated in 4 subjects before and after the surgical excision of temporal lobe epileptogenic lesions. An ample ablation of the cortical area involved has produced in 3 of these patients an improvement in their ability to form conditioned responses and in particular in their capacity to discriminate between positive and negative conditioning stimuli. This confirms Morrell's hypothesis that this kind of negative influence demonstrated by irritative cortical lesions is related to their specifically epileptogenic character and not as a simple consequence of the destruction of nervous tissue due to scarring.

32. Study of the effect of Mogadon on the visual cortical responses to photic stimuli in the cat. — J. Zattoni (Genoa).

Twenty-seven adult cats have been studied (22 acute and 5 chronic preparations). The responses evoked by single visual stimuli were recorded from two or more electrodes placed on the dura overlying cortical areas 17 and 18; both bipolar and unipolar montages (reference electrode on the mandibular bone) were recorded simultaneously. The evoked responses were recorded on magnetic tape and electronically summated in groups of 30–50. Single evoked responses were also recorded on an oscilloscope and photographed. The effects produced by an i.v. injection of Mogadon (1–2 mg and in some cases 2.2–4 mg) were as follows: (1) the response recorded bipolarly from cortical areas 17 and 18 showed a decrease in amplitude in 80% of the cases; (2) the response unipolarly recorded from area 17 showed an increase in amplitude in 70% of the cases; from area 18 there was a decrease in amplitude in 76% of cases; (3) there were no significant changes in the latency of the initial components of the response but there was an increase in the latency of the late components.

The following paper was inadvertently omitted from the Proceedings of the meeting held in Rome on October 21, 1967.

Modifications of the evoked responses during the conditioning process. — C. Morocutti and J. A. Sommer-Smith (Siena).

The potentials evoked by acoustic stimuli recorded from the acoustic, visual and sensori-motor cortices, from the medial geniculate body, from the hippocampus, from the centro-median nucleus of thalamus and from the mesencephalic reticular formation were studied during the stages of the conditioning process (habituation, reinforcement and extinction) in a series of cats with chronically implanted electrodes, using a Mnemotron CAT 400 computer.

During habituation the voltage of the secondary component of these responses usually appeared to be correlated with the EEG voltage. In some cases reductions of amplitude were observed in the cortical responses and in the responses of the centro-median nucleus. During reinforcement an increase of voltage was recorded in some cases when an alarm reaction occurred, mainly from the cortex. This increase was greater in the cortical area receiving the afferent impulses from the unconditioned stimulus (sensori-motor cortex). During extinction an inconstant diminution of the voltage of the evoked potentials was observed, more evident in the acoustic and sensori-motor cortices and in the centro-median nucleus.

No significant correlation between the morphology of the evoked potentials and the state of learning was recorded. Rather, the modifications of voltage appeared to be correlated with the state of alarm and with the characteristics of the basal EEG. With reference to these data, the authors discussed the significance that the modifications of the evoked potentials can have in the neurophysiological mechanisms of the learning process.

Electroenceph. clin. Neurophysiol., **1969,** *27*: 96–103

Electroencephalography and Clinical Neurophysiology
Elsevier Publishing Company, Amsterdam – Printed in The Netherlands

JOINT MEETING OF L'ASSOCIATION D'EEG ET DE NEUROPHYSIOLOGIE CLINIQUE SUISSE and LA SOCIÉTÉ D'ÉLECTROENCÉPHALOGRAPHIE ET DE NEUROPHYSIOLOGIE CLINIQUE DE LANGUE FRANÇAISE

Basel, October 1–2, 1968

Secretaries: DR. H. J. BEIN
Biologische Abteilung, Ciba, A.G., 4000 Basel (Switzerland)

and

DR. G. C. LAIRY
Hôpital Henri-Rousselle, 1, rue Cabanis, Paris 14 (France)

1. Some aspects of the biochemical pharmacology of psychotropic drugs. — L. Maître (Basel, Switzerland).

A review is given of the metabolism of noradrenaline and its alterations by some typical psychoactive drugs, such as reserpine, chlorpromazine, imipramine and chlorodiazepoxide.

Noradrenaline uptake-release experiments were carried out *in vitro* on isolated nerve amine storage granules or *in vivo* by estimating the fate of intravenously or intracisternally administered [^{3}H]noradrenaline. These techniques allow to differentiate clearly between an inhibition of the noradrenaline uptake by the nerve cell membrane and an inhibition of the noradrenaline uptake at the level of subcellular amine storage granules.

The relationship between the *in vivo* effects of these drugs on the noradrenaline uptake by isolated nerve granules, and the effects observed *in vivo*, is outlined. Furthermore, it is shown that many *in vivo* effects of psychotropic drugs, such as the noradrenaline depleting action of reserpine or the inhibition of the noradrenaline uptake through the nerve cell membrane caused by imipramine, are in many respects similar in peripheral and central sympathetic adrenergic neurones.

Methods for studying the turnover rate of catecholamines in the brain are presented, such as the rate of transformation of tyrosine into catecholamines, the rate of disappearance of the endogenous catecholamine stores after blockade of their biosynthesis and the rate of disappearance of radioactive amines after labelling the endogenous stores. Chlorpromazine is shown as a typical example of a drug affecting the catecholamine turnover, without greatly impairing uptake or storage mechanisms. The estimation of the turnover rate in the brain is emphasized, since it reflects at least partly the nervous impulse flow in the central catecholaminergic neurones.

2. Usefulness and prospects of EEG in psychopharmacology. — G. Verdeaux (Paris, France).

For the last 15 years the progress of psychiatric therapy has been closely related with that of psychopharmacology. EEG was naturally used at the beginning of this period to test the action of psychotropic drugs and then, as their different actions gradually became known, to define possible contra-indications and try to determine their dosage. At present the EEG in psychopharmacology is a means of daily control and experience is sufficient to define its usefulness and propose some principles. At the same time, as the drugs multiply and become more specific, there develop investigations, the prospects and values of which will be considered.

3. Pharmacological differentiation of sedative drugs. — K. Dixon and M. Taeschler (Basel, Switzerland).

Activity profiles were constructed for thioridazine, diazepam, phenobarbital and promethazine on the basis of their action in the mouse and rat. Tests adopted in the mouse were: (a) impairment of rota-rod performance; (b) inhibition of spontaneous locomotor activity; (c) inhibition of amphetamine-induced excitation; (d) antagonism to pentylenetetrazol tonic convulsions; and in the rat (e) modification of amphetamine induced stereotypy; (f) facilitation of, and (g) inhibition of, a conditioned avoidance response; (h) inhibition of emotional defaecation.

Evaluation of the four drugs showed that each possessed a characteristic pattern of sedation. Thus, thioridazine exerted its sedative action predominantly through an anti-excitatory component, together with a certain anti-emotional effect. Promethazine, on the other hand, exhibited a non-specific over-all sedation. Considerable overlap occurred between diazepam and phenobarbital, both of which exerted an anticonvulsant action and facilitated the conditioned avoidance response in low doses. The latter property is probably attributable to the phenomenon of "disinhibition" and suggests that the particular form of sedation induced by these two compounds is based on a "disinhibiting" effect. The possible significance of the "disinhibitory" phenomenon and its relationship to anticonvulsant and anti-anxiety properties is discussed.

4. Electrographic and behavioural effects of several psychodysleptic drugs on free cats. — A. Rougeul, J. Verdeaux and A. Letalle (Paris, France).

Electrical and behavioural effects of two groups of hallucinogenic drugs were compared on free implanted cats. (a) Anticholinergics like atropine and Ditran (ethotrimeprazine) elicited a typical ECoG of slow sleep, in spite of uninterrupted pacing. (b) On the other hand, drugs like mescaline, psilocybin and LSD-25 induced a typical ECoG of the drowsy state, with suppression of slow sleep (*i.e.*, sustained rhythms at 4–7/sec, without the appearance of spindles at 12–18 c/sec) in spite of hyperattentive behaviour. A tentative study was also performed to correlate psychodysleptic action of the second type with chemical structure. Six drugs were synthesized, with structures intermediate between mescaline and psilocybin. Two of them (CT 4719 and 5172) had approximately the same effects on ECoG and behaviour as these three classical psychodysleptics. On the other hand, the four others (CT 5126, 4864, 4820) were inactive, in spite of their very similar structure.

5. Organization of sleeping and waking in the cat during the 24 hours: pharmacological changes. — M. Baldy-Moulinier, G. Dapres and P. Passouant (Montpellier, France).

A study of the action of various pharmacodynamic substances on the organization of waking and sleeping was made in 12 cats with indwelling electrodes by continuous recording for several days (6–20). To evaluate the pharmacological changes the organization of sleeping and waking was first studied in the normal cat. The total durations during the 24 hours of waking, slow sleep and fast sleep were practically identical for all the animals. The organization of these three states varied from one animal to another but some indication of periodicity was nevertheless found. The substances studied were: 5-HT, reserpine, nialamide, chlorimipramine and hydergine. The effects were as follows: (1) increase in the duration of waking with decrease in the durations of both types of sleep (reserpine) or only of slow sleep (hydergine); (2) decrease or suppression of fast sleep (5-HT, nialamide, chlorimipramine) with increase of slow sleep and secondary rebound of fast sleep with 5-HT. With nialamide and chlorimipramine prolonged suppression of fast sleep did not result in disturbances of behaviour, and recovery from fast sleep was progressive without rebound. The organization of sleeping and waking during the 24 hours in the cat was discussed. The changes obtained for each of the five different pharmacological substances showed the value of prolonged studies during the 24 hours to demonstrate the effect of drugs on waking and sleeping and to separate the action of each of the drugs on the central nervous system.

6. Modification of spontaneous and evoked activity of hippocampal and lateral geniculate neurones by nitrazepam and phenobarbital. — F. A. Steiner and P. Hummel (Basel and Zurich, Switzerland).

An attempt was made to differentiate the effects of nitrazepam (1,3-dihydro-7-nitro-5-phenyl-[2H]-1,4-benzodiazepin-2-one) and phenobarbital, locally and systemically applied, on single unit activity and single unit response to visual stimulation in the hippocampal formation and in the lateral geniculate body of cats anaesthetized with chloralose–urethane. On *local application* (micro-electrophoresis) in both regions nitrazepam had no depressant effect, but influenced the pattern of spontaneous discharge: a tendency to form bursts of spikes was noted; whereas phenobarbital strongly depressed neuronal activity. On *systemic application* (i.v. injection) nitrazepam had a short (0.5–2.5 min) transitory depressing action on spontaneous activity in both regions and phenobarbital depressed spontaneous activity for a relatively long time (up to more than 60 min). Nitrazepam abolished unit responses to visual stimulation in the hippocampal formation; after phenobarbital, in contrast, no abolition but gradually reduction was seen. In the lateral geniculate body after nitrazepam the unit responses to visual stimulation remained uninfluenced or were somewhat reduced; after phenobarbital the extent of this sensory response was gradually reduced.

It is concluded that nitrazepam reduces the sensory input to the hippocampal formation by specifically depressing the projecting systems for afferent sensory information. Phenobarbital, in contrast, unspecifically depresses the neuronal activity in both examined structures.

7. Demonstration by a screening method of the exceptional anti-convulsant properties of a new benzodiazepine. — H. Gastaut, J. Catier, C. Dravet and J. Roger (Marseille, France).

Four new benzodiazepines synthetized by Hoffman-La Roche (RO 5–4200, RO 5–4023, RO 5–3453 and RO 5–3350) were compared with diazepam (Valium) and nitrazepam (Mogadon) for their effects (by the i.v. route) on the epileptic outbursts: (a) provoked by slow i.v. injection of Cardiazol; (b) provoked by flicker in photosensitive epileptics; and (c) spontaneously recorded in epileptics in the intervals between attacks or during status. The duration of action against Cardiazol, photo-convulsions, epilepsy and status was evaluated for each product. The results showed that RO 5–4023 was the most effective drug (5 times more effective than Valium and Mogadon) and the best tolerated, which gives it a great future in the treatment of status epilepticus. As, furthermore, it has been shown to have a definite action on epileptic attacks when given by mouth, it can be accepted that it represents a particularly effective weapon against chronic epilepsy as well as against status epilepticus.

8. Dyskinetic reactions to phenothiazine drugs and cryptotetany. — H. R. Müller and H. E. Kaeser (Basel, Switzerland).

Based on the observation of Schaaf and Payne that in patients with hypoparathyroidism there were constantly dystonic and dyskinetic reactions to small doses of prochlorperazine, the authors investigated a group of patients presenting similar side-effects of neuroleptic drugs, with special regard to the presence of tetanic signs.

The series consists of 7 subjects between 19 and 36 years of age; 6 had shown dystonic reactions to thiethylperazine and one to thiopropazate. The side-effects in question had been observed 3 months to 3 years before the present investigation. On examination there were no neurological signs .The values of calcium, magnesium and phosphate were within normal limits; in each case, however, the EMG of m. abductor digiti V during hyperventilation showed doublets, triplets or multiplets, so that the diagnosis of hyperventilation-tetany could be made.

9. Comparative experimental electrographic study of the anticonvulsant properties of a new derivative of the benzodiazepines RO 5-4023. — R. Poiré and J. Royer (Nancy, France).

In their researches in man on the possible anticonvulsant properties of many substances by studying possible changes in the paroxysmal photic responses in the EEG, natural or not (1962) the authors were particularly interested in the benzodiazepine derivatives injected i.v. RO 5–0690 (chlordiazepoxide, 1962), which was found to be active against evoked paroxysms in a dose 10 times less than that of trimethadione (taken as reference), was rapidly followed by other derivatives active in doses still approximately 10 times less without increase of toxicity, particularly RO 5–2807 (diazepam, 1963), RO 4–5360 (nitrazepam, 1965). Among the derivatives at present being studied RO 5–4023 is particularly interesting since it consistently blocks the evoked paroxysms and the associated clinical changes at a dose 10 times less than that of diazepam (of the order of a mg) with an equally low toxicity. In the EEG, as with the previous derivatives, low voltage fast rhythms appear and sometimes secondary slow activity at the same time as a lowering of behavioural alertness. As could be predicted from the experimental study, the immediate action of RO 5–4023 on spontaneous epileptic paroxysms is particularly striking in relation to generalized attacks and in status epilepticus.

10. The treatment of generalized epilepsy by Acrisuxine. — A. Beaumanoir and F. Martin (Geneva, Switzerland).

Acrisuxine, the combination of a synthetized quinine with a succinimide, was used for 9 months in 6 cases of particularly severe Lennox syndrome. A homologous group of subjects in the same conditions received a placebo. An analytical and statistical study of the attacks was carried out by a well-trained team. Simultaneously with diurnal and nocturnal EEGs, psychotechnical and biochemical investigations were made. With average doses of 3 capsules daily (equivalent to 450 mg of Suxinutine per day) control was obtained, very satisfactorily in comparison with all other drugs previously prescribed, of the non-convulsive attacks, such as true absences or the absences of petit mal variant. Thus, in cases of severe epileptogenic encephalopathy with frequent non-convulsive epileptic attacks, Acrisuxine at the present time seems to us to be a suitable drug, well tolerated and effective in smaller doses than the Suxinutine which is one of its components. Our tests make it possible to recommend for the Lennox syndrome a therapy consisting principally of Acrisuxine, of derivatives of diazepam (Valium or Mogadon) and of barbiturates associated with belladona or with a psycho-amine.

11. The value of the EEG in the treatment of behavioural disturbances in children. — R. Kuhn (Münsterlingen, Switzerland).

200 children suffering from disturbed behaviour were examined by EEG. A hundred of them seemed to have clinically mainly organic damage; 100 others mainly depressive. Feeble-minded children and those whose mentally disturbed conduct could easily be explained by the clinical picture, were not taken into consideration.

Among the children with rather organic damage one-third of the cases presented unequivocal pathological EEGs, partly epileptic, partly unspecific diffuse alterations. In most cases these patients showed a favourable reaction when an anti-epileptic treatment was applied, even when there were no clinical symptoms of epilepsy. Normal EEGs were found in one-third of the 100 children showing depressive states. These patients gave the best reaction to anti-depressive therapy. In the remaining cases the EEGs showed mental retardation and unspecific abnormalities. It was not possible to derive from the EEGs evidence for the kind of treatment which might give the most successful result.

These investigations show that a normal EEG can have — for diagnosis and treatment of a sick child — exactly the same importance as an abnormal or pathological one.

12. Changes in the EEG during metabolic disturbances. — M. F. Radvanyi and C. Dreyfus-Brisac (Paris, France).

The material studied consisted of: 4 cases of Schwartz-Bartter syndrome, 4 cases of hypernatraemia, 7 cases of dyskalaemia and 13 cases of acute renal insufficiency.

A significant hyponatraemia (118–130 mequiv/l) was well tolerated in the Schwartz-Bartter cases from the clinical and EEG points of view. On the other hand, dehydration, with return of the biochemical values to normal, twice led to electro-clinical disturbances. This emphasizes the danger of a rapid biochemical readjustment.

Hypernatraemia (163–174 mequiv/l) was equally well tolerated, except in a case of acute accidental overdose leading to a reversible coma (in the EEG diffuse slow waves disappeared progressively in 15 days).

The dyskalaemias, in 4 cases out of 7, led to disturbances of the EEG characterized by triphasic slow waves and superimposed sharp waves.

The acute renal insufficiencies (13 cases of which 12 were due to post-operative collapse and one to Osler's endocarditis) were divided into 2 groups according to whether or not they were treated with large doses of penicillin. Among the untreated subjects, all after operation (6 cases), 5 had EEGs characterized by increased slow activity. Among the treated subjects (7 cases) of which 6 were after operation, 6 showed a special EEG picture: diffuse sharp theta and delta activity of large amplitude, 3 times accompanied by irregular clonus or generalized attacks. The toxic role of penicillin was confirmed in 2 cases by cessation of the paroxysmal changes after stopping penicillin, although the blood urea remained at a high level.

13. Histamine as a waking factor (Validity of evoked potentials in psychopharmacology). — M. Monnier and R. Sauer (Basel, Switzerland).

Extracorporeal haemodialysis, performed according to the technique of Monnier and Hösli (1964), showed that histamine is to be found in different proportions in the dialysates of experimentally induced sleep and arousal. This fact led to the study of the action of histamine on wakefulness.

A solution of *histamine* di-hydrochloride at a concentration of 1 mg/30 ml was infused into the jugular vein of conscious rabbits during 30 min. The delta activities were automatically analysed and the evoked potentials averaged by a Mnemotron computer (CAT).

A decrease of the spontaneous delta activities was observed, symptomatic of an arousal reaction. Furthermore, an increase in amplitude of the first component of the potentials evoked by stimulation of the reticulo-cortical, hippocampo-cortical and thalamo-cortical systems suggests an activating reticular and hippocampal mechanism, similar to that resulting from infusion of amphetamine and opposed to that of chlorpromazine. The waking effect of histamine is not due to primary visceral reactions (as shown by recordings of the blood pressure, ECG and EPG), but possibly to stimulation of visceral afferent systems, acting on the reticular formation and hippocampus.

Analysis of the cortical potentials evoked by stimulation of certain subcortical systems is of practical use in psychopharmacology provided that the variations of the first positive component be clearly distinguished from those of the second negative component. Therefore, the evoked potentials should never be measured from peak to peak. This specification of Tissot and Monnier (1959) concerning the thalamo-cortical evoked response and the reticular excitatory mechanism of the first component is confirmed by the present computer analysis.

14. The prognostic value of the EEG during the first two years of life. — N. Monod and P. Ducas (Paris, France).

The results of a systematic longitudinal study of 161 children born at term were presented. These children were followed from the clinical, psychological and EEG points of view from the neonatal period to an age varying from 3 to 11 years. Two aspects of this study will be discussed: the prognostic value of the normal EEG and the electrical abnormalities found during the first years.

1. *The prognostic value of the neonatal record* of the child born at or before term should not be ignored. In fact, out of a total of 313 records taken during the first days, 93 % of the very pathological records were recorded in children who subsequently had an unfavourable evolution (severe neuro-psychic sequelae or even death) whereas 72 of the newborns who had normal records had a satisfactory clinical evolution. However, severe disorders such as mongolism or kernicterus were not accompanied by significant electrical abnormalities during the neonatal period. Furthermore, there was no obvious relationship between neonatal electrical disturbances and the appearance of a late isolated epilepsy or of minor sequels. The prognostic value of the neonatal EEG is maximal during the first week and diminishes after the end of the second week.

2. *Paroxysmal abnormalities of the first two years* (hypsarrhythmia, spikes and focal spikes and waves) and the absence of maturation are related to the abnormalities of the neonatal period and have a bad prognostic significance. However, no special electrical or maturational abnormalities appeared during the first 2 years in a small group of children who subsequently became epileptic. Some paroxysmal abnormalities were recorded in normal children followed for more than 8 years.

15. Neuropathy and hyperthyroidism. — H. P. Ludin, J. Spiess and M. P. Koenig (Berne, Switzerland).

Thirteen patients presenting clinically and biochemically unquestionable hyperthyroidism underwent neurological and EMG examination. Eight of these patients showed slight to marked weakness of proximal muscles, 3 of them had in addition mild atrophies of these muscles. The distal muscles in the lower extremities were slightly paretic in 4 cases, in 2 of them with mild atrophies. No significant sensory disturbance could be found and the tendon reflexes were diminished in only one case. EMG showed definite signs of myopathy in proximal muscles of 10 patients. In these muscles no indications of neurogenic lesions could be observed. In the small foot muscles, however, such changes were found in 8 cases. No slowing of motor nerve conduction velocity has been observed. Six out of 7 patients with a neurogenic EMG had normal sensory conduction times and normal nerve action potentials in the distal segment of the ulnar nerve. Only in one case was this potential of low voltage and highly polyphasic. Besides the well-known myopathic changes in patients with hyperthyroidism, the number of neurogenic lesions found in this study is surprisingly high. The authors suppose that it is the expression of subclinical polyneuropathy associated with thyrotoxicosis.

16. Aetiology of the carpal tunnel syndrome. — J. Lefebvre, S. de Seze, J. L. Lerique, C. Hamonet, P. Chaumont, B. Bigot and P. Dreyfus (Paris, France).

A complete electrical examination, consisting of motor and sensory conduction studies of the median nerve in the forearm and the hand, was made on 115 hands in 88 subjects with compression of the median nerve at the carpal tunnel. Our results showed that, in a first group of 54 hands exhibiting a carpal tunnel syndrome with neurological deficit in the median territory of the hand, the electrical examination demonstrated slowing of the motor and sensory conduction, or both, in 90.7% of the cases. In the second group of 61 carpal tunnel syndromes with acroparaesthesiae alone this slowing was present in 25.6% of the cases. Electrical examination is a guide to therapy (a distal motor latency of more than 8 msec is an absolute indication for operation) and a control of the results; there is, therefore, in addition to its reliability and its diagnostic value a certain medico-legal interest.

17. Radiotelemetric EEG study of adult epileptics. — L. Vidart and S. Geier (Paris, France).

The authors summarized the results obtained from the study of 61 radiotelemetric EEG records from adult epileptics of both sexes. These recordings lasted 6 h, representing a working day in a Day Hospital for epileptics. Four conclusions were reached: the temporal distribution of the diffuse paroxysms was not always random but very often responded to variations in the subject's situation; for identical electrical discharges the disturbances of consciousness were variable, very often absent; the disturbances of tonic and motor control were as significant as the paroxysms; slowness is a variable phenomenon which constitutes the major handicap of the epileptic at work.

The authors reintroduce the concept of resistance to explain the above results. The central nervous system develops an active resistance, either permanent with slowness as a result, or at the moment of discharge. It is the variation of this resistance which explains variations in disturbances of consciousness for a given discharge. The authors conclude by defining epilepsy, not as a series of attacks but as an adjustment between the possibility of an attack and the variable resistance opposed by the subject to this instability.

18. Dynamic aspects of the human EEG. First results of a radiotelemetric study. — G. Arfel, C. Casanova and M. Coulmance (Paris, France).

The 47 subjects of this examination were selected, not according to clinical criteria, but on purely EEG grounds, based on a previous conventional EEG (peculiarities of frequency, of distribution and of reactivity of the components; occurrence of "unusual" wave forms, such as spikes and spikes and waves, paroxysmal episodes of slow waves, etc.). The procedure for this examination, the average duration of which was 3 h, was according to a simple experimental protocol. No attempt at diagnosis was made and only the "dynamic" properties of the cerebral rhythms were investigated. Their variations during the various tests were relatively limited, with special features in some of them (puzzles, listening to music). The behaviour of the open-eyed alpha rhythm depended on its various types, the underlying psychophysiological causes of which were not elucidated (occipital alpha rhythm, propagated alpha rhythm, bursts of alpha rhythm). The occurrence of the "unusual" wave forms did not seem to be particularly favoured by the chosen experimental procedure; however, some examples of facilitation of these wave forms were reported. In spite of the relatively limited findings, this first investigation was sufficiently fruitful to justify continuing the research.

19. Neuromyotonia. — H. E. Kaeser and F. Corbat (Basel, Switzerland).

Description of a 60-year-old male with generalized muscle hypertrophy, clumsiness, increased fatigability and continuous fasciculations in all muscles. On EMG examination continuous fasciculations, either single or at high repetition rates, and of various shapes and durations, a normal interference pattern on voluntary effort and a delayed relaxation with after-discharges are noted. All clinical and EMG symptoms disappear during administration of Tegretol or diphenylhydantoin. The syndrome is likely to be identical with those described as "continuous muscle fibre activity" or "syndrome fibrillaire", although those cases were described in children or young adults who developed also contractures.

20. Recording sensory action potentials of the finger nerves by use of a special needle electrode. — H. R. Müller and G. Muheim (Basel, Switzerland).

A special needle electrode was used for bipolar recording of the sensory action potentials of single finger nerves. It consists of two platinum needles fixed vertically 10 mm apart in a plastic plate, with an exposed length of 2.5 mm. The two needle points are stuck into the middle phalanx lengthwise to the volar finger nerve. The whole electrode is then fixed with adhesive plaster to the finger.

The innervation of the fingers was studied in 20 hands of healthy subjects by antidromic stimulation of the median and ulnar nerves at the wrist. In 18 cases the 4th finger proved to be innervated by both the median and ulnar nerves, the action potential of the radial side showing a larger amplitude when the median nerve was stimulated, and that of the ulnar side when stimulation of the ulnar nerve was done. In 3 cases this double innervation concerned also the third finger.

In a separate series the authors checked 61 finger nerve lesions at the finger base or in the palm 2–8 years after the accident. Most nerves had been sutured. In only 2 cases the sensory nerve action potential reached its normal value; in 25 cases it was strongly reduced, and in 23 cases it could not be recorded at all. Comparison with the ninhydrin reaction and with two point discrimination showed that the evoked action potential of the finger nerves was more sensitive for functional testing.

21. Separation of the various independent phenomena among the slow potential changes (contingent negative variations). — M. Dongier (Liège, Belgium).

In the phenomenon first described by Walter (1964) the slow deflection is by definition contingent on the association of two stimuli, of which the first is imperative. It has been designated the E wave (expectancy wave). Although fairly often visible at the vertex in the primary record without summation, it escapes detection by the routine EEG technique because of the need to use a very long time constant to demonstrate it. The "Bereitschaftspotential" or I wave (intention wave) of Kornhuber and Deecke (1965) does not depend on the association of stimuli but *precedes* (by about a second) a voluntary action.

We propose to separate, under the name of C wave, (conflicting wave) a wave, also surface negative, seen electivity in psychiatric patients after the imperative stimulus. It can be demonstrated in the classical experiment for investigating the E wave, appearing as a prolongation of it, but also when averaging sequences which only include a single stimulus (imperative), as shown by Timsit *et al.* in our laboratory. It is then different from the E wave and in fact a minority of subjects without visible E waves have a well developed C wave. It is as if the act of responding adequately and rapidly to the imperative stimulus does not lead to the normal return to the baseline after action or decision, a phenomenon which could be related either to the inter-personal conflict (the response, though objectively satisfying, is not so subjectively because of the ambivalence of the subject and of the difficulty of fitting it into the symbolic scheme) or to a neurophysiological disturbance hitherto undetermined.

The diagnostic value of the C wave in psychiatry appears to be very high, superior to that of the E wave. (The latter in fact is more closely linked to transitory psychophysiological factors such as attention and motivation, than to the psychiatric diagnosis.) A combined study of the E and C waves (very easy in the same experiment) gives still better results and in our view constitutes the best neurophysiological test at present available in the psychiatric clinic (Timsit *et al.* 1968).

22. Study of vestibular habituation in the pendular test. — M. Collard, C. Conraux and M. S. Thiebaut (Strasbourg, France).

A very general physiological phenomenon in the living being, habituation is defined for the vestibular apparatus as a diminution in responses following repeated stimulation. After reviewing the different classical stages of this habituation (acquisition, retention and transfer) the authors mention that numerous experimental works have shown that it is a central phenomenon. Its investigation in disease can easily be carried out thanks to the pendular rotation test. In making two successive tests an important change in the electronystagmographic response is seen in a number of cases, both quantitatively (diminution of amplitude, increase in frequency of the nystagmus, change in the slope of the slow component, reduction of tonic movement and increase of threshold) and qualitatively (irregularity of the ENG, disturbance of sensation). Habituation is never found in normal subjects. It is very rare in peripheral lesions. On the other hand, it is frequent and significant with central lesions, notably vertebro-basilar insufficiencies, cranial trauma and drug intoxications.

23. Choice of binocular and monocular derivations in electronystagmography. III. Linear, oblique and circular nystagmus. — V. Gabersek (Paris, France).

In ENG the simultaneous use of 10 derivations (2 binocular and 8 monocular) shows three types of behaviour of the eyeballs, which have been defined in terms of the graphic elements recorded during well-defined voluntary eye movements. (1) The first type is the pure classical horizontal or vertical nystagmus, which we have called linear nystagmus and which appears with identical amplitude in the two monocular horizontal (upper or lower) or vertical (nasal and temporal) traces from the same eye. (2) The second type, oblique nystagmus, is defined by the association of horizontal and vertical components. The low right or high left direction leads to diminution or even disappearance of deflections in the upper left horizontal monocular derivation and, on the contrary, in the upper right horizontal monocular derivation for a high right or low left direction. (3) The third type, circular nystagmus, represents an external or internal rotation of the eyes (around the corneo-macula axis). Its clockwise direction, defined by deflections in the horizontal and vertical binocular derivations, results in an increase of amplitude of the deflections in the upper left and lower right horizontal monocular derivations, whereas the anti-clockwise direction gives deflections of increased amplitude in the upper right and lower left horizontal monocular derivations. Each type of nystagmus can occur simultaneously in the two eyes or, of course, in one eye alone; it is also possible to see different types of nystagmus in the two eyes. Lastly, these types of nystagmus can change and follow one another during the course of a given thermal or pendular stimulus.

Electroencephalography and Clinical Neurophysiology
Elsevier Publishing Company, Amsterdam – Printed in The Netherlands

BOOK REVIEWS

Edited by H. Petsche *and* John R. Hughes

Structure and function of the limbic system. — W. R. Adey and T. Tokizane (Editors). (Elsevier, Amsterdam, 1967, 489 p., $28.00).

In a series of books on progress in brain research this one deals with the structure and function of the limbic system and consists of 25 papers which were presented by well known investigators at the symposium held at Hakone, Japan in September 1965. This collection of papers may have limited interest for those who are already acquainted with much of the material which is presented. However, it will be of special interest to those who have not had time to keep up with the literature. It is unfortunate that there is no discussion or attempt to synthesize the presentations in order to arrive at an over-all concept of the role of the limbic system in brain function. In the state of our knowledge, it may be a little premature trying to make such an attempt; however, it certainly would have been worthwhile in relation to redirecting some of our research concepts and efforts. In some instances the number of illustrations may be excessive and not of very much value, especially in relation to the additional expense which they add to the price of the book. Some of the papers are rather verbose and lengthy. The subject index would have made the book more utilizable if more attention were given to improved organization and more detail. The major theme which holds these papers together, although not stated, is to further understand the role of the limbic system in behavior in terms of its neural and chemical correlates. The variety of techniques utilized in the various investigations consists of: micro-electrode recordings, evoked potentials, cortical and subcortical EEGs, computerization, conditioning, histochemistry, pharmacologic manipulation, direct and remote brain stimulation and recording, cinephotography and gross behavioral descriptions. The following is a brief résumé of each paper by the respective authors.

Y. Oomura *et al.* found by electrophysiologic technique that the limbic system, as represented by the amygdala and septum, inhibited the lateral hypothalamus (feeding center) and facilitated the medial-ventral hypothalamus (satiation center). C. D. Clemente and M. B. Sterman, by electrical stimulation of the preoptic basal forebrain, demonstrated behavioral sleep and synchronization of the cortical EEG, typical of sleep patterns. J. M. R. Delgado stressed the feasibility of utilizing remote stimulation techniques in freely moving animals with chronically implanted electrodes. M. Kawakami *et al.* demonstrated a positive feedback control in the hippocampus and a negative feedback control in the amygdala upon ovarian progesterone formation. It was found that during estrogen dominance the hippocampal afferents to the arcuate nucleus of the hypothalamus are inhibited whereas amygdaloid afferents are facilitated. During progesterone dominance the opposite was true. R. W. Hunsperger and V. M. Bucher demonstrated flight reaction in the freely moving cat as occurring from the stimulation of stria medullaris, the bed nucleus of stria medullaris, the anterior hypothalamus and preoptic regions. H. Nakao described "switch-off behavior" in which an animal learns to press a bar in order to turn off an electrical stimulus (applied to the hypothalamus or mesencephalon), associated with flight reactions. He found that electrical stimulation of the amygdala and hippocampus even to the point of eliciting an after-discharge inhibited this switch-off behavior. J. Olds observed that hippocampal neurons responded in a control fashion prior to the emergence of the discriminated operant response. M. Egger and J. P. Flynn emphasized localization of function in the amygdala by demonstrating suppression of hypothalamically induced attack behavior during stimulation of the large celled portion of the basal amygdaloid nucleus and the antero-medial portion of the lateral nucleus. A. Costin *et al.* demonstrated that labyrinthine stimulation by clockwise rotation of the animal resulted in prolongation of hippocampal after-discharges whereas counterclockwise rotation reduced the duration of the discharges. M. R. Covian demonstrated prolonged blood pressure depression in the chloralosed cat following electrical stimulation of the septum. Vagotomy and atropine did not affect the response and it was concluded that inhibition of vaso-constrictor fibers probably was responsible. L. Pickenhain and F. Klingberg found that hippocampal slow waves appeared in all behavioral situations in which motivated behavior existed, but not in that behavior which was automatized. The more strongly motivated behavior was correlated with frequencies up to 12 c/sec whereas slightly motivated movements were related to 6–8 c/sec. W. R. Adey dealt with the general subject of hippocampal states and functional relations with cortico-subcortical systems in attention and learning. K. Lissák and E. Endröczi demonstrated that electrical stimulation of the hippocampus and amygdala interfere with the goal-directed motor activity, rather than decoding of memory mechanisms. S. S. Fox *et al.* demonstrated interaction of auditory and visual responses at the cerebellar single cell level by stimulation of the hippocampus and amygdala. Y. Yamaguchi *et al.* observed theta waves in the neocortex which were in synchrony with those in the hippocampus and postulated their hippocampal origin. The theta waves were predominantly in the occipital area and during their presence there was facilitation of the cortical evoked responses from stimulation of the medial and lateral geniculate bodies. E. S. Airapetyants and T. S. Sotnichenko emphasized the relative independence of the cingulate gyrus from the rest of the limbic system. They demonstrated efferents from the anterior cingulate to the anterior and lateral cortical region and from the posterior cingulate to the occipital cortical area. H. Niki demonstrated that hippocampectomy in the rat interfered with mechanisms of inhibition which were associated with a learned response. K. H. Pribram presented a neurologic model which included the limbic system in information processing. In this process the hippocampus may function as an inhibitory mechanism to cortical recurrent inhibition. E. F. Domino *et al.* presented further studies on cholinergic mechanisms in neocortical and limbic activating systems. Dissociation between neocortical and limbic activating systems was induced by ventricular injection of hemicholinium. R. Kido *et al.* investigated the effects of morphinan hydrobromide, a histamine-releasing compound, on behavior and EEG changes. Behaviorally, it induced sedation and sleep in cats, excitation in dogs and an intermediate effect in monkeys. K. F. Killam and E. K. Killam suggested that the role of cholinergic mechanisms in modulating sensory and motor function may take place through interactions between limbic and lemniscal systems. Anti-cholinergic drugs which block conditioned behavior, simultaneously reduced 40 c/sec activity in the amygloid complex. P. Andersen and T. Lomo demonstrated that hippocampal cell firing is in part dependent upon the frequency of the input. Frequencies of 10–12 c/sec were found to be optimal for maximal numbers of discharging hippocampal cells whereas less than 6 c/sec and greater than 15 c/sec appeared to decrease or abolish hippocampal cell firing. P. L. Parmeggiani, by studying theta rhythms, identified the thalamic nuclei where interaction takes place between hippocampal and ascending reticular system activity. The hippocampus also may influence the neocortex, without interacting with ascending reticular systems at thalamic levels, by way of the anterior ventral, the medial dorsal and the lateral dorsal nuclei of the thalamus. J. A. Gergen demonstrated that the hippocampal neuron appears to be more directly affected by afferent systems originating in the subcortical centers which project to it by way of the septal-fornix system rather than via the entorhinal area. The last paper, by P. Passouant and C. Pternitis, demonstrated that the hippocampus was more resistant to hypoxia than the cortex and that the hippocampus of the adult cat was more resistant than that of the infant.

O. J. ANDY
University of Mississippi Medical Center, Jackson, Miss. 39216 (U.S.A.)

Electroenceph. clin. Neurophysiol., **1969,** *27*: 110–111

The brain stem of the cat. — A. L. Berman. (University of Wisconsin Press, Madison, 1968, 175 p., $50.00, 477 sh.).

This will be the definitive cell atlas of the cat's brain-stem. It is too large and too lavish to be otherwise, having probably the greatest dimensions of any book in the medical sciences published in many a year: 17 by 23 inches. There are 80 large plates, 40 of which are double-page spreads. All illustrations are from photographs of cell-stained microscopic sections of the cat's brain-stem: 30 in the frontal plane, 25 sagittals and 25 horizontals. There are no fiber-stained sections or drawings. The magnification in all is 22×, and each is surrounded by a frame divided into millimeters corresponding to stereotaxic coordinates.

The photographs are virtually cell-distribution maps, and are printed without a background screen, each cell becoming a black spot. This was achieved with an electronic-scanning photo-intensifying machine. Thus, there is no distinction between light cells and dark cells, so that the solitary nucleus appears darker than the hypoglossal, and the numerous glial nuclei silt up the background much more than would the regular pattern of the 160-line halftone screen.

The various nuclei are designated by 3-letter abbreviations which are only 2 mm high, and nuclear boundaries are not drawn. Thus, the purity of the photograph is virtually unsullied.

There is no preliminary or summarizing illustrative material, no mid-sagittally cut skull with the brain included, no X-rays to project bony topography, no view of the whole head or skull. Positions of illustrated sections from the other planes are not indicated by lines on section photographs.

For witness marks, wires were placed in the brain on stereotaxic coordinates, with the head held in the machine. The brain was then removed, fixed in formalin, dehydrated (and hence demyelinated), then sectioned in celloidin. This ordinarily results in shrinkage of 20–25%, and the tract regions shrink more than the cellular masses. No statement is made of what steps were taken to compensate for this. Some stereotaxic atlas makers take great pains to compensate for shrinkage, either by photographing sawn slices of the frozen head, or by slicing the brain as it sits in the opened skull, with a razor blade held in the machine, and reading the coordinates of check points with the machine itself.

The thalamic and hypothalamic nuclei are identified in the sagittal series only, but the other series do not include the diencephalon. We understand that the expertise of Dr. Jerzy Rose was called in here, which accounts for the accuracy of the results. We cannot find what has become of nucleus reuniens and nucleus submedius, unless they are engulfed in the "ventromedial complex".

Of course, this mammoth atlas far transcends others in the detailed depiction of the brain-stem, yet nuclei have not been subdivided as far as in some papers. The large illustrations enable comparisons of sections and hence have great documentary and scientific value. If one wanted merely sets of coordinates for ordinary stereotaxic work, one of the smaller atlases, or even such papers as that of Jiminez-Castellanos would be adequate—making here no judgment on their comparative accuracies. If one wanted to know what cells might have been involved in some electrode placement, this atlas would be useful; yet without the corresponding fiber picture, one could not arrive at a complete answer.

Electroenceph. clin. Neurophysiol., **1969,** *27*: 111–112

It is difficult to escape the conclusion that such a large and expensive atlas should have included more than the cell arrangement of the cat's brain-stem below the diencephalon. Reducing the sagittals and horizontals to half a dozen each, cutting down somewhat on the dimensions and the blank paper, would have produced the savings that would permit inclusion of fiber-stained sections, cellular blow-ups, and orientation illustrations. Nevertheless, the atlas stands as a monument that will cast a long shadow.

Since the cerebral hemispheres are not included in the illustrations, it may not be so useful to the researches of electroencephalographers as to brain-stem electrophysiologists.

WENDELL J. S. KRIEG
Northwestern University Medical School, Chicago, Ill. 60611 (U.S.A.)

Electroenceph. clin. Neurophysiol., **1969,** *27*: 111–112

Neurologie des Neugeborenen.—G. Joppich und F. J. Schulte. (Springer-Verlag, Berlin–Heidelberg–New York, 1968, 648 p., 153 Fig., DM 138.00, $34.50).

This is the first full length textbook on the neurology of the newborn infant and the authors must be congratulated on their excellent work. Nineteen well balanced and clearly written chapters describe the neurophysiology of prematures and full-term babies, techniques of clinical examination of the nervous system, inborn errors of metabolism, endocrine aspects, diseases of the peripheral nerves, muscle diseases, malformations, chromosomal defects, brain tumours, electrolyte problems, brain damage occurring during the pre- and perinatal periods and pre- and post-natal infections. Despite the tremendous number of references (4342) which are quoted in the text, the authors give their own views on many problems as well. In contrast to previous books on pediatric neurology full attention is paid to EEG, evoked potentials, electromyography and nerve conduction velocity. In recent years, many contributions have been made applying these techniques to the assessment of the baby's gestational age, the early diagnosis of brain dysfunction and in studies on the effects of endocrine, metabolic and electrolyte disorders upon the nervous system. A considerable number of these important investigations has been made by one of the authors (Schulte) himself.

This book is to be highly recommended to all who are interested in the normal and abnormal nervous system of infants in their first four weeks of life.

H. F. R. PRECHTL
Department of Developmental Neurology, Groningen (The Netherlands)

Electroenceph. clin. Neurophysiol., **1969,** *27*: 112

RELATIONSHIP OF SLOW POTENTIAL CHANGES TO RESPONSE SPEED AND MOTIVATION IN MAN[1,2]

MICHAEL WASZAK, PH.D.[3] AND WALTER D. OBRIST, PH.D.

Department of Psychiatry, Duke University, Durham, N.C. 27706 (U.S.A.)

(Accepted for publication: November 1, 1968)

In 1964 Walter *et al.* presented their original observations on the "contingent negative variation" (CNV) in man, a phenomenon that has been repeatedly confirmed by subsequent experimentation (Cohen and Walter 1966; Irwin *et al.* 1966; Low *et al.* 1966; Hillyard and Galambos 1967; Walter *et al.* 1967). The usual method for eliciting this surface-negative shift employs a classical reaction time paradigm, where a warning signal (the "conditional stimulus") is followed by an imperative stimulus that serves as a signal for response. Because of the well-established fact that reaction time is shortened appreciably by the presence of a warning signal (Teichner 1957), the question arises whether the speed of response in such situations is related to the magnitude of this slow negative potential. Walter *et al.* (1964) noted a consistent reduction in reaction time during the developing phase of the CNV. This finding was later confirmed and extended by Hillyard and Galambos (1967). On the other hand, Irwin *et al.* (1966) failed to obtain significant correlations between reaction time and CNV amplitude, although a trend in the expected direction was observed.

The present investigation was designed to shed further light on the relationship between reaction time and CNV, particularly the extent to which differences in CNV amplitude are associated with variations in response speed. An attempt was made to control several variables that were left uncontrolled in earlier studies; namely, the influence of anticipation, the effects of practice, and the motivational quality of the instructions.

Unlike traditional reaction time studies, previous CNV experiments have employed a constant foreperiod, which makes it possible for the subject to anticipate precisely the time of the imperative stimulus and to initiate a response before the stimulus actually occurs. This anticipatory factor was minimized in the present study through the use of a disjunctive reaction task, in which the imperative stimulus could either be positive (respond) or negative (do not respond). Thus, for a particular warning signal, the subject had no advanced knowledge of whether a response was required or not. Prior practice was given in the CNV reaction time task in order to reduce the possibility that the observed relationship is merely a function of the parallel development of behavioral and electrical responses over time. Motivational factors influencing the correlation were tested by comparing two sets of instructions which are known to have different effects upon response speed.

METHODS

Subjects

The data of ten male college students, 18–22 years of age, are included in this report. None of the experimental subjects had any knowledge of the problem under investigation.

Procedure

The subject was seated at a table before a telegraph key which he was required to press in response to auditory stimuli delivered from a speaker 1.5 m away. An attempt was made to minimize bodily movement by placing the head

[1] Supported by Grants MH-30678 and HD-00668 from the United States Public Health Service.

[2] Based on a dissertation submitted by the senior author in partial fulfillment of requirements for the Ph.D. degree in psychology at Duke University.

[3] Present address: Department of Anatomy, University of California, Los Angeles, Calif. 90034.

in a headholder, by taping the dominant (responding) arm to a board, and by instructing the subject to press the key as lightly as possible. These precautions were taken after preliminary experiments had shown that bodily movements could significantly influence the form of the post-response slow potentials recorded from the scalp.

In early experiments the subjects performed with their eyes closed. Because this procedure often resulted in eye movement contamination of vertex potentials, later subjects were tested with their eyes open. Of the ten subjects included in this report, four gave acceptable recordings with eyes closed, while six performed with eyes open and fixated on a spot 2 m away.

An irregularly spaced series of tone pairs was presented in which a 1000 c/sec warning signal (S_1) was followed after a constant 1.0 sec interval by a second stimulus (S_2). The latter consisted of either a high (1200 c/sec) or a low (350 c/sec) frequency tone. Half of the subjects were instructed to press the key in response to the high tone and to make no movement when they heard the low tone, while the other half were told to respond only to the low and not to the high tone. The signals calling for a response (Yes-Tones) and those requiring no response (No-Tones) were presented randomly in a 3 to 2 ratio. The duration of each auditory stimulus was 150 msec.

A series of 20 practice trials was followed either by a "Speed" or a "Relax" Condition, each Condition coming first for half of the subjects. In the Speed Condition an attempt was made to motivate the subject to react as fast as possible by praising his performance and by telling him that the speed of his reactions will be compared with that of other subjects. In the Relax Condition, the subject was told that his reaction times would not be measured and that he should relax as much as possible, while continuing to respond appropriately. Eighty stimulus pairs were presented in each of the two conditions, there being 48 "Yes-Trials" and 32 "No-Trials" per condition.

Apparatus

Two Ag–AgCl electrodes with less than 100 μV standing potential between them were prepared by chloriding conventional Grass silver cup electrodes. These were filled with Sandborn Redux paste and attached to the vertex (Cz) and mastoid process by collodion. The potentials were recorded on a Grass Model 5 Polygraph. They were amplified by a 5P1 DC pre-amplifier, using a capacity-coupled input with a time constant of 1.35 sec, and by a driver amplifier with a high frequency cut-off at 15 c/sec. The latter was coupled through a Grass R5 DC reverter to one channel of a Mnemotron tape recorder and to a Nuclear-of-Chicago Data Retrieval Computer for on-line averaging. A computer sweep of 4.0 sec was triggered 0.5 sec before the onset of the first stimulus. Each sweep thus included 0.5 sec of pre-stimulus activity, a 1.0 sec inter-stimulus interval, and 2.5 sec of post-stimulus activity.

Eye movements were recorded from two EEG cup electrodes placed diagonally above and below the right eye. The potentials were amplified by a second 5P1 DC pre-amplifier and driver amplifier, whose output was fed into another channel of the tape recorder. Signals from the stimulus generator and telegraph key were also recorded on tape to indicate the onset of stimuli and responses. A recording convention was used, such that a negative polarity (upward pen deflection) indicated electro-negativity at the vertex relative to the mastoid electrode, or at the superior relative to the inferior eye placement.

Analysis of data

All trials containing artifact were deleted by careful editing of the original polygraph records. Using tape playbacks, the following potentials were separately summated and plotted for each subject on a Moseley X–Y recorder: vertex activity for all Yes-Trials and for all No-Trials both in the Speed and Relax Conditions; eye potentials for the same four groups of trials; and vertex activity for the 10 trials containing the subject's fastest reactions and for the 10 trials containing his slowest responses under both motivational conditions. Reaction times were measured to the nearest 4 msec from slow-speed tape playbacks into an EEG machine.

A baseline was obtained for each plot of the summated potentials by averaging with a ruler 10 pre-stimulus points spaced 50 msec apart. All amplitude measurements were made relative to this baseline. The amplitude of the CNV was estimated by averaging 5 equispaced points in the

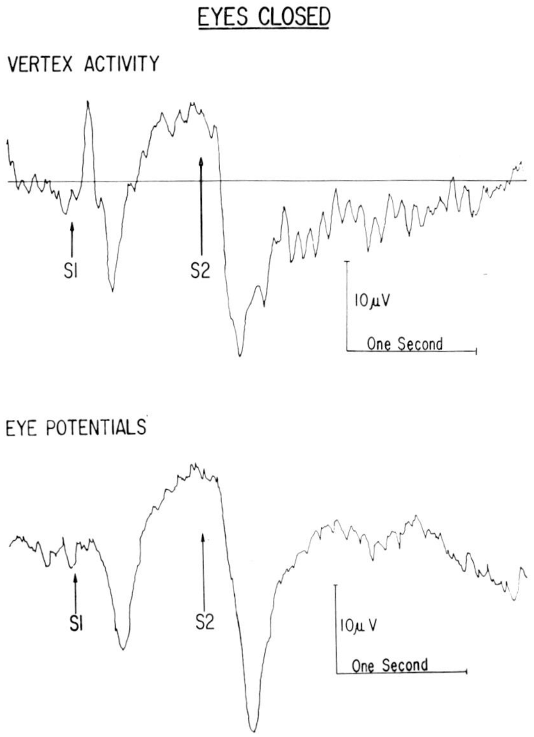

Fig. 1

Top: Summation of 46 trials in speed condition from vertex of subject with closed eyes. *Bottom*: Summation of eye potentials of same subject over same trials. S_1 = first tone; S_2 = second tone. Upward deflection indicates negativity at the vertex or superior eye electrode.

0.2 sec preceding the second stimulus. Amplitudes of the vertex-negative evoked potentials following S_1 and S_2 were estimated by measuring the highest point between 120 and 140 msec after each of the stimuli. The amplitude of the vertex-positive potential (R+) following S_2 was also determined. Because this potential was often ill-defined in the Yes-Trials, a positive peak was selected that occurred closest in time to the more easily identifiable response in the No-Trials. Fig. 3 illustrates the various measurements made of the CNV and evoked potentials.

RESULTS

Slow potentials of the type described by Walter *et al.* (1964) as CNVs were recorded from all subjects under the several conditions employed. It was found necessary, however, to distinguish such responses from potentials associated with eye movements.

Influence of eye movements upon vertex potentials

Fig. 1 shows the summated vertex activity during 46 Yes-Trials of the Speed Condition for one subject who had his eyes closed (*top*) and his eye potentials summated over the same group of trials (*bottom*). Whereas the vertex-negative evoked potential following S_1 does not appear in the graph obtained from the eyes, a marked positive potential following S_1 and S_2 and a negative shift in the S_1-S_2 interval can be seen in both records. It was concluded that electrical potentials generated by eye movements probably exerted a major influence upon vertex potentials in this subject. Consequently, he was excluded from the study. Six additional subjects performing with closed eyes were excluded for the same reason.

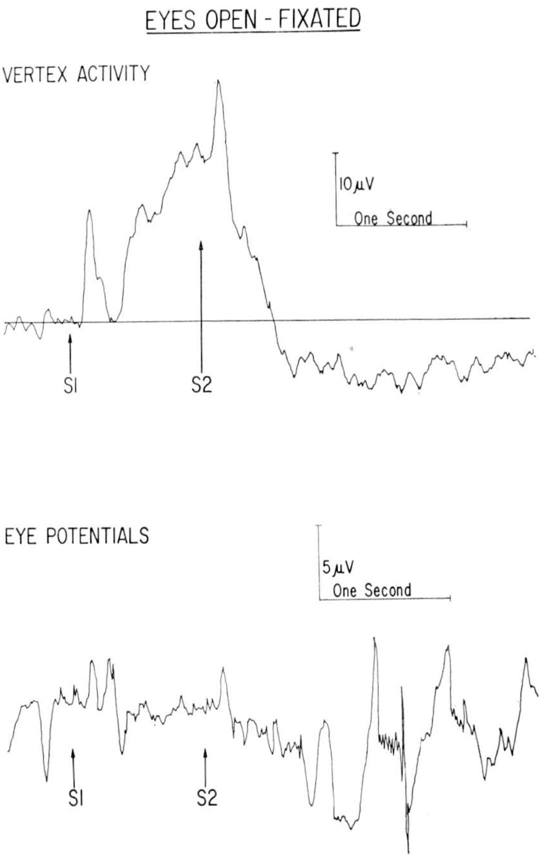

Fig. 2

Top: Summation of 37 trials in speed condition from vertex of subject with eyes open and fixated. *Bottom*: Summation of eye potentials of same subject over same trials. S_1 = first tone; S_2 = second tone. Polarity is the same as in Fig. 1.

Only four out of eleven subjects with closed eyes did not reveal any eye potentials occurring in a constant relationship to the stimuli, and these cases were included in the study.

Fig. 2 shows the summation of vertex activity over 37 Yes-Trials in the Speed Condition for one subject who had his eyes open and fixated (*top*) and the corresponding recordings from the eye electrodes (*bottom*). Although the eye potentials were amplified twice as much as the vertex activity, no eye movements can be detected until about 700 msec after S_2 when the subject began to blink. The absence of a consistent temporal relationship between eye movements and stimulation

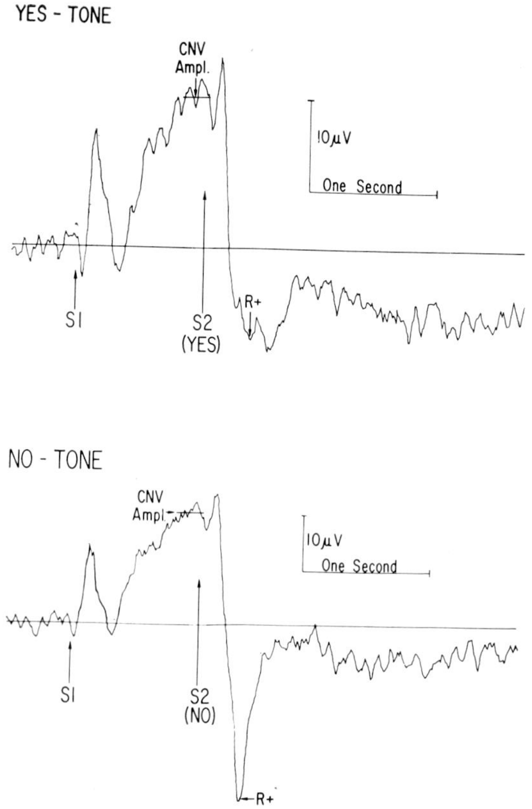

Fig. 3

Top: Summation of 46 trials in speed condition recorded from one subject while second stimulus was Yes-Tone. *Bottom*: Summation of 29 trials from same subject in same condition while second stimulus was No-Tone. Note difference in voltage calibration. S_1 = first tone; S_2 = second tone; CNV Ampl. = average amplitude of CNV during 200 msec preceding S_2; R+ = positive potential following S_2 (see text for details of measurement). Polarity is the same as in Fig. 1.

TABLE I

Mean amplitude (in μV) of the positive peak following Yes-Tones and No-Tones in the Speed and the Relax Condition

	Yes-Tones	No-Tones	Difference	*t*	*d.f.*	*P*
Speed	4.18	17.17	12.99	4.27	8	< 0.005
Relax	4.87	13.91	9.04	4.60	8	< 0.005

was characteristic of all six subjects who performed with open and fixated eyes in this study.

Differences in potentials following Yes- and No-Tones

Fig. 3 illustrates the summated vertex activity for one subject under the Speed Condition. The top graph represents the potentials recorded from 46 Yes-Trials, while the bottom graph shows the potentials from 29 No-Trials. Note the difference in amplitude calibration between the two graphs. A sharp wave of deep positivity (R + No) follows the negative evoked potential to the No-Tone, while a broader wave of much smaller positivity (R + Yes) follows the Yes-Tone. Such a configuration was consistently found in the records of eight out of nine subjects[1], although not all of them showed a positive peak of such large amplitude in the No-Trials. None of these potentials appeared in the summated eye recordings.

The difference in magnitude of the positive potentials following Yes- and No-Tones was tested statistically by comparing their mean amplitudes. Table I reveals that the difference is highly significant in both the Speed and Relax Conditions. In order to show that this difference is not due to the way in which R + Yes was selected (see Methods), R + No was also compared with the maximum positive potential occurring anywhere in the 800 msec following the onset of a Yes-Tone. This comparison also yielded significant differences for the two motivational conditions, similar to those in Table I.

Vertex potentials and reaction time

Within subjects, the mean CNV amplitude

[1] R+ was not measured for one subject whose summated eye potentials indicated consistent eye movements after S_2, but whose recordings were otherwise free of artifact.

TABLE II

Mean amplitude (in μV) of the CNV for the ten fastest and the ten slowest of the subjects' 48 reaction times during the Speed and the Relax Condition

	Fastest reactions	Slowest reactions	Difference	t	$d.f.$	P*
Speed	16.90	11.53	5.37	2.79	9	< 0.05
Relax	12.99	8.39	4.60	2.84	9	< 0.02

* Two-tailed test.

associated with the 10 fastest reaction times was significantly higher than the mean CNV amplitude preceding the 10 slowest reactions. Table II indicates the extent of this difference, which occurred in both motivational conditions. Neither the amplitude of the negative evoked potentials to S_1 and S_2, nor the positive potentials following Yes- and No-Tones were significantly different for the fastest and slowest reactions.

Between subjects, mean reaction time was not significantly correlated with CNV amplitude or with either of the two negative evoked potentials. When the amplitude of the positive potential following S_2 was correlated with response speed, however, significant coefficients ($P < 0.05$) did emerge. For R+Yes, $r = -0.74$ in the Relax Condition; for R+No, $r = -0.79$ in the Speed and -0.67 in the Relax Condition. Thus, subjects with faster mean reaction times tended to have larger R+ potentials, even during those trials when they were not responding.

Motivation and vertex potentials

The effectiveness of the differential instructions in the Speed and Relax Conditions is indicated by the difference in reaction time. In the Speed Condition the mean reaction time was 252 msec, as compared with 355 msec in the Relax Condition ($t = 2.98$, $d.f. = 9$, $P < 0.02$).

No statistically significant differences for CNV amplitude, the negative evoked potential to S_2, R + Yes, or R+No were obtained between the two conditions. The negative evoked potential to the warning signal (S_1), however, was significantly higher during the Speed than during the Relax Condition (11.06 μV *vs.* 9.56 μV; $t = 2.95$, $d.f. = 9$, $P < 0.02$). In an additional test, the difference between each subject's mean reaction time in the Speed and the Relax Condition was correlated with the corresponding difference between his vertex potentials. Significant correlations were found for CNV amplitude ($r = +0.79$, $P < 0.01$) and for the amplitude of the negative evoked potential to S_2 ($r = +0.77$, $P < 0.01$). Thus, subjects whose reaction times showed greater improvement in the Speed as compared with the Relax Condition, also developed greater differences in CNV and evoked response amplitudes between the two conditions.

DISCUSSION

The present experiment demonstrates that CNVs can be recorded during the fixed foreperiod of a disjunctive reaction task. Within subjects, the fastest 10 reaction times were preceded by CNVs of significantly larger amplitude than were the 10 slowest. This relationship held true during induced states of both high and low motivation. Because the subjects had no prior knowledge of whether or not they were required to respond to the imperative stimulus, it is unlikely that anticipatory reactions could account for these findings. Practice effects are also an unlikely explanation, since they were minimized by the administration of practice trials. The relationship between CNV amplitude and reaction time obtained within subjects suggests that physiological events responsible for the slow potential shift may have functional significance in increasing the speed with which a subject can respond to a stimulus.

The results differ in some respects from those obtained earlier with simple reaction tasks. Irwin *et al.* (1966) failed to find a significant difference between amplitude of the CNVs associated with the subjects' fastest and slowest reactions, although a trend in the expected direction was observed. Hillyard and Galambos (1967), however, demonstrated statistically significant correlations between reaction time and CNV both within and between subjects. In the present study, the only significant correlation obtained between subjects involved differences in motivational state. Those subjects whose mean reaction time improved most in the Speed over the Relax Condition tended to have correspondingly larger differences in CNV amplitude and the negative potential evoked by S_2.

Evoked potentials and response speed have been found to be correlated in a number of studies (Dustman and Beck 1965; Morrell and Morrell 1966; Wilkinson and Morlock 1967). The failure to find a relationship in this experiment between response speed and amplitude of the evoked potentials to S_1 and S_2 might be accounted for by the particular methods employed; namely, the smaller number of trials, the fact that only potentials slower than 15 c/sec were faithfully recorded, the presence of a warning signal, and the use of a disjunctive reaction task. Furthermore, the evoked responses to S_2 differed from those of earlier studies in that they were superimposed on CNVs.

The finding that the evoked potential to S_1 was significantly larger in the Speed than during the Relax Condition agrees with previously reported correlations between motivation and evoked potential amplitude (Spong *et al.* 1965; Donchin and Cohen 1967). On the other hand, the small non-significant difference in CNV amplitude obtained between the Speed and Relax Conditions is not consistent with the hypothesis that motivational state is a primary determinant of the CNV (Irwin *et al.* 1966; Walter 1966).

The large difference in the form of the potentials following Yes- and No-Tones is noteworthy. After a Yes-Tone, the negative evoked potential to S_2 was followed by a broad positivity of moderate amplitude. When the subject was required to withhold his response (after a No-Tone), a short but high amplitude positivity appeared. Although a small positive potential following the CNV might be expected as a function of the relatively short (1.35 sec) time constant used, this factor is not sufficient to account for the amplitude of the observed potentials, their time course, or the consistent difference between Yes- and No-Trials. It seems unlikely that the latter difference is an artifact due to performing or withholding a motor response, since overt movements were minimized by the precautions described in Methods. The influence of eye movement was also ruled out by the examination of records from the eye leads. In a control experiment employing the same procedure as the one described here, except that a warning signal was not used, no difference in the configuration of the potentials following Yes- and No-Tones could be detected. It thus appears that the observed differences in positive potential may reflect different processes in the brain following the two types of stimuli.

Previous animal studies have shown positive potential shifts in a variety of behavioral situations (Rowland and Goldstone 1963; Wurtz 1966). In human subjects, Cohen and Walter (1966) observed slow positive potentials following semantic stimulation, which they considered significant. Donchin and Smith (1969) noted the occurrence of positive potentials approximately 300 msec after task-relevant imperative stimuli, a latency similar to that found in the present study.

Although a physiological interpretation of these positive potentials cannot be made in the absence of data on their electrogenesis, it may be possible to speculate about their psychological significance. Subjects in the present experiment were asked to report their subjective feelings in a post-experimental interrogation. A categorization of the responses showed that during the inter-stimulus interval the subjects experienced a state of excitation, accompanied by eagerness to make a fast and correct response. After a Yes-Tone they felt relieved that the trial was over and were satisfied that they had performed correctly. Following a No-Signal they had to exert great effort to inhibit a response which they had been preparing to perform. The subjective state of "relief" was thus accompanied by positive potentials of a different kind than was the conscious effort to inhibit the response.

In most cases, instructions to the subject to keep his eyes open and fixated and to avoid blinking during the inter-stimulus interval effectively reduced contamination of vertex activity with eye potentials. When a subject performs with closed eyes, it seems necessary not only to monitor eye potentials on a polygraph, but also to summate them on a computer over the same trials as the vertex activity. This is important since the eye potentials, like the CNV, may not be of large enough amplitude to be detected in a single trial. Yet when they occur in constant time relationship to the stimuli, they may contribute significantly to the summated vertex activity, as in Fig. 1.

SUMMARY

Slow potential changes were recorded from the scalp of ten adult subjects during performance of a disjunctive reaction task. Tones separated by a constant 1.0 sec interval were employed for the conditional and imperative stimuli. The subject was instructed to execute or withhold a digital response, depending upon the frequency of the imperative stimulus. Motivational state was manipulated by two different sets of instructions.

1. Contingent negative variations (CNVs) were obtained in all subjects under conditions of both high and low motivation.

2. In a majority of subjects performing with closed eyes, potentials originating from the eyes were seen to contaminate activity recorded from the vertex. This problem was not encountered in subjects who had their eyes open and fixated.

3. Within subjects, the fastest reaction times were preceded by CNVs of significantly larger amplitude than were the slowest responses. A comparable relationship was not found between subjects.

4. Reaction times were shorter, and the negative evoked potential to the warning stimulus had a significantly greater amplitude when the subjects were in a state of high motivation than when they were urged to relax. Other potentials, including the CNV, did not show this difference between motivational conditions.

5. Trials in which subjects were required to respond were followed by a broad positive wave of moderate amplitude, whereas trials in which they withheld a response were followed by a short positive wave of much greater amplitude. The height of both potentials was significantly correlated with mean reaction time across subjects.

RÉSUMÉ

RELATIONS ENTRE MODIFICATIONS DE POTENTIELS LENTS, VITESSE DE RÉPONSE ET MOTIVATION CHEZ L'HOMME

Des modifications de potentiels lents sont enregistrées à partir du scalp chez dix sujets adultes pendant la réalisation d'une tâche impliquant une réaction de discrimination. Des sons séparés par un intervalle constant de 1 sec ont été utilisés pour les stimuli conditionnels et impératifs. On demande aux sujets d'exécuter ou de refuser une réponse digitale suivant la fréquence du stimulus impératif. L'état de motivation est obtenu par deux séries différentes d'instructions.

1. Les variations contingentes négatives sont obtenues chez tous les sujets que les conditions de motivation soient élevées ou basses.

2. Chez la plupart des sujets travaillant les yeux fermés, les potentiels qui prennent leur origine au niveau des yeux contaminent l'activité enregistrée au niveau du vertex. Ce problème ne se rencontre plus chez les sujets qui gardent les yeux ouverts et fixes.

3. Chez un même sujet, on note que les temps de réaction les plus rapides sont précédés par des variations contingentes négatives d'amplitude nettement plus grande que les réponses les plus lentes. On n'observe pas cette relation si on compare les sujets entre eux.

4. Les temps de réaction sont plus courts, et les potentiels évoqués négatifs au stimulus de renforcement d'amplitude nettement plus grande quand les sujets sont dans un état de motivation élevée que lorsqu'il leur est demandé de se détendre. D'autres potentiels, parmi lesquels la variation contingente négative, n'ont pas montré ces différences entre les conditions de motivation.

5. Les séquences au cours desquelles il est demandé au sujet de répondre sont suivies d'une large onde positive d'amplitude modérée, tandis que celles au cours desquelles ils refusent de répondre sont suivies d'une onde positive brève, d'amplitude beaucoup plus grande. La hauteur de ces deux potentiels a une corrélation significative avec le temps moyen de réaction des sujets.

REFERENCES

COHEN, J. and WALTER, W. G. The interaction of responses in the brain to semantic stimuli. *Psychophysiology*, **1966**, *2*: 187–196.

DONCHIN, E. and COHEN, L. Averaged evoked potentials and intramodality selective attention. *Electroenceph. clin. Neurophysiol.*, **1967**, *22*: 537–546.

DONCHIN, E. and SMITH, D. D. B. The CNV and the "late positive wave" — two sides of the same coin. *Electroenceph. clin. Neurophysiol.*, **1969**, *27* (in press).

DUSTMAN, R. E. and BECK, E. C. Phase of alpha brain waves, reaction time and visually evoked potentials. *Electroenceph. clin. Neurophysiol.*, **1965**, *18*: 433–440.

HILLYARD, S. A. and GALAMBOS, R. Effects of stimulus and response contingencies on a surface negative slow potential shift in man. *Electroenceph. clin. Neurophysiol.*, **1967,** *22*: 297–304.

IRWIN, D. A., KNOTT, J. R., MCADAM, D. W. and REBERT, C. S. Motivational determinants of the "contingent negative variation". *Electroenceph. clin. Neurophysiol.*, **1966,** *21*: 538–543.

LOW, M. D., BORDA, R. P., FROST, J. D. and KELLAWAY, P. Surface-negative, slow-potential shift associated with conditioning in man. *Neurology (Minneap.)*, **1966,** *16*: 771–782.

MORRELL, L. and MORRELL, F. Evoked potentials and reaction time: a study of intra-individual variability. *Electroenceph. clin. Neurophysiol.*, **1966,** *20*: 567–575.

ROWLAND, V. and GOLDSTONE, M. Appetitively conditioned and drive-related bioelectric baseline shift in cat cortex. *Electroenceph. clin. Neurophysiol.*, **1963,** *15*: 474–485.

SPONG, P., HAIDER, M. and LINDSLEY, D. B. Selective attentiveness and cortical evoked responses to visual and auditory stimuli. *Science*, **1965,** *148*: 395–397.

TEICHNER, W. H. Effects of foreperiod, induced muscular tension, and stimulus regularity on simple reaction time. *J. exp. Psychol.*, **1957,** *53*: 277–284.

WALTER, W. G. Expectancy waves and intention waves in the human brain and their application to the direct cerebral control of machines. *Electroenceph. clin. Neurophysiol.*, **1966,** *21*: 616.

WALTER, W. G., COOPER, R., ALDRIDGE, V. J., MCCALLUM, W. C. and WINTER, A. L. Contingent negative variation: an electrical sign of sensory-motor association and expectancy in the human brain. *Nature (Lond.)*, **1964,** *203*: 380–384.

WALTER, W. G., COOPER, R., CROW, H. J., MCCALLUM, W. C., WARREN, W. J., ALDRIDGE, V. J., STORM VAN LEEUWEN, W. and KAMP, A. Contingent negative variation and evoked responses recorded by radiotelemetry in free-ranging subjects. *Electroenceph. clin. Neurophysiol.*, **1967,** *23*: 197–206.

WILKINSON, R. T. and MORLOCK, H. C. Auditory evoked response and reaction time. *Electroenceph. clin. Neurophysiol.*, **1967,** *23*: 50–56.

WURTZ, R. H. Steady potential correlates of intracranial reinforcement. *Electroenceph. clin. Neurophysiol.*, **1966,** *20*: 59–67.

Reference: WASZAK, M. and OBRIST, W. D. Relationship of slow potential changes to response speed and motivation in man. *Electroenceph. clin. Neurophysiol.*, **1969,** *27*: 113–120.

Electroencephalography and Clinical Neurophysiology
Elsevier Publishing Company, Amsterdam – Printed in The Netherlands

ACOUSTIC EVOKED RESPONSES IN NEWBORN INFANTS: THE INFLUENCE OF PITCH AND COMPLEXITY OF THE STIMULUS

H. G. LENARD[1], H. VON BERNUTH AND S. J. HUTT[2]

Department of Developmental Neurology, University Hospital, Groningen (The Netherlands)

(Accepted for publication: November 28, 1968)

The present study was preceded by a polygraphic investigation of autonomic and electromyographic responses to acoustic stimuli in newborn infants (Hutt *et al.* 1968a,b). In these experiments it was shown that human newborns react more frequently and more strongly to square wave tones than to pure sine wave tones of equal sound pressure. Square wave sounds with low frequency fundamentals were the most potent stimuli. Human voices were slightly less effective than square wave tones of 125 and 250 c/sec, but produced more reactions than either square wave tones with high frequency fundamentals or sine wave stimuli. From these observations the question arose as to whether stimuli of different wave forms and frequencies evoke quantitatively different electroencephalographic responses. To examine this question we selected five sound stimuli whose capacity to evoke differential autonomic and electromyographic responses was already known: a female human voice; a sine and a square wave tone whose fundamental was approximately that of the voice (125 c/sec); and a sine and a square wave tone with a fundamental 3 octaves higher (1000 c/sec). The latter frequency is known to be in the band of maximum loudness for adult subjects (Wever 1949). On the basis of the earlier study (Hutt *et al.* 1968b) it was hypothesized that evoked responses would be greatest to a 125 c/sec square wave tone and of decreasing amplitude to a human voice, a 1000 c/sec square wave tone, a 125 c/sec sine wave and a 1000 c/sec sine wave tone, respectively.

If the first hypothesis were substantiated, a further question would be: what is the determining factor that makes a 125 c/sec square wave tone the most potent of the tested stimuli? Is it merely the band-width or does the patterned frequency power spectrum of this stimulus play the main role? In our previous study it was hypothesized that, in human newborns, the greater the length of basilar membrane displaced (measured from the oval window) the higher the probability of eliciting a behavioural response. Thus, white noise whose band-width is identical with that of the 125 c/sec square wave tone should be equally effective in eliciting a response. In order to examine this problem evoked responses to a 125 c/sec square wave tone were compared with evoked responses to white noise of the same band-width (10,000 c/sec). High band pass and low band pass noise stimuli were also tested, with the hypothesis that they should produce smaller evoked responses. Since stimuli of 1000 c/sec had been used in the first experiment, this was used as the cut-off point for dividing the white noise into high and low bands.

METHODS

Fourteen healthy full-term newborn infants, aged 4–8 days, were studied for 2–3 h between feeds. The infants were placed lying on their sides in a basinette in a climate chamber (30° C, 50–60% humidity). The first six infants (Group I) were stimulated with square wave tones of 125 c/sec and 1000 c/sec, sine wave tones of 125 c/sec and 1000 c/sec, and a female human voice. In the

[1] Present address: Universitäts-Kinderklinik, 34 Göttingen, Humboldtallee 38, W. Germany.

[2] Present address: Human Development Research Unit, University of Oxford and St. Catherine's College, Oxford, England.

other eight infants (Group II) a 125 c/sec square wave tone and three bands of filtered white noise were used as stimuli.

Grass EEG electrodes were fixed with collodion at C_z, T_5 and T_6. Bipolar recordings were obtained from T_5–C_z and from T_6–C_z, but only the lead of the side that was turned towards the sound source was analysed. The EEG, together with EKG, heart rate, respiration, the trigger signal and the stimulus (picked up with a microphone) were monitored on an Offner-Beckmann Type R Dynograph. Data were stored on an Ampex FR 1800 magnetic tape for off-line analysis.

Symmetrical square and sine waves of 125 and 1000 c/sec were produced by a Peekel Type 013V electronic oscillator. The sound envelopes were rhomboid with rise times varying between 25 msec (for the 125 c/sec square wave tone) and 10 msec (for the 1000 c/sec sine wave tone). The word "baby", spoken by a female voice, was reproduced from a tape loop, using a Kudelski Nagra III recorder. The voice had a fundamental frequency of 200 c/sec with significant high frequency components up to 8000 c/sec. For the second part of the study white noise, produced by a General Radio Type 1390A noise generator, was filtered with a SKL variable electronic filter Type 380A, which produced a cut-off of 24 dB per octave. The filter settings were: 200 c/sec high pass—5000 c/sec low pass for "broad band" noise, 200 c/sec high pass—500 c/sec low pass for "low band" noise, and 2000 c/sec high pass —5000 c/sec low pass for "high band" noise.

All signals were reproduced, after amplification, from a Philips Type Ad 3800 loudspeaker. The loudspeaker was suspended above the basinette, 40 cm from the baby's ear, its axis in the same straight line as the external auditory meatus. The sound reproducing system gave a linear frequency response, rising 4 dB per octave from 100 to 2000 c/sec and a flat response from 2000 to 10,000 c/sec. The sound production equipment was calibrated with a General Radio Sound pressure meter Type 1881A to give a sound pressure level of 80 dB *re* 0.0002 μbar at the baby's ear for all stimuli. The ambient noise level in the climate chamber was 50 ± 2.5 dB. The duration of the stimulus was 2 sec. Since other investigators have found that the amplitude of evoked responses varies with the EEG sleep stages (Williams *et al.* 1962) the different stimuli were given in a predetermined sequence, one after the other, to ensure that each type of stimulus would appear equally often in each state. The orders of presentation were: 125 c/sec square, 125 c/sec sine, 1000 c/sec square, 1000 c/sec sine, voice, 125 c/sec square etc. for Group 1; 125 c/sec square, low band noise, high band noise, broad band noise, 125 c/sec square etc. for Group II. The interval between successive stimuli was 10–15 sec; sequential effects were therefore unlikely. Stimuli were presented *only* when the axes of the loudspeaker and the baby's exposed ear were in the same straight line. No stimulus was given when the baby was moving, sucking or crying, or when artefacts were seen in the write-out.

The evoked responses to 40 stimuli of each quality were summed off-line on a TMC Computer of Average Transients Type 400B. The computer was triggered 80–100 msec prior to the onset of the tones and noise bands and simultaneously with the onset of the voice stimulus. The read-out of the computer was displayed on a Moseley X–Y plotter.

RESULTS

The idealized response obtained with our electrode setting consisted successively of: a positive, a negative and another positive deflection (Fig. 1). Following the designation of Weitzman *et al.* (1965) and of Ornitz *et al.* (1967), the deflections were named P_2, N_2 and P_3.

The average of the evoked responses of the

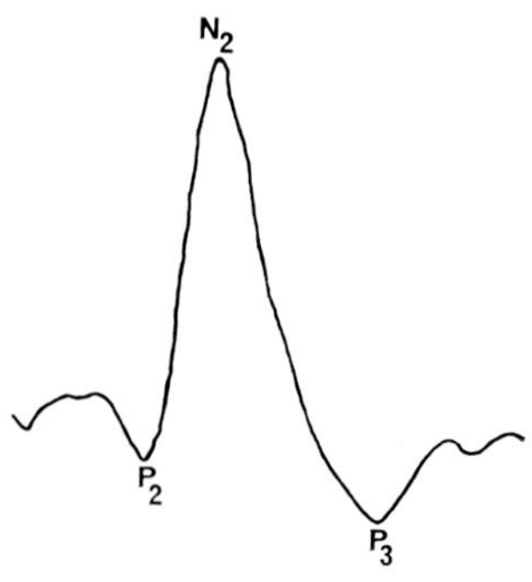

Fig. 1
Idealized evoked response with designation of the deflections (Weitzman *et al.* 1965).

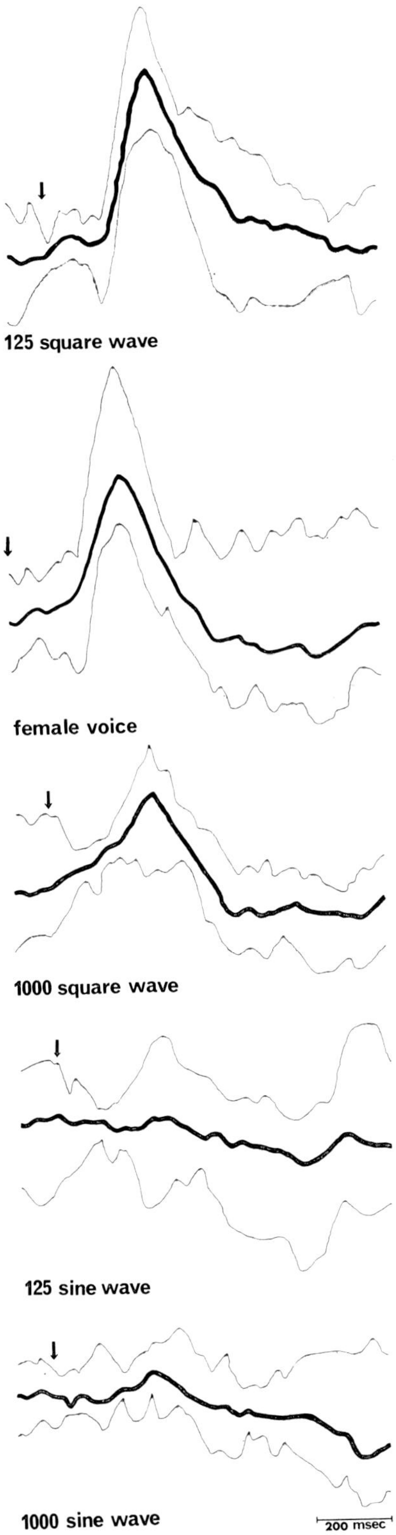

six infants in Group I and of the eight infants in Group II to each stimulus was obtained by superimposition of the 6 (or 8) evoked responses on transparent paper and successive computation of mean values 20 msec apart. The resulting

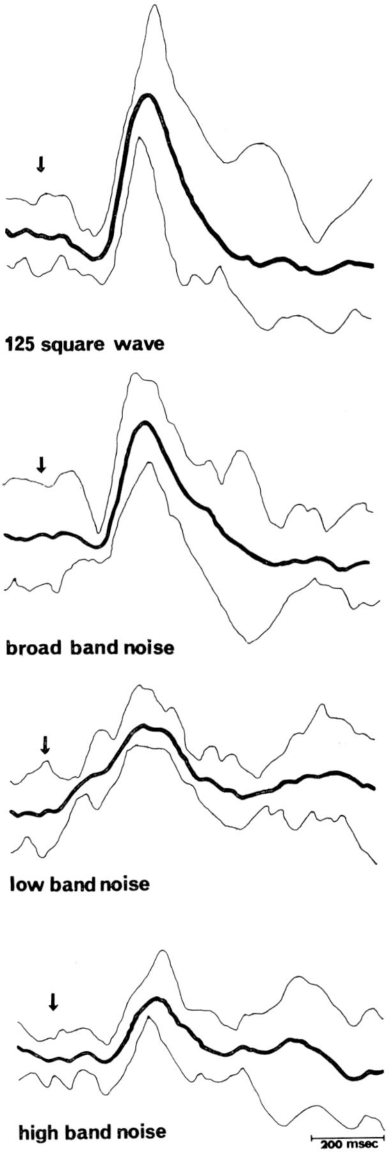

Fig. 3

Mean and range of averaged evoked responses of eight infants (Group II). Calibration: 200 msec.

← Fig. 2

Mean and range of averaged evoked responses of six infants (Group I). Calibration: 200 msec.

TABLE I

Amplitude of N_2 in mm: Group I

Baby	125 c/sec square wave	Female voice	1000 c/sec square wave	125 c/sec sine wave	1000 c/sec sine wave
1	85	98	50	0	44
2	138	110	77	30	0
3	115	50	81	23	42
4	78	63	0	0	0
5	178	193	62	51	32
6	188	95	55	24	0

curves for all stimuli in both groups, together with the range of the evoked responses to each stimulus, are given in Fig. 2 and 3. From these averaged average curves it is evident that only wave N_2 is consistent enough to be subjected to statistical analysis. Wave P_2 is only visible in average curves of the responses to the more potent stimuli, and wave P_3 cannot be demonstrated at all. Statistical analysis was therefore confined to wave N_2. Peak-to-peak amplitudes of N_2, measured from the EEG pen write-out, were in the range of 15–30μV for the 125 c/sec square wave and were correspondingly smaller for the other sounds. As amplifiers with continuously variable "gain" controls were used, it was not possible to replicate precisely the same recording conditions between babies; for this reason parametric statistical tests were not applied. Since, however, the same gains were always employed *within* babies, it was legitimate to make comparisons amongst responses to different sounds using non-parametric statistics. The units of measurement used were mm on the X–Y plot.

TABLE II

Amplitude of N_2 in mm: Group II

Baby	125 c/sec square wave	Broad band	Low band	High band
1	180	119	32	41
2	133	107	40	68
3	113	155	83	62
4	160	92	79	41
5	90	69	47	53
6	132	66	70	57
7	140	92	75	40
8	115	105	80	85

Data are given in Table I (for Group I) and in Table II (for Group II). Considerable differences in peak amplitudes between individuals are in part due to real inter-individual differences and are in part caused by the fact that the time spent in regular (NREM) sleep—the period when the evoked responses were greatest—varied considerably between different babies. Non-parametric statistics were therefore further necessitated to avoid a disproportionate effect of very large evoked responses from any one subject.

To test the hypothesis that evoked responses of decreasing amplitude would be obtained when the stimuli were: a 125 c/sec square wave, a human voice, 1000 c/sec square wave, a 125 c/sec sine wave and a 1000 c/sec sine wave, respectively, the trend analogue of Friedman's test was applied (de Jonge 1963). The null hypothesis that the 5 experimental stimuli had no differential effect upon the magnitude of the evoked response was rejected at the 0.001 level of confidence ($T=4.32$, one-tailed test.) No significant differences could be demonstrated between the response amplitude rankings of the 125 c/sec square wave and voice stimuli ($T=0.80$) or between those of the responses to the 125 c/sec and 1000 c/sec sine wave stimuli ($T=0.40$). On the other hand, the rankings of the 1000 c/sec square wave differed from those of the voice at almost the 0.05 level of confidence ($T=1.6$) and from those of the 125 c/sec sine wave at the 0.025 level ($T=2.0$, all one-tailed tests). It is thus clear that the response magnitude rankings of the N_2 wave are in close conformity with the original hypothesis.

An over-all test of trend on the data from Group II also resulted in rejection of the null hypothesis ($T=3.8$, $P<0.001$, one-tailed test). The response amplitudes to the 125 c/sec square wave obtained significantly higher rankings than those to the broad band white noise stimuli ($T=2.20$) which in turn were ranked significantly higher than the responses to high band noise ($T=2.20$). The differences in rankings between broad band and low band responses and between low band and high band responses were not statistically significant.

DISCUSSION

The size of acoustic evoked potentials in infants is known to be related to the EEG sleep stages (Appleby 1965; Barnet 1965; Barnet and Goodwin 1965; Weitzman *et al.* 1965; Ornitz *et al.* 1967; Rapin and Graziani 1967; Schulte *et al.* 1967) and to the intensity of the stimulus (Rapin 1964; Goodman *et al.* 1964; Appleby 1965; Barnet 1965; Barnet and Goodwin 1965; Cody and Bickford 1965). The influence of the pitch, band width and wave form of the stimulus has, as yet, been little studied.

Clicks and pure tone pips are the stimuli most generally employed in studies of acoustic evoked responses. Although the duration of our stimuli was unusually long for a study of evoked responses, this factor is unlikely to account for any differences between our results and those from studies using briefer stimuli. Stimuli of long duration are known to produce an on-effect which is comparable in all parameters with a click-evoked response (Chatrian *et al.* 1960) and only this on-effect was analysed in the present study.

In practice, our own results for the two pure tone stimuli are in close agreement with studies employing shorter duration stimuli. Goodman *et al.* (1964) found no differences in the evoked responses to tone pips from 600 to 4800 c/sec. Rapin and Graziani (1967) used clicks and pure tone pips between 250 and 3000 c/sec, but did not observe any systematic differences dependent upon the frequency of the stimulus.

On the other hand, frequency specific effects were found in the present study when square wave tones were used, the evoked response to the 125 c/sec tone being in every case greater in amplitude than that to the 1000 c/sec tone. The difference cannot be attributed to vibration effects, since control experiments with the babies' ears stopped showed a marked diminution in responsiveness irrespective of the stimulus characteristics. Goodman *et al.* (1964) have stressed the critical importance of the rise time of the stimulus in determining the size of the evoked response. In general, the amplitude of the evoked response bears an inverse relationship to rise time. Since, in the present study, the rise time of the sound envelope of the low frequency sounds was longer than that of the high frequency sounds, results opposite to those obtained would have been expected if rise time were an important factor.

Vibration and rise time, furthermore, cannot be critical factors in explaining the differences between the responses to the three types of stimulus in Group I: sine wave, square wave and voice. Responses to all stimuli were suppressed when the babies' ears were stopped. Moreover, owing to a peculiarity of our sound producing equipment, the rise time of the sound envelope of the square wave tones was not faster than that of the sine waves, and the rise time of the voice was longer than that of either.

A more plausible factor in explaining the differences both amongst the three types of stimulus and between frequencies, is band width. Zwicker *et al.* (1957) have demonstrated a direct relationship, in adult subjects, between judgements of loudness and critical band width of the sound stimulus. In the present case the band widths of the stimuli were related to the magnitude of their evoked responses. It might be argued therefore that the amplitudes of the evoked responses simply reflected the loudness of the stimuli. It is clear, however, from the results of the second part of the study that band width alone is not the critical factor. There was no significant difference between the rankings of the low band and high band evoked responses even though the band width of the latter stimulus exceeded that of the former by a factor of 10. Similarly, the band width of the broad band white noise was identical with that of the 125 c/sec square wave tone, whilst its evoked response was significantly smaller than that to the square wave. The evoked responses to the human voice were not significantly different from those to the 125 c/sec square wave, even though the band width of the latter was some 2000 c/sec greater. It is thus clear that more than band width is involved in determining the magnitude of the evoked response.

Our own earlier hypothesis (Hutt *et al.* 1968b) was that in human newborns, the greater the length of the basilar membrane displaced (measuring from the oval window) the greater the probability of behavioural and autonomic responses to the sound. Assuming a parallel with these responses, the hypothesis would account for the order of magnitude of all the evoked electroencephalographic responses with the exception of that to broad band noise. It was predicted that this would be equally effective to the 125 c/sec square wave. The fact that this prediction was not fulfilled suggests that more complex mechanisms of pattern recognition may be involved than that originally postulated. The results certainly offer support to Eisenberg's theory (1969) that the auditory system of the human neonate is differentially tuned to react to the carrier frequencies of language.

Though the present study was not designed with audiometric testing in mind, the results may have some implications for testing hearing in newborn infants. They show clearly that pure tones are not the optimal stimuli to elicit reactions in newborns. It seems that the human infant has a lower threshold for biologically meaningful sounds than for pure tones. If stimuli having properties similar to the former are used, intensities as high as those commonly used in neonatal audiometry may be unnecessary.

SUMMARY

1. Averaged evoked responses were recorded bipolarly from T_5–C_z and T_6–C_z in groups (I, II) of human newborns during acoustic stimulation.

2. Group I was stimulated with five sounds: sine and square wave tones at 125 and 1000 c/sec, respectively, and a recorded female voice saying "baby". Group II was stimulated with four sounds: the 125 c/sec square wave, white noise of approximately equal band width ("wide band") and two filtered components of it ("low band" and "high band"), respectively.

3. The response most consistently present following stimulation was the N_2 wave. In Group I evoked N_2 responses of decreasing amplitude were obtained to: the 125 c/sec square wave, the voice, the 1000 c/sec square wave, the 125 c/sec and 1000 c/sec sine waves, respectively. In Group II the order of magnitude from greatest to smallest was: 125 c/sec square wave, wide band noise, low band noise and high band noise.

4. The results support the hypothesis proposed in an earlier publication, that the degree of behavioural and physiological response to sound in a newborn infant is proportional to the length of basilar membrane excited by the stimulus.

RÉSUMÉ

RÉPONSES ÉVOQUÉES ACOUSTIQUES CHEZ LES ENFANTS NOUVEAU-NÉS: INFLUENCE DU TON ET DE LA COMPLEXITÉ DU STIMULUS

1. Les réponses évoquées moyennes à une stimulation acoustique sont enregistrées en bipolaire sur les dérivations T_5–C_z et T_6–C_z chez deux groupes (I et II) de nouveau-nés.

2. Le groupe I est stimulé au moyen de cinq sons: ondes sinusoïdales et carrées à 125 et 1000 c/sec respectivement, plus une voix féminine enregistrée disant "bébé". Le groupe II est stimulé au moyen de quatre sons: ondes carrées à 125 c/sec, bruit d'une largeur de bande approximativement égale ("bande large") et deux de ses composantes filtrées (respectivement "bande basse" et "bande haute").

3. La réponse la plus constamment observée après la stimulation est l'onde N_2. Dans le groupe I l'amplitude des réponses évoquées N_2 suit un ordre de grandeur décroissant pour: l'onde carrée à 125 c/sec, la voix, l'onde carrée à 1000 c/sec, les ondes sinusoïdales à respectivement 125 et 1000 c/sec. Dans le groupe II cette décroissance suit l'ordre suivant: onde carrée 125 c/sec, bruit à bande large, bruit à bande basse et bruit à bande haute.

4. Ces résultats sont en faveur de l'hypothèse proposée dans une publication antérieure, suggérant que le degré de réponse comportementale et physiologique au bruit chez un enfant nouveau-né est proportionnel à la longueur de la membrane basilaire excitée par le stimulus.

The authors want to express their sincere thanks to Dr. H. F. R. Prechtl for providing the opportunity to carry out this study and for his advice and encouragement during the course of the experiments. They are also greatly indebted to Dr. H. Schaafsma and to Drs. W. J. Muntjewerff for their help with statistical and technical problems, and to Prof. H. Huizing for lending part of the equipment.

REFERENCES

Appleby, S. V. The slow vertex maximal sound evoked response in infants. *Acta oto-laryng. (Stockh.)*, **1965,** *Suppl. 206*: 146–152.

Barnet, A. B. Averaged evoked electroencephalographic responses to clicks in the infant. *Acta oto-laryng. (Stockh.)*, **1965,** *Suppl. 206*: 134–146.

Barnet, A. B. and Goodwin, R. S. Averaged evoked electroencephalographic responses to clicks in the human newborn. *Electroenceph. clin. Neurophysiol.*, **1965,** *18*: 441–450.

Chatrian, G. E., Petersen, M. C. and Lazarte, J. A. Responses to clicks from the human brain: some depth electrographic observations. *Electroenceph. clin. Neurophysiol.*, **1960,** *12*: 479–489.

Cody, D. T. R. and Bickford, R. G. Cortical audiometry: an objective method of evaluating auditory acuity in man. *Mayo Clin. Proc.*, **1965,** *40*: 273–287.

Eisenberg, R. B. The organisation of auditory behaviour: auditory competence in adult life may depend on central nervous system specialisations present at birth. *Int. Audiol.*, **1969** (in press).

Goodman, W. S., Appleby, S. V., Scott, J. W. and Ireland, P. E. Audiometry in newborn children by electroencephalography. *Laryngoscope (St. Louis)*, **1964,** *74*: 1316–1328.

Hutt, C., von Bernuth, H., Lenard, H. G., Hutt, S. J. and Prechtl, H. F. R. Habituation in relation to state in the human neonate. *Nature (Lond.)*, **1968**a, *220*: 622–624.

Hutt, S. J., Hutt, C., Lenard, H. G., von Bernuth, H. and Muntjewerff, W. J. Auditory responsivity in the human neonate. *Nature (Lond.)*, **1968**b, *218*: 888–890.

Jonge, H. de. *Medische statistiek.* Verhand. Ned. Inst. Praev. Geneesk., No. 41, 2nd ed., Leiden, **1963.**

Ornitz, E. M., Ritvo, E. R., Carr, E. M., Panman, E. M. and Walter, R. D. The variability of the auditory averaged evoked response during sleep and dreaming in children and adults. *Electroenceph. clin. Neurophysiol.*, **1967,** *22*: 514–524.

Rapin, I. Evoked responses to clicks in a group of children with communication disorders. *Ann. N.Y. Acad. Sci.*, **1964,** *112*: 182–203.

Rapin, I. and Graziani, L. J. Auditory evoked potentials in normal, brain-damaged, and deaf infants. *Neurology (Minneap.)*, **1967,** *17*: 881–894.

Schulte, F. J., Akiyama, Y. and Parmelee, A. H. Auditory evoked responses during sleep in premature and fullterm newborn infants. *Electroenceph. clin. Neurophysiol.*, **1967,** *23*: 97.

Weitzman, E. D., Fishbein, W. and Graziani, L. Auditory evoked responses obtained from the scalp electroencephalogram of the full-term human neonate during sleep. *Pediatrics*, **1965,** *35*: 458–462.

Wever, E. G. *Theory of Hearing.* Wiley, New York, **1949,** 484 p.

Williams, H. C., Tepas, D. I. and Morlock, H. C. Evoked responses to clicks and electroencephalographic stages in man. *Science*, **1962,** *138*: 685–686.

Zwicker, E., Flottorp, G. and Stevens, S. S. Critical band widths in loudness summation. *J. acoust. Soc. Amer.*, **1957,** *29*: 548–557.

Reference: Lenard, H. G., von Bernuth, H. and Hutt, S. J. Acoustic evoked responses in newborn infants: the influence of pitch and complexity of the stimulus. *Electroenceph. clin. Neurophysiol.*, **1969,** *27*: 121–127.

Electroencephalography and Clinical Neurophysiology
Elsevier Publishing Company, Amsterdam – Printed in The Netherlands

EEG SLEEP PATTERNS IN MENTAL RETARDATION[1]

I. FEINBERG, M. BRAUN AND E. SHULMAN

Department of Psychiatry, State University of New York, Downstate Medical Center, Brooklyn, N.Y. 11203 (U.S.A.)

(Accepted for publication: November 26, 1968)

INTRODUCTION

Previous studies have demonstrated significant correlation coefficients between intellectual level and EEG sleep variables, especially those measuring REM sleep, within groups of subjects suffering from the mild cognitive deficit of normal old age and the more severe impairment of chronic brain syndrome (Feinberg *et al.* 1967). The present investigation attempted to test the generality of the relations between sleep variables and intellectual deficit found in the aged by study of patients with mental retardation due to mongolism, phenylketonuria, brain damage and undifferentiated etiologies. In at least the first three of these conditions the pathology responsible for the cognitive impairment may be presumed different from that involved in aging. The design of the study included independent assessments of the EEG sleep pattern and the intelligence of these adult retardates. In addition to certain theoretical implications, the data obtained contribute to the empirical description of sleep in mental retardation on which there have been but two other publications (Petre-Quadens and Jouvet 1966; Goldie *et al.* 1968). Preliminary reports of the present study have been presented elsewhere (Feinberg 1968; Feinberg *et al.* 1968).

MATERIALS AND METHODS

A. *Subjects*

Subjects were selected for study from the Letchworth Village population by Dr. G. Jervis. Four diagnostic groups were included:

1. *Mongoloids (MONG): (N=9).* Ten subjects were initially studied. Their mean age was 36 (range: 23–49) years. One atypical subject with severe insomnia (mean sleep time over 5 nights =88 min) was eliminated from the study since he might have represented an instance of premature senility in mongolism (Jervis 1948).

2. *Phenylketonurics (PKU): (N = 6).* The mean age of these subjects was 45 (range: 18–60) years.

3. *Brain-damaged (BD): (N = 6).* The mean age of these subjects was 32 (range: 21–50) years. In most cases the diagnosis of brain damage as the responsible agent for the retardation was presumptive and based upon the history.

4. *Undifferentiated retardates (UNDIFF): (N = 11).* The mean age of these subjects was 31 (range: 20–50) years. Some subjects in this group probably would fall into the category of simple familial retardation; for others the etiology of retardation was unknown.

With the exception of one 50-year-old PKU patient, all of the subjects were male.

The sleep patterns of these retardates were compared with those previously recorded in two reference groups (Feinberg *et al.* 1967):

5. *Young normal adults (YN): (N = 15).* These subjects ranged in age from 19 to 36 years (mean: 26). They were actively engaged in their usual occupations during the period of the study.

6. *Chronic brain syndrome patients (CBS): (N = 15).* These elderly subjects ranged in age from 65 to 92 years (mean: 78). They suffered from intellectual deficit (especially of recent memory) but did not manifest delusions or hallucinations.

B. *Drugs and daytime naps*

Six of the thirty-two retardates were receiving drugs known to affect the central nervous system. Since the ingestion of these drugs was chronic,

[1] This work was supported in part by Research Grant No. MH 10927 from the National Institute of Mental Health, National Institutes of Health.

and since the duration of withdrawal effects is unknown, it seemed simpler, for the purposes of this preliminary investigation, to continue the drugs in their usual dosage rather than to discontinue them. None of the sleep results of patients receiving drugs diverged significantly from those found in drug-free subjects of the same subgroup.

In view of the importance of preventing daytime naps, special instructions were issued to the nursing staff. Reports of the staff and of the patients themselves suggest that daytime sleep was rare. The data obtained were consistent with these reports, for by the third night of study the subjects manifested total sleep times which were normal or high for their ages.

C. *Procedure*

Recording techniques were identical with those described previously (Feinberg *et al.* 1967). EEG and eye movements (EM) were monitored on an Offner Type T machine run continuously throughout the night at a paper speed of 15 mm/sec and a gain of 8 mm/50 μV. Left parietal and left occipital EEG derivations were referred to joined bilateral mastoid electrodes. EMs were recorded in two channels: electrodes placed at the outer canthus of each eye were each referred to a forehead electrode placed just above the nasion. This method detects both horizontal and vertical EMs (Feinberg *et al.* in press). Thirty subjects were studied for 5 consecutive nights, two for 4 nights each.

Psychometric testing with the Wechsler Pre-School and Primary Scale of Intelligence (WPPSI, Wechsler 1967) was attempted on each subject for whom sleep data were obtained. The testing was carried out without knowledge of the sleep results by consultant psychologists, Dr. J. Gorelick and Mr. Z .Weiss, experienced in the field of mental retardation. Similarly, the scoring of the sleep tracings was done without awareness of the test results by a rater who had had no contact with the subjects themselves.

Scoring of the sleep EEG

The methods used in scoring the sleep tracings have been presented in detail elsewhere (Feinberg *et al.* 1967). The Dement and Kleitman (1957) system for classifying the EEG stages of sleep was employed. Rapid eye movement (REM) sleep refers to paradoxical sleep generally and non-REM (NREM) sleep refers to EEG sleep stages 2, 3 and 4 combined. The unit of analysis for the EEG tracings was a 20 sec epoch or one page of record. Brief definitions of the sleep measures to be reported here follow: (1) *Total sleep time*: determined by the disappearance of alpha, reduction of tonic muscle activity, and the occurrence of sleep spindles, K complexes, and other slow waves. (2) *Awakenings*: determined by the reappearance of alpha, and other waking frequencies, and muscle activity for at least 40 sec. (3) *Sleep latency*: the time required for the onset of a sleep period lasting at least 5 min. (4) *Stage 1 latency*: amount of sleep recorded prior to the first epoch containing emergent stage 1 EEG. (5) *Emergent stage 1 EEG*: time occupied by low voltage, irregular EEG after the onset of slow wave sleep. The stage 1 EEG occurring at the onset of sleep is not included. The method of scoring stage 1 EEG is modified from Dement (1962). (6) *Eye movement activity* (EM_{20}): number of 20 sec epochs showing evidence of EMs. A second measure, the number of 4 sec epochs with EM, gave similar results and will not be reported here. (7) *EM density*: the percentage of pages of stage 1 EEG with EM (EM_{20}/stage 1 $\times$ 100). (8) *Percent* EM_{20}: the percentage of sleep pages with EM. (9) *Sleep spindles*: the number of bursts, at least 0.5 sec in duration, of sinusoidal, 12–14 c/sec waves. Bursts occurring simultaneously in both EEG leads were counted once. (10) *Stage 3 EEG*: the number of 20 sec epochs which showed at least 10, but no more than 15 delta waves (<4 c/sec) at least 50 μV in amplitude. (11) *Stage 4 EEG*: the number of 20 sec epochs with 16 or more delta waves or in which over one-half the epoch was occupied by delta activity. (12) *Percent stage 3 and percent stage 4*: stage 3 and stage 4 EEG scores divided by total sleep time.

Because of the laboriousness of their analysis, spindling and EEG stages 3 and 4 were scored for only one night — that with median EM_{20} score. The remaining variables were scored for all nights.

RESULTS

All significance tests to be reported here are two-tailed.

A. "*First-night*" *effects*

It is known that subjects participating in laboratory studies of sleep tend initially to show disturbed sleep manifested by a larger number of awakenings and a lower percentage of REM sleep than on subsequent nights ("first-night effect", Rechtschaffen and Verdone 1964; Dement *et al.* 1965; Agnew *et al.* 1966). In normal adults, these effects are relatively slight and have usually disappeared by the second night of study. Fig. 1 indicates that the retardates manifested similar but more pronounced difficulty in adapting to the sleep laboratory and that apparent adaptation was not achieved until the third night of study. Whereas all 4 subgroups showed a marked reduction in total sleep time on the first 2 nights, the tendency toward a disproportionate reduction in REM sleep was most marked in the MONG and PKU subjects (Fig. 2). To minimize these adaptation effects, data to be presented for the retardate and CBS groups are based upon means of nights 3–5 (nights 2–4 for subjects studied 4 nights). Since the adaptation effects for the YN subjects were relatively slight, the data presented for this group include all nights of study.

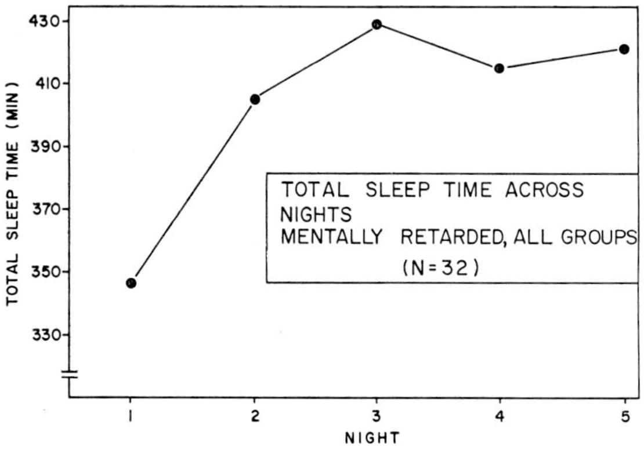

Fig. 1
Mean total sleep time for each night of study. Low values for the first 2 nights constitute an adaptation ("first-night") effect.

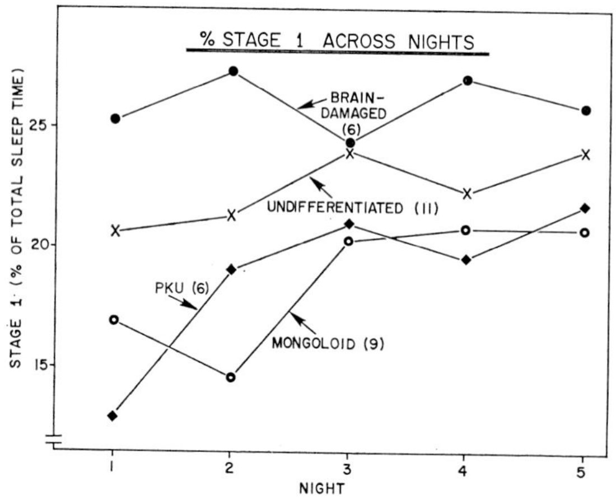

Fig. 2
Mean percentage emergent stage 1 EEG for each night of study.

B. *Total sleep time and awakenings*

Table I gives results for total sleep time and related measures. Compared with YN and retardate groups, CBS patients showed reduced total sleep time associated with prolonged sleep latency and an increase in the number and extent (percent time awake) of awakenings. In contrast, the retardates showed total sleep times at least equal to those found in the YN group. Only one retardate group, the PKU, showed a sleep latency significantly longer than that of the YN group. The number of awakenings was not significantly increased beyond the YN level in any subgroup of retardates. However, Table I indicates that compared with YN values, 3 of the 4 subgroups showed a significant increase in average duration of awakenings and in percent time awake[1].

C. *Stage 1 EEG and eye movement*

Table II gives the results for the two measures of REM sleep, emergent stage 1 EEG and EM activity, employed here. Stage 1 latency scores were significantly lower in CBS subjects than in each of the other groups. In contrast, MONG and PKU patients tended to have latencies longer than those of young normal adults. BD and UNDIFF retardates showed latency values similar to those of the YN group.

The number of REM periods ranged from 3.9 in the MONG subjects to 4.6 in the BD group. No statistically significant differences were found among any of the groups under consideration.

[1] This latter finding may have resulted from the institutional practice of early bedtime and, consequently, an amount of time in bed in excess of sleep need. Whatever the basis of the slight increase in awakening among the retardates, the present data show clearly that the *extreme* fragmentation of sleep which characterizes both normal and pathological old age is not associated with these retardation syndromes.

TABLE I

Group scores for total sleep time and amount of waking
Mann-Whitney U test (Siegel 1956)

Group (*N*)		Sleep latency (min)	Total sleep time (min)	Time awake/ time in bed (%)	Awakenings per subject (No.)	Average duration of awakenings (min)
YN	Mean	10.4	393.9	6.1	3.1	4.6
(15)	Range	2–26	345–432	2–12	2–5	1–9
CBS	Mean	26.2*	309.0**	30.7**	9.3**	15.6**
(15)	Range	2–74	225–379	18–51	3–21	9–25
MONG	Mean	37.6	420.0++	17.3**,++	2.9++	20.0**
(9)	Range	4–99	348–491	5–30	1–10	7–31
PKU	Mean	33.9*	406.9++	15.8*,+	2.0*,++	19.9**
(6)	Range	14–74	363–451	7–28	1–3	8–30
BD	Mean	19.5§	409.5+	14.4+	2.9+	12.5
(6)	Range	9–54	327–497	4–34	0–9	0–33
UNDIFF	Mean	14.0	432.9*,++	10.2*,++,†	3.0++	13.2*
(11)	Range	4–54	353–524	4–20	1–8	3–39

*$P < 0.05$, **$P < 0.01$ Significantly different from YN.
+$P < 0.05$, ++$P < 0.01$ Significantly different from CBS.
†$P < 0.05$ Significantly different from MONG.
§$P < 0.05$ Significantly different from PKU.

TABLE II

Group scores for measures of REM sleep
Mann-Whitney U test

Group (*N*)		Stage 1 latency (min)	Stage 1 (min)	Stage 1 % total sleep	EM_{20} (epoch)	% total sleep with EM	% EM density
YN	Mean	66.9	98.9	25.0	162.7	13.8	55.5
(15)	Range	51–92	64–132	17–32	97–226	9–20	37–71
CBS	Mean	38.7**	62.4**	20.0*	99.5**	10.8	56.2
(15)	Range	8–82	27–111	12–30	19–187	2–17	21–80
Mong	Mean	93.4*,++	89.0+	20.6*	88.9**	6.9**,+	33.3**,++
(9)	Range	50–139	44–117	11–25	34–129	3–10	25–44
PKU	Mean	95.0*,++	86.1	20.9*	121.0*,†	10.0*,†	49.8†
(6)	Range	71–117	43–106	12–24	71–160	5–13	24–72
BD	Mean	65.1+	105.9++,§	25.4+,†,§	164.6+,††,§§	13.2††,§§	52.7††
(6)	Range	38–97	69–133	20–29	119–213	12–14	48–59
UNDIFF	Mean	73.6++	104.1+	23.4	146.7+,††	11.0††	48.2†
(11)	Range	54–113	45–164	12–34	71–241	7–17	32–59

* $P < 0.05$, ** $P < 0.01$ Significantly different from YN.
\+ $P < 0.05$, ++ $P < 0.01$ Significantly different from CBS.
† $P < 0.05$, †† $P < 0.01$ Significantly different from MONG.
§ $P < 0.05$, §§ $P < 0.01$ Significantly different from PKU.

The relative constancy of this periodicity among such diverse states of brain function was noteworthy.

Table II shows that, in general, absolute and percentage values for both emergent stage 1 EEG and EM activity were lower than YN levels for CBS, MONG and PKU subjects, although these differences did not reach statistical significance in every comparison. BD and UNDIFF groups did not differ significantly from the YN subjects on these measures. However, the difference between YN and UNDIFF groups in percentage EM_{20} scores approached statistical significance ($P \sim 0.05$). The heterogeneity of the scores of the UNDIFF subjects shown in these tables is consistent with the assumption that this group includes a variety of brain disorders.

It is of interest to note that differences from YN levels for stage 1 EEG and EM activity did not necessarily occur to the same degree. Thus, MONG subjects had a reduction of 50% in percentage EM activity, whereas their percentage stage 1 EEG was only 20% lower than that found in the YNs.

D. *Spindling, stage 3 and stage 4 EEG*

Table III gives results for spindle counts and amounts of stage 3 and stage 4 EEG. Spindle scores for CBS, MONG and PKU subjects were significantly lower than in the YN group. BD and UNDIFF subjects also showed considerably lower values than YN subjects, although these differences did not achieve statistical significance. However, when the data from the one YN subject with zero spindle scores were omitted (this subject consistently showed spindle bursts whose frequency, 11 c/sec, was below our criterion), the differences in spindle counts between young normal adults and the BD and UNDIFF group became statistically significant ($P < 0.05$).

Absolute and percentage values for stage 3 EEG in the UNDIFF group tended to be higher than for the YN and BD subjects. For stage 4 EEG, CBS patients had lower values than YN subjects, a finding consistent with the changes now known to occur with age (Agnew *et al.* 1967; Feinberg *et al.* 1967; Kales *et al.* 1967; Feinberg and Carlson 1968). Among the retardates, the BD subjects showed low absolute and percentage values for stage 4 EEG, values differing from those of young adults at a high level of confidence ($P < 0.01$). In addition, the percentage of stage 4 EEG in the BD group was significantly lower than in MONG, PKU and UNDIFF subjects.

It has long been recognized that stage 3 and 4 EEG activity are maximal in the early hours of sleep, declining steadily across the night. Fig. 3

TABLE III

Spindling, Stage 3 and Stage 4 activity
Mann-Whitney U test

Group (*N*)		Spindles (No.)	Stage 3 (20 sec epoch)	Stage 3 (% total sleep)	Stage 4 (20 sec epoch)	Stage 4 (% total sleep)
YN	Mean	76.4	116.0	9.6	156.9	13.0
(15)	Range	0–164	12–239	1–19	0–311	0–24
CBS	Mean	23.5**	153.8	16.5	42.9**	4.6**
(15)	Range	2–70	7–357	1–44	0–133	0–14
MONG	Mean	31.4*	123.4	9.7	158.3++	11.9+
(9)	Range	3–75	83–176	6–13	25–310	2–20
PKU	Mean	21.2*	119.0	10.3	106.0	9.2
(5)	Range	2–68	23–163	2–16	1–234	0–21
BD	Mean	35.8	77.8	6.1	28.2**,†	2.0**,†,⊕
(6)	Range	2–63	0–160	0–12	0–87	0–5
UNDIFF	Mean	47.6+	170.1*,§	13.6§	130.1+,§	9.9+,§
(11)	Range	8–119	23–289	2–23	0–250	0–20

* $P < 0.05$, ** $P < 0.01$: Significantly different from YN.
\+ $P < 0.05$, ++ $P < 0.01$: Significantly different from CBS.
† $P < 0.05$ Significantly different from MONG.
⊕ $P < 0.05$ Significantly different from PKU.
§ $P < 0.05$ Significantly different from BD.

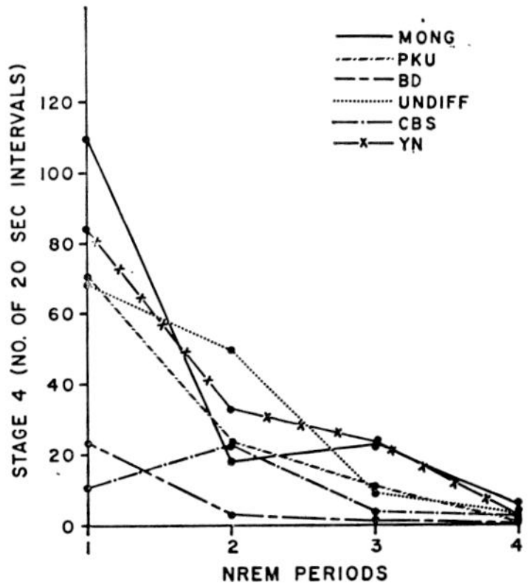

Fig. 3
Mean absolute stage 4 EEG as a function of successive periods of NREM sleep within a single night.

illustrates these changes as a function of successive NREM periods for the absolute amount of stage 4 EEG. Data were included only from subjects who completed at least 4 NREM periods on the night of study[1].

E. *Sleep cycles*

Fig. 4 presents the sequences of NREM and REM sleep for each group. Data were included in this figure only for nights in which at least 4 cycles were completed; data for individual subjects were included in group means only if based upon 2 or more nights with at least 4 cycles.

Certain differences among groups are apparent. The first NREM periods of the CBS and BD subjects were relatively short, perhaps because of the low stage 4 values in these groups. MONG and, to a lesser extent, PKU subjects, tended to show lengthy first NREM periods. NREM periods in all groups tended to decline in duration during the latter part of the night. An abbreviated first REM period, which is characteristic of young adults, was not apparent in CBS and PKU groups. However, this trend was present in MONG, BD and UNDIFF patients.

F. *Intercorrelation of sleep variables, age and psychometric scores*

1. *Relation of sleep variables to age*. Previously we reported the results of a regression analysis of sleep variables on age in normal subjects ranging in age from 4 to 96 years (Feinberg and Carlson 1968). The age range of the thirty-two retardates described here was considerably more narrow (from 18 to 60 years, with only 3 subjects over 50 years). Nevertheless, as may be observed in the correlation matrix of Table IV, the same age trends found for normal subjects were apparent in the retardates. Correlation coefficients for stage 3 and stage 4 EEG, while not statistically significant, revealed the same trends previously found in normals. Stage 4 EEG tended to decline with age, and stage 3 to increase.

Psychometric scores were not significantly correlated with age in these subjects. Nevertheless, in view of this first application of the WPPSI to retarded subjects, it is of interest to note that the Verbal and Performance scores on this test showed the same age trends as those found in the Wechsler Adult Intelligence Scale in normals (Doppelt and Wallace 1955). Thus Verbal scores showed a correlation coefficient with age which was close to zero, whereas Performance scores showed a negative relation which approached statistical significance ($r = -0.30$; 0.35 being required for significance at the 5% level).

2. *Relation of sleep variables to psychometric scores*. Psychometric scores showed statistically significant associations with a number of sleep variables. Verbal scores were correlated at the 1% level with each of the measures of eye movement employed ($r \geq 0.63$). WPPSI Performance scores were correlated at similar confidence levels with these variables, and, in addition, at the 5% level, with sleep latency (−0.41), total sleep time (0.40), percent time awake (−0.47) and the absolute value of stage 1 (0.41).

Thus, these data indicate that the level of intellectual function in this group of retardates

[1] An analysis of variance for the regressions of stage 3 and 4 EEG on successive NREM periods was carried out by Dr. V. R. Carlson of the National Institute of Mental Health. The slopes of these regressions were significantly different from zero ($P < 0.001$), and also differed among groups ($P < 0.001$). The slopes for stage 3 differed from those for stage 4 ($P < 0.01$). The curvature apparent in the figure was significant since a quadratic fit produced a reliable reduction in deviations beyond those obtained with a linear fit ($P < 0.001$). These results indicate that variations may occur in the rate of production of delta sleep across the night. The fact that the trends are curvilinear has implications for sleep models which consider NREM and REM processes as competitive.

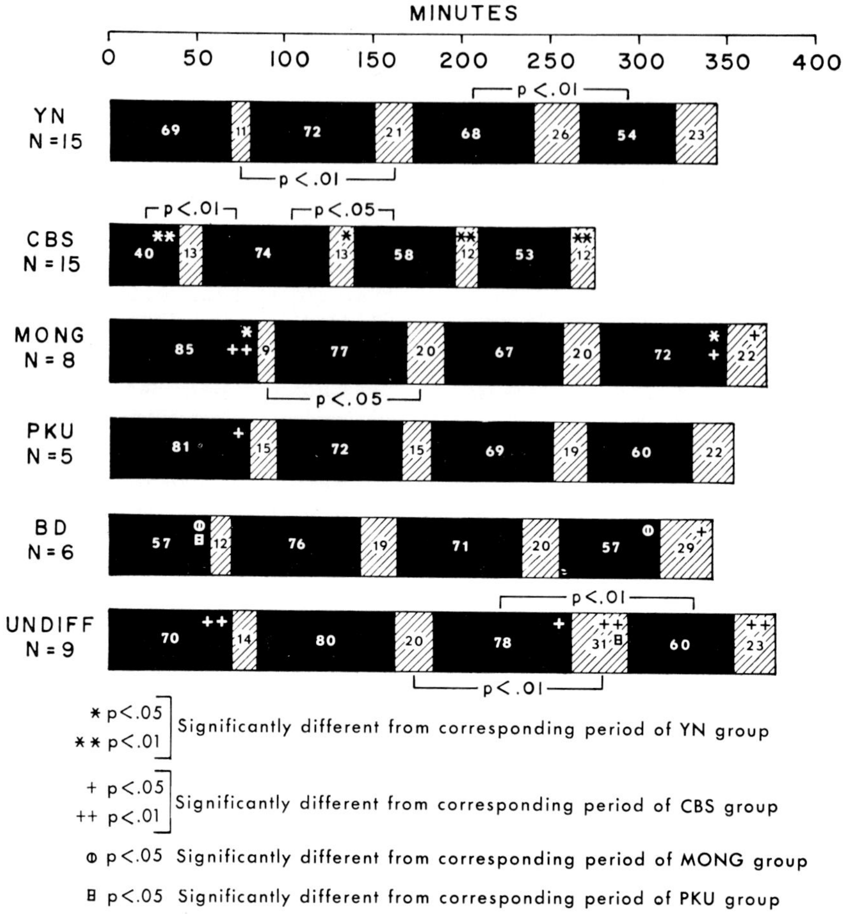

Fig. 4

Durations of successive NREM (black) and REM (striped) sleep periods for each group. The first 4 cycles are shown. Values for individual subjects were based on means for at least 2 nights on which 4 REM periods were completed. Since not all subjects completed 4 REM periods on 2 nights, the *N*'s for some subgroups differ from those shown in the tables.

was positively correlated with estimates of REM sleep provided by measures of emergent stage 1 EEG and EM activity. These relations were not attributable to age. For example, the correlations of WPPSI Verbal and Performance scores with EM_{20}, with the correlation to age partialled out, were 0.74 and 0.64 ($P<0.01$). The finding in the retardates of a relation between REM sleep measures and psychometric performance parallels earlier results for patients with cognitive deficit due to age (Feinberg *et al.* 1967). However, in the aged subjects, stage 1 EEG and EM_{20} showed equally good correlations with psychometric scores. In the retardates, these correlations were consistently higher for EMs perhaps because this phasic activity reflects the intensity of REM processes, as the evidence of Evarts (1962) and Berger and Oswald (1962) would suggest.

One further observation testifies to the strength of the relation between eye movement activity and intellectual function in the retardates. Stanford-Binet scores, taken from hospital records at the conclusion of the study, showed a rank-order correlation of 0.77 with percent EM_{20}, although these IQ tests had been administered years earlier by several different psychologists.

Total sleep time and percentage time awake were significantly correlated with WPPSI Performance scores. This finding may reflect the special sensitivity of both Performance skills and these sleep variables to age. However, it is of interest to note that the correlations of the sleep variables with Performance scores were statistically significant, whereas the correlations of age itself with these scores were somewhat lower and failed to reach significance. These results suggest that the cognitive skills which diminish with age in normals are similarly affected in the mentally retarded. It also appears that for these latter subjects, as well as for the normal elderly, sleep variables provide a quantitative index of these effects at least as reliable as that provided by age itself.

A scattergram of the relation of EM_{20} to WPPSI total scores is presented in Fig. 5. It may be seen that among the 4 subgroups the association between these variables was most evident for the UNDIFF group, which also had the largest number of subjects. No apparent relation was seen in the PKU subjects; however, three of these subjects were over 50 years of age and two of these subjects were receiving drugs. A moderate relation was apparent among the MONG and BD groups. Obviously, more definite conclusions must await the study of a larger number of cases within each subgroup.

A correlation matrix for the variables shown in Table IV was computed separately for each subgroup of retardates. In general, the patterns of these results were similar to those in the group as a whole. However, it was interesting to note

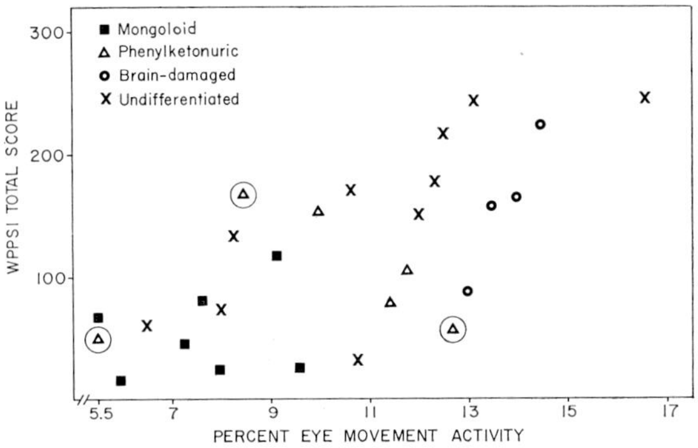

Fig. 5

Percentage eye movement activity (% EM_{20}) plotted against WPPSI Total scores. Data points for subjects over 50 years of age are circled. These subjects do not contribute disproportionately to the correlation.

that the BD group who were distinguished from the other retardates by low scores for stage 4 EEG, were the only group to show positive correlations between stage 4 EEG and WPPSI scores.

Qualitative observations

The EEG stages of sleep in these retardates were often difficult to score. These difficulties stemmed, in part, from the low levels of eye movement, less clear-cut flattening of the EEG during REM sleep, and from the paucity of sleep spindles. In addition, K complexes were usually quite atypical in wave form and were less abundant than normal. One MONG, three PKU and five UNDIFF subjects were rated as showing typical K complexes; the remainder of the subjects in this study had atypical K complexes. Since the K complex of sleep and the evoked response appear to be similar phenomena (Davis 1939; Davis *et al.* 1939), the present observations would predict abnormalities in evoked response wave forms in these mental retardation syndromes. Findings indicating the presence of such abnormalities in mongoloid infants have already been reported by Barnet and Lodge (1967).

Extremely low voltage records, such as frequently occurred in both the normal and pathological aged subjects (Feinberg *et al.* 1965, 1967) were not common among the retardates. Only four of the thirty-two subjects were rated as having abnormally low voltage tracings. Paroxysmal discharges were frequent in the PKU and BD subjects but were rare in MONG and UNDIFF patients.

A prominent feature of the sleep tracings of the MONG subjects was relatively high voltage beta activity. Medium or high levels of beta activity were found in all MONG subjects and moderate but less marked levels in PKU subjects. In contrast, this activity was uncommon in the BD and UNDIFF groups. The beta activity of the MONG subjects, while most prominent during REM periods, invaded the other stages of sleep as well. One wonders whether some of this activity is related to the "extreme spindle" which Gibbs and Gibbs (1962) described in some retardates. However, these latter authors state that such spindles were never seen over age 12 years, whereas the youngest subject in the present group was 18 years.

TABLE IV

Intercorrelations for age, sleep variables and psychometric scores+

	(*N*)	1	2	3	4	5	6	7	8	9	10	11	12	13	14	15	16	17
1. Age	(32)																	
2. Sleep latency	(32)	20																
3. Total sleep time	(32)	—47**	—56**															
4. Total NREM	(32)	—26	—61**	86**														
5. No. awakenings	(32)	42*	—12	—22	—08													
6. % Time awake	(32)	50**	74**	—87**	—80**	29												
7. Stage 1 latency	(32)	12	—10	12	39*	—04	—11											
8. Total stage 1	(32)	—54**	—27	77**	33	—30	—61**	—28										
9. % Stage 1	(32)	—46**	—11	51**	C0	—25	—36*	—43*	94**									
10. Spindle counts	(32)	—55**	—23	14	11	09	—22	—18	12	08								
11. % Stage 3	(31)	27	—36*	—10	20	24	—13	19	—43*	—54**	08							
12. % Stage 4	(31)	—24	—27	37*	57**	—13	—35	40*	—02	—23	10	17						
13. EM_{20}	(32)	—44*	—28	58**	22	—19	—52**	—31	79**	75**	02	—25	—08					
14. % EM_{20}	(32)	—35*	—18	35*	—03	—11	—32	—43*	68**	73**	01	—29	—23	96**				
15. EM density	(32)	04	—24	—03	—03	13	—08	—18	—01	—01	—08	22	—08	56**	65**			
16. WPPSI Verbal	(28)	—02	—26	11	—07	—06	—17	—23	31	33	—11	—04	—28	67**	71**	63**		
17. WPPSI Perf.	(28)	—30	—41*	40*	25	—13	—47*	—13	41*	28	04	02	00	68**	61**	51**	81**	
18. WPPSI Total	(27)	—19	—36	33	15	—15	—39*	—15	43*	36	—05	00	—16	73**	69**	57**	94**	97**

* $P < 0.05$.
** $P < 0.01$.
+ Decimal points omitted.

Alpha activity was poorly organized and low in abundance in the MONG group. Alpha frequencies tended to be low in all groups, most clearly so in the MONG subjects. The mean and ranges for alpha frequencies (in c/sec) were as follows: MONG 8.6 (7–11); PKU 9.4 (8–11); BD 9.3 (8–12); UNDIFF 9.3 (7–11); CBS 8.9 (7.5–10.5).

DISCUSSION

A. *REM sleep*

The present results indicate that REM sleep measures are quantitatively related to level of intellectual function in mentally retarded subjects. This relation is independent of age. The correlation coefficient of 0.73 for the relation of WPPSI scores to percentage eye movement not only possesses a high degree of statistical reliability ($P < 0.001$), but also accounts for a large proportion ($\sim 50\%$) of the variance[1].

What is the basis for the positive relation between REM sleep processes and intelligence? One possibility, first suggested by Jackson (1958), is that during sleep the brain carries out certain active processes required for adequate waking function. This view, the sleep-cognition hypothesis, has more recently been advanced by ourselves (Feinberg 1964; Feinberg *et al.* 1967; Feinberg and Carlson 1968; Feinberg and Evarts 1968) and others (Evans and Newman 1964; Gaarder 1966; Greenberg and Leiderman 1966; Moruzzi 1966; Breger 1967; Shapiro 1968). Evidence which has been cited as consistent with this view includes ontogenetic changes in human sleep, the parallel variations of cerebral oxygen uptake and sleep across age and in chronic brain syndrome, and the correlation coefficients between sleep variables and psychometric performance in CBS and aged normal subjects.

The present data, in extending the range of conditions in which REM sleep is correlated with intellectual function, lend further support to the sleep-cognition hypothesis. However, this support, as well as that noted above, is indirect. Thus it is possible that brain pathology impairs sleep mechanisms and intelligence in the absence of any direct relation between the latter two variables. Ellingson (1966) put forward this interpretation for the apparent correlations between waking EEG and psychometric performance. Applied to the present data, this view would predict that the correlation coefficients between psychometric scores and REM sleep would be lowest in subjects with least evidence of brain pathology. However, it was this group, the undifferentiated retardates, who showed the highest correlation between these measures. Nevertheless, since it remains possible that some patients diagnosed as undifferentiated retardates actually suffer from unrecognized types of brain disease, the latter evidence can only be considered suggestive.

If the relationship between REM sleep and intelligence is causal, toward what neural processes might REM sleep contribute? In view of the paucity of evidence, only brief speculation seems warranted. It does seem clear that sleep is a highly active process (Evarts 1967; Kety 1967) and that the brain does not rest, in Sherrington's (1953) sense, during sleep. It also seems apparent that synaptic growth and decay play vital roles in intelligence and learning (Eccles 1966; Moruzzi 1966). For this reason, it seems probable to us (as it was to Jackson 1958) that during sleep the brain carries out repair or erasure of synapses, or both. Further discussion of the psychological and physiological evidence relevant to this issue may be found in Feinberg and Evarts (1968).

The findings described above are consistent with the few observations on the REM sleep of retardates reported thus far. Petre-Quadens and Jouvet (1966) studied forty-two retardates for 1 or 2 nights each but analyzed only the data of the first night. While these results may therefore be heavily affected by adaptation effects, their direction — low percentages of REM sleep in the retardates — was the same as in the present study. Goldie *et al.* (1968) described decreased REM sleep in a small group of mongoloid infants. More recently Castaldo (1968) reported low values for REM sleep in sixteen mongoloid subjects and noted that, within this group, lower values were associated with more severe intellectual deficit.

B. *NREM sleep, effects of age*

Spindling activity was low in abundance in all 4 retardate groups. The amount of spindling is also reduced in the normal and senile aged (Feinberg *et al.* 1967). It seems reasonable to pro-

[1] See also "Note added in proof" on page 138.

pose that intellectual deficit in general is associated with a reduction in the number of spindle bursts or with a slowing of spindle frequencies (either change would give low spindle scores with the measure we employed). However, in neither the retarded nor the aged subjects have spindle scores shown consistent correlations with psychometric performance. The failure to find such relations may reflect limitations of the methods employed thus far to measure spindle activity. Alternatively, this failure may indicate that the tests used have been insensitive to the type of cognitive impairment associated with damage to spindle mechanisms. Whichever the case, it appears that almost complete absence of spindles may occur in subjects, such as aged normals, with only mild degrees of cognitive deficit.

The finding of low stage 4 in the brain-damaged retardates suggests that although brain damage predisposes toward slow wave activity in the waking EEG, it diminishes the slow waves of normal sleep. The same changes occur in normal old age and in chronic brain syndrome where stage 4 sleep is reduced in the presence of slow waves in the waking EEG (Feinberg *et al.* 1967). These observations suggest that the slow waves of sleep are functionally dissimilar to the pathological slowing of the waking EEG, an interpretation supported by the differences in brain metabolic rate associated with the two conditions (Mangold *et al.* 1955; Obrist *et al.* 1963). The finding of low stage 4 in brain-damaged subjects is also of interest in view of the hypothesis that stage 4 EEG reflects the activity of plastic neurons (Feinberg *et al.* 1967). Since it is reasonable to assume that plastic neurons have high metabolic rates and are therefore specially vulnerable to damage by anoxia and infection, the present result is consistent with this speculation.

The same changes in sleep pattern associated with age in normal subjects occurred in the retardates. The clear age-relations found in these subjects in the face of a relatively narrow age range and of the variability contributed by heterogeneous brain conditions testifies to the profound effects of age on the brain activity of sleep. It also raises the possibility that these effects may be even more pronounced in patients with brain impairment than in normal subjects.

Whereas aging exerts common effects on the sleep patterns of patients with quite different brain conditions, the brain conditions studied here produce a variety of patterns of abnormal sleep. These differences are summarized in Table V. The diverse patterns of abnormality rule out the possibility that these changes are artifacts of factors common to all groups, such as institutionalization or anxiety. In addition, the quite distinctive patterns observed in some subgroups (such as the MONG) raise the possibility that the sleep EEG may ultimately prove diagnostic of certain retardation syndromes. Such a finding could have application in the study of such behavioral syndromes as infantile autism, where a subgroup of patients is believed to suffer from retardation due to organic brain disease. Abnormalities of the sleep EEG might prove useful in distinguishing this group from those whose abnormal behavior results from other causes. While the few studies of EEG sleep patterns in autism and childhood schizophrenia carried out thus far have revealed normal sleep patterns (Onheiber *et al.* 1965; Ornitz *et al.* 1965), the number of patients studied was too small to test this suggestion.

Note added in proof: Neurological examinations being carried out by one of us (I.F.) have revealed a high incidence of visual disturbance (oculomotor imbalance, nystagmus, lens opacities) in the mongoloid subjects. This finding raises the possibility that the low eye movement scores in this group are related to a specific disorder of the visual system rather than (or perhaps as well as) to low IQ. This question is being actively pursued. The rank-order correlation between EM_{20} and WPPSI total, omitting the mongoloid subjects, was 0.53 ($P<0.02$, two-tailed).

SUMMARY

EEG and eye movement were recorded continuously during sleep in thirty-two adult subjects with mental retardation. Included were patients with mongolism, phenylketonuria (PKU), brain damage and undifferentiated retardation. The intellectual level of these patients was independently evaluated with the Wechsler Pre-School and Primary Scale of Intelligence (WPPSI). Sleep measures in the retardates were compared with

TABLE V

Differences from the EEG sleep pattern of young normal adults found in five groups with cognitive impairment

	Chronic brain syndrome	MONG	PKU	BD	UNDIFF
Total sleep time	reduced	N	N	N	N
Number of awakenings	marked increase	N	N	N	N
% Time awake	marked increase	? increase	N	? increase	? increase
REM sleep					
Stage 1 EEG (tonic)	moderate decrease	moderate decrease	slight decrease	N	slight decrease
EM activity (phasic)	moderate decrease	marked decrease	slight decrease	N	slight decrease (wide range)
NREM sleep					
Stage 4 EEG (amount)	marked decrease	N	N	marked decrease	N
Spindles	decreased	decreased	decreased	decreased	decreased
K complex wave form	abnormal	abnormal	abnormal	abnormal	abnormal
Sleep cycle					
Duration of $NREM_1$	short	long	long	short	? N
Normal abbreviation of REM_1	absent	N	? absent	N	N
Other					
Beta	occasionally prominent	markedly prominent	N	N	N
Epileptiform activity	occasional	absent	prominent	occasional	absent

N = no clear difference.

data available for normal adults and for elderly patients with chronic brain syndrome.

WPPSI scores were positively correlated with emergent stage 1 EEG and with rapid eye movement (REM) activity, findings consistent with the sleep-cognition hypothesis. Compared with normal adults, mongoloid subjects showed low amounts of REM sleep, with an extreme reduction in the amount of eye movement, and quite prominent beta activity. PKU subjects showed a trend toward low values for REM and their sleep tracings manifested much epileptiform activity. Brain-damaged subjects had normal amounts of REM sleep but little stage 4 EEG compared to normal controls or to other retardates. Undifferentiated patients showed widely varying amounts of REM activity, ranging from extremely low to quite high values. Total sleep time was not reduced below normal levels in any of the retardate groups. All four groups showed atypical K complexes and a paucity of sleep spindles. The effects of age on the sleep patterns of the retardates were similar to those previously found in normals.

The results suggest that investigation of the sleep EEG pattern in conditions of altered brain function may prove of diagnostic value and may lead to new insights into such fundamental questions as the neurobiology of intelligence, the effects of aging on the central nervous system, and the nature and function of sleep itself.

RÉSUMÉ

PATTERNS EEG DE SOMMEIL ET ARRIÉRATION MENTALE

L'EEG et les mouvements oculaires ont été enregistrés de façon continue pendant le sommeil chez trente-deux adultes arriérés mentaux. Ces sujets comportaient des cas de mongolisme, de phénylpyruvie, de lésions cérébrales et de retard indifférencié. Le niveau intellectuel de ces malades a été évalué de façon indépendante au moyen du test de WPPSI. Les quantifications du sommeil des sujets arriérés ont été comparées aux données existantes chez les adultes normaux et chez des malades âgés avec syndromes cérébraux organiques chroniques.

Les scores au WPPSI sont en relation positive avec l'activité EEG rapide et les mouvements oculaires rapides, donnée en rapport avec l'hypothèse d'une relation entre sommeil et cognition. Par comparaison aux adultes normaux on trouve chez les sujets mongoliques une faible proportion de sommeil avec mouvements oculaires, et une extrême réduction de la quantité des mouvements oculaires, et une prédominance de l'activité beta. Chez les sujets avec phénylpyruvie on observe une tendance à des valeurs basses de sommeil rapide et une forte proportion d'activité épileptiforme dans les tracés de sommeil. Les sujets avec lésions cérébrales organiques ont des proportions normales de sommeil rapide, mais peu de stade IV par comparaison aux contrôles normaux ou aux autres catégories de sujets arriérés. Les cas d'arriération indifférenciée montrent des quantités très variables d'activité rapide, allant de valeurs extrêmement basses à des valeurs tout à fait élevées. Le temps total de sommeil n'est inférieur au temps normal dans aucun de groupes de sujets arriérés. On observe dans les quatre groupes des complexes K atypiques et des spindles apauvris. Les effets de l'âge sur les patterns EEG de sommeil des sujets arriérés sont semblables à ceux qui ont été précédemment définis chez les normaux.

Il découle de ces résultats que les investigations EEG du sommeil dans certaines conditions d'altération de la fonction cérébrale peuvent apporter un élément diagnostique et aboutir à des nouvelles perspectives dans des domaines aussi fondamentaux que la neurobiologie de l'intelligence, les effets de l'âge sur le système nerveux central, la nature et la fonction du sommeil lui-même.

We are indebted to Dr G. Jervis, former Director of Research, Letchworth Village, N. Y., for selection of patients and advice throughout the study. We are also grateful to Dr. J. Schneider, Superintendent, for permission to carry out this research.

REFERENCES

AGNEW JR., H. W., WEBB, W. B. and WILLIAMS, R. L. The first night effect: an EEG study of sleep. *Psychophysiology*, **1966**, *2*: 263–266.

AGNEW JR., H. W., WEBB, W. B. and WILLIAMS, R. L. Sleep patterns in late middle-aged males: an EEG study. *Electroenceph. clin. Neurophysiol.*, **1967**, *23*: 168–171.

BARNET, A. B. and LODGE, A. Click evoked EEG responses in normal and developmentally retarded infants. *Nature (Lond.)*, **1967**, *214*: 252–255.

BERGER, R. J. and OSWALD, I. Eye movements during active and passive dreams. *Science*, **1962**, *137*: 601.

BREGER, L. Function of dreams. *J. abnorm. Psychol.*, **1967**, *72* (2, Whole No. 641).

CASTALDO, V. *EEG study of sleep patterns in adolescent mongoloids (Down's syndrome)*. Presented at Ass. Psychophysiol. Study Sleep, Denver, Colo., **1968**.

DAVIS, H., DAVIS, P. A., LOOMIS, A. L., HARVEY, E. N. and HOBART, G. Electrical reaction of the human brain to auditory stimulation during sleep. *J. Neurophysiol.*, **1939**, *2*: 500–514.

DAVIS, P. A. Effects of acoustic stimuli on the waking brain. *J. Neurophysiol.*, **1939**, *2*: 494–499.

DEMENT, W. C. *A manual for scoring dream time*. Presented at Ass. Psychophysiol. Study Sleep, Chicago, Ill., **1962**.

DEMENT, W. C., KAHN, E. and ROFFWARG, H. P. The influence of the laboratory situation on the dreams of the experimental subject. *J. nerv. ment. Dis.*, **1965**, *140*: 119–131.

DEMENT, W. and KLEITMAN, N. Cyclic variations in EEG during sleep and their relation to eye movements, body motility, and dreaming. *Electroenceph. clin. Neurophysiol.*, **1957**, *9*: 673–690.

DOPPELT, J. E. and WALLACE, W. L. Standardization of the Wechsler Adult Intelligence Scale for older persons. *J. abnorm. soc. Psychol.*, **1955**, *51*: 312–330.

ECCLES, J. C. Conscious experience and memory. In J. C. ECCLES (Ed.), *Brain and conscious experience*. Springer, New York, **1966**: 314–344.

ELLINGSON, R. J. Relationship between EEG and test intelligence: a commentary. *Psychol. Bull.*, **1966**, *65*: 91–98.

EVANS, C. R. and NEWMAN, E. A. Dreaming: an analogy from computers. *New Scientist*, **1964**, *24*: 577–579.

EVARTS, E. V. Activity of neurons in visual cortex of the cat during sleep with low-voltage fast EEG activity. *J. Neurophysiol.*, **1962**, *25*: 812–816.

EVARTS, E. V. Activity of individual cerebral neurons during sleep and arousal. *Res. Publ. Ass. nerv. ment. Dis.*, **1967**, *45*: 319–336.

FEINBERG, I. *Current studies on sleep and dreaming*. Presented at Ass. Psychophysiol. Study Sleep, Palo Alto, Calif., **1964**.

FEINBERG, I. Eye movement activity during sleep and intellectual function in mental retardation. *Science*, **1968**, *159*: 1256.

FEINBERG, I., BRAUN, M. and KORESKO, R. L. Vertical eye-movement during REM sleep: effects of age and electrode placement. *Psychophysiology*, (In press).

FEINBERG, I., BRAUN, M. and SHULMAN, E. Electrophysiological sleep patterns in mongolism and phenylpyruvic oligophrenia (PKU). *Psychophysiology*, **1968,** *4*: 395 (Abstract).

FEINBERG, I. and CARLSON, V. R. Sleep variables as a function of age in man. *Arch. gen. Psychiat.*, **1968,** *18*: 239–250.

FEINBERG, I. and EVARTS, E. V. *Changing concepts of the function of sleep*. Presented at Soc. Biol. Psychiat., Washington, D.C., June **1968**. (To be published)

FEINBERG, I., KORESKO, R. L. and HELLER, N. EEG sleep patterns as a function of normal and pathological aging in man. *J. psychiat. Res.*, **1967,** *5*: 107–144.

FEINBERG, I., KORESKO, R. L. and SCHAFFNER, I. Sleep electroencephalographic and eye-movement patterns in patients with chronic brain syndrome. *J. psychiat. Res.*, **1965,** *3*: 11–26.

GAARDER, K. A conceptual model of sleep. *Arch. gen. Psychiat.*, **1966,** *14*: 253–260.

GIBBS, E. L. and GIBBS, F. A. Extreme spindles: correlation of electroencephalographic sleep pattern with mental retardation. *Science*, **1962,** *138*: 1106–1107.

GOLDIE, L., CURTIS, J. A. H., SVENDSEN, U. and ROBERTON, N. R. C. Abnormal sleep rhythms in mongol babies. *Lancet*, **1968,** *1*: 229–230.

GREENBERG, R. and LEIDERMAN, P. H. Perceptions, the dream process and memory: an up-to-date version of notes on a mystic writing pad. *Comprehens. Psychiat.*, **1966,** *7*: 517–523.

JACKSON, J. H. Selected writings of Hughlings Jackson. In J. TAYLOR *et al.* (Eds.), *Selected writings of Hughlings Jackson*. Basic Books, New York, **1958,** 2: 117–118.

JERVIS, G. A. Early senile changes in mongoloid idiocy. *Amer. J. Psychiat.*, **1948,** *105*: 102–107.

KALES, A., WILSON, T., KALES, J. D., JACOBSON, A., PAULSON, M. J., KOLLAR, E. and WALTER, R.D. All-night sleep measurements in normal elderly subjects: effects of aging. *Amer. Geriat. Soc.*, **1967,** *15*: 405–414.

KETY, S. S. Relationship between energy metabolism of the brain and functional activity. *Res. Publ. Ass. nerv. ment. Dis.*, **1967,** *45*: 39–47.

MANGOLD, R., SOKOLOFF, L., CONNER, E., KLEINERMAN, J., THERMAN, P. O. and KETY, S. S. The effects of sleep and lack of sleep on the cerebral circulation and metabolism of normal young men. *J. clin. Invest.*, **1955,** *34*: 1092–1100.

MORUZZI, G. The functional significance of sleep with particular regard to the brain mechanisms underlying consciousness. In J. C. ECCLES (Ed.), *Brain and conscious experience*. Springer, New York, **1966:** 345–388.

OBRIST, W. D., SOKOLOFF, L., LASSEN, N. A., LANE, M. H., BUTLER, R. N. and FEINBERG, I. Relation of EEG to cerebral blood flow and metabolism in old age. *Electroenceph. clin. Neurophysiol.*, **1963,** *15*: 610–619.

ONHEIBER, P., WHITE, P. T., DEMYER, M. K. and OTTINGER, D. R. Sleep and dream patterns of child schizophrenics. *Arch. gen. Psychiat.*, **1965,** *12*: 568–571.

ORNITZ, E.M., RITVO, E. V. and WALTER, R. D. Dreaming sleep in autistic and schizophrenic children. *Amer. J. Psychiat.*, **1965,** *122*: 419–424.

PETRE-QUADENS, O. and JOUVET, M. Paradoxical phase of sleep in the mentally retarded. *J. neurol. Sci.*, **1966,** *3*: 608–612.

RECHTSCHAFFEN, A. and VERDONE, P. Amount of dreaming: effect of incentive, adaptation to laboratory and individual differences. *Percept. mot. Skills*, **1964,** *19*: 947–958.

SHAPIRO, A. A theoretical model for empirical data on the psychophysiology of sleep and dreaming. *Psychophysiology*, **1968,** *4*: 375–376 (Abstract).

SHERRINGTON, C. *Man on his nature*. Cambridge Press, Cambridge, **1953,** 478 p.

SIEGEL, S. *Nonparametric statistics for the behavioral sciences*. McGraw-Hill, New York, **1956,** 312 p.

WECHSLER, D. *Manual for the Wechsler Pre-School and Primary Scale of Intelligence*. Psychological Corp., New York, **1967,** 85 p.

Reference: FEINBERG, I., BRAUN, M. and SHULMAN, E. EEG sleep patterns in mental retardation. *Electroenceph. clin. Neurophysiol.*, **1969,** *27:* 128–141.

Electroencephalography and Clinical Neurophysiology
Elsevier Publishing Company, Amsterdam – Printed in The Netherlands

AVERAGED VISUAL EVOKED POTENTIALS IN HUMANS: MECHANISM OF DICHOPTIC INTERACTION STUDIED IN A SUBJECT WITH A SPLIT CHIASMA[1]

D. LEHMANN AND D. H. FENDER

Smith-Kettlewell Institute of Visual Sciences, Pacific Medical Center, San Francisco, Calif. 94115 and Computing Center, California Institute of Technology, Pasadena, Calif. 91109 (U.S.A.)

(Accepted for publication: November 19, 1968)

In a previous paper (Lehmann and Fender 1968) we examined averaged EEG potentials evoked by monocular flashes of constant parameters when the other eye viewed continuously illuminated targets containing different amounts of structure. Increasing the structure of the steady-light target resulted in a progressive decrease of the root mean square (RMS) value of the evoked potential. We suggested that the cause of this effect was direct interaction between the dichoptic stimuli in the central neural processors.

We had recently the opportunity to examine a young subject with a traumatic split of the chiasma, a condition which ensured that the primary visual cortex does not include units receiving binocular input (Fisher *et al.* 1968), and which permitted us to test our hypothesis of the mechanism of dichoptic interaction. If change of the evoked potential does not occur in this subject, then input from corresponding retinal areas to central binocular units is an essential condition for the interaction.

METHOD

The experimental method is described in detail elsewhere (Lehmann and Fender 1968). One eye viewed stroboscope flashes, while the other eye observed one of three targets in steady illumination (a small central black dot, an erect cross, and an erect grid of 15 equally spaced lines). Four experiments were conducted with the following viewing conditions: (1) flashes seen by right eye, target seen by left eye; (2) flashes left, target right; (3) flashes and target right, left eye dark; and (4) flashes and target left, right eye dark. The three targets were used in each experiment. The subject was instructed to keep his gaze directed at the center of the target during the recording. Two to four recordings were obtained with each target.

EEG electrodes were attached at P_z and over

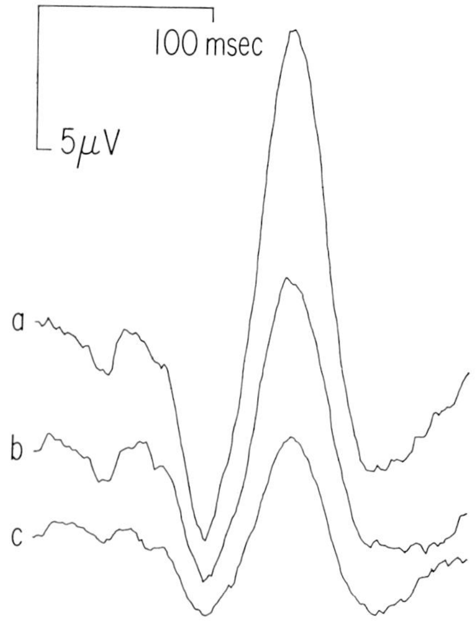

Fig. 1
Mean averaged evoked potentials. Flash seen by right eye, left eye sees steadily illuminated cross target. a: O_2 to O_1; b: O_2 to P_z; c: P_z to O_1. Upward deflection indicates positivity in the first mentioned electrode of each pair.

[1] This research was supported by the National Institutes of Health U.S. Public Health Service Grants NB 06038 and NB 03627.

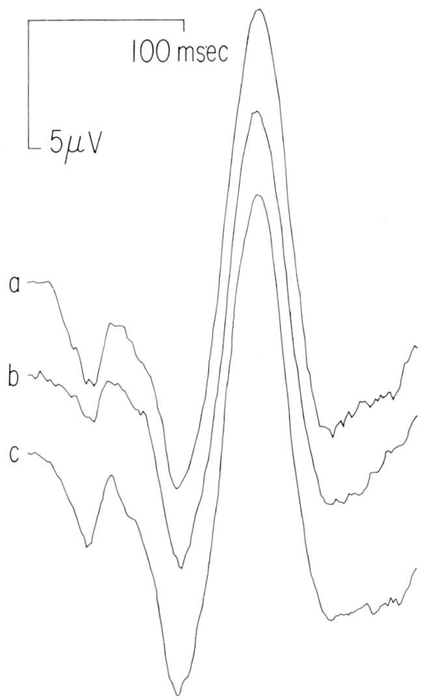

Fig. 2
Mean averaged evoked potentials, O_2 to O_1. Viewing condition as in Fig. 1. a: grid target; b: cross target; c: dot target.

both occipital areas 5 cm lateral from the midline and 4 cm frontal of the inion (close to O_1 and O_2). Three channels of a CAT 1000 were used to summate 100 EEG flash responses of each experimental run from the three electrode combinations. The analysis time was 250 msec after each flash. For purposes of illustration, the data from all experimental runs representing the same electrode combination and target condition were averaged together to form the mean response.

RESULTS

In previous experiments with this subject (Lehmann *et al.* 1969) we have shown that the potential evoked by a monocular flash arises almost entirely from a single locus of electrical activity situated in the occipital region of the hemisphere ipsilateral to the flashed eye. If a single source of electrical activity is generated in the slightly different experimental conditions of this paper, then all electrode combinations in the field of the source should give wave forms of the same shape, differing only in amplitude. This is confirmed by the three curves of Fig. 1 which shows that the results obtained from various

TABLE I

Comparison of the RMS values of the evoked potentials

Target condition: Left eye	Target condition: Right eye	Mean* R.M.S.	Variance	D.F.	*P* (two tailed)	
A. In dichoptic viewing conditions						
Dot	Flash	1.0247	0.0044	8	} > 0.2	} > 0.4
Cross	Flash	0.9670	0.0072	5	} > 0.4	
Grid	Flash	1.0000	0.0014	5		
Flash	Dot	1.0225	0.0052	8	} > 0.15	} > 0.4
Flash	Cross	0.9613	0.0099	8	} > 0.3	
Flash	Grid	1.0000	0.0046	8		
B. When one eye sees the flash superposed on the continuously illuminated structured target						
Dark	Dot & Flash	1.7417	0.0230	8	} < 0.01	} < 0.001
Dark	Cross & Flash	1.4712	0.0142	8	} < 0.001	
Dark	Grid & Flash	1.0000	0.0689	11		
Dot & Flash	Dark	1.6045	0.0436	11	} < 0.001	} < 0.001
Cross & Flash	Dark	1.3276	0.0060	11	} < 0.001	
Grid & Flash	Dark	1.0000	0.0119	11		

* This Table represents the observations from four separate experiments; to facilitate intercomparison of the results, the data from each experiment have been scaled so that the value for the grid condition is equal to unity.

electrodes differ only by a scaling factor except for a small interval between 165 and 215 msec; we may therefore pool the observations from all electrodes in any manipulation of the data. In addition, Fig. 2 shows that there is no change in the shape of the responses recorded from the same electrode combination as the steady-light target contralateral to the stimulated eye is changed; the size of the curve may thus be characterized by the RMS value of the response about its arithmetic mean. Table I, *A* shows that the RMS values remain constant in all target conditions. This is in contrast with our previous findings on normal subjects (Lehmann and Fender 1968).

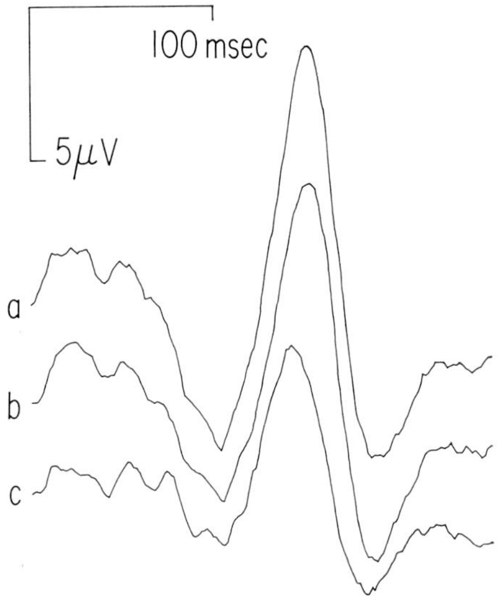

Fig. 3
Mean averaged evoked potentials, O_2 to P_z. Right eye viewing the flash superposed on the continuously illuminated structured target. a: dot target; b: cross target; c: grid target.

As a control we have changed the experimental conditions and presented the structured target in continuous illumination superposed on the flash illumination to the same eye. Typical curves are shown in Fig. 3, and the results are given in Table I, *B*; the structured target now reduces the RMS value of the evoked potential.

DISCUSSION

The evoked potentials recorded from a subject with sagittal interruption of the chiasma show no evidence of interaction between dichoptic stimuli. The dichoptic interaction is easily recorded in normal subjects with direct binocular input to each hemisphere. This indicates that dichoptic modification of evoked potentials in normal subjects depends on the central interaction of input from corresponding retinal areas.

One possible alternative schema of interaction can be excluded. Our results show that structure presented to a non-corresponding retinal area does not modify the evoked potential; hence there is no general process whereby the sensitivity of one entire retina or the responsiveness of the visual cortex is changed as a function of the structure shown to a portion of the contraocular visual field.

SUMMARY

EEG evoked potentials were averaged from a subject with a sagittal split of the chiasma. Light flashes of constant parameters were shown to one eye while the other eye saw continuously illuminated targets containing different amounts of visual structure. Contrary to earlier results obtained with normal subjects, the pathological subject exhibited no change of the monocularly evoked potentials with increasing amounts of contraocular target structure. This suggests that the change of evoked potentials in dichoptic stimulus conditions in normal subjects reflects the interaction in the visual cortex between afferents from corresponding retinal areas, and does not reflect general changes of retinal or cortical excitability as a function of input to non-corresponding retinal areas.

RÉSUMÉ

POTENTIELS ÉVOQUÉS VISUELS MOYENS CHEZ L'HOMME: ÉTUDE DES MÉCANISMES D'INTERACTION DES DEUX YEUX SÉPARÉS CHEZ UN SUJET AVEC CHIASMA DIVISÉ

Les potentiels évoqués EEG sont moyennés chez un sujet avec discission sagittale du chiasma. Des éclairs lumineux de paramètres constants sont projetés à un seul oeil pendant que l'autre oeil regarde de façon continu des champs illuminés contenant des structures visuelles en proportions variables. Contrairement aux résul-

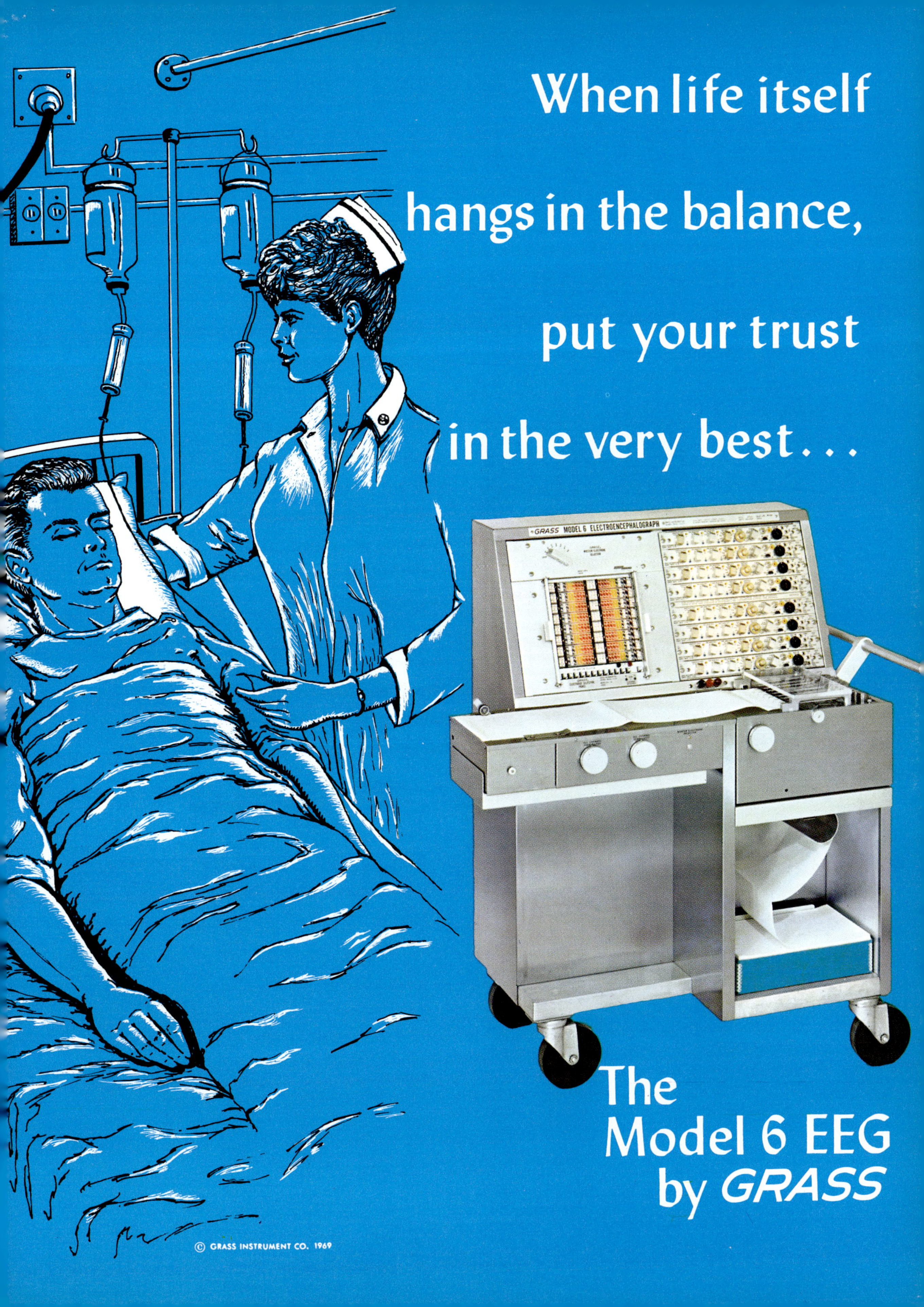
When life itself
hangs in the balance,
put your trust
in the very best...
GRASS MODEL 6 ELECTROENCEPHALOGRAPH
The
Model 6 EEG
by GRASS
© GRASS INSTRUMENT CO. 1969

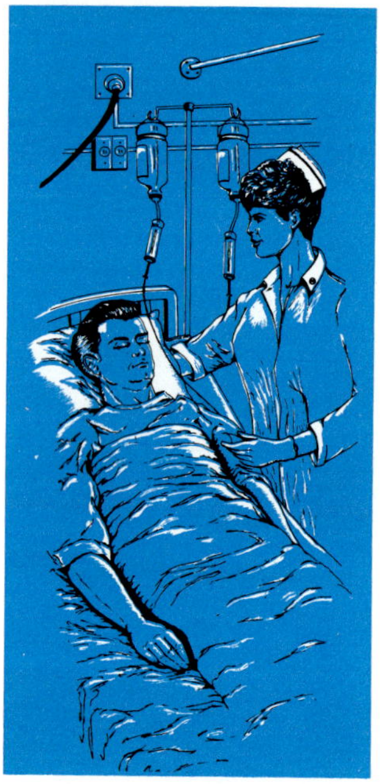

tats antérieurs obtenus chez les sujets normaux, le sujet pathologique ne montre aucune modification des potentiels évoqués monoculaires avec les quantités croissantes de structures controlatérales. Ceci suppose que la modification de ces potentiels évoqués dans des conditions de stimulations différentielles des deux yeux chez les sujets normaux reflète l'interaction au niveau du cortex visuel d'afférences provenant des aires rétiniennes correspondantes, mais ne reflète pas de modifications générales de la rétine ou de l'excitabilité corticale en fonction des afférences allant aux aires rétiniennes non correspondantes.

REFERENCES

Fisher, N. F., Jampolsky, A. and Scott, A. Traumatic bitemporal hemianopsia. I. Diagnosis of macular splitting. *Amer. J. Ophthal.*, **1968,** *65*: 237–242.

Lehmann, D. and Fender, D. H. Component analysis of human averaged evoked potentials: Dichoptic stimuli using different target structure. *Electroenceph. clin. Neurophysiol.*, **1968,** *24*: 542–553.

Lehmann, D., Kavanagh, R. N. and Fender, D. H. Field studies of averaged visually evoked EEG potentials in a patient with a split chiasm. *Electroenceph. clin. Neurophysiol.*, **1969,** *26*: 193–199.

Reference: Lehmann, D. and Fender, D. H. Averaged visual evoked potentials in humans: mechanism of dichoptic interaction studied in a subject with a split chiasma. *Electroenceph. clin. Neurophysiol.*, **1969,** *27*: 142–145.

Electroencephalography and Clinical Neurophysiology
Elsevier Publishing Company, Amsterdam – Printed in The Netherlands

COMPARISON OF EVOKED GROSS AND UNIT RESPONSES IN ASSOCIATION CORTEX OF WAKING CAT[1]

RICHARD F. THOMPSON, PH.D., LEWIS A. BETTINGER[2], PH.D., HERMAN BIRCH, PH.D. AND PHILIP M. GROVES, M.A.

Department of Psychobiology, University of California, Irvine, Calif. 92664 (U.S.A.)

(Accepted for publication: November 6, 1968)

INTRODUCTION

Gross responses evoked by sensory stimuli in association areas of the cortex of the unanesthetized cat have been described by several groups (Buser and Borenstein 1959; Albe-Fessard and Fessard 1963; Thompson and Shaw 1965; Bignall 1967; Petřek *et al.* 1968). Goldring *et al.* (1967) recently reported failure to obtain gross evoked association responses in normal waking cats and questioned some of the earlier studies (see Discussion) on the basis of the referential recording methods used. It would seem that the study by Goldring *et al.* (1967) is the only negative report to date concerning the occurrence of evoked responses in association cortex of unanesthetized cat. They suggested that the cortical "dipole" seen in association areas of the chloralosed cat is substantially altered or non-existent in the normal waking animal. The fundamental issue is perhaps not so much the extent to which gross evoked responses can be recorded from association areas of the cortex in the waking preparation but rather the extent to which such responses are locally generated in association cortex. The fact that single cell responses can be evoked is not in itself sufficient to demonstrate local generation of the gross evoked response. However, if a close and invariant correspondence can be shown to exist between the temporal pattern of evoked cellular discharge and the gross evoked response following a peripheral stimulus, it may be considered presumptive evidence for local generation of the latter. There have been several reports of such correspondence between evoked unit and gross activity in the primary visual system (Fox and O' Brien 1965; Dill *et al.* 1968; Verzeano *et al.* 1968). In this paper we apply the same type of analysis to association cortex of the normal waking cat.

[1] Supported in part by Research Grant NB-02161 from the National Institutes of Health and Research Scientist Award MH-06650 from the National Institute of Mental Health.

[2] Current address: Department of Psychology, Vanderbilt University, Nashville, Tenn.

METHODS

A chronic micro-manipulator system of the same general type described by Hubel (1959) and Evarts (1960) was used. A permanent receptacle chamber was affixed to the skull surrounding a trephine hole over the posterior middle suprasylvian association area (PMSA), using Nembutal anesthesia. Animals were studied for periods up to 3 weeks following implantation. The region of implanted cortex was subsequently sectioned and stained for localization of electrode tracks.

During a recording session a remotely controlled hydraulic micro-manipulator system was inserted into the receptacle chamber and a micro-electrode (glass-coated tungsten, of 1–3 μ tip diameter with impedances ranging from 5 to 20 mΩ) advanced through the cortex. Recording was against a distant reference placed variously in skull overlying frontal bone sinus, skull immediately adjacent to recording chamber, wire sutured through cut edge of scalp or wire sutured through skin of forepaw. Reference electrode location had no effect on responses. Individual evoked gross and unit responses were recorded on film; unit activity was also transcribed on tape. On-line averages of gross evoked responses were

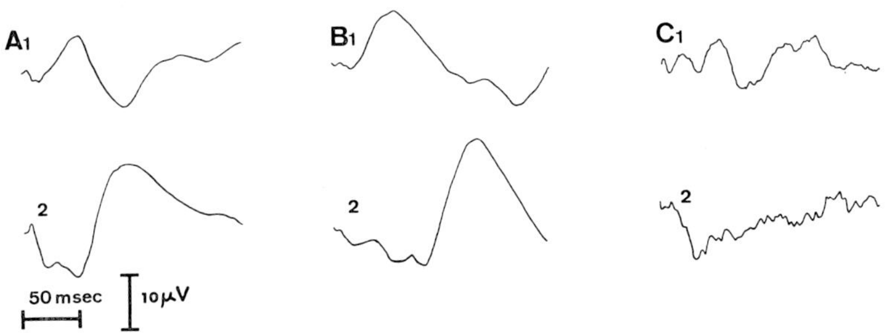

Fig. 1
Averaged gross evoked responses recorded from the surface (1) and approximately 2.4 mm below the surface (2) of cortex in association area PMSA in waking cat to click (*A*), light flash (*B*) and ipsilateral forepaw shock (*C*). Each tracing is the average of 256 successive responses. In this and subsequent figures, positivity is up and the stimulus always occurs at onset of trace.

obtained with a Fabri-Tek Model 1062 computer. Post-stimulus histograms were computed both on-line and subsequently from tape records using a Nuclear-Chicago Model 7100 computer. Gross and unit activity was recorded simultaneously from the same micro-electrode using a high input impedance pre-amplifier (Roveti MPA-20). The output from this was delivered to two Tektronix 122 amplifiers whose filters were respectively set to pass gross and unit activity. A Spencer-Kennedy variable electronic filter completed the elimination of any trace of gross activity in the unit channel. This filter system did not introduce any significant phase shift in the evoked responses. Cell spikes were separated for post-stimulus histogram analysis using a Schmitt-trigger discriminator. The gross evoked association responses, which are of small amplitude in the waking cat when recording referentially, did not produce any baseline shift in the filtered unit channel, even when averaged, and hence did not contaminate the post-stimulus histogram analysis of the unit data. All data were obtained when the cats were awake but "inattentive"; *i.e.*, sitting quietly or lying down (head on forepaws) with eyes open.

RESULTS

Examples of averaged gross evoked responses to click, light flash and ipsilateral forepaw shock recorded from association area PMSA are shown in Fig. 1, at the surface (A_1, B_1, C_1) and at about 2 mm depth; here the polarity of the initial component reverses and exhibits a clear initial negativity (A_2, B_2, C_2).

Individual examples of unit activity in area PMSA evoked by various peripheral stimuli are shown in Fig. 2. The majority of units tended to fire at relatively slow and variable spontaneous rates in the absence of stimulation. The largest unit in Fig. 2 (marked by dot) is clearly evoked; it

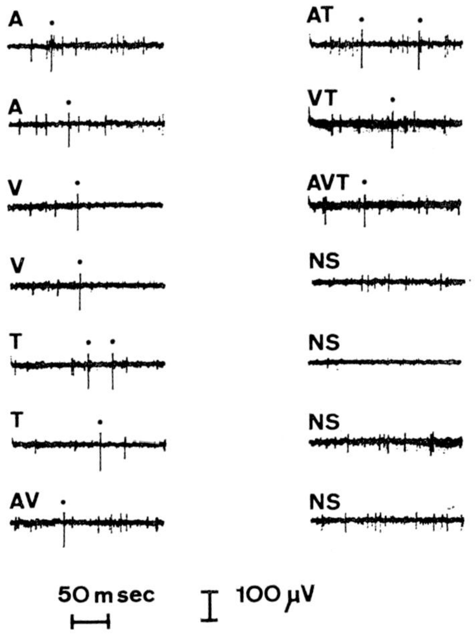

Fig. 2
Examples of unit responses (largest evoked unit marked by dot) in area PMSA in waking cat to click (A), light flash (V), ipsilateral forepaw shock (T) and simultaneous combinations of these (AV = click–flash, AT = click–shock, VT = flash–shock, AVT = click–flash–shock). Spontaneous activity is indicated in tracings with no stimuli (NS). Stimuli, both singly and in combinations, always occur at onset of trace.

responds within a particular restricted latency range for each type of stimulus and does not fire in the absence of stimulation. Note that where combined stimuli are given, the stimulus yielding the shortest latency response predominates (*e.g.*, response to click–flash–shock and click have similar shorter latencies than response to flash–shock). This same predominance of shortest response latency stimulus occurs for polymodal cells in area PMSA of the chloralosed preparation (Bettinger *et al.* 1967). The smaller units shown in Fig. 2 appear to have much broader latency ranges. In fact, of many cases it is not possible to distinguish between spontaneous unit activity and unit responses evoked by the stimulus on the basis of this type of individual response data.

The records shown in Fig. 2 are illustrative of the multi-unit data used for computation of post-stimulus histograms. Note that two relatively large separate unit responses are clearly distinguishable on the basis of amplitude. In addition, there are a number of smaller amplitude spikes merging into the background "noise" level that cannot be identified individually.

Comparisons of averaged gross evoked potentials and unit post-stimulus histograms in association area PMSA to peripheral stimuli are shown in Fig. 3. Note that the periods of maximum probability of unit discharge (peaks of post-stimulus histograms) tend to occur at or just after the peaks of the negative components of the evoked responses. This close correspondence between negative components of the evoked response and peaks of post-stimulus unit histogram in area PMSA was uniformly obtained in a total of 34 determinations made on five animals.

Effect of stimulus repetition rate for light flash is illustrated in Fig. 3, *A* and *B*. Note that the faster repetition rate (*B*) results in a marked depression of the amplitude of the gross response and the amplitude of the post-stimulus unit histogram. Response to click stimulation is illustrated in Fig. 3, *C* and response to a simultaneous light flash-click stimulus is shown in Fig. 3, *D*. Note that the post-stimulus histogram shows a later peak corresponding to a later negativity in the averaged gross response to the combined visual-auditory stimulus. In all cases there is a close and consistent relationship between the gross evoked response wave forms and the periods of maximum unit activity following the stimulus, the histogram peaks occurring at (*B*), or more commonly just beyond (*A*, *C*, *D*), the negative peaks of the gross responses when only the largest amplitude spikes are included in the analysis.

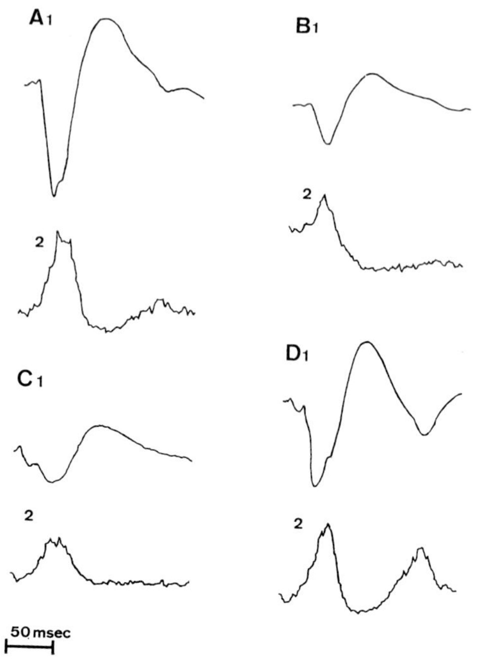

Fig. 3
Comparisons of simultaneously recorded averaged gross evoked responses (1) and unit post-stimulus histograms (2) from area PMSA in normal waking cat; micro-electrodes approximately 1 mm below surface of cortex. *A*: response to light flashes at 2 sec interval. *B*: same at 0.5 sec interval. *C*: response to click (2 sec intervals). *D*: response to simultaneous click–flash (2 sec intervals). Only the largest spikes were included in the unit analysis. Each tracing is the average of 1,024 successive responses.

Fox and O'Brien (1965) reported a close correspondence between peak of a unit histogram and the positive peak of the evoked potential in visual cortex. More recently, Verzeano *et al.* (1968) and Dill *et al.* (1968) have presented evidence indicating that in lateral geniculate body and visual cortex, if only the largest amplitude spikes are included in the analysis, the unit histogram peaks occur a few milliseconds after the negative peak of the first derivative of the gross potential, sometimes on the negative peak of the gross response, but most frequently on its positive slope; however, if both larger and smaller

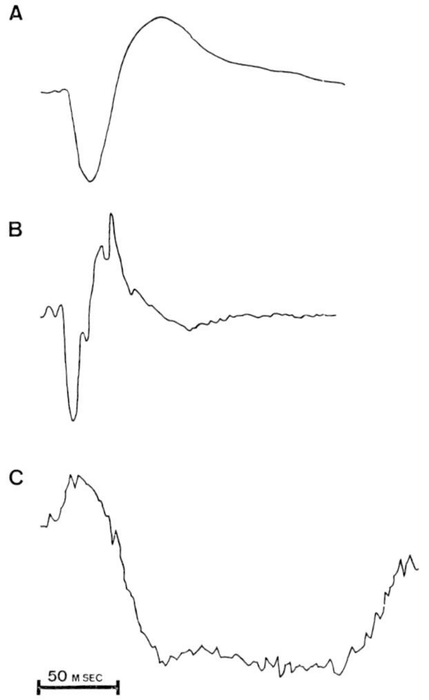

Fig. 4
Comparison of gross evoked association response (*A*), first derivative of gross response (*B*) and post-stimulus unit histogram (*C*) to light flash. Both larger and smaller spikes included in unit analysis. Each tracing is the average of 1,024 successive responses.

amplitude spikes are included in the unit analysis, the histogram peaks correspond closely to the negative peaks of the first derivative of the gross potential. We completed a comparable analysis for unit activity in association area PMSA to light flash stimulation. Data were obtained under identical conditions to those for the data of Fig. 3, except that the discriminator level was lowered to include both smaller and larger spikes. Fig. 4 illustrates the gross evoked response (*A*), the first derivative (*B*), and the post-stimulus histogram (*C*) obtained. Note that the region of maximum unit response probability corresponds to the region of maximum negative peak of the first derivative of the evoked potential. Note also that there is a more pronounced and longer duration decrease in unit activity following the period of maximum response under these conditions.

DISCUSSION

Evidence presented here and in previous studies supports the view that gross association responses evoked by peripheral stimuli are generated in cortex of the middle suprasylvian gyrus of the normal waking cat. This evidence may be summarized as follows:

(1) Gross response latency, wave form and polarity on suprasylvian gyrus are comparable in the waking and chloralosed preparations (Albe-Fessard and Rogeul 1958; Buser and Borenstein 1959; Buser *et al.* 1959; Albe-Fessard and Fessard 1963; Thompson *et al.* 1963a; Shaw and Thompson 1964b; Thompson and Shaw 1965; Bignall 1967).

(2) Areal distributions of gross responses on the posterior middle suprasylvian gyrus appear similar in the chloralosed and waking states, being essentially comparable for auditory, visual and tactile stimuli (Thompson *et al.* 1963a; Thompson and Shaw 1965).

(3) Depth distribution in suprasylvian cortex of polarity reversal of the initial component of the gross response is comparable in the waking and chloralosed preparations (see Fig. 1 and Thompson *et al.* 1963a).

(4) Single cell discharges in suprasylvian cortex, having similar latencies, are evoked by peripheral stimuli in the chloralosed and waking preparations (see Fig. 2 and Bental and Bihari 1963; Shimazono *et al.* 1963; Dubner and Rutledge 1964; Bettinger *et al.* 1967).

(5) A close and essentially invariant relationship obtains between the probability of single cell discharges and the form of the gross potential evoked by peripheral stimuli in the suprasylvian association cortex of the normal waking cat (Fig. 3 and 4). (A similar relationship was found in the chloralosed cat, Thompson *et al.* 1963a.) Such results are in agreement with those obtained in the lateral geniculate body and visual cortex (Dill *et al.* 1968; Verzeano *et al.* 1968).

Comparison of recording techniques used in the study by Goldring *et al.* (1967), where no association responses were observed, and in our studies indicates several differences:

(a) Goldring *et al.* used a transcortical electrode with an extradural silver ball and a depth electrode inserted in white matter (no depth indicated). Our bipolar transcortical electrodes in previous studies, where gross evoked association responses were obtained in normal waking cats

(Thompson and Shaw 1965), were implanted after removal of the dura; the surface electrode was placed directly on the pia and the small wire depth electrode was placed at a depth of 1.8 mm directly below the surface electrode (the depth at which the "sink" response is maximum for association responses in the chloralosed animal, Thompson *et al.* 1963a). In the present study, the micro-electrodes were within the region of the active cortical field. It is possible that responses recorded by Goldring *et al.* were attenuated because their transcortical electrodes were considerably further from the source-sink than was the case in our experiments.

(b) Goldring *et al.* used a 0.5 sec inter-stimulus interval; we have commonly used a longer one (2 sec or more). Both gross evoked responses and evoked single neuron activity in association areas are markedly attenuated when short inter-stimulus intervals are used, both in the chloralosed (Thompson *et al.* 1963b; Bettinger *et al.* 1967) and the waking preparation (see Fig. 3, *A* and *B*).

(c) Goldring *et al.* do not discuss the behavioral states of their animals. Yet these variables were found to be very important for the presence or absence of cortical association responses (Shaw and Thompson 1964a; Thompson and Shaw 1965; Thompson and Bettinger 1969). Any increase in behavioral "arousal" or degree of attentiveness reduced or abolished the association response for a period of time.

The close correspondence between amplitude of the gross evoked response and probability of evoked unit discharge in association cortex reported here implies that the reduction in gross evoked potential amplitude during "attention" will be accompanied by a reduced probability of evoked single cell responses. In a recent discussion of the neural factors underlying behavioral attention, data were presented suggesting that activity of neurons in posterior association cortex of cat increases whenever a novel or significant stimulus is presented (Thompson and Bettinger 1969). We suggest the following hypothesis: neurons in posterior association areas of the cortex of cat are specifically concerned with processing of information of significance for the organism. Thus when an animal attends to a novel or significant stimulus, ongoing cellular activity in posterior association cortex increases; this in turn will result in reduced probability of evoked unit discharges and reduction in amplitude of the gross evoked potential to a repeated stimulus.

SUMMARY

Averaged evoked gross and unit responses to auditory, visual and tactile stimuli were recorded from association cortex (posterior middle suprasylvian area) of the normal waking cat using a chronically implanted micro-manipulator system. Surface appearance and depth distribution of gross responses evoked by peripheral stimuli resembled such responses in the chloralosed preparation. There was a close and relatively invariant relationship between the gross response and the post-stimulus histogram of unit responses; the largest unit spikes tended to occur at or just beyond the peak of the depth negativity and smaller units tended to fire at the period of maximum negative slope of the gross depth potential. The data are interpreted as supporting the view that the gross evoked association response is generated in association cortex in the normal waking cat.

RÉSUMÉ

COMPARAISON DES RÉPONSES ÉVOQUÉES GLOBALES ET UNITAIRES SUR LE CORTEX ASSOCIATIF DU CHAT ÉVEILLÉ

Les réponses évoquées moyennes globales et unitaires à des stimuli auditifs visuels et tactiles ont été enregistrées au niveau du cortex d'association (aire suprasylvienne postérieure médiane) du chat normal éveillé à l'aide d'une système chroniquement implanté à micro-manipulation. L'apparition en surface et la distribution en profondeur des réponses globales évoquées par les stimuli périphériques ressemblent aux réponses obtenues en préparation chloralosée. Il y a une relation étroite et relativement invariable entre la réponse globale et l'histogramme post-stimulus des réponses unitaires; les pointes unitaires les plus grandes tendent à survenir au moment du maximum de négativité en profondeur ou tout de suite après, et les unités les plus petites tendent à pulser à la période de la descente négative maximum du potentiel global de profondeur. Ces faits constituent des arguments en faveur de l'hypothèse suivant laquelle les réponses évoquées globales d'association prennent leur naissance dans le cortex associatif chez le chat normal éveillé.

The authors wish to express their gratitude to Dr. M. Verzeano for his invaluable advice and encouragement. The technical assistance of Mrs. S. Beydler and Miss M. Westwell is gratefully acknowledged.

REFERENCES

ALBE-FESSARD, D. and FESSARD, A. Thalamic integrations and their consequences at the telencephalic level. G. MORUZZI *et al.* (Eds.), *Progress in brain research. Brain mechanisms.* Elsevier, Amsterdam, **1963,** *1*: 115–148.

ALBE-FESSARD, D. et ROGEUL, A. Activités d'origine, somesthésique évoquées sur le cortex nonspécifique du chat anesthésié au chloralose: rôle du centre médian du thalamus. *Electroenceph. clin. Neurophysiol.*, **1958,** *10*: 131–151.

BENTAL, E. and BIHARI, B. Evoked activity of single neurons in sensory association cortex of the cat. *J. Neurophysiol.*, **1963,** *26*: 207–214.

BETTINGER, L. A., DAVIS, J. L., MEIKLE, M. B., BIRCH, H., KOPP, R., SMITH, H. E. and THOMPSON, R. F. "Novelty" cells in association cortex of cat. *Psychonom. Sci.*, **1967,** *9*: 421–422.

BIGNALL, K. E. Effects of subcortical ablations on polysensory cortical responses and interactions in the cat. *Exp. Neurol.*. **1967,** *18*: 56–67.

BUSER, P. et BORENSTEIN, P. Réponses somesthésiques, visuelles et auditives, recueillies au niveau du cortex "associatif" suprasylvien chez le chat curarisé non anesthésié. *Electroenceph. clin. Neurophysiol.*, **1959,** *11*: 285–304.

BUSER, P., BORENSTEIN, P. et BRUNER, J. Étude des systèmes "associatifs" visuels et auditifs chez le chat anesthésié au chloralose. *Electroenceph. clin. Neurophysiol.*, **1959,** *11*: 305–324.

DILL, R. C., VALLECALLE, E. and VERZEANO, M. Evoked potentials, neuronal activity and stimulus intensity in the visual system. *Physiol. Behav.*, **1968,** *3*: 797–801.

DUBNER, R. and RUTLEDGE, L. T. Recording and analysis of converging input upon neurons in cat association area cortex. *J. Neurophysiol.*, **1964,** *27*: 620–634.

EVARTS, E. V. Effects of sleep and waking on spontaneous and evoked discharge of single units in visual cortex. *Fed. Proc.*, **1960,** *19*: 828–837.

FOX, S. S. and O'BRIEN, J. H. Duplication of evoked potential waveform by curve of probability of firing of a single cell. *Science*, **1965,** *147*: 888.

GOLDRING, S., SHEPTAK, P. and KARAHASHI, Y. Averaged responses from association areas in waking cat. *Electroenceph. clin. Neurophysiol.*, **1967,** *23*: 241–247.

HUBEL, D. H. Single unit activity in striate cortex of unrestrained cats. *J. Physiol. (Lond.)*, **1959,** *147*: 226–238.

PETŘEK, J., GOLDA, V. and LISONĚK, P. Cortical response amplitude changes produced by rhythmic acoustic stimulation in cats. *Exp. Brain Res.*, **1968,** *6*: 19–31.

SHAW, J. A. and THOMPSON, R. F. Dependence of evoked cortical association responses on behavioral variables. *Psychonom. Sci.*, **1964**a, *1*: 153–154.

SHAW, J. A. and THOMPSON, R. F. Inverse relation between evoked cortical association responses and behavioral orienting to repeated auditory stimuli. *Psychonom. Sci.*, **1964**b, *1*: 399–400.

SCHIMAZONO, Y., TORII, H., ENDO, M., IHARA, S., HARUKAWA, H. and MATSUDA, M. Convergence of thalamic and sensory afferent impulses to single neurons in the cortical association area of cats. *Folia psychiat. neurol. jap.*, **1963,** *17*: 144–155.

THOMPSON, R. F. and BETTINGER, L. A. Neural substrates of attention. In D. MOSTOFSKY (Ed.), *Attention: A behavioral analysis.* Appleton-Century-Crofts, New York, **1969,** in press.

THOMPSON, R. F., JOHNSON, R. H. and HOOPES, J. Organization of auditory, somatic sensory, and visual projection to association fields of cerebral cortex in cat. *J. Neurophysiol.*, **1963**a, *26*: 343–364.

THOMPSON, R. F. and SHAW, J. A. Behavioral correlates of evoked activity recorded from association areas of the cerebral cortex. *J. comp. physiol. Psychol.*, **1965,** *60*: 329–339.

THOMPSON, R. F., SMITH, H. E. and BLISS, D. Auditory, somatic sensory, and visual response interactions and interrelations in association and primary cortical fields of the cat. *J. Neurophysiol.*, **1963**b, *26*: 365–378.

VERZEANO, M., DILL, R. C., VALLECALLE, E., GROVES, P. and THOMAS, J. Evoked responses and neuronal activity in the lateral geniculate. *Experientia (Basel)*, **1968,** *24*: 360–362.

Reference: THOMPSON, R. F., BETTINGER, L. A., BIRCH, H. and GROVES, P. M. Comparison of evoked gross and unit responses in association cortex of waking cat. *Electroenceph. clin. Neurophysiol.*, **1969,** *27*: 146–151.

Electroencephalography and Clinical Neurophysiology
Elsevier Publishing Company, Amsterdam – Printed in The Netherlands

SLOW POTENTIAL CHANGES IN CAT BRAIN DURING CLASSICAL APPETITIVE AND AVERSIVE CONDITIONING OF JAW MOVEMENT[1]

CHARLES S. REBERT[2] AND DONALD A. IRWIN[3]

Department of Psychiatry, The University of Iowa, Iowa City, Iowa 52241 (U.S.A.)

(Accepted for publication: November 1, 1968)

INTRODUCTION

One of the problems to which a great deal of recent research effort has been directed is that of understanding the central nervous system processes involved in the acquisition of new behaviors. The measurement of electrical activity from the brain has provided a wealth of information concerning this general problem, and recent investigations of slow potentials (SPs) in the cerebral cortex of animals indicate that such potentials may reflect changes in cortical functioning related to learning or motivation. Chiorini (1969) and Rowland and Goldstone (1963) have specifically implicated motivational events in the genesis of slow potentials, and Morrell (1960) has interpreted the occurrence of SPs in the cortex during the development of conditioned responding as indicating a dendritic locus of "closure".

Whereas SP responses have been recorded from subcortical regions during non-learning situations (Hayward *et al.* 1966), the occurrence of SPs in the depths of brain during behavioral conditioning has not previously been reported. In light of conclusions which have been drawn from investigations of SPs in the cerebral cortex, it is pertinent to ask certain questions regarding the significance of subcortically generated SPs. Will such potentials also change in a systematic way during the elaboration of conditioned responses? Do some subcortical regions exhibit SPs in response to conditioning procedures, while others do not, and do those which react exhibit distinct response profiles over the course of training? Do systematic changes in SPs during the course of conditioning represent motivational or associative events? If some SP changes occur which appear to represent motivational changes, are they a function of the rewarding or punishing character of "reinforcing" stimuli?

In order to answer these questions, the following brain regions were selected for study during classical conditioning of jaw movement: medial geniculate, ventralis postero-medialis of the thalamus, lateral and ventro-medial nuclei of the hypothalamus, cingulate gyrus, and extradural motor cortex. The thalamic areas constitute relay nuclei for the conditioned (auditory) and unconditioned (gustatory) stimuli (CS and UCS). The hypothalamic regions are related to feeding and emotional behavior, while the motor cortex relates to movement of the striate musculature. Cingulate gyrus apparently mediates autonomic responses as stimulation there induces changes in heart rate, salivation, and other responses.

METHODS

Electrodes were stereotaxically implanted in thirty mature cats under Nembutal anesthesia using the atlases of Jasper and Ajmone Marsan (1954) and Snider and Niemer (1961). The electrode described by Rowland (1961) was modified for both cortical and subcortical recording. Glass

[1] This paper is based on a dissertation submitted by the senior author to the Department of Psychology, The University of Iowa, in partial fulfillment of the requirements for the Ph. D. degree.

[2] Present address: Department of Biobehavioral Sciences, Stanford Research Institute, Menlo Park, Calif. 94025.

[3] Present address: Department of Psychophysiology-Neurophysiology, The Fels Research Institute, Yellow Springs, Ohio.

tubes, 0.7–1.0 mm O.D., filled with agar-saline were implanted and their exposed portion covered by glass tubes, 1 cm in length and 4 mm O.D., which were filled with powdered silver chloride surrounding a chlorided coil of No. 30 wire. Lead wires from the electrodes were attached to a U.S. Components UMI series 9-pin female connector. "Duz-All" and "Grip" dental acrylics were used to cement the electrode assembly firmly to the skull. The reference electrode was on midline interparietal bone.

Because corneal-retinal potentials associated with eye movements are sufficiently large to be recorded by electrodes placed in virtually any part of the cat brain (unpublished observations) the eyes were enucleated.

For delivery of fluid into the mouth, a polyethylene tube (P.E. 260) was routed beneath the skin of the jaw, through the buccal mucosa and through a hole which was drilled in the lateral aspect of the upper rear molar. The external end of the tube was anchored with acrylic to the side of the head plug.

During training sessions the cat was held in a restraining device which was housed in a 23″ × 23″ × 35″ wooden box. Head movement was prevented by fastening bolts, which were embedded in the acrylic head plug, to a metal plate above the animal's head.

The presentation of CS and UCS was timed by pulses from Tektronix type 161 and 162 pulse generators, and Grass S-4 stimulators. A complex tone of square pulses at 1250 p/sec (CS) was presented via a small speaker mounted in the conditioning box 20 cm in front of and 20 cm below the cat's face. Intensity was 28 dB above ambient noise of 50 dB.

A homogenized and strained mixture of concentrated milk, ground horsemeat and water, or 0.07 *N* acetic acid constituted the appetitive and aversive UCS. These were delivered to the jaw fistula via a Hunter solenoid valve. Duration of valve opening was controlled by a Grass S-4 stimulator, and adjusted so that 0.8 ml of fluid was delivered.

Jaw movements were recorded with a Giannini 85111 micro-torque potentiometer by taping the small metal arm of the potentiometer to fur on the animal's chin. Resistance changes produced by rotation of the potentiometer were transformed to voltage changes by a Wheatstone bridge circuit, and amplified and traced on the moving paper of a Grass model 7 polygraph.

Electrical activity of the brain was amplified and displayed by a Grass model 7 polygraph utilizing chopper stabilized 7P-1 pre-amplifiers. A pre-stimulus voltage calibration signal (Emde 1964) was imposed in series with the recording leads 240 msec prior to each trial, and was summated along with the brain responses. Taped records of EEG samples were made with a Precision Instruments model 6108, 8-channel FM tape recorder. A Mnemotron CAT 400B was used to summate brain responses. Plots of summated SPs were made from the CAT memory on a Houston Instruments Corp. HR-80 T–Y plotter.

Magnitude of SPs in μV were obtained from plots of summated SPs for each session (15 trials). For purposes of scoring, "best fit" lines were visually determined for the pre-calibration baseline, calibration pulse amplitude, and SP amplitude during the last 200 msec of the inter-stimulus interval.

After a post-operative recovery period of at least 2 weeks, or until normal feeding habits were re-established, animals were subjected to daily training for 1 h and fed immediately afterward. Fifteen trials were given each day in habituation, training and extinction sessions with an inter-trial interval of 1–3 min for experimental animals, and 0.5–1.5 min for pseudoconditioning controls. Three days of habituation, which consisted of the presentation of CS alone (2 sec duration) were given. Training, which for the experimental groups consisted of paired presentation of CS and UCS in a forward classical delay conditioning paradigm with 1 sec inter-stimulus interval and overlap of CS and UCS for 1 sec, was continued for 13 days. Control animals were presented unpaired CS and UCS unsystematically with the restriction that no more than 3 CS or UCS could occur in succession. Extinction consisted of presentation of the 2 sec CS alone for 6 sessions (only those responses occurring in the initial 1 sec being counted as CRs).

RESULTS

Histological data

Histological study of the brains showed that all motor cortex (MC) placements were accurate.

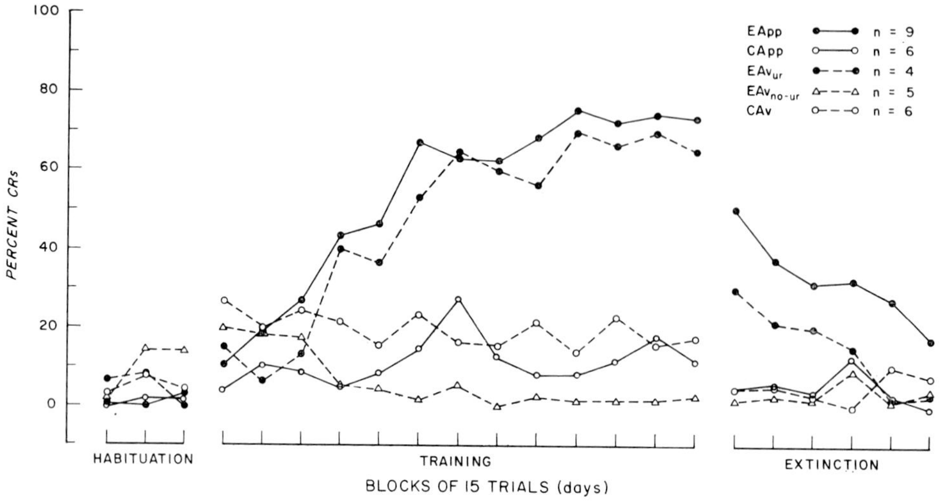

Fig. 1

Per cent conditioned jaw responses during habituation, training, and extinction for experimental appetitive (EApp), control appetitive (CApp), experimental aversive animals which emitted UCRs (EAv_{ur}), experimental aversive animals which did not emit UCRs ($EAv_{no\text{-}ur}$), and control aversive (CAv) groups.

Twenty-eight of the 30 medial geniculate (MG) placements were in MG. Twenty-eight animals had electrodes correctly placed in the lateral hypothalamus (LH), while only 7 placements were in the ventro-medial nucleus (VMH). However, 4 placement categories could be formed of the 27 electrodes in the general region of ventral hypothalamus (VH). These placements were: VMH, $N = 7$; peri-VMH, electrodes which were close to but not within VMH, $N = 8$; mammillary region, $N = 7$; and electrodes which penetrated the base of the brain, $N = 5$. All electrodes aimed at the cingulate gyrus were in splenial sulcus or gyrus (SPG).

Behavioral data

The percentages of conditioned responses (CRs) emitted by various groups each day are shown in Fig. 1. Results of Mann-Whitney "U" tests applied to those data are presented in Table I. During learning, there were significant differences between the mean level of conditioned responding of the experimental appetitive (EApp) group and both its control group (CApp) and the experimental aversive (EAv) group. An acquisition function was generated by EApp cats but not by EAv animals (not shown) nor any other group. The percentage of CRs in the EApp group increased rather consistently up to day 6 of training, then leveled off to approach asymptote. During extinction EApp cats were still responding significantly more than their controls, although a decline to near control levels did occur.

The low level of conditioning the EAv group is linked to the fact that five of the nine animals in that group either failed to emit unconditioned responses (UCRs) to the acid at any time, or initially gave such responses but discontinued jawing within 2–3 days of the start of training. Cats in the EAv group which did continue to respond to the acid (EAv/ur animals) also developed CRs. Non-responding (EAv/no-ur animals) did not develop CRs (Fig. 1). The rate of increase of CRs in the EAv/ur group was also fairly consistent up to the middle of training (day 7) where there was then an inflection in the acquisition function similar to that seen in EApp animals at day 6 of training.

Electrophysiological data

Slow potential changes elicited by the CS were recorded at various times from all of the brain regions sampled. An example of an SP elicited from LH during training is presented in Fig. 2. In general, when an SP occurred it was fully developed within the inter-stimulus interval, and endured

TABLE I

Results of Mann-Whitney U tests applied to mean differences of conditioned jaw movement for the various treatment groups*

Conditions and groups	n_1, n_2	U	P
Habituation			
EApp–CApp	9, 6	25.5	NS
EApp–EAv	9, 9	19.6	NS
EApp–EAv/ur	9, 4	11.0	NS
EApp–EAv/no-ur	9, 5	11.0	NS
EAv–CAv	9, 6	25.0	NS
EAv/ur–CAv	4, 6	11.5	NS
EAv/no-ur–CAv	5, 6	12.5	NS
EAv/ur–EAv/no-ur	4, 5	8.0	NS
Training			
EApp–CApp	9, 6	0.0	< 0.0005
EApp–EAv	9, 9	15.5	< 0.05
EApp–EAv/ur	9, 4	15.0	NS
EApp–EAv/no-ur	9, 5	1.0	< 0.002
EAv–CAv	9, 6	22.0	NS
EAv/ur–CAv	4, 6	3.0	< 0.04
EAv/no-ur–CAv	5, 6	7.0	NS
EAv/ur–EAv/no-ur	4, 5	0.0	< 0.0005
Extinction			
EApp–CApp	9, 6	11.0	< 0.05
EApp–EAv	9, 9	22.5	NS
EApp–EAv/ur	9, 4	15.0	NS
EApp–EAv/no-ur	9, 5	0.0	< 0.0005
EAv–CAv	9, 6	19.0	NS
EAv/ur–CAv	4, 6	2.0	< 0.02
EAv/no-ur–CAv	5, 6	21.00	NS
EAv/ur–EAv/no-ur	4, 5	2.0	< 0.04

* Abbreviations refer to the various treatment groups, experimental and control appetitive (EApp and CApp) and aversive (EAv and CAv), and EAv animals which did or did not give UCRs to the acid (EAv/ur and EAv/no-ur).

for as long as the tone was presented (2 sec) and quite frequently lasted 3 or more sec.

a. *Placement comparisons*

Analysis of variance of the combined SP scores of all groups and conditions (habituation, training and extinction) indicated that over-all, the several placements reacted differently to the tone ($F=4.4$, $df=5/95$, $P<0.005$). This effect was due primarily to the fact that the MG and VPM placements were, on the average, more negative than the others. Mean SP amplitude in μV for the various placements were: MG $= -8.3$; LH $=6.7$; VH $= -1.9$; MC $=0.0$; SPG $=2.7$; and VPM $= -12.8$. Changes in SP amplitude from habituation to training to extinction also varied from one placement to the other (over-all interaction of placements and conditions, $F=6.6$, $df=10/190$, $P<0.005$). Means of MG and LH increased in positivity from habituation to extinction, while MC and VH became more positive during training than they were in habituation, but exhibited an increased degree of negativity in extinction. Splenial gyrus increased in negativity across conditions, whereas VPM remained essentially the same. The above changes across conditions were statistically significant for MG, LH, MC and SPG.

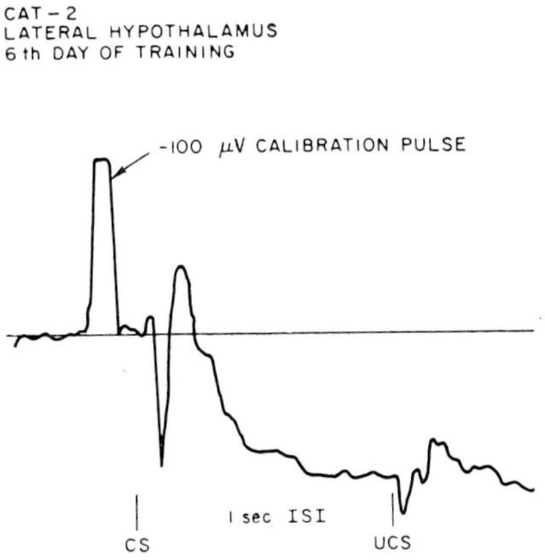

Fig. 2

Slow potential record of lateral hypothalamus of cat number 2. A positive potential at the active electrode appears as a downward deflection in the tracing.

b. *Treatment comparisons*

Motor cortex. With respect to comparisons between treatment groups and days during the various conditions, this region was unreactive. It showed no statistically significant differences between groups, nor systematic changes during the training period.

Ventral hypothalamus. Differences between the histologically defined placement categories in this general region were analyzed with all treatment groups combined. Analysis of variance indicated that there was an over-all difference among the means ($F=3.2$, $df=3/23$, $P<0.05$). The mammillary and extra-brain placements did

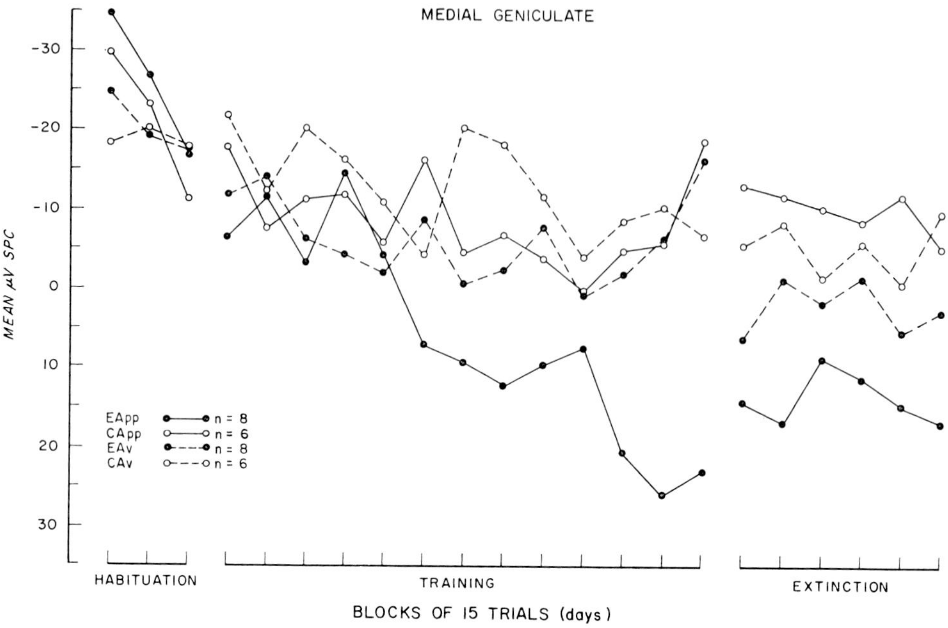

Fig. 3
Daily mean SP amplitude of medial geniculate in the several treatment groups.

not respond statistically differently from zero, whereas the VMH shifted negatively (−15.2 μV) and closely surrounding tissue shifted in a positive direction (11.5 μV). There were no systematic changes in any of these placements in habituation, training or extinction.

Medial geniculate. When scores of all animals were combined a significant change in the positive direction of SP amplitude over days was found during habituation and training, but not during extinction. When reinforcement groups were considered separately (Fig. 3), a statistical comparison involving EApp and CApp animals indicated only that there was a change of SP amplitude over days, marginally significant in habituation, but significant in training ($F=2.0$, $df=12/144$, $P<0.05$). The divergence of EApp and CApp means during training, although dramatic graphically, was not significant. The EApp and CApp groups did differ significantly on the last day of training, however ($t=2.32$, $df=12$, $P<0.05$ two tailed). During extinction there was a marginally significant effect of type of paradigm (experimental or control) used for the appetitive animals, EApp cats giving more positive shifts than CApp cats ($F=3.9$, $df=1/12$, $P<0.08$). There were no reliable differences between EAv and CAv, or EAv/ur and EAv/no-ur groups.

Lateral hypothalamus. Because there were no major effects of the reinforcement variable (appetitive or aversive UCS) in the region of lateral hypothalamus, the SP data from the two experimental groups were combined, as were the data from the two control groups. Plots of daily mean SP amplitudes for these two groups (Exp and Cont) are shown in Fig. 4. For these combined groups there were no mean differences between experimental and control animals, nor any differences in the manner in which these groups changed across days during habituation. However, during training, analysis of variance indicated that amplitude of SPs in the Exp and Cont groups changed differently across days ($F=2.7$, $df=12/312$, $P<0.01$). The control animals showed little systematic change in SP amplitude over the course of training, while the experimental animals exhibited a gradual increase in positive amplitude of the SP. The apparent interaction of days and groups during extinction was not significant, and there were no differences in SPs between

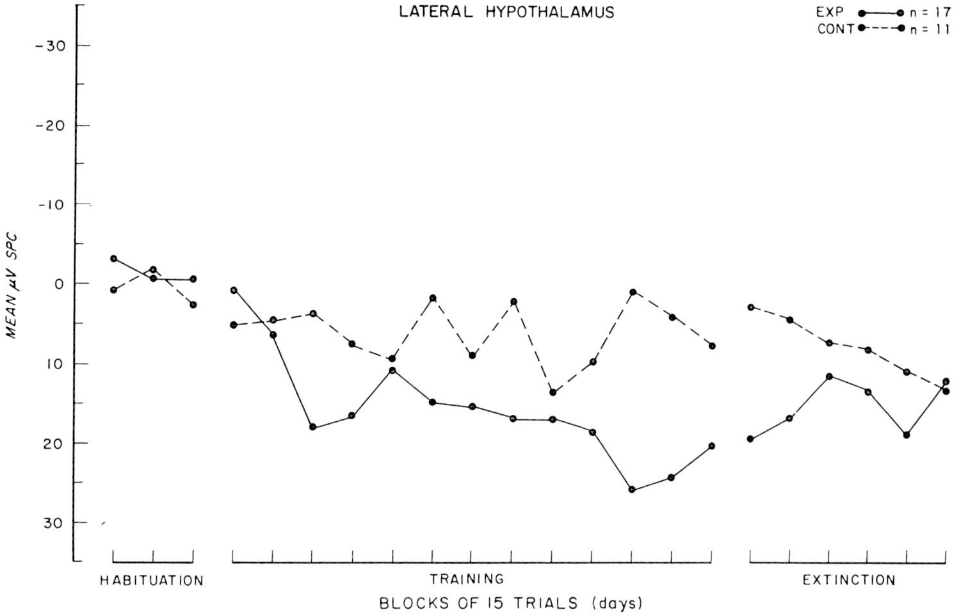

Fig. 4

Daily mean SP amplitude of lateral hypothalamus in the combined experimental and combined control groups.

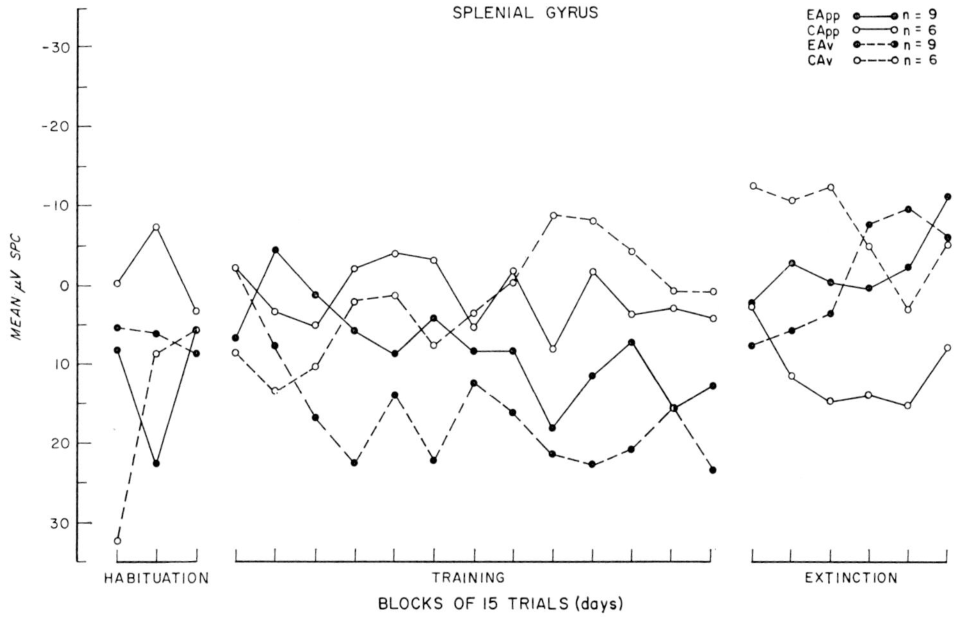

Fig. 5

Daily mean SP amplitude of splenial gyrus in the several treatment groups.

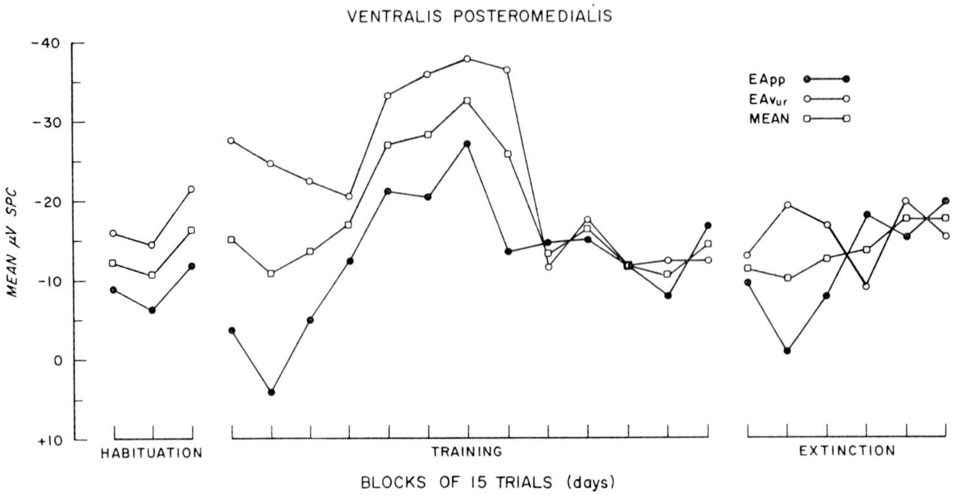

Fig. 6

Daily mean SP amplitude of ventralis posteromedialis for EApp and EAv_{ur} groups and the daily means of these groups combined (*i.e.*, all experimental animals that emitted UCRs).

EAv/ur and EAv/no-ur animals.

Splenial gyrus. In SPG Exp and Cont groups exhibited different profiles of SP changes across days during habituation ($F=3.3$, $df=2/52$, $P<0.05$). However, the groups were very similar at the end of habituation. During training there was only a near significant difference in such profiles ($F=1.7$, $df=12/312$, $P<0.07$). The control animals exhibited a slight increase of SP amplitude in the negative direction over the course of training, while experimental animals showed the reverse. Separate consideration of appetitive and aversive groups (Fig. 5) indicated that the EApp and CApp groups were not different during training, whereas SP amplitudes of EAv and CAv cats did act differently ($F=1.9$, $df=12/156$, $P<0.05$ for the Days × Group interaction). EAv animals showed an early increase in positive SP amplitude while their controls showed a more gradual increase in the negative direction.

Treatment comparisons yielded few meaningful results for the VPM placement, but as seen in Fig. 6, experimental animals which responded consistently to the UCS (*i.e.*, EApp and EAv/ur animals) exhibited SPs which increased in negative amplitude up to day 7 of training. The potentials dropped off rapidly thereafter to the value seen in habituation. An interesting aspect of these changes is their relationship to the behavioral learning curves seen in Fig. 1. As noted before, the learning curves for responding animals showed a rather distinct tendency to level off at days 6 and 7 of training, the same general period during which the negative SPs in VPM showed a sharp decline.

DISCUSSION

The results of this investigation indicate that SP events which are related to behavioral conditioning occur in the depths of brain as well as in the cerebral cortex. Unless an appropriate control group is employed, however, it is not clear whether such events are related specifically to associative factors in the situation or not. There were apparently very general factors in the experimental situation which produced SP changes in MG and MC which were unrelated to associative mechanisms; *i.e.*, these regions responded in a similar manner in both experimental and control groups.

In MG there were also marginal effects of the training paradigm used with appetitive animals, suggesting that associative mechanisms specific to appetitive reinforcement were involved to some extent in the geniculate reaction. Substantial variability between cats precluded demonstrating that possibility more concretely. During training the trend of changes in EApp animals was in the same direction as that seen during habituation. It appears as if habituation of the geniculate was accentuated by systematically pairing the CS with appetitive reinforcement. This is not, of course, what generally seems to occur, and more information about SPs in MG in needed to clarify these findings.

The absence of negative SPs at the cortical surface in frontal brain regions in these animals, in contrast to reports of other investigators (Rowland and Goldstone 1963; Chiorini 1969), could be due to several technical differences. The most obvious source of difference between this and other studies lies in the absence of any contribution from corneal-retinal potentials in the present study. In light of the necessity of high deprivation reported by Rowland and Goldstone (1963), it might be possible to attribute differences between this study and others to the state of deprivation or reward magnitude.

Slow potentials developed early in training in LH and became progressively more positive in experimental animals as training proceeded, indicating a role of this structure in the mediation of learned behavior. Since these data were obtained from differently motivated animals, it is also apparent that the LH function is not specifically related to the hedonic character of reinforcement.

In apparent contrast to this interpretation, other investigators indicate that the LH is involved specifically in food related reactions but not defensive CRs (Kalyuzhnyi *et al.* 1968). However, when the hedonic character of reinforcing stimuli is varied, there is often a concomitant variation of the relevant response system (Kalyuzhnyi *et al.* 1968; Rowland *et al.* 1967). In the present study, the masticatory-salivary system was involved in the reaction to both positive and negative reinforcers. However, since jaw movements were not seen in some animals in which SPs occurred, the SPs recorded from the LH in this study may reflect primarily changes related to the salivary functions of the region (Hainsworth and Epstein 1966). It is also plausible that lateral hypothalamic SPs indicate the occurrence of conditioned emotional responses elicited by the pairing of CS and UCS, as electrical stimulation of LH produces reactions characteristic of sympathetic nervous system activity, and the region is related anatomically to both limbic and midbrain-activating systems (Crosby *et al.* 1962; Truex and Carpenter 1964).

In contrast to the non-specific relationship of lateral hypothalamic SPs to reinforcement type, SPG reacted such that the different training procedures (experimental and control) had an effect on SPs only when an aversive reinforcer was used. The relationship of the anterior regions of SPG (and sulcus) to many neuronal areas, or to psychobehavioral phenomena is largely unknown. Functionally, posterior and lateral splenial areas have been found to respond to many kinds of sensory input and have come to be regarded as polysensory non-primary cortex (Buser and Bignall 1967). It is likely that anterior splenial regions share many of the characteristics of posterior areas. It is possible, also, that since anterior splenial cells are so closely related to cingulate gyrus anatomically, they might also be related functionally.

Whereas SPs can be shown to change systematically in response to experimental treatments, their exact physiological significance has yet to be determined. It is generally assumed that the cytoarchitecture of cortex plays a role in the determination of cortical SPs, and while the vertical arrangement of many cortical cells provides a convenient point of departure for the discussion of SP genesis, it is clear from depth recording that a systematic arrangement of cells is not necessary to SP occurrence. However, the lack of definitive cellular arrangement in many non-cortical regions makes it especially difficult to specify the relationship that might hold between SPs and unit activity in such areas.

In general, this study confirms other investigations (Morrell 1960; Rowland and Goldstone 1963; Low *et al.* 1966; Chiorini 1969) which indicate that slow potential phenomena reflect events in brain which are significantly related to associative and motivational changes.

With respect to questions posed earlier, it can be concluded that certain regions (*e.g.*, VMH and peri-VMH areas) while responsive to sensory stimulation, do not change in response to conditioning. Other regions do show altered responses as conditioned behavior develops, yet some areas (*e.g.*, MG and MC) apparently react to general conditions in the experimental situation. Other regions like LH and SPG appear to change in response to specific environmental contingencies. There was a similarity in the profile of SP amplitude changes across days of MG, LH and SPG, in that experimental groups exhibited changes in the direction of greater positivity, although showing different amplitude or polarity of response early in training. VPM, on the other hand, showed a brief period of increasing negative SPs during early portions of conditioning, which declined rapidly at the midpoint of training. In general, there was little influence of "reinforcement" type upon the SP responses. However, potentials in MG appeared to change more with appetitive reinforcement, while changes recorded from SPG occurred primarily in the context of negative reinforcement

SUMMARY

Slow potentials were recorded from several subcortical nuclei and from dura over motor cortex of thirty cats during classical conditioning of jaw movement using tone as conditioned stimulus, and acid or a meat-milk mix as unconditioned stimulus. Potentials in medial geniculate grew more positive during habituation and training. Slow potentials measured from lateral hypothalamus and splenial gyrus in experimental groups changed differently over the course of training than slow potentials measured from control groups. In splenial gyrus the foregoing effect was specific to groups receiving aversive reinforcement. No significant effects of treatment variables were found in motor cortex or medial ventral hypothalamus. The thalamic relay for gustatory input (VPM) appeared to be related to early development of behavioral conditioned responses, while being of little importance during response stabilization.

RÉSUMÉ

MODIFICATIONS DES POTENTIELS LENTS DANS LE CERVEAU DU CHAT PENDANT LE CONDITIONNEMENT APPÉTITIF CLASSIQUE DES MOUVEMENTS DE LA MÂCHOIRE ET LE CONDITIONNEMENT D'AVERSION

Sur trente chats, les potentiels lents ont été enregistrés au niveau de plusieurs noyaux sous-corticaux et au niveau de la dure-mère recouvrant le cortex moteur pendant le conditionnement classique du mouvement de la mâchoire, en utilisant un son comme stimulus conditionnel et un acide ou un mélange de viande et de lait comme stimulus inconditionnel. Au niveau du corps genouillé médian, les potentiels deviennent plus positifs pendant l'habituation et l'entraînement. Au niveau de l'hypothalamus latéral et du gyrus cingulaire, les potentiels lents mesurés dans les groupes expérimentaux se modifient au cours de l'entraînement, d'une façon différente des potentiels mesurés dans les groupes de contrôle. Au niveau du gyrus cingulaire, cet effet est spécifique aux groupes qui reçoivent des renforcements d'aversion. Aucune efficacité particulière des différents traîtements n'a été notée au niveau du cortex moteur ou de l'hypothalamus ventral médian. Le relai thalamique des afférences gustatives (VPM) paraît être en relation avec le développement précoce des réponses conditionnées comportementales, tandis qu'il paraît de peu d'importance lors de la stabilisation des réponses.

The authors thank Drs. J. R. Knott and D. W. McAdam for their support and encouragement, and for the use of animals and facilities of the Department of Psychiatry at the State Psychopathic Hospital, University of Iowa. Appreciation is also expressed to Dr. W. W. Kaelber for his assistance with histological verification of electrode placements, to Mrs. D. Walker for her careful histological work, and to Mr. A. Rudell for his perfection of the jaw fistula technique.

REFERENCES

Buser, P. and Bignall, K. E. Nonprimary sensory projections on the cat neocortex. *Int. Rev. Neurobiol.*, **1967**, *10*: 111–165.

Chiorini, J. R. Slow potential changes from cat cortex and classical aversive conditioning. *Electroenceph. clin. Neurophysiol.*, **1969**, *26*: 399–406.

Crosby, E. C., Humphrey, T. and Lauer, E. W. *Correlative anatomy of the nervous system.* Macmillan, New York, **1962**, 731 p.

Emde, J. W. A time locked, low level calibrator. *Electroenceph. clin. Neurophysiol.*, **1964**, *16*: 616–618.

Hainsworth, F. R. and Epstein, A. N. Severe impairment of heat induced saliva spreading in rats recovered from lateral hypothalamic lesions. *Science*, **1966**, *153*: 1255–1257.

Hayward, J. N., Fairchild, M. D. and Stuart, D. G. Hypothalamic and cortical D–C potential changes induced by stimulation of the midbrain reticular formation. *Exp. Brain Res.*, **1966**, *1*: 205–219.

JASPER, H. and AJMONE MARSAN, C. *A stereotaxic atlas of the diencephalon of the cat*. Nat. Res. Council of Canada, Ottawa, **1954.**

KALYUZHNYI, L. V., NEKRASOVA, L. I. and ZAKHAROVA, I. N. Changes in electrical and conditioned-reflex activity after destruction of lateral hypothalamus in rabbits. *Neurosci. Transl.*, **1968,** *1*: 131–135.

LOW, M. D., BORDA, R. P. and KELLAWAY, P. "Contingent Negative Variation" in rhesus monkeys: an EEG sign of a specific mental process. *Percept. Mot. Skills*, **1966**, *22*: 443–446.

MORRELL, F. Microelectrode and steady potential studies suggesting a dendritic locus of closure. *Electroenceph. clin. Neurophysiol.*, **1960,** *Suppl. 13*: 65–79.

ROWLAND, V. Simple non-polarizable electrode for chronic implantation. *Electroenceph. clin. Neurophysiol.*, **1961,** *13*: 290–291.

ROWLAND, V., BRADLEY, H., SCHOOL, P. and DEUTSCHMAN, D. Cortical steady-potential shifts in conditioning. *Cond. Reflex*, **1967,** *2*: 3–22.

ROWLAND, V. and GOLDSTONE, M. Appetitively conditioned and drive-related bioelectric baseline shift in cat cortex. *Electroenceph. clin. Neurophysiol.*, **1963,** *15*: 474–485.

SNIDER, R. S. and NIEMER, W. T. *A stereotaxic atlas of the cat brain*. Univ. Chicago Press, Chicago, **1961.**

TRUEX, R. C. and CARPENTER, M. B. *Human neuroanatomy*. Williams and Wilkins, Baltimore, **1964,** 591 p.

Reference: REBERT, C. S. and IRWIN, D. A. Slow potential changes in cat brain during classical appetitive and aversive conditioning of jaw movement. *Electroenceph. clin. Neurophysiol.*, **1969,** *27*: 152–161.

Electroencephalography and Clinical Neurophysiology
Elsevier Publishing Company, Amsterdam – Printed in The Netherlands

THE INFLUENCE OF INTRA-HIPPOCAMPAL GAMMA-AMINOBUTYRIC ACID ON THE ORIENTING REFLEX

R. Rogozea, J. Ungher and V. Florea-Ciocoiu

The Institute of Neurology of the Academy, Bucharest (Rumania)

(Accepted for publication: November 4, 1968)

The present study was suggested on the one hand by the fact that the hippocampus has been said to play a significant role in the orienting reflex (Green and Arduini 1954; Grastyán *et al.* 1959 etc.) and, on the other, by the great number of observations which have already demonstrated that gamma-aminobutyric acid (GABA) plays a role in neuronal regulation (Iwama and Jasper 1957; Purpura and Grundfest 1957; Dasgupta *et al.* 1958; Crighel 1966). Based on these data we thought it of interest to ascertain the extent to which local intra-hippocampal administration of GABA induces changes in the orienting reflex (behaviour and EEG).

MATERIAL AND METHOD

The experiments were carried out on eleven adult cats. The EEG and behavioural investigations were performed in chronic experiments, the animals being awake, free or semi-restrained, for electrical recording.

The cats were anaesthetized with hexobarbital sodium (Evipan) and silver electrodes in bipolar arrangement were implanted stereotaxically (Jasper and Ajmone Marsan 1954) in the medial ectosylvian gyrus, posterior ectosylvian gyrus, anterior suprasylvian gyrus, mesencephalic reticular formation (MRF) and posterior hypothalamic area. The cortical and deep electrodes were implanted unilaterally. For local administration of the drug and electrical recording at this level, a stainless steel electrode-cannula was introduced into the dorsal hippocampus. The cannula was implanted unilaterally in seven cats and bilaterally in four. The investigations started only after the animals had fully recovered.

In animals thus prepared the orienting responses to repetitive auditory stimulation were tested behaviourally and electroencephalographically before administration of the drug, after intra-hippocampal injection of inactive carbon (Norit) (both being control tests) and, finally, after intra-hippocampal GABA administration. The criteria for the orienting responses were the appearance of the somatic and EEG responses (starts, complex motor orienting responses, neocortical and hippocampal arousal reactions) evoked by repetitive sensory stimuli. Their aspect, dynamics and habituation were studied. In order to time the GABA effects the orienting reflex was observed for 45 min before and after the administration of the drug. The orienting responses were elicited by a variety of repetitive auditory stimuli which had different physical parameters (frequency, intensity, duration), their sequential order depending on the process of extinction of the orienting reflex which began after the same stimulus had been repeated a number of times. For example, when the orienting reaction was extinguished by repeated application of a tone of 1000 c/sec, 10 dB, 3 sec duration it was replaced by a tone of 1500 c/sec, 15 dB, 2 sec duration and so forth. The physical parameters of the repetitive auditory stimuli varied within rather close limits, in order to obtain the closest possible degrees of loudness (a fact confirmed by control tests). The same stimuli were used before and after administration of the drug. We also used as auditory stimulus the appellative "pss-pss".

Besides the orienting reflex, the spontaneous behaviour and bioelectrical activity were observed before and after the administration of the drug. The animals were tested in an electrically and acoustically insulated box. The records were made with an 8-channel Kaiser EEG apparatus.

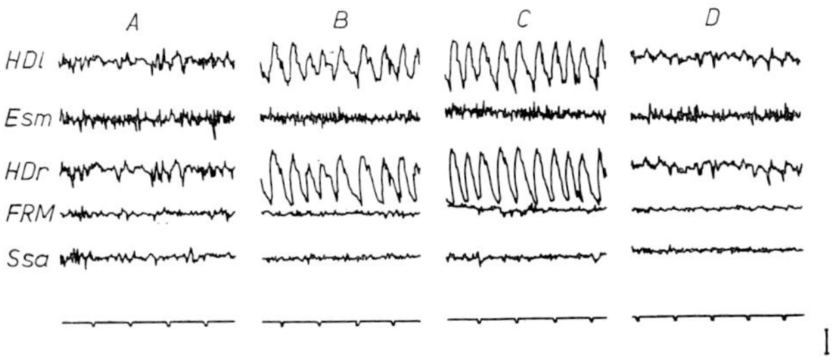

Fig. 1

Early alterations in hippocampal electrical activity after bilateral intra-hippocampal administration of GABA. Cat CH 1. *A*: before GABA; *B*: 5 sec following GABA: high voltage slow hippocampal activity (3 c/sec, 200 μV); *C*: 5 sec following inactive carbon (control): same slow activity; *D*: 2 min following GABA. In this and subsequent figures: Esm = medial ectosylvian gyrus; Esp = posterior ectosylvian gyrus; Ssa = anterior suprasylvian gyrus; FRM = mesencephalic reticular formation; Hip. p = posterior hypothalamic area; HD = dorsal hippocampus; HDr = right dorsal hippocampus; HDl = left dorsal hippocampus. Bipolar recordings. Calibration = 100 μV. Time in seconds at the bottom of the diagram.

Drug administration. Crystals of GABA were administered intra-hippocampally, through the cannula. The dose used was 0.7–0.8 mg/cannula, as established by previous control experiments in which the drug had been marked by dye (fuchsin) to establish the amount ensuring the best diffusion of GABA in the hippocampus and confining it within this structure.

Histological verification of the electrode placements was made.

RESULTS

1. *Effect of GABA on spontaneous behaviour and bioelectrical activity*

Intra-hippocampal administration of GABA was not followed by any particular change in the animal's spontaneous behaviour (we considered as "spontaneous" the animal's behaviour in the absence of any stimuli applied by the experimenter). The drug did not induce any obvious changes in the animal's responsiveness to extraneous stimuli. In two cases drowsiness, with the accompanying electrical changes, was noted 8–10 min after drug administration. It did not appear to be a constant phenomenon, however.

The spontaneous electrical changes following the administration of the drug were more significant. Thus, immediately after GABA administration a high voltage slow activity (200–300 μV, 2–3 c/sec) occurred, strictly confined to the hippocampus (Fig. 1). Subsequently this activity, observed in six of the animals studied, diminished progressively and disappeared within 1–2 min. In a seventh animal, this type of activity appeared 3 min after GABA and disappeared in the 4th minute. In two of the above mentioned animals, however, the same type of activity was observed also in control experiments after intra-hippocampal administration of inactive carbon (Fig. 1).

Besides this early and transient change in spontaneous electrical activity after GABA further alterations in hippocampal activity were noted: on the one hand the disappearance in eight cases of the 4–7 c/sec spontaneous synchronization, a phenomenon observed 2–7 min following administration (Fig. 2), and, on the other, a slight increase

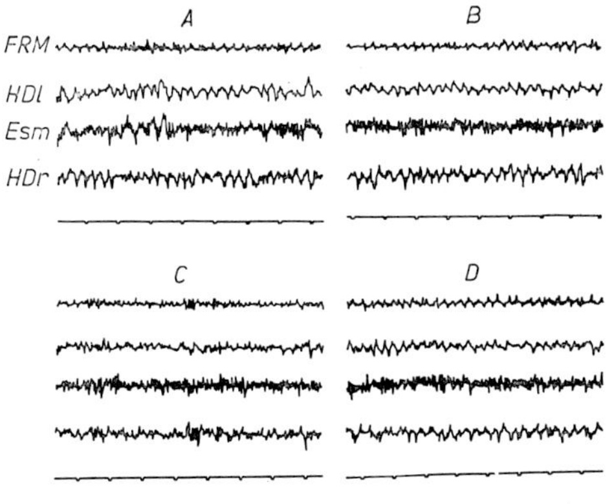

Fig. 2

Between 2 and 7 min following GABA: the spontaneous hippocampal synchronization is suppressed. Cat CH 5. *A*: before GABA; *B*: 2 min following inactive carbon; *C*: 2 min following GABA; *D*: 8 min following GABA.

in amplitude of the electrical activity of this structure, which could be observed up to 35–40 min (Fig. 3). No changes in amplitude or frequency of the neocortical spontaneous activity were noted.

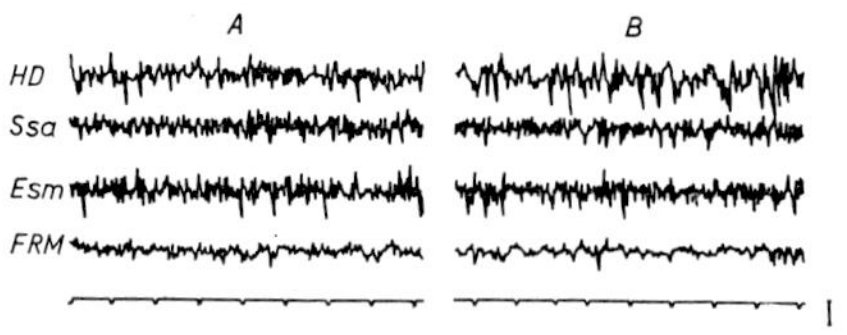

Fig. 3
Increase in hippocampal activity following GABA. Cat CH 12. *A*: before GABA; *B*: following GABA.

Intra-hippocampal administration of GABA bilaterally in two and unilaterally in one animal induced the appearance of some convulsive discharges in MRF 2 min after administration of the drug (Fig. 4); the reticular discharges lasted 22, 12 and 10 min, respectively. The frequency of these discharges was higher during the first minutes and decreased progressively afterwards. The fact that convulsive activity was not seen in these animals in control experiments should be emphasized. All the above changes in spontaneous electrical activity also appeared in animals in which administration of the drug did not induce immediately high voltage slow activity in the hippocampus.

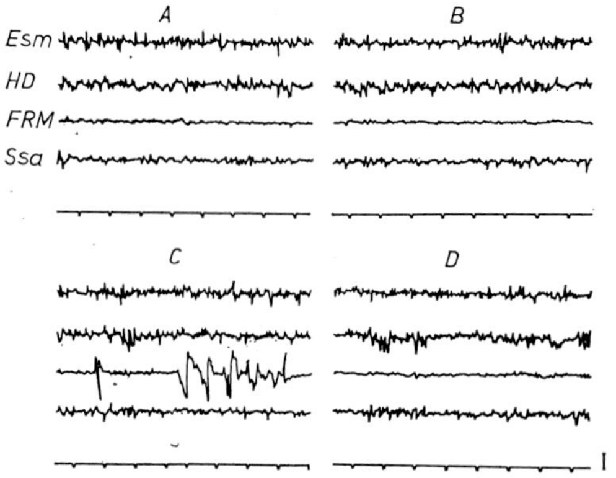

Fig. 4
Discharges appear in MRF 2 min after intra-hippocampal GABA. Cat CH 6. *A*: before GABA; *B*: 2 min following inactive carbon; *C*: 2 min after GABA; *D*: 13 min after GABA.

2. *Effect of GABA on behavioural and bioelectrical components of the orienting reflex*

After intra-hippocampal GABA constant changes in the orienting behaviour appeared. These concerned in the first place the orienting behaviour dynamics, in that extinction of orienting responses, following within 2–7 min the administration of the drug, occurred later than in control experiments (Fig. 5). The late extinction of the orienting behaviour was more evident after bilateral administration of GABA. Secondly, the changes concerned the somatic aspect of the orienting reflex in that administration of the drug was followed within the above interval mostly by starts, complex motor reactions being less often observed than in control experiments.

Significant alterations of the EEG orienting component were noted after administration of the drug. Thus, it was observed that dorsal hippocampal evoked potentials to repetitive auditory stimuli were extinguished after GABA administration earlier than in control experiments. In contrast, potentials elicited in the auditory primary and associative neocortical areas by repetitive auditory stimulation did not differ from responses recorded at this level in control experiments.

The depression, or even the suppression, of the hippocampal arousal reaction to auditory stimuli was the most constant and significant effect of intra-hippocampal administration of GABA upon the EEG component of the orienting reflex (Fig. 6). Such depression or suppression of theta rhythm was evident especially during the first 2–6 min following administration of the drug and it coincided with the behavioural period of delayed extinction of the orienting somatic responses. Subsequently the hippocampal arousal reaction tended to reappear progressively. Moreover, in one animal a spontaneous theta rhythm appeared 9 min after administration of GABA and it was impossible to interrupt it for 4 min by various sensory stimuli (Fig. 6). It is noteworthy that intra-hippocampal administration of GABA depressed or suppressed temporarily the arousal reaction in this structure but failed to alter the neocortical arousal reaction to repetitive auditory stimuli (Fig. 6).

Furthermore, the behaviour and the EEG component of the orienting reflex were both af-

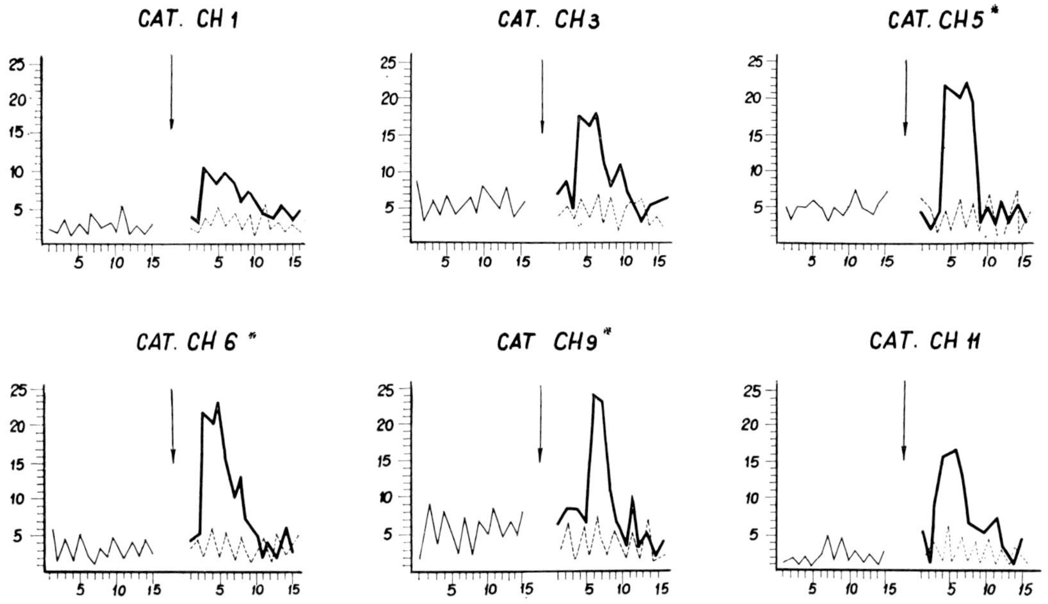

Fig. 5

The dynamics of extinction of the orienting reflex following GABA. Ordinate = number of repetitive applications of stimuli; abscissa = time scale in minutes. Continuous line = extinction of orienting activity before GABA. Dashed line = extinction after inactive carbon. Thick line = extinction following GABA. Arrow = GABA.

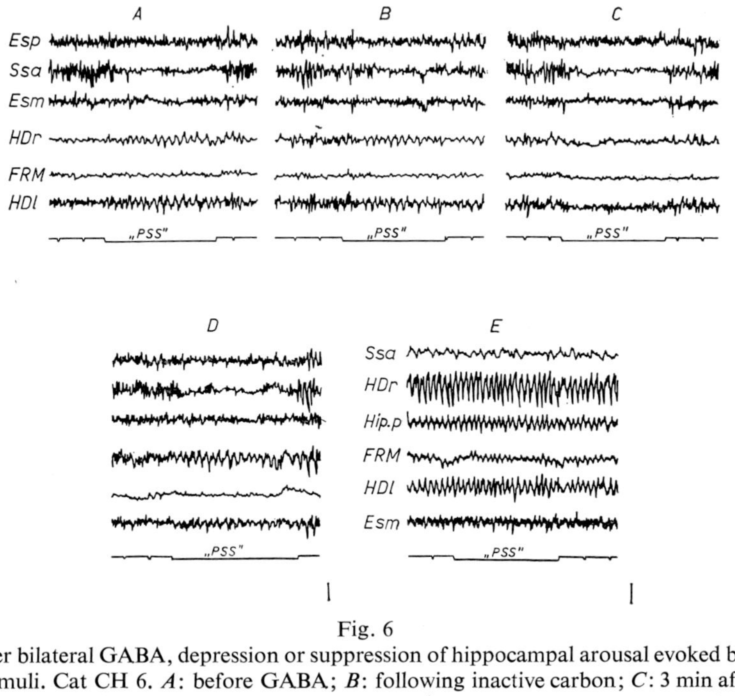

Fig. 6

2–7 min after bilateral GABA, depression or suppression of hippocampal arousal evoked by repetitive auditory stimuli. Cat CH 6. *A*: before GABA; *B*: following inactive carbon; *C*: 3 min after GABA; *D*: 8 min after GABA; *E*: 9 min after GABA in cat CH 9. Persistent spontaneous theta rhythm.

fected even when administration of the drug did not immediately induce high voltage slow activity in the hippocampus.

DISCUSSION

The above behavioural and EEG data show that the effects of local uni- or bilateral intra-hippocampal administration of GABA appear from the second minute of administration, consisting in depression or suppression of the spontaneous or evoked hippocampal synchronization to a sensory stimulus, in a slight increase of the activity in this structure, in orienting behavioural alterations, etc. The most marked effects are noted between 2 and 7 min after administration; subsequently slight alterations of the spontaneous electrical activity continue to appear up to 35–40 min. The fact that in our experiments the effects of intra-hippocampal administration of the drug appeared with more readiness than in the experiments of some other authors who used parenteral administration (Marazzi *et al.* 1958; Takahashi *et al.* 1959; Monnier and Romanowski 1962) could be explained by avoidance of the blood-brain barrier and, therefore, by greater concentrations of GABA, obtained exclusively in this structure in a shorter time interval. It is true that the first electrical changes after administration of the drug are immediate and appear as high voltage slow hippocampal activity. However, bearing in mind that this type of activity was encountered also in control experiments during which inactive carbon was administered it might be regarded as a result of irritation of the hippocampus and not as a specific pharmacodynamic effect of the drug.

From our data it appears that the uni- or bilateral intra-hippocampal administration of GABA induces alterations neither in spontaneous behaviour nor in neocortical electrical activity. On comparing these data with those reported by other authors after parenteral (intravenous, intracarotid and even intracisternal) administration of GABA (Csok and Lang 1955; Marazzi *et al.* 1958; Takahashi *et al.* 1959; Monnier and Romanowski 1962), *viz.*, slight motor restlessness with facilitation of neocortical electrical activity, local intra-hippocampal administration of GABA seems to have no influence on neocortical electrogenesis and spontaneous behaviour, its action being exclusively exerted at the hippocampal level. This assumption is supported also by the persistence at the neocortical level of the electrographic arousal reaction and of the evoked potential to auditory stimulation following intra-hippocampal administration of GABA.

The local effect of the drug is marked by consecutive changes in the spontaneous electrical activity in this structure, by changes in its hippocampal arousal reaction and in hippocampal potentials evoked by repetitive auditory stimulation, by alteration of the orienting behaviour and, finally, by the discharges induced in MRF. The mechanism whereby GABA induces changes in the orienting reflex (behaviour and EEG) is hard to specify, however. Are these due to an inhibitory or to an excitatory effect of the drug on hippocampal neurones? Arguments can be found to support both hypotheses. We believe that the above-mentioned alterations are more likely to be the result of an inhibiting effect of GABA and we base our assumption on the following facts: (1) the hippocampal arousal reaction, which, according to Green and Arduini (1954), Bremner (1964) etc., expresses a state of hippocampal excitation, is depressed or suppressed, denoting that the effect of the drug is inhibitory; (2) extinction of the evoked potential to repetitive auditory stimulation occurs earlier after GABA administration, denoting that the ability of the neurones to develop the evoked response is reduced. In this connection there are many further observations proving that topical neocortical application of GABA induces a depression of the responses evoked by stimulation of the specific and nonspecific afferent systems and by direct cortical stimulation (Iwama and Jasper 1957; Purpura and Grundfest 1957; Yamamoto *et al.* 1959; Monnier and Romanowski 1962; Crighel 1966). Our data and those available in the literature enable us to infer that the mechanism whereby the drug depresses the hippocampal evoked potential is similar. The evoked potential might be depressed following GABA also on account of the effect exerted by the drug on the pattern of the background activity, the attenuation of the evoked potentials being likely to be a consequence of such change; the fact that after intra-hippocampal administration of GABA the depression of the hippocampal EEG component of the orienting reflex (evoked potential and theta activity) is accompanied by lateness of extinction of orienting behaviour (including the somatic aspect of such behaviour) supports the assumption that the neuronal depressing effect of GABA would suppress the modulating action exerted by hippocampus upon the MRF and, implicitly, upon the orienting reflex. This assumption is also supported by the fact that the reticular discharges following GABA administration appeared after a time interval equal to that necessary for the development of the above mentioned electrical and behavioural alterations.

We believe that the discharges in MRF are generated by chronic local irritation due to the electrode implanted in this structure and facilitated by temporary depression by GABA of the modulating influence of the hippocampus upon MRF. Our assumption that GABA administered intra-hippocampally fails to develop the suppressive hippocampal influence on the orienting reflex is also supported by our observations (Rogozea and Ungher 1968) in which chronic lesions of hippocampus induce the same alterations, but of persistent character.

The above phenomena are more marked after bilateral administration of the drug, thus demonstrating that the depression induced by unilateral administration of GABA is more or less compensatable, whereas that induced by bilateral administration is not.

Our data confirm, therefore, the role played by the hippocampus in inhibiting some mesencephalic physiological mechanisms, the orienting reflex specifically. They raise again the question of the functional significance of the theta rhythm. The dissociative effect of intra-hippocampal GABA, expressed by delay of habituation of the orienting behaviour simultaneously with depression or suppression of the theta rhythm, suggests, in contrast to what has been suggested by Grastyán *et al.* (1959) and in agreement with the data of Green and Arduini (1954), that this pattern of activity expresses an active functional state of the hippocampus requisite to the habituation of the orienting reflex.

SUMMARY

The spontaneous electrical background and evoked orienting EEG activities were tested before and after intra-hippocampal administration of gamma-aminobutyric acid (GABA) to eleven adult cats with electrodes chronically implanted in the ectosylvian and suprasylvian gyri, mesencephalic reticular formation (MRF), posterior hypothalamic area and dorsal hippocampus. Concomitantly the spontaneous and auditorily induced behaviour were observed. The results were as follows:

1. The effects of intra-hippocampal GABA appeared 2 min following uni- or bilateral administration, were, mostly evident between 2 and 7 min and disappeared after 35–40 min. The rapid effect of the drug was due to its intra-hippocampal administration, which permitted avoidance of the blood-brain barrier and thus immediately induced a high concentration of GABA.

2. No changes in the animals behaviour and in the electrical activity of the neocortex were observed (the neocortical arousal reaction and the potentials evoked by repetitive auditory stimulation were not altered). Thus intra-hippocampal GABA exerts its influence exclusively upon the hippocampus.

3. Intra-hippocampal GABA induced changes in hippocampal activity (slight increase of spontaneous electrical activity, faster extinction of the hippocampal evoked response to repetitive auditory stimulation and depression, or even suppression, of the spontaneous or evoked arousal reaction), delayed extinction of orienting behaviour and convulsive activity in MRF. The EEG and behavioural changes were simultaneous.

4. The authors assume that the alterations are due to a depressing action of the drug on hippocampal neurones. The local depressing effect is responsible for suppression of the modulating effect of the hippocampus on the MRF and therefore upon the orienting reflex.

RÉSUMÉ

L'INFLUENCE DE L'ACIDE GAMMA-AMINOBUTYRIQUE INTRA-HIPPOCAMPIQUE SUR LE RÉFLEXE D'ORIENTATION

L'activité électrique de fond spontanée et les activités EEG évoquées d'orientation ont été testées avant et après administration intra-hippocampique de GABA à onze chats adultes avec électrodes chroniquement implantées dans les gyri ectosylvien et suprasylvien, le FRM, l'aire hypothalamique postérieure et l'hippocampe dorsal. Concomitament, le comportement spontané et induit par voie auditive a été observé. Les résultats ont été les suivants:

1. Les effets du GABA intra-hippocampique s'expriment 2 min après l'administration uni- ou bilatérale, sont particulièrement évidents entre 2 et 7 min et disparaissent après 35–40 min. L'effet rapide de la drogue est du à son administration intra-hippocampique, qui permet d'éviter la barrière hémato-cérébrale et provoque ainsi immédiatement une concentration élevée de GABA.

2. Aucun changement du comportement de l'animal ni de l'activité électrique du néo-cortex n'a été observé (la réaction d'arousal néo-corticale et les potentiels évoqués par stimulation auditive répétitive ne sont pas altérés). Ainsi, le GABA intra-hippocampique exerce son influence exclusivement sur l'hippocampe.

3. Le GABA intra-hippocampique entraîne des changements de l'activité hippocampique (légère augmentation de l'activité électrique spontanée, expansion plus rapide des réponses évoquées hippocampiques à des stimulations auditives répétitives et dépression ou même suppression de la réaction d'arousal spontanée ou évoquée), l'extinction tardive du comportement d'orientation et une activité convulsive dans le MRF. Les modifications EEG et comportementales sont simultanées.

4. Les auteurs supposent que ces altérations sont dues à une action dépressive de la drogue sur les neurones hippocampiques. L'effet dépresseur local est responsable de la suppression de l'effet modulant de l'hippocampe sur le MRF et par conséquent sur le réflexe d'orientation.

REFERENCES

BREMNER, F. J. Hippocampal activity during avoidance behaviour in the rat. *J. comp. Physiol.*, **1964,** *58*: 16–22.

CRIGHEL, E. The effects of GABA and strychnine on neocortical structures involved in the onset mechanism of epileptic activity. *Epilepsia (Amst.)*, **1966,** *7*: 283–290.

CSOK, G. UND LANG, K. Über einige Wirkungen von L-Glutaminsäure, D-Glutaminsäure und -Aminobutersäure. *Naunyn-Schmiedeberg's Arch. exp. Path. Pharmak.*, **1955,** *227*: 214–220.

DASGUPTA, S. R., KILLAM, E. K. and KILLAM, K. F. Drug action on rhinencephalic seizure activity in the cat. *J. Pharmacol. exp. Ther.*, **1958,** *122*: 16A.

GRASTYÁN, E., LISSAK, K., MADARÁSZ, I. and DONHOFFER, H. Hippocampal electrical activity during the development of conditioned reflexes. *Electroenceph. clin. Neurophysiol.*, **1959,** *11*: 409–430.

GREEN, J. D. and ARDUINI, A. Hippocampal electrical activity in arousal. *J. Neurophysiol.*, **1954,** *17*: 532–557.

IWAMA, K. and JASPER, H. H. The action of gamma aminobutyric acid upon cortical activity in the cat. *J. Physiol. (Lond.)*, **1957,** *138*: 365–380.

JASPER, H. H. and AJMONE MARSAN, C. *A stereotaxic atlas of the diencephalon of the cat.* Nat. Res. Council of Canada, Ottawa, **1954,** 15 p.

MARAZZI, A. S., HART, E. R. and RODRIQUEZ, J. M. Action of bloodborne gamma-aminobutyric acid on central synapses. *Science*, **1958,** *127*: 284–285.

MONNIER, M. et ROMANOWSKI, W. Les systèmes cholinoceptifs cérébraux—actions de l'acétylcholine, de la physostigmine, pilocarpine et de GABA. *Electroenceph. clin. Neurophysiol.*, **1962,** *14*: 486–498.

PURPURA, D. P. and GRUNDFEST, H. Physiological and pharmacological consequences of different synaptic organizations in cerebral and cerebellar cortex of cat. *J. Neurophysiol.*, **1957,** *20*: 494–522.

ROGOZEA, R. and UNGHER, J. Changes in orienting activity of cat induced by chronic hippocampal lesions. *Exp. Neurol.*, **1968,** *21*: 176–186.

TAKAHASHI, H., MATSUZAKI, H., KUMEI, K. and TAKAHASHI, H. EEG arousal by GABA in the rabbit under anesthesia, cyanpoisoning or asphyxia. *Jap. J. Physiol.*, **1959,** *9*: 207–217.

YAMAMOTO, Ch., YUYAMA, T. and IWAMA, K. Suppressing effects on electrocortical activity of GABA in cats. *Jap. J. Physiol.*, **1959,** *9*: 160–170.

Reference: ROGOZEA, R., UNGHER, J. and FLOREA-CIOCOIU, V. The influence of intra-hippocampal gamma-aminobutyric acid on the orienting reflex. *Electroenceph. clin. Neurophysiol.*, **1969,** *27*: 162–168.

Electroencephalography and Clinical Neurophysiology
Elsevier Publishing Company, Amsterdam – Printed in The Netherlands

VARIATIONS IN HUMAN PHYSIOLOGICAL FINGER TREMOR, WITH PARTICULAR REFERENCE TO CHANGES WITH AGE

C. D. Marsden, J. C. Meadows, G. W. Lange and R. S. Watson

Departments of Medicine and Neurology, St. Thomas's Hospital, London, S. E. 1 and the National Physical Laboratory, Teddington (Great Britain)

(Accepted for publication: November 22, 1968)

Physiological tremor has intrigued neurophysiologists ever since Schäfer demonstrated a 10 c/sec rhythm in the normal human voluntary myogram (Schäfer *et al.* 1886). Finger tremor limits our finesse of motor control as, for instance, is apparent when we attempt to thread a needle or wield a soldering iron. It is possible that analysis of this phenomenon might yield clues to the mechanisms of human voluntary motor control, yet despite many investigations the origin of physiological tremor is still uncertain. Tremor varies considerably in different subjects and in the same subject at different times. Experimental studies on tremor must take into account such normal variation. The purpose of this paper is to establish the extent to which tremor of the outstretched finger may vary in the individual and in a group of normal subjects. It is hoped that these data may aid in the interpretation of tremor studies in various clinical disorders and in the evaluation of the effects of drugs on tremor.

The techniques of spectrum analysis have been applied to tremor recorded from the outstretched index finger in eighty-eight subjects with ages between 3 and 85 years. Distinctive changes in tremor with age have been observed, and their significance is discussed.

METHODS

Subjects

The subjects studied were either colleagues (34) or volunteer patients in hospital for minor surgery or investigation of unrelated diseases (54), none of whom had evidence of disease of the central, peripheral or autonomic nervous systems. None of the patients was taking drugs, other than hypnotics administered at least 12 h previously.

Data collection

All studies were conducted in a quiet room with the subject sitting in a comfortable chair. Tremor was recorded from the right hand alone in seventy subjects, and from both hands simultaneously in eighteen subjects. The subject was instructed to adduct the arm at the shoulder and flex the elbow so that the pronated forearm lay comfortably on a rigid surface supported down to the wrist. During each period of tremor recording the subject was asked to extend the wrist and adduct the fingers actively so that they were in line with the forearm, and to maintain this posture throughout a period of 2 min without direct visual reference.

Tremor was detected by an accelerometer (Ether BLA 2, weight 2.25 g) taped over the dorsal surface of the terminal interphalangeal joint of the index finger. The output of the accelerometer was amplified and passed through a filter acting as an integrator above 1 c/sec so as to obtain a signal corresponding to velocity. This was fed to an analogue to digital converter to obtain punched tape (at 110 characters/sec) for subsequent computer analysis.

The velocity signal was chosen as the measured parameter since it is likely that velocity is most closely related to force in an isotonic task in the region of peak frequency, although the two are related strictly by a characteristic frequency response function.

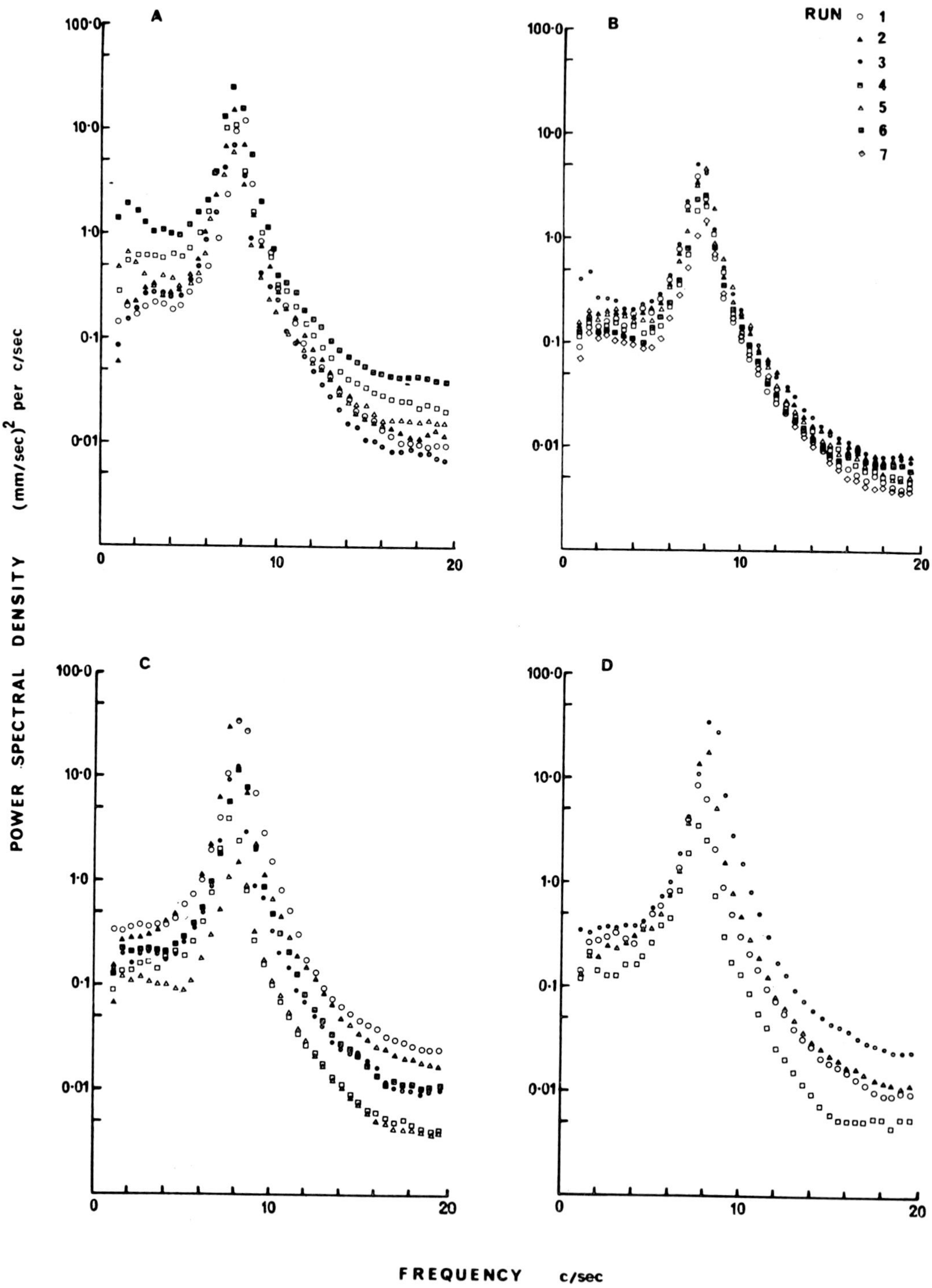

Fig. 1
The spectrum of finger tremor recorded from the right hand in subject J.M. at intervals over varying periods of time: *A*: for 1 min at 3 min intervals for 15 min; *B*: for 2 min at 10 min intervals for 1 h; *C*: for 2 min at 1 h intervals for 6 h, and *D*: for 2 min daily for 4 days.

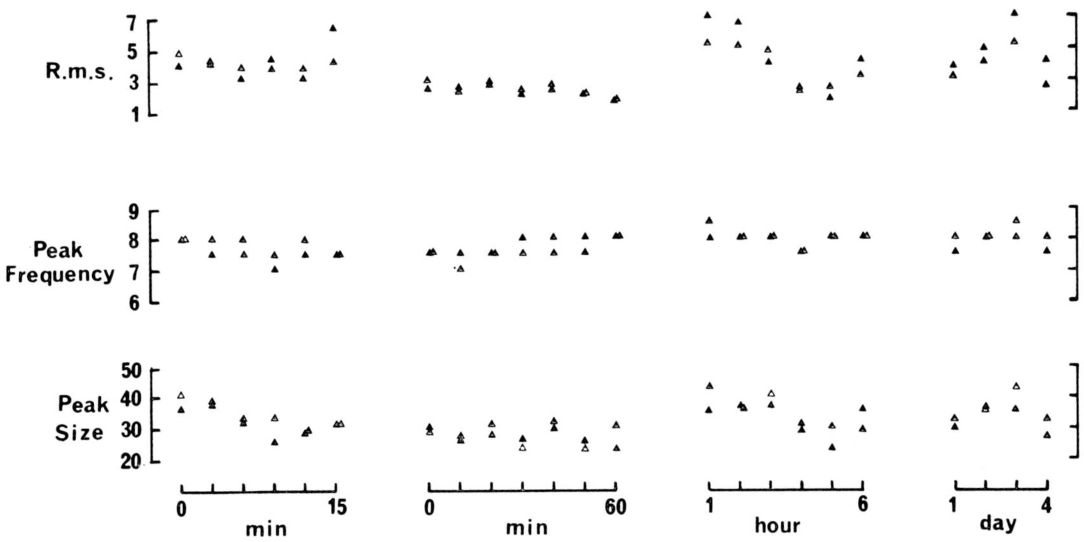

Fig. 2

Changes in RMS velocity between 1 and 20 c/sec (mm/sec), peak frequency (to the nearest 0.5 cycle), and relative peak size, expressed as the percentage of total RMS velocity between 1 and 20 c/sec in the 0.5 cycle band at peak frequency. Tremor was recorded in subject J.M. from the right (▲) and left (△) hands at intervals over the varying periods of time detailed in the legend to Fig. 1.

Data analysis

The data were analysed with the National Physical Laboratory "Hermes" computer. The spectrum was estimated by first calculating the auto-covariance function (mean and trend removed). A Hanning lag window was then applied, followed by Fourier transformation (Blackman and Tukey 1959). Estimates were first computed at 0.25 cycle intervals and later smoothed in the frequency domain to obtain reasonably independent values at 0.5 c/sec intervals. The over-all smoothing corresponded to a filter with equivalent "noise band-width" of 0.6 c/sec. Each record was analysed in sections of approximately 30 sec duration. Histograms and spectra of individual sections were compared to ensure consistency of variance and spectral shape during each record. Each result comprised an ensemble average of at least four sections, representing approximately 2 min total recording.

Data presentation

Tremor spectra, as shown in Fig. 1 and subsequent figures, have been plotted as power spectral density in $(mm/sec)^2$ per c/sec on a logarithmic scale (ordinate) against frequency in c/sec on a linear scale averaged in 0.5 c/sec bands (abscissa). Total tremor has been expressed as root mean square (RMS) error velocity between 1 and 20 c/sec in mm/sec, which is the square root of the variance of the subject in performing the test. Peak frequency has been calculated to the nearest 0.5 cycle. The size of

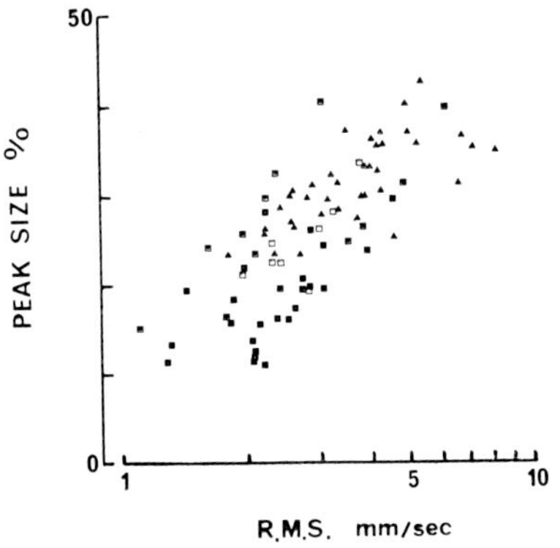

Fig. 3

Relation between the relative size of the peak (ordinate) and total RMS velocity (abscissa) obtained from C.M.'s right (■) and left (▲) hands, and that obtained from J.M.'s right (□) and left (△) hands. Relative peak size increases as tremor increases ($r = +0.33$, $P < 0.01$).

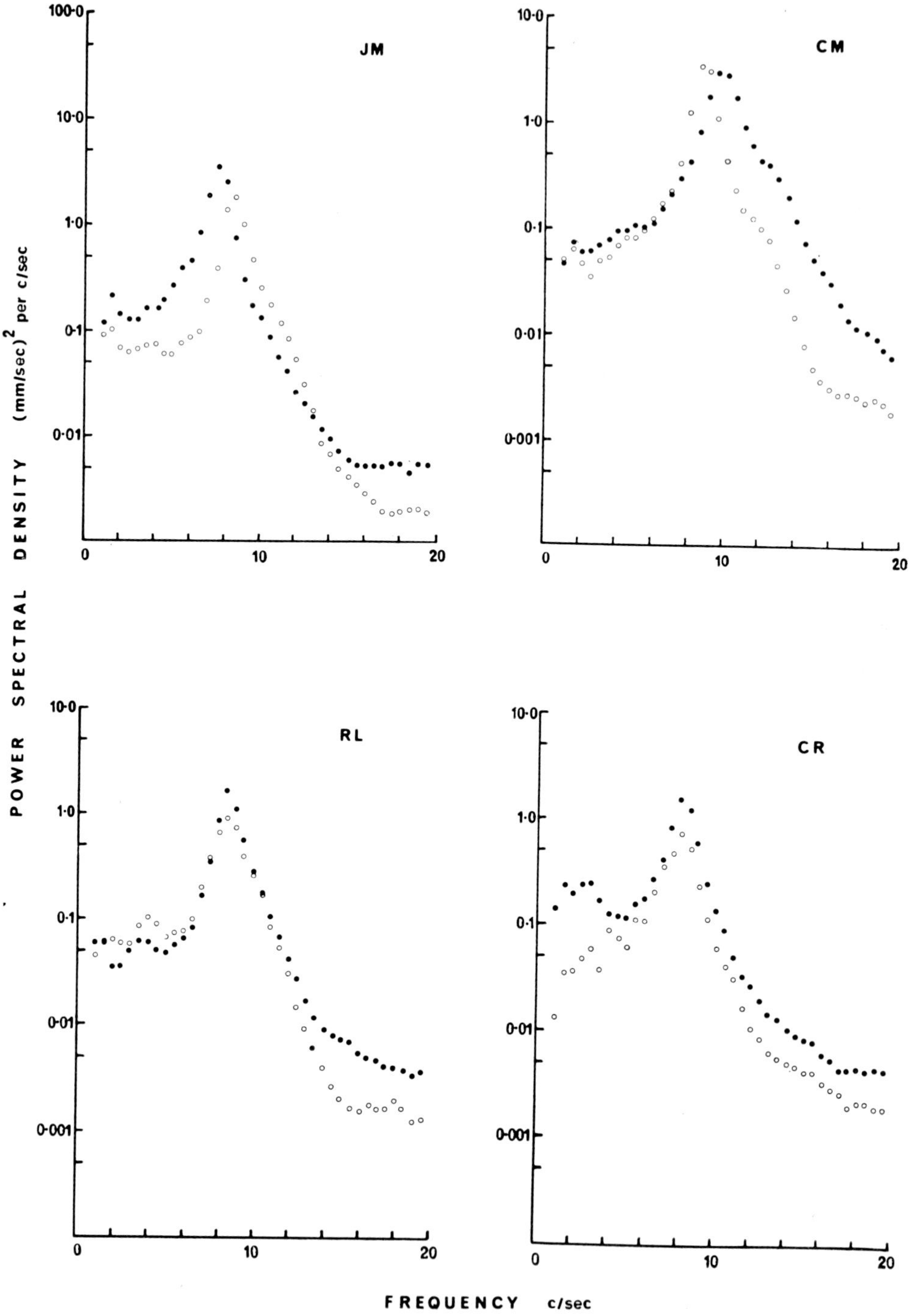

Fig. 4

Tremor spectra recorded from subjects J.M. and C.M. at an interval of 16 months and from subjects R.L. and C.R. at an interval of 10 months. (Initial spectrum, open circle; subsequent spectrum, closed circle.)

the peak, relative to tremor at other frequencies between 1 and 20 c/sec, has been expressed as a percentage of the total error velocity between 1 and 20 c/sec in the 0.5 cycle band at peak frequency. Statistical analysis of differences between mean values was by Student's *t* test, using a two-tailed test of significance.

RESULTS

Typical tremor spectra, as shown in Fig. 1, show error at all frequencies between 1 and 20 c/sec. Three portions of the spectrum are recognizable; low frequency error between about 1 and 5 c/sec, a well-defined peak around 9 c/sec (see Halliday and Redfearn 1956) and error above about 12 c/sec which rapidly decreases as frequency increases.

Variation of tremor in the individual subject

Tremor was recorded at regular intervals from both hands over periods of 15 min, 1 h, 6 h and 4 or 5 days in two trained subjects. Details of the experimental protocols are shown in the legend to Fig. 1, which shows the results obtained in subject J.M. The variations in total tremor, peak frequency and relative size of the peak for subject J.M. are shown in Fig. 2.

Total tremor varied from run to run, but the coefficient of variation—(SD/mean) × 100—for each of the two subjects was approximately 30%. The shape of the tremor spectrum remained constant and peak frequency rarely altered by more than 1 c/sec. Relative peak size was proportional to total tremor ($r = +0.33$, $P < 0.01$) (Fig. 3).

In four adult subjects tremor was analysed at intervals of 10 or 16 months (Fig. 4). It is striking that even at these long intervals, the shape of the tremor spectrum and amplitude of tremor remained very similar in each of the four subjects.

Variation of tremor between subjects

Tremor of the right hand was recorded over a period of 2 min in eighty-eight subjects aged between 3 and 85 years. Twenty-seven children (16 male, 11 female), with ages less than 16 years, and sixty-one adults (32 male, 29 female) were studied.

TABLE I

Differences between the tremor spectra of children and adults. Mean values are shown with statistical significance of differences or correlations

<table>
<tr><th rowspan="2"></th><th colspan="2">Children ($N = 27$)</th><th colspan="2">Adults ($N = 61$)</th><th rowspan="2">Significance</th></tr>
<tr><th>with peak $N = 16$</th><th>with no peak $N = 11$</th><th>with peak $N = 58$</th><th>with no peak $N = 3$</th></tr>
<tr><td rowspan="2">Total RMS velocity between 1 and 20 c/sec (mm/sec)</td><td colspan="2">2.70</td><td colspan="2">3.00</td><td>$t = 0.79$ (N.S.)</td></tr>
<tr><td>2.82</td><td>2.54</td><td></td><td></td><td>$t = 0.66$ (N.S.)</td></tr>
<tr><td rowspan="2">RMS velocity between 1 and 5 c/sec (mm/sec)</td><td colspan="2">1.07</td><td colspan="2">0.34</td><td>$t = 5.38$***</td></tr>
<tr><td>0.82</td><td>1.43</td><td></td><td></td><td>$t = 2.29$*</td></tr>
<tr><td>Size of peak, as % of total RMS velocity between 1 and 20 c/sec</td><td>11.8</td><td></td><td>18.9</td><td></td><td>$t = 3.51$***</td></tr>
<tr><td>Correlation between RMS velocity between 1 and 5 c/sec and size of peak</td><td colspan="2">$r = -0.53$*</td><td colspan="2">$r = -0.30$*</td><td></td></tr>
<tr><td>Correlation between RMS velocity between 1 and 20 c/sec and size of peak</td><td colspan="4">$r = +0.63$*** (children and adults)</td><td></td></tr>
<tr><td>Peak frequency</td><td>8.9</td><td></td><td>8.5</td><td></td><td>$t = 0.86$ (N.S.)</td></tr>
</table>

N.S. = not significant; * = $P < 0.05$; ** = $P < 0.01$; *** = $P < 0.001$.

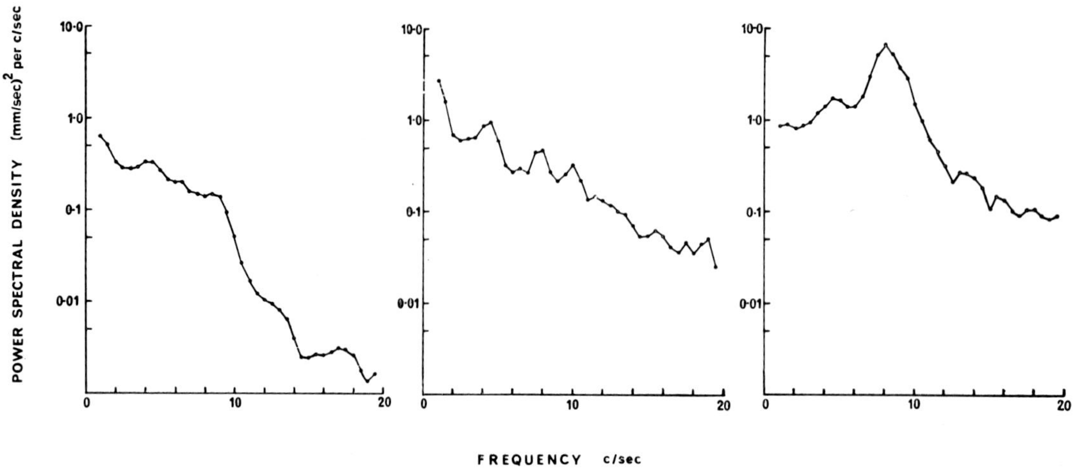

Fig. 5
Tremor spectra recorded from a child (M.H., 5 years) showing no definite peak, a child (D.D., 5 years) showing multiple small peaks and a child (P.D., 7 years) showing a well-defined peak.

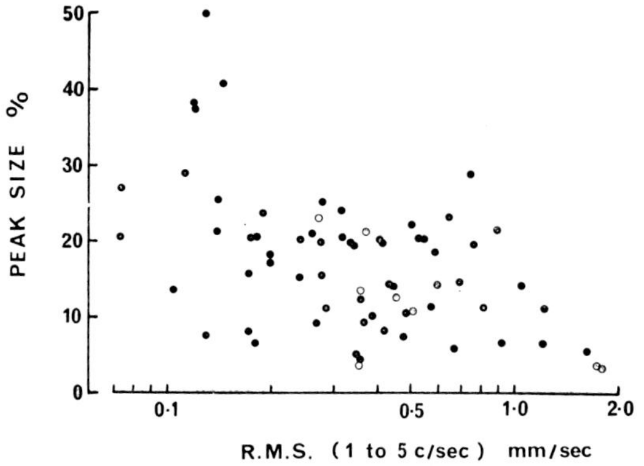

Fig. 6
Relation between the relative size of the peak (ordinate) and RMS velocity between 1 and 5 c/sec (abscissa) in children (○) ($r = -0.53$, $P < 0.05$) and adults (●) ($r = -0.30$, $P < 0.05$). Peak size decreases as low frequency tremor increases in both groups.

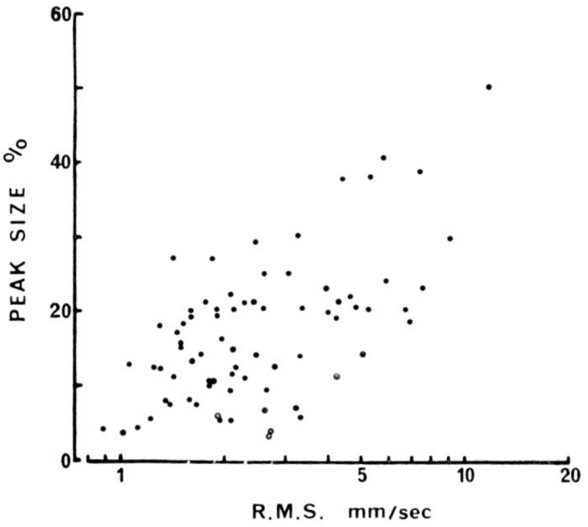

Fig. 7
Relation between relative size of the peak (ordinate) and RMS velocity between 1 and 20 c/sec (abscissa) in children (○) and in adults (●). Peak size increases as tremor increases ($r = +0.63$, $P < 0.001$).

There were no significant differences in tremor between males and females. Children differed from adults in a number of respects, which are summarized in Table I. The most notable difference was the frequent absence of a well-defined tremor peak in children, whose spectra ranged from those with no definite peak, to those with multiple peaks, and to those with single well-defined peaks such as were seen in most adults (Fig. 5). When present, the peaks in children were smaller than in adults, peak size being inversely proportional to low frequency tremor (Fig. 6). However, the greater the total tremor, the larger was the relative size of the peak (Fig. 7).

Although the peak frequency did not differ in children from that in adults, it did appear to decrease over the age of about 50 years. Mean peak frequency in individuals aged between 20 and 40 years (9.0 c/sec) was significantly higher than that in subjects aged over 60 years (7.7 c/sec) ($t = 4.07$, $P < 0.001$).

DISCUSSION

The fluctuations in tremor observed in two trained subjects during periods ranging from minutes to months were not great, and the shape of the tremor spectrum was very similar at different times. Many factors are known to contribute to fluctuations in tremor amplitude, including anxiety (Graham 1945; Redfearn 1957), alcoholism (Carrie 1965), thyrotoxicosis (Lippold *et al.* 1959; Marsden *et al.* 1968) and fatigue (Eagles *et al.* 1953). Some of the fluctuation of tremor amplitude that occurs in the normal subject may be due to variations in catecholamine secretion, for adrenaline infusion has also been found to increase tremor considerably (Marsden *et al.* 1967a). In addition, the amplitude of tremor is dependent upon the force exerted (Sutton and Sykes 1967b) and, in certain tasks, upon visual feedback (*e.g.*, Sutton and Sykes 1967a; Merton *et al.* 1967). All these factors must be taken into account when planning experiments on physiological tremor and when evaluating the results.

In the population studied a number of interesting points have emerged, particularly with reference to changes in tremor with age. One of the more widely quoted theories of origin of physiological tremor is that it represents the effect of delay in operation of the stretch reflex loop (Halliday and Redfearn 1956; Hammond *et al.* 1956; Lippold *et al.* 1957). These authors suggest that delay between spindle response and muscle contraction is compatible with the typical 9 c/sec peak frequency of physiological tremor. A number of workers have observed that mean tremor frequency calculated visually from analogue records of tremor is lower in children than in adults (Marshall and Walsh 1956; Marshall 1959; van Buskirk and Fink 1962). This fact has been one of the chief arguments advanced against the servo-loop hypothesis, for a higher frequency of tremor might be expected in children with shorter neuronal pathways than adults. However, the present study does not confirm this observation; the frequency of the peak in children, where present, was not significantly different from that in adults. It is possible that this discrepancy might be due to the relatively small number of children studied; Marshall (1959), for example, examined 287 children. However, only one of our children showed a peak frequency less than the mean values quoted by Marshall (Fig. 8), and there is a significant difference between the mean peak frequency of tremor in children in this series (8.9 c/sec) and that calculated from Marshall's data (7.0 c/sec) ($t = 4.05$, $P < 0.001$), even though the mean age of the children in this series (8.5 years) was less than that of Marshall's (10.3 years).

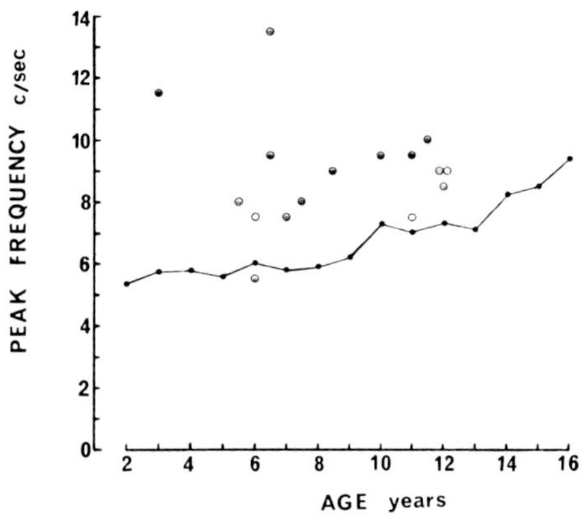

Fig. 8

Changes in peak frequency (ordinate) with age (abscissa) in children. The sixteen children with definite tremor peaks in the present series (○) are compared with the mean values obtained by Marshall (1959) (●), who calculated tremor frequency visually from analogue records.

An alternative explanation is that the selection in this series of only those children whose spectra exhibited a definite peak excluded eleven children in whom no peak was obvious. In the latter group, calculation of mean tremor frequency from visual records would have given substantially lower figures in view of the predominance of low frequency components in all tremor spectra. By this means a figure for mean frequency may be obtained from records in which spectral analysis reveals no dominant frequency component to tremor. It is known that it is possible to derive a mean frequency (as the interval between successive maxima or axis cross-overs) for a band-limited random noise signal, which has no dominant frequency components (*cf.*, Bendat 1958).

The lower mean frequency of tremor in childhood, when calculated by visual inspection of analogue records, probably reflects no more than the frequent *absence* of significant tremor peaks in children rather than a significant difference in peak frequency between children and adults. Although this analysis casts doubt on one of the objections to the muscle length-servo hypothesis of tremor, another more compelling observation argues against it, namely, that a well-defined 9 c/sec peak has been observed in a totally deafferented human arm (Marsden *et al.* 1967b).

There is, however, little doubt that physiological tremor in children differs from that in adults. The present findings indicate that a dominant tremor peak is present in only about 60% of children under the age of 16 (whereas about 95% of adults have an obvious tremor peak), and that when present it is significantly smaller than in adults. The size of the peak is inversely related to tremor at low frequencies; *e.g.*, between 1 and 5 c/sec as examined in this study. Thus the small or absent peak characteristic of childhood is related to significantly greater tremor at low frequencies in children compared with adults. This suggests that tremor is less random, that is to say more organized, at a particular frequency in adults. Children are obviously clumsy in performing fine movements, which may be related to the more random nature of their motor activity. The nature of the neuronal pathways responsible for adult motor finesse is unknown, but it is tempting to relate their development to the appearance of an organized rhythm in the force of muscle contraction.

Another feature of interest is the decline of tremor frequency in elderly adults, a finding that confirms Marshall's earlier observation (1961). It is difficult to equate this with an increasing delay in the stretch reflex due to the known fall in nerve conduction velocity with age (Norris *et al.* 1953), which in any case is only of the order of 8–9 m/sec between the ages of 30 and 80 years. Such a fall in conduction velocity would only add about 6 msec to the total delay between spindle and muscle which would shift the peak by less than 1 c/sec, on the basis of the muscle length-servo hypothesis. An alternative explanation seems more likely, but none is obvious at this time.

SUMMARY

1. The spectrum of physiological tremor has been recorded from the outstretched index finger of eighty-eight healthy subjects with ages between 3 and 85 years, and at frequent intervals over long periods of time in two trained subjects.

2. The shape of the velocity spectrum remained very constant in the individual, although the total root mean square (RMS) error velocity between 1 and 20 c/sec varied from time to time. For the two subjects studied the coefficient of variation averaged about 30%. A well-defined peak at around 9 c/sec was always present in both subjects. Peak frequency rarely shifted by more than 1 c/sec. The relative size of the peak was related to the RMS velocity between 1 and 20 c/sec, peak size increasing as tremor increased.

3. A definite peak was only present in about 60% of the spectra recorded from twenty-seven children with ages less than 16 years, while a peak was obvious in about 95% of the spectra recorded from sixty-one adults. The relative size of the peak was significantly smaller in children than in adults.

4. The relative size of the peak was inversely related to the RMS velocity between 1 and 5 c/sec, peak size increasing as low frequency tremor decreased. The smaller peak size in children, when present, was related to significantly greater low frequency tremor in children compared with adults. It appears that tremor is more commonly organized around a peak frequency in adults than in children.

5. As in the individual, in the group of subjects studied there was a significant relationship between relative peak size and total RMS velocity between 1 and 20 c/sec, peak size increasing as over-all tremor increased.

6. There was no significant difference between peak frequency in children and adults, but peak frequency decreased over about the age of 50 years. Previous reports of a lower peak frequency in children, when calculated visually from analogue tremor records, probably reflect the frequent absence of a peak in childhood. The predominance of low frequency tremor in all

spectra would then give the visual impression of a low frequency peak.

RÉSUMÉ

VARIATION DU TREMBLEMENT PHYSIOLOGIQUE DES DOIGTS CHEZ L'HOMME AVEC ÉTUDE PARTICULIÈRE DE SES MODIFICATIONS SUIVANT L'ÂGE

1. Le spectre du tremblement physiologique a été enregistré au niveau de l'index étendu chez quatre-vingts-huit sujets bien portants dont l'âge varie entre 3 et 85 ans et, chez deux sujets entraînés, à de fréquents intervalles sur de longues périodes de temps.

2. La forme du spectre de vitesse reste très constante pour un individu, bien que la racine carrée moyenne totale de la vitesse de l'erreur entre 1 et 20 c/sec varie d'une fois à l'autre. Pour les deux sujets étudiés, le coëfficient de variation se situe autour d'une moyenne de 30%. Un pic bien défini à environ 9 c/sec s'observe toujours chez les deux sujets. Le pic de fréquence varie rarement de plus de 1 c/sec. La taille relative de ce pic est liée à la racine carrée moyenne de la vitesse entre 1 et 20 c/sec et croit lorsque le tremblement augmente.

3. Un pic marqué ne s'observe que dans chez environ 60% des spectres enregistrés chez vingt-sept enfants âgés de moins de 16 ans, tandis qu'il est net dans environ 95% des spectres enregistrés chez soixante-et-un adultes. La taille relative de ce pic est nettement plus petite chez l'enfant que chez l'adulte.

4. La taille relative du pic est inversement liée à la racine carrée moyenne de la vitesse entre 1 et 5 c/sec et augmente lorsque la fréquence lente du tremblement diminue. Le fait que le pic soit moindre chez l'enfant, quand il existe, est lié au fait que le tremblement de basse fréquence est nettement plus intense chez l'enfant que chez l'adulte. Il semble que le tremblement soit plus habituellement organisé autour d'un pic de fréquence chez l'adulte que chez l'enfant.

5. Comme pour le sujet individuel, dans le groupe de sujets étudiés, on note une relation significative entre la taille relative du pic et la racine carrée moyenne totale de vitesse entre 1 et 20 c/sec, la taille du pic augmentant lorsque le tremblement global augmente.

6. Il n'y a pas de différence significative entre la fréquence du pic chez l'enfant et chez l'adulte, mais la fréquence du pic diminue vers la cinquantaine. Les données antérieures qui font état d'un pic de fréquence plus bas chez l'enfant quand il est calculé visuellement à partir de tracés analogiques de tremblements, reflètent probablement l'absence fréquente d'un pic dans l'enfance. La prédominance d'un tremblement de basse fréquence dans tous les spectres donnerait alors l'impression visuelle d'un pic à basse fréquence.

We should like to thank Dr. John Marshall for his helpful comments on this paper. The Endowment Fund of St. Thomas's Hospital and the National Fund for Research into Crippling Diseases kindly provided funds to support the work. The facilities and support provided by the National Physical Laboratory, and later the Warren Springs Laboratory, are also gratefully acknowledged.

REFERENCES

BENDAT, J. S. *Principles and applications of random noise theory.* Wiley, New York, **1958,** 431 p.

BLACKMAN, R. B. and TUKEY, J. W. *The measurement of power spectra.* Dover Publications, New York, **1959,** 190 p.

BUSKIRK, C. VAN and FINK, R. A. Physiologic tremor, an experimental study. *Neurology (Minneap.)*, **1962,** *12*: 361–370.

CARRIE, J. R. G. Finger tremor in alcoholic patients. *J. Neurol. Neurosurg. Psychiat.*, **1965,** *28*: 529–532.

EAGLES, J. B., HALLIDAY, A. M. and REDFEARN, J. W. T. The effects of fatigue on tremor. In W. F. FLOYD and A. T. WELFORD (Eds.), *Symposium on fatigue.* Lewis, London, **1953**: 41–58.

GRAHAM, J. D. P. Static tremor in anxiety states. *J. Neurol. Neurosurg. Psychiat.*, **1945,** *8*: 57–60.

HALLIDAY, A. M. and REDFEARN, J. W. T. An analysis of the frequencies of finger tremor in healthy subjects. *J. Physiol. (Lond.)*, **1956,** *134*: 600–611.

HAMMOND, P. H., MERTON, P. A. and SUTTON, G. G. Nervous gradation of muscular contraction. *Brit. med. Bull.*, **1956,** *12*: 214–218.

LIPPOLD, O. C. J., REDFEARN, J. W. T. and VUČO, J. The rhythmical activity of groups of motor units in the voluntary contraction of muscle. *J. Physiol. (Lond.)*, **1957,** *137*: 473–487.

LIPPOLD, O. C. J., REDFEARN, J. W. T. and VUČO, J. The frequency analysis of tremor in normal and thyrotoxic subjects. *Clin. Sci.*, **1959,** *18*: 587–595.

MARSDEN, C. D., FOLEY, T. H., OWEN, D. A. L. and MCALLISTER, R. G. Peripheral β-adrenergic receptors concerned with tremor. *Clin. Sci.*, **1967**a, *33*: 53–65.

MARSDEN, C. D., GIMLETTE, T. M. D., MCALLISTER, R. G., OWEN, D. A. L. and MILLER, T. N. Effect of β-adrenergic blockade on finger tremor and Achilles reflex time in anxious and thyrotoxic patients. *Acta endocr. (Kbh.)*, **1968,** *57*: 353–362.

MARSDEN, C. D., MEADOWS, J. C., LANGE, G. W. and WATSON, R. S. Effect of deafferentation on human physiological tremor. *Lancet*, **1967**b, *2*: 700–702.

MARSHALL, J. Physiological tremor in children. *J. Neurol. Neurosurg. Psychiat.*, **1959,** *22*: 33–35.

MARSHALL, J. The effect of ageing upon physiological tremor. *J. Neurol. Neurosurg. Psychiat.*, **1961,** *24*: 14–17.

MARSHALL, J. and WALSH, E. G. Physiological tremor. *J. Neurol. Neurosurg. Psychiat.*, **1956,** *19*: 260–267.

MERTON, P. A., MORTON, H. B. and RASHBASS, C. Visual feedback in hand tremor. *Nature (Lond.)*, **1967,** *216*: 583–584.

NORRIS, A. H., SHOCK, N. W. and WAGMAN, I. H. Age changes in the maximum conduction velocity of motor fibres of human ulnar nerves. *J. appl. Physiol.*, **1953,** *5*: 589–593.

REDFEARN, J. W. T. Frequency analysis of physiological and neurotic tremors. *J. Neurol. Neurosurg. Psychiat.*, **1957,** *20*: 302–313.

SCHÄFER, E. A., CANNEY, E. L. and TUNSTALL, J. O. On the rhythm of muscular response to volitional impulses in man. *J. Physiol. (Lond.)*, **1886,** *7*: 111–117.

SUTTON, G. G. and SYKES, K. The effect of withdrawal of visual presentation of errors upon the frequency spectrum of tremor in a manual task. *J. Physiol. (Lond.)*, **1967**a, *190*: 281–293.

SUTTON, G. G. and SYKES, K. The variation of hand tremor with force in healthy subjects. *J. Physiol. (Lond.)*, **1967**b, *191*: 699–711.

Reference: MARSDEN, C. D., MEADOWS, J. C., LANGE, G. W. and WATSON, R. S. Variations in human physiological finger tremor, with particular reference to changes with age. *Electroenceph. clin. Neurophysiol.*, **1969,** *27*: 169–178.

Electroencephalography and Clinical Neurophysiology
Elsevier Publishing Company, Amsterdam – Printed in The Netherlands

THE RELATION BETWEEN PHYSIOLOGICAL TREMOR OF THE TWO HANDS IN HEALTHY SUBJECTS

C. D. MARSDEN, J. C. MEADOWS, G. W. LANGE AND R. S. WATSON

Departments of Medicine and Neurology, St. Thomas's Hospital, London, S. E. 1 and the National Physical Laboratory, Teddington (Great Britain)

(Accepted for publication: November 22, 1968)

It is of some practical importance to know the relation of tremor of one hand to that of the other. Our ability to perform tasks involving manual dexterity is limited by fluctuations in the force of muscle contraction and variations in the position of the hand and fingers which we term physiological tremor. If these fluctuations were totally asynchronous delicate operations involving the use of both hands would be even more frustrated than if tremor of the two hands were synchronized. By holding a pencil in each hand and trying to keep the points in light contact, it is apparent that the involuntary movements of the two hands are not perfectly synchronous. This paper attempts to establish the statistical relationship between tremors of the two hands.

METHODS

A group of eighteen healthy subjects (9 male, 9 female, with ages between 19 and 81 years) has been investigated, and repeated studies have been performed on two trained subjects (C.M. and J.M.). Details of the methods of recording tremor and analysis of the data were presented in the previous paper (Marsden *et al.* 1969). In all experiments tremor was recorded over a 2 min period, simultaneously from the index fingers of both hands, while the subject attempted to maintain the fingers outstretched without direct visual reference. The outputs of the two accelerometers used to detect tremor were fed through a 2-channel converter so that they could be punched into paper tape for subsequent computer analysis. Since the punching speed was 110 characters/sec each channel was punched at a rate of 55 characters/sec.

In the previous paper the power spectrum of tremor of one hand was considered. The analysis has been extended to derive the statistical relation between the tremors of both hands; this corresponds to a cross-spectrum between two variables, as distinct from the analysis of tremor of one hand which provides an auto-spectrum of a single variable. To derive the auto-spectrum, the auto-covariance function was computed from the record of tremor and subsequently Fourier transformed. The record of tremor of one hand was first cross-multiplied by itself, and then by the same signal delayed by time lags of τ, 2 τ, 3 τ, ... up to 220 τ, so as to build up the auto-covariance function. In the present analysis of tremor of both hands, τ corresponded to an interval of 18 msec, providing covariance functions over 4 sec (*i.e.*, less than 5% of the total duration of the tremor record).

The cross-spectrum was derived in similar fashion, except that the record of tremor from one hand was multiplied by that from the other hand over a series of ± 220 τ lags, to yield a cross-covariance function. This was subsequently Fourier transformed, giving estimates of the cross-spectrum, in terms of magnitude and phase at each frequency. The magnitude represented the cross-power of related components at each frequency [$(mm/sec)^2$ per c/sec] and the phase represented their phase relationship.

The significance of the relation between

tremors of the two hands has been expressed as their coherence, *i.e.*

$$\frac{(\text{Cross-spectral power})^2}{\text{Auto-spectral power (right hand)} \times \text{Auto-spectral power (left hand)}}$$

The coherence indicated the proportion of the tremor power of one hand which might be "explained" by tremor of the other hand. A coherence of 1 indicated a completely deterministic relation between the two hands, a coherence of 0 represented complete statistical independence.

RESULTS

Tremor correlation in the group of eighteen subjects

There was no significant difference between the two hands in respect of total RMS error velocity between 1 and 20 c/sec, peak frequency, or relative size of peak. Definite peaks were present in the tremor spectra of both hands in all but one of the eighteen subjects. The dominant hand was established in fourteen subjects and was the right hand in all but one individual. No significant differences between tremors of the dominant and non-dominant hands were seen. There was a significant positive correlation between total RMS error velocities between 1 and 20 c/sec of the two hands ($r = +0.86$, $P < 0.001$), tremor of one hand being of about the same magnitude as that of the other (Fig. 1). Similarly, the peak frequency and relative size of the peak of tremor of one hand were correlated with those of the other (for peak frequency, $r = +0.76$, $P < 0.001$; for relative size of the peak, $r = +0.78$, $P < 0.001$) (Fig. 2 and 3).

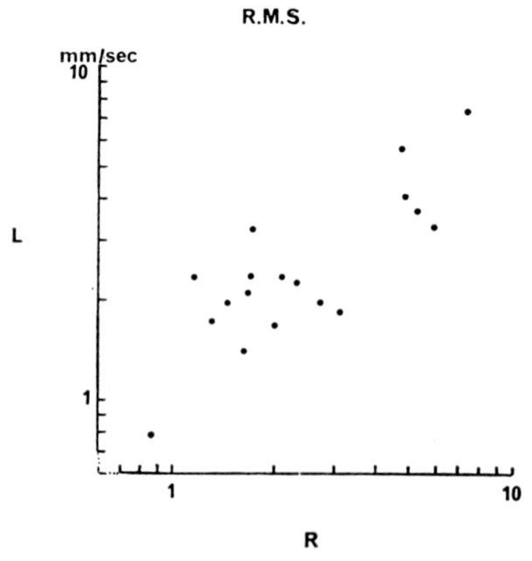

Fig. 1
Relation of total RMS error velocity (mm/sec) between 1 and 20 c/sec of left hand (ordinate) and that of right hand (abscissa) in eighteen healthy subjects. In this and all subsequent figures RMS velocity is plotted on a logarithmic scale ($r = +0.86$, $P < 0.001$).

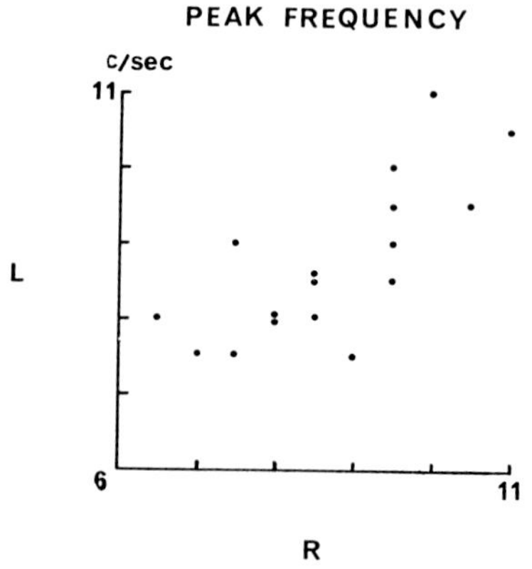

Fig. 2
Relation of peak frequency (to the nearest 0.5 cycle) of tremor of left hand (ordinate) to that of right hand (abscissa) in the seventeen subjects with single well-defined peaks in tremor spectra from both hands ($r = +0.76$, $P < 0.001$).

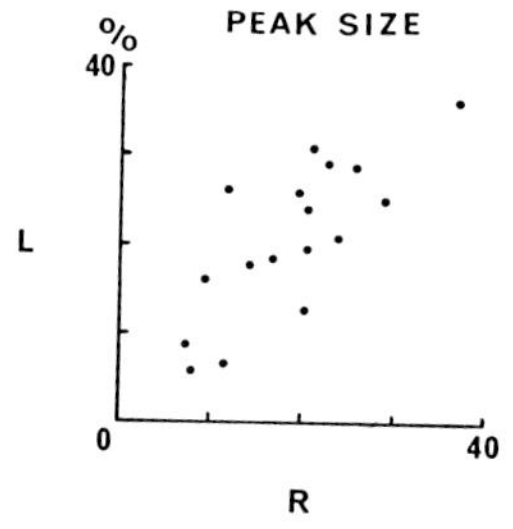

Fig. 3
Relation of relative size of peak (expressed as the percentage of total RMS error velocity between 1 and 20 c/sec contained in the 0.5 cycle band at peak frequency) of tremor of the left hand (ordinate) to that of right hand (abscissa) in seventeen healthy subjects ($r = +0.78$, $P < 0.001$).

Fig. 4 shows representative tremor spectra from the right and left hands of three individuals. In most subjects the spectrum of tremor of one hand was very similar to that of the other. The spectra shown in Fig. 4 range from an example of the greatest difference between the two hands (subject I.C.) to an example of almost identical spectra (subject J.M.). The shape of the cross-

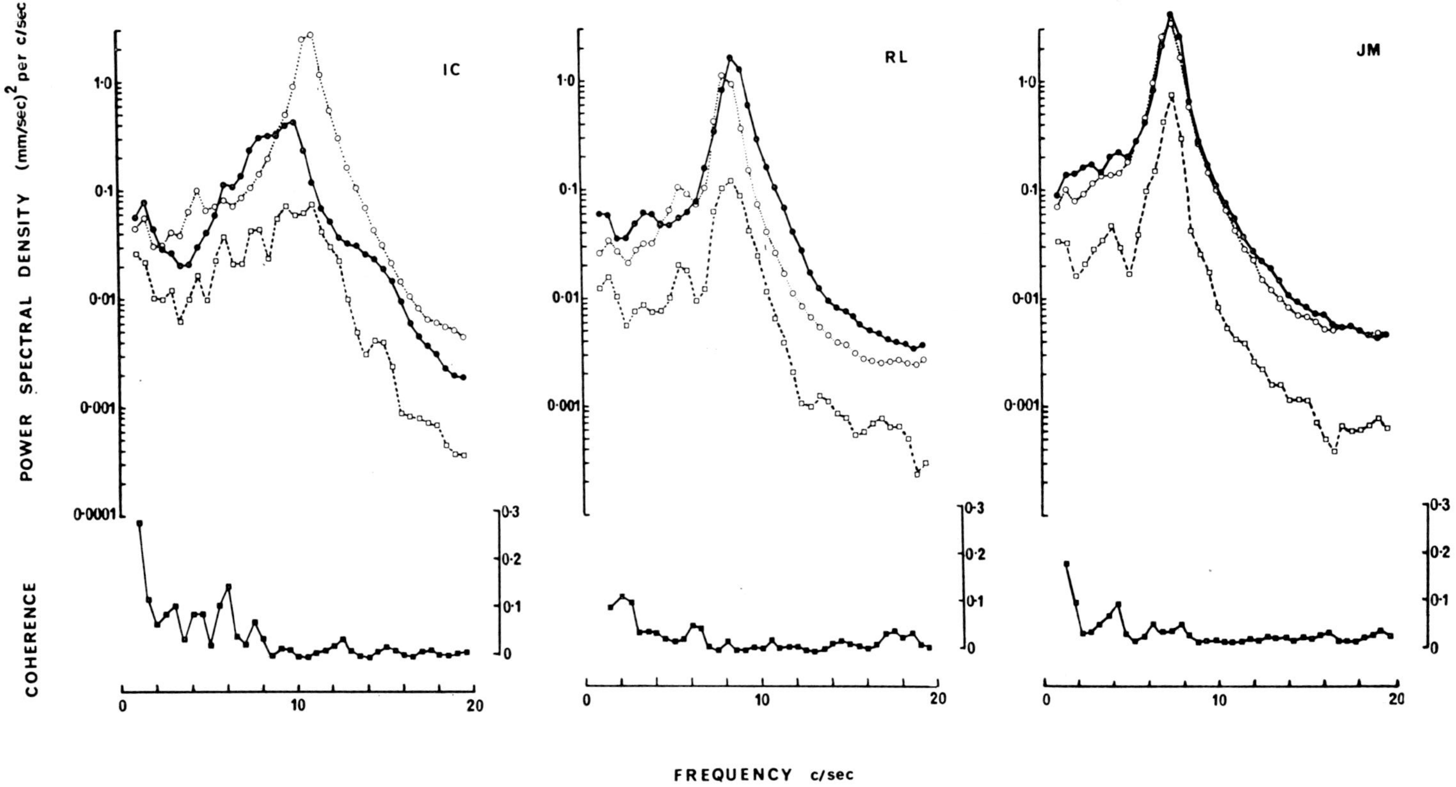

Fig. 4

Representative tremor spectra from three subjects, showing examples of marked difference (I.C. 40 years, female), slight difference (R.L. 37 years, male) and close similarity between the two hands (J.M. 28 years, male). Each spectrum shows: above, the spectra of tremor of the right (●) and left (○) hands; middle, the cross-spectrum between hands (□), and below, the coherence between hands (■).

spectrum was similar to that of the auto-spectra, and the cross-spectral power, although considerably less than the auto-spectral power, was proportional to mean auto-spectral power ($r = +0.97$, $P < 0.001$).

The over-all coherence between hands was small, averaging 0.033 (range 0.108–0.008) between 1 and 20 c/sec. As is seen in Fig. 4 the coherence between hands varied at different frequencies, but there was no significant increase in coherence at peak frequency. Thus the coherence in the 1.5 cycles around peak frequency also averaged 0.033 (range 0.148–0.002). Although the magnitude of the cross-spectral power increased as over-all tremor increased, coherence was not related to mean tremor amplitude ($r = -0.07$, $P > 0.1$).

Correlation between tremor of the two hands in the individual

As has been described in the previous paper, tremor of the outstretched finger varies from time to time in the individual subject. Totals of 22 tremor records from subject C.M. over a period of 5 days, and 19 tremor records from subject J.M. over a period of 4 days were available for analysis.

RMS error velocity between 1 and 20 c/sec of the right hand was consistently related to that from the left hand in both subjects (C.M. $r = +0.77$, $P < 0.001$; J.M. $r = +0.73$, $P < 0.001$). There was a significant correlation for peak frequency between hands in C.M. ($r = +0.82$, $P < 0.001$) but not in J.M. ($r = +0.32$, $P > 0.1$). There was a significant correlation for relative size of the peak between hands for J.M. ($r = +0.68$, $P < 0.001$) but not for C.M. ($r = +0.22$, $P > 0.1$).

The coherence between hands was always small in the two subjects, averaging 0.043 (range 0.006–0.086) in C.M. and 0.024 (range 0.004–0.051) in J.M.

Phase relation between tremors of the two hands

Phase relations were examined in records of tremor obtained simultaneously from both hands in four subjects. Fig. 5 shows phase relations of tremors of the two hands against frequency at 0.25 cycle intervals for one subject. No consistent phase relation is evident in this subject. Concordant results were obtained in the other three subjects.

Significance of observed coherence

The question arises as to the significance of the observed small degree of coherence between hands. Some coherence between two totally independent signals is an inevitable statistical effect, since only a finite sample can be analysed. The extent of this spurious coherence depends on sample size (the smaller the sample the greater the spurious cross-power and coherence) and also the characteristic shape of the spectrum analysed (Bendat and Piersoll 1966). Studies have therefore been undertaken to estimate the extent of spurious coherence inherent in analysis of the present data.

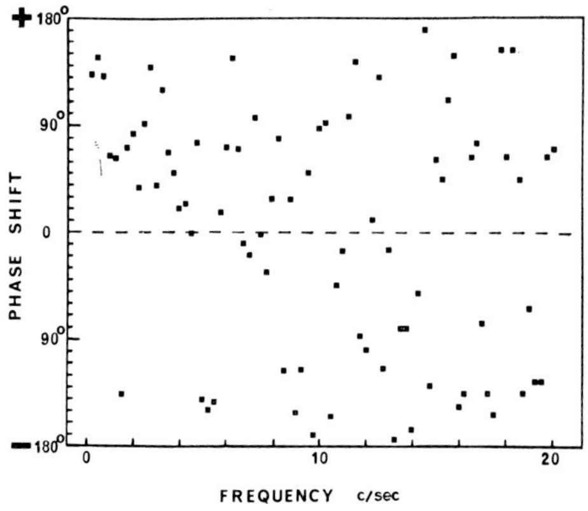

Fig. 5
Phase relation between tremors of the two hands in subject J.M. A positive phase shift indicates that the left hand leads the right hand.

It is reasonable to assume that the fine structure of the tremor wave form from the right hand is unrelated to that from the left hand one minute later. In fact, the calculated covariance functions for tremor of the two hands decayed to negligeable quantities within at most 8 sec. Accordingly, tremor of the right hand during the first minute of a 2 min record was analysed in relation to tremor of the left hand during the last minute of the record, and *vice versa*. The resulting spurious cross-power and coherence for data from subjects are shown in Table I, in comparison to the true values for cross-power and coherence obtained from the data. Spurious

TABLE I

Comparison of observed values for RMS error velocity between 1 and 20 c/sec (for auto- and cross-spectra) and coherence, with spurious values obtained when tremor of the right hand was compared with that of the left hand one minute later

Subject	Observed			Spurious		
	Auto-spectral RMS (mm/sec)	Cross-spectral RMS (mm/sec)	Coherence	Auto-spectral RMS (mm/sec)	Cross-spectral RMS (mm/sec)	Coherence
J.M.	4.65 3.24	1.54	0.025	4.74 3.15	1.56	0.027
H.R.	3.14 1.82	0.88	0.018	2.90 1.83	0.84	0.019
R.L.	1.77 1.39	0.55	0.016	1.80 1.42	0.54	0.013
A.R.	0.86 0.78	0.47	0.108	0.92 0.86	0.36	0.028
M.A.	4.82 5.44	2.21	0.035	4.62 5.05	1.82	0.020
I.C.	1.32 2.31	0.63	0.017	1.94 2.36	0.74	0.015
S.S.	1.75 3.11	1.28	0.090	1.75 3.14	0.93	0.024
T.F.	1.46 1.92	0.64	0.021	1.43 1.92	0.63	0.021

coherence amounted to values of between 0.013 and 0.028 and was indistinguishable from true coherence in six of the eight subjects. True coherence between the tremor of both hands exceeded the value of 0.030 in only six of the eighteen subjects studied.

DISCUSSION

It has been impossible to demonstrate any significant coherence between tremors of the two hands in most subjects in the present study. Barlow (1967) gave a figure of 0.25 for the cross-correlation coefficient between tremors of the two hands of one normal subject, corresponding to a coherence of about 0.06, which is close to the figures obtained in this investigation. It remains possible that a very small degree of coherence does exist, but if so it usually lies within the range of spurious coherence inherent in the sample chosen for analysis. Even in the few subjects in whom coherence values exceeded the latter they were very small.

The lack of marked coherence between hands indicates that there is virtually no moment to moment link between the shapes of the tremor wave forms of the two hands. It is therefore unlikely that the amplitude and frequency of tremor of the two hands are determined by some common source of activation. A number of authors have suggested that "normal tremor" merely represents oscillations due to ballisto-cardiac impulses (Brumlik 1962; Wachs 1964; Yap and Boshes 1967). The absence of significant coherence between tremors of the two hands is incompatible with the hypothesis that tremor arises from a common source such as cardiac thrust. For the same reason it is unlikely that a single portion of the central nervous system—a hypothetical tremor "pacemaker"—is responsible for driving anterior horn cells at a certain frequency to produce tremor during muscle contraction; such a system would give rise to at least partially coherent tremor of the two hands, even though the nervous input to muscles is heavily filtered by the dynamics of the musculo-skeletal system (*cf.*, Marshall and Walsh 1956).

In the previous paper (Marsden *et al.* 1969) it was shown that the measured parameters of tremor of one hand (total RMS velocity, peak frequency and peak size) vary from subject to subject and from time to time in the same individual. Although there appears to be no single driving influence common to the two hands, the present study indicates that these parameters are usually similar on the two sides, and that they usually alter together. Thus the over-all magnitude of tremor, peak frequency and the relative size of the peak of tremor of one hand are related to those of tremor of the other hand, both in the group of subjects studied and usually in the individual subject. This is not surprising when one considers some of the factors that may influence the frequency and amplitude of tremor. For example, the amplitude of tremor is markedly affected by changes in the dynamic properties of muscle. The faster muscle twitch characteristic of thyrotoxicosis and produced by adrenaline is accompanied by alteration of the frequency transfer properties of muscle, leading to increased tremor (unpublished observations). Hormones and other blood-borne agents affecting tremor will affect both arms to the same degree, producing similar changes in the measured parameters of tremor, whether they act on the muscles concerned with tremor or their nervous inputs. There is no reason why other factors which affect tremor, such as temperature or fatigue, should affect the two arms differentially. The lack of coherence between tremors of the two hands demonstrated in this study indicates that many of the factors responsible for fluctuations in tremor act as on two distinct systems, which, because they share the same environment, have similar properties.

SUMMARY

1. The techniques of cross-spectral analysis have been applied to tremor of the outstretched fingers recorded simultaneously from both hands of eighteen healthy subjects and at repeated intervals in two trained subjects.

2. The coherence between the tremor wave forms of the two hands was negligeable, averaging only about 0.03 in the group of subjects studied. There was no consistent phase relationship between the tremors of the two hands.

3. The observed coherence between hands rarely exceeded the spurious coherence inevitable in statistical analysis of a finite sample.

4. The absence of significant coherence between the tremor wave forms of the two hands is incompatible with the hypothesis that tremor arises from a common source such as cardiac thrust, or from a single tremor "pacemaker" in the central nervous system.

5. There was a significant relationship between the over-all amplitudes of tremor, peak frequencies and relative sizes of peak of tremor of the two hands in the group of subjects studied and usually in the individual. Such similarities are not the result of a common origin for tremor, but suggest that many of the factors affecting tremor act on both arms to the same degree.

RÉSUMÉ

RELATION ENTRE TREMBLEMENT PHYSIOLOGIQUE DES DEUX MAINS CHEZ DES SUJETS BIEN PORTANTS

1. Des techniques d'analyse cross-spectrale ont été appliquées à l'étude du tremblement des doigts étendus enregistrés simultanément au niveau des deux mains chez dix-huit sujets bien portants et à intervalles répétés chez deux sujets entraînés.

2. La concordance entre la forme des ondes de tremblement des deux mains est faible, n'atteignant en moyenne qu'environ 0.03 dans le groupe des sujets étudiés. Il n'y a pas de relation de phase constante entre les tremblements des deux mains.

3. La concordance observée entre les deux mains excède rarement la concordance de hasard, inévitable dans les analyses statistiques d'un échantillonnage défini.

4. L'absence de concordance significative entre les ondes de tremblement des deux mains est incompatible avec l'hypothèse suivant laquelle le tremblement viendrait d'une source commune, telle que l'impulsion cardiaque, ou d'un pacemaker unique de tremblement dans le système nerveux central.

5. On note une relation significative entre l'amplitude globale du tremblement, les pics de fréquences et la taille relative du pic de tremblement des deux mains dans le groupe de sujets étudiés et de façon habituelle chez un sujet donné. De telles similarités ne sont pas le résultat d'une origine unique du tremblement, mais suggèrent que plusieurs des facteurs qui affectent le tremblement agissent sur les deux bras à un même degré.

Electroenceph. clin. Neurophysiol., **1969**, *27*: 179–185

The Endowment of St. Thomas's Hospital and the National Fund for Research into Crippling Diseases kindly provided funds to support the work. The facilities and support provided by the National Physical Laboratory, and later the Warren Springs Laboratory, are also gratefully acknowledged.

REFERENCES

BARLOW, J. Correlation analysis of EEG–tremor relationships in man. *Electroenceph. clin. Neurophysiol.*, **1967,** *Suppl. 25*: 167–177.

BENDAT, J. S. and PIERSOLL, A. G. *Measurement and analysis of random data.* Wiley, New York, **1966,** 390 p.

BRUMLIK, J. On the nature of normal tremor. *Neurology (Minneap.)*, **1962,** *12*: 159–179.

MARSDEN, C. D., MEADOWS, J. C., LANGE, G. W. and WATSON, R. S. Variations in human physiological tremor, with particular reference to changes with age. *Electroenceph. clin. Neurophysiol.*, **1969,** *27*: 169–178.

MARSHALL, J. and WALSH, E. G. Physiological tremor. *J. Neurol. Neurosurg. Psychiat.*, **1956,** *19*: 260–267.

WACHS, H. Studies of physiologic tremor in the dog. *Neurology (Minneap.)*, **1964,** *14*: 50–61.

YAP, C. B. and BOSHES, B. The frequency and pattern of normal tremor. *Electroenceph. clin. Neurophysiol.*, **1967,** *22*: 197–203.

Reference: MARSDEN, C. D., MEADOWS, J. C., LANGE, G. W. and WATSON, R. S. The relation between physiological tremor of the two hands in healthy subjects. *Electroenceph. clin. Neurophysiol.*, **1969,** *27*: 179–185.

Electroencephalography and Clinical Neurophysiology
Elsevier Publishing Company, Amsterdam – Printed in The Netherlands

EEG RESPONSE TO PHOTIC STIMULATION AS A FUNCTION OF COGNITIVE STYLE[1]

WILLIAM VOGEL, DONALD M. BROVERMAN, EDWARD L. KLAIBER AND KAROLY J. KUN

Research Institute of Life Sciences, Worcester State Hospital; Clark University; Worcester Foundation for Experimental Biology; and Wrentham Research Foundation, Worcester, Mass. 01604 (U.S.A.)

(Accepted for publication: November 7, 1968)

The automatization cognitive style is an index of the ability to automatize behaviors; *i.e.*, to overlearn repetitive tasks via practice so that minimums of conscious effort are required for their successful, efficient performance. Persons with a relatively high degree of this ability are termed "strong automatizers"; individuals who are relatively deficient in this ability are termed "weak automatizers" (Broverman *et al.* 1966). Recently, differences were reported between the EEGs of strong and weak automatizers under conditions of rest and of mental effort (Vogel *et al.* 1968).

Broverman *et al.* (1968) have argued that differences in automatization ability are a function of the balance between central adrenergic and central cholinergic neural processes, with strong automatization reflecting a relatively greater degree of adrenergic activity. A number of studies suggest that the phenothiazines, which induce a central cholinergic state by impairing central adrenergic mechanisms, increase alpha driving and paroxysmal responses to photic stimulation (Jörgensen and Wulff 1958; Wilson and Glotfelty 1958; Mišurec and Náhunek 1964; Killam *et al.* 1967). Conversely, Ostfeld *et al.* (1960) and Floru *et al.* (1962) found that driving responses are decreased by substances which produce an adrenergic state, either by impairing central cholinergic mechanisms (*e.g.*, atropine) or by enhancing central adrenergic mechanisms (*e.g.*, noradrenaline).

Those behaviors regulated by the central cholinergic system (*e.g.*, rest, relaxation) have been termed "trophotropic", while those regulated by the central adrenergic system (*e.g.*, motor activity, alertness, etc.) have been termed "ergotropic" (Hess 1954). As might be expected, increased driving is associated with trophotropic behaviors, and decreased driving is associated with ergotropic behaviors (Ulett and Gleser 1952; Carels 1962, 1965; Demeter and Nestianu 1965).

Consequently, if the argument is correct that strong automatizers are relatively adrenergic dominant compared to weak automatizers (Broverman *et al.* 1968), then it may be hypothesized that strong automatizers should show fewer EEG driving responses to photic stimulation than should weak automatizers. The purpose of this study was to test such a hypothesis.

METHOD

Subjects

The subjects (*S*s) were thirty-six normal male college students.

Cognitive tests

All *S*s were individually administered a battery of 17 cognitive tasks used to assess the automatization cognitive style as described in a previous article (Vogel *et al.* 1968).

A factor analysis of the within-individual variance yielded an automatization factor similar to those described in previous analyses of similar cognitive batteries (Broverman 1964; Broverman *et al.* 1966; Vogel *et al.* 1968). Each individual was assigned an automatization index score which represented his ability to perform better or less

[1] This work was supported by Research Grants HD 01798 and 02557 from the Institutes of Child Health and Human Development, U.S. Public Health Service.

well on simple, repetitive tasks than might be expected on the basis of his general level of ability. In this manner, each person was classified as a strong or weak automatizer.

The strong and weak automatizer groups each contained eighteen *S*s. For procedural reasons to be discussed below, two *S*s were dropped from each group. The mean ages of the sixteen strong and sixteen weak automatizers who finally constituted each group were, respectively, 21.2 $\pm$0.5 years and 21.4 $\pm$0.6 years; their mean Wechsler Adult Intelligence (Verbal) IQ scores were respectively 127.0 $\pm$8.0 and 131.0 $\pm$12.0. The age and IQ differences between the groups did not approach statistical significance. Since the scores on the automatization index served as the criterion for the categorization of *S*s as strong or weak automatizers, there is no overlap on this index between the two groups. The mean automatization index of the strong automatizers was 2.4 $\pm$1.5; that of the weak automatizers was -3.1 ± 2.3.

The cognitive test administration, analysis of the cognitive data, and classification of *S*s as strong or weak automatizers were performed by different individuals than those who worked with the EEG aspects of the experiment. The cognitive information was withheld from the EEG workers until after the EEG data were collected and scored.

EEG techniques

The EEG data were obtained on a Grass model 5D polygraph, with Grass model 5P5E EEG pre-amplifiers and Grass 5P5 amplifiers. The time constant was 0.2 sec. The sensitivity used was 30 μV/cm pen deflection. Grass EC2 electrode cream was applied under Grass E5 gold disc electrodes. The EEG data employed for this report were obtained from one pair of occipital electrodes with each electrode placed 3 cm above the inion and 2 cm from the midline.

Recordings were obtained at rest for a period of 5 min, and during photic stimulation. This was performed while the subject kept his eyes closed, using a Grass PS 2 photostimulator which was placed parallel to the plane of the face 30 cm from the eyes, so that both visual fields were equally stimulated. Stimulation started at intensity "2" for 10 sec for trials of 10, 15, 20, 25 and 30 f/sec, with 10 sec rest between trials. Similar series of trials were then given at intensity steps "4", "8" and "16". Thus, each subject was exposed to 20 photic stimulation trials.

Since the frequency of the background rhythm is likely to affect the EEG driving phenomenon (Ostow 1949; Mundy-Castle 1953; Montagu 1967) it appeared necessary to equate the strong and weak automatizer samples for alpha index, and alpha frequency at rest. A 120 sec EEG sample during rest was employed. It was found that the two groups of subjects could be equated by eliminating two strong and two weak automatizers. The mean alpha frequency of the remaining sixteen strong automatizers was 10.4 c/sec, compared to 10.3 c/sec of the remaining sixteen weak automatizers. The mean alpha index percentages of the strong and weak automatizers were 40% and 39%, respectively. The differences between the two groups were not statistically significant.

An EEG "driving" response to photic stimulation was defined as two consecutive seconds of EEG waves at the fundamental frequency of the photic stimulation, or at one of its harmonics or subharmonics. "Driving" was scored only if the entire response, as defined, occurred within the limits of the duration of the photic signal, and only if activity from one frequency band and no other was present during a 2 sec period; *i.e.*, superimposed activity (*e.g.*, beta upon alpha) was not scored.

Theoretically, driving could be scored more than once for any given 10 sec stimulation under two circumstances: (1) if two distinctly discontinuous driving responses appeared; *e.g.*, 2 sec of driving at 10 c/sec, followed by a definite cessation of driving, and then a resumption of driving; (2) if two consecutive but qualitatively different driving responses occurred; *e.g.*, a response at the fundamental frequency of the photic stimulation followed by a response at one of its harmonics or subharmonics. However, only one subject evidenced two scorable driving responses during a single 10 sec stimulation period.

EEG records were scored twice; interscorer reliabilities in regard to the presence or absence of driving, and type of driving, were both 0.95+.

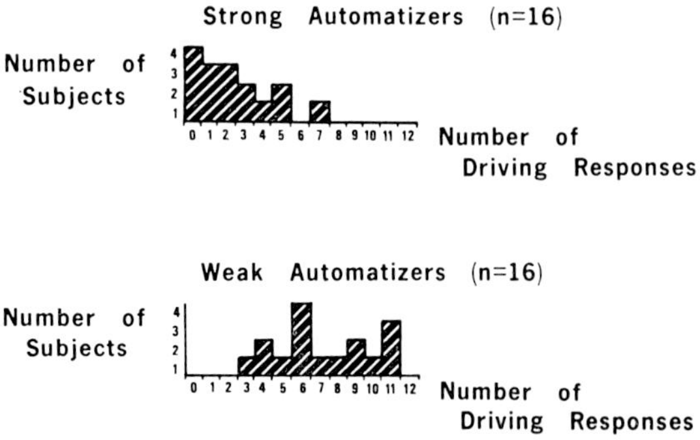

Fig. 1
Frequency distributions of driving responses of strong and weak automatizers.

RESULTS

Number of driving responses to photic stimulation of strong and weak automatizers

The distributions of driving responses of strong and weak automatizers are shown in Fig. 1. Half of the thirty-two *S*s made 4 or less driving responses; the other half of the *S*s made 5 or more responses. A chi-square analysis comparing strong and weak automatizers showed that thirteen strong and three weak automatizers were below the group median for all thirty-two *S*s; three strong and thirteen weak automatizers were above the group median for all thirty-two *S*s. The chi-square of 12.50 ($P < 0.001$) indicates that significantly more weak than strong automatizers gave greater than the median number of responses.

The mean number of driving responses of the strong automatizers was 2.25, $\sigma = 2.1$; the mean of the weak automatizers was 7.25, $\sigma = 2.7$. An analysis of variance indicates that the difference between these two means is statistically significant ($F = 34.48$, $P < 0.001$, with 1/30 df).

Characteristics of photic stimulation which produce driving

Strong and weak automatizers differed sharply in regard to the photic stimulus frequencies which produced driving (see Table I): 67% of the driving responses of the strong automatizers, but only 43% of the driving responses of the weak automatizers, were evoked by photic stimulation of 15 f/sec or slower. The frequency count on which these percentages are based

TABLE I

Distribution of EEG driving responses of strong and weak automatizer groups

Photic stimulation (f/sec)	Weak: Alpha	Weak: 15 c/sec	Weak: 20 c/sec	Weak: 25 c/sec	Weak: 30 c/sec	Weak: 35 c/sec	Weak: 40 c/sec	Weak: Total No. of responses	Weak: % of total responses	Strong: Alpha	Strong: 15 c/sec	Strong: 20 c/sec	Strong: 25 c/sec	Strong: 30 c/sec	Strong: 35 c/sec	Strong: 40 c/sec	Strong: Total No. of responses	Strong: % of total responses
10	27	—	—	—	—	—	—	27	23.3	8	—	1	—	—	—	—	9	25.0
15	7	16	—	—	—	—	—	23	19.8	1	14	—	—	—	—	—	15	41.6
20	14	—	15	—	—	—	—	29	25.0	3	—	3	—	—	—	1	7	19.4
25	10	—	—	8	—	—	—	18	15.5	1	—	—	—	—	—	—	1	2.7
30	12	—	1	1	5	—	—	19	16.4	1	—	—	—	3	—	—	4	11.1
Total number of responses	70	16	16	9	5	—	—	116	—	14	14	4	—	3	—	1	36	—
% of total responses	60.3	13.7	13.7	7.7	4.3	—	—	—	—	38.9	38.9	11.1	—	8.3	—	2.8	—	—

yields a statistically significant chi-square ($\chi^2 = 6.11$, $P < 0.02$).

Characteristics of driving responses evoked by photic stimulation

Table I indicates that the weak automatizers display two predominant types of EEG driving responses; *i.e.*, a tendency to drive at the frequency of the photic stimulation, and a tendency to drive at alpha frequencies regardless of the frequency of the photic stimulation. A similar dual response tendency is not apparent among the strong automatizers.

Finally, there was no significant tendency for the number of driving responses of strong, as contrasted with weak, automatizers to vary as a function of stimulus intensity.

DISCUSSION

The results of the study support the hypothesis that the EEGs of weak automatizers will respond more to photic stimulation than the EEGs of strong automatizers. Since, as we have noted previously, EEG driving responses to photic stimulation have been reported to be increased by enhancement of central cholinergic states and decreased by induction of central adrenergic states, the results of this study reinforce the notion that weak and strong automatization are behavioral manifestations of central cholinergic *vs.* adrenergic dominant states, respectively.

The present paper suggests that the cholinergic linked alpha driving responses to photic stimulation may represent Class I inhibition (see Vogel *et al.* 1968) wherein the organism seeks to terminate responses to noxious, neurally fatiguing, stimuli.

The results also indicate that weak automatizers tend to yield two different alpha "driving" responses to photic stimulation: alpha provocation, or the tendency of alpha to be elicited regardless of the frequency of the flickering light, and alpha "following", or a tendency of alpha to be evoked at the frequency of the flickering light. It is possible that one or the other of these types of responses may be more intimately associated with Class I inhibition, and, therefore, decreased adrenergia and increased cholinergia. This question appears to be a promising area for future research.

SUMMARY

The automatization cognitive style is defined as greater ability (strong automatization) or lesser ability (weak automatization) to perform simple repetitive tasks than might be expected from an individual's general level of intellectual performance. Strong automatizers were found to be less responsive to photic stimulation of the EEG than were weak automatizers.

These findings were interpreted to mean that strong automatizers possess a relatively greater degree of central adrenergic dominance than do weak automatizers.

RÉSUMÉ

RÉPONSES EEG À LA STIMULATION PHOTIQUE EN FONCTION DU STYLE COGNITIF

Le style cognitif d'acquisition d'automatismes est défini comme une capacité plus grande (automatisation forte) ou moins grande (automatisation faible) à effectuer des tâches répétitives simples que ce qui pourrait être attendu d'un individu étant donné le niveau général de ses performances intellectuelles. Les sujets qui acquièrent rapidement des automatismes se montrent moins réactifs à la stimulation photique de l'EEG que ne le sont les sujets à automatisation faible.

On peut interpréter ces données dans le sens que les sujets à "automatisation forte" possèdent un degré de dominance centrale adrénergique relativement plus grand que les sujets à "automatisation faible".

REFERENCES

Broverman, D. M. Generality and behavioral correlates of cognitive styles. *J. consult. Psychol.*, **1964,** *28*: 487–500.

Broverman, D. M., Broverman, I. K. and Klaiber, E. L. The ability to automatize and the automatization cognitive style: a validation study. *Percept. mot. Skills*, **1966,** *23*: 419–437.

Broverman, D. M., Klaiber, E. L., Kobayashi, Y. and Vogel, W. Roles of activation and inhibition in sex differences in cognitive styles. *Psychol. Rev.*, **1968,** *75*: 23–50.

Carels, G. Facilitation et inhibition des réponses corticales visuelles chez l'homme. *Electroenceph. clin. Neurophysiol.*, **1962,** *14*: 714–723.

CARELS, G. Facilitation et inhibition des paroxysmes électroencéphalographiques induit par la stimulation lumineuse intermittente. *Electroenceph. clin. Neurophysiol.*, **1965,** *18*: 415–418.

DEMETER, A. and NESTIANU, V. The dynamics of photic driving undei conditions of effort in athletes. *Electroenceph. clin. Neurophysiol.*, **1965,** *18*: 635.

FLORU, R., COSTIN, A., NESTIANU, V. and STERESCU-VOLANSCHI, M. Researches concerning the effect of noradrenaline upon the electrical activity of the central nervous system and upon the evoked rhythm of intermittent photic stimulation in cats with chronic electrodes. *Electroenceph. clin. Neurophysiol.*, **1962,** *14*: 566.

HESS, W. R. *The diencephalon, autonomic and pyramidal functions.* Grune and Stratton, New York, **1954,** 153 p.

JÖRGENSEN, R. S. and WULFF, M. H. The effect of orally administered chlorpromazine on the electroencephalogram of man. *Electroenceph. clin. Neurophysiol.*, **1958,** *10*: 325–329.

KILLAM, K. F., KILLAM, E. K. and NAQUET, R. An animal model of light sensitive epilepsy. *Electroenceph. clin. Neurophysiol.*, **1967,** *22*: 497–513.

MIŠUREC, J. and NÁHUNEK, K. Changes in photo-Metrazol (photomyoclonic) threshold in treatment with some psychopharmacological drugs. *Electroenceph. clin. Neurophysiol.*, **1964,** *17*: 607.

MONTAGU, J. D. The relationship between the intensity of repetitive photic stimulation and the cerebral response. *Electroenceph. clin. Neurophysiol.*, **1967,** *23*: 152–161.

MUNDY-CASTLE, A. C. An analysis of central responses to photic stimulation in normal adults. *Electroenceph. clin. Neurophysiol.*, **1953,** *5*: 1–22.

OSTFELD, A. M., MACHNE, X. and UNNA, K. R. The effects of atropine on the electroencephalogram and behavior in man. *J. Pharmacol. exp. Ther.*, **1960,** *128*: 265–272.

OSTOW, M. Flickered light as a provocative test in electroencephalography. *Electroenceph. clin. Neurophysiol.*, **1949,** *1*: 245.

ULETT, G. A. and GLESER, G. The effect of experimental stress upon the photically activated EEG. *Electroenceph. clin. Neurophysiol.*, **1952,** *4*: 251.

VOGEL, W., BROVERMAN, D. and KLAIBER, E. L. EEG and mental abilities. *Electroenceph. clin. Neurophysiol.*, **1968,** *24*: 166–175.

WILSON, W. P. and GLOTFELTY, J. S. Effect of intravenous promazine on arousal responses in man. *Dis. nerv. Syst.*, **1958,** *19*: 307–309.

Reference: VOGEL, W., BROVERMAN, D. M., KLAIBER, E. L. and KUN, K. J. EEG response to photic stimulation as a function of cognitive style. *Electroenceph. clin. Neurophysiol.*, **1969,** *27*: 186–190.

CLINICAL AND LABORATORY NOTES

EEG PATTERNS IN JUVENILE CEREBRAL LIPIDOSIS[1]

ROBERT J. ELLINGSON AND RICHARD J. SCHAIN[2]

Nebraska Psychiatric Institute, University of Nebraska Medical Center, Omaha, Nebr. 68105 (U.S.A.)

(Accepted for publication: December 6, 1968)

Juvenile cerebral lipidosis (juvenile amaurotic family idiocy, Spielmeyer-Vogt disease, cerebromacular degeneration) is one of the hereditary neuronal lipidoses. The age of onset, usually at 5–8 years, and the course of the disease are relatively uniform (Jervis 1941, 1959). The usual initial manifestation is rapidly progressive loss of visual acuity. Funduscopic examination initially reveals narrowing of retinal vessels with yellowish pigmentation in the disc. Later, the findings of retinitis pigmentosa are prominent. Convulsions may appear at any time after onset of the disease. Generalized neurological signs appear relatively late, and include ataxia, tremors, rigidity, and pathological reflexes indicative of upper motor neuron disease. Progressive mental deterioration with behavioral disturbances are often associated with the neurological findings. The evolution of a characteristic speech abnormality consisting of repetitive speech, discoordination of sounds, and frequent breakdown of speech patterns has been described (Schain and Wiley 1965). Death usually occurs 10–15 years after onset of the initial symptoms. Histological examination reveals a characteristic lipid infiltration of neurons in the retina and central nervous system.

Five children with diagnoses of juvenile cerebral lipidosis were followed for periods of 2–9 years, and a sixth was seen on one occasion. This report presents the electrographic–clinical correlations found in this disease.

CASE REPORTS

Patient J. P.: 18-year-old white female. Onset of visual disturbances at 5 years with progression to blindness by age 7. Onset of seizures at age 11. The patient displayed retinitis pigmentosa, dementia, and marked emotional disturbances. Motor dysfunction was equivocal, and speech remained almost normal at last examination.

Nine EEGs were recorded between ages 8 and 16 years. There was a clear progression of EEG abnormality, starting with bursts of diffuse 4–5 c/sec waves at age 8. Bursts of diffuse 2.5–3 c/sec waves with occasional spike-and-wave complexes were seen at the time of onset of seizures at age 11. The amplitude and amount of spike- and-wave activity increased significantly over the subsequent 5 years. There was no evidence of "driving" or any other response to repetitive photic stimulation.

Patient G.K.: 17-year-old white female. Onset of visual disturbances at 7 years, progressing to blindness at 8 years. Onset of seizures at 8 years. The patient displayed retinitis pigmentosa, repetitive speech, motor dysfunction, and dementia. Karyotype was normal.

Seven EEGs were recorded between ages 9 and 16 years. Again there was a clear parallel between increasing EEG abnormality and clinical deterioration. At age 9 the EEG showed bursts of diffuse 2.5–3 c/sec slow waves with occasional spike-and-wave complexes (Fig. 1). At age 15 on a day when the patient was having a series of seizures the EEG showed almost continuous diffuse wave-and-spike activity (Fig. 2); a generalized tonic-clonic seizure was also recorded. On days when seizures were under control the EEG was not so abnormal; polyspike-and-wave complexes were often seen. The last 2 EEGs before the patient died at age 16 showed progressive deterioration of background activity with progressively more prominent

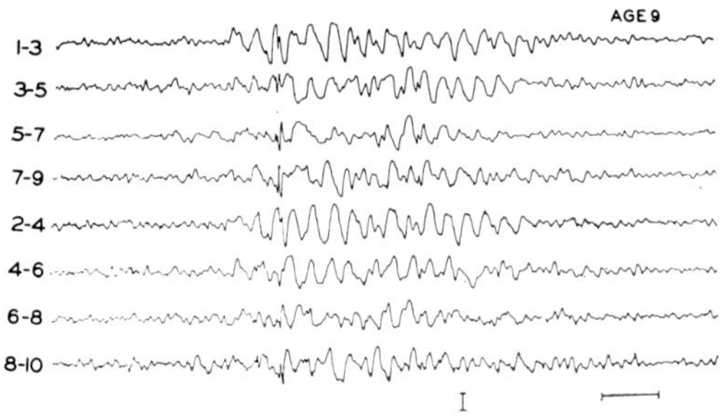

Fig. 1
Patient G. K. EEG No. 1. This record was made available through the courtesy of Dr. R. Bickford, Mayo Clinic, Rochester, Minn. The electrode code system is that used at the Mayo Clinic. Electrode positions approximate those of the International 10–20 System as follows: 1 = Fp_1, 2 = Fp_2, 3 = F_3, 4 = F_4, 5 = C_3, 6 = C_4, 7 = P_3, 8 = P_4, 9 = O_1, 10 = O_2. The vertical and horizontal calibration lines indicate 100 μV and 1 sec, respectively.

[1] Supported by NIH Grant No. HD 00370 from the National Institute of Child Health and Human Development.

[2] Present address: Division of Pediatric Neurology, U.C.L.A. Center for the Health Sciences, Los Angeles, Calif. 90024.

irregular slow waves and fewer and less well formed spike-and-waves complexes (Fig. 3). The diagnosis was confirmed at autopsy.

Patient L. K.: 20-year-old white male; the brother of Patient G. K. Progression of the disease was much slower than in his sister. Onset of visual disturbance at 8 years, with progression to blindness by age 11. Onset of seizures at 10 years. The patient displayed retinitis pigmentosa and repetitive speech, but no significant motor dysfunction and only mild dementia. Later his speech slowed, and he displayed sporadic emotional outbursts. He died at age 20. Immediate cause of death was given as bronchopneumonia. Autopsy was not permitted.

Eight EEGs were recorded between ages 15 and 20 years. The first EEG showed diffuse bursts and runs, up to 8 sec in duration, of 2.5–3 c/sec spike-and-wave complexes with mild slow background activity. There was little change over the subsequent 52 months except for increasingly greater irregularity of the background activity. The final EEG 3 months before death showed a considerable increase of irregular theta and delta activity in the background and a decrease in the number and clarity of wave form of the spike-and-wave complexes. Repetitive photic stimulation elicited no "driving" response or any change in abnormal activity.

In this relatively well-preserved patient there was only a slight deterioration in the EEG picture over a period of 52 months, during which there was likewise only slowly progressing clinical deterioration, and then a more rapid deterioration in the EEG during the last 8 months before death.

Patient C. T.: 16-year-old white male. Onset of visual disturbances at 5 years, progressing to blindness at 8 years. Onset of seizures at 8 years. The patient displayed retinitis pigmentosa, repetitive speech, motor dysfunction, and dementia. Karyotype was normal.

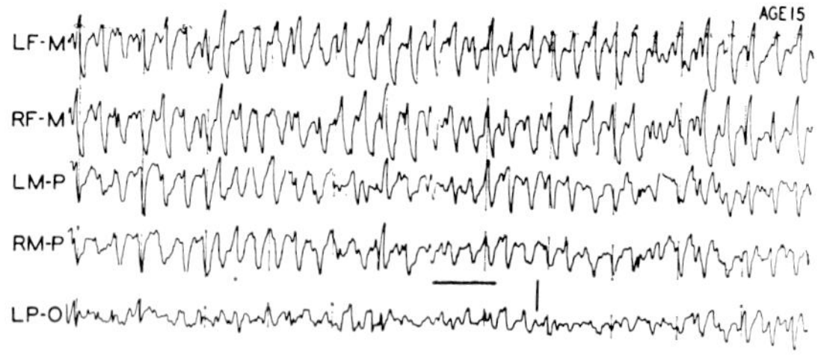

Fig. 2
Patient G. K. EEG No. 3. The spike-and-wave activity shown was present almost continuously. Later in the record a generalized convulsion was recorded. The electrode code system is as follows: L = left, R = right, F = frontal, M = motor (precentral), P = parietal, O = occipital, AT = anterior temporal, PT = posterior temporal. The vertical and horizontal calibration lines indicate 100 μV and 1 sec, respectively.

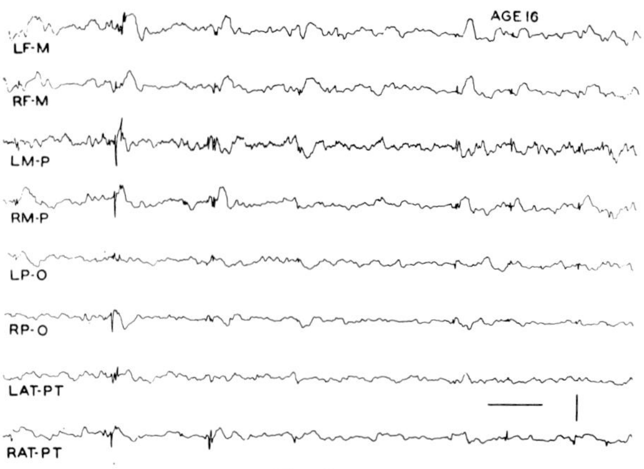

Fig. 3
Patient G. K. EEG No. 7, recorded 2 months before death. Note the deterioration of both background activity and spike-and-wave forms typical of the terminal stages of the disease. Electrode code same as for Fig. 2. The vertical and horizontal calibration lines indicate 100 μV and 1 sec, respectively.

Six EEGs were recorded between ages 14 and 16 years. The first showed a dominant rhythm at 6–7 c/sec and diffuse bursts of 2–4 c/sec slow waves with occasional spike-and wave complexes and rare multifocal spikes and sharp waves. The EEG picture subsequently showed a moderate deterioration, especially between the third and fourth EEGs at age 15, with the development of more frequent spike-and-wave and polyspike-and-wave complexes and deterioration of background activity. These EEG changes coincided with a period of marked clinical deterioration. The patient died of pneumonia at age 16. Autopsy was not permitted.

EEGs were also obtained on the patient's father, age 52, mother, age 45, and two sisters, ages 17 and 10; all were in good health. All EEGs were normal.

Patient D. P.: 17-year-old white male. Onset of visual disturbances at 5 years, progressing to blindness at 11 years. Onset of seizures at 10 years. The patient displayed retinitis pigmentosa, repetitive speech, but no motor dysfunction or dementia. Clinically, he was the most intact of the five cases initially, but later deteriorated.

Four EEGs were recorded between the ages of 14 and 16 years. The first showed only a mild diffuse slow abnormality. Two small spike-and-wave complexes were seen in the second EEG 8 months later. The third EEG showed runs of high voltage 2–3 c/sec waves and 2 isolated spike-and-wave complexes. The fourth EEG showed a striking deterioration of pattern which paralleled an exacerbation of clinical signs. Here there was a distinct increase in EEG abnormality paralleling clinical deterioration over the span of 30 months.

Patient W. W.: 7-year-old white male. Onset of visual disturbances at age 5; at the time of EEG only light-dark vision remained. The patient displays retinitis pigmentosa, explosive repetitive speech, but no other neurological signs. Intellect has been well-preserved until recent

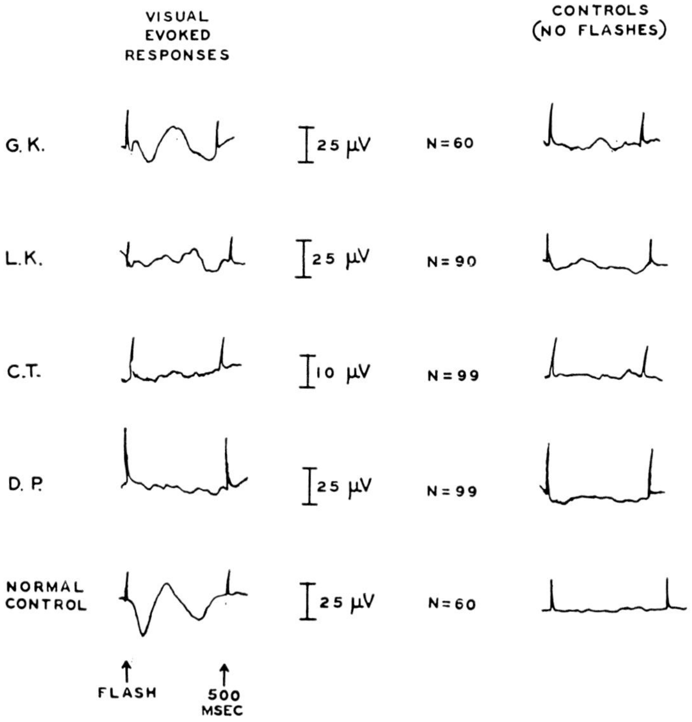

Fig. 4
Summated visual evoked responses recorded between an electrode just above the inion and a reference electrode on the left earlobe in four patients with juvenile cerebral lipidosis and one normal control. An analog summating device was used. Evoked responses (not shown) were recorded on a sixth patient using a digital instrument. The first spike artifact in each tracing in the left-hand column coincides with the presentation of the single flash stimulus; in the right-hand ("Controls") column it signals the start of randomly chosen epochs. The second spike artifact in both columns is a time marker 500 msec later. A downward deflection indicates relative positivity at the inion electrode. The number of epochs (N) over which summation was accomplished in each case is indicated. Age at recording was 16 years in all cases except L.K., who was 18. The evoked response in the case of patient G. K. is simpler than those usually seen in humans; the response of the normal control subject was deliberately chosen to show that such simple responses can be recorded from normals.

months. An EEG showed marked diffuse slow wave and spike-and-wave abnormality. These EEG abnormalities were greater than usually seen at this age.

Attempts were made to record occipital evoked responses to light flashes by means of response summating computers in five of the six cases. No responses could be recorded in four of the five (Fig. 4). Patient G. K., however, yielded a clear response despite her condition of advanced deterioration and severe loss of visual function.

DISCUSSION

Many cases of heredo-degenerative disorders of the central nervous system associated with blindness have been reported in the EEG literature, but only fifteen can be clearly identified as juvenile cerebral lipidosis (Levy and Little 1940; Lubin and Marburg 1943; Radermecker 1952; Hoffman 1956; Crawley 1957; Jefferson and Rutter 1958; Meyer and Manning 1961; Edgar and Post 1963). Thirteen of the fifteen displayed the type of paroxysmal EEG patterns described in the previous section of this paper. The three exceptions showed random diffuse slow activity (Lubin and Marburg 1943; Jefferson and Rutter 1958). Jefferson and Rutter's two patients were siblings who showed less clinical deterioration than usual at ages 16 and 19 years.

Of ten cases with 2 or more EEGs recorded at intervals, four showed a progressive increase of abnormality (Levy and Little 1940; Radermecker 1952; Crawley 1957; Meyer and Manning 1961), four failed to show such an increase over relatively brief intervals of 6–12 months (Radermecker 1952; Crawley 1957), none showed a decrease in abnormality, and Hoffman's (1956) two cases showed variable changes over several-month periods of ACTH treatment, which was ineffective. Of the three siblings reported by Crawley, the 14-year-old displayed the greatest EEG abnormality, the 12-year-old the next greatest amount, and the 9-year-old the least.

Our data, together with previous reports, indicate that EEG patterns in patients with juvenile cerebral lipidosis are relatively uniform, consisting mainly of diffuse bursts of 2.5–4 c/sec slow waves and spike-and-wave complexes. Occasionally there is a variable asymmetry between hemispheres, and sporadic focal spikes may occur, but the foci do not remain constant. The data further indicate that there is a progression of EEG abnormality paralleling clinical deterioration. Early EEG abnormality consists largely of bursts of slow waves with or without occasional spikes. This may be the only abnormality seen for a long time in slowly developing cases, especially in the absence of seizures. With time, the incidence and amplitude of the paroxysms increase, and more spike-and-wave complexes are seen. Late in the course of the disease background activity becomes slower and more irregular, and spike-and-wave complexes may also deteriorate.

The EEG pattern seen in this disease is different from that reported in Tay-Sachs disease (Cobb *et al.* 1952; Schneck 1965), which is earlier in onset, displays generally a more or less regular and lower frequency spike-and-wave activity, and a greater tendency toward inter-areal asymmetry. In juvenile cerebral lipidosis we have not seen the sharp and slow wave complexes at 1–2 c/sec or the triphasic forms so common in Tay-Sachs disease.

The EEG pattern seen in juvenile cerebral lipidosis is definitely not pathognomonic, since it is indistinguishable from patterns seen in many patients with idiopathic epilepsy and other diffuse brain diseases, such as phenylketonuria. The EEG may, however, assist in arriving at a diagnosis of juvenile cerebral lipidosis in children displaying progressive loss of visual acuity prior to the appearance of signs suggestive of a diffuse neurological disease.

The finding in a patient with markedly deteriorated visual function of a visual evoked response, which was similar to that of a normal control, illustrates an important point. A normal-looking evoked response cannot be taken as evidence of lack of sensory deficit, but only as evidence that *some* sensory function is present. It should be noted, however, that the converse is not asserted; abnormal-appearing evoked responses may give clues to abnormal function in a sensory system.

SUMMARY

EEG and visual evoked response observations have been presented in six patients, of whom five were followed for periods of 2–9 years. An EEG pattern has been observed, consisting of diffuse 2.5–4 c/sec slow waves and spike-and-wave complexes, with occasional variable asymmetries and inconsistent focal sporadic spikes. Evidence is presented that the progression of EEG abnormality parallels clinical deterioration.

RÉSUMÉ

PATTERNS EEG DE LA LIPOÏDOSE CÉRÉBRALE INFANTILE

Les auteurs présentent leurs observations sur l'EEG et les réponses évoquées visuelles obtenues chez six malades dont cinq ont été suivis sur des périodes de 2–9 ans. Ils ont observé un pattern EEG consistant en ondes lentes diffuses de 2.5–4 c/sec et en complexes pointe-ondes avec asymétrie occasionnelle variable et pointes focales sporadiques inconstantes. La progression des anomalies EEG parallèlement à la détérioration clinique est illustrée.

REFERENCES

COBB, W., MARTIN, F. and PAMPIGLIONE, G. Cerebral lipidosis: An electroencephalographic study. *Brain*, **1952**, *75*: 343–357.

CRAWLEY, J. Three cases of the juvenile form of amaurotic familial idiocy (Vogt–Spielmeyer disease) with electroencephalographic findings. *J. Pediat.*, **1957**, *51*: 571–579.

EDGAR, G. W. F. and POST, P. J. J. Amaurotic idiocy and epilepsy. *Epilepsia (Amst.)*, **1963**, *4*: 241–260.

HOFFMAN, J. Pigmentary retinal lipoid neuronal heredodegeneration (Spielmeyer–Vogt disease). *Electroenceph. clin. Neurophysiol.*, **1956**, *8*: 506–512.

JEFFERSON, M. and RUTTER, M. L. A report of two cases of the juvenile form of amaurotic familial idiocy (cerebromacular degeneration). *J. Neurol. Neurosurg. Psychiat.*, **1958**, *21*: 31–37.

JERVIS, G. A. Juvenile amaurotic family idiocy. Six cases of its occurrence in siblings. *Amer. J. Dis. Child.*, **1941**, *61*: 327–338.

JERVIS, G. A. Juvenile amaurotic family idiocy. *Amer. J. Dis. Child.*, **1959**, *97*: 663–667.

LEVY, S. and LITTLE, O.A.G. Juvenile familial amaurotic idiocy (Vogt–Spielmeyer disease). *Arch. Neurol. Psychiat. (Chic.)*, **1940**, *44*: 1274–1289.

LUBIN, A. J. and MARBURG, O. Juvenile amaurotic idiocy. *Arch. Neurol. Psychiat. (Chic.)*, **1943**, *49*: 559–573.

MEYER, H. and MANNING JR., G. C. Juvenile cerebral lipoidosis in two siblings. *Arch. Neurol. (Chic.)*, **1961**, *4*: 430–440.

RADERMECKER, J. Relations anatomocliniques et électroencéphalographiques dans le groupe des idioties amaurotiques. *Dtsch. Z. Nervenheilk.*, **1952**, *169*: 236–254.

SCHAIN, R. J. and WILEY, J. Evolution of a characteristic speech disorder in juvenile cerebral lipidosis. *Trans. Amer. neurol. Ass.*, **1965**, *90*: 290–291.

SCHNECK, L. The early electroencephalographic and seizure characteristics of Tay-Sachs' disease. *Acta neurol. scand.*, **1965**, *41*: 163-171.

Reference: ELLINGSON, R. J. and SCHAIN, R. J. EEG patterns in juvenile cerebral lipidosis. *Electroenceph. clin. Neurophysiol.*, **1969**, *27*: 191–194.

Electroencephalography and Clinical Neurophysiology
Elsevier Publishing Company, Amsterdam – Printed in The Netherlands

THE AUDITORY EVOKED RESPONSE IN BABIES DURING REM SLEEP[1]

EDWARD M. ORNITZ, M.D., EDWARD R. RITVO, M.D., Y. H. LEE, M.D., LEE M. PANMAN, B.A., RICHARD D. WALTER, M.D. AND ANNE MASON

Neuropsychiatric Institute, U.C.L.A. Center for the Health Sciences, Los Angeles, Calif. 90024 (U.S.A.)

(Accepted for publication: October 30, 1968)

INTRODUCTION

Young autistic children show an EEG pattern during rapid eye movement (REM) sleep suggestive of earlier maturational levels (Ornitz *et al.* 1969). The purpose of the present paper is to determine to what extent the tendency to increased amplitude of the auditory averaged evoked response during REM sleep in autistic children (Ornitz *et al.* 1968) might also reflect an earlier maturational level. Therefore, the findings on a group of normal babies are presented.

METHODS

Twelve normal babies, eleven boys and one girl, (age range 6–12 months, mean 8.2 months) were studied one night each. 251–419 min (mean 332 min) of sleep including an average of 4.4 REM sleep periods were recorded per subject night. Details of data sampling and analysis, and auditory stimulation and recording techniques are described in Ornitz *et al.* (1968).

RESULTS

The general characteristics of the auditory average evoked response (AER) in the normal baby are illustrated in Fig. 1. The latencies of wave N_2 during Stage 2 (mean 298 msec, S.D. ± 31.2) were not significantly greater than those reported for normal children (Ornitz *et al.* 1968). However, the latencies of wave N_2 during REM sleep (mean 262 msec, S.D. ± 70.8) were significantly greater than those reported for normal children ($P = 0.047$, $t = 2.14$ with 16.6° of freedom).

In the twelve normal babies (see Table I) the amplitude of wave N_2 during REM sleep was greater than that during Stage 2 sleep in eight and less in four. When amplitudes of wave N_2 during REM sleep were compared with amplitudes during Stage 2 sleep, subject by subject, the mean of the resulting ratios indicated a relative increase in amplitude during REM sleep in the group of babies (unweighted mean = 1.16; weighted

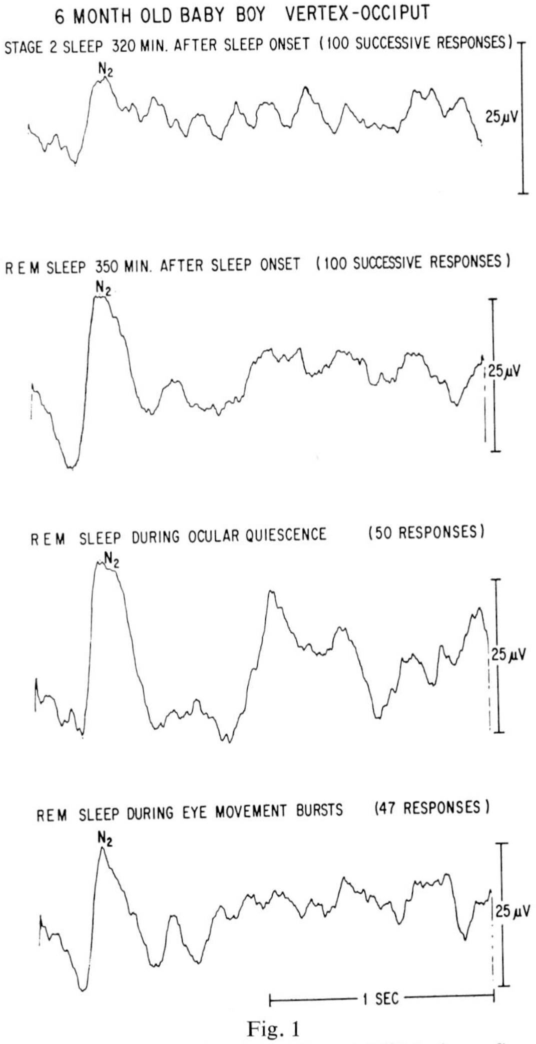

Fig. 1
Auditory AERs during Stage 2 and REM sleep. Summations during ocular quiescence and eye movement bursts are not consecutive responses. Upward deflection indicates negativity in respect to the vertex electrode.

[1] Supported by Grant No. USPHS-MH-13517, Grant No. USPHS-NB-02808, and the McGregor Fund.

TABLE I

Averaged evoked response amplitudes in babies 6–12 months old

Age (months)	Sex	Number of AERs sampled				Mean amplitude wave N_2 (μV)				Ratio of amplitude wave N_2		
		Stage 2 sleep	REM sleep	Ocular quiescence	Eye movement bursts	Stage 2 sleep	REM sleep	Ocular quiescence	Eye movement bursts	During REM sleep/stage 2 sleep	During ocular quiescence/stage 2 sleep	During eye movement bursts/stage 2 sleep
6	M	16	12	3	2	10.1	9.0	7.7	11.0	0.89	0.76	1.09
6	M	3	9	3	5	36.3	42.6	45.7	40.2	1.17	1.26	1.11
6	M	12	11	4	6	7.6	6.0	10.2	11.2	0.79	1.34	1.47
6	M	18	11	4	3	15.4	21.4	26.8	18.0	1.39	1.74	1.17
7	M	19	6	6	4	8.0	11.0	8.8	15.5	1.38	1.10	1.94
8	F	26	8	5	2	11.4	7.5	7.8	8.5	0.66	0.68	0.74
8	M	16	18	9	10	12.4	16.1	13.6	14.7	1.30	1.10	1.19
9	M	21	14	4	13	8.2	10.3	12.7	11.4	1.26	1.55	1.39
9	M	18	6	3	4	9.0	10.8	14.3	12.5	1.20	1.59	1.39
9	M	5	5	4	3	7.6	12.4	19.0	13.0	1.63	2.50	1.71
11	M	15	16	10	8	15.0	15.3	20.4	13.0	0.96	1.28	0.82
12	M	15	13	8	2	18.8	24.3	25.6	14.5	1.29	1.36	0.77

mean[1] = 1.13). The probability that this ratio was greater than 1.0[2] was, for the unweighted mean ratio, $P = 0.073$ ($t = 1.98$ with 11° of freedom), and for the weighted mean ratio, $P = 0.119$ ($t = 1.69$ with 11° of freedom).

When the auditory AER was summed separately during the eye movement bursts of REM sleep, the amplitude of wave N_2 was greater than that during Stage 2 sleep in nine out of the twelve babies (see Table I). The amplitudes of wave N_2 during the eye movement bursts were compared with the amplitudes during Stage 2 sleep, subject by subject, and the mean of the resulting ratios indicated a relative increase in amplitude during the eye movement bursts (unweighted mean = 1.23; weighted mean = 1.24). For the difference between this mean ratio and 1.0, $P = 0.057$ ($t = 2.13$ with 11° of freedom) for the unweighted mean and $P = 0.039$ ($t = 2.34$ with 11° of freedom) for the weighted mean.

Ten of the twelve babies also had larger responses during the ocular quiescent epochs of REM sleep than during Stage 2 sleep (see Table I). For the twelve subjects, the mean of the ratios of amplitudes of wave N_2 during the ocular quiescent epochs of REM sleep relative to Stage 2 sleep (unweighted mean = 1.36; weighted mean = 1.29) was significantly greater than 1.0 ($P = 0.023$, $t = 2.65$, for the unweighted mean; $P = 0.033$, $t = 2.44$, for the weighted mean).

[1] Individual ratios were weighted according to the number of AERs in each sleep stage (see Table I) and weighted means of the ratios were computed as previously described (Ornitz *et al.* 1968).

[2] A ratio of 1.0 would indicate no difference between amplitudes in the two sleep stages.

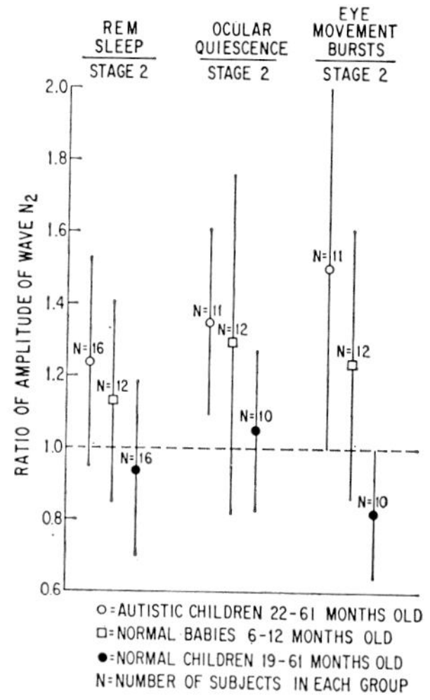

Fig. 2

Group means and standard deviations of ratios of amplitude of wave N_2 during different phases of sleep in babies compared with normal and autistic children.

Fig. 2 compares amplitudes of wave N_2 in normal babies, normal children and autistic children. Data for the latter 2 groups were derived from Ornitz *et al.* (1968). Although the ratios of amplitudes for the babies tended to be between those of the autistic and normal children, there were no significant differences between these normal babies and the autistic children. On the other hand the REM sleep/Stage 2 and Eye movement burst/Stage 2 ratios for the babies were significantly higher than for the normal children ($P = 0.032$ and $P = 0.006$, respectively).

DISCUSSION

The major finding of this report is that 6–12-month-old normal babies fail to show the depression of auditory AERs characteristic of normal children during the eye movement bursts of REM sleep. Furthermore, these normal infants show enhanced auditory AERs during both the ocular quiescent and the eye movement burst phases of REM sleep and their response amplitudes during the ocular motility are similar to those of autistic children and significantly distinct from those of normal children. This finding has significance both for the concept of *phasic inhibition* during REM sleep and for previous findings in autistic children (see discussion in Ornitz *et al.* 1967; Ornitz *et al.* 1968).

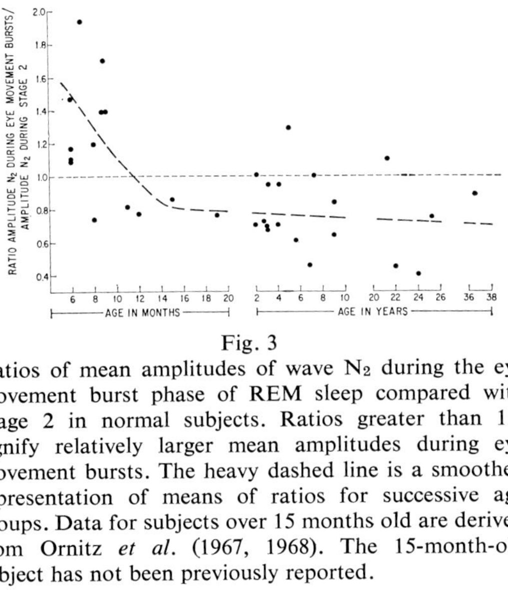

Fig. 3

Ratios of mean amplitudes of wave N_2 during the eye movement burst phase of REM sleep compared with Stage 2 in normal subjects. Ratios greater than 1.0 signify relatively larger mean amplitudes during eye movement bursts. The heavy dashed line is a smoothed representation of means of ratios for successive age groups. Data for subjects over 15 months old are derived from Ornitz *et al.* (1967, 1968). The 15-month-old subject has not been previously reported.

Fig. 3 suggests that during REM sleep the *phasic inhibition* of auditory evoked responses is not present initially but develops toward the end of the first year of life and that a tendency toward increasing inhibition is progressive with further maturation. It is of interest that the greatest increment of phasic inhibition seems to develop at about the same age as the greatest decrement of REM sleep time occurs (compare Roffwarg *et al.* 1966). Thus, phasic inhibition may represent a maturational step in the developmental physiology of REM sleep, providing greater functional differentiation within REM sleep as total REM sleep time is reduced. Roffwarg *et al.* (1966) proposed that *in utero* REM sleep may serve as an endogenous source of stimulation to the developing nervous system and that the decrement in REM sleep time post-natally may signify a decreased need for endogenous excitation. The counterpart of such a developmental shift might be the maturation of an inhibitory system within the REM sleep state to protect the exogenously stimulated post-natal organism from the effects of excessive endogenous excitation.

These results also suggest that the large AERs during the ocular motility of REM sleep in younger autistic children (Ornitz *et al.* 1968) are due to a delay in the normal development of phasic inhibition during REM sleep in such patients. This interpretation is consistent with other neurophysiologic findings (Ornitz *et al.* 1969) and with clinical observations (Bender and Freedman 1952; Ornitz and Ritvo 1968b) suggestive of maturational delay in autistic children. The absence of phasic inhibition of sensory input during the early years of life in autistic children may reflect an inadequate protection against the excitatory effects of the REM state (Ornitz and Ritvo 1968a).

SUMMARY

1. The auditory averaged evoked response (AER) was measured at the vertex in twelve 6–12-month-old normal babies during Stage 2 and rapid eye movement (REM) sleep and during the ocular quiescent and eye movement burst phases of REM sleep. Amplitudes and latencies of wave N_2 of the auditory AER were compared during the different sleep stages and to previously reported values for normal and autistic children.

2. The latencies of wave N_2 in the babies were similar to those of the normal children during Stage 2. However, latencies during REM sleep and during both the eye movement burst and ocular quiescent epochs of REM sleep were significantly longer in the babies.

3. The babies showed a tendency toward greater amplitudes of wave N_2 during both the eye movement burst and ocular quiescent phases of REM sleep than during Stage 2 sleep. In the group of babies, the relative amplitudes of wave N_2 during both REM sleep and the eye movement bursts of REM sleep (relative to Stage 2 sleep) were significantly greater than in a group of normal children, but were similar to those of a group of young autistic children.

4. These findings suggest that the normal phasic inhibition of evoked responses accompanying the ocular activity of REM sleep may not be present in the very young organism and that the development of phasic inhibition may be related to maturational factors underlying the post-natal reduction of REM sleep time.

RÉSUMÉ

RÉPONSES ÉVOQUÉES AUDITIVES DU BÉBÉ PENDANT LE SOMMEIL AVEC MOUVEMENTS OCULAIRES

1. Les réponses évoquées moyennes auditives ont été mesurées au niveau du vertex chez douze bébés normaux de 6 à 12 mois pendant le stade II et le sommeil avec mouvements oculaires; dans ce dernier cas les réponses ont été mesurées pendant et en dehors des bouffées de mouvements oculaires. Les amplitudes et les latences de

l'onde N_2 de la réponse évoquée moyenne auditive sont comparées au cours des différents stades de sommeil ainsi qu'aux valeurs précédemment rapportées chez les enfants normaux et autistiques.

2. Les latences de l'onde N_2 observées chez les bébés sont semblables à celles des enfants normaux pendant le stade II. Par contre, les latences sont nettement plus longues chez les bébés pendant le sommeil avec mouvements oculaires rapides que ce soit pendant les bouffées de mouvements oculaires ou pendant les époques de tranquillité oculaire.

3. On note chez les bébés que l'amplitude de l'onde N_2 est légèrement plus grande pendant les bouffées de mouvements oculaires et les phases de tranquillité oculaire du sommeil rapide que pendant le stade II. Chez les bébés, les amplitudes de l'onde N_2 pendant le sommeil rapide et pendant les bouffées de mouvements oculaires de ce sommeil sont (par comparaison au stade II) nettement plus grandes que celles qui ont été mesurées dans un groupe d'enfants normaux, mais qu'elles sont semblables à celles d'un groupe de jeunes enfants autistiques.

4. Ces données suggèrent que l'inhibition phasique normale des réponses évoquées accompagnant l'activité oculaire du sommeil rapide peu ne pas être présente dans l'organisme très jeune et que le développement de l'inhibition phasique peut être reliée à ces facteurs maturationnels soustendant la réduction post-natale du temps de sommeil rapide.

The authors are grateful for the generous statistical consultation of Dr. A. B. Forsythe, Dr. M. B. Brown and the Health Sciences Computing Facility supported by National Institute of Health Grant FR 3.

REFERENCES

BENDER, L. and FREEDMAN, A. M. A study of the first 3 years in the maturation of schizophrenic children. *Quart. J. Child Behav.*, **1952,** *4*: 245–272.

ORNITZ, E. M. and RITVO, E. R. Neurophysiologic mechanisms underlying perceptual inconstancy in autistic and schizophrenic children. *Arch. gen. Psychiat.*, **1968**a, *19*: 22–27.

ORNITZ, E. M. and RITVO, E. R. Perceptual inconstancy in early infantile autism. *Arch. gen. Psychiat.*, **1968**b, *18*: 76–98.

ORNITZ, E. M., RITVO, E. R., BROWN, M. B., LA FRANCHI, S., PARMELEE, T. and WALTER, R. D. The EEG and rapid eye movements during REM sleep in normal and autistic children. *Electroenceph. clin. Neurophysiol.*, **1969,** *26*: 167–175.

ORNITZ, E. M., RITVO, E. R., CARR, E. M., PANMAN, L. M. and WALTER, R. D. The variability of the auditory averaged evoked response during sleep and dreaming in children and adults. *Electroenceph. clin. Neurophysiol.*, **1967,** *22*: 514–524.

ORNITZ, E. M., RITVO, E. R., PANMAN, L. M., LEE, Y. H., CARR, E. M. and WALTER, R. D. The auditory evoked response in normal and autistic children during sleep. *Electroenceph. clin. Neurophysiol.*, **1968,** *25*: 221–230.

ROFFWARG, H. P., MUZIO, J. N. and DEMENT, W. C. Ontogenetic development of the human sleep-dream cycle. *Science*, **1966,** *152*: 604–619.

Reference: ORNITZ, E. M., RITVO, E. R., LEE, Y. H., PANMAN, L. M., WALTER, R. D. and MASON, A. The auditory evoked response in babies during REM sleep. *Electroenceph. clin. Neurophysiol.*, **1969,** *27*: 195–198.

Electroencephalography and Clinical Neurophysiology
Elsevier Publishing Company, Amsterdam – Printed in The Netherlands

TECHNICAL CONTRIBUTIONS

Z-AXIS MODULATION IN NEURAL SPIKE DISPLAY

CHRISTOPHER J. CONWAY AND WILLIAM E. BRADLEY

Department of Neurology, University of Minnesota Medical Center, Minneapolis, Minn. 55455 (U.S.A.)

(Accepted for publication: November 5, 1968)

The photographing of unit spikes from an oscilloscope screen is often difficult to accomplish satisfactorily since the brightness of the image is inversely proportional to the velocity of the spot over the phosphor.

If the intensity of the beam were modulated to vary with the velocity of the spot on the screen, an image of even brightness could be displayed, and the quality of photographs improved.

An instrument has been desciibed which performs spike intensification as one of its functions (Kellett *et al.* 1965). The major drawback of this device is that intensification is not proportional to beam velocity, but is done

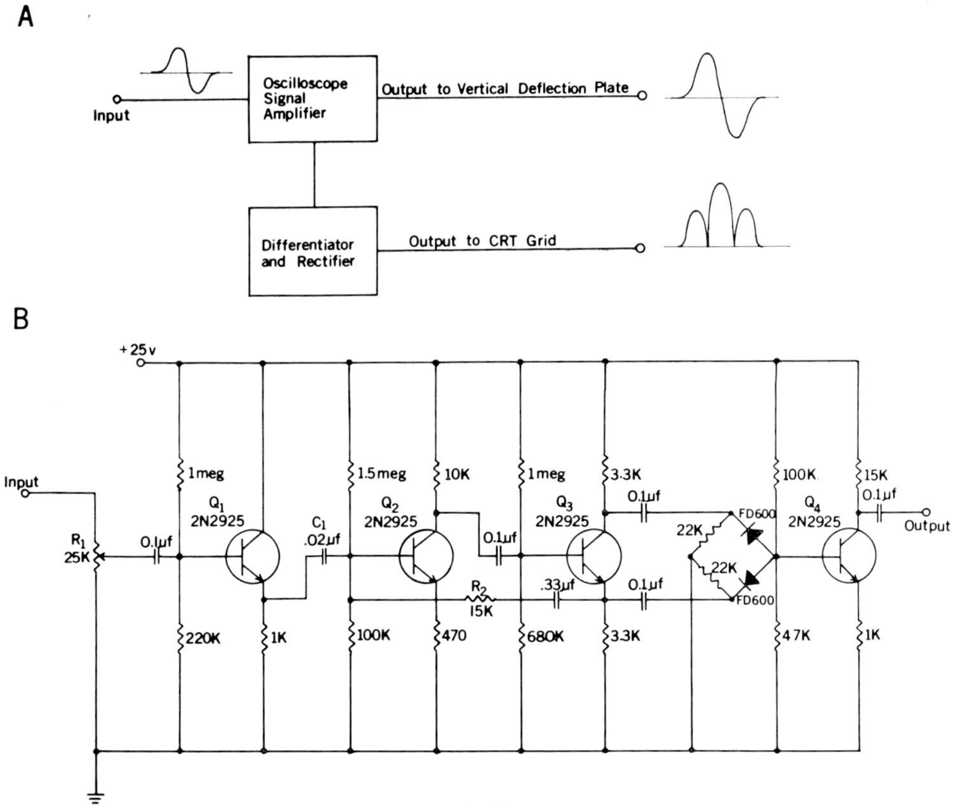

Fig. 1

A: Principle of operation. The input signal to the oscilloscope determines the vertical velocity of the CRT spot. The intensity of the spot is regulated by the rectified time-derivative of the input signal, providing maximum intensification when spot velocity is greatest. *B*: Circuit developed for use with Tektronix 565 oscilloscope. Input is taken from "Vertical Signal Out" BNC connector on rear panel of oscilloscope. Output is connected to appropriate "CRT Grid" jack. FD600 diodes are manufactured by Fairchild Semiconductor Inc. For further explanation see text.

by a square pulse from a Schmitt trigger circuit. The result is that brightening is uneven and the peaks of spikes may be over-intensified and defocussed. In addition the circuit is considerably more complex than the one described below and utilizes a number of vacuum tubes.

This report describes a circuit constructed in our laboratory to vary the intensity of the CRT beam in proportion to beam velocity. The device was designed for use with a Tektronix 565 oscilloscope, and is very simple and inexpensive.

DESCRIPTION OF INSTRUMENT

The principle of operation, illustrated in Fig. 1, *A*, is as follows. The vertical position of the scanning spot is controlled by the input signal to the oscilloscope amplifier; therefore, the vertical velocity of the spot at any given time is directly proportional to the time derivative of the input signal. By passing the input signal through a differentiating circuit, an output equivalent to the time derivative of the input is obtained. This signal cannot be used directly to vary the intensity of the beam, because it has positive and negative phases, corresponding to the rising and falling phases of the input, and would therefore result in alternate brightening and blanking of the image on the screen. The Tektronix 565 oscilloscope requires a positive signal applied to the CRT grid to brighten the trace (Tektronix Engineering Staff), so the output of the differentiator must be rectified to provide a signal which is always positive. This signal can in turn be amplified and applied to the CRT grid. The circuit used is shown in Fig. 1, *B*. This particular circuit was designed for the Tektronix 565, but the principles would be similar for other oscilloscopes, and minor modifications would suffice.

The signal to be displayed is connected to the oscilloscope in the normal manner, and the input to the device is taken from the "Vertical Signal Out" connector on the rear of the oscilloscope cabinet. The potentiometer R_1 in the diagram regulates the input level to the device, thereby controlling the output level and the degree of intensification. Transistor Q_1 is an emitter follower to provide high input impedance to the device. Transistors Q_2 and Q_3 form a high gain amplifying stage and perform the differentiating function.

Transistor Q_3 also acts as a phase-splitter in addition to being part of the differentiator enabling full wave rectification at the diode bridge. The output of the diode bridge is connected directly to the base of Q_4, which amplifies the signal to the desired output level, reaching a maximum of +20 V. Output of the circuit is connected to the appropriate CRT grid jack on the rear panel.

The circuit is extremely simple, and will, therefore, not perform without phase-shift over a very wide frequency range. However, its performance is entirely satisfactory in the frequency range of neural spikes, that is 500 c/sec to 5 kc/sec. Should it be necessary to use it outside that range, phase-shift can be corrected by adjusting the value of R_2.

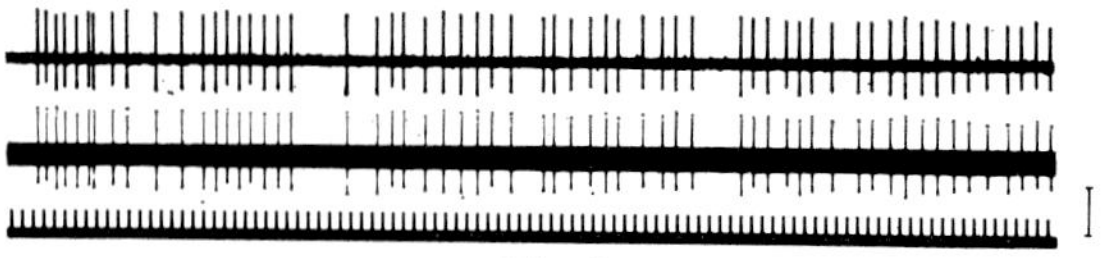

Fig. 2

Performance of device. Units from reticular formation of cat. Upper trace has CRT intensity controlled by device; note the equal sharpness of baseline and spikes. Lower trace is the identical signal except that the intensity has manual adjustment only. Note that the spikes photograph poorly even though the intensity is turned up so high that the baseline is obliterated. Bottom trace is time marker at 100 msec. Calibration: 500 μV.

Total current drain of the device is 8 mA, so it may be operated from a battery without difficulty.

An example of the application of the device is shown in Fig. 2. The signal to be photographed was fed to both upper and lower beams of the oscilloscope simultaneously. The difference in image quality between the two traces is apparent in the illustration.

When units must be photographed at very slow sweep speeds this device is of great assistance.

SUMMARY

A device has been described which automatically controls the intensity of the CRT spot to provide even brightness for a slow moving baseline and fast vertical spikes. The device operates in the frequency range of neural unit spikes and provides great improvement in the quality of negatives photographed from the CRO screen. It is in addition very inexpensive and easy to build.

RÉSUMÉ

UTILISATION DE LA MODULATION D'INTENSITÉ DU FAISCEAU CATHODIQUE (AXE Z) DANS LA PRÉSENTATION DES POINTES NEURONIQUES

Les auteurs décrivent un dispositif qui contrôle automatiquement l'intensité du spot du tube à rayons cathodiques, afin d'obtenir une brillance égale pour une ligne de base à déplacement lent et pour des pointes verticales rapides. Ce dispositif fonctionne dans la gamme de fréquence des pointes neuroniques unitaires et permet une nette amélioration de la qualité des négatifs photographiés à partir de l'écran oscillographique. Il est de plus très peu coûteux et facile à construire.

REFERENCES

Kellet, R. C., Phillis, J. W. and Veale, J. L. A spike intensifier and single trigger generator for identification of ventral root axons. *Electroenceph. clin. Neurophysiol.*, **1965**, *18*: 82–84.

Tektronix Engineering Staff. *Instruction manual for type RM565 oscilloscope*. Tektronix, Inc., P. O. Box 500, Beaverton, Ore.

Reference: Conway, C. J. and Bradley, W. E. Z-axis modulation in neural spike display. *Electroenceph. clin. Neurophysiol.*, **1969**, *27*: 199–200.

MULTI-BARRELED COAXIAL MICRO-PIPETTES WITH INDEPENDENT CONTROL OF THE CENTRAL RECORDING BARREL[1]

R. SPEHLMANN

VA Research Hospital and Department of Neurology and Psychiatry, Northwestern University Medical School, Chicago, Ill. 60611 (U.S.A.)

(Accepted for publication: November 13, 1968)

Electrophysiological investigation of drug action upon CNS neurons has been greatly advanced by the introduction of multi-barreled micro-pipettes (Curtis and Eccles 1958). These permit electrophoretic application of drug ions from the orifices of various drug barrels positioned in the vicinity of a single neuron whose electrical activity is simultaneously recorded through another barrel of the compound pipette. Two types of electrodes predominate. One type consists of several adjoining pipettes, which end separately at a common level, forming the electrode tip. When drugs are applied to the outside of cells, recording of neuronal activity will, of necessity, be extracellular. Electrodes of this type having tip diameters of 1 μ or less are difficult to handle (Spehlmann 1963) because the high electrical resistance of the barrels limits their recording and current passing capabilities. Recording is further impaired by marked resistive and capacitative coupling between drug and recording barrels. These drawbacks can be partly overcome by increasing the diameter of drug barrel orifices to 1–2 μ each. At this diameter, spontaneous diffusion of drug ions from the orifices can be controlled by a retaining voltage of a polarity opposite to the one used for ion ejection (Del Castillo and Katz 1955; Curtis 1964). However, electrode tips with such large orifices become quite bulky if one wishes to use a greater number of drug barrels, and can produce significant trauma if one attempts to approach cerebral cells so as to be close enough to isolate signals from one neuron.

Another type of multi-barreled micro-electrode has a small-tipped recording barrel which protrudes over the drug barrel endings. This reduces trauma in the recording area and facilitates the approach to smaller neurons. Larger neurons can be impaled with the recording barrel while the drug barrels remain in an extracellular position. Earlier pharmacological investigations of this type (Curtis *et al.* 1959) used a "concentric" or "coaxial" (Tomita 1956) arrangement of an inner recording pipette protruding through the orifice of an outer drug-filled pipette. Because of marked electrical coupling and difficulties in the control of drug release, this arrangement has more recently been abandoned in favor of a recording barrel cemented to the side, with its tip protruding beyond the end, of a single (Werman *et al.* 1967, 1968) or multi-barreled (Curtis 1968) drug pipette. The use of a recording pipette threaded through the center barrel of a 5-barreled electrode has been proposed (Salmoiraghi and Weight 1967). For work in the visual cortex of cats with its comparatively small cells, we have developed another sort of electrode which combines the advantages of previous electrode types with each other and, especially, affords axial movement of the recording barrel relative to the drug barrels during the experiment.

DESCRIPTION

This electrode consists of an assembly of from 6 to 10 drug barrels which surround a central recording barrel. The mantle of drug barrels was made from Pyrex brand glass tubing of 2 or 3 mm outer diameter, cut into lengths of 10 cm each and fire polished at the ends. The middle parts of these pieces of tubing were heated in a gas-oxygen flame and fused side-to-side over a distance of from 2 to 5 cm so as to form the wall of a hollow cylinder. The middle of the fused section was then heated evenly and stretched to about half the diameter of the original bundle by gently pulling on the ends of the bundle. The transition from the thicker part on the left end to the thinner part in the middle of the bundle was heated again and glass was pulled away towards the right side. This maneuver was repeated several times to gradually shape a tip whose taper was determined by the degree of heat and pulling force applied during each step. Shaping of the thinner parts of the tip was facilitated by the use of a micro-forge. Very little heat and force were used for the final pull which separated the last thin strands of glass capillaries, resulting in a tip of 3–10 μ in total diameter. The right half of the original bundle was treated in a like way to shape a tip of the same dimensions, thus resulting in a second electrode. At the tip, the orifices of all barrels lay in the same plane. The cross section of drug barrels was round in the stem but appeared to be half-circular or elliptical where they

[1] Supported by Public Health Service Research Grant NB06820.

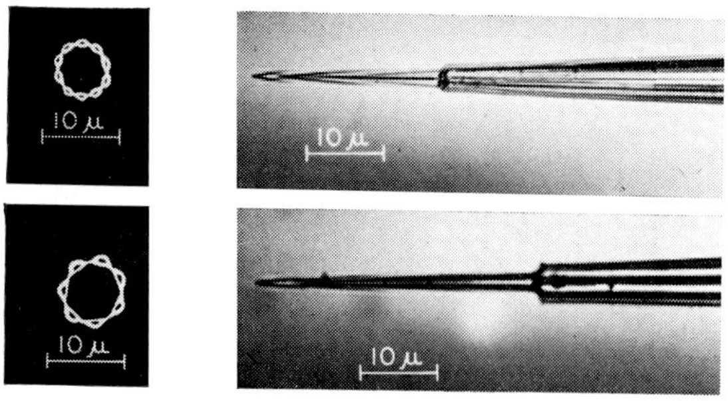

Fig. 1
Photomicrographs of electrode tips with ten (upper part) and seven (lower part) drug barrels. *Left*: End view of drug barrels only, light being transmitted within glass of drug barrel assembly. *Right*: Side view of complete electrodes with smaller drug barrel tips than shown on left side; conventional microscope illumination.

had been stretched to form the tip (Fig. 1, *left*). The long diameter of the orifices measured up to 2 μ in bundles formed of six lengths of 3 mm glass tubing and having tips of 10 μ. Smaller orifices were obtained by using smaller tips, a larger number of barrels or smaller diameter glass tubing.

In our experience, this technique of controlling tip size was more satisfactory than the alternative procedure of producing a finer tip and subsequently increasing its diameter. Whereas finer tips were easily obtained by using sufficient heat and pulling force, we found it difficult to enlarge the electrode tip. In an attempt to control tip diameter, we broke electrode tips by bumping them against smooth or rough glass or metal surfaces, or ground them with a fast turning diamond cutting wheel or etched them with hydrofluoric acid. In our hands, all these techniques resulted in comparatively ragged tips with the individual barrels ending at levels differing by 1 μ or more. Besides, the taper of such tips was not suitable for insertion of a single central pipette.

Satisfactory barrel assemblies were filled by boiling in distilled water at 40° C under reduced atmospheric pressure. The water was then withdrawn from the shafts with a polyethylene tube and replaced by drug solutions of suitable concentration and pH. At least 48 h were allowed for diffusion of drugs into the barrel tips during storage in a humid environment. A conventional single barreled micro-pipette, with a tip of less than 1 μ in diameter, was used as a recording barrel. It was drawn from 2 mm Pyrex glass tubing. When 3 mm tubing was used, some effort (Frank and Becker 1964) had to be made to keep the taper slim enough to permit insertion of the recording barrel through the drug barrel assembly. Recording barrels were filled with suitable electrolytes in the conventional manner. Control over the movement of the recording tip relative to the drug barrel orifices was accomplished with a micro-manipulator of high resolution. For this purpose, a hydraulic manipulator was constructed using rolling diaphragms and other materials indicated in a recent report (Lutz and Wagman 1965). The slave cylinder of this manipulator was connected, through a "Y" connector, to two micrometer driven master cylinders. One of them had the same diameter as the slave cylinder and therefore provided for a 1:1 transmission of the micrometer movement of the master piston to the slave piston. The other master cylinder had a smaller diameter. One micrometer revolution, advancing the master piston by 0.5 mm, resulted in 15 μ of slave piston travel over a total range of 120 μ of slave movement. The drug barrel assembly was rigidly clamped in a clip which was attached to the body of the slave cylinder with setscrews, permitting lateral adjustment of the axis of the drug barrel assembly. The slave cylinder was tilted horizontally for microscopic inspection of the electrode tip during the following procedures. The single barreled pipette was introduced by hand into the central space of the drug barrel assembly and gently pushed forward until its tip could be distinguished within about 1 cm of the drug barrel endings. Further movement was controlled with the manipulator. The movement of the slave piston was transmitted to the central pipette by means of a short metal rod connected to a locking ball joint, which in turn was locked to the piston shaft with a setscrew. This rod was positioned behind the end of the central electrode. The coarse drive was used to push the tip of the central electrode to the level of the ends of the drug barrels. Protrusion of the recording tip over these ends was adjusted with the fine drive. The taper of the inner pipette and of the inside of the central space of the drug barrel assembly usually permitted the inner tip to protrude over the outer orifices by a distance approximating 10 times the total diameter of the end of the drug barrel assembly (Fig. 1, *right*). If this value could not be obtained, or if lateral deviation resulted from axial movement of the central barrel, electrodes were usually discarded. In some instances, the recording tip was fixed at a protrusion of from 15 to 60 μ by cementing its shaft to the shafts of drug barrels by means of sticky wax. Such electrodes were removed from the hydraulic micro-manipulator and, for the experiment, attached to a conventional micro-electrode manipulator. If, on the other hand, protrusion of the central barrel was satisfactory, the rod on the cylinder piston was withdrawn from the end of the central barrel and, with the help of the setscrews, positioned very close to the side of that barrel and cemented to it with a drop of sticky wax (Fig. 2).

For the experiment, protrusion of the inner barrel was adjusted to 15–30 μ. The slave cylinder was attached to a conventional micro-manipulator which was used to advance the entire electrode assembly through the cortex until signals from a neuron could be first distinguished. Then the fine control of the hydraulic manipulator was used to advance the recording barrel relative to the drug barrels and brain tissue. If this did not increase the amplitude of neuronal action potentials, the recording barrel was withdrawn to its initial position. The entire electrode was then advanced about the same distance as that which the recording barrel had been withdrawn, and the recording barrel was again protruded. This approach often resulted in recordings of spike potentials of several millivolts in amplitude. Some of the larger spikes were

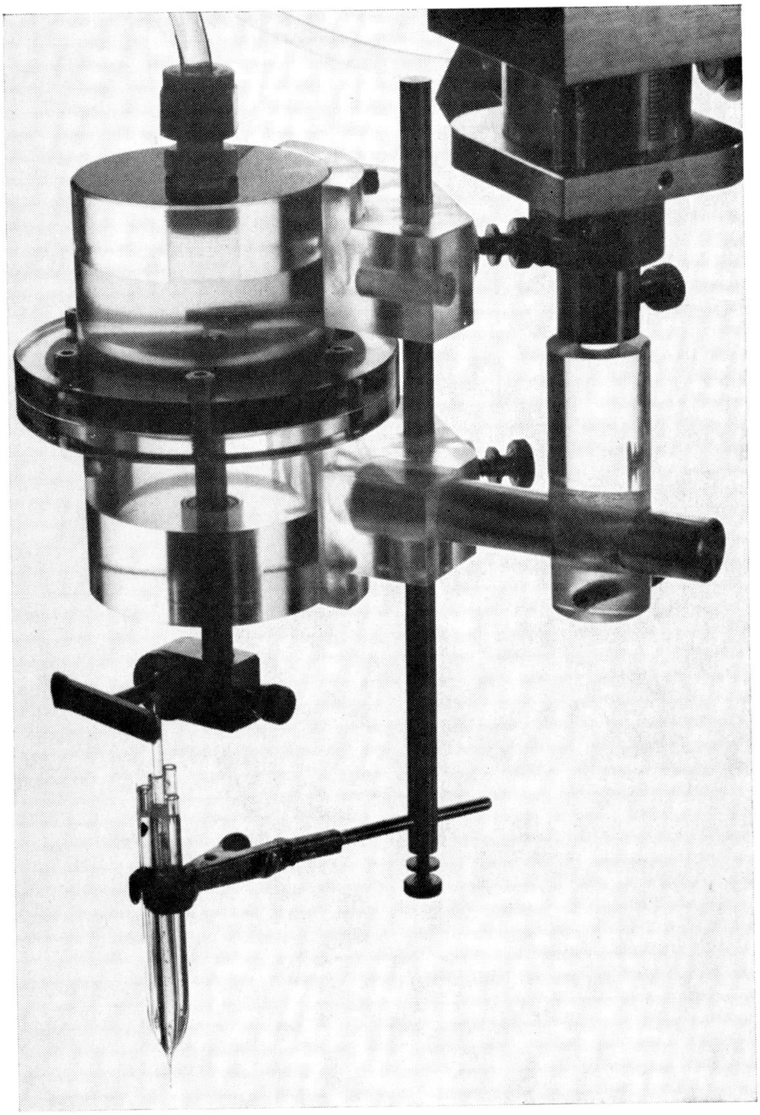

Fig. 2
Slave cylinder of hydraulic micro-manipulator holding electrode with seven drug barrels. Central recording barrel is connected to metal rod on locking ball joint attached to piston shaft. Slave cylinder is held in conventional micro-electrode manipulator (right and upper part of picture).

accompanied by slow waves of such polarity and relation to spike discharges as to indicate that they reflected neuronal membrane potential (Fig. 3). These recordings, made in the visual cortex, often resembled the "quasi-intracellular" derivations obtained with single micro-pipettes in cerebral neurons (McIlwain and Creutzfeldt 1967). The stability of recordings in regard to respiratory and circulatory movement of the brain was at least as good for multi-barreled micro-electrodes as it was for single electrodes in a given preparation. The drug barrels presumably stabilize the tissues penetrated by the recording barrel.

Drugs were liberated while recording action potentials with tip protrusions of up to 60 μ. Within this limit, the latency of the drug effect and minimum effective electrophoretic current intensity seemed independent of the degree of protrusion. For instance, the excitant and depressant actions of L-glutamate and gamma-aminobutyric acid were typically obtained within one second of the onset of electrophoretic currents of $1\text{–}5 \cdot 10^{-8}$ A. Longer latencies and stronger minimum effective currents were observed in trial recordings with tip protrusions of 100 μ. Even under this condition, the firing rates of some neurons were altered by currents

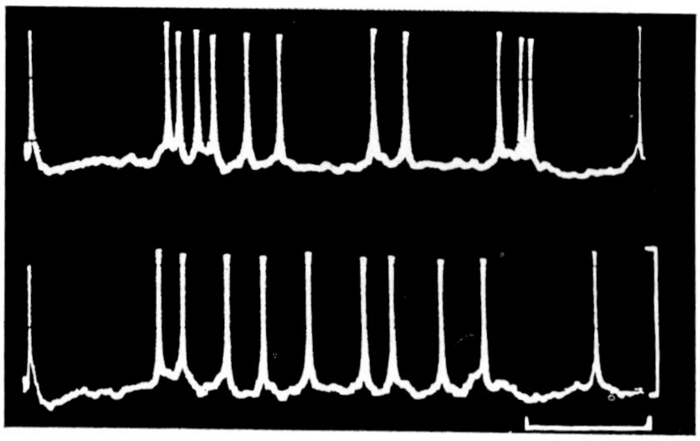

Fig. 3
Neuron in cat visual cortex firing in response to electrical stimulation of the optic radiation. Stimulus coincides with onset of each sweep. Action and resting potentials recorded through the center barrel of a composite electrode with ten drug barrels. Calibrations: 100 msec and 10 mV.

of 10^{-7} A or less passed through an NaCl filled drug barrel. It is impossible to interpret this phenomenon because of the unknown spatial relationship of the electrically excitable structure, and the recording and polarizing barrels.

Electrical coupling between drug and recording barrels depended, within certain limits, upon the protrusion of the recording barrel. Coupling resistance between any one drug barrel and the recording barrel was rarely above 50 kΩ and usually below 10 kΩ, a potential change of less than 1 mV being induced in the recording barrel as a result of a current flow of 10^{-7} A, the strongest intensity used for drug electrophoresis in our experiments. No attempt was made to measure or compensate for capacitative coupling because electrophoretic currents were always altered gradually. The recording input had the conventional features of high impedance, neutralization of tip potentials and capacitative losses and a bridge circuit for electrical polarization through the recording barrel.

SUMMARY

The action of several different drugs upon the electrical activity of single neurons can be studied with an electrode composed of 6–10 drug barrels surrounding a central recording barrel. Controlled independent protrusion of the latter during the experiment facilitates atraumatic approach to smaller, cerebral, neurons.

RÉSUMÉ

MICRO-PIPETTES À MULTI-RÉSERVOIRES COAXIAUX AVEC CONTRÔLE INDÉPENDANT DU RESERVOIR D'ENREGISTREMENT CENTRAL

L'action de plusieurs drogues différentes sur l'activité électrique des neurones unitaires peut être étudiée au moyen d'une électrode composée de 6–10 réservoirs de drogues entourant une électrode centrale d'enregistrement. La saillie indépendante et controlable de cette dernière pendant l'expérimentation facilite l'approche sans traumatisme de neurones cérébraux plus petits.

The author thanks Mr. J. Pacourek from the Instrumentation Laboratory of the VA Research Hospital for the expert construction of the hydraulic micro-manipulator and Mrs. J. Gordon and Messrs. F. Hartman, R. Hawkinson and D. Henley from the Medical Illustrations Laboratory for their help in preparing the illustrations.

REFERENCES

CURTIS, D. R. Microelectrophoresis. In W. L. NASTUK (Ed.), *Physical techniques in biological research.* Academic Press, New York, **1964,** *5*: 144–190.

CURTIS, D. R. A method for assembly of "parallel" micro-pipettes. *Electroenceph. clin. Neurophysiol.*, **1968,** *24*: 587–589.

CURTIS, D. R. and ECCLES, R. M. The excitation of Renshaw cells by pharmacological agents applied electrophoretically. *J. Physiol. (Lond.)*, **1958,** *141*: 435–445.

CURTIS, D. R., PHILLIS, J. W. and WATKINS, J. C. The depression of spinal neurones by γ-amino-n-butyric acid and β-alanine. *J. Physiol. (Lond.)*, **1959,** *146*: 185–203.

DEL CASTILLO, J. and KATZ, B. On the location of acetylcholine receptors. *J. Physiol. (Lond.)*, **1955,** *128*: 157–181.

FRANK, K. and BECKER, M. C. Microelectrodes for recording and stimulation. In W. L. NASTUK (Ed.), *Physical techniques in biological research.* Academic Press, New York, **1964,** *5*: 22–87.

LUTZ, A. and WAGMAN, I. H. A rolling diaphragm hydraulic micro-manipulator. *Electroenceph. clin. Neurophysiol.*, **1965,** *18*: 184–186.

MCILWAIN, J. T. and CREUTZFELDT, O. D. Microelectrode study of synaptic excitation and inhibition in the lateral geniculate nucleus of the cat. *J. Neurophysiol.*, **1967,** *30*: 1–21.

SALMOIRAGHI, G. C. and WEIGHT, F. Micromethods in neuropharmacology; an approach to the study of anesthetics. *Anesthesiology*, **1967,** *28*: 54–64.

SPEHLMANN, R. Acetylcholine and prostigmine electrophoresis at visual cortex neurons. *J. Neurophysiol.*, **1963,** *26*: 127–139.

TOMITA, T. The nature of action potentials in the lateral eye of the horseshoe crab as recorded by simultaneous intra- and extracellular recording. *Jap. J. Physiol.*, **1956,** *6*: 327–340.

WERMAN, R., DAVIDOFF, R. A. and APRISON, M. H. Inhibition of motoneurons by iontophoresis of glycine. *Nature (Lond.)*, **1967,** *214*: 681–683.

WERMAN, R., DAVIDOFF, R. A. and APRISON, M. H. Inhibitory action of glycine on spinal neurons in the cat. *J. Neurophysiol.*, **1968,** *31*: 81–95.

Reference: SPEHLMANN, R. Multi-barreled coaxial micro-pipettes with independent control of the central recording barrel. *Electroenceph. clin. Neurophysiol.*, **1969,** *27*: 201–204.

A TECHNIQUE FOR THE CHRONIC IMPLANTATION OF MULTIPLE MOVABLE MICRO-ELECTRODES

E. ROY JOHN AND PILAR P. MORGADES

Brain Research Laboratory, Department of Psychiatry, New York Medical College, New York, N. Y. 10029 (U.S.A.)

(Accepted for publication: November 19, 1968)

This paper describes a newly developed technique to record simultaneously from adjacent micro-electrodes implanted in the same brain region, over periods of weeks or months, in unrestrained performing animals. The device is simple and inexpensive and permits a wide range of precisely controllable movement of the implanted micro-electrodes. A number of devices have been previously described which are intended for chronic studies of neural units but which have one or several of the following disadvantages: (a) do not carry multiple micro-electrodes; (b) require removal of the electrode after a recording session; (c) are too bulky to permit more than one unit to be mounted on the head of a cat; (d) are difficult to construct; or (e) are too expensive (Davies 1956; Gusel'nikov 1957; Hubel 1957, 1958; Ricci *et al.* 1957; Strumwasser 1958; Katsuki *et al.* 1959; Kogan 1959; Evarts 1960, 1968; Fuster 1961; Sawa and Delgado 1963; Hayward *et al.* 1964; Davis and Tollow 1966; Goldberg and Greenwood 1966; MacLean 1967; Oomura *et al.* 1967).

METHOD

Several views of the present device are shown in Fig. 1 and a detailed drawing is presented in Fig. 2.

(1) The base is a stainless steel spool with a Teflon core through its center, a screw thread at one end, and a flange which can be imbedded in acrylic resin to hold the base over a hole in the skull. The Teflon core contains a hole 0.0415 in. in diameter. The drive shaft (0.042 in. in diameter) fits into this hole so tightly that considerable effort is required to move it manually, although it can easily be moved by the micro-drive.

(2) The drive shaft consists of a 19 gauge seamless stainless steel tube, 1.500 in. long (0.042 O. D., 0.030 I.D.; obtained from Becton Dickinson, Rutherford, N. J.), with a 1.050 × 0.250 mm thread extending 1/16 in. along the upper end of the shaft. The shaft contains ceramic tubing (1.531 in. long, 0.030 in. O. D.) pierced by two holes (0.005 in. I. D.; 125 μ apart), which protrudes slightly below the shaft. (Double bore insulation No. AP35; obtained from McDanel Refractory Porcelain Co., 510 9th Ave., P. O. Box 560, Beaver Falls, Pa. A four-hole ceramic is also available, with the holes located at the corners of a square, 125μ on a side, No. AR4T005132. Since the O. D. of this ceramic is 0.034 in. the drive shaft must be constructed of slightly larger tubing.)

(3) The two micro-electrodes are made of 0.005 in. diameter 70% Pt – 30% Ir wire (obtained from Medwire Corp., an affiliate of Sigmund Cohn Corp., 121 South Columbus Ave., Mt. Vernon, N.Y.), inserted into the ceramic, and protruding about 1/8 in. at the top and 3/8 in. at the bottom of the shaft. The ceramic locates the two electrodes a known distance apart and insulates them. A plastic cap is then threaded over the upper end of the shaft and cemented into position with Epoxylite (Epoxylite Electrode Insulator No. 6001-M and Epoxylite Solvent, obtained from the Epoxylite Corp., South El Monte, Calif.). The bare ends of the two wires are bent 90° so that they lie in two grooves which constitute a diameter on the top of the cap. Next, a larger contact cap is screwed firmly over the first one. On its top are two threaded holes (1 mm) located so that the electrode wires underneath are visible, and two clearance holes (No. 78 drill). A flexible wire (FO 5–9860 Tensolite, obtainable from Medwire Corp.) is brought through a clearance hole in the base and is passed through each clearance hole in the cap. Insulation is removed at the upper end. Finally, a 0.132 in. long, 1 mm diameter filister head screw is placed in each threaded hole and tightened so that the lead wire is under the head of the screw and the tip of the screw makes contact with the electrode below. A steel snap cover protects these contact screws. The two lead wires are then connected to a subminiature plug (such as Winchester No. SM3S; when two drives are implanted, a Continental No. MM–5–22 SSGD is used) for eventual input to a recording device after implant. A third contact will be connected to a ground lead from some appropriate point on the animal. This completes the assembly of the drive. After the electrodes are properly sharpened (Wolbarsht *et al.* 1960), they are insulated and sealed into the ceramic by coating the assembly with molten glass. The glass extends over the ceramic onto the steel shaft, waterproofing the entire assembly[1].

[1] Glass-insulated Pt–Ir micro-electrodes were selected because it was felt that they might be most durable for very long-term implantation. We see no reason why varnish-insulated stainless steel or tungsten micro-electrodes could not be used in this drive if the insulation would remain intact after long immersion in brain tissue (Grundfest *et al.* 1950; Hubel 1957).

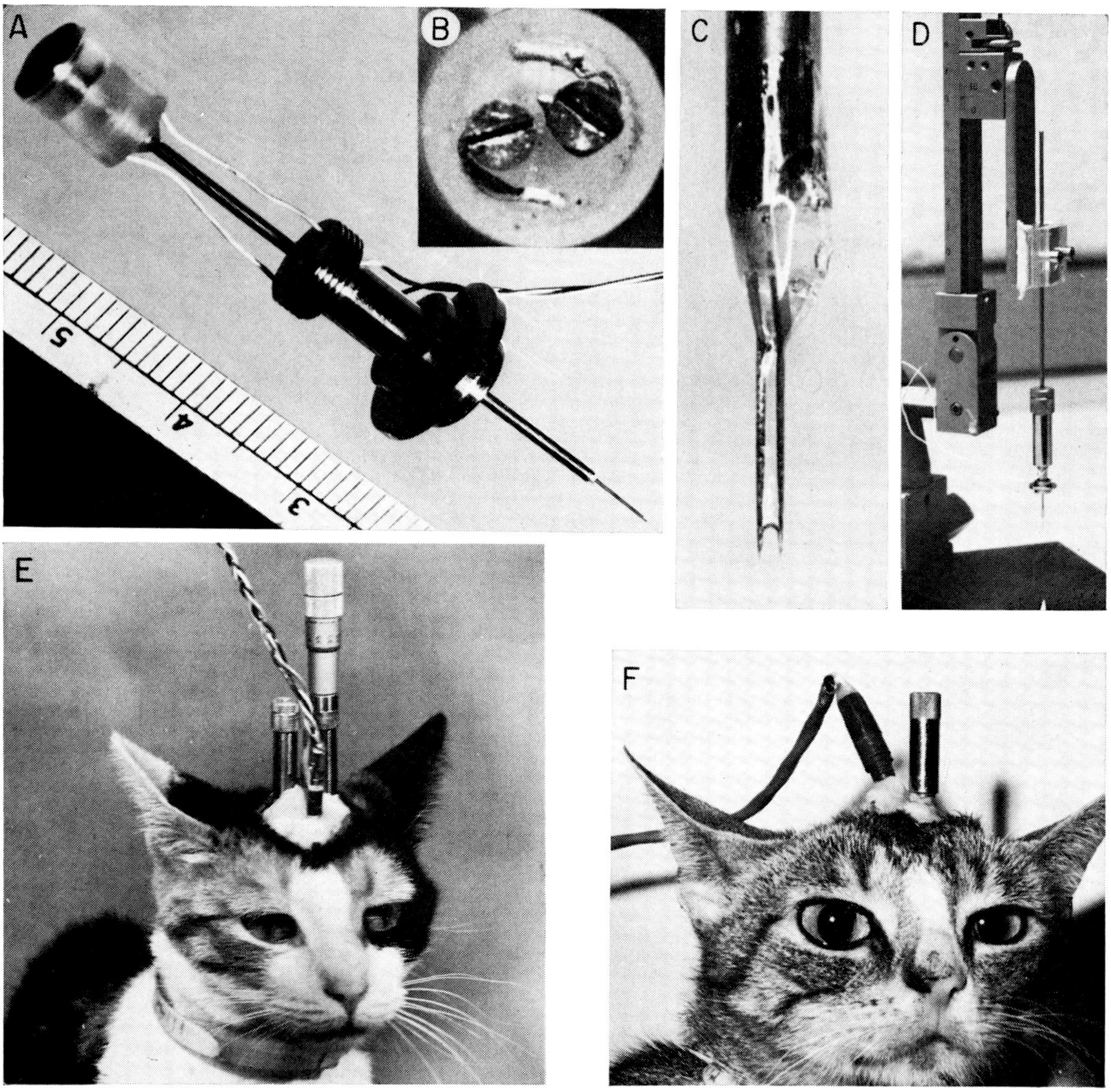

Fig. 1

A: This figure shows the drive base carrying the drive shaft. Two unsharpened electrodes can be seen projecting from the ceramic at the right end of the shaft. The contact cap is in place on the left end of the shaft, connecting the white lead wires to the upper end of the electrodes. *B*: End view of the contact cap with the snap cover removed, exposing the two contact screws and leads. *C*: Two microelectrode tips, insulated with glass which also covers ceramic and end of drive shaft. *D*: View of assembled drive, with protective cover in place, held in stereotaxic holder ready for implantation. Total weight is 9.5 g. *E*: Micro-drive attached to base of left side drive ready to advance electrodes after implantation. Subminiature plug, recording cable, and right side drive can also be seen. *F*: Another cat, showing covered assembly as used for routine recording with stationary electrodes.

(4) The shaft, electrode contacts, and lead wires are then enclosed by a stainless steel cover which screws to the thread on the base. The cover protects the drive shaft from being accidentally jarred and carries a screw plug at its upper end. Removal of the plug permits insertion of a post for attachment to a stereotaxic carrier during implan-

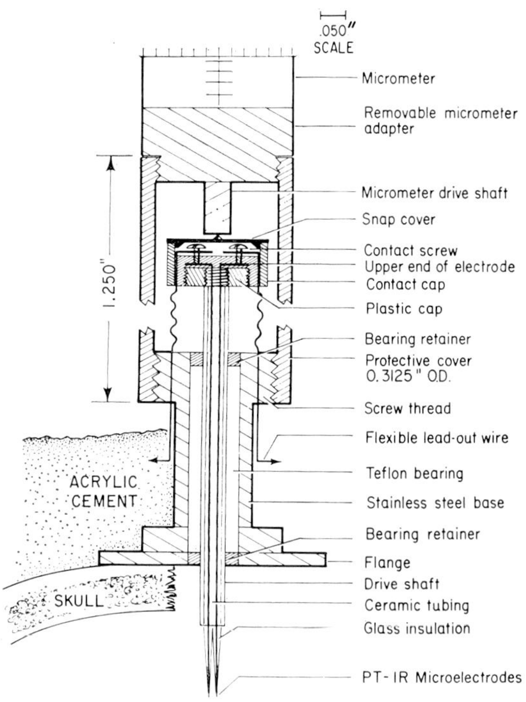

Fig. 2

Detailed cross-sectional drawing of the assembled drive. Scale in inches.

tation. The cover also provides the foundation into which the micro-drive itself is screwed whenever it becomes necessary to move the electrodes.

(5) The micro-drive is a Lufkin 10 mm (20 turns) micrometer, weighing 26 g and fitted with an adapter ring so that it can be screwed into the cover. It is also covered with a Teflon sleeve at the tip to maintain insulation from the electrodes themselves. To move the electrodes, the micrometer is attached to the cover and advanced so as to press against the end of the drive shaft, while the electrode outputs are monitored on an oscilloscope. Once satisfactory neural units are found, the micrometer is carefully removed and the plug reinserted into the cover. At present, no provision exists for mechanical retraction of the electrodes. However, the drive shaft has been manually withdrawn and good unit records obtained on a second penetration[1].

Fig. 3 illustrates single and multiple unit activity recorded at time intervals ranging from 30 to 50 days after implantation.

DISCUSSION

This micro-drive has been used in four animals for periods averaging about 7 months each. We have found it to be of great utility in investigations of behavioral electrophysiology. Specific single cells have been observed for varying periods of time, ranging from a few minutes up to as much as 6 days. Using larger amplification, multiple unit responses of about 40 μV amplitude can be studied for very long periods without the necessity to move the electrode. Pulse height discrimination techniques are used to analyze such activity. We have obtained data with extremely reproducible characteristics from such populations for periods as long as 6 weeks. Preliminary results have already been reported (John and Morgades 1968; Morgades and John 1967, 1968).

SUMMARY

A technique is described for the chronic implantation of multiple movable micro-electrodes. This method permits study of the activity of single or multiple units in the unrestrained animal over long periods of time.

RÉSUMÉ

TECHNIQUE D'IMPLANTATION CHRONIQUE DE MICRO-ÉLECTRODES MULTIPLES ET MOBILES

Une technique est décrite pour l'implantation chronique de micro-électrodes multiples et mobiles. Cette méthode permet l'étude de l'activité d'unités isolées ou multiples

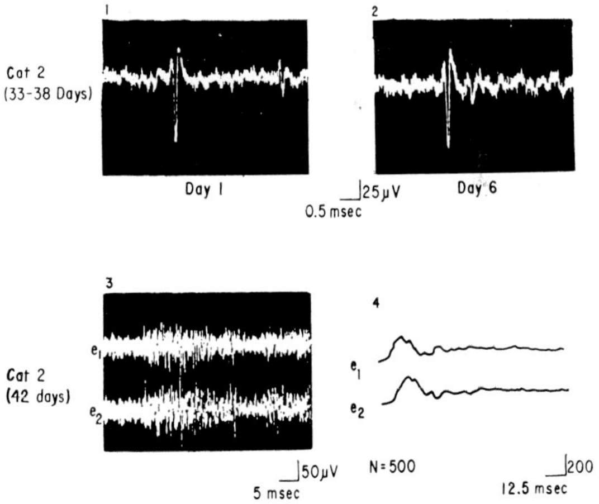

Fig. 3

Results obtained from two micro-drives in the same cat, during performance of conditioned responses. Oscilloscope tracing showing response to light flash of a single unit from the superior colliculus: on the 33rd day (*1*) and on the 38th day (*2*) after implantation. Wave shape and firing patterns (not shown) monitored during these 6 days convince us that these records came from the same cell. (*3*) Multiple unit responses to light flash from two microelectrodes (e_1 and e_2) in medial geniculate body on 42nd day. (*4*) Post-stimulus time histogram ($N = 500$) of multiple unit responses.

[1] Further construction details of the device will be provided to interested researchers upon request.

chez l'animal non maintenu sur des périodes de temps prolongées.

This work was supported by N.I.M.H. Grant MH 08579. We wish to express our appreciation to Dr. M. Verzeano for his great help in the initial stages of this project. We thank Mr. S. Pischinger for his assistance in the design and Mr. L. Keiper for his assistance in the construction of the micro-drive.

REFERENCES

DAVIES, P. W. Chamber for microelectrode studies in the cerebral cortex. *Science*, **1956**, *124*: 179–180.

DAVIS, R. and TOLLOW, A. S. Adjustable stimulating and recording electrodes in brain of the unrestrained animal. A study of red nucleus. *Electroenceph. clin. Neurophysiol.*, **1966**, *21*: 196–200.

EVARTS, E. V. Effects of sleep and waking on spontaneous and evoked discharge of single units in visual cortex. *Fed. Proc.*, **1960**, *19*: 828–837.

EVARTS, E. V. A technique for recording activity of subcortical neurons in moving animals. *Electroenceph. clin. Neurophysiol.*, **1968**, *24*: 83–86.

FUSTER, J. M. Excitation and inhibition of neuronal firing in visual cortex by reticular stimulation. *Science*, **1961**, *133*: 2011–2012.

GOLDBERG, J. M. and GREENWOOD, D. D. Response of neurons of the dorsal and posteroventral cochlear nuclei of the cat to acoustic stimuli of long duration. *J. Neurophysiol.*, **1966**, *29*: 72–93.

GRUNDFEST, H., SENGSTAKEN, R. W., OETTINGER, W. H. and GURRY, R. W. Stainless steel micro-needle electrodes made by electrolytic pointing. *Rev. sci. Instrum.*, **1950**, *21*: 360–361.

GUSEL'NIKOV, V. J. Methods of recording encephalograms in small animals in chronic experiments with the help of microelectrodes. *Zh. vyssh. nerv. Deyat. Pavlova*, **1957**, *7*: 626–628.

HAYWARD, J. N., FAIRCHILD, M. D., STUART, D. G. and DEEMER, J. A. A stereotaxic platform for micro-electrode studies in chronic animals. *Electroenceph. clin. Neurophysiol.*, **1964**, *16*: 522–524.

HUBEL, D. H. Tungsten microelectrode for recording from single units. *Science*, **1957**, *125*: 549–550.

HUBEL, D. H. Cortical unit responses to visual stimuli in nonanesthetized cats. *Amer. J. Ophthal.*, **1958**, *46*: 110–121.

JOHN, E. R. and MORGADES, P. P. Chronic microelectrode studies of conditioned responses in cats. *Fed. Proc.*, **1968**, *27*: 277.

KATSUKI, J., MURATA, K., SUGA, N. and TAKENAKA, T. Electrical activity of cortical auditory neurons of unanaesthetized and unrestrained cat. *Proc. Jap. Acad.*, **1959**, *35*: 571–574.

KOGAN, A. B. A method of electrode implantation in unrestrained animals. *Electroenceph. clin. Neurophysiol.*, **1959**, *11*: 812–813.

MACLEAN, P. D. A chronically fixed stereotaxic device for intracerebral exploration with macro- and micro-electrodes. *Electroenceph. clin. Neurophysiol.*, **1967**, *22*: 180–182.

MORGADES, P. P. and JOHN, E. R. A technique for the chronic implantation of multiple movable microelectrodes. *Physiologist*, **1967**, *10*: 254.

MORGADES, P. P. and JOHN, E. R. Multiple unit and evoked potential correlations with behavior in the trained cat. *Proc. Int. Union physiol. Sci.*, XXIV Int. Congr., Abstracts, **1968**, *7*: 304.

OOMURA, J., OOYAMA, H., NAKA, F. and YAMAMOTO, T. Microelectrode positioners for chronic animals. *Physiol. and Behavior*, **1967**, *2*: 89–91.

RICCI, G., DOANE, B. et JASPER, H. H. Étude du conditionnement au moyen de microélectrodes: Techniques et résultats préliminaires. *4th Int. Congr. Electroenceph. clin. Neurophysiol.*, Abstracts, **1957**: 90–92.

SAWA, M. and DELGADO, J. M. R. Amygdala unitary activity in the unrestrained cat. *Electroenceph. clin. Neurophysiol.*, **1963**, *15*: 637–650.

STRUMWASSER, F. Long term recording from single neurons in brain of unrestrained mammals. *Science*, **1958**, *127*: 469–470.

WOLBARSHT, M. L., MACNICHOL JR., E. F. and WAGNER, H. G. Glass insulated platinum microelectrode. *Science*, **1960**, *125*: 1309–1310.

Reference: JOHN, E. R. and MORGADES, P. P. A technique for the chronic implantation of multiple movable micro-electrodes. *Electroenceph. clin. Neurophysiol.*, **1969**, *27*: 205–208.

Electroencephalography and Clinical Neurophysiology
Elsevier Publishing Company, Amsterdam – Printed in The Netherlands

A PRINTED CIRCUIT SWIVEL FOR RECORDING FROM FREELY MOVING ANIMALS[1]

A. EDELSON AND T. L. HOLDSTOCK

Department of Psychology, University of the Witwatersrand, Johannesburg (South Africa)

(Accepted for publication: November 11, 1968)

When central nervous and autonomic (*e. g.*, heart rate) activities are to be recorded from freely moving animals, swivel devices are called for to prevent the twisting of recording cables. These devices are also necessary when freely moving animals are to be stimulated through chronically implanted electrodes. To cope with these needs, basically two designs for coupling the animal to the electronic equipment have been proposed. In the one, ball races are used as suspension elements and as rotating contacts (Simpson and Valenstein 1963; Johnson *et al.* 1966). In the other kind, concentric grooves filled with some conducting medium, and small tubes dipping into it, are used (Sutton and Miller 1963; Ballintijn 1965; Berkley and Kling 1967; Mundl 1967; Anschel 1968).

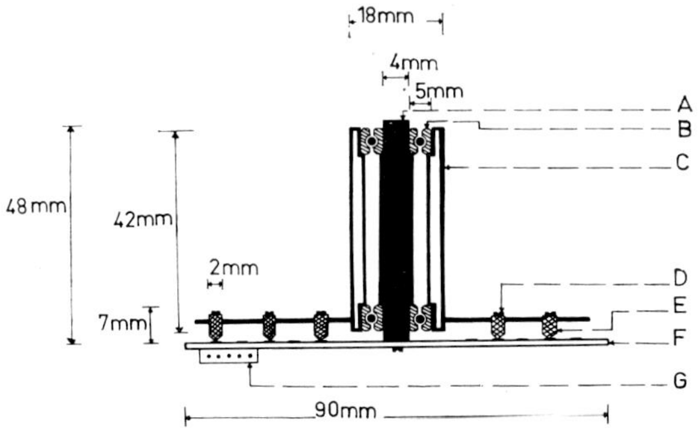

Fig. 1
Cross-section of swivel. A, aluminium shaft, 5 mm × 48 mm (shouldered to 4 mm for 7 mm at both its ends); B, ball bearing, 4 mm bore, 13 mm outside diameter; C, plexiglass block, 18mm × 18 mm × 48 mm (the shaft diameter of 13.5 mm is slightly widened for 5 mm at both ends to allow press-fit of ball bearing); D, brush retaining screw; E, nickel-plated brush of braided copper wire ("Monogram" toy racing car contacts); F, epoxy glass printed circuit board (0.035 mm copper on one side); G, 5-pin connector (Amphenol).

A third kind of design is presented in Fig. 1 and 2. It is easily constructed, inexpensive and has low electrical noise in stimulating and recording. The design, furthermore, is flexible and lends itself readily to modification.

The basic component of the swivel consists in a printed circuit board (F). The center of the board is screwed on to an aluminium shaft (A) which runs in two small ball bearings (B). The bearings are press-fitted at the bottom and top of a plexiglass block (C). Concentric circuits, five in this instance, are printed on the board (H). The circuits are drawn with Maruzen wonder ink and ammonium persulphate is used to dissolve the copper not covered by the ink. During rotation of the board the concentric circuits provide continuous contact with nickel-plated brushes of braided copper wire (E). The copper brushes are mounted on a plexiglass bar which is attached to the block by means of a mounting bracket. Each circuit is separately connected to a 5-pin connector (G), mounted on the underside and towards the edge of the printed circuit board. By mounting it towards the edge, the least amount of torsion on the connecting cable causes the disk to rotate freely. It thus does not depend on wire twist to transmit turning torque to the coupler. However, a coiled spring of

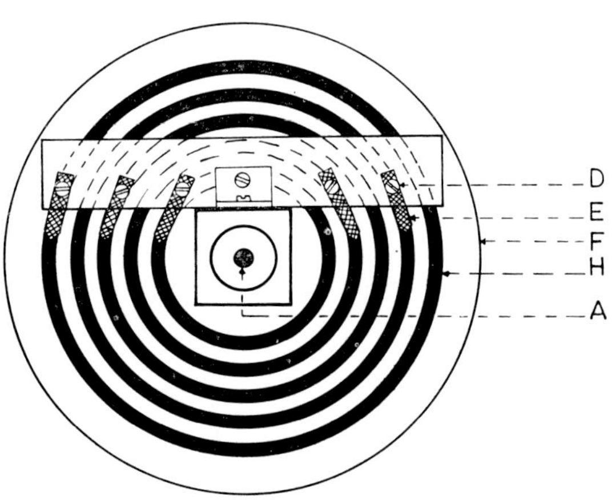

Fig. 2
Plan view of swivel. H, printed circuit. Other symbols as before.

[1] The development of this apparatus was supported by the South African Council for Social Research and by the American Psychological Foundation.

No. 2 guitar wire has been used as the core of the connecting cable, primarily for the purpose of taking up the slack as the animal moves about. With this arrangement thermal potentials of 5–10 μV, as well as a variation in resistance of 2 Ω, were measured between the leads from the animal and the output from the printed circuit board. Further reduction of noise can be obtained by gold-plating the tracks and the brushes as well as by using a sliding contact lubricant. It is also suggested that low-noise[1] cables be used between the animal and swivel to assure artifact-free transmission of low level signals.

By slightly modifying the design an alternative method, similar to that proposed by Berkley and Kling (1967), can be used to take up the slack in the recording cable. In this case, the printed circuit board is the fixed element and the brush holder is the part that rotates. The pin connector is attached to one end of the brush holder and a pulley to the other end. The cable from the test subject runs over the pulley and is looped below the rotating bar before being inserted into the pin connector. The loop in the connecting cable is maintained with a counter-weight and provides movement compensation.

None of the dimensions of the swivel appears to be critical. By reducing the width and the distance between circuits (2 mm), as well as staggering the brushes on alternate tracks, many circuits can be accommodated in a relatively small space. Although we have used the swivel primarily to record EEG activity, heart rate and muscle potentials in white rats, the device lends itself readily to use with other species.

SUMMARY

The twisting of electric cables is a major problem when physiological signals are recorded from freely moving animals. A new design for a swivel to overcome this problem is described. As the animal moves about, concentric printed circuits fixed to a rotatable shaft provide continuous contact with nickel-plated brushes of braided copper wire. The swivel has low electrical noise, it is easy to construct, inexpensive, and lends itself readily to modification.

[1] Mininoise Cable, No. 50–3804, Microdot Inc., Pasadena, Calif.

RÉSUMÉ

ROTULE À CIRCUIT IMPRIMÉ POUR L'ENREGISTREMENT DES SIGNAUX PHYSIOLOGIQUES CHEZ DES ANIMAUX LIBRES

Lorsqu'on enregistre des signaux physiologiques sur des animaux libres, un problème important est posé par la torsion du câble électrique. Pour résoudre ce problème, l'auteur décrit un nouveau modèle de rotule. Lorsque l'animal bouge, un arrangement de circuits imprimés concentriques montés sur un arbre rotatif permet la continuité du contact avec des faisceaux de fil de cuivre tressé. La rotule elle-même a peu d'effets électrostatiques, est simple à construire, peu coûteuse, et se prête aisément à des modifications.

REFERENCES

Anschel, S. A commutator and cable for squirrel monkeys. *Physiol. Behav.*, **1968,** *3*: 591–592.

Ballintijn, C. M. Electric recording from unnarcotized unrestrained small animals. *Med. Electron. biol. Engng.*, **1965,** *3*: 71–73.

Berkley, M. A. and Kling, J. W. A small animal cable complex with vertical movement compensation. *Physiol. Behav.*, **1967**, *2*: 315–316.

Johnson, R. N., Trehub, A. and Pietskowski, E. An easily constructed cable swivel device for brain stimulation experiments. *J. exp. Anal. Behav.*, **1966,** *9*: 17–18.

Mundl, W. J. An improved swivel for recording from behaving subjects. *Electroenceph. clin. Neurophysiol.*, **1967,** *23*: 483–485.

Simpson, R. and Valenstein, E. S. An inexpensive swivel-device for electrical stimulation of unrestrained animals. *Electroenceph. clin. Neurophysiol.*, **1963,** *15*: 900–901.

Sutton, D. and Miller, J. M. Implanted electrodes: cable coupler for elimination of movement artifact. *Science*, **1963,** *140*: 988–989.

Reference: Edelson, A. and Holdstock, T. L. A printed circuit swivel for recording from freely moving animals. *Electroenceph. clin. Neurophysiol.*, **1969**, *27*: 209–210.

Electroencephalography and Clinical Neurophysiology
Elsevier Publishing Company, Amsterdam – Printed in The Netherlands

SOCIETY PROCEEDINGS

ÖSTERREICHISCHE GESELLSCHAFT FÜR ELECTROENCEPHALOGRAPHIE

Vienna, November 25, 1967

Secretary: Dr. Erich Scherzer

Allgemeine Unfallversicherungsanstalt, 2, Webergasse, A–1200 Vienna (Austria)

1. EEG investigations in measles encephalitis. — S. Enge (Graz).

Our investigations relate to 18 former patients who were acutely ill with measles encephalitis in the years 1949–1965. The average age at the time of the illness was little more than 6 years and at the control investigation the figure was 13.5 years; the interval between the illness and the time of the control investigation was on the average 7.5 years. In 14 children it was possible to record the EEG in the acute stage of the disease. In only one case was the record unremarkable (clinically a predominantly spinal affection); in all the remaining 13 cases there were pathological records, mostly with marked diffuse generalized changes. The time taken for restoration of normality was relatively short; at the times of discharge, out of 12 EEGs 6 were already normal. The more severe the acute illness, the longer a pathological EEG persisted. At the time of the control investigation (1966), out of the total of 18 cases 8 had normal EEGs and in 10 the EEG was pathological, in which a remarkably high percentage (8 cases) of epileptic activity was observed (in 6 cases generalized and in 2 focal). In comparison with the findings at discharge, in 5 cases there was a new development, the recurrence of pathological activity, mostly in the form of specific changes. It was demonstrated, in correlation with the clinical deficits, that in the younger children the encephalitis took a more severe course, and in these children both neurological and psychic deficits, and also pathological EEGs, were much more frequently noted at the control investigation. The more severe the course the encephalitis took at the time, the earlier were there consequential appearances, and thus the latent time for the younger children was relatively short. The significance of electroencephalographic longitudinal studies is underlined, in order to uncover cerebral complications early, *e.g.* residual damage, before this manifests itself clinically.

2. Psychomotor status epilepticus. — C. Förster, A. Ross and J. Kugler (Munich, Germany).

During the last 10 years we examined 100 patients suffering from status epilepticus. One third of these patients showed grand mal status, one third petit mal status and one third status of partial seizures. Only 2 of the patients were proved to have a temporal focal discharge during the status. The clinical symptoms consisted of repeated psychomotor seizures. The percentage of epileptic patients without status and with unilateral temporal alterations in the EEG, however, amounts to more than 20%. Clinical and electrical symptoms correspond to a psychomotor status in the two cases we described. Obviously a rapid clinical or electrical generalization occurs in most of the patients showing partial seizures when they are in status. Therefore the existence of local abnormalities and clinical manifestations of psychomotor status can rarely be observed. A critical objection to a method, frequently used, of interpreting an EEG results from these observations: generalized abnormalities in a patient showing status cannot rule out an origin of seizures strictly localized to a certain region of one hemisphere. We add to the cases of psychomotor status previously published by other authors two of our observations showing a well defined form of temporal lobe status.

3. Siblings with Unverricht-Lundborg myoclonic epilepsy; a familial and longitudinal investigation. — G. S. Barolin and K. Pateisky (Vienna).

A brother and sister displayed with photographic uniformity the same courses of disease: grand mal with visual aura as the first manifestation after puberty —myoclonic episodes 1 year later—increase in attacks and a progressive psychic syndrome—death 3 years after the beginning of the illness. Typical myoclonic bodies were demonstrated in the brain, liver and cardiac muscle.

The EEG findings in the early stage after the first grand mal attacks were: uncharacteristic bilaterally synchronous theta and spike outbursts; in the myoclonic stage: typical rhythmic recurrent short groups of irregular spikes; in the final stage: severe disturbance of background rhythm and irregular groups with high voltage spikes. Flicker exerted a strong stimulating effect on the cerebral electrical pattern as well as clinically on the myoclonus. In polygraphic recording the muscle twitches were by no means always synchronous with the cerebral spikes. Nitrazepam suppressed the myoclonic cerebral and clinical patterns and the photosensitivity. The irregular slow background activity then remained without rhythmic spike discharges.

Investigation of all available members of the family produced normal results clinically, neurologically and electroencephalographically. Notably, chromosome analyses in the patients and their family were unexceptional.

4. Beta activity and older age. — C. Spunda (Vienna).

The frequency of occurrence of strongly expressed or dominant beta activity was studied in a group of 5010 cases. This group included 660 hemisphere tumours, 529 psychiatric illnesses, 571 head injuries and 3250 cerebrovascular cases. The average frequency of beta activity was 16.5%, being lowest with the tumours (10.6%) and highest with the vascular cases (18.1%).

The whole group of patients was divided into those of up to 60 years of age and those older than this. There were significant statistical differences only in the psychiatric and head injury cases, in which beta increases were two to three times as frequent in the older cases. The rest, including vascular cases, showed only minor differences. The practical significance of an increase of beta activity as a sole pathological finding must, therefore, be doubted.

5. Retrograde amnesia in experimental anaesthesia. A contribution to memory theories. — J. Kugler, M. Laub and A. Doenicke (Munich, Germany).

Eight healthy volunteers were anaesthetized twice. First, they received Epontol (propanidid) 7 mg/kg i.v. in 5 sec. One week later the same dose was injected in 20 sec. The persons were asked a simple question, to be answered by yes or no, 10 sec before starting the injection, at the first moment of injecting the substance and 10 sec after starting the injection. Anaesthesia was produced within 20 sec after starting a rapid injection and within 30 sec if the substance was given slowly. Depth of anaesthesia, EEG changes and interval to the first clinically observable awakening reactions showed no significant differences. Serum determination of Epontol yielded incomplete degradation 10 min after rapid and 20 min after slow injection. At the 25th min after rapid injection the persons were able to reproduce all test questions correctly; a retrograde amnesia of a maximal duration of 10 sec cannot be ruled out. At the 25th min after slow injection almost no single question of the third group was remembered, but half the questions of the second group and all but one of the first group. There was a retrograde amnesia persisting for an average of 25 sec. The differences in duration of retrograde amnesia corresponded with differences in the velocity of degradation of Epontol, in contrast to the depth and duration of anaesthesia, in which no differences could be observed. We suppose that a functional disturbance of brain cells outlasted the interval of anaesthesia without showing any significant changes in the EEG. This disturbance is important for fixation of psychic processes and retrograde extinction of memory. How these results are consistent with theories of memory based on specific induction and with new theories of specific excitation is discussed (Rohracher).

6. Electronystagmographic findings in disturbances of the optokinetic reaction. — E. Scherzer (Vienna).

Electronystagmography offers us two methods of detecting an optokinetic disturbance: (1) the release of nystagmus by means of an optokinetic stimulus pattern and (2) recording of the smooth pursuit movements by the eyes of a sinusoidal visual stimulus (pendular movement).

Disturbances of the optokinetic reaction can be caused by reduced attentiveness or psychogenic inhibition. In these cases we demonstrate optokinetic nystagmus best by rotation of the patient in the rotating chair, with constant angular velocity and open eyes. Furthermore, there are also organically caused optokinetic disturbances which always point to a central lesion and consist in a reduction of the physiological reaction. Such disturbances, in our experience, are best recognized by decrease of the angular velocity of the slow phase of nystagmus (threshold value 20% for horizontal lateral differences). Coarser disturbances frequently lead to disintegration of nystagmus, which occurs especially with rapidly moving stimulus patterns.

The most severe disturbance in patients is represented by the complete absence of optokinetic reaction. Most frequently we found horizontal optokinetic disturbances: contralateral decrease with lesions in the cerebrum and thalamic region, ipsilateral decrease with lesions in the midbrain and pons. Disturbances of vertical optokinetic nystagmus were rare and were related to bilateral lesions in the midbrain. Optokinetic disturbances in all directions, provided that psychogenic inhibition and blindness were excepted, were related to sizable bilateral cerebral foci or to severe bilateral lesions of the midbrain and pons.

Aetiologically all central affections come into question, but also cases with congenital fixation nystagmus. In this, electronystagmographically there is often an inversion of the optokinetic response besides its reduction and irregularity. Bilateral horizontal disturbances of the optokinetic reaction were at times difficult to establish and showed themselves most distinctly by isolated testing of ocular pursuit movements in response to a sinusoidal stimulus. This resulted in saccades in the otherwise regular curves on both sides.

7. The diagnostic possibilities of the EMG in tetany. — E. Lorenzoni (Graz).

198 patients who might have had tetany were examined electromyographically. Of these, 63 had positive EMG signs of tetany in the form of doublets or multiplets. Recording was from the relaxed hand musculature, with arterial occlusion and hyperventilation for 3 min.

No correlation could be found between the EMG and the potassium/calcium levels in the blood. A disturbance of potassium or calcium level was found in 41 % of the patients with positive EMG signs of tetany and in 43 % of those with negative EMGs. Hypokalaemia was most frequent, followed by hypercalcaemia; hypocalcaemia was in only the third place, with other alterations of the potassium/calcium ratio last. Signs of tetany in the EMG can be considered as expressions of a neuromuscular over-excitability generated by disturbances of potassium or calcium levels, but they are not necessarily produced in these conditions. The EMG shows a better correlation with the electrical excitability of peripheral nerves, as demonstrated by the cathodal-break twitch. In the majority of patients with positive signs of tetany in the EMG the electrical excitability was raised, while in those with negative EMGs it was normal in most cases. In establishing the clinical diagnosis the EMG was taken into account extensively and the diagnosis of tetany was made in the great majority of cases by positive tetanic signs in the EMG, as well as on clinical grounds. Thus it follows that the EMG is the most sensitive method of investigation in tetany.

8. EEG computer audiometry. — K. Burian, G. F. Gestring and S. Hruby (Vienna).

Perception of sensory excitation causes EEG desynchronization; with the aid of averaging computers stimuli approaching threshold intensities can be detected. This 16 mm colourfilm demonstrates and explains a clinical technique of applying this phenomenon to determine the functional threshold of the ear, independent of the patient's cooperation. Following a basic explanation of the simple averaging computer the clinical arrangement is shown schematically and explained in detail. A patient is examined and the result interpreted. In a clinically deaf child the negative screening test is demonstrated; the following EEG computer audiometry shows the ear and acoustic nerve to be intact. In some children with gross EEG abnormalities the simple tone stimulus is inadequate for threshold evaluation; by interaction between two sensory stimuli at predetermined intervals between 70 and 200 msec, objective audiograms with an accuracy of ± 5 dB can be achieved. The child demonstrated shows normal ECA findings and was referred to psychiatric treatment, where it is responding very well. Prescription of a hearing aid in cases of clinical deafness associated with normal ECA findings is, in the authors' opinion, contraindicated.

9. Clinical application of the EEG analysis of intersensory interaction. — K. Burian, G. F. Gestring and S. Hruby (Vienna).

The EEG analysis of 2 sensory stimuli at a given interval permits the authors an indirect evaluation of minute sensory excitation. While perceived stimuli of all modalities will evoke a wave complex in the normal EEG, near-threshold stimulation frequently fails to evoke such a complex in the pathological EEG with reproducible accuracy. In these cases the proof of peripheral perception can be obtained by observing the effect which a stimulus of this intensity has on the response to a second, stronger and clearly visible, stimulus given at an interval of a few milliseconds. This second stimulus need not be of the same modality: non-interaction proves the first stimulus to be unperceived. Algebraic summation of both responses is shown not only if the same modality is used for both stimuli, but also if, for instance, acoustic and visual signals are offered at an interval of 150 msec.

In the clinic the authors use intersensory interactions for children when acoustic threshold determinations cannot be achieved by the conventional method.

10. Determination of sensitivity by EEG analysis. — H. Jantsch and G. F. Gestring (Vienna).

Sensory perception evokes alterations in the EEG rhythms. Event-linked computer analysis permits not only near-threshold evaluation of sensory stimuli but also determination of the over-all conduction time required for impulse transmission from the stimulated organ to the brain. EEG computer audiometry is based on this phenomena (Burian *et al.*, *Wien. klin. Wschr.*, 1967, *79*: 535). If an electrical impulse is applied to a cutaneous area and time-linked EEG analysis is performed, a characteristic bi- or triphasic wave complex appears 150–300 msec later in an unspecific (vertex-mastoid) derivation only if the stimulus is perceived by the patient. The amplitude of the second positive peak increases to a certain extent with increased stimulation but fails to appear if an anaesthetic area is stimulated, thus permitting an objective determination of diminution of sensation.

By comparative right–left cutaneous stimulation unilateral conduction time increases were seen following peripheral nerve transplantations (ulnar) even after sensation had returned to the affected area.

In a patient suffering from a herniated nucleus pulposus, mapping stimulation showed the most pronounced response delay to occur on stimulating the cutaneous area representing L4; surgery confirmed the exact location of the lesion. This method does not depend on patient cooperation, permitting its use in comatose or anaesthetized patients and small children.

11. Computer analysis of cortical responses to stimulation of specific thalamic nuclei in man. — J. A. Ganglberger, G. F. Gestring, E. Groll-Knapp, G. Guttmann and M. Haider (Vienna).

Routine controls necessary to assure accurate placement of intracerebral electrodes during stereotactic surgery enabled the authors to stimulate specific and non-specific thalamic nuclei in the human brain. Subperiosteal and cortical electrodes fed the potentials into a Mingograf EEG apparatus for direct visible tracings and "on line" into a CAT 1000. Simultaneously an

FM analogue magnetic tape recorder was used for storage and subsequent evaluation. The cortical response to thalamic stimulation consists in a reproducible wave complex whose main characteristics are detectable by conventional EEG techniques. Following the stimulus artefact a first wave component is described in the literature with a peak latency of 20–25 msec, which is followed by two much slower waves. One of us previously described phase reversal of this first component over the motor region on stimulation of specific thalamic motor nuclei, while the last slow wave remains in-phase throughout the hemisphere. With our method we were able to detect much faster positive components, appearing 2.5–5.5 msec (deflection time) after the stimulus. We feel that this early component is the so-called primary response of the motor cortex to specific thalamic stimulation. Although this early component was previously postulated from neuroanatomical evidence, this seems to be the first electrophysiological proof of the existence of the primary motor response in man. Further analysis in progress will elucidate the involvement and relationship of specific and non-specific projection systems in the formation of this complex cortical response.

12. Expectancy, readiness and orienting potentials from thalamic and cortical leads in man. — M. Haider, J. A. Ganglberger, G. F. Gestring, E. Groll-Knapp and G. Guttmann (Vienna).

Computer analyses of slow potential changes associated with orienting, motor readiness and expectancy reactions were performed during electrophysiological controls of the intracerebral electrode position in stereotactic surgery. It was found that clicks applied to the patient regularly at a constant interval of 1.1 sec always evoked a response in the cortical and scalp leads, while the potentials recorded from the motor nuclei of the thalamus showed wide variations in amplitude and even totally failed to appear in some patients. On the other hand if irregular clicks were interspersed randomly between the regular clicks a pronounced wave complex appeared in the thalamic leads preceding the late components of cortical evoked potentials. If the patient was asked to push a button every time he heard an irregular click, this thalamic potential was greatly augmented and followed by a slowly rising motor readiness potential in the cortex. The authors show that long lasting expectancy waves in the cortex are likewise preceded by a positive change appearing in the thalamic motor nuclei.

Electroenceph. clin. Neurophysiol., **1969,** *27*: 211–214

NEDERLANDSE VERENIGING VOOR ELEKTRO-ENCEFALOGRAFIE EN KLINISCHE NEUROFYSIOLOGIE

Utrecht, November 2, 1968

Secretary: S. L. Visser

94, Keizer Karelweg, Amstelveen (The Netherlands)

SYMPOSIUM ON THE SIGNIFICANCE OF EEG FOR "STATEMENT ON DEATH"

1. Introduction. — W. Storm van Leeuwen (Utrecht).

The "Statement on death" which was accepted by the General Assembly of the World Medical Association in August of this year in Sydney was discussed. Moreover, part of a declaration on heart transplantation, as stated at a Conference of C.I.O.M.S. in June of this year in Geneva, was considered. The recommendations were thought to be generally agreeable.

Concerning the significance of EEG for the diagnosis of death it was generally agreed that cerebral death cannot be pronounced so long as any EEG potential differences, however feeble, can be recorded. The problem turns around the conditions in which no electrical brain activity can be recorded at the scalp and has the following aspects:

a. Terminology; terms in use are: electrical silence, isoelectric EEG, rectilinear curve. Proposed is the use of isoelectric EEG.

b. Recording techniques. Proposed is the use of: (1) derivations with large inter-electrode distances; (2) minimal time constant 1 sec; (3) minimal HF response 30 c/sec; (4) minimal amplification 30 μV/cm. If the investigation cannot be carried out at these parameters, increased caution is necessary.

c. Significance of duration of isoelectric EEG. No specific agreement was reached. The matter depends too much on other factors.

d. Significance for cerebral function of isoelectric

EEG. Its meaning is disappearance of at least part of the function of the cortex. It does not mean that subcortical function is absent. A case was presented showing an isoelectric EEG in a patient in whom many brain-stem reflexes were present.

2. Cerebral death and the isoelectric EEG. (Review of literature). — E. J. Jonkman (Wassenaar).

Before making the decision that an EEG is to be considered as isoelectric certain technical criteria have to be met. It appears that these criteria are ill-defined in the literature. Recording times of at least 1 h, amplifications of 2–3 μV/mm and the use of a time constant of at least 0.3 sec are considered to be necessary. The question arises whether an isoelectric EEG can be a transitory phenomenon. Apart from short lasting anoxia and deep hypothermia this can occur in rare cases of barbiturate poisoning (Bird) and possibly in some cases of encephalitis (Bental, Hamlin).

The criteria for the diagnosis of cerebral death, as given by several authors, can be summarized as follows: (1) absence of all response to stimulation, areflexia, generalized hypotonia; (2) loss of regulation of blood pressure and body temperature; (3) absence of spontaneous respiration; (4) an EEG which is isoelectric during at least 24 h; (5) absence of changes of heart rate on ocular compression, carotid sinus massage and i.v. atropine; (6) normal values of blood sugar and serum electrolytes; (7) satisfactory information concerning the cause of the coma (exclude barbiturate poisoning). The presence of an EEG is compatible with the diagnosis of cerebral death.

Two cases were presented in which the isoelectric EEG was not a sign of cerebral death. (1) In a case of congenital external hydrocephalus no EEG could be recorded. After removal of the extracerebral fluid by surgical procedures, an EEG appeared. Mental development of the child was only mildly impaired. (2) In a child of 2 years an acute encephalopathy of unknown origin gave rise to a massive cerebral oedema. This led to a state of decortication. Subcortical functions, spontaneous swallowing and reflexes were preserved. The EEG remained isoelectric during the observation period of 5 months. Cortical biopsy showed severe anoxic damage to ganglion cells. With a depth electrode subcortical activity could be found. This case will be published in detail elsewhere.

3. A retrospective investigation of the clinical symptoms and course of patients with a complete or incomplete isoelectric EEG. — H. Leenstra-Borsje, S. Boonstra, E. J. Blokzijl and S. L. H. Notermans (Groningen).

From EEG reports were selected 45 patients with complete (35) or incomplete (10) isoelectric records. All patients were in deep coma; almost all of them were treated with mechanical ventilation and antihypotensive medicines. All patients died except in 2 cases of barbiturate intoxication. Of the 35 patients with a completely isoelectric EEG, 28 showed all signs of clinical cerebral death (absence of spontaneous respiration, total areflexia and hypotonia, dilated pupils without reactivity), whereas 7 had one or more remaining symptoms of clinical CNS activity (some tendon reflexes, some spontaneous respiration and, in 1 case, a positive pupillary reaction). Of the 10 patients with an incompletely isoelectric EEG 3 had all the signs of clinical cerebral death (only a few alpha and theta waves of low voltage in the EEG), the remaining 7 having one or more "positive" clinical CNS signs. The survival time after a completely or incompletely isoelectric EEG was determined: 30 of the 45 patients died within the first 24 h, 6 during the second 24 h. Only 3 patients with a completely isoelectric EEG survived beyond 48 h; they succumbed on the 3rd, 8th and 9th days, respectively. In patients with a completely isoelectric EEG, during 0.5 h recording, the presence of some "positive" clinical CNS sign did not appear to influence the survival time. In 2 cases with a completely isoelectric EEG a follow-up showed some cerebral electrical activity after 7 h and 2 days respectively, but these patients still expired.

Amongst other conclusions it was stated that an isoelectric EEG is not an absolute proof of cerebral death, that it should always be dealt with in the context of the findings of the clinical physician and that, at least in cases with ethical or legal problems, an EEG should be indicated as an additional means for the correct diagnosis of cerebral death.

4. Two cases of isoelectric EEGs ("Apparent exceptions proving the rule"). — S. L. Visser (Amsterdam).

1. Woman, 27 years. Coma for 47 days. Initially slow (theta and delta) activity in the EEG. Clinically no spontaneous respiration but persistence of some muscular reflexes. The EEG remained isoelectric from the 12th to the last day. Nevertheless recording with depth electrodes on the 37th day showed theta and delta activity in bursts bilaterally in the thalamic region. On the 47th day cardiac arrest.

2. Woman, 76 years. Coma for 7 days. From the beginning of the coma to the end an isoelectric EEG. Clinically there were no reflexes, yet the respiration remained (after a short initial arrest) spontaneous. It may be wondered whether this could be caused by the hypothyroidism from which the patient suffered. The EEG remained isoelectric. On the 7th day sudden cardiac and respiratory arrest.

Both cases demonstrate the unfavourable prognosis of the isoelectric EEG in spite of reflexes or spontaneous respiration. A silent scalp EEG does not mean that subcortical regions are also always isoelectric. Therefore it is better to speak in terms of statistics (the chance of a fatal prognosis is 100%) rather than in philosophical terms such as "cerebral death".

Electroenceph. clin. Neurophysiol., **1969**, *27*: 214–215

Electroencephalography and Clinical Neurophysiology
Elsevier Publishing Company, Amsterdam – Printed in The Netherlands

ISRAEL SOCIETY FOR ELECTROENCEPHALOGRAPHY AND NEUROPHYSIOLOGY

Jerusalem, May 5, 1968

Secretary: Dr. S. Lavy

Mayer de Rothschild Hadassah University Hospital, P.O. Box 499, Jerusalem (Israel)

1. Hypsarrhythmia. — P. Lerman (Petah Tikwa).

The clinical manifestations characteristic of hypsarrhythmia were recognized as long as 120 years ago. The EEG changes in this disorder, first described by Gibbs and Gibbs, assume different forms, varying according to the heterogeneous aetiology and the patient's age. In this presentation EEG samples from 12 infants, 6 weeks to 3 years old, with hypsarrhythmic tracings are shown and analysed. The case histories are briefly presented. Aetiological factors are discussed as well as the clinical and electrical aspects. The results of ACTH therapy are shown and commented upon. The clinical and EEG evolution is illustrated in cases with a long follow-up.

The cases are clinically classified into 2 main groups: (a) those displaying evidence of primary brain damage; (b) those lacking evidence of primary brain damage.

The tracings are classified into the following categories: (1) diffuse dysrhythmia; (2) unilateral dysrhythmia; (3) prevalent slow hypersynchrony; (4) prevalent sharp transients — synchronous and asynchronous spike discharges. An EEG pattern, called pre-hypsarrhythmia by some authors, is described as seen in very young infants (under 3 months of age). The variations between sleep and waking tracings are described. The prognostic value of EEG studies in patients suffering from infantile spasms is discussed.

2. Electroencephalographic changes in anovulatory cycles. — E. Bental, B. Sharf, M. Sharf and T. Kuzminsky (Haifa).

An EEG survey was performed on 45 women, aged 20–41 years, suffering from anovulatory cycles. All of them had previous clinical, hormonal, cytological and endoscopic examinations and were thereupon treated with clomiphene citrate. EEG examinations were performed on each of them before, during and after this treatment. The same standard procedures of examination were applied to all, namely: waking record and hyperventilation for 3 min, as well as photic stimulation.

The EEG examinations gave the following results: 20 (45%) were classified as within normal limits and 25 (55%) as abnormal. In 19 cases the abnormality consisted of irregular background activity and diffuse theta waves at 5–7 c/sec, bilateral, mainly temporo-parietal. In 7 cases there were short general bursts of slow activity and in 5 other cases delta waves at 3 c/sec The abnormalities appeared mainly during overbreathing and photic stimulation. Of the 25 cases with abnormal EEGs before treatment with clomiphene, 13 (52%) showed reversal to normal after the treatment. All of these women had ovulation and in 4 cases pregnancy occurred.

The high percentage of abnormal EEGs in our group seems to justify the assumption that the EEG disturbances probably indicate a diencephalic-hypothalamic disturbance. The fact that clomiphene, which is supposed to act on the median eminence and anterior hypothalamus, caused reversal of the EEG abnormalities seems further to support this hypothesis. In view of this preliminary observation it seems justified to perform an EEG examination of all cases with anovulatory cycles.

3. Petit mal-like discharge in the electroencephalograms of adults. — M. Elian (Petah Tikwa).

There is general agreement as to the age specificity of the 3–4 c/sec generalized spike and wave discharge, which appears most frequently between the ages of 4–16 years and tends to disappear around the end of the second decade. Experiments in animals confirm the concept that the petit mal-like discharge is more closely related to age than to any other aetiological factor. Since it is an easily recognizable pattern, its appearance for the first time in an adult becomes noteworthy. Two patients are described in whom somewhat irregular generalized spike and wave discharges were seen on several occasions. Clinically, one had only grand mal seizures (which had begun at the age of 26, with the petit mal-like discharge first noted 3 years later). The other had one episode of confusion, lasting several hours, at the age of 55 and on one occasion rhythmic eyelid flutter was noted during a typical electrical discharge. In both these patients the neurological examination, laboratory tests and pneumoencephalography were all normal. The concept of secondary synchrony and the relation of the abnormality to various intracranial tumours, to pubertas praecox and other hormonal changes, and to a genetic determination are discussed. The nature and cause of the age dependency of the petit mal-like discharge is as yet unknown, and there is no answer to the question of why this relationship to youth was not preserved in a few patients.

4. EEG changes in uraemic patients undergoing regular haemodialysis. — S. Lavy and A. Aviram (Jerusalem).

Six patients with chronic renal failure treated by regular haemodialysis with the Kiil artificial kidney were examined. Five patients had already attended the program for 8–18 months and one was only starting. All of them were fairly rehabilitated. Blood chemistry was similar in all patients, revealing before dialysis moderate uraemia (80–160 mg%, creatinine 12–19 mg%), slight elevation of serum potassium and mild acidosis. These parameters became almost normal after 12 h of dialysis, only blood creatinine sustained at a relatively high level (4–6 mg%).

EEGs were obtained twice in each patient, before and 24 h after dialysis. In 5 cases diffuse EEG abnormalities were noted before the dialysis, consisting of absence of alpha activity and the appearance of a large amount of irregular large amplitude 2–6 c/sec activity, more accentuated in the posterior areas. During overbreathing additional slowing of the background activity was noted. The tracings of the same patients obtained 24 h after haemodialysis showed additional deterioration of the background, manifested by an increase of the slow activity already noted in the pre-dialysis record and accentuated in the posterior cerebral areas. Only in one case were the pre- and post-dialysis EEGs normal.

The high incidence of EEG abnormalities found in patients with chronic renal failure under regular haemodialysis showed no correlation with the biochemical state. The delayed clearance of uraemic products from the CSF and the osmotic disequilibrium between the CSF and the blood following haemodialysis may be considered to be the cause of the EEG disturbances.

5. Changes in the electroretinogram (ERG) in lesions of the optic nerve. — M. Feinsod and E. Auerbach (Jerusalem).

There are reports in the literature concerning cerebral control of retinal activity by an inhibitory influence through centrifugal optic nerve fibres. Optic nerve injury may involve these centrifugal fibres (lately described also in man) and abolish the inhibitory influence, resulting in supernormal retinal responses. However, the expected supernormal ERG was not always found. Measurements of the ERG and the visual evoked responses of patients with optic nerve lesions indicated that a supernormal ERG is but one of the results of abolished centrifugal influence. The present study makes it likely that the kinetics of the mechanisms governing ERG recovery are also involved.

While ERG recovery in the normal visual system is completed after 20–30 min, in optic nerve lesions the ERG generally continues to grow beyond this period of time in the dark, as observed in 3 patients. Repeated ERG tests during two attacks of retrobulbar neuritis were carried out in one patient. These tests make it seem more likely that the centrifugal fibres are more sensitive to pathological conditions of the optic nerve than the centripetal, because of the delayed return of the ERG to normal values after each attack. In one of the cases described the ERG became supernormal before optic nerve involvement was detectable by ophthalmoscopy.

6. EEG changes in subacute encephalopathy (Creutzfeldt–Jakob disease). — Y. Goldhammer and J. Braham (Tel Hashomer).

During the space of one year, 4 patients between the ages of 42 and 67 years were examined who presented clinical features compatible with this diagnosis. The initial symptoms were neuropsychiatric in nature, with depression, delusions, headaches, disturbances of vision. After a few weeks mental deterioration was evident, with the advent of akinetic mutism and the emergence of occasional myoclonus. From then on the illness pursued a rapid downhill course with coma and rigidity of the limbs, generally held in a flexed position. Myoclonic jerks were then widespread, irregularly involving the whole body.

In all patients a similar EEG pattern was seen, and was present in the early stages. Normal background rhythms gave place to an irregular dysrhythmia on which were superimposed high voltage 2–3 c/sec waves, sometimes in the form of grouped general discharges. In particular, triangular sharp waves appeared every few seconds in all leads, occasionally with clear temporal relationship to a myoclonic jerk. These features taken as a whole made a characteristic and easily recognizable picture. When necropsy of the first case established the diagnosis of Creutzfeldt–Jakob disease, similar EEG patterns were recalled in 3 other patients, and reexamination of the clinical and histological material enabled the correct diagnosis to be made, in one during life. The triad of mental deterioration, myoclonus and EEG changes as described, makes it possible for this disorder to be clearly defined within the group of pre-senile dementias.

7. Penicillin convulsions. — S. Lavy and H. Stein (Jerusalem).

The use of i.v. penicillin is accompanied sometimes by the appearance of epileptic attacks. The convulsive properties of penicillin were first described in patients in 1945, and were supported by experimental studies. The appearance of epileptic attacks in a patient under i.v. penicillin therapy raises various diagnostic and therapeutic problems. The EEG examination might be very useful in differentiating between penicillin-induced epilepsy and an inflammatory epileptic focus.

The case histories of 3 patients suffering from gram-negative bacteraemia and septicaemia who developed convulsive episodes under i.v. penicillin were summarized. The penicillin was given in large doses of 40–70 mill. units for a period of 24 h. Grand mal or Jacksonian epileptic attacks appeared between 12 and 96 h after the beginning of the penicillin administration. Neurological examination did not reveal any abnormalities, but the EEGs, recorded immediately after the episodes of convulsions, showed large amounts of diffuse sharp and slow activity over all brain areas, together with absence of alpha rhythm. The penicillin was discontinued and EEG follow-ups after 24 and 72 h showed complete recovery, and reappearance of alpha rhythm.

These diffuse EEG changes suggest that the epileptic attacks were induced by the toxic effect of penicillin on the cerebral cortex. However, a focal EEG abnormality should be considered to be compatible with a localized inflammatory brain lesion.

8. Uncommon EEG findings in hepato-lenticular degeneration. — A. Mera (Zrifin).

The EEG in hepato-lenticular degeneration (HLD) is abnormal in more than 50%. The most common pathological findings are: dysrhythmia, continuous generalized slow activity, asymmetry and bursts of slow waves. Two cases of HLD are presented in which unusual epileptic patterns were found.

A girl aged 9 with HLD had an EEG with diffuse disturbances. After 10 months of treatment with penicillamine and potassium sulphide the patient was admitted again in status epilepticus. This time the EEG showed focal disturbances, 1.5–2 c/sec, in the right posterior region. After 2 weeks diffuse slowing, poly-spikes and slow wave complexes in the right hemisphere were found. It is known that penicillamine may cause pyridoxine deficiency, which may induce convulsive seizures. Pyridoxine was added to her treatment with penicillamine, and for 4 months she had no seizures, but the EEG continued to show epileptic patterns.

Our second case, a girl aged 11, was under treatment since 5 years, first with BAL, then with penicillamine. In two recent EEG records paroxysmal activity with frequent biphasic spikes in the left hemisphere were found. She never had epileptic fits.

Both epilepsy and spike and wave patterns are uncommon in HLD. The pathological changes in HLD may involve, besides the basal ganglia, the cortex and the cerebellum. In our 2 cases the epileptic patterns had a focal character which was probably caused by lesions due to HLD. Considering the focal character of the lesion, the familial factor may be questioned in our first case, whereas the pyridoxine deficiency may have had a facilitating role in the causation of the clinical seizures. In our second case HLD seems to be the only aetiological factor.

9. Petit mal status without impairment of consciousness. — M. I. Assael (Jerusalem).

The paper presents long-term records of petit mal seizures without loss or impairment of consciousness. The recorded paroxysmal outbursts of spike and wave complexes are reproducible by hyperventilation. The patient is a girl aged 17 who, after the death of her mother, apparently in the wake of emotional stress, suddenly exhibited peculiarities in her behaviour and, owing to this condition, was referred by the consultant psychiatrist to the EEG laboratory for investigation. Records were made on an 8-channel Alvar standard apparatus, applying unipolar and bipolar techniques. Routine recording was done at rest and after overbreathing and photic stimulation by stroboscope light flashes at various freqencies. In the course of several recording sessions blood samples were taken for biochemical investigation. During paroxysmal outbursts of 3 c/sec spike and slow wave complexes the patient was subjected to various psychological and intelligence tests to ascertain the state of her consciousness.

EEGs and biochemical findings showed a close connection, which definitely confirmed the assumed interdependence between petit mal attacks and variations in the pH of the blood and in acid–base metabolism. The results suggest that changes in acid–base metabolism (low pH and high CO_2 levels) constitute an autogenic defence mechanism against the occurrence of petit mal seizures, or rather an autogenic healing system which tends to prevent the occurrence of, and to obliterate, attacks of petit mal.

10. Valium administration in status epilepticus and EEG follow-up. — S. Lavy and M. Assael (Jerusalem).

Over the past years, diazepam was found to be the first choice in the treatment of status epilepticus or continued seizure activity. The dramatic effect of i.v. administration of diazepam on the electrical seizures was observed by continuous EEG recording in 3 adult patients suffering from status epilepticus. The patients, aged from 30 to 36 years old, were admitted to the emergency room of Hadassah University Hospital in status epilepticus. Before their admission they received paraldehyde, chloral hydrate and i.v. barbiturates without any effect. They all showed signs of respiratory depression after these various therapeutic attempts. On admission their EEGs showed bursts of spikes and slow waves of high voltage intermingled with a large number of low voltage spindles. Taking into consideration the high frequency of the epileptic attacks and the poor general condition of the patients, i.v. diazepam was administered under continuous EEG recording. This method permitted us to minimize the amount of the drug in order to control the clinical features and to stop electrical discharges. The patients received 20–30 mg diazepam by i.v. injection at a slow rate for 5–10 min, with complete cessation of the epileptic attacks. The continuous EEG recording permitted us to avoid additional undesirable effects in patients already suffering from central nervous system depression by repeated epileptic attacks and inefficient therapeutic experiences.

11. Pathways involved in caudate nucleus effects on the posterior hypothalamus. — S. Feldman and N. Dafny (Jerusalem).

Previous studies have shown that the caudate nucleus causes a decrease in the rate of firing of single cells in the anterior hypothalamus in cats. In the present study the responsiveness of units in the posterior hypothalamus, as changes in the rate and pattern of firing following caudate stimulation, and the effects of brain lesions, were evaluated. The analysis of the relationship between the effects of caudate stimuli and sensory responsiveness of single cells has demonstrated that the caudate affected mainly units which were facilitated by peripheral stimuli. Single caudate stimuli inhibited both the spontaneous activity of the unit and, when applied 25 msec before a photic, acoustic or sciatic stimulus, also inhibited the subsequent sensory response. The inhibitory effect, which was particularly marked during the first 1000 msec, diminished gradually and the changes in firing rate were accompanied by alterations in the pattern of the histogram.

In animals with bilateral lesions of the globus pallidus the spontaneous activity of the majority of the responsive cells was facilitated by caudate stimulation. Pallidal lesions also reduced the percentage of hypothalamic units responsive to caudate stimulation; however, they increased the number of cells facilitated by the caudate stimulus following caudate-peripheral interaction. Midbrain reticular formation lesions reduced the inhibitory effects of the caudate exerted on the hypothalamus. These studies indicate that the globus pallidus and reticular formation participate in the inhibitory effects of the caudate on single cells in the hypothalamus, and that the presence of the former may modify the responsiveness of hypothalamic units to peripheral stimuli.

12. Effects of extra-hypothalamic structures on single cell activity in the posterior hypothalamus. — N. Dafny and S. Feldman (Jerusalem).

Experiments were performed on cats to determine the role of the midbrain reticular formation, dorsal hippocampus and septum on the spontaneous activity and on the responsiveness of posterior hypothalamic neurones to photic, acoustic and sciatic nerve stimulation. The data were statistically evaluated as to change in the rate and pattern of firing. Single reticular stimuli affected 80% of the 102 cells examined, by changing the spontaneous and evoked activity when a conditioning reticular stimulus was applied at an interval of 25 msec. While the spontaneous activity was affected in the first 1000 msec after reticular stimulation, the reticular-peripheral interaction caused a late inhibition. Analysis of the data shows a high level of significance ($P=0.001$) for those units in which a change in the pattern of firing occurred. Therefore these units determined the pattern of the compound histogram. The spontaneous and evoked activity of about 50% of posterior hypothalamic units in another group of 77 cells was affected by the dorsal hippocampus, the majority of cells being inhibited. Similar inhibitory effects were exerted by the septum in a third group of 72 cells in the posterior hypothalamus. The interaction between the hippocampus or septum and the sensory stimuli abolished, in the 2000 msec histogram, the triple peak response of the sensory stimulus alone. The study of the interaction between the central and peripheral stimuli, at different time intervals, has shown that, following a conditioning reticular stimulus, complete recovery was attained at 200 msec, following a septal stimulus at 100 msec, and following a hippocampal stimulus the beginning of recovery was observed at 300 msec. These results demonstrate the important role played by extra-hypothalamic structures on the spontaneous and evoked single cell activity in the hypothalamus.

13. The influence of high oxygen pressure on the electrical activity of the brain. — D. Harel, J. Kerem and S. Lavy (Jerusalem).

In the present study the origin and site of hyperbaric oxygen convulsions was investigated. The electrical activity of intact rabbit brain in curarized animals was studied with the help of electrodes implanted in cortical and subcortical areas and the EEG was continuously recorded before during and after seizures.

Early abnormal cerebral activity, consisting of runs of slow waves or bursts of sharp waves, was most frequently recorded from cortical leads. There was no constant focus in any particular cortical area examined, nor was their appearance simultaneous in several structures. In half of the animals the early abnormal activity developed into generalized discharge. Occasionally, early changes were first recorded in subcortical areas, spreading to cortex and other adjacent subcortical areas.

In conformity with previous experimental work carried out by other investigators our results show that no brain structure plays a particular role in the genesis and development of hyperbaric oxygen seizures; neither could any area be demonstrated as particularly sensitive in their production. Our studies appear to imply that, in the intact brain of curarized rabbits, these seizures have a random origin or develop simultaneously in many brain structures.

14. Regulation of transmitter release at the neuromuscular synapse: the cooperative hypothesis. — R. Rahamimoff and F. A. Dodge Jr. (Jerusalem).

There are only two necessary requirements for obtaining increased probability of quantal release of transmitter from the pre-synaptic nerve fibre; *viz.*, depolarization of the nerve terminal and the presence of calcium ions in the bathing medium. This communication deals with a quantitative analysis of the action of calcium ions. There are indications that Ca ions combine with specific sites on the nerve membrane. If the quantal release was simply proportional to the number of sites occupied by Ca, one would expect that the kinetics would reveal a rectangular hyperbola. However, the quantitative relationship between Ca and number of quanta released by the nerve impulse (quantal content, m) is highly non-linear. Plotting of the same results on log–log scales produces a straight line with a slope of four (3.78 in 28 experiments), indicating that there is a fourth power relation between Ca and m. Addition of a constant amount of Mg reduces m, without altering the slope of the logarithmic relation. The results are explained quantitatively on the hypothesis that Ca ions combine with a specific site X on the nerve terminal, forming CaX, and that the number of m is proportional to the fourth power of CaX.

15. Psychopharmacological activity of some substances extracted from *Cannabis sativa* L. (hashish). — Y. Grunfeld and H. Edery (Ness-Ziona).

The psychopharmacological actions of (I) 1-tetrahydrocannabinol, (II) 1(6)-tetrahydrocannabinol-C_6, (III) 1(6)-tetrahydrocannabinol, (IV) 1-hydroxy hexahydrocannabinol, (V) L-ethoxy hexahydrocannabinol, (VI) 1(6)-tetrahydrocannabinolic acid methyl ester, Isomer I, (VII) 1(6)-tetrahydrocannabinolic acid methyl ester, Isomer II, (VIII) cannabigerol, (IX) hexyl-hashish, (X) cannabinchromene (natural) and (XI) cannabinchromene (synthetic) have been studied in a battery of animal tests described previously (1), as well as on the general behaviour of dogs.

I and II (100 mg/kg i.v.) caused ataxia, fearfulness, "absences", pronounced sedation and "catatonic stupor" in monkeys and the animals adopted a typical posture ("thinker position"). These changes lasted approximately 3 h. Dogs and rats showed ataxia and a catatonic-like state. This latter state could be reversed in rats by administration of amphetamine. III brought about similar effects to those elicited by I, but only after higher doses, and the changes lasted a shorter time. None of the other compounds produced any obvious effects in monkeys and dogs at doses up to 7 mg/kg.

It is suggested that the rhesus monkey might serve as a suitable model for assessing the psychopharmacological activity of hashish-extracted substances.

16. Changes in the electrical activity of the brain following pinealectomy. — I. Nir, K. Behroozi, M. Assael, I. Ivriani and F. G. Sulman (Jerusalem).

EEGs of pinealectomized and sham-operated rats were studied. Each animal served as its own control, by recording the EEG before and after operation. Eight female albino rats weighing 150±10 g each were used in each group. Four monopolar ball-pointed permanent silver electrodes were stereotaxically placed on the dura over the cortex in the left and right anterior and posterior areas; a free needle was used to record the temporal area. The electrocortical findings were: The pinealectomized rats showed a basic electrical activity of permanent monorhythmic waves, while those in the intact controls and sham-operated animals were notched, monstrous, polyrhythmic and polymorphic. A shift from low frequency (2–3 c/sec), in the controls and sham-operated rats, to high frequency (8–11 c/sec), in the pinealectomized animals, was observed. Amplitudes in the pinealectomized rats (35–75 μV) were much smaller than in the sham-operated and intact controls. Over and above this background activity a clear tendency to synchronization and hypersynchronization, with sporadic general paroxysmal outbursts of slow waves (2–4 c/sec) of large amplitude (150–200 μV), of centrencephalic origin, was observed in the pinealectomized rats. The electrical effects may be explained by the endocrine changes known to occur after ablation of the gland.

17. Electrocortical reactions of pinealectomized and intact rats to lethal doses of pentobarbital. — K. Behroozi, M. Assael, I. Ivriani and I. Nir (Jerusalem).

This communication presents changes observed in electrical activity of the brain in pinealectomized rats following administration of lethal doses of pentobarbital, as compared with sham-operated and intact controls. EEGs and ECGs were recorded simultaneously. Eight female albino rats weighing 170±10 g each, were used in each group. Four monopolar ball-pointed silver electrodes were stereotaxically placed on the dura over the cortex in the left and right anterior and posterior regions, and a free needle in the temporal area. After 3 min spindles from all EEG electrodes appeared in pinealectomized animals, while no electrical changes were apparent in either the sham-operated or intact controls. After 5 min the EEG in the pinealectomized group was synchronized, regular and symmetrical, whereas in the controls there was slowing of the background rhythm with the appearance of 1–3 c/sec waves in the delta and theta ranges. After 7 min spiky waves were derived from all electrodes in the pinealectomized animals. After 8 min, in the controls, electrical activity disappeared apart from single, slow, sporadic waves, whereas in the pinealectomized group waves appeared regularly at 6–8 c/sec and 5–10 μV. After 9 min the electrical activity of the brain and heart ceased in the controls, whereas in the pinealectomized animals it continued until the 15th min. These results indicate that the pineal gland affects the electrical activity of the brain.

18. A combination narcosis suitable for acute neurophysiological experiments. — J. E. Steiner (Jerusalem).

A new combination narcosis is proposed, based on the synergistic effect of chloralose and chlordiazepoxide HCl (Librium, Roche). This narcotic procedure was found suitable for acute neurophysiological experiments. It was possible to maintain both cats and rabbits in a sufficient surgical anaesthesia for 6–12 h. The average dose ensuring optimal conditions was: 20–25 mg/kg chloralose and 3.5–4 mg/kg chlorodiazepoxide HCl. Chloralose was dissolved in a mixture of equal parts of absolute ethanol and pure glycerol in a concentration of 10 or 20 mg/ml. Before injection the desired amount was diluted with an equal volume of saline. This mixture produced optimal anaesthesia by i.v. injection (induction time about 1 h) in cats and by i.v. injection (induction time 1–3 min) in rabbits. For i.v. administration in cats we used a short ether induction.

By combination of the two drugs a marked lowering of the usual doses of the components was possible. The hyper-reflexia often observed in chloralose anaesthesia could be completely eliminated. The electrocorticogram showed a "sleep pattern" similar to the records in natural sleep. Administration of analeptic drugs during the anaesthesia evoked typical electrographic changes, with minor convulsive effects. No changes in the heart rate or in the ECG were observed. No respiratory disorders were observed. The intrinsic electrical activity of the phrenic nerve remained unchanged during 6 h. No marked hypnotic effect was noted. The gross electrogram of afferent (sensory) impulses was not affected. This was demonstrated on the evoked activity of the chorda tympani nerve (in cats) after adequate (chemical) stimulation of the tongue.

19. Organization of the giant axons in the ventral nerve cord of the American cockroach (*Periplaneta americana*). — M. Spira, I. Parnas and F. Bergmann (Jerusalem).

According to Roeder (1948) the sensory cercal nerve of the cockroach forms its first synapse at the 6th abdominal ganglion (A6), from which giant fibres ascend directly to the metathoracic ganglion (T3). Part of the ascending pathways continues towards the meso- (T2) and prothoracic ganglion (T1) and finally to the suboesophageal ganglion (S0). Roeder's claim that separate giant fibres subserve descending impulses was supported by the degeneration experiments of Hess (1958).

Since neurophysiological evidence for the descending pathways is still missing, we have tried to clarify this problem by the following experiments. (1) Stimulation of the connective S0–T1 produced potentials in abdominal giant fibres which were always composed of more than 2 spikes. (2) The average delay of the descending impulses at each thoracic ganglion was 0.66 msec, *i.e.*, equal to the delay of ascending potentials (Roeder 1948). (3) Simultaneous stimulation in both directions gave evidence for interaction of ascending and descending impulses, implying the use of common pathways. (4) Application of nicotine (5 μg/ml) to the isolated nervous system blocked both ascending and descending impulse conduction at the thoracic ganglia.

Two models will be presented to explain bidirectional conduction along the same pathway.

20. Histological and electrophysiological studies of normal and degenerated giant axons of the American cockroach. — F. Bergmann, M. Spira and I. Parnas (Jerusalem).

Roeder (1948) and Hess (1958) described grouping of the abdominal giant axons into dorsal and ventral groups. These groups could not be identified in serial sections above the metathoracic ganglion (T3). After cutting the abdominal connective A5–A6, all abdominal giant axons degenerated except 2 ventral fibres; therefore, conduction of descending impulses was attributed to the latter. No degeneration was found in the thorax, *i.e.*, above T3. It was concluded that the giant axons terminate at T3.

In the present study we succeeded in identifying the whole ventral group of giant axons in the thorax also. After cutting at A5–A6, all fibres underwent degeneration, but this process was much slower in the 2 ventral fibres described by Hess. Degeneration extended into the thorax, implying a continuous structure of the giant fibres from A6 to T1. The fibre diameter decreased from distal to proximal. The fibres become specially narrow when passing through the thoracic ganglia. Stimulation at various stages of degeneration revealed that the process advanced from T1 in the caudal direction, towards A6. Both histological and neurophysiological evidence thus support the conclusion that ascending and descending impulses are conducted by the same fibres. The absence of synapses is in accord with the first model, presented in the foregoing communication. The blocking effect of nicotine can be explained by the greater susceptibility of the narrow intra-ganglionic portions (the "isthmuses") of the giant axons.

21. Micro-electrode studies of the giant fibres of the American cockroach. — I. Parnas, M. Spira, R. Werman and F. Bergmann (Jerusalem).

Micro-electrodes, inserted into the giant axons at different locations, recorded both ascending and descending impulses, in accordance with the observations reported in the two preceding communications. By proper spacing of an ascending and a descending impulse, the second potential could be blocked by the first one. High frequency stimulation (60–80 c/sec) caused blockade of cercal nerve impulses at A6 and of potentials, evoked from thoracic sites, at thoracic ganglia. The site of the first thoracic block varied from one experiment to another, but in each case the thoracic structure that was first fatigued, and showed the lowest safety margin, was also the first to undergo inhibition by nicotine.

These results lead again to the conclusion that the giant fibres are continuous from A6 to T1 and that the heterogeneous response of various parts of the giant axons to a variety of conditions is due to the progressive narrowing of the diameter and to the formation of isthmuses in the thoracic ganglia.

22. Electrical and mechanical properties of the abdominal extensor muscles of the prawn, *Polaemon elegans*. — D. Dagan and I. Parnas (Jerusalem).

Electrical and mechanical properties of the deep, medial (DEAM), lateral (DEAL) and superficial lateral (SEAL) abdominal muscles were studied. The DEAM muscle responds to direct intracellular and indirect stimulation, with a transient membrane depolarization which exhibits the properties of a propagated non-decremental action potential, with an amplitude of 60–80 mV. It is followed by a fast all-or-none twitch with a duration of 30 msec at 20° C. The membrane potential is K dependent, but is affected also by Na and Cl ions. The DEAL muscle is slower and responds to intracellular stimulation with spikes or local responses. The SEAL muscle responds only with local responses. The I–V curve shows that the three muscle bundles are composed of heterogeneous fibre populations. Nerve-induced responses varied from junction potentials showing facilitation and post-tetanic potentiation to all-or-some spikes.

Electroenceph. clin. Neurophysiol., **1969**, *27*: 216–221

Electroencephalography and Clinical Neurophysiology
Elsevier Publishing Company, Amsterdam – Printed in The Netherlands

BOOK REVIEWS

Edited by H. PETSCHE *and* JOHN R. HUGHES

Physiological basis of the alpha rhythm. — P. Andersen and S. A. Andersson. (Appleton-Century-Crofts, New York, 1968, 235 p., $12.00).

Few subjects are more relevant to the central interests of the general reader of this Journal than that considered in this monograph. For it would be surprising indeed if the thoughtful electroencephalographer did not daily wonder about the origin of brain waves in general and the basis of the alpha rhythm in particular. The authors of this monograph, both prominent experimental neurophysiologists, have gone well beyond the wondering stage in their treatment of these subjects. They have presented a personal testament of the power of extended hypothesis in order to provide a provocative account of a possible physiological basis of the alpha rhythm. The reader is alerted to this in the Introduction which clearly defines the basis for the proposed hypothesis: the discovery of a powerful recurrent inhibitory system in the thalamus. With this and the assumption that the barbiturate spindle activity in animals is analogous to the human alpha rhythm, the authors proceed to describe the experimental work upon which the new theory of the alpha rhythm has been based.

The development of ideas on the rhythmicity of brain waves considers the fundamental controversy concerning "autorhythmicity *versus* circus movement". Retrospectively the authors find it difficult to understand how anyone could have seriously held to the reverberating circuit notion for so long when contrary evidence seemed so compelling. This impatience with history is further reflected in the rather cursory treatment of additional significant concepts such as those developed by Bishop and his associates. The main thrust of the brief historical survey of ideas on brain rhythmicity is not intended to provide the reader with a clear perspective but to prepare him for a critical attack upon the so-called midline thalamic pacemaker theory of Dempsey and Morison. Every reader of this Journal is familiar with the work of the latter investigators, as well as of Jasper and his associates, who demonstrated the important role of medial and intralaminar thalamic nuclei in the production of synchronized electrocortical activity. The authors contend that the Dempsey–Morison theory of a general thalamic pacemaker or rhythmic oscillator influencing wide cortical areas was "so satisfying that many subsequent experimenters were more inclined to confirm the original supposition than to test it critically". The fact that many workers recorded typical spindle activity in specific relay nuclei indicated that distinctions between specific and non-specific "pacemakers" might not be as clear as originally proposed in the Dempsey–Morison–Jasper hypothesis. Evidently the authors have considered this observation the major point of departure for their test of the general midline pacemaker hypothesis. What follows in this book is evidence for a new view called the *facultative pacemaker theory* which holds that: (1) all major thalamic nuclei have the ability to produce rhythmic activity and to control an appropriate part of the cortex; (2) rhythmicity resides in a particular thalamic mechanism that is dependent upon a powerful recurrent inhibitory process, and (3) a cellular mechanism is responsible for the rhythmic thalamo-cortical activity.

Attempts to establish the independent and sometimes restricted nature of spindle activity in different thalamic nuclei and cortex draw upon a vast amount of published and unpublished work. Approximately 20–30 of the nearly 100 figures in this monograph do not have courtesy citations and thus must be considered unpublished. This substantiates the authors' forecast in the Introduction that "Of necessity, the description will be somewhat colored by our own experience. It may seem to the reader that somewhat more emphasis is placed upon experiments by our own group than is justified". To the extent that the reader clearly recognizes this work to be a vehicle for the development of a new hypothesis there would hardly be any reason for the authors to claim otherwise.

Two types of experiments are described in support of the facultative pacemaker hypothesis: simultaneous recording from a number of thalamic nuclei during barbiturate-induced spindle activity and the production of localized lesions within the thalamus. Although no microphotographs of the extent of the lesions in the thalamus are presented, findings of persistent localized spindle activity after widespread ablations of medial thalamus lend support to the authors' thesis of facultative pacemakers. Additional findings indicate that spindle activity in postcruciate areas is not affected by medial thalamic lesions but is abolished by lateral thalamic ablations. It has also been shown that a small area of VPL (approx. 200 μ in diameter) may be rhythmically linked with a small region of postcruciate cortex. This presumably underlies the congruence of spindle activity in a restricted specific thalamocortical projection area and a thalamic locus. The data are considered indicative of a "parcellation of the thalamic control of cortical rhythm" and are supported by detailed analysis of independent intra-spindle frequencies and inter-spindle periods in activities recorded from several electrodes. Some attempt to relate new findings to the wealth of data pointing to a high priority system for effecting generalized synchronization is noted in the statement that "synchrony occurs because all thalamic nuclei have a capacity to produce rhythmic activity and that this independent ability may be brought together by an intrathalamic synchronizing mechanism".

A large part of this monograph is devoted to defining

the basic mechanisms underlying spontaneous and evoked thalamic rhythms. The recurrent inhibition and post-anodal exaltation hypotheses are viewed as critical factors in the generation of the 10 c/sec thalamic rhythm. The theory, derived from the earlier experiments of Andersen and Eccles, is elaborated and documented by new and unpublished data. The concept of post-anodal exaltation is developed in accordance with the Hodgkin–Huxley hypothesis. The authors' treatment of voltage clamp data leads to the startling conclusion that "the IPSP presumably increases the sodium conductance of the membrane. Therefore, a seemingly paradoxical situation develops. Although the cell is inhibited because of the large hyperpolarization, this process also causes the membrane to become more excitable". The reader will judge for himself whether this argument is at all convincing or meaningful as an explanation for the depolarization that generally succeeds IPSPs observed in thalamic neurons during rhythmic activity. Suffice it to say this reviewer has held that such post-anodal exaltation leading to impulse initiation is a property of depolarized thalamic neurons. The authors counter this by illustrating (Fig. 9.15) findings from a neuron exhibiting 10 mV *intracellular spikes* in which hyperpolarization is succeeded by anode break responses. In point of fact the new data amply confirm the conclusion of the reviewer, who would even question whether the new data were obtained with intracellular recording as indicated in the legend of Fig. 9.15.

One feature of this monograph is the inclusion of a chapter dealing with the histological substrate for thalamic-rhythmic activity. The chief concern here is with the identification of cells with recurrent axon collaterals and elements that could subserve the role of inhibitory interneurons. The authors rely heavily upon recent Golgi findings of Tömböl in building their story on the nature of thalamic interneurons and the distribution of recurrent axon collaterals of presumed relay cells. Identification of a neuron with a long axon that makes contact with neurons in different thalamic nuclei has presumably been made by Tömböl and the Scheibels. The authors refer to this as a distributor neuron and effectively incorporate it into their hypothesis. However, they claim that intrathalamic interactions are mainly directed from non-specific to specific nuclei when in fact recent work suggests the opposite to be the case.

The later chapters in this monograph are concerned with the analysis of recruiting potentials in thalamus and cortex and effects of pharmacological agents on spontaneous rhythmic thalamocortical activity. The studies of recruiting activities adequately consider the findings of others in the field. Attention is also focused on the PSP theory of electrocortical potentials, a subject that has been repeatedly treated in a number of reviews and original papers in this Journal.

A final chapter deals with models of rhythmic activity and the use and limitations of such models as applied to physiological studies. There can be no question but that work along these lines will continue to be an important adjunct to biological experimentation. In this context the authors have come up with a simulated computer network that shows much of the rhythmic behavior observed in thalamic neuronal organizations. The fact that this model incorporates features of recurrent inhibition as a major element serves to emphasize a final statement that "it is not unlikely that the thalamic inhibition serves a particular purpose". Whatever the fate of the recurrent inhibition hypothesis of thalamic rhythmicity, it is an established fact that inhibition plays an important role in thalamic synchronization. The authors and their colleagues have indeed contributed greatly to this discovery as well as others of fundamental importance for the understanding of the genesis of brain waves. The hypothesis detailed in this monograph will undoubtedly be discussed and tested for several years to come. The issues considered are by no means trivial. This should be sufficient reason for the clinical and experimental neurophysiologist to study this monograph with more than casual interest.

DOMINICK P. PURPURA
Department of Anatomy,
Albert Einstein College of Medicine,
Bronx, N. Y. 10461 (U.S.A.)

Electroenceph. clin. Neurophysiol., **1969,** *27*: 222–223

An atlas of pathological pneumoencephalographic anatomy. — G. di Chiro, M. M. Schecter and I. Wickbom. (C. C. Thomas, Springfield, 1967, 555 p., $ 49.50).

This atlas, written to complement the authors' previous classical work in normal pneumoencephalography, consists of abnormal ventriculograms and pneumoencephalograms with occasional angiograms. The reproductions generally are of the same size as the original films, and are of excellent quality and detail, with few exceptions. A selected bibliography at the end of the volume includes both excellent general references and significant specific ones. Lesions are presented via sequential anatomic regions, beginning at the foramen magnum and ascending. The nature of neuroradiology results in the book being oriented mainly toward space-occupying lesions but various degenerative and congenital abnormalities are also present.

The volume of pathological entities discussed is impressive, as is the depth of coverage regarding any specific type of lesion; thus, in the posterior fossa there are numerous films merely to demonstrate different types of aqueductal kinking, whereas other studies are presented to demonstrate the fourth ventricle displacements, impingements and obstructions. Certainly, posterior fossa tumors with their characteristic air study changes are well covered. Other areas exceptionally well described include (1) several excellent examples of tentorial meningiomas, (2) multiple studies of pinealomas, colloid cysts and third ventricle ependymomas, (3) comparison of chromophobe adenomas and retro-suprasellar aneurysms, and (4) numerous examples of both upward and downward tentorial herniations. Corpus callosum agenesis is well demonstrated with multiple films contrasting complete and partial agenesis.

Each reproduction is adequately described and is usually supplemented with appropriate arrows on the film.

Electroenceph. clin. Neurophysiol., **1969,** *27*: 223–224

A basic grasp of normal pneumoencephalography is presumed. (Such a need can be well filled by the authors' previous work.)

The cost of this Atlas will probably limit individual purchases but it would certainly be of considerable help to students or board candidates in neurosurgery, neurology or radiology. This is especially true now that air studies are being used increasingly less. Predictably this will result in a decreasing familiarity with the more subtle air study changes. The Atlas is strongly recommended for departmental libraries in neurosurgery, neurology and radiology. It is an excellent presentation and will undoubtedly become a classic volume in neuroradiology.

EUGENE D. GEORGE and PAUL C. BUCY
Northwestern University Medical Center, Chicago, Ill. 60611 (U.S.A.)

Electroenceph. clin. Neurophysiol., **1969**, *27*: 223–224

Hypothalamus und Thalamus. Experimental-Dokumente. — W. R. Hess. (Thieme, Stuttgart, 2nd edition, 78 p., 207 Fig., DM 48.00).

This is the second edition of the short summary of the experimental work of W. R. Hess. The effects of diencephalic electrical stimulation on autonomic responses and behaviour are documented in 207 figures, many of them including several stills from movies. The appropriate stimulus points are shown in histological slides and stimulus maps are attached which combine the stimulus points for different symptoms. A short description of each experiment shown in the photograph is attached. Although this text is in German, non-German-speaking readers can collect sufficient information on stimulus parameters etc.

It is a good idea of the author and the publisher to make this valuable experimental material, which is spread throughout many individual papers and out of print monographs, available. This is a purely documentary work. The conclusions which Hess drew from his experiments on the diencephalon are summarized in two papers (W. R. Hess: Cerebrale Organisation somatomotorischer Leistungen. *Arch. Psychiat. Nervenkr.*, 1965, *207*: 33 and 1966, *208*: 209). The book also includes a bibliography of the publications on brain-stem stimulation by Hess and his pupils.

O. CREUTZFELDT
Max-Planck-Institut für Psychiatrie, Munich (Germany)

Electroenceph. clin. Neurophysiol., **1969**, *27*: 224

ANNOUNCEMENT

THIRD EUROPEAN SYMPOSIUM ON EPILEPSY

This symposium is arranged by the International Bureau for Epilepsy, the International League against Epilepsy and the Danish Epilepsy Association.

The symposium will take place at Hotel Marienlyst, Elsinore (near Copenhagen), Denmark, on the 21st–23rd June, 1970.

The medical topics will be: Etiological factors in the epilepsies: (a) genetic factors; (b) prenatal and perinatal factors.

The social and psychological topics will be: (a) Life insurance and disability pension. (b) The interaction between the epileptic child and teenager and the milieu.

The symposium will be activated by panel discussions and group discussions.

Further information and preliminary application: DIS Congress Service, 36 Skindergade, DK-1159 Copenhagen K, Denmark.

Electroenceph. clin. Neurophysiol., **1969**, *27*: 224

Electroencephalography and Clinical Neurophysiology
Elsevier Publishing Company, Amsterdam – Printed in The Netherlands

ASPECTS DYNAMIQUES DE L'ÉLECTROENCÉPHALOGRAMME HUMAIN. PREMIERS RÉSULTATS D'UNE ÉTUDE RADIO-TÉLÉMÉTRIQUE

G. ARFEL, C. CASANOVA ET M. COULMANCE

Unité de Neurophysiologie Chirurgicale de l'I.N.S.E.R.M., 42, rue Richemond-Desbassayns, 92 Suresnes (France)

(Accepted for publication: December 24, 1968)

L'objet de ce travail était de voir si l'EEG humain obtenu par radio-télémétrie révèle une "dynamique" des rythmes cérébraux aussi évidente que celle démontrée chez l'animal par Storm van Leeuwen *et al.* (1963a, b; 1967a, b).

Des investigations télémétriques ont été pratiquées chez l'homme dans des circonstances particulières: pilotes, au cours des diverses séquences du vol normal (Blanc *et al.* 1967) ou acrobatique (Nestianu *et al.* 1964); enfants énurétiques dans le sommeil nocturne (Weinmann 1968); joueur de football, lors des phases successives du jeu (Hughes et Hendrix 1968); sujets soumis à une expérimentation pour étude des "variations contingentes négatives" et des potentiels évoqués (Walter *et al.* 1967); épileptiques en voie de réadaptation pour réinsertion dans des circuits professionnels (Vidart et Geier 1967, 1968); enfants présentant des absences petit mal et soumis à diverses épreuves (Bureau *et al.* 1968).

Notre intention était d'envisager l'évolution globale de l'EEG chez une population de sujets variée, dans un certain cadre expérimental, évolution concernant aussi bien les activités physiologiques que des éléments inhabituels (dont certains considérés dans l'appréciation courante comme franchement anormaux). Cette évolution serait interprétée dans la perspective d'une étude de "réactivité", au sens que lui attribue Lairy (1956): "possibilités et modalités nouvelles d'organisation de l'activité électrique corticale" sous l'effet de divers facteurs; recherche d'interférences éventuelles avec certains faits de comportement (Lairy 1964). Notre étude s'est finalement réduite à des confrontations plus modestes dont nous apportons les premiers résultats.

MATÉRIEL ET MÉTHODE

Les quarante-sept sujets (32 adultes, 15 enfants de 6–16 ans), chez lesquels a été pratiqué un examen télémétrique entre Octobre 1967 et Juin 1968, avaient été préalablement soumis à un EEG conventionnel dans nos laboratoires de routine. Cinq d'entre eux, pilotes-essayeurs d'une Société de Construction Automobile, étaient adressés à l'EEG dans le seul but d'un contrôle systématique.

La sélection des sujets en vue de la télémétrie s'est basée sur des critères essentiellement EEG, faisant abstraction de la pathologie éventuelle. Ainsi ont été choisis des patients pour lesquels l'EEG antérieur révélait certaines particularités: par exemple, dans la fréquence, la répartition, les modalités réactionnelles des activités physiologiques; figures "paroxystiques" s'extériorisant dans des conditions définies (attention, distraction, fléchissement vigile); états de vigilance précaires, etc.

Les trente-deux adultes comportaient, outre les cinq conducteurs déjà cités, quatorze épileptiques connus et deux malades porteurs de tumeurs cérébrales; les autres patients présentaient des troubles divers (céphalées, syndromes subjectifs post-traumatiques, etc.). Parmi les quinze enfants, trois etaient des épileptiques avérés; deux présentaient des séquelles d'encéphalopathies avec signes neurologiques et arriération mentale; les dix autres avaient été conduits à l'EEG pour instabilité psychomotrice, retard scolaire, troubles caractériels mineurs, troubles du sommeil.

L'examen a été réalisé par transmission hertzienne, au moyen de Televars, avec réception de 10–12 dérivations simultanées sur un électroencéphalographe Duplex à transistors.

Les émetteurs utilisés se présentent sous forme de capsules cylindriques compactes (diamètre, 25 mm; hauteur, 12 mm; poids, 12 g, y compris l'alimentation par piles Mallory au mercure de 1,2 V/3 mA). L'autonomie d'émission effective est d'environ 20 h. L'amplificateur subminiature à transistors a pour caractéristiques: bande passante de 0,5–5.000 c/sec; constante de temps de 0,1 sec; gain en tension, 1.000; bruit de fond de 1,0 μV lorsque l'entrée est fermée sur 5.000 Ω; impédance d'entrée de 300.000 Ω.

L'oscillateur H.F. émet sur la bande F.M. de radio-

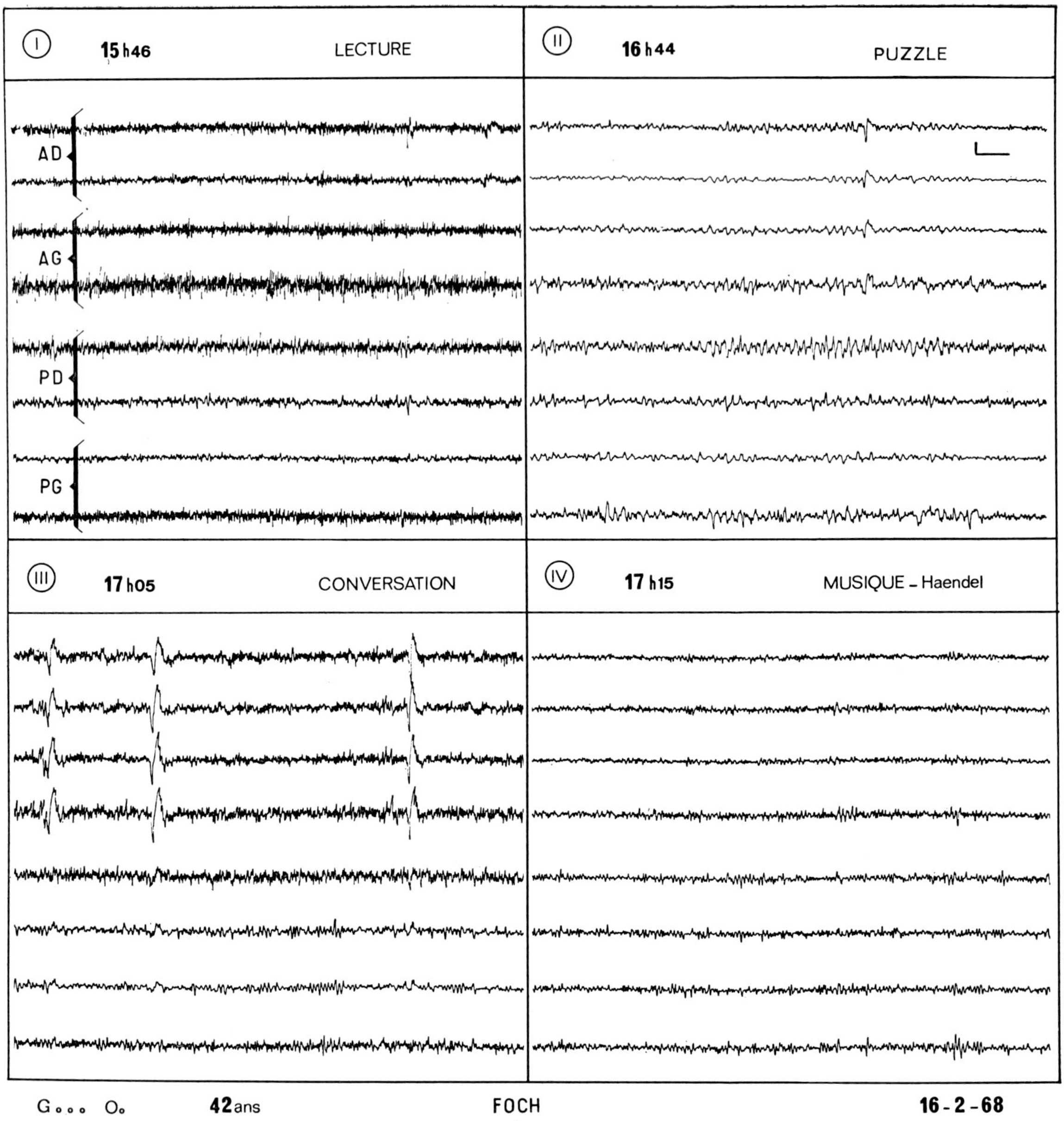

Fig. 1

Variations selon l'épreuve.
I: patiente de 42 ans, intellectuellement peu évoluée; les sérieuses difficultés provoquées par la lecture s'accompagnent d'un myogramme intense sur toutes les régions (15 h 46). *II* (16 h 44): pendant le puzzle, exécuté avec application, survenue d'ondes théta pointues, rythmiques à 5 c/sec essentiellement temporo-occipitales (5e et 8e lignes). *III* (17 h 05): conversation; quelques groupes d'ondes alpha à 9 c /sec apparaissent sur les dérivations postérieures (4 lignes inférieures). *IV* (17 h 15): audition musicale: remarquable "uniformisation" des rythmes: activités diffuses de 9–11 c/sec un peu plus amples sur les dérivations postérieures (4 dernières lignes).
Pour chaque fragment de cette figure et pour les figures 4 et 6: ligne 1 – fronto-temporal droit; 2 – fronto-rolandique droit; 3 – fronto-rolandique gauche; 4 – fronto-temporal gauche; 5 – temporo-occipital droit; 6 – rolando-occipital droit; 7 – rolando-occipital gauche; 8 – temporo-occipital gauche. Pour les autres figures (2, 2 bis, 3 et 5) FV = frontal médian-vertex; VO = vertex-occipital médian.
Calibrage: sur toutes les figures: 1 sec et 50 μV.

diffusion: gamme 87/108 Mc/sec (longueur d'onde 3 m). La puissance émise est inférieure au mW. L'antenne d'émission, d'une longueur de 5 cm, est incorporée dans le boîtier de l'oscillateur; la portée est d'environ 20 m. L'émetteur se trouve à un potentiel flottant par rapport à la masse, éliminant l'induction de 50 périodes. La fréquence d'émission de chaque émetteur peut être règlée par un noyau d'antenne. Les électrodes de détection sont directement reliées à l'émetteur par un câble bipolaire.

L'antenne réceptrice est une antenne 1/4 d'onde. Le récepteur "tunner" type radio-diffusion, comporte à l'entrée un étage séparateur d'antenne. Un haut-parleur permet le réglage du ou des récepteurs juxtaposés sur les différentes voies de l'émission. (Sortie du récepteur, 100 mV.)

Le nombre de dérivations est réduit par les moyens techniques: la bande de fréquence d'émission est limitée, chaque émetteur devant être séparé des autres d'un mégacycle au moins pour éviter les interférences entre chaines. L'examen est facilité par le blindage de la salle de télémétrie, portes et fenêtres comprises.

Les électrodes utilisées, fixées au collodion, sont du type Capsulex Alvar, en acier inoxydable (diamètre de 5 mm); dans notre technique actuelle, l'enregistrement est effectué en douze dérivations, dix d'entre elles dévolues à l'EEG, une au rythme respiratoire et une à l'electrocardiogramme. L'enregistrement EEG, en technique bipolaire, explore de façon symétrique les régions fronto-temporales, fronto-rolandiques, temporo-occipitales, rolando-occipitales droites et gauches, ainsi que la ligne médiane dans le sens antero-postérieur (fronto-vertex, vertex-occiput); le rythme respiratoire est capté à partir d'une micro-thermistance de 15 kΩ montée dans un pont de Wheatstone et fixée sous une narine. Le rythme cardiaque est obtenu en dérivation type D2.

L'examen a lieu dans une vaste pièce (70 m^2), sous la surveillance d'un ou deux observateurs. L'enregistrement dure environ 3 h, selon un protocole autant que possible identique d'un sujet à l'autre. Il comporte une première période pendant laquelle le patient est allongé, yeux ouverts puis yeux fermés, afin d'obtenir un tracé comparatif avec l'EEG conventionnel. La durée de cette partie de l'examen est plus ou moins longue selon que s'installe ou non le sommeil; elle excède rarement une heure. Ultérieurement, le sujet est soumis à une série d'épreuves simples: dessin libre, lectures, puzzles de difficultés variables ou autres jeux de patience, audition musicale d'un disque qu'il choisit lui-même, conversations. Dans ces divers temps, il lui est, évidemment, laissé toute liberté corporelle. La durée de chaque épreuve varie de 10–15 min avec des intervalles d'environ 5 min entre chacune d'elles. Une évaluation du comportement est faite par l'observation constante du sujet au cours des situations successives.

RÉSULTATS

1. *Variations selon l'épreuve*

L'aspect habituel de l'EEG est évidemment retrouvé lorsque le sujet est allongé, yeux fermés, en état de relaxation psycho-sensorielle et motrice; des variations ont pu être observées, par ailleurs, pendant le déroulement des diverses épreuves. Parmi les adultes, 22 sur 32 tracés ont ainsi montré une différenciation "circonstantielle", sinon pour toutes les épreuves, du moins nettement pour certaines d'entre elles; le même fait a été noté chez onze enfants sur quinze.

Ces modifications, toutefois, couvrent un registre assez peu varié et il n'a pas été possible de rapporter une activité spécifique à une situation donnée. Tout au plus note-t-on que l'émergence d'ondes pointues postérieures, au niveau de la ligne médiane ou des portions adjacentes (Fig. 1, 16 h 44; Fig. 2, 17 h 33) est surtout fréquente pendant la réalisation de puzzles ou autres jeux de patience comportant de multiples pièces et sollicitant vivement la recherche visuelle. Ces figures, ondes lambda vraisemblables, se manifestent par salves alors que la pièce adéquate est recherchée activement dans la boîte contenant le jeu et cessent brusquement dès que la pièce valable est enfin trouvée.

L'audition musicale suscite, dans un certain nombre de cas, un aspect singulier, "uniformisé", c'est-à-dire avec réduction de la différenciation topographique (compte-tenu des montages utilisés). Pendant cette épreuve (Fig. 1, 17 h 15; Fig. 2, 18 h 04; Fig. 3, 16 h 51), des activités fusiformes dont la fréquence est souvent autour de 9–12 c/sec s'extériorisent, semble-t-il, au niveau du vertex et des régions voisines. Il n'est pas possible de dire s'il s'agit de figures apparentées aux rythmes mu ou de rythmes alpha issus de régions postérieures et propagés; pour ne pas modifier le déroulement spontané de l'épreuve, nous n'avons soumis aucun des sujets de cette série aux tests usuels permettant de différencier ces divers types d'activités.

Pendant la lecture, l'appréciation du rythme cérébral est gênée par l'interférence d'artefacts dus aux déplacements latéraux des globes oculaires et s'étendant largement aux dérivations postérieures.

L'aspect peut varier d'un instant à l'autre au cours d'une même épreuve (Fig. 2 bis).

2. *Dynamique du rythme alpha*

Parmi les activités recueillies, le rythme alpha est le mieux différencié et le plus connu dans ses

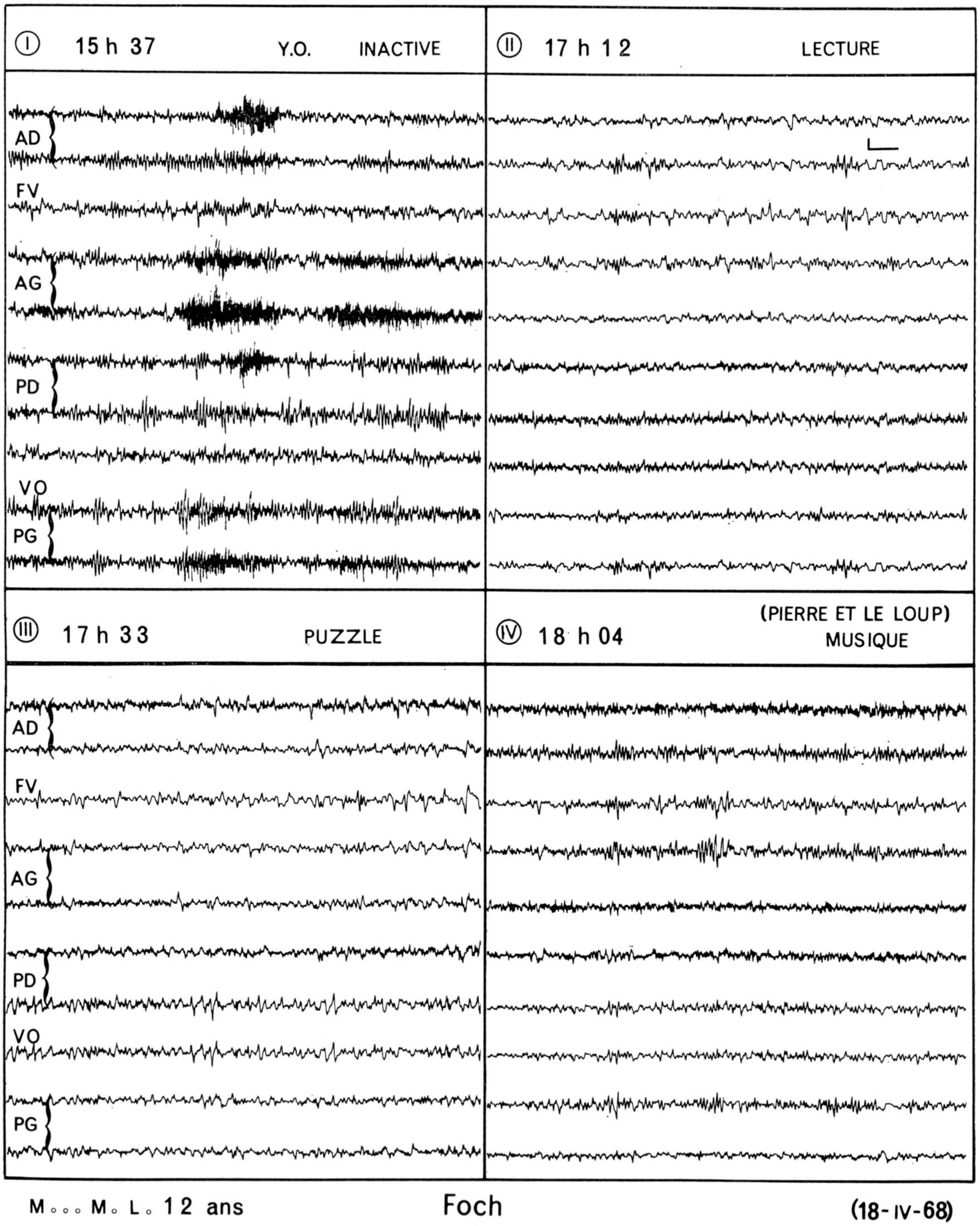

Fig. 2

Variations selon l'épreuve.
I (15 h 37): jeune patiente inactive, yeux ouverts. Alpha (9–10 c/sec), abondant, non seulement postérieur (PD, VO, PG), mais largement propagé aux dérivations antérieures (AD, FV, AG). *II* (17 h 12): oscillations lentes antérieures observées pendant la lecture (5 premières lignes) et correspondant aux mouvements de latéralité des globes oculaires. Quelques fuseaux d'activités à 9 c/sec. *III* (17 h 33): présence d'éléments pointus à 4 c/sec, postérieurs (visibles surtout au niveau des 7ème et 8ème lignes: dérivation rolando-occipitale droite et vertex-occipitale médiane). *IV* (18 h 04): "uniformisation" partielle des rythmes pendant l'audition musicale.

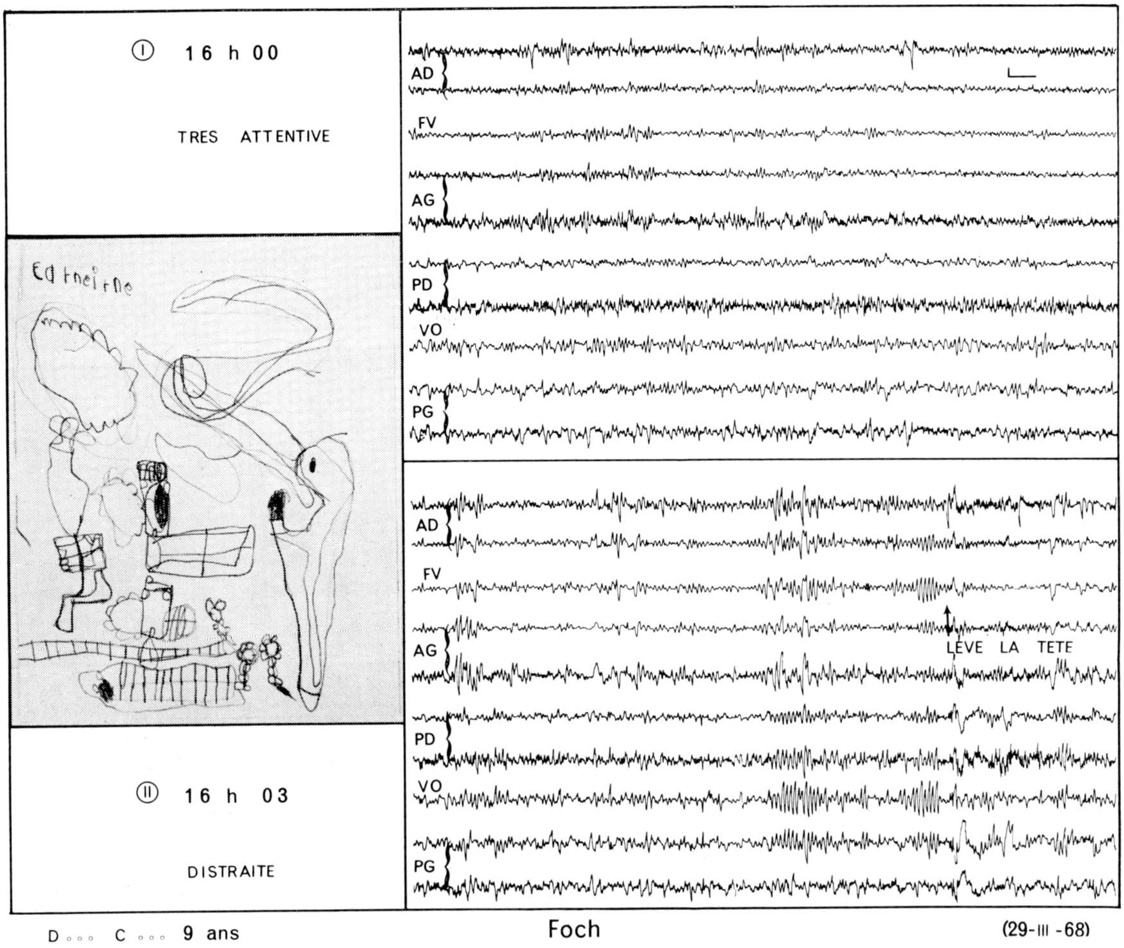

Fig. 2 bis

Variations au cours d'une épreuve de dessin selon l'état d'attention (*I*: 16 h 00) ou de distraction (*II*: 16 h 03); dans cette dernière circonstance, survenue de bouffées sinusoïdales au niveau du vertex (particulièrement en VO) et des régions voisines, bloquées lorsque l'enfant lève la tête vers l'observateur.

particularités morphologiques, topographiques et ses aptitudes réactionnelles. Son évolution est donc suivie avec le plus de facilité.

A. Chez le sujet yeux-ouverts, plusieurs modalités d'extériorisation ont été discernées dans une première approximation (Fig. 2–4).

(i) Activités s'inscrivant dans la gamme des fréquences alpha et de même topographie que celles-ci (Fig. 1, 17 h 05). Elles s'en distinguent dans certains cas par une organisation moins régulière, une moindre amplitude, une fréquence différant de 2–3 c/sec (comparativement au rythme alpha observé chez le même sujet yeux fermés). L'intrication de fréquences diverses oscillant entre 8 et 12 c/sec est également possible.

(ii) Activités ayant une forme tout à fait comparable à celle du rythme alpha yeux-fermés, mais de topographie plus diffuse: une large propagation se fait alors vers les régions antérieures où ces activités prennent volontiers un aspect pointu (alpha "propagé"). Là encore, possibilité d'interférences avec des rythmes mu (Fig. 2, 15 h 37; Fig. 3, 17 h 22).

(iii) Séquences de rythme alpha de brève durée (quelques secondes ou une fraction de seconde), ayant strictement la même morphologie et le

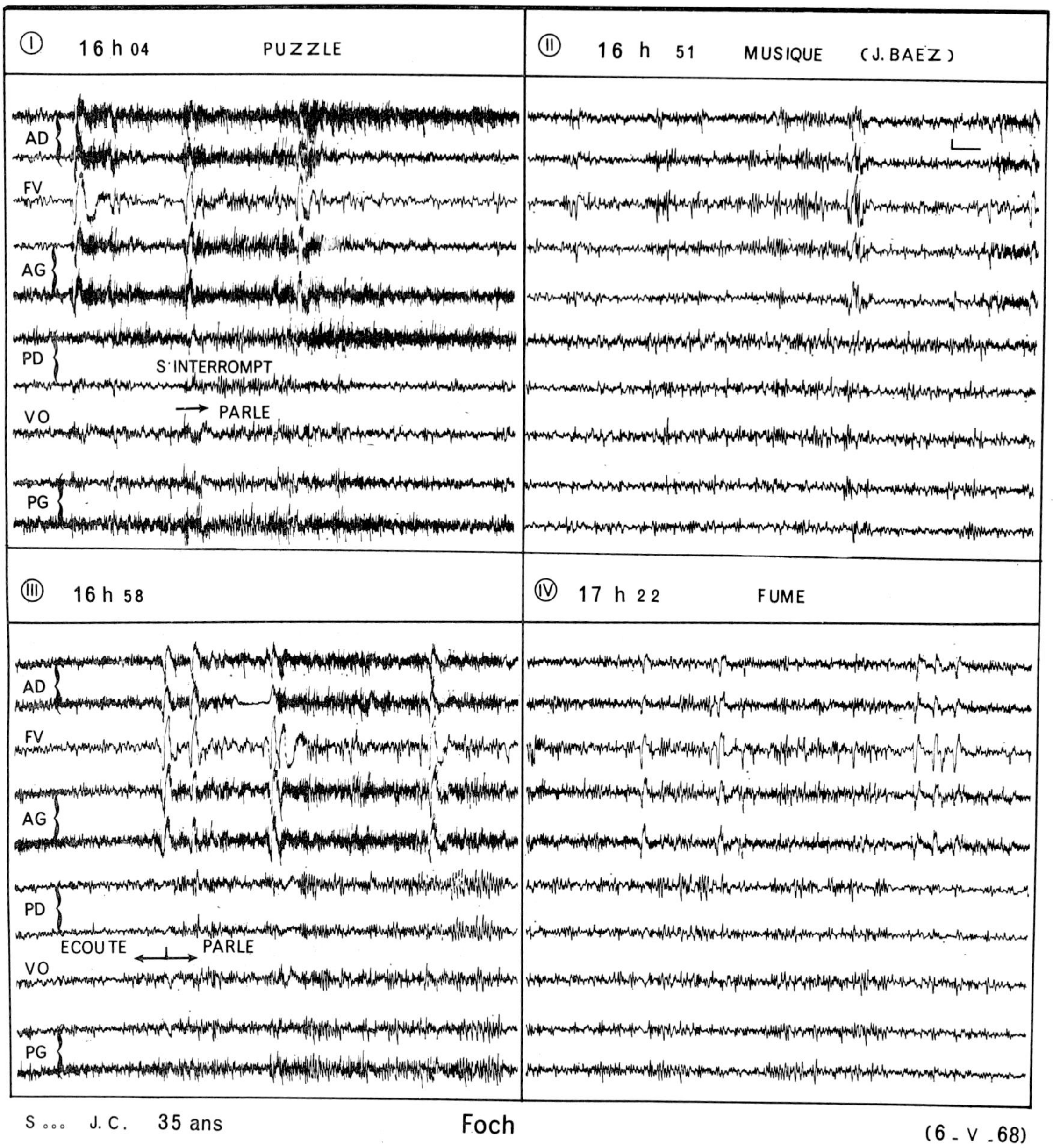

Fig. 3

Dynamique des activités alpha.
Exemple de rythmes alpha se manifestant chez le sujet *yeux-ouverts* (pilote-automobile; examen systématique). *I* (16 h 04): en cours de puzzle, le sujet interrompt sa recherche pendant quelques secondes et parle: libération d'une bouffée d'alpha au niveau des dérivations postérieures. Après 3 sec, reprise du jeu: alpha bloqué. *II* (16 h 51): audition musicale; aspect partiellement "uniformisé" (avec quelques éléments "paroxystiques"). *III* (16 h 58): conversation; dans l'exemple choisi, reprise de l'activité alpha postérieure (PD, VO, PG) lorsque le sujet répond à son interlocuteur. Au même moment, recrudescence du clignement palpébral et des myogrammes frontaux (les 5 premières lignes). *IV* (17 h 22): sujet inactif; alpha "propagé". Aspect rappelant celui du fragment de 16 h 51, avec un clignement palpébral plus actif et une amplitude des activités alpha plus élevée sur les dérivations postérieures.

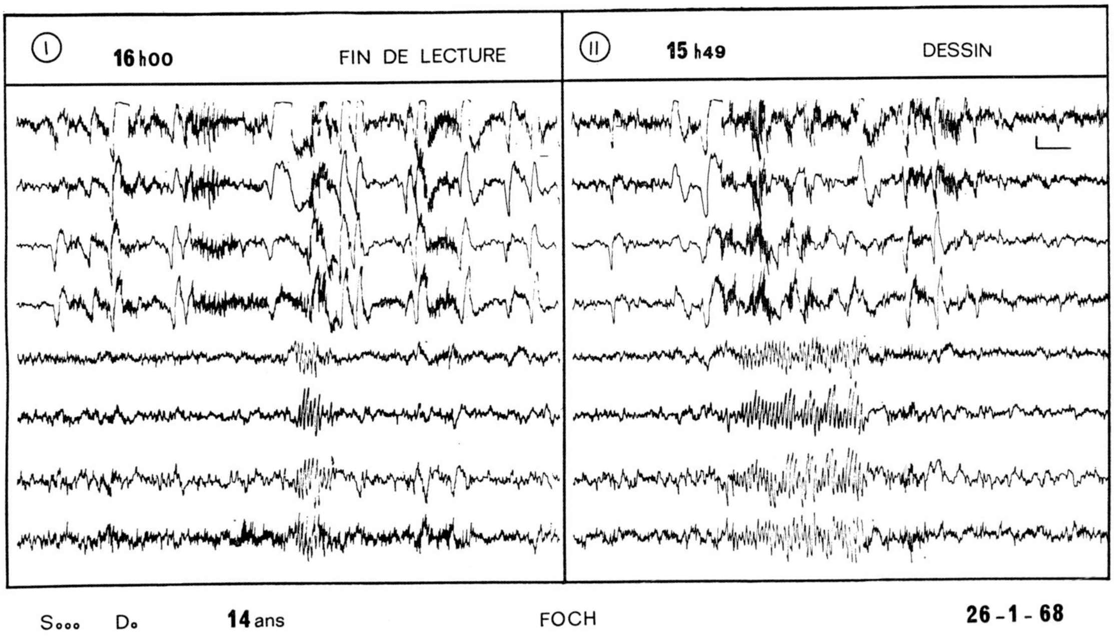

Fig. 4

Dynamique des activités alpha: exemples d'"échappement d'alpha" (E.A.). Remarquer sur les fragments prélevés pendant la lecture (*I*: 16 h 00) et le dessin (*II*: 15 h 49), la simultanéité de l'E.A. et des mouvements oculo-palpébraux se manifestant sur les dérivations antérieures (les 4 premières lignes).

même siège que le rythme alpha yeux-fermés, s'extériorisant et disparaissant de façon soudaine (Fig. 3, 16 h 04 et 16 h 58; Fig. 4). Ces bouffées, que nous dénommons "échappement d'alpha", sont liées de façon évidente dans la plupart des cas à un clignement ou une série de clignements palpébraux, ou de mouvements oculaires, sans qu'une relation chronologique exacte puisse être établie.

Quel que soit le type d'activité alpha, sa survenue yeux-ouverts reste un fait assez rare; elle n'a constitué une particularité marquante que chez sept adultes (sur 32) et trois enfants (sur 15). Cette extériorisation du rythme alpha yeux-ouverts se produit plus fréquemment chez les patients montrant un rythme alpha abondant yeux-fermés. Les diverses modalités d'extériorisation peuvent successivement s'observer chez un même sujet (Fig. 3).

La première variété se voit essentiellement dans les phases inactives, telle la partie initiale de l'examen, alors que le sujet déambule librement ou est allongé, ou encore dans l'intervalle de deux épreuves "actives".

La deuxième variété est indifféremment rencontrée chez le sujet actif ou inactif et cela est, par exemple, le fait des épileptiques sous forte imprégnation médicamenteuse. Pour d'autres sujets, un rythme alpha de ce type ne s'extériorise qu'au cours des épreuves jugées sans intérêt ou trop astreignantes, alors qu'un blocage complet se produit dès qu'ils participent vraiment à l'expérience proposée. Ce rythme alpha "propagé" est sans doute celui rencontré au cours de l'audition musicale.

La troisième variété se voit plus volontiers dans les phases actives, au cours du dessin, du jeu, de la conversation. Elle se produit lorsque le sujet abandonne, pour un instant très bref, l'activité en cours (Fig. 3, 16 h 04; Fig. 4, 15 h 49 et 16 h 00), ou lorsqu'il en est brusquement détourné. Elle semble parfois traduire une réponse à plusieurs sollicitations extérieures *ou* à l'alternance de celles-ci; par exemple, au cours de

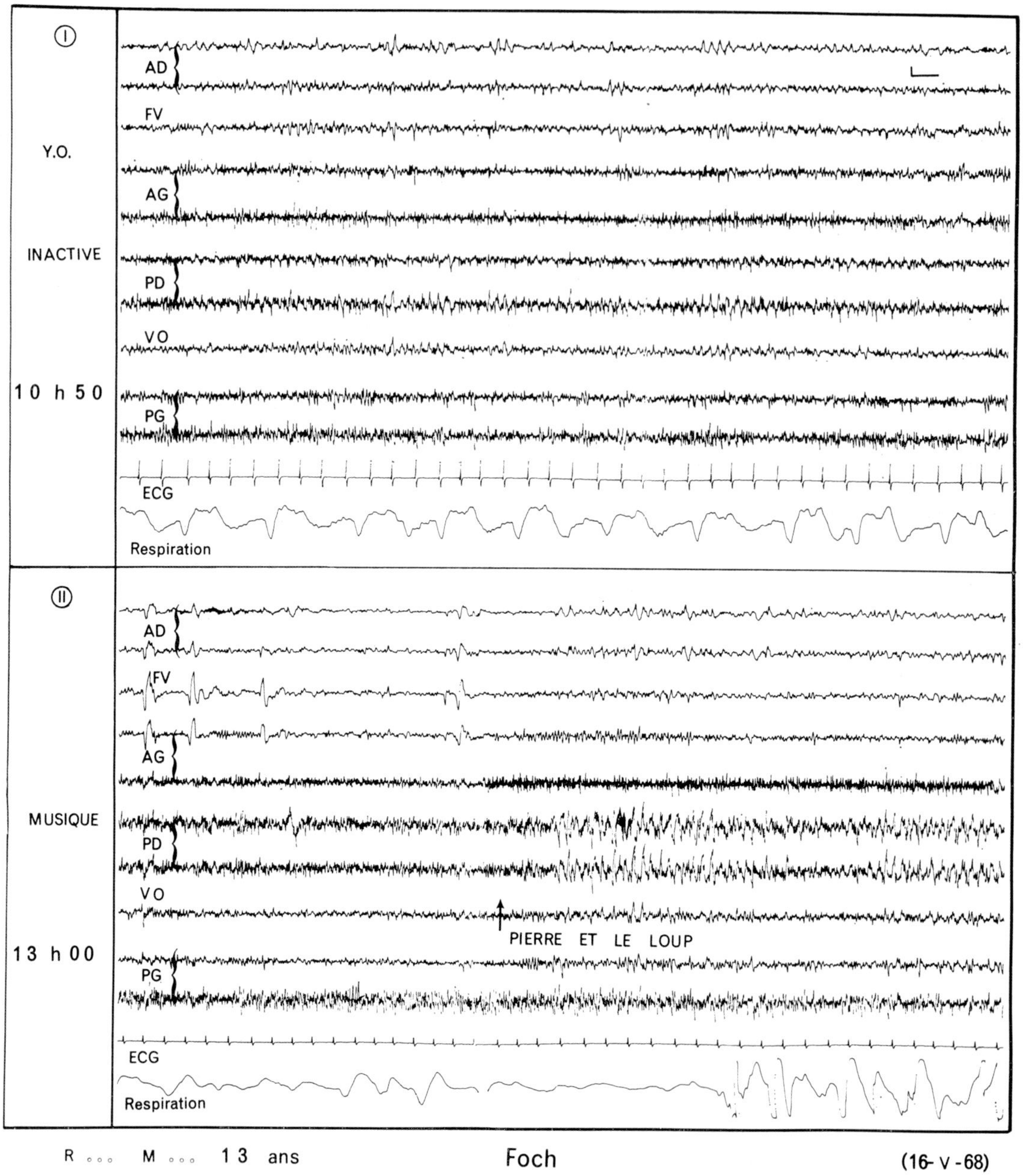

Fig. 5

Facilitation des "figures inhabituelles".

Enfant de 13 ans, présentant des myoclonies continues de la commissure labiale gauche. *I* (10 h 50): yeux ouverts, inactive: oscillations régulières de 3.5–4 c/sec au niveau de l'hémisphère *droit* (AD et PD), notamment régions temporales et parieto-occipitales. *II* (13 h 00): musique: dès que débute l'audition de "Pierre et le Loup" (Prokofiev), brusque recrudescence des anomalies *droites* au niveau des régions postérieures (PD). L'élément émotif se manifeste par des variations de la courbe respiratoire (12ème ligne, en bas). Sur les 5è et 10è lignes, empâtement du trait dû à la présence de myogrammes temporaux du côté des myoclonies.

la conversation, l'"échappement d'alpha" peut se situer tour à tour au début de l'"écoute" et de la réponse (Fig. 3, 16 h 04 et 16 h 58).

B. Chez le sujet yeux-fermés: la valeur de la méthode est attestée par le fait qu'un rythme alpha exactement semblable à celui de l'EEG conventionnel préalable s'établit. Assez rapidement dans certains cas, s'observent une dé-différenciation topographique et bientôt une discontinuité du rythme alpha, préludant à l'installation de fluctuations de la vigilance ou d'un sommeil franc. Mentionnons à ce propos la fréquence de survenue du sommeil: treize adultes sur trente-deux se sont endormis, deux jusqu'au stade IV, onze jusqu'aux stades II et III; chez seize autres, apparition de stades liminaires entre veille et sommeil, avec intermittence du rythme alpha, intrication à des bouffées diffuses de rythmes plus lents. De même dix enfants sur quinze sont entrés dans un sommeil confirmé, six abordant les stades III et IV.

3. *Figures inhabituelles*

Nous désignons par ce vocable certains éléments qui se distinguent de la normalité classique, qu'il s'agisse de figures bien caractérisées telles que les pointes et pointes-ondes, ou d'ondes lentes de fréquences diverses survenant avec une abondance inhabituelle ou montrant une tendance paroxystique. Ces activités sont soit diffuses, soit localisées.

Parmi les sujets de notre groupe expérimental, des figures "inhabituelles" répondant à la définition choisie avaient été observées chez *treize* adultes lors de l'examen conventionnel; elles n'ont été retrouvées par radio-télémétrie que chez *huit* d'entre eux. Pour les enfants, neuf EEG "inhabituels" préalables; *cinq* seulement sous télémétrie. Chez deux patients, des crises électriques ou électro-cliniques localisées se sont manifestées, alors que les EEG de routine antérieurs en étaient indemnes. Inversement, une épileptique adulte, dont le tracé conventionnel montrait d'innombrables complexes pointes-ondes, n'en a révélé aucun pendant deux examens télémétriques consécutifs.

C'est seulement chez quatre sujets que les circonstances de l'examen ont eu quelque influence sur l'extériorisation des figures inhabituelles: trois épileptiques (ayant un EEG abondamment

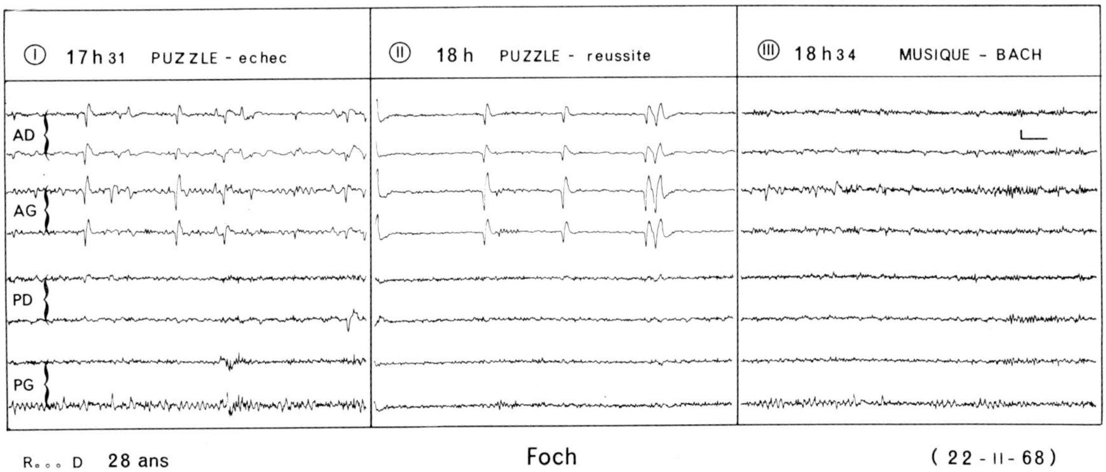

Fig. 6

Facilitation des figures "inhabituelles". Jeune femme ingénieur-pilote subissant un examen systématique. Aucun fait pathologique notable. Oscillations lentes rythmiques, à 5 c/sec, se manifestant par intermittence sur les régions temporo-frontales *gauches*. *I* (17 h 31): puzzle difficile, non résolu malgré une recherche active: les figures lentes, mêlées à quelques éléments pointus, s'établissent alors de façon *continue* en temporo-frontale gauche (3ème, 4ème et 8ème lignes). *II* (18 h 00): autre type de puzzle ne posant à la jeune femme aucune difficulté; disparition totale des ondes lentes. *III* (18 h 34): elles se manifestent à nouveau pendant l'audition musicale (8ème ligne) mais avec des intermittences.

pourvu en pointes et pointes-ondes) et une jeune femme, ingénieur-pilote, subissant un examen systématique. Chez l'une des trois épileptiques, remarquable facilitation des décharges paroxystiques observée dans la période précédant immédiatement sa décision d'abandonner un jeu de patience difficile. Sur le tracé d'une autre de ces trois malades, âgée de 13 ans, multiplication des éléments pointus au cours de l'attention angoissée qu'elle apporte à l'audition de "Pierre et le Loup" (Fig. 5, 13 h 00). La troisième, présentant une épilepsie temporale, se heurte au cours d'un puzzle à des difficultés qu'elle juge bientôt insurmontables ("je n'y arriverai jamais"); pendant cette période, foisonnement de pointes sur le lobe temporal droit; celles-ci se résorbent dès que la patiente est autorisée à choisir une épreuve plus simple.

La jeune femme ingénieur-pilote avait été conduite en télémétrie en raison de l'existence d'ondes lentes (3–4 c/sec) rythmiques, se manifestant par brusques séquences sur sa région temporale gauche. En télémétrie, ces éléments, à peu près indifférents aux divers autres temps de l'examen, montrent une nette recrudescence au cours d'un puzzle non réussi, contrastant avec leur extinction quasi complète pendant un autre puzzle facilement résolu (Fig. 6, 17 h 31 et 18 h 00).

En dehors de ces quatre exemples, certaines figures inhabituelles n'ont montré d'accentuation significative qu'au cours des fluctuations de la vigilance ou pendant le sommeil léger; ce fait ne mérite mention que dans la mesure où les circonstances de l'examen télémétrique favorisent l'endormissement.

4. *Artefacts*

L'incidence et la signification des divers artefacts rencontrés (clignements palpébraux, mouvements oculaires de lecture, myogrammes, etc.) a été provisoirement négligée. Mentionnons simplement les variations considérables de fréquence du clignement palpébral chez la plupart des patients au cours des diverses phases de la procédure expérimentale. Les artefacts du type myogramme renseignent sur l'état de tension psychomotrice du sujet et leurs variations d'intensité peuvent être un appoint utile dans une étude comportementale; mais l'appréciation du rythme cérébral sous-jacent nécessite l'application de filtres les éliminant partiellement.

DISCUSSION

Faisant abstraction de toute préoccupation diagnostique et même d'une simple distinction entre normalité et non-normalité, ce travail avait donc pour seul objet l'appréciation d'une dynamique éventuelle des rythmes hors du cadre habituel de l'EEG.

Les recherches expérimentales de Storm van Leeuwen *et al.* (1967a, b) ont montré de façon frappante la coïncidence, l'alternance ou l'indépendance des activités recueillies dans les structures explorées, selon le comportement de l'animal. Des différenciations temporelles et topographiques remarquablement précises sont observées. Au sein d'une même structure existent parfois plusieurs points d'émergence d'une activité donnée (par exemple: le rythme théta hippocampique) liés au type d'attention exercée.

Contrastant avec cette mosaïque d'aspects fonctionnels intriqués ou alternés l'EEG transcrânien, obtenu par télémétrie chez l'homme ayant sa liberté corporelle, fournit des informations d'une relative pauvreté. Cela tient d'abord au fait bien connu (rappelé justement par Storm van Leeuwen *et al.*) que l'EEG de surface ne reproduit qu'une partie extrêmement réduite des activités électriques cérébrales; en outre, sont intervenus dans notre recherche des problèmes techniques et méthodologiques.

Techniques: le nombre restreint de dérivations et, surtout, la fixité du montage initialement choisi, imposent à l'exploration une "rigidité" qui limite l'abondance et l'exactitude de l'information. Aucune analyse topographique réelle ne peut être envisagée du fait de l'application d'un seul montage bipolaire longitudinal à grandes distances inter-électrodes; tout au plus peut-on juger de variations globales ou intéressant de larges secteurs. Par ailleurs, le nécessité de filtrer les myogrammes élimine vraisemblablement certains types d'activités cérébrales, de même que l'usage de la constante de temps très courte (0,1 sec) des oscillateurs. (Malgré cela, les fragments de l'examen télémétrique comparables à l'EEG conventionnel ne révèlent aucune distorsion majeure: tous les types d'activités, des plus lentes aux plus rapides, sont retrouvés.)

Méthodologiques: le cadre dans lequel se déroulent nos examens a été fixé arbitrairement et représente un contexte artificiel dépourvu, sans doute, de contenu suggestif pour la plupart des patients. Le facteur "stress", dont le rôle fondamental est démontré par les expériences de Storm van Leeuwen *et al.* (1967b) et par les travaux de Lairy (1967) est ici très amoindri. La majorité des sujets se disent parfaitement détendus et soulignent la différence avec la sensation de contrainte que leur avait donnée l'EEG conventionnel; la facilité de l'assoupissement témoigne, partiellement, de ce sentiment de sécurité et de confort. Beaucoup de sujets participent à l'examen comme à une expérience divertissante; seules certaines épreuves paraissent fastidieuses ou créent des difficultés, telles que le dessin (pour lequel les adultes sont très peu inspirés) ou les jeux de patience que certains s'irritent de ne pouvoir instantanément réaliser. Il s'agit de "traumatismes" mineurs, ne justifiant pas ces excessives "décharges d'énergie génératrice d'angoisse", dont les figures paroxystiques seraient le corollaire (Lairy 1967).

Le cadre arbitraire et "bénin" choisi pour cette première série expérimentale peut expliquer que la dynamique des pointes et des pointes-ondes ne montre pas les remarquables variations observées par Vidart et Geier (1967, 1968), étudiant les épileptiques au travail, pendant de longues journées qui comportent l'alternance d'activités intellectuelles et manuelles plus ou moins élaborées avec des phases récréatives. Le confort et l'agrément relatif de l'examen télémétrique semblent, chez nos sujets, réduire de façon manifeste l'extériorisation des figures paroxystiques (le contraste avec les anomalies majeures de l'EEG conventionnel est frappant pour certains d'entre eux). A l'exemple de Bureau *et al.* (1968) nous nous proposons de réaliser nos examens ultérieurs dans des conditions plus complexes (tests d'efficience, épreuves projectives, etc.).

Dans notre procédure expérimentale nous avons vu, cependant, quelques exemples de facilitation des éléments "inhabituels"; cette facilitation est, sans doute, une modalité plus expressive que les autres de différenciation "circonstantielle". Car, bien que leur registre soit peu étendu, des variations s'observent à travers l'accomplissement des diverses tâches; incertaines pendant plusieurs phases de l'examen, elles peuvent prendre soudain, chez un sujet donné, une physionomie particulière pour l'une des épreuves; celle-ci, neutre aux yeux de l'observateur, peut avoir un contenu spécialement suggestif pour le sujet et susciter des états psychologiques extrêmement divers. Nous n'avons pas cherché à les appréhender dans ce premier travail: notre étude préliminaire avait pour but la recherche d'aspects "évolutifs"; leur évidence s'impose malgré le caractère sommaire du cadre technique et du programme expérimental.

L'évolution du rythme alpha chez le sujet yeux-ouverts suggère des interprétations diverses. Les phénomènes d'attention, d'émotion, d'anxiété sont classiquement impliqués dans le blocage des activités alpha; à l'inverse, l'extériorisation de celles-ci serait facilitée par la "distraction diffuse", aussi bien à l'égard du milieu ambiant que des propres sensations du patient. Dans certains de nos cas, l'apparition de rythme alpha yeux-ouverts (surtout de la première et de la deuxième variété décrites) nous a paru relever de façon évidente de processus de ce type: inattention ou inintérêt; l'inhibition du rythme alpha était alors obtenue par les épreuves sollicitant une participation active du sujet. Chez des pilotes-automobiles pour lesquels la persistance de rythmes alpha yeux-ouverts avait fait craindre un déficit de vigilance ou d'attention, l'existence et la constance du blocage dans les épreuves éveillant l'intérêt, nous ont semblé être le signe d'une disponibilité adéquate face aux difficultés éventuelles.

Cependant, d'autres facteurs se répercutent vraisemblablement sur les modalités d'extériorisation du rythme alpha; on rejoint alors les situations "facilitatrices" créées dans certaines procédures expérimentales et évoquées par divers auteurs (Williams 1940; Kreitman et Shaw 1965; Mulholland 1965, 1968). L'émergence d'activités alpha yeux-ouverts (observées dans 7–13% des cas selon Williams), serait favorisée par les manoeuvres suscitant un état d'alerte ou d'attention et par certains tests de discrimination sensorielle. Cette facilitation du rythme alpha suggèrerait les notions de "variations psychologiques globales", d'"efficience comportementale", d'effets adaptateurs (dans le sens homeostasie); elle se verrait lors du passage d'une situation à une autre, que ce soit, par exemple, de la relaxation à des états d'alerte ou l'inverse. Une interprétation de ce type peut être avancée pour certains de nos sujets chez lesquels la mobilisation du rythme alpha est observée dans un contexte actif tel que la conversation, l'éclosion de ce rythme (en général, soudaine) se faisant alors au début de la réponse à une question posée, ou au début du silence attentif suscité par une autre question. La raison pour laquelle ces faits se manifestent chez certains sujets et non chez d'autres est totalement obscure.

Enfin, la coïncidence de brèves bouffées d'"échappement d'alpha" et du clignement palpébral évoque certaines études expérimentales cherchant à établir (Fenwick 1966; Dewan 1968; Fenwick et Walker 1968; Kris 1968) les relations du rythme alpha avec la position des globes oculaires. Dans nos observations, il n'est pas douteux qu'un battement de paupières ou un mouvement oculaire, précède parfois l'extériorisation d'une brève séquence d'activité alpha (levée passagère d'un effet inhibiteur?); il faut noter que ce rythme reste alors strictement occipital ce qui pourrait être en faveur de sa nature essentiellement "visuelle".

Aux quelques commentaires qui viennent d'être faits, il nous faut ajouter que l'exploitation des données expérimentales que nous avons recueillies n'a comporté que la simple inspection visuelle; l'adjonction de méthodes du traitement de l'information sera, tôt ou tard, nécessaire pour appréhender vraiment l'intimité des faits observés, dégager leur signification éventuelle dans les études de comportement ou leur contribution diagnostique en clinique humaine.

RÉSUMÉ

1. Ce travail étudie les variations éventuelles de l'EEG humain recueilli par radio-télémétrie. Les sujets soumis à cet examen ont été sélectionnés non pas sur des critères cliniques mais selon des critères purement EEG se référant à un EEG conventionnel préalable (particularités de fréquence, de répartition et de réactivité des éléments physiologiques; survenue de figures "inhabituelles" du type pointes et pointes-ondes, séquences paroxystiques d'ondes lentes, etc.). Un protocole expérimental simple sert de cadre à ces examens dont la durée moyenne est de 3 h.

2. Toute préoccupation diagnostique est exclue et seule est considérée la "dynamique" des rythmes cérébraux; leurs variations au cours des diverses épreuves sont relativement limitées avec quelques aspects particuliers pour certaines d'entre elles (puzzles, audition musicale).

3. La dynamique du rythme alpha *yeux-ouverts* se présente selon des modalités variées (alpha occipital; alpha "propagé"; bouffées d'"échappement d'alpha") dont le substratum psychophysiologique suggère diverses remarques mais n'est pas élucidé.

4. L'extériorisation des figures "inhabituelles" ne semble pas spécialement favorisée par la procédure expérimentale choisie; quelques exemples de "facilitation" de ces éléments sont, cependant, rapportés.

SUMMARY

DYNAMIC ASPECTS OF THE HUMAN EEG. FIRST RESULTS OF A RADIOTELEMETRIC STUDY

1. This is a study of the possible variations of the human EEG recorded by radiotelemetry. The subjects examined were not selected on clinical criteria but according to purely EEG criteria derived from a previous conventional EEG (frequency, distribution and reactivity of the components, occurrence of "unusual" wave forms such as spikes, spikes and waves, paroxysmal bursts of slow waves, etc.). A simple experimental protocol formed the basis of these examinations, the average duration of which was 3 h.

2. No attempt at diagnosis was made and only the dynamic behaviour of the cerebral rhythms was considered. Their variations during various tests were relatively limited, with special features in some of them (puzzles, listening to music).

3. The behaviour of the open-eyed alpha rhythm depended upon its various types (occipital, "propagated", bursts of "alpha release"), the psychophysiological substratum of which suggested some comments but was not elucidated.

4. The occurrence of the "unusual" wave forms did not seem to be specially favoured by the chosen experimental procedure; however, some examples of "facilitation" of these wave forms are reported.

Electroenceph. clin. Neurophysiol., **1969**, *27*: 225–237

BIBLIOGRAPHIE

BLANC, C., GRAVIER, H. and GEIER, S. Radiotelemetric recordings of the electroencephalograms of civil aviation pilots during flight. *Electroenceph. clin. Neurophysiol.*, **1967,** *23*: 580P.

BUREAU, M., GUEY, J., DRAVET, C. et ROGER, J. Étude de la répartition des absences petit mal chez l'enfant en fonction de ses activités. *Rev. neurol.*, **1968,** *118*: 493–494.

DEWAN, E. M. A demonstration of the effect of eye position and accommodation on the occipital alpha rhythm. *Electroenceph. clin. Neurophysiol.*, **1968,** *24*: 188P.

FENWICK, P. B. C. The effects of eye movements on alpha rhythm. *Electroenceph. clin. Neurophysiol.*, **1966,** *21*: 618P.

FENWICK, P. B. C. and WALKER, S. The effects of eye position on the alpha rhythm. *Electroenceph. clin. Neurophysiol.*, **1968,** *25*: 508P.

HUGHES, J. R. and HENDRIX, D. E. Telemetered EEG from a football player in action. *Electroenceph. clin. Neurophysiol.*, **1968,** *24*: 183–186.

KREITMAN, N. and SHAW, J. C. Experimental enhancement of alpha activity. *Electroenceph. clin. Neurophysiol.*, **1965,** *18*: 147–155.

KRIS, C. EOG and EEG measurement while learning to position the eyes when the lids are open and closed. *Electroenceph. clin. Neurophysiol.*, **1968,** *24*: 189P.

LAIRY, G. C. Organisation de l'électroencéphalogramme normal et pathologique. *Rev. neurol.*, **1956,** *94*: 749–801.

LAIRY, G. C. Quelques remarques sur le problème "EEG et physiologie du comportement". *Electroenceph. clin. Neurophysiol.*, **1964,** *16*: 130–135.

LAIRY, G. C. L'EEG comme moyen d'investigation des modalités individuelles d'adaptation aux situations de stress. *Electroenceph. clin. Neurophysiol.*, **1967,** *Suppl. 25*: 282–298.

MULHOLLAND, T. B. Occurrence of the electroencephalographic alpha rhythm with eyes open. *Nature (Lond.)*, **1965,** *206*: 746.

MULHOLLAND, T. B. The concept of attention and the EEG alpha rhythm. *Electroenceph. clin. Neurophysiol.*, **1968,** *24*: 188P.

NESTIANU, V., BENGULESCU, D., IONESCU, V., DANELIUC, E., BONCIOCAT, C., AVRAMESCU, C. and TIRON, V. Study of EEG and EKG by tele-transmission in airmen during acrobatic flights. *Electroenceph. clin. Neurophysiol.*, **1964,** *17*: 598P.

STORM VAN LEEUWEN, W., KAMP, A., KOK, M. L., QUARTEL, F. DE, LOPES DA SILVA, F. H. et TIELEN, A. M. Relations entre les activités électriques cérébrales du chien, son comportement et sa direction d'attention. *Actualités neurophysiol.*, **1967**a: 167–186.

STORM VAN LEEUWEN, W., KAMP, A., KOK, M. L., QUARTEL, F. DE and TIELEN, A. EEG of unrestrained animals under stressful conditions. *Electroenceph. clin. Neurophysiol.*, **1967**b, *Suppl. 25*: 212–225.

STORM VAN LEEUWEN, W., KAMP, A., KOK, M. L. et TIELEN, M. Relation entre l'activité électrique de certaines structures cérébrales et le comportement du chien. *Rev. neurol.*, **1963**a, *109*: 258–259.

STORM VAN LEEUWEN, W., KAMP, A., KOK, M. L. and ZAAL, J. Monitoring states of alertness by telemetering the EEG. *Electroenceph. clin. Neurophysiol.*, **1963**b, *15*: 164P.

VIDART, L. et GEIER, S. Enregistrements téléencéphalographiques chez des sujets épileptiques pendant le travail. *Rev. neurol.*, **1967,** *117*: 475–480.

VIDART, L. et GEIER, S. Le travail, la fatigue et l'état psychique chez les malades épileptiques: étude télé-EEG. *Rev. neurol.*, **1968,** *118*: 473.

WALTER, W. G., COOPER, R., CROW, H. J., MCCALLUM, W. C., WARREN, W. J., ALDRIDGE, V. J., STORM VAN LEEUWEN, W. and KAMP, A. Contingent negative variation and evoked responses recorded by radiotelemetry in free-ranging subjects. *Electroenceph. clin. Neurophysiol.*, **1967,** *23*: 197–206.

WEINMANN, H. M. Telemetric recording of sleep rhythms in enuretic children. *Electroenceph. clin. Neurophysiol.*, **1968,** *24*: 391P.

WILLIAMS JR., A. C. Facilitation of the alpha rhythm of the electroencephalogram. *J. exp. Psychol.*, **1940,** *25*: 413–422.

Référence: ARFEL, G., CASANOVA, C. et COULMANCE, M. Aspects dynamiques de l'électroencéphalogramme humain. Premiers résultats d'une étude radio-télémétrique. *Electroenceph. clin. Neurophysiol.*, **1969,** *27*: 225–237.

Electroencephalography and Clinical Neurophysiology
Elsevier Publishing Company, Amsterdam – Printed in The Netherlands

SELECTIVE SUPPRESSION OF CEREBRAL EVOKED POTENTIALS TO PATTERNED LIGHT IN AMBLYOPIA EX ANOPSIA[1]

C. T. Lombroso, M.D., F. H. Duffy, M.D. and R. M. Robb, M.D.

Division of Clinical Neurophysiology, Department of Neurology, Children's Hospital Medical Center, and Departments of Neurology and of Ophthalmology, Harvard Medical School, Boston, Mass. 02115 (U.S.A.)

(Accepted for publication: December 27, 1968)

INTRODUCTION

The neurophysiology of the visual defect in amblyopia ex anopsia and the site of primary pathology are still poorly understood. As early as 1921 Ammann noted that the visual acuity of the amblyopic eye was not altered by wearing dark glasses, whereas the acuity of the normal eye was decreased (see also Von Noorden and Burian 1959a). Wald and Burian (1944) interpreted the condition as a selective impairment of pattern vision while light perception remained undisturbed. More than pattern vision was implicated when Feinberg (1956) showed that flicker fusion is distinctly reduced in amblyopic eyes. Von Noorden and Burian (1959b) provided a quantitative demonstration that at low levels of illumination the acuity of the amblyopic eye is equal to, or frequently better, than the acuity of the normal eye of the same individual. They suggested that the effects of low levels of illumination might be to reduce the levels of contrast. The same authors (1960) showed that blanking time was significantly longer for the amblyopic eye, suggesting that the cerebral integration of visual information received from the amblyopic eye was either slower or more vulnerable. Perceptual blanking is defined by Lindsley and Emmons (1958) as the obliteration of tachistoscopically presented information by a brief flash of light following the initial tachistoscopic presentation by a short interval. This has been considered as the result of interference at the cortical level. Blanking time is defined as the minimal separation between information carrying flash and blanking flash, where the blanking flash is successful in destroying data carried in the information flash. Von Noorden (1961) illustrated that the reaction time was prolonged in amblyopic eyes especially under binocular stimulation and at low levels of illumination. In this case, it is of interest to note that in the presence of stimulation of the normal eye, the amblyopic eye showed a degradation in performance.

Enoch (1959) presented evidence that disturbances of the spatial orientation of retinal receptor elements could account for at least part of the decreased acuity in strabismic amblyopia. On the other hand, Burian and Lawwill (1966) and Nawratzki *et al.* (1966) failed to demonstrate significant abnormalities in the electroretinogram (ERG) following discrete foveal stimulation in children with amblyopia ex anopsia. It is known, however, that the ERG may be normal in the presence of known macular disease (Burian and Lawwill 1966).

It is the purpose of this paper to present electrophysiological data in a study of children with amblyopia ex anopsia. This study is based on the evaluation of the computer enhanced visual evoked response (VER) recorded from the occipital scalp. Fishman (1966) has shown that the VER can be obtained when the level of illumination is such that no ERG can be recorded. In addition, Vaughan and Silverstein (1968) have shown that the VER is to a large extent the result of foveal activity and that even when the parafoveal retina is stimulated, the VER may in large part be attributed to stray light impinging upon the fovea.

[1] This work was assisted in part by a National Institute of Neurological Diseases and Blindness Grant (NB-07926-01) and a National Institute of Health General Research Grant (FR-05482-05), allocated through the Children's Hospital Medical Center, and in part by a Burt Wolbach Award.

METHOD AND MATERIAL

The VERs of twenty-two amblyopic children from 4 to 16 years of age and of ten normal subjects were evaluated. Of the amblyopic children, eight had strabismic amblyopia with foveal fixation in the amblyopic eye, nine had strabismic amblyopia with eccentric fixation and four had refractive amblyopia from marked anisometropia.

Recordings were made from a 3 cm diameter rosette of four bipolar pairs as shown in Fig. 2 (see Clynes 1965). Simultaneous recordings were also made from O_z – mastoid, O_z – C_z, neck muscles, and DC eye electrodes. Silver–silver chloride discs were applied to the scalp with collodion and fed into a Grass Model-7 Polygraph with a 0.1–75 c/sec response characteristic. Raw EEG was recorded on an FM tape deck for subsequent off-line analysis on a CAT 1000 or CAT 400. Care was taken to avoid those trials associated with eye blink, eye movement or muscle artifact. By permitting the subject to rest his head on a pillow while sitting upright, almost all muscle artifact was removed from the EEG. This was accompanied by the virtual absence of contributions to the VER from muscle micro-reflexes (see Bickford 1966). The stimulus was "cool white light" from three digitally controlled Iconix fluorescent lamps with 1 msec rise times fixed in a 35 × 50 cm stimulus box. A plain translucent screen or a patterned translucent screen was placed before the lamps 50 cm in front of the subject. The pattern was a black-white checkerboard with high light-dark interface index (Spehlmann 1965; Harter and White 1968). Check size was 1 cm square. Radiant light energy was held at identical levels (3 log units above threshold) for both plain and patterned stimulation by means of a calibrated light meter. The stimulus was a 500 or 1000 msec square pulse of light which allowed examination of the "on" response alone and not the inconstant mixture of "off" and "on" response seen with pulses of shorter duration (Efron 1964). Inter-stimulus intervals ranged from 250 to 2250 msec in a pseudo-random (flat, non-Gaussian) distribution as programmed on punched paper tape. This permitted a minimum number of trials to be given in a short period of time, and insured a flat baseline by averaging randomly over a potentially non-random EEG segment (*e.g.*, those with unusually long "off" responses). Preliminary investigation revealed no interaction between the "off" and "on" responses for inter-stimulus intervals of 200 msec or greater. The stimulus was delayed 50 msec from onset of the analysis sweep. Averages in which the baseline period was not flat were considered invalid. 150–300 trials were taken to form each average. "Attention" was controlled not only by the random appearance of the stimulus but by having subjects count the number of flashes seen with frequent interrogation to assure diligence. Requesting the children to look at the screen was very successful in reducing the amount of alpha activity in the raw EEG (see Mulholland, in press). Pupils were dilated with 1% cyclopentolate to avoid changes attributable to long-term pupillary constriction (see Bergamini *et al.* 1965). Subjects were refracted and their corrected acuity measured on the day of their evoked potential examination. Full spectacle corrections were worn to provide an accurate focus on the screen. Each eye was stimulated individually with both plain and patterned light, the unused eye being carefully patched. The size of the field, being 60° horizontally and 40° vertically, was sufficient to insure foveal stimulation in cases of: (a) eccentric fixation,

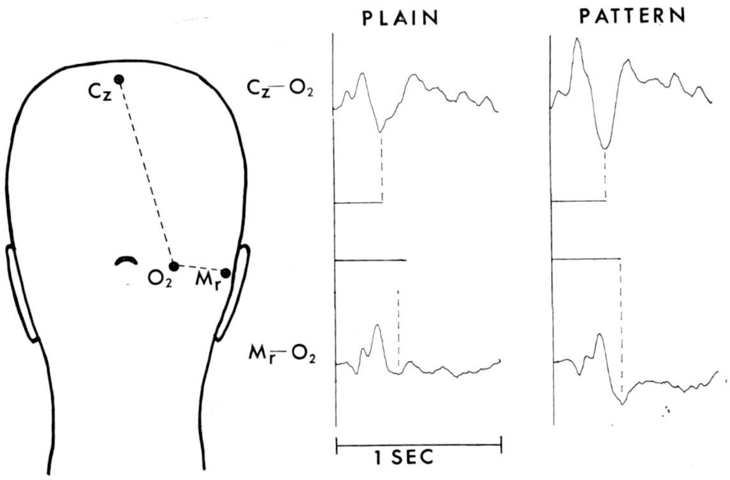

Fig. 1

Standard electrode configurations C_z–O_2 and M_r–O_2 are shown with the simultaneously recorded evoked responses to plain (first column) and to patterned (second column) light. Note that the latency to component showing most change (as shown by the dotted line) is a function of electrode placement. Note that the change in ER produced by pattern is more marked in the C_z–O_2 electrode configuration.

and (b) children whose young age precluded prolonged cooperation in controlling direction of gaze. A review of the extensive VER literature revealed marked variability in wave shapes obtained by different investigators. This may be due, in part, to: (a) lack of a standard electrode montage, and (b) to the erroneous assumption that wave shape is largely independent of electrode position. Fig. 1 shows that not only are wave shapes different for different electrode positions, but that, when experimental conditions are altered, the change which occurs in the VER may be a function of the recording axis.

The evoked potential is spatially three-dimensional as generated. When projected onto the scalp from the brain, a 3-space to 2-space transformation is made and one dimension of information is lost to those recording from the scalp. The problem is not to lose further information by inadequate scalp electrode montages.

At a given point within the 2-space of scalp, two recording axes (*i.e.*, two bipolar pairs at 90° separation) are necessary and sufficient. However, the 3 cm inter-electrode spacing of the rosette is not negligible. Scalp curvature, field polarization, or highly localized sources may cause apparent electric field anisotropy (polarization). To avoid losing a component the simplest solution is to add an additional orthogonal set of bipolar electrodes skewed 45° to the first set. This is the arrangement originally described by Clynes (1965) and Clynes and Kohn (1967) in which the scalp overlying the occipital cortex was surrounded with a circular array of four bipolar electrode pairs, forming two orthogonal sets (0°–90°, 45°–135°; see Fig. 2). The column CAT 1000 represents four simultaneously derived VERs obtained from the rosette array and are termed the input quadruplet. Inspection reveals that the individual curves appear different from one another and point up, again, the importance of electrode orientation in obtaining the VER. Despite the over-all dissimilarity, there appear to be VER components with representation in each curve. For example, there is (I) with maximum value at 185 msec and another (II) at 270 msec. It is to be noted that component I appears to be maximally represented at 135° (isopotential line at 45°) and component II maximally represented at 90°.

To reduce the volume of VERs per experiment, an IBM 7094 program was developed in conjunction with the Harvard Computing Center to further analyze the input quadruplet. A principal component analysis was employed using multiplication and subtraction in a manner intuitively similar to that employed to solve simultaneous algebraic equations by factoring. Principal components were separated by their differing percent contributions to each of the input quadruplet curves. As the differing contribution was a function of differing electric field orientations, the output components of the analysis program are separated on the basis of having different spatial orientations. By the nature of the factoring analysis the principal components may be considered independent but not necessarily unique.

In Fig. 2 under heading "IBM 7094" are calcomp plots of the output traces, representing results of this principal component analysis. A separate print out shows that the Max. (largest) component would be maximally displayed by a bipolar electrode pair at 136°, first difference curve (next largest component) at 60°, second difference curve (next largest ouput component) at 24° and that the third difference curve (smallest output component) is not significant. Note that Max. is identical to component I and the first difference is component II. In a sense, this may be considered a form of data reduction permitting one to examine one, two or three "pure" curves rather than four mixtures. The example of Fig. 2 is such that rapid separation of components by visual

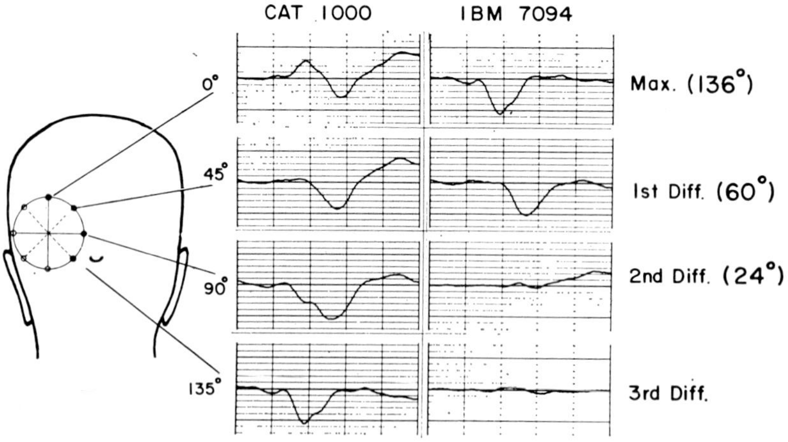

Fig. 2

A rosette of 4 bipolar pairs is shown applied to the left occipital area with grid 1 as black and grid 2 as open circles. Under CAT 1000 are the 4 VERs and under IBM are the 4 curves representing output of a factoring analysis performed on the 4 VERs (see text). Time window in each case is 500 msec and each major vertical dimension represents 10 mV.

inspection is a simple matter. The greatest application of this program, of course, is to large volumes of work, especially where these components are not so obvious. This "principal component analysis technique" bears no direct relation to the "factoring analysis technique" of Lehmann and Fender (1968).

Peak voltage measurements are generally employed to describe the magnitude of an evoked potential. When wave shapes are no longer similar, this technique becomes inadequate as only one point is sampled per curve. V_{rms}, calculated as

$$\left[\frac{1}{T}\int_T V^2(t)dt\right]^{\frac{1}{2}}$$

is preferred, since it represents average deviation from baseline independent of sign. Since at least one orthogonal pair of bipolar electrodes is required to include all evoked potential contribution one cannot take V_{rms} at 0° or 90° alone as representative of response magnitude. They cannot be simply added together as voltage is a vector. By squaring each, we may then sum them for voltage squared has the units of power, a scalar quantity. Thus, response magnitude (power) equals power 0° plus power 90°. A further complication, however, is the necessity of one additional orthogonal pair to insure inclusion of all components in their proper proportion. A solution is that the principal output components are essentially independent (non-redundant) and as an intuitive approximation one may add the power (V_{rms}^2) of each of these to obtain the total power. This usually checks well with the alternative solution of adding the power along the orthogonal axis.

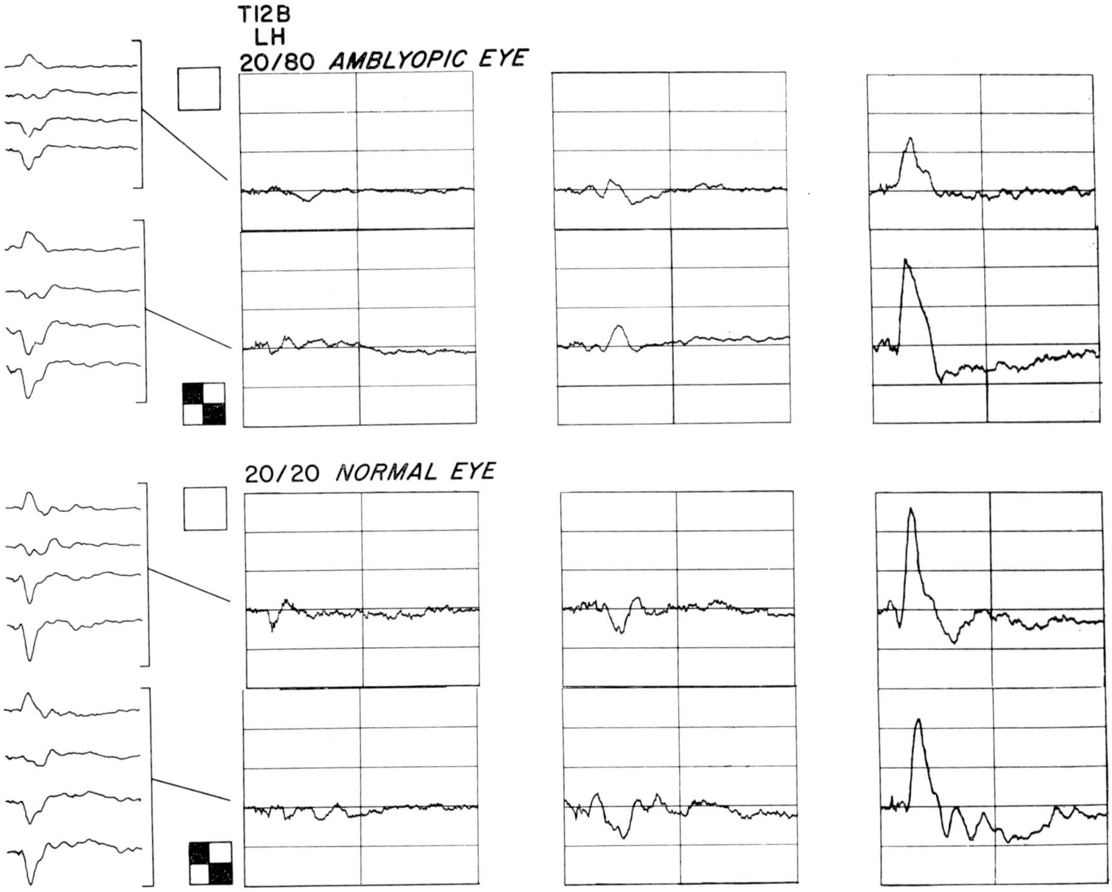

Fig. 3

VER analysis from the left hemisphere of a 17-year-old with amblyopia ex anopsia. For each condition, the 4 input VERs from the rosette are displayed to the left for reference. The 3 significant curves of the IBM 7094 analysis are displayed horizontally to the right in rows. The upper two rows are the responses of the amblyopic eye to plain (plain marker) light and patterned (checkered marker) light. The lower two rows refer to the same two conditions of stimulation for the normal eye. Each major vertical division is 5 mV and total time scale is 1000 msec. Note that display convention between input and output curves is reversed. Each curve represents 300 trials. Visual acuity is that obtained using full spectacle corrections.

RESULTS

Evoked potentials from the unipolar electrodes, the rosette array (input quadruplet), and the principal component analysis were all examined for each case. Although the same information could frequently be obtained by inspection of any one of these, the unipolar arrays were least useful and the principal component analysis most useful. To reduce the amount of data displayed in our results (see Fig. 3–6) the unipolar curves are omitted and the input quadruplets are displayed on diminished scale to the left of each row. For each figure, the upper two rows pertain to stimulation of the amblyopic eye, and the lower two of the normal eye. From the input quadruplets on the left, lines lead to the three significant principal components as determined by the factoring analysis program. In most cases, the fourth and smallest output component (3rd diff. curve) was not significant and was, therefore, not displayed. The earliest computer program displayed components arbitrarily at one of two equivalent angles; *i.e.*, positive at 10° or negative at 190°. Although later programs have been corrected, outputs of the early version (see Fig. 5) have apparent sign reversal from one quadruplet to another.

The twenty-two subjects divided themselves into two groups of eleven each. A typical result of the first group is seen in Fig. 3, the response of a 17-year-old boy with refractive amblyopia. In examining the Max. component (right-hand column), one sees that in comparison with the normal eye, the amblyopic eye shows slightly attenuated amplitude to plain light and responds by increased amplitude but with no increase in complexity of wave form to patterned light. The second com-

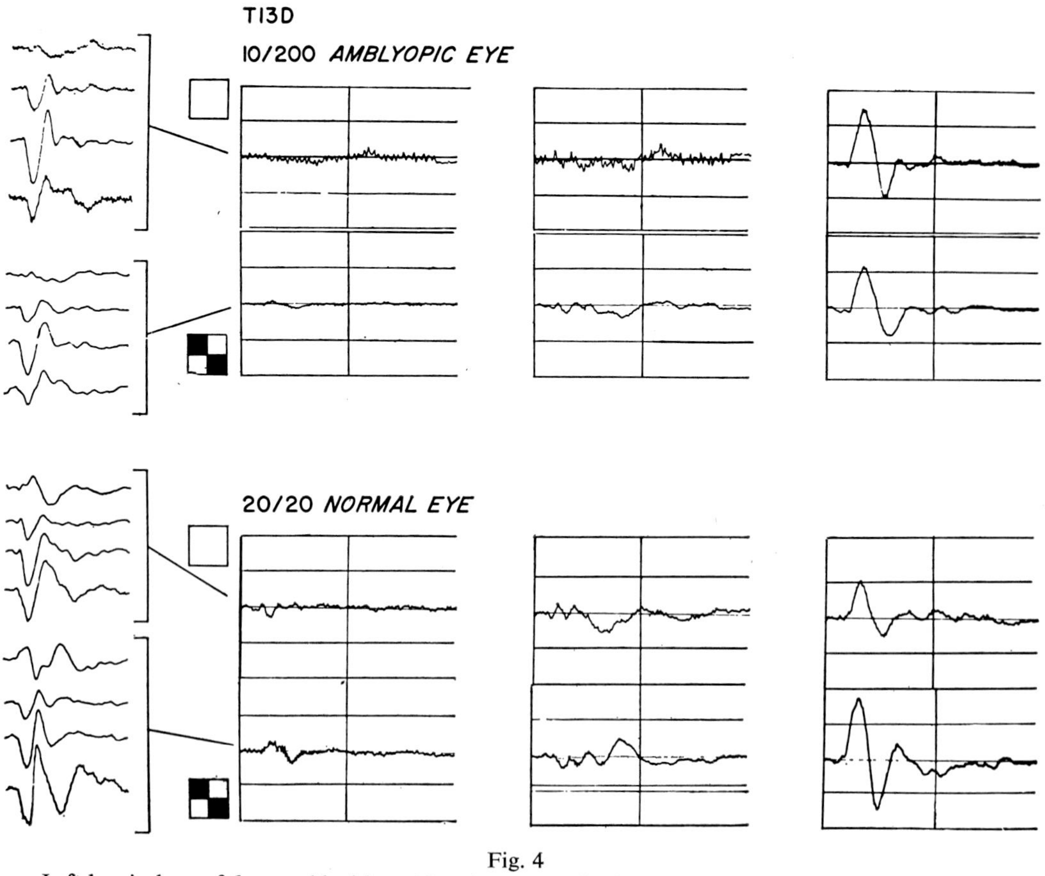

Fig. 4
Left hemisphere of 6-year-old with amblyopia ex anopsia. Same display and scale as Fig. 3. Here and in Fig. 5 and 6 note the reduced response to pattern in the amblyopic eye.

ponents (middle column) are larger in each case for the normal eye. The remaining ten children in this first group showed responses which were similar, although not all showed a larger amplitude of the response to patterned light in the amblyopic eye. Among the eleven, there was no correlation with visual acuity (after optical correction) and no difference in the responses of the four children whose amblyopia was on the basis of anisometropia rather than strabismus. In the entire study, there was no significant difference between right and left hemispheres.

On the other hand, the other group of eleven showed responses similar to those illustrated in Fig. 4–6. The response to plain light was normal or slightly more complex in the amblyopic eye than in the normal eye, but there appeared to be a marked decrease in the amplitude and wave form complexity of the principal output component of the VER to pattern in the amblyopic eye. Note that this suppression of VER in pattern vision was unrelated to visual acuity (compare subject T13C with T18E) or to the type of amblyopia (strabismic eccentric fixation, T13D; strabismic with central fixation, T13C), and refractive (T18E). Thus, while the first group of children with amblyopia showed, mainly, poor development (lesser complexity) of the VER to patterned light on their bad eye, the second group showed a definite reduction in amplitude and wave form complexity of the VER to pattern.

Fig. 7 examines the change in power of the VERs when the conditions of stimulation are changed from plain to patterned light. The upper

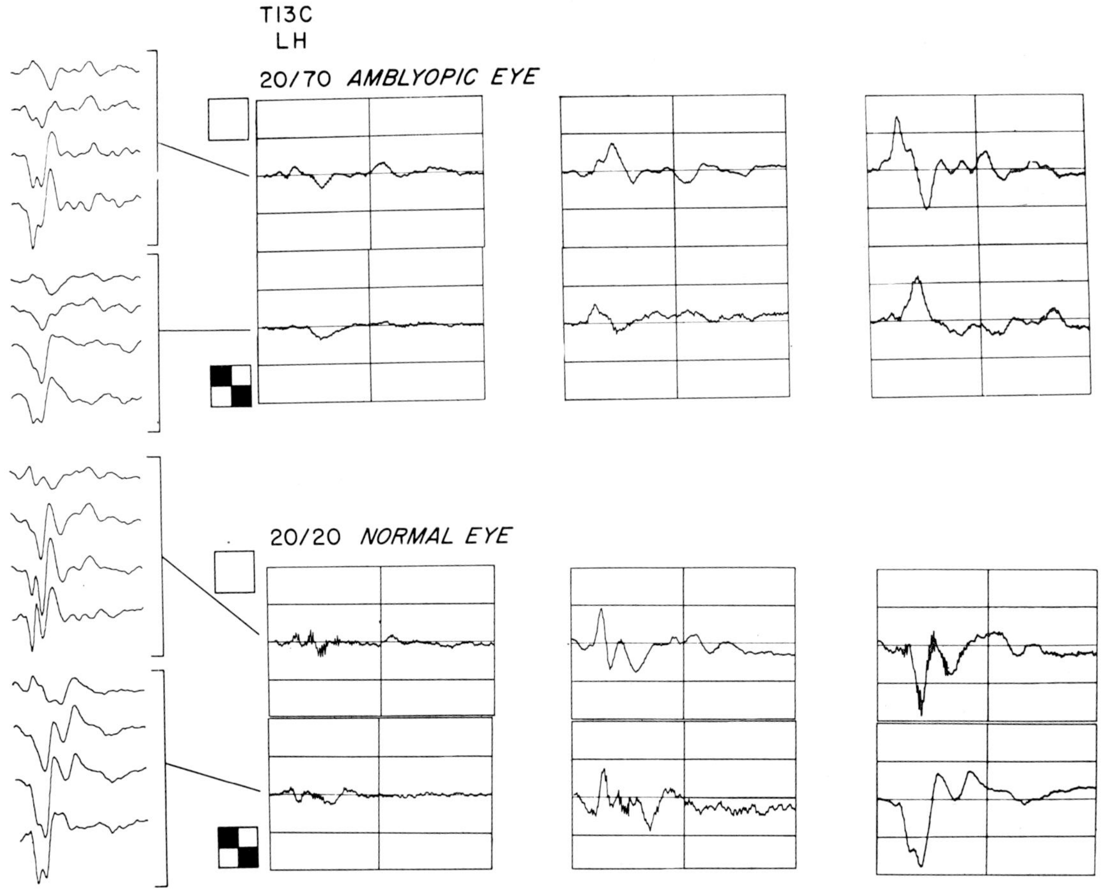

Fig. 5

Left hemisphere of a 7-year-old with amblyopia ex anopsia. Same display and scale. Input and output curves are displayed with the same convention, except that "normal eye" curves appear inverted due to unusual display convention (see text).

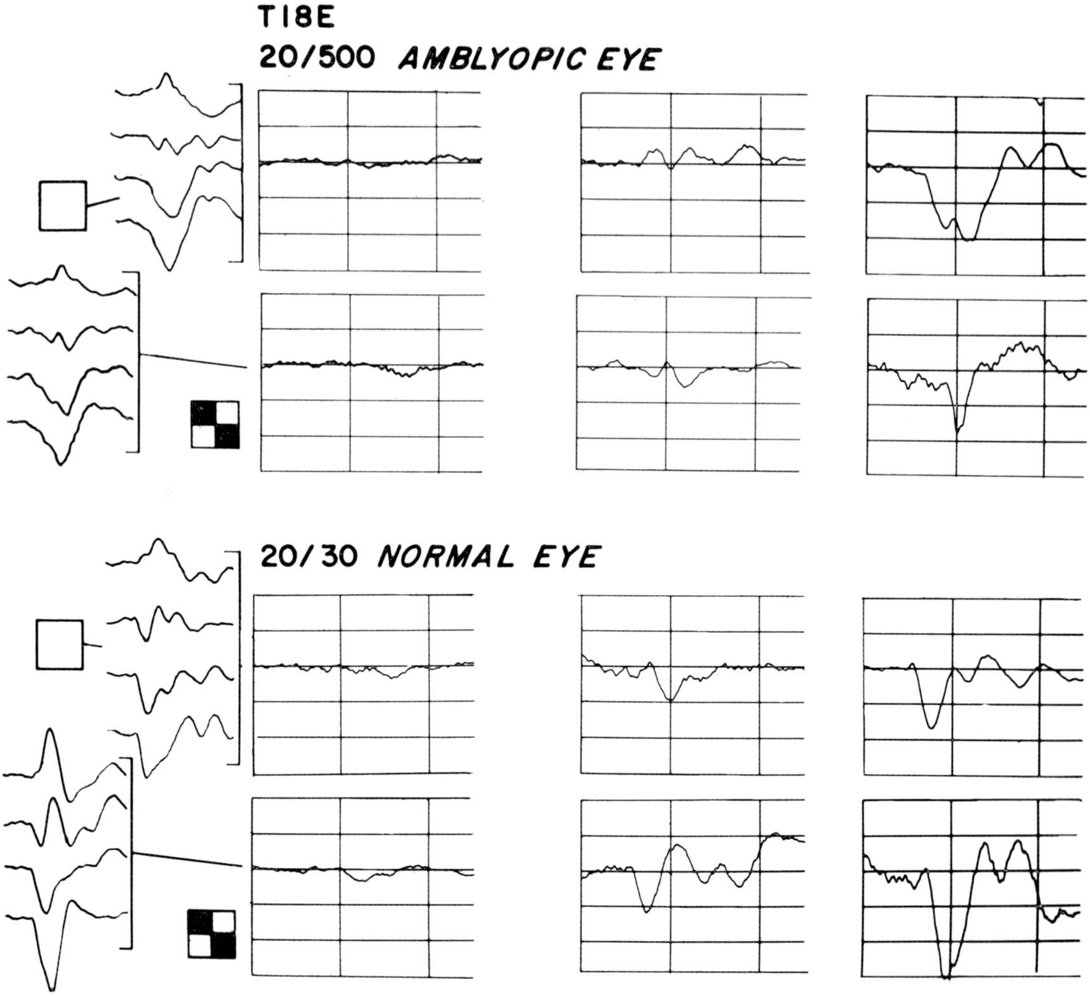

Fig. 6
Left hemisphere of a 10-year-old with amblyopia ex anopsia. Same display and scale as in Fig. 4. Note, again, the marked reduction in response to pattern in the amblyopic eye.

graph shows that 47% of the fifteen subjects so examined showed an increase and 53% a decrease with pattern stimulation of the amblyopic eye. However, 67% showed an increase and 33% a decrease for stimulation of the normal eye as seen in the second graph. For each subject the calculation, % increase power (normal eye) − % in-

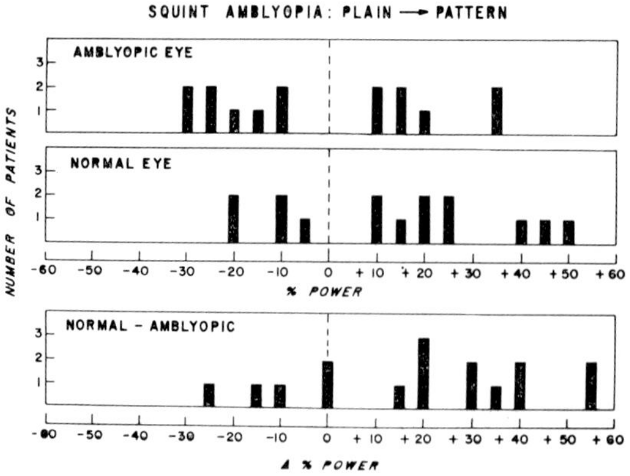

Fig. 7
The lower graph shows that more power was employed in the normal eye than in the amblyopic eye per patient when viewing a patterned image (see text for explanation).

crease power (amblyopic eye) $= \Delta$ % power, was performed and shown in the third graph. Here it is to be noted that for 78 % of the subjects, more power was seen in the VER produced by stimulation with pattern of the normal as opposed to the amblyopic eye.

DISCUSSION AND CONCLUSIONS

Hubel (1959, 1960), Hubel and Wiesel (1963, 1965) and Wiesel and Hubel (1963, 1965) approached the enigma of amblyopia as an extension of their work on the basic neurophysiology of the visual system. They found that in the normal newborn cat, the single cortical cell response to light is similar to that in the cortex of the adult cat; namely, that single cells are sensitive to light, pattern and movement and that many single cell units are driven by both eyes. They produced an experimental amblyopia by two differing techniques: (1) unilateral eyelid suture at birth, and (2) unilateral extra ocular muscle surgery at birth to produce strabismus. With the first method, almost no cortical cells would respond when the resulting amblyopic eye was stimulated at a subsequent time. With the second method, the clinical condition of alternating fixation occurred and cortical unit responses were abnormal. Single cortical cells could be driven by just one eye or the other but not by both eyes—suggesting a disassociation of the eye at a cortical level paralleling the clinical alternating fixation.

As important as these results are to basic visual neurophysiology, their analogy to humans with amblyopia ex anopsia is uncertain. In human strabismic amblyopia, the turned eye is not deprived of all formed images as in condition (1) above. In addition, loss of visual acuity is characteristically associated with preferred fixation with one eye and not alternating fixation as in condition (2) above. In children, the image from the turned eye appears to be suppressed to avoid diplopia, and this suppression eventually is associated with the loss of formed vision measurable even when the turned eye is tested alone (*cf.* Von Noorden and Burian 1959b).

It was the purpose of this paper to present electrophysiological data in the child with amblyopia. In our series of twenty-two children, a normal response to both plain and patterned light was found in the unaffected eye. The amblyopic eye showed a slight increase in some children (36 %), and in others a slight decrease (42 %) and no change (22 %) in the amplitude of the evoked response to plain light. In all cases, the complexity of the VER to plain light in the amblyopic eye was similar to that in the normal eye. The response to pattern in the amblyopic eye was of greater interest. Fifty percent of the children showed a lack of wave form complexity which one usually associated with pattern stimulation. Of even greater interest was the fact that, for the remaining 50 %, there was actual degradation of both amplitude and wave form complexity in response to patterned stimulation of their amblyopic eye (see Fig. 4–6). Our results may appear to contradict those of Fishman and Copenhaver (1967) who found no abnormality of VER in amblyopes. However, these authors used only plain light, conventional electrode placement, and looked mainly at amplitude and latency differences. In contrast to other investigators (*cf.* De Voe *et al.* 1968 and Nawratzki *et al.* 1966), we found measurements of latency and peak amplitude of the VER to be variable and inconclusive from subject to subject and from experiment to experiment.

However, if one accepts average power of the VER as an indicator of underlying cortical activity, then there would appear to be cortical suppression of electrical activity induced by patterned images when the amblyopic eye is stimulated (see Fig. 7).

At the geniculate level, there is little known binocular interaction making this an unlikely site for visual inhibition or electrical suppression. The majority of cortical cells, however, are known to be driven by both eyes. It would seem that the degradation of acuity under binocular condition noted by Von Noorden and Leffler (1966) must, therefore, take place at the cortical level. Neither this nor our results can exclude some degree of defect in amblyopia at the peripheral levels of the visual system (*cf.* Enoch 1959).

Now, if the findings of this paper (namely, that there is a selective defect in the VER to patterned images which is not present under conditions of stimulation of plain light) are coupled with the report by Hubel and Wiesel (1963, 1965) that only in the visual cortex does one find single cells uniquely sensitive to pattern, then the evidence that the cortex is a major site of the defect in amblyopia ex anopsia appears most probable.

SUMMARY

Experimental evidence is presented to show that there is an abnormal depression of the computer derived visual evoked response to patterned images when they are presented to the amblyopic eye in a significant number of children with amblyopia ex anopsia. In contrast, no differences of significance were seen in the VERs obtained by stimulating the normal and amblyopic eyes individually with plain light. A specific inhibition of pattern vision is postulated. When this evidence is evaluated in the light of the known fact that cells uniquely sensitive to shape are found only in the cortex, then the cortex (rather than the retina or geniculate body) appears to be the most likely site of the defect in human amblyopia ex anopsia.

RÉSUMÉ

SUPPRESSION SELECTIVE DES POTENTIELS ÉVOQUÉS CÉRÉBRAUX À UN PATTERN LUMINEUX DANS L'AMBLYOPIE EX ANOPSIA

Les auteurs présentent des résultats expérimentaux montrant qu'il existe une dépression anormale de la réponse évoquée visuelle obtenue par calculateur à des patterns visuels lorsqu'ils sont présentés à l'oeil amblyope sur un nombre significatif d'enfants atteints d'amblyopie ex anopsia. À l'opposé, aucune différence significative n'a été observée dans les réponses évoquées visuelles obtenues en stimulant individuellement l'oeil normal et l'oeil amblyope avec une lumière simple. Ils font l'hypothèse qu'il existe une inhibition spécifique de la vision des formes. Si on considère cette donnée à la lumière des faits connus suivant lesquels les cellules uniquement sensibles aux formes ne sont trouvées que dans le cortex, alors le cortex (plutôt que la rétine ou le corps genouillé) semble être le siège le plus vraisemblable du déficit dans l'amblyopie ex anopsia humaine.

REFERENCES

AMMANN, E. Einige Beobachtungen bei "Zentrales" Sehen — Sehen der Glaukomatosen — Sehen der Amblyopen. *Klin. Mbl. Augenheilk.*, **1921**, *66*: 564–573.

BERGAMINI, L., BERGAMASCO, B., MOMBELLI, A. M. and GANDIGLIO, G. Visual evoked potentials in subjects with congenital aniridia. *Electroenceph. clin. Neurophysiol.*, **1965**, *19*: 394–397.

BICKFORD, R. G. Human "microreflexes" revealed by computer analysis. *Neurology (Minneap.)*, **1966**, *16*: 302–314.

BURIAN, H. M. and LAWWILL, T. Electroretinographic studies in strabismic amblyopia. *Amer. J. Ophthal.*, **1966**, *61*: 422–430.

CLYNES, M. Brain space analysis of evoked potential components applied to chromaticity waves. *6th Int. Conf. med. Electron. biol. Eng. (Tokyo)*, **1965**: 460P.

CLYNES, M. and KOHN, M. Spatial visual evoked potentials as physiologic language elements for color and field structure. *Electroenceph. clin. Neurophysiol.*, **1967**, *Suppl. 26*: 82–86.

DE VOE, R. G., RIPPS, H. and VAUGHAN, H. G. Cortical responses to stimulation of the human fovea. *Vision Res.*, **1968**, *8*: 135–147.

EFRON, R. Artificial synthesis of evoked responses to light flash. *Ann. N. Y. Acad. Sci.*, **1964**, *112*: 292–304.

ENOCH, J. M. Receptor amblyopia. *Amer. J. Ophthal.*, **1959** (Sept. Pt. II), *48*: 262–273.

FEINBERG, I. Critical flicker frequency in amblyopia ex anopsia. *Amer. J. Ophthal.*, **1956**, *42*: 473–482.

FISHMAN, R. S. The visual-evoked cortical response in night blindness. *Amer. J. Ophthal.*, **1966**, *62*: 1166–1770.

FISHMAN, R. S. and COPENHAVER, R. M. Macular disease and amblyopia. The visual-evoked response. *Arch. Ophthal. (Chic.)*, **1967**, *77*: 718–725.

HARTER, M. and WHITE, C. Effects of contour, sharpness and check-size on visually evoked cortical potentials. *Vision Res.*, **1968**, *8*: 701–711.

HUBEL, D. H. Single unit activity in striate cortex of unrestrained cats. *J. Physiol. (Lond.)*, **1959**, *147*: 226–238.

HUBEL, D. H. Single unit activity in lateral geniculate body and optic tract of unrestrained cats. *J. Physiol. (Lond.)*, **1960**, *150*: 91–104.

HUBEL, D. H. and WIESEL, T. N. Receptive fields in cells of striate cortex of very young visually inexperienced kittens. *J. Neurophysiol.*, **1963**, *26*: 994–1002.

HUBEL, D. H. and WIESEL, T. N. Binocular interaction in striate cortex of kittens reared with artificial squint. *J. Neurophysiol.*, **1965**, *28*: 1041–1059.

LEHMANN, D. and FENDER, D. H. Component analysis of human averaged evoked potentials: dichoptic stimuli using different target structure. *Electroenceph. clin. Neurophysiol.*, **1968**, *24*: 542–553.

LINDSLEY, D. B. and EMMONS, W. H. Perceptual blanking, evoked potentials, and perception time. *Electroenceph. clin. Neurophysiol.*, **1958**, *10*: 359–368.

MULHOLLAND, T. Concept of attention and the electroencephalographic alpha rhythms. *Conf. Concept of Attention in Neurophysiology*, Teddington, England, October 3, **1967**. Butterworth, London. In press.

NAWRATZKI, I., AUERBACH, E. and ROWE, H. The electrical response in retina and occipital cortex following photic stimulation of normal and amblyopic eyes. *Amer. J. Ophthal.*, **1966,** *61*: 432–435.

SPEHLMANN, R. The averaged electrical responses to diffuse and patterned light in the human. *Electroenceph. clin. Neurophysiol.*, **1965,** *19*: 560–569.

VAUGHAN, H. G. and SILVERSTEIN, L. Metacontrast and evoked potentials: a reappraisal. *Science*, **1968,** *160*: 207–208.

VON NOORDEN, G. K. Reaction time in normal and amblyopic eyes. *Arch. Ophthal. (Chic.)*, **1961,** *66*: 695–701.

VON NOORDEN, G. K. and BURIAN, H. M. Visual acuity in normal and amblyopic patients under reduced illumination. I. Behavior of visual acuity with and without neutral density filter. *Arch. Ophthal. (Chic.)*, **1959**a, *61*: 533–535.

VO NOORDEN, G. K. and BURIAN, H. M. Visual acuity in normal and amblyopic patients under reduced illumination. II. The visual acuity at various levels of illumination. *Arch. Ophthal. (Chic.)*, **1959**b, *62*: 396–399.

VON NOORDEN, G. K. and BURIAN, H. M. Perceptual blanking in normal and amblyopic eyes. *Arch. Ophthal. (Chic.)*, **1960,** *64*: 817–822.

VON NOORDEN, G. K. and LEFFLER, M. B. Visual acuity under monocular and binocular conditions. *Arch. Ophthal. (Chic.)*, **1966,** *76*: 172–177.

WALD, G. and BURIAN, H. M. The dissociation of form vision and light perception in strabismic amblyopia. *Amer. J. Ophthal.*, **1944,** *27*: 950–963.

WIESEL, T. N. and HUBEL, D. H. Single cell responses in striate cortex of kittens deprived of vision in one eye. *J. Neurophysiol.*, **1963,** *26*: 1003–1017.

WIESEL, T. N. and HUBEL, D. H. Receptive fields and functional architecture in two non striate visual areas (18 and 19) of the cat. *J. Neurophysiol.*, **1965,** *28*: 229–289.

Reference: LOMBROSO, C. T., DUFFY, F. H. and ROBB, R. M. Selective suppression of cerebral evoked potentials to patterned light in amblyopia ex anopsia. *Electroenceph. clin. Neurophysiol.*, **1969,** *27*: 238–247.

Electroencephalography and Clinical Neurophysiology
Elsevier Publishing Company, Amsterdam – Printed in The Netherlands

CHANGES INDUCED IN STABILIZED IMAGE VISIBILITY BY EXPERIMENTAL ALTERATION OF THE ONGOING EEG[1,2]

ULKER TULUNAY KEESEY AND DENNIS J. NICHOLS

Medical School, University of Wisconsin and Laboratory Computer Facility, University of Wisconsin, Madison, Wis. 53706 (U.S.A.)

(Accepted for publication: December 11, 1968)

INTRODUCTION

When a target is observed under stabilized image conditions, *i.e.*, when a target image is made to remain stationary with respect to the retina despite the ever present movements of the eye, lines and borders gradually fade, leaving a uniform, perceptually empty field. This effect is transitory, and the target comes back into view intermittently in parts or in total. Even though the fading or disappearance and reappearance of a stabilized image has been demonstrated many times, the physiological basis of these events is not well understood. It was originally assumed that disappearance is due to retinal adaptation incurred by the stationary image (Riggs *et al.* 1953; Ditchburn 1955) and reappearance was regarded as the result of a disturbance in the adaptation state by an uncontrolled change in the position of the retinal image (Cornsweet 1966). For reviews of this problem see Heckenmueller (1965), Keesey and Nichols (1967) and Gerrits *et al.* (1966).

That at least disappearance is more than a retinal adaptation phenomenon has been suggested by data showing disappearance of targets in "meaningful" units (Pritchard *et al.* 1960), lesser disappearance when a sensory system other than visual is stimulated (Pritchard 1964), and the interocular transfer effects of image fading (Krauskopf and Riggs 1959; Cohen 1961). Recently considerable attention has been directed toward the regularity of stabilized image reappearance (Fiorentini and Ercoles 1963; Pritchard 1964; Lehmann *et al.* 1965; Keesey and Nichols 1967), and it has been suggested that the origin of stabilized disappearance and reappearance is a physiological event with a recurrent activity pattern. There are data (Evans and Smith 1964; Lehmann *et al.* 1965; Keesey and Nichols 1967) indicating that spontaneous fluctuations in cortical activity might influence the timing of the fading and subsequent reappearance of the stabilized image. For example, the onset of the alpha component of the EEG was found to precede the report of image disappearance and alpha termination to anticipate the report of reappearance (Lehmann *et al.* 1965; Keesey and Nichols 1967). In addition, when sampled over many observation periods, the components of EEG were found to be distributed across time in such a way that percentage of alpha occurrence was maximum at approximately the same point in time a minimum level in stabilized target visibility was obtained. No such temporal relation between the probability of alpha occurrence and probability of image fading could be found under various normal (unstabilized) viewing conditions (Keesey and Nichols 1967).

The present set of experiments is an extension of these studies. Our main purpose is to determine

[1] Part of this study was reported at the March 1966 meetings of the Optical Society of America. The abstract is published in *J. opt. Soc. Amer.*, 1966, *56*: 543 (WG14).

[2] This project was conducted under the sponsorship of National Institutes of Mental Health, Grant NB-06151. It received partial support from a General Research Support Grant to the University of Wisconsin Medical School from the National Institutes of Health, Division of Research Facilities and Resources, Bethesda, Md. and from the University of Wisconsin Research Committee. Part of the data analysis was made possible through the Laboratory Computer Facility, University of Wisconsin.

whether or not the time at which disappearance or reappearance occurs can be controlled by inducing changes in the probability of alpha occurrence normally found under stabilized viewing conditions.

APPARATUS AND PROCEDURE

The experimental situation was similar to that reported previously (Keesey and Nichols 1967). Briefly, the target was a circular field rendered stationary on the retina by the contact lens-collimator method described by Pritchard (1961). With this instrument the image was viewed at infinity with relaxed accommodation. The magnification factor of the collimator was approximately 30, so that a circular aperture of 1.4 mm occupied about 7° in the visual field. The beam falling on the target plate was measured to be 13 foot-lamberts. One of the important features of this arrangement was that one of the lenses was imaged on the plane of the pupil, giving an effective artificial pupil with a diameter of 1.5 mm. The target was presented in complete darkness, and viewed monocularly, the right eye being used. The left eye was occluded in the main part of the experiment. At the beginning of each observation period the target appeared to the subject as a bright field against a dark background. The subject was instructed to report when the target disappeared into the background leaving a subjectively uniform dark grey or black field, and also when it reappeared as a bright field. Such variations in the visibility of the target were signalled by closing a hand-held switch when the target was clearly seen and opening the switch when it faded.

We attempted to alter the ongoing EEG pattern by presenting an "arousing" auditory stimulus either after the onset of alpha activity or randomly within the observation period. For this purpose, the EEG was derived from two electrodes, one placed on the vertex and one slightly above and to the right of the inion, and recorded continuously on a Beckmann Dynograph. The EEG signal was also sampled by a Control Data 160-A computer. An adaptive closed-loop program could recognize alpha activity while it was occurring and deliver the auditory stimulus 0.4 sec (for subject UTK) and 0.25 sec (for subject DJN) after each alpha onset[1]. These times were chosen so that the auxiliary stimulus could be presented within the interval—corrected for reaction time (RT)—by which alpha onset was found to precede image disappearance[2]. The auditory stimulus was a burst of white noise delivered binaurally through ear phones. The intensity of the stimulus was adjusted so that alpha blocking could be obtained reliably for each subject. There were four sessions for the alpha dependent presentation of the white noise, each consisting of 50 observation periods of 16 sec. Subsequently, four more sessions again totalling 200 observation periods were used to present the auditory stimulus semi-randomly, where the average number of presentations was determined according to the number of alpha dependent presentations of the white noise in the previous four sessions.

As a check on the results, the experiment was repeated with a visual auxiliary stimulus. This was a stroboscopic flash presented to the left, the contralateral, eye. With appropriate lenses and baffles the flash appeared to subtend the same area as the target. Care was taken so that no light from the strobe could fall on the right eye viewing the stabilized image.

Throughout the experiment the subject's EEG, his signals of image disappearance and reappearance, beginning and end of trials, and the

[1] The computer program for this study employed a cycle-by-cycle recognition described by Farley *et al.* (1962). Each cycle of the EEG signal was used to define the average amplitude-versus-frequency relationship. The amplitude data were kept in a table and updated every 48 sec. Each update consisted of multiplying all previous entries in the table by 0.5, thereby causing the oldest data to be weighted the least. Three criteria were used to judge the alpha activity: (1) minimum burst length, which was constant for each subject; (2) minimum amplitude, and (3) frequency range. It was the program's job to constantly recalculate the last two criteria, recognize the alpha activity and present a stimulus with each alpha onset.

[2] RT to the fading of a target was estimated by noting the time elapsed between the experimenter dimming or defocusing the normally viewed target and the subject reporting these events. RT to disappearance was found to be 0.49 sec for UTK and 0.52 sec for DJN. Under stabilized viewing alpha onset preceded report of image disappearance by 1.0 sec for UTK and 0.75 sec for DJN. These times were obtained by determining modes of interval histograms relating alpha onset to image disappearance (Keesey and Nichols 1967).

time of auxiliary stimulus presentation were monitored on the Beckmann Dynograph and recorded on analog tape. The subject was placed in a light tight, electrically shielded room, some distance away from the recording equipment. His heavily padded ear phones which were used for the auditory stimulus presentation also sealed out incidental room noise, and served as a means of communicating, by presenting a short duration pure tone, the beginning and end of trials.

The characteristics of individual EEG for the two subjects, the authors, were determined in previous sessions (see Keesey and Nichols 1967). UTK had well defined spindles of 10 c/sec with a maximum amplitude of 20 μV, in darkness with the eyes open. Subject DJN had an alpha activity of 40 μV, about 9.8 c/sec which became continuous with passage of time regardless of presence or absence of light. Pressing or releasing a switch did not interfere with ongoing EEG activity for either subject.

The previous study (Keesey and Nichols 1967)

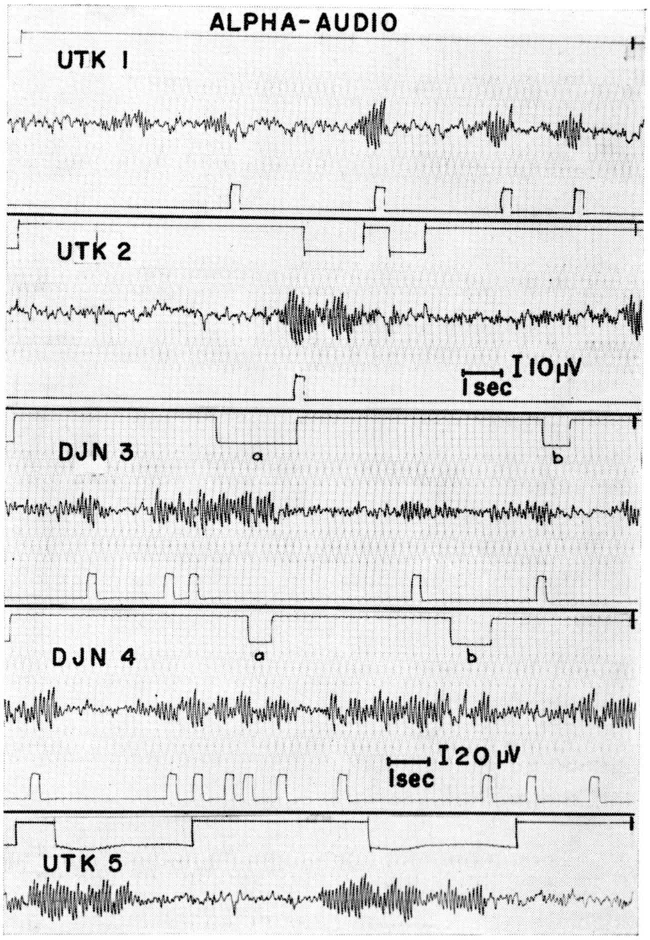

Fig. 1
Sample recordings. The first trace in each block of three traces is the subject's designation o stabilized target visibility. Downward stroke signifies disappearance, upward stroke clear visibility of the target. The second trace is the EEG, the third the computer controlled presentation of the auxiliary stimulus. The first four blocks are from the alpha-audio condition when the white noise was presented 0.4 sec (UTK) and 0.25 sec (DJN) after alpha onset while viewing the stabilized image. The last block is from the control experiment in which the stabilized image is viewed without the auditory stimulus presentation.

where the stabilized target was viewed without the auxiliary stimulus served as a control experiment for the present set of studies.

RESULTS

The effect of the alpha dependent and random presentations of an auxiliary stimulus on stabilized viewing was assessed mainly in three ways: (1) the average duration and number of disappearance events, and the percentage of time the image disappeared under the two conditions of delivery of the auxiliary stimulus were compared with each other and with the same measures obtained under the control condition where no auxiliary stimulus was presented; (2) the temporal relation of alpha occurrence, that is its proximity to the disappearance and reappearance events, was examined; (3) the probability of alpha occurrence and the probability of image disappearance as a function of time under the conditions of the alpha dependent and random presentation of the auxiliary stimulus were compared with each other and with the same measure obtained under the control condition.

The control experiment had shown that a stabilized target viewed without an auxiliary stimulus presentation would disappear typically 2 times with a mean duration of 2.2 sec in a 16 sec observation period. Alpha onset tended to precede image disappearance by 1.0 (UTK) or 0.75 (DJN) sec. Similarly image disappearance was preceded by alpha termination by an interval of approximately 1.0 (UTK) or 0.9 (DJN) sec. These intervals were found to be longer than the measured reaction time, approximately 0.5 sec to a slowly fading and reappearing image.

Fig. 1 gives an indication of how an auxiliary stimulus affected stabilized viewing. This figure contains four sample recordings taken during the main part of the experiment when the stabilized image was viewed with the white noise presented shortly after computer recognition of each alpha burst (alpha-audio condition). A trace from the control experiment when the image was viewed without any auxiliary stimulus presentation is also included (UTK 5). It can be seen that presentation of noise 0.4 (UTK) or 0.25 (DJN) sec after alpha onset (presumably before image disappearance can take place) sometimes resulted in reports of seeing the stabilized image continuously for the 16 sec of the viewing period (UTK 1). Whereas the percentage of observation periods in which no disappearance took place was low (26% for UTK and 4% for DJN), in each such period the alpha rhythm was either blocked successfully each time or none occurred. When the alpha rhythm could not be blocked (UTK 2, DJN 3a, DJN 4b) a disappearance of long duration (1.5 sec or longer) was reported. This accounted for 5% (UTK) and 40% (DJN) of all disappearances. It should be noted that for UTK noise was effective in blocking the alpha rhythm 95% of the time while for DJN the percentage of unblocked alpha was as high as 20. The most common occurrence for both subjects was a disappearance of short duration, relative to the control condition, in close temporal proximity to an alpha burst (UTK 2; DJN 3a, b; DJN 4a). Frequency histograms (Fig. 2 UTK*a* and DJN*b*) relating alpha onset to image disappearance show that alpha onset preceded image disappearance most frequently by an interval of

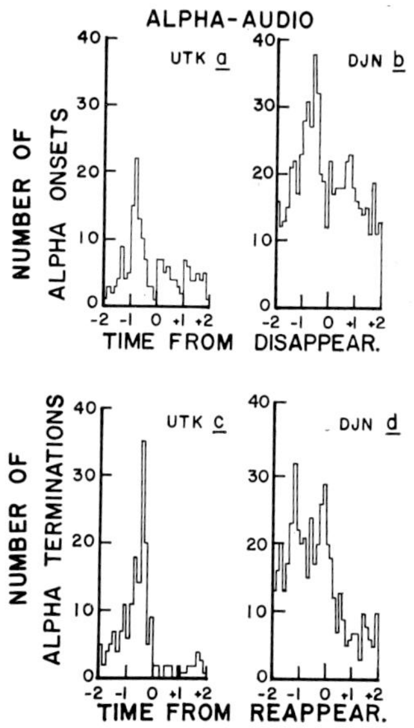

Fig. 2

Interval histograms. Alpha-audio condition. Subject's signal of image disappearance is related to alpha onset (UTK*a* and DJN*b*) and subject's signal of image reappearance to alpha termination (UTK*c* and DJN*d*). For these histograms, the interval between each alpha onset and report of image disappearance; and each alpha termination and report of image reappearance was measured for each of the 200 trials. 0 time is the subject's signal, (−) means alpha onset of termination preceding, (+) following the signal. 2 sec around the signal is shown.

TABLE I

Effect of auxiliary stimulus on disappearance of stabilized image and alpha occurrence

	Stabilized				
	1 control: no aux. stimulus	2 alpha-audio	3 random-audio	4 alpha-visual	5 random-visual
Subject UTK					
% Disappearance	23.6	10.4	19.8	10.9	13.8
Mean duration of disappearance (sec)	2.3	0.8	1.9	1.2	1.4
Mean number of disappearances	2.0	1.0	1.1	1.2	1.4
% Alpha	16.2	10.6	9.5	9.1	9.2
Subject DJN					
% Disappearance	20.9	16.6	25.5	16.0	18.0
Mean duration of disappearance (sec)	2.0	1.5	2.4	1.4	2.1
Mean number of disappearances	1.6	1.6	1.7	1.6	1.5
% Alpha	28.9	30.9	37.7	32.7	29.4

This table shows (1) the mean length of time occupied by disappearance expressed as a percentage of 224 trials (control UTK) and 200 trials (for all other conditions for both UTK and DJN) of 16 sec duration each, (2) mean duration of disappearance in seconds reflecting a random sample of $n = 50$ for UTK and $n = 200$ for DJN, (3) mean number of disappearances $n = 200$ for UTK and DJN, (4) the mean length of time occupied by alpha, $n = 224$ trials of 16 sec duration for UTK control, $n = 200$ trials of 16 sec duration for UTK and DJN under all other conditions. The data under column 1 were derived from Keesey and Nichols (1967).

0.6 sec (UTK) or 0.8 sec (DJN). Similarly Fig. 2 UTK*c* and DJN*d* show that a reappearance was most likely to be reported 0.5 sec (UTK) or 1.25 sec (DJN) after an alpha termination. An examination of the records revealed that in over 60% of all cases a reappearance was initiated by a noise presentation which was followed by 0.2 sec by an alpha termination. Thus a reappearance most frequently occurred 0.7 sec (UTK) or 1.45 sec (DJN) after the presentation of the auditory stimulus.

Table I summarizes the effects of the alpha dependent (alpha-audio and alpha-visual) and random (random-audio and random-visual) presentation of both of the auxiliary stimuli on percentage of image disappearance and alpha occurrence during stabilized viewing. The 1st column of the table contains results of the control experiment when the stabilized image was viewed without the auxiliary stimulus.

A comparison of columns 2 and 4 with column 1 shows that for subject UTK the delivery of either of the auxiliary stimuli after each onset of the alpha rhythm reduced the mean percentage of time the target disappeared to a level significantly lower than obtained under the control condition ($P < 0.02$)[1]. Random presentation of either stimulus (columns 3 and 5), where the number of presentations matched those given under the alpha dependent condition, also reduced image disappearance relative to the control condition where the target was viewed without any auxiliary stimulus presentation ($P < 0.02$). The low disappearance level obtained under all stimulus delivery conditions was due to both fewer disappearances and shorter duration of the individual disappearance events. Here a comparison of the alpha-audio with random-audio and of the alpha-visual with random-visual conditions is of importance. It shows that white noise or a flash presented shortly after alpha onset yielded shorter disappearances giving a significantly

[1] Significance of difference between percentages was computed according to Garret (1953).

lower ($P < 0.02$) percentage of disappearance than found where noise or flash was presented randomly.

For UTK, the percent alpha present under either the alpha dependent or random presentation of either of the auxiliary stimuli was found to be lower than obtained under the control condition ($P < 0.02$).

For subject DJN the stabilized target disappeared for a lower percentage of time under the alpha-audio, alpha-visual and random-visual conditions than the control condition ($P < 0.02$). Reduced disappearance of the target seemed to be due to the short duration of disappearance events, rather than to a reduction in the number of them. A randomly presented auditory stimulus however allowed for longer disappearance events, contributing to higher percentage image fading than obtained when the target was viewed without any auxiliary stimulus ($P < 0.02$).

As with subject UTK, the presentation of the auditory or the visual stimulus when contingent on the onset of alpha rhythm, yielded target disappearances of shorter duration giving a lower disappearance level than found when either of the stimuli was presented randomly ($P < 0.02$). This finding emphasizes the critical temporal relation of the auxiliary stimulus to alpha occurrence in effectively reducing disappearance of the stabilized image.

For this subject, the alpha level in the presence of the auxiliary stimulus was either significantly higher than (random-audio, alpha-visual, $P < 0.02$) or the same as (alpha-audio, random-visual) found under the control condition. This reflects the fact that for DJN, the subject with abundant alpha, the auxiliary stimuli were not good blocking agents. In addition, for this subject, the alpha block response, the small amplitude fast activity, was of short duration, alpha recurring soon after an auxiliary stimulus presentation (see Fig. 1, DJN 4).

The question of the effect of auxiliary stimulus presentation on both the temporal distribution of alpha activity and the temporal pattern of stabilized image disappearance and reappearance still remains. One way of assessing the time course of alpha occurrence and target visibility is to determine the probability of these events as a function of time. For this purpose, the tapes from each session were played back to the computer which, using a program employed in the previous experiment (Keesey and Nichols 1967), divided each 16 sec observation period into 1/8 sec intervals. Each interval was assigned two scores; one, representing the presence of alpha rhythm and the other showing whether or not the image was reported as seen. The 200 trials were stacked in this manner, with the scores in each interval representing the percentage of trials the alpha rhythm was present and the target was seen for each 1/8 sec interval. Fig. 3 shows the time course of the probability of alpha occurrence and image disappearance for the alpha-audio and random-audio condition for both subjects. Such patterns obtained under the control experiment when the image was viewed without the auditory stimulus are also included for comparison purposes.

For subject UTK (Fig. 3, UTK*a*), the temporal pattern of alpha distribution under the control condition showed well defined peaks around the 4th and 12th sec of observation. Corresponding to the high probability of alpha occurrence at these points in time were the points of high probability of image disappearance. In contrast, alpha dependent presentation of the auditory stimulus had the effect of distributing alpha across the whole trial at a low level with only small cyclical variations. The image disappearance pattern, after an initial rise, showed a flat distribution around a low level of 10%, that is, disappearance of a short duration seemed to be equally likely to occur at any point in time during the 16 sec observation period. For subject DJN (Fig. 3, DJN*b*), viewing a stabilized image without an auditory stimulus produced an alpha pattern which showed a high probability of occurrence around the 7th sec of viewing. On the other hand, the presentation of white noise after the onset of the alpha rhythm yielded an alpha pattern which showed a peak of activity at about the 5th sec of viewing. In the latter case, after a decline of alpha activity to a minimum at about the 7th sec, alpha became oscillatory around a mean level of 35%. The disappearance pattern under the alpha-audio condition, as under the control condition, showed good correspondence to the temporal alpha pattern. That is, probability of image disappearance increased within the first 5 sec with a subsequent

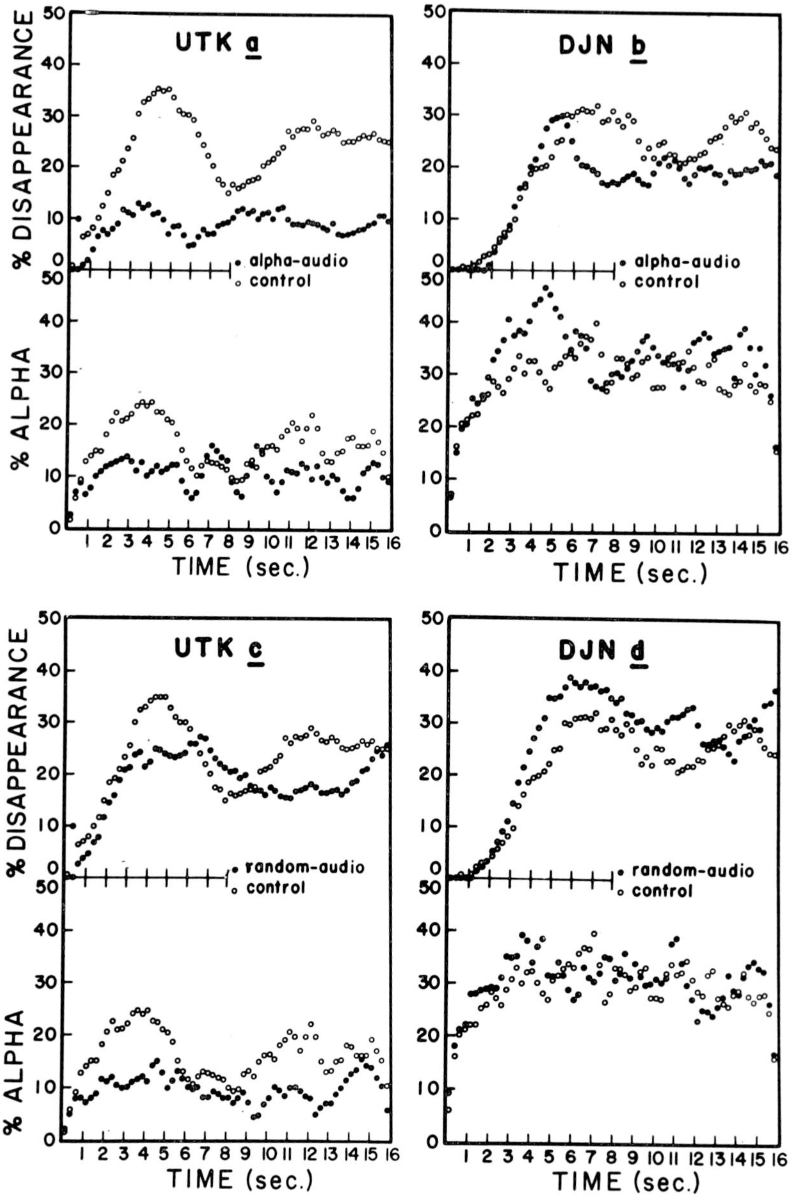

Fig. 3

Patterns of alpha occurrence and image disappearance. Solid dots: alpha-audio condition. Temporal pattern of stabilized image disappearance and alpha activity compiled over 200 trials. UTK*a*, white noise presented 0.4 sec after each alpha onset; DJN*b*, white noise presented 0.25 sec after each alpha onset; UTK*c*, white noise presented randomly within the trial; DJN*d*, white noise presented randomly within the trial. Open circles: control — no auxiliary stimulus during stabilized image viewing; temporal pattern of stabilized image disappearance and alpha activity —224 trials for UTK, 200 trials for DJN. These data were derived from Keesey and Nichols (1967).

decline around the 7th sec. After this, probability of a disappearance to occur was low but equal at any point in time.

Contrary to the alpha dependent presentation of the stimulus, randomly presented white noise did not seem to affect the distribution of alpha occurrence found under stabilized viewing without noise (Fig. 3, UTK*c*, DJN*d*). Correspondingly, the image disappearance patterns obtained under the random-audio condition seemed to be similar to the patterns produced under the control condition. The alpha dependent and random presentation of the visual stimulus gave essentially the same results.

The results indicate that visibility of a stabilized image can be enhanced by presenting a generally excitatory stimulus shortly after alpha onset. However, a burst of white noise might cause blinks, variations in pupil size or accommodation resulting in changes respectively in placement, luminance, and quality of the retinal image. To assess the contribution of blinks to image reappearance, EOGs were taken for 50 consecutive trials during the main part of the experiment. The recordings showed that for the first three or four trials each presentation of white noise was followed by a large eye movement or a blink. Such blinks might have resulted in mechanical disturbance of stabilization and helped to prevent or shorten image disappearance during these early trials. However, reports of continuous seeing persisted after blinks ceased to appear in conjunction with white noise. Actually, only 35% of blinks occurred within a 1 sec period after the noise presentation. Moreover, reappearances of the image were largely independent of blinks or large eye movements as only 20% were found to be preceded, by 1 sec or less, by blinks or eye movements occurring alone or accompanied by white noise[1].

DISCUSSION

The two subjects used in the present experiment belong to the segment of the population whose EEG shows well developed alpha rhythm and its blocking when presented with an excitatory stimulus. This limits the generality of our discussion. The two subjects, however, showed widely differing EEG characteristics. As pointed out in the procedure and result sections, DJN had abundant alpha activity which became continuous in a relaxed situation. With this subject the arousal response upon auxiliary stimulus presentation was of a shorter duration and adaptation to an alpha blocking stimulus was much more evident than exhibited by UTK's EEG. In the case of DJN the auxiliary stimulus was presented 0.25 sec after each alpha onset; for UTK the stimulus was given 0.4 sec after the onset of the alpha rhythm. This might have contributed further to the lesser alpha blocking effects observed with DJN. Nevertheless there are similarities between the data obtained from the two subjects permitting us to speculate on the effects of a generally excitatory stimulus on both alpha occurrence and stabilized image visibility.

The present results essentially agree with an earlier report (Pritchard 1964) which showed improved visibility of a stabilized target upon periodic presentation of an auditory stimulus. The present study shows that only the alpha dependent presentation of the stimulus improves image visibility consistently and effectively. Indeed, in the case of DJN, image disappearance was actually higher upon random presentation of the auditory stimulus than when no auxiliary stimulus was used. On the other hand, for both subjects alpha contingent presentation of either the auditory or the visual stimulus reduced image disappearance by a significantly higher percentage than the random presentation of the same stimulus. Most importantly, for both subjects alpha contingent presentation of a generally "excitatory" stimulus manipulated the time of occurrence of the alpha component and the "arousal" response of the EEG, and imposed changes in the temporal patterning of stabilized image disappearance and reappearance which were correlated with the new EEG pattern. A randomly presented auxiliary stimulus, while it depressed or elevated visibility and alpha levels according to the subject, tended not to produce any changes in the temporal patterning of image disappearance and alpha occurrence.

The possibility of the auditory or the visual stimulus enhancing image visibility through peripheral channels cannot be excluded irrefutably.

[1] The possibility of variations in pupil size affecting variations in retinal illuminance, therefore a change in stabilized image visibility, was circumvented by a feature of the apparatus which provided a constant size artificial pupil. Changes in image quality due to accommodative variations is still a consideration since small hyperopic, 0.15 D, changes in accommodation due to sudden onset of white noise have been reported (Roth 1966). However, in the present situation, choice of the target, a 7° circular field, and the nature of the response, complete fading and reappearance of a light field made it unlikely that a sharpening of edges due to such a small change in accommodation could be reported.

However, this possibility was minimized in this study (see results) and the improved visibility of the stabilized image obtained under the alpha dependent presentation of the auxiliary stimuli seems to be largely due to a regulatory function of central events.

Does evidence indicating (Krauskopf and Riggs 1959; Cohen 1961; Pritchard 1964; Lehmann *et al.* 1965; Keesey and Nichols 1967; and the present results) central involvement in producing disappearance and reappearance of a stabilized image necessarily imply the absence of retinal adaptation with a motionless image? Various attempts assessing adaptive changes in peripheral neural activity during stabilized image viewing have given results showing no differences in ERGs or VEPs obtained under the normal or stabilized conditions (Lehmann *et al.* 1967; Riggs and Whittle 1967). On the other hand, it has been established in vertebrate and mammalian visual systems that neural activity at both the peripheral and cortical levels loses strength upon steady stimulation (Hartline 1938; Riggs and Graham 1940; Burns *et al.* 1962), while flickering or moving the target on receptors gives rise to vigorous cortical activity (Burns *et al.* 1962). Although there is as yet no direct physiological evidence for it, some adaptation must go on in the human visual system during viewing of a steadily illuminated stationary target as shown by some psychophysical experiments (Burkhart 1966). An attractive hypothesis for stabilized disappearance and reappearance of the target such as used in the present studies would state that peripheral and cortical activity generated by the onset of the stabilized image becomes progressively weak during lengthy viewing of the immobile and steadily illuminated target. In this case the cortical activity may revert to a spontaneous pattern, large amplitude rhythmical activity signalling the reduced peripheral activity level, therefore the functional absence of light; and low level fast activity, whether spontaneously produced or induced by an excitatory stimulus, signalling the presence of light.

The present studies cannot identify the structures mediating such interaction of neural activity. However, some micro-electrode studies investigating the mutually regulatory functions of various structures in the visual pathways bear close parallels to the present studies. For example, Arden and Söderberg (1961) noted changes in the firing rate of the geniculate in response to a steady or flickering visual stimulus when the auditory input caused a desynchronization of slow wave activity of the ongoing EEG. Recently, Spinelli *et al.* (1965) demonstrated efferent control of receptor events by showing that a response to an auditory stimulus can be initiated in the optic nerve. Since these non-optically induced responses were abolished after optic tract section, their origin seemed to be central, perhaps due to the generally excitatory function of the reticular formation. The present experiments demonstrate once more the possibility of centrifugal control of stabilized disappearance and reappearance and allow us to speculate further on the possible involvement of structures such as the reticular formation in stabilized image disappearance and reappearance.

SUMMARY

Continuous EEG recordings were taken while judgments of stabilized image disappearance and reappearance were being made. On-line use of a computer executing a closed-loop program made it possible to detect the alpha rhythm while it was occurring, and to present a burst of white noise shortly after each onset of alpha activity. The stimulus could also be presented in random order. It was found that alpha dependent presentation of the stimulus both lengthened the time the stabilized image stayed visible and changed the temporal patterns of alpha occurrence and image disappearance and reappearance in comparison to the condition where the stabilized image was viewed without any white noise presentation.

RÉSUMÉ

CHANGEMENTS INDUITS DANS LA VISIBILITÉ DE L'IMAGE STABILISÉE PAR L'ALTÉRATION EXPÉRIMENTALE DE L'EEG ACTUEL

Pendant l'enregistrement EEG continu, sont effectués des jugements de disparition et de réapparition d'une image stabilisée. L'utilisation en ligne d'un calculateur exécutant un programme bouclé donne la possibilité de détecter le rythme alpha au moment où il survient, et de déclencher une bouffée de bruit blanc peu après chaque survenue d'activité alpha. Le stimulus peut également être présenté dans un ordre aléatoire. On observe que la présentation du stimulus dépendante de l'alpha augmente le temps pendant lequel l'image stabilisée reste visible en même temps qu'elle modifie le pattern temporel de la survenue de l'alpha et de la disparition et de la réapparition de l'image par comparaison à ce qui se passe quand l'image stabilisée est vue sans aucune présentation de bruit blanc.

These experiments were carried out at the Behavioral Cybernetics Laboratory, University of Wisconsin. We gratefully acknowledge the help of Dr. K. U. Smith of the Department of Psychology and the director of the Behavioral Cybernetics Laboratory who donated advice, computer time and space to this project. We also thank Dr. E. Johnson of Madison, Wis. for fitting the tight limbal seating scleral contact lenses used in these experiments.

REFERENCES

ARDEN, G. B. and SÖDERBERG, U. The transfer of optic information through the lateral geniculate body of the rabbit. In W. ROSENBLITH (Ed.), *Sensory communication.* M.I.T. Press, Cambridge, Mass., **1961,** *27*: 521–544.

BURKHART, D. A. Brightness and the increment threshold. *J. opt. Soc. Amer.*, **1966,** *56*: 979–981.

BURNS, B. D., HERON, W. and PRITCHARD, R. Physiological excitation of visual cortex in cats' unanaesthetized isolated forebrain. *J. Neurophysiol.*, **1962,** *25*: 165–181.

COHEN, H. B. The effect of contralateral visual stimulation on visibility with stabilized retinal images. *Canad. J. Psychol.*, **1961,** *15*: 212–219.

CORNSWEET, T. N. Stabilized image techniques. In M. A. WHITCOMB (Ed.), *Recent developments in vision research.* Armed Forces NRC Committee on Vision, Publ. 1272, Nat. Acad. of Sciences–Nat. Res. Council, Washington, D. C., **1966:** 171–184.

DITCHBURN, R. W. Eye movements in relation to retinal action. *Opt. Acta*, **1955,** *1*: 171–176.

EVANS, C. R. and SMITH, G. K. Alpha-frequency of electroencephalogram and a stabilized retinal image. *Nature (Lond.)*, **1964,** *204*: 303–304.

FARLEY, B. G., CLARK JR., W. A. and GOLMIRE JR., J. T. Computer techniques for the study of patterns in the electroencephalogram. *IRE Trans.*, **1962,** *BME-9*: 4–12.

FIORENTINI, A. and ERCOLES, A. M. Fluctuations of response to a stabilized visual stimulus. *Atti Fond. G. Ronchi*, **1963,** *18*: 548–560.

GARRET, H. E. *Statistics in psychology and education.* Longmans, Green and Co., New York, **1953,** 236 p.

GERRITS, H. J. M., DE HAAN, B. and VENDRIK, A. J. H. Experiments with retinal stabilized images. Relations between the observations and neural data. *Vision Res.*, **1966,** *6*: 427–440.

HARTLINE, H. K. The response of single optic nerve fibres of the vertebrate eye to illumination of the retina. *Amer. J. Physiol.*, **1938,** *121*: 400–415.

HECKENMUELLER, E. G. Stabilization of the retinal image: A review of method, effects and theory. *Psychol. Bull.*, **1965,** *63*: 157–169.

KEESEY, U. T. and NICHOLS, D. J. Fluctuations in target visibility as related to the occurrence of the alpha component of the electroencephalogram. *Vision Res.*, **1967,** *7*: 859–879.

KRAUSKOPF, J. and RIGGS, L. A. Interocular transfer in the disappearance of stabilized images. *Amer. J. Psychol.*, **1959,** *72*: 248–252.

LEHMANN, D., BEELER, G. W. and FENDER, D. H. Changes in patterns of the human electroencephalogram during fluctuations of perception of stabilized retinal images. *Electroenceph. clin. Neurophysiol.*, **1965,** *19*: 336–343.

LEHMANN, D., BEELER, G. W. and FENDER, D. H. EEG responses to light flashes during the observation of stabilized and normal retinal images. *Electroenceph. clin. Neurophysiol.*, **1967,** *22*: 136–142.

PRITCHARD, R. M. A collimator stabilizing system. *Quart. J. exp. Psychol.*, **1961,** *13*: 181–183.

PRITCHARD, R. M. Physiological nystagmus and vision. In M. B. BENDER (Ed.), *The oculomotor system.* Harper and Row, New York, **1964,** *15*: 321–332.

PRITCHARD, R. M., HERON, W. and HEBB, D. O. Visual perception approached by the method of stabilized images. *Canad. J. Psychol.*, **1960,** *14*: 67–77.

RIGGS, L. A. and GRAHAM, C. H. Some aspects of light adaptation in a single photoreceptor unit. *J. cell. comp. Physiol.*, **1940,** *16*: 15–23.

RIGGS, L. A., RATLIFF, F., CORNSWEET, J. C. and CORNSWEET, T. N. The disappearance of a steadily fixated visual test object. *J. opt. Soc. Amer.*, **1953,** *44*: 315–321.

RIGGS, L. A. and WHITTLE, P. Human occipital potentials evoked by subjectively faded visual stimulus. *Vision Res.*, **1967,** *7*: 441–451.

ROTH, N. Startling noise and resting refractive state. *Brit. J. physiol. Opt.*, **1966,** *23*: 223–231.

SPINELLI, D. N., PRIBRAM, K. N. and WEINGARTEN, M. Centrifugal optic nerve responses evoked by auditory and somatic stimulation. *Exp. Neurol.* **1965,** *12*: 303–319.

Reference: KEESEY, U. T. and NICHOLS, D. J. Changes induced in stabilized image visibility by experimental alteration of the ongoing EEG. *Electroenceph. clin. Neurophysiol.*, **1969,** *27*: 248–257.

Electroencephalography and Clinical Neurophysiology
Elsevier Publishing Company, Amsterdam – Printed in The Netherlands

MODIFICATIONS DES ACTIVITÉS ÉVOQUÉES CORTICALES ET THALAMIQUES AU COURS D'UN CONDITIONNEMENT SENSORIEL. I. LOCALISATION DES RÉPONSES ET VARIATIONS AVEC LA VIGILANCE

G. Lelord[1] et C. Maho

Laboratoire de Physiologie des Centres Nerveux, Faculté des Sciences, 4, avenue Gordon-Bennet, Paris 16e (France)

(Accepted for publication: December 30, 1968)

De nombreux travaux publiés au cours de ces dernières années ont montré l'existence de variations importantes des potentiels évoqués recueillis au cours du conditionnement chez l'animal. C'est ainsi que des potentiels évoqués auditifs provoqués par un stimulus conditionnel auditif (clic, pip, son) présentent des variations d'amplitude tant au niveau de l'aire auditive primaire que du corps genouillé médian dans des conditionnements alimentaires (Hearst *et al.* 1960), défensifs (Galambos *et al.* 1956; Naumova *et al.* 1966) ou même sensoriels (Jouvet et Hernández-Peón 1957). Il en est de même pour les activités évoquées ou les rythmes entraînés recueillis dans des structures associatives comme la formation réticulée (John et Killam 1959; Jouvet et Hernández-Peón 1957), le centre médian (Yoshii *et al.* 1956; John *et al.* 1964), l'hippocampe (Grastyán *et al.* 1959) etc.

Certains auteurs cependant (Popov 1948; Jouvet et Hernández-Peón 1957) ont montré que le conditionnement fait apparaître des modifications particulières au niveau de l'aire primaire du cortex cérébral correspondant au stimulus inconditionnel. Dans le cas d'un conditionnement associant une stimulation auditive à une stimulation appliquée sur un nerf sensitif de la peau, c'est au niveau de l'aire somatique primaire que ces modifications sont observées (Buser et Roger 1957; Lelord 1967). On les retrouve également dans la région du relais primaire thalamique de la sensibilité (Lelord, voir Albe-Fessard et Fessard 1963; Maho 1968).

Ces données électrophysiologiques rejoignent les observations d'auteurs différents effectuant des expériences d'ablations et pour lesquels les structures primaires correspondant au stimulus conditionnel (Pavlov 1929) ou au stimulus inconditionnel (Konorski 1948, 1960) jouent un rôle prédominant dans la formation du conditionnement.

C'est pourquoi nous avons tout d'abord recueilli les activités évoquées dans différentes structures corticales et sous-corticales avant d'effectuer l'étude systématique des modifications observées sur l'aire primaire somatique et dans la région du noyau ventral-postéro-latéral (VPL) du thalamus au cours d'un conditionnement associant une stimulation auditive à une stimulation appliquée sur un nerf sensitif de la peau.

TECHNIQUE

Vingt chats, porteurs d'électrodes implantées à demeure suivant une technique utilisant des points d'ancrage (Libouban et Aleonard 1960) ont été examinés. Les électrodes superficielles sont des fils d'argent dont l'extrémité arrondie est posée sur la dure-mère. Les électrodes profondes, bipolaires concentriques en acier, sont descendues sous contrôle stéréotaxique. Leur axe correspondant à la partie focale, mobile dans le sens vertical par rapport à la gaine d'acier, peut être déplacé dans les jours qui suivent l'intervention (Aleonard 1962). Toutes les mises en

[1] Chargé de Recherches au C.N.R.S.

place et descentes d'électrodes sont effectuées non seulement à l'aide de repères anatomiques mais en fonction de l'aspect des réponses observées extemporanément sur l'écran d'un oscilloscope. Ultérieurement, un contrôle histologique est effectué sur des coupes réalisées sous congélation et colorées par la méthode de Nissl.

Le stimulus conditionnel est un son dont la durée est de 4 msec pour une intensité de 15 dB au dessus du seuil d'audibilité et une fréquence de 2500 c/sec. Le stimulus inconditionnel est appliqué directement sur la branche superficielle du nerf radial où sont fixées deux électrodes, reliées par de longs fils glissés sous la peau au soquet fixé sur le crâne. La durée (0,2 msec) et le voltage (0,5 V) de cette stimulation sont trop faibles pour faire apparaître un mouvement réflexe, mais suffisent pour obtenir de façon régulière un potentiel évoqué sur l'aire primaire somatique. Le stimulus conditionnel et le stimulus inconditionnel sont séparés par un intervalle de temps de 300 msec.

Le local où l'animal évolue librement est constitué par une cage vitrée de 1 m de côté,

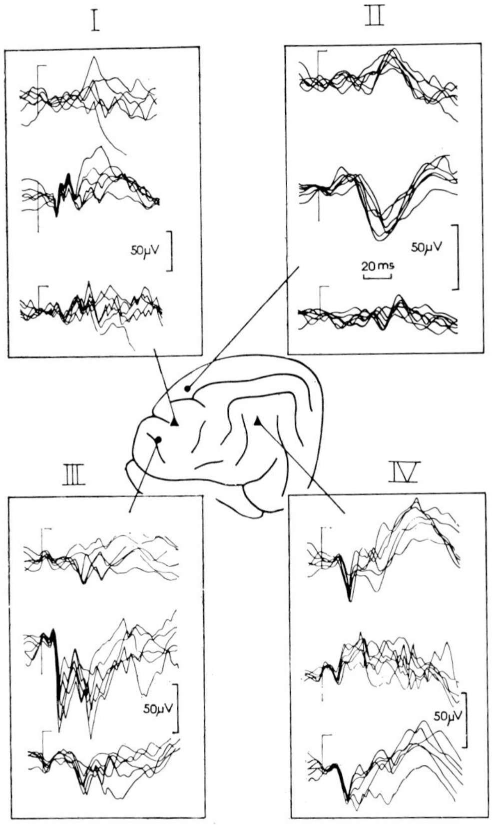

Fig. 1

Réponses évoquées par le son sur différentes aires corticales avant et après une série d'expériences. Réponses superposées par une méthode graphique: Les signets indiquent les artefacts des sons, les traits, les artefacts des stimulations du nerf. Chaque cadre résume le résultat d'une série d'expériences d'association chez un animal différent. Tracé supérieur: réponse au son avant association; tracé moyen: réponse à la stimulation du nerf; tracé inférieur: réponse au son après association. *I*: aire primaire somatique; *II*: partie antérieure du gyrus marginal; *III*: cortex prémoteur; *IV*: aire primaire auditive.

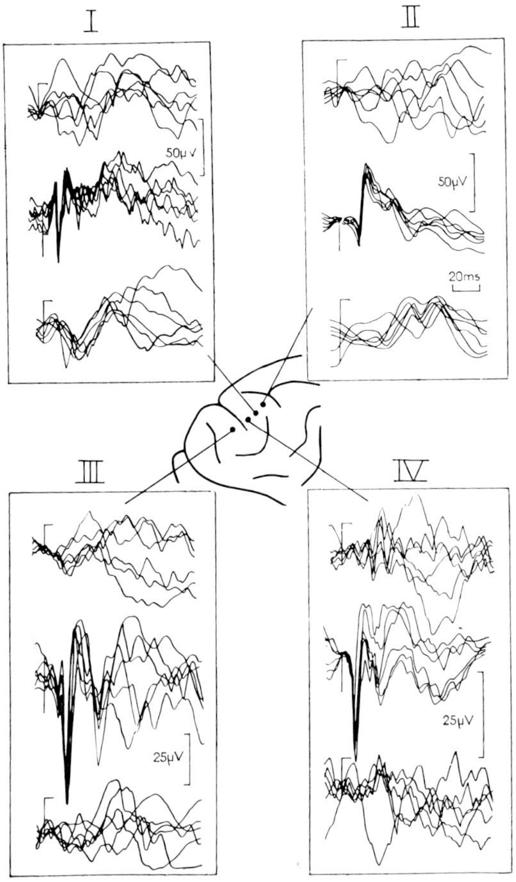

Fig. 2

Réponses évoquées par le son sur l'aire sensorimotrice avant et après le conditionnement. Même représentation que sur la Fig. 1. Chaque cadre résume ici le résultat d'une série d'expériences de conditionnement chez un animal différent: *I* et *II*: les électrodes sont placées très en arrière du sillon cruciatus, et même, près du sillon ansiforme (*II*). *III* et *IV*: les électrodes sont placées à proximité, immédiatement en avant et en arrière, du sillon cruciatus.

étanche aux bruits, légèrement éclairée par une veilleuse permettant l'observation facile du comportement. La cage est elle-même placée dans une pièce de faibles dimensions, qui communique avec la salle où se trouve l'expérimentateur par une orifice percé dans la cloison et fermé par une glace sans tain. Les fils qui relient l'animal aux appareils passent à travers les différentes parois. Les variations de potentiels sont transmises à un pré-amplificateur différentiel dont la sortie est reliée d'une part aux entrées d'un scripteur à plumes (8 pistes), d'autre part à l'entrée d'un oscilloscope cathodique permettant de photographier les réponses une par une avant de les superposer à l'aide d'une méthode graphique, et d'un appareil à mémoire magnétique qui effectue directement le calcul des potentiels évoqués moyens pour un nombre de stimulations déterminé. Chaque expérience dure environ 90 min et comporte l'application de 100–150 couples de stimulations à des intervalles de temps variant de 15 sec à 1 min et demie. Au total 318 expériences ont été effectuées.

RÉSULTATS

Exploration de l'aire corticale sensorimotrice, du noyau VPL et des structures adjacentes

1. *Aire sensorimotrice.* Dans un conditionnement associant un son à une stimulation du nerf, c'est au niveau de l'aire sensorimotrice que les réponses au son présentent les modifications les plus importantes comme le montre la Fig. 1. Chaque cadre résume le résultat de 10–20 expériences d'association. Le tracé supérieur montre la réponse au son lorsque cette stimulation est donnée seule au cours des 2 ou 3 premières séances, le tracé moyen la réponse à la

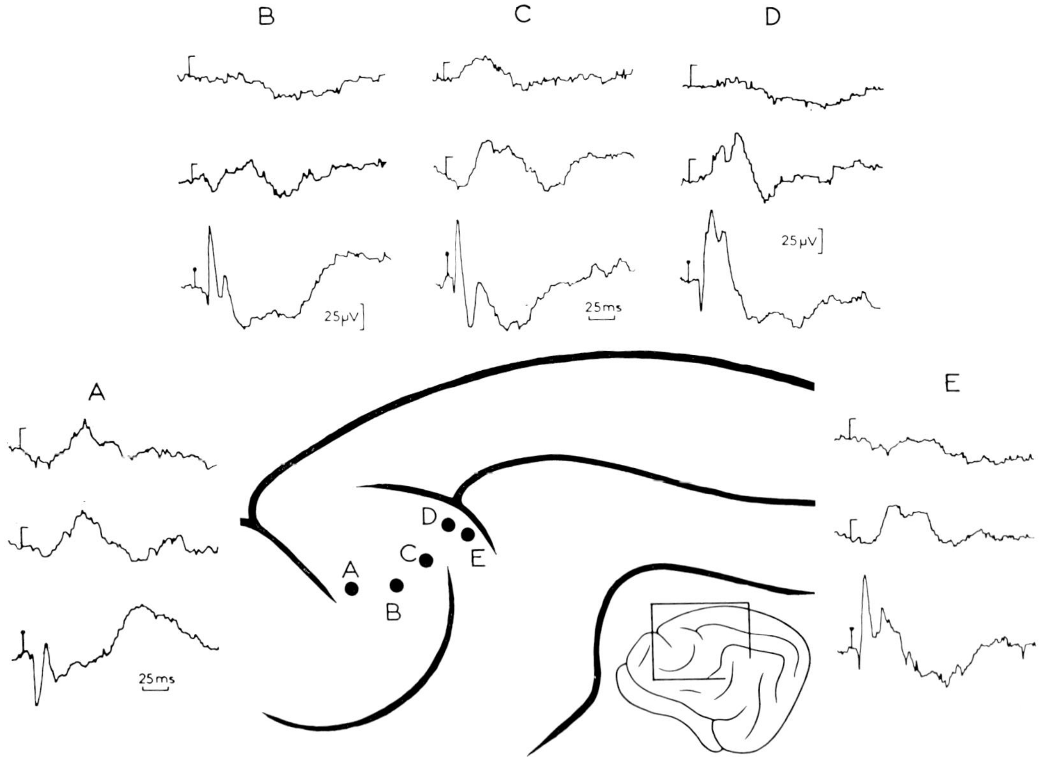

Fig. 3

Réponses évoquées par le son sur l'aire sensorimotrice avant et après conditionnement. Chaque cadre montre les réponses moyennes à 25 stimulations. En haut, réponse au son avant conditionnement. En dessous, réponse au son après conditionnement. Sur la ligne inférieure la réponse à la stimulation du nerf. Les modifications les plus apparentes concernent les réponses recueillies dans la région la plus postérieure du gyrus sigmoïde.

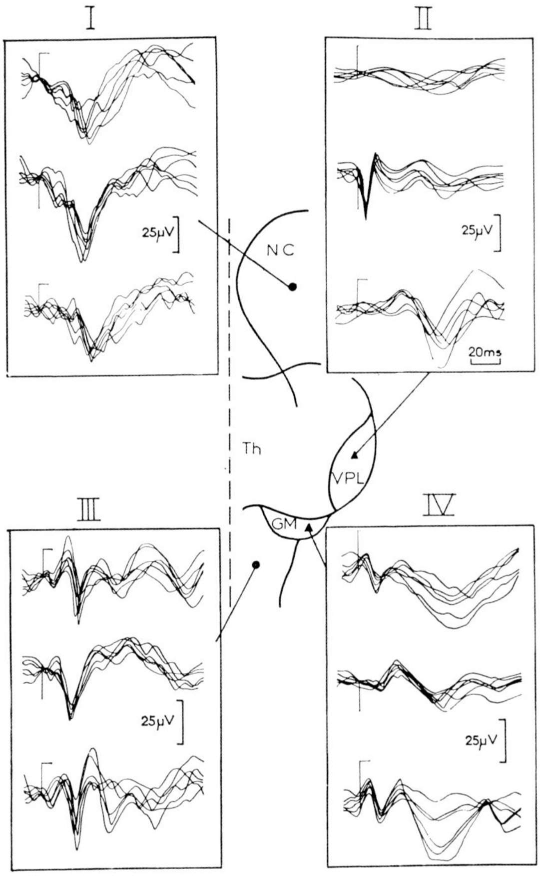

Fig. 4
Réponses évoquées par le son dans différentes structures sous-corticales avant et après conditionnement. Réponses superposées par la méthode graphique: Chaque cadre résume le résultat d'une série d'expériences de conditionnement. Tracé supérieur et inférieur: réponse au son avant et après conditionnement; tracé moyen: réponse à la stimulation du nerf. *I*: noyau caudé; *II*: région du VPL; *III*: formation réticulée; *IV*: corps genouillé médian.

stimulation du nerf appliquée seule, et le tracé inférieur la réponse au son modifiée par les expériences d'association des deux stimulations. Ces modifications, très apparentes sur l'aire primaire somatique, semblent peu marquées non seulement sur l'aire auditive primaire, mais au niveau des aires corticales associatives (gyrus marginal antérieur, aire prémotrice).

Une étude plus précise de l'aire primaire somatique est résumée sur la Fig. 2 qui montre le contraste entre le caractère discret des modifications observées de part et d'autre et à proximité du sillon crucié (en bas), et l'importance des remaniements enregistrés en arrière de ce sillon (en haut et à gauche) et même à proximité du gyrus ansiforme (en haut et à droite). Une analyse systématique du gyrus sigmoïde postérieur permet de comparer sur la Fig. 3 les réponses au son seul (tracé supérieur) avec les réponses au son après conditionnement (tracé moyen) tandis que le tracé inférieur indique la réponse à la stimulation du nerf. Il apparaît ici que les réponses conditionnées les plus caractéristiques sont recueillies dans la région la plus postérieure de ce gyrus.

2. *Noyau VPL et structures adjacentes.* L'exploration de différentes structures sous-corticales (corps genouillé médian, noyau caudé, centre médian, noyau ventro-latéral du thalamus, noyau VPL) est résumée sur la Fig. 4 et paraît confirmer les observations déjà effectuées au niveau du cortex. En effet, dans le corps genouillé médian comme sur le cortex auditif (en bas à droite), les modifications apportées par le couplage des stimulations sont peu apparentes. Il en est de même dans les structures associatives comme la formation réticulée du tronc cérébral (en bas et à gauche) et le noyau caudé (en haut et à gauche) et dans les noyaux thalamiques associatifs, comme le centre médian et le noyau ventrolatéral où les réponses au son, amples avant toute association, sont peu modifiées par elles. Par contre, le conditionnement est apparent au niveau du noyau ventral-postéro-latéral du thalamus (en haut et à droite) où il se traduit par des modifications importantes de la réponse évoquée par le son après le couplage des stimulations.

Une étude plus précise de ce noyau et des structures adjacentes permet de reconnaître les zones où le conditionnement est le plus manifeste. Ces zones occupent une certaine étendue comme l'indiquent les résultats condensés sur Fig. 5 et 6. Les colonnes correspondent à des expériences effectuées chez des animaux différents. La Fig. 5 indique trois enregistrements du noyau VPL effectués chez trois animaux différents à différentes antériorités (9,5; 8,5 et 7,5) de l'atlas de Jasper et Ajmone Marsan (1954), tandis que la Fig. 6 montre trois autres animaux examinés à une antériorité semblable, mais à des hauteurs différentes: limite ventrale du VPL, base du

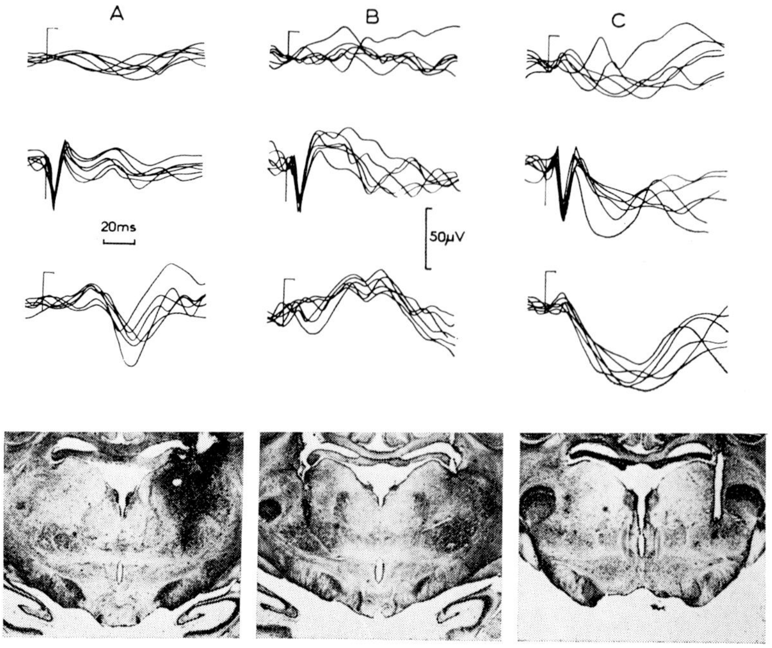

Fig. 5
Réponses évoquées par le son dans la région du VPL avant et après conditionnement. Réponses superposées par une méthode graphique. Les signets indiquent les artefacts du son, les traits, les artefacts des stimulations du nerf. Chaque colonne (*A*, *B*, *C*) résume le résultat d'une série d'expériences de conditionnement chez un animal différent. De haut en bas: Réponse au son avant conditionnement, réponse à la stimulation du nerf, réponse au son après conditionnement, contrôle histologique. Les modifications apportées par le conditionnement sont observées pour des plans antérieurs différents (*A*: 9,5; *B*: 8,5; *C*: 8), le plan latéral étant 6,5 et le plan horizontal 0,5 pour les trois animaux.

VPL et limite dorsale de ce noyau. La moitié inférieure de la figure indique la position exacte de l'extrémité inférieure de l'électrode focale telle qu'elle apparaît sur la coupe histologique. La partie supérieure de la figure résume les séries de 15–25 expériences effectuées chez chaque animal, avant (tracé supérieur) et après le conditionnement (tracé moyen), le tracé inférieur indiquant l'aspect de la réponse à la stimulation du nerf radial contralatéral (la présence d'un accident positif précoce de latence très brève confirme le siège de l'électrode focale dans le VPL). Dans tous les cas, il apparaît que le conditionnement modifie la latence et l'amplitude de la réponse au son, la morphologie de cette réponse variant avec le siège de l'électrode.

On peut observer en effet sur la Fig. 5 pour les animaux *A*, *B* et *C* examinés à des antériorités différentes, une augmentation considérable de l'amplitude et un remodelage morphologique qui caractérise les activités évoquées conditionnées. Sur la Fig. 6, la technique des moyennes permet de comparer avec précision l'aspect des tracés avant et après conditionnement suivant le niveau du noyau examiné. Pour une région très ventrale, la réponse, tardive et faiblement négative, devient très précoce et très ample. De même pour une autre région ventrale du VPL la réponse observée présente également une augmentation d'amplitude mais ici, la latence est réduite des deux tiers. Enfin, il faut noter que l'exploration de la limite dorsale du noyau met en évidence l'apparition d'une réponse totalement nouvelle au cours du conditionnement. Cette réponse, là encore, possède une morphologie bien nette.

En dépit de cette étendue relative des zones où le conditionnement est manifeste, une localisation assez précise peut être proposée.

En effet les modifications de réponses apportées par le conditionnement sont d'autant plus importantes que l'électrode qui les recueille est située dans les régions périphériques du

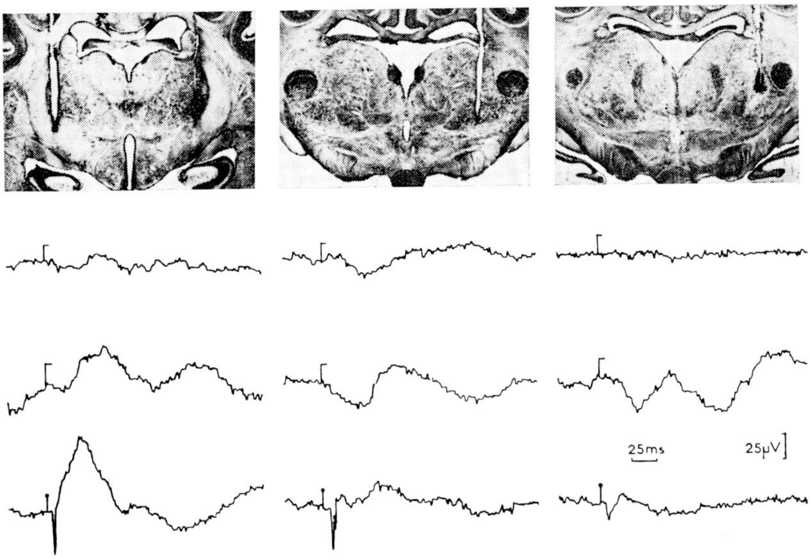

Fig. 6
Réponses évoquées par le son dans la région du VPL avant et après conditionnement. Chaque image correspond à une moyenne de 25 réponses. Chaque colonne résume le résultat d'une série d'expériences de conditionnement chez un animal différent. De haut en bas: réponse au son avant conditionnement, réponse au son après conditionnement, réponse à la stimulation du nerf, contrôle histologique. Les modifications apportées par le conditionnement sont observées pour des plans antérieurs sensiblement identiques, mais à des hauteurs différentes: —1; 0; +1,5.

noyau VPL. Ces modifications consistent essentiellement en un accroissement de l'amplitude pour les réponses de la région dorsale de ce noyau, tandis qu'elles se manifestent surtout par une forte réduction de la latence pour les réponses recueillies dans la partie ventrale du VPL. Au niveau d'une zone très postérieure correspondant au groupe postérieur décrit par Poggio et Mountcastle (1960), les modifications observées sont très importantes et concernant aussi bien l'amplitude que la latence (Fig. 5). Une précision supplémentaire est apportée par la descente de deux électrodes à biseau court (distance inter-électrode inférieure à 0,5 mm), l'une immédiatement au-dessus (hauteur 1) l'autre en plein VPL (hauteur 0). Il apparaît alors que seule l'électrode supérieure permet de recueillir des modifications caractéristiques du conditionnement alors que les réponses au son obtenues par l'électrode inférieure restent discrètes aussi bien

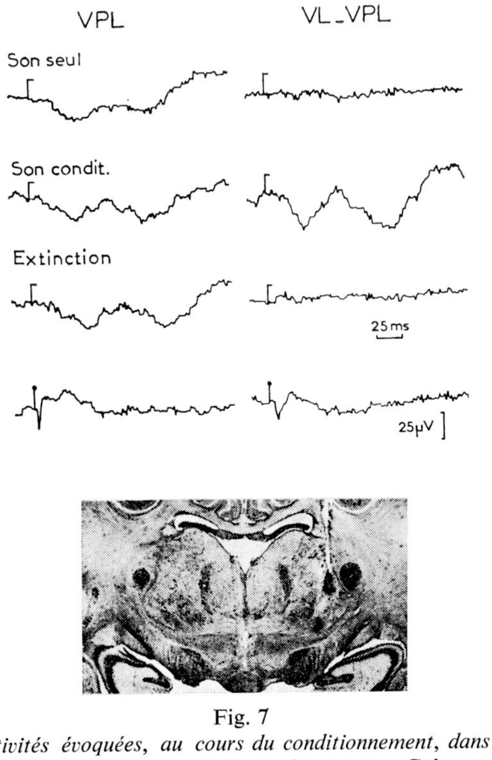

Fig. 7
Activités évoquées, au cours du conditionnement, dans le VPL et immédiatement au dessus de ce noyau. Colonne de gauche: région ventrale du VPL. Colonne de droite: partie supérieure de ce noyau à la limite du VL. Image inférieure: emplacement des électrodes réceptrices. De haut en bas: son seul; son conditionné; son après extinction; stimulation du nerf contralatéral.

après qu'avant le conditionnement (Fig. 7). Le Tableau I récapitule les modifications d'amplitude et de latence des activités évoquées par le son au cours du conditionnement. Si les accroissements d'amplitude peuvent être notés aussi bien pour les réponses corticales que pour les réponses thalamiques, les réductions de latence concernent surtout les réponses de la région ventrale et postérieure du VPL, tandis que dans la zone dorsale ce sont des réponses nouvelles qui apparaissent.

Variations des réponses avec les états de vigilance

Les zones d'enregistrement des activités évoquées conditionnées ayant été choisies, il restait à préciser les variations de ces activités avec la vigilance (Lelord et Kummer 1962). En

TABLEAU I

Modifications d'amplitude et de latence des réponses évoquées par le son avant et après conditionnement, sur le cortex SI, et à deux niveaux du VPL, chez des animaux différents

	Amplitude (μV)		Latence (msec)	
Cortex SI	13	33	28	25
	12	35	26	25
	13	23	22	19
VPL région ventrale	12	35	40	15
	9	22	25	8
	12	25	30	12
VPL limite dorsale	—	22	—	17
	—	22	—	17
	—	35	—	15

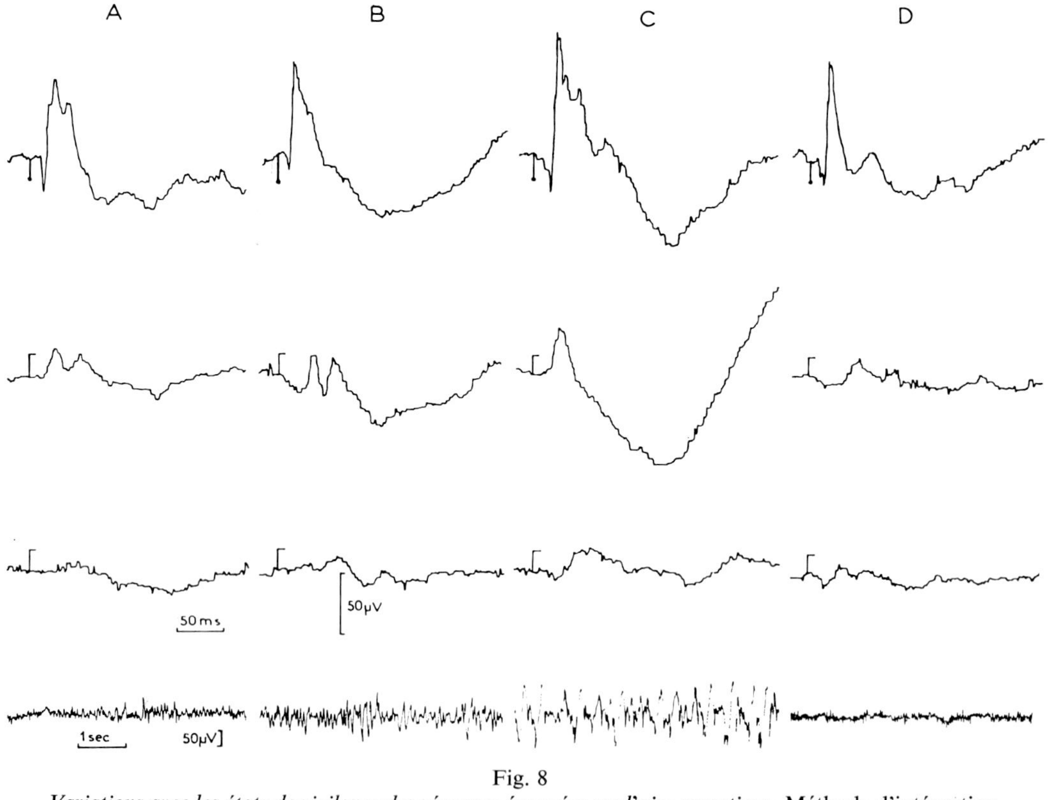

Fig. 8

Variations avec les états de vigilance des réponses évoquées sur l'aire somatique. Méthode d'intégration automatique. Ligne supérieure: potentiels évoqués par la stimulation du nerf; ligne moyenne: réponse au son conditionné; ligne inférieure: réponse au son après extinction; en bas: tracé électroencéphalographique. Colonne *A*: éveil; *B*: vigilance moyenne; *C*: sommeil à ondes lentes; *D*: sommeil à rythmes rapides.

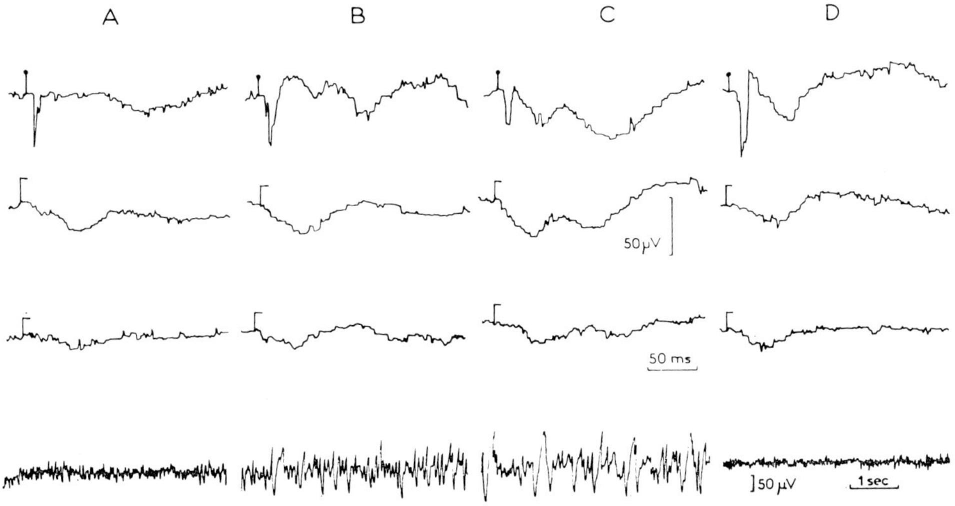

Fig. 9

Variations avec les états de vigilance des réponses évoquées dans la région du VPL. Méthode d'intégration automatique. Ligne supérieure: potentiel évoqué par la stimulation du nerf; ligne moyenne: réponse au son conditionné; ligne inférieure: réponse au son après extinction; en bas: tracé électroencéphalographique. Colonne *A*: éveil; *B*: vigilance moyenne; *C*: sommeil à ondes lentes; *D*: sommeil à rythmes rapides.

effet, ces variations sont si importantes qu'elles rendent nécessaire le choix d'un état de vigilance déterminé pour permettre l'observation exacte des modifications apportées par le conditionnement.

Sur le cortex. Lorsque l'animal est éveillé et que son tracé EEG est rapide, les réponses évoquées conditionnées sont de faible amplitude (25 μV), constituées par une composante négative bifide (latence 25 msec, durée 70 msec) suivie d'une onde lente positive peu marquée (Fig. 8). L'amplitude de ces réponses augmente lorsque l'animal est somnolent, qu'il se tient allongé les yeux mi-clos, et que son tracé EEG présente des oscillations régulières de 7–10 c/sec. Tout en augmentant d'amplitude, les deux accidents de la composante précoce se distinguent plus nettement, tandis que l'onde positive se creuse davantage.

Tout différents sont les aspects des réponses observées au cours du sommeil avec des ondes lentes sur le tracé EEG. Les réponses présentent alors un seul accident négatif de même amplitude que pendant la phase d'éveil (25 μV) et de même latence. Mais cet accident est suivi d'une onde positive tardive qui peut atteindre une grande amplitude (60 μV) et durer 160 msec.

Au cours de la phase de sommeil à rythmes rapides, la réponse se modifie totalement. L'onde négative ne comporte plus qu'un accident de faible amplitude (20 μV) et l'onde positive, si importante dans la phase de sommeil à ondes lentes disparaît ici totalement.

Dans le thalamus. Si le passage de la phase de l'éveil à celui de la vigilance moyenne n'entraîne pas de modifications notables des réponses, le passage à la phase de sommeil à ondes lentes se traduit, comme pour les réponses corticales, par des transformations importantes. Cependant, il faut noter que celles-ci concernent surtout les phases tardives de la réponse, et que ces modifications n'interviennent que pour les enregistrements recueillis à la partie ventrale du VPL (Fig. 9). La réponse conditionnée, constituée d'une seule onde positive au cours des phases d'éveil et de vigilance moyenne se transforme pendant la phase de sommeil et présente deux ondes positives successives (durée totale 150 msec, amplitude 60 μV) séparées par un accident négatif de faible amplitude.

Au cours du sommeil à rythmes rapides, la réponse reprend l'aspect qu'elle avait pour les phases d'éveil et de somnolence, tandis que son amplitude diminue beaucoup.

DISCUSSION

Les résultats obtenus dans cette étude mettent en évidence des caractères topographiques et morphologiques précis des activités évoquées conditionnées.

En effet, ces activités sont observées dans des zones bien délimitées, contrairement à ce qui est généralement signalé dans les travaux de conditionnement électrophysiologique. La plupart de ces travaux signalent en effet une diffusion importante des réponses évoquées au cours des expériences de conditionnement. En fait, il semble que les réponses observées correspondent au type de conditionnement effectué. Lorsque celui-ci met en jeu des comportements d'ensemble, comme les réactions motrices et posturales qui accompagnent le conditionnement salivaire, il n'est guère de structures dont l'activité ne soit modifiée par le conditionnement (Yoshii et Maeno 1958).

Il en est de même lorsque sont utilisées des stimulations rythmiques qui ont la propriété particulière d'entraîner l'activité de structures nombreuses et complexes (Livanov et Polyakov 1945; Morrell et Jasper 1956; John *et al.* 1964).

Au contraire, si le stimulus inconditionnel évoque une réponse caractéristique bien localisée, le stimulus conditionnel donne également des modifications localisées (Lelord *et al.* 1965). Bien plus ces modifications prédominent au niveau de l'aire de projection corticale et du relais thalamique des voies afférentes correspondant au stimulus inconditionnel (Lelord 1967; Maho 1968).

Cette topographie particulière des activités évoquées corticales caractéristiques du conditionnement a déjà été observée par différent auteurs (Livanov et Ryabinorskaya 1947; Popov 1948; Buser et Roger 1957; Jasper *et al.* 1960). Dans les expériences effectuées ici, les modifications les plus importantes sont observées sur une zone située très en arrière du sillon cruciatus et que différents travaux (Buser et Imbert 1961; Jankowska et Albe-Fessard 1961; Salmon-Legagneur 1966) considèrent comme l'aire sensitive proprement dite. Ces modifications, contrairement aux activités recueillies sur l'aire motrice, sont très sensibles aux variations de vigilance, comme le sont les réflexes conditionnés classiques (Maho 1968). Bien plus, leur localisation très postérieure s'accorde avec les résultats obtenus à l'aide d'ablations (Stepien *et al.* 1961) ou de stimulations (Tarnecki 1962) effectuées chez le chien et montrant le rôle prédominant de l'aire sensitive proprement dite dans la formation d'un conditionnement instrumental. Ainsi, les aires correspondant à l'"analyseur" (Pavlov 1929) de la sensibilité joueraient dans tous les conditionnements mettant en jeu des afférences somesthétiques, un rôle essentiel.

L'importance des voies afférentes est confirmée par l'étude des activités évoquées conditionnées dans le thalamus puisque ces activités prédominent dans la région du noyau ventral postéro-latéral dont la partie périphérique constitue une zone privilégiée où sont électivement retrouvées les réponses conditionnées (Lelord, voir Albe-Fessard et Fessard 1963).

Différents auteurs ont individualisé cette zone périphérique comme une coque recouvrant le VPL dans sa partie dorsale et rostrale (Kruger et Albe-Fessard 1960; Jankowska et Albe-Fessard 1961; Mallart *et al.* 1961; Massion *et al.* 1963; Albe-Fessard et Bowsher 1965). Cette zone répond essentiellement aux afférences somatiques contralatérales, mais également aux afférences ipsilatérales et, pour certaines cellules seulement, aux stimulations hétérosensorielles (zone P.O. de Poggio et Mountcastle 1960). Cette coque est donc considérée comme associative à somatotopie préférentielle.

Effectivement, c'est à ce niveau que sont observées les modifications les plus apparentes provoquées par le conditionnement. Cependant ces modifications ne sont pas homogènes: à la partie inférieure de la coque, elles sont sensibles aux variations de vigilance et leur latence est brève; au contraire, à la partie supérieure de la coque elles sont insensibles aux variations de vigilance et leur latence est longue.

Quant aux réponses observées à la partie centrale du VPL, elles sont peu modifiées par le conditionnement. Elles sont même totalement absentes chez l'un des animaux (Fig. 8). Peut-être dans ce cas l'électrode était-elle placée dans la région du VPL recevant des afférences musculaires (Andersson *et al.* 1966; Mallart 1964, 1967). Cette localisation expliquerait pourquoi un conditionnement sensoriel cutané ne modifierait pas les réponses au son recueillies à ce niveau. C'est pour les mêmes raisons que la région du gyrus sygmoïde antérieur postcrucié, région décrite comme étant une zone de projection d'afférences motrices et sensorielles (Albe-Fessard *et al.* 1961; Buser et Imbert 1961; Andersson *et al.* 1966, Oscarsson et Rosen 1966) ne présenterait également que de faibles modifications conditionnées. De toutes façons des précisions complémentaires nécessiteront l'emploi de méthodes microphysiologiques.

Quoiqu'il en soit, cette étude a contribué à mettre en évidence l'existence de zones préférentielles du conditionnement. Sur le cortex, ces zones coïncident avec l'aire primaire de projection des voies afférentes du stimulus inconditionnel. Dans le thalamus, elles ne correspondent ni au relais purement primaire, ni aux structures associatives, mais elles contribuent à individualiser des zones faiblement associatives à somatotopie préférentielle (Albe-Fessard 1961).

Ces différents résultats, obtenus à l'aide d'une méthode directement inspirée par les principes de Pavlov (1929) (isolement de réponses précises et facilement mesurables), amènent à proposer une définition de la réponse conditionnée reposant non plus nécessairement sur les épreuves classiques de l'extinction ou de la différenciation, mais sur des caractères morphologiques et topographiques particuliers de cette réponse.

RÉSUMÉ

Ce travail porte sur l'étude de modifications des réponses évoquées au cours d'un conditionnement sensorisensoriel. Le stimulus conditionnel est un son bref, le stimulus inconditionnel une stimulation brève et de faible intensité de la branche cutanée du nerf radial. Aucun mouvement n'étant observé, ce sont uniquement les modifications des réponses électrophysiologiques qui sont étudiées. Au total 318 expériences ont été effectuées chez le chat libre.

Les modifications apparaissent électivement sur l'aire corticale (SI) et dans la région du relais thalamique primaire (VPL) des voies afférentes correspondant au stimulus inconditionnel. Elles sont localisées au niveau du cortex SI sur une zone très postérieure correspondant à l'aire primaire somatique proprement dite, et dans le thalamus, à la périphérie du noyau VPL, zone associative à somatotopie préférentielle.

Les modifications corticales consistent en un accroissement d'amplitude, un remaniement morphologique et une faible diminution de latence tandis que les réponses thalamiques présentent, à côté des modifications d'amplitude et de morphologie, une importante réduction des latences. L'effet des variations du niveau de vigilance, important sur les réponses évoquées conditionnées corticales est peu marqué sur les réponses thalamiques, tout au moins sur leur phase précoce.

Ainsi se trouvent individualisées des zones préférentielles du conditionnement qui peuvent contribuer à la définition des principaux caractères du conditionnement électrophysiologique.

SUMMARY

CHANGES IN CORTICAL AND THALAMIC EVOKED ACTIVITY DURING SENSORY CONDITIONING. I. LOCALIZATION OF THE RESPONSES AND VARIATION WITH VIGILANCE

Modifications of evoked responses in the freely moving cat were studied during sensory conditioning, using a brief tone as conditioned stimulus and brief stimulation of weak intensity to the cutaneous branch of the radial nerve as the unconditioned stimulus. No movement was observed; only modifications of electrophysiological responses were studied. Altogether 318 experiments were carried out.

Changes occurred specifically in the cortical area (SI) and in the primary thalamic relay (VPL) of the afferent pathways concerned with the unconditioned stimulus. In cortical area SI they were localized in a posterior zone corresponding to the actual primary somatic area, and in the thalamus at the periphery of VPL, an associative region with somatotopic preference.

The cortical changes consisted in an increase of amplitude, change of configuration and slight decrease of latency, whereas the thalamic responses underwent significant reductions of latency in addition to change of amplitude and form. Variations in level of vigilance had significant effects on the conditioned evoked cortical responses but little effect on thalamic responses, at least on their initial phases.

Electroenceph. clin. Neurophysiol., **1969,** *27*: 258–269

Thus preferential zones for conditioned changes were defined which may assist in the understanding of the main features of electrophysiological conditioning.

BIBLIOGRAPHIE

ALBE-FESSARD, D. Nouvelles données sur l'origine des composantes des potentiels évoqués somesthésiques. In A. M. MONNIER (Ed.), *Actualités neurophysiol.*, **1961,** *3*: 24–60.

ALBE-FESSARD, D. and BOWSHER, D. Responses of monkey thalamus to somatic stimuli under chloralose anaesthesia. *Electroenceph. clin. Neurophysiol.*, **1965,** *19*: 1–15.

ALBE-FESSARD, D., DUMONT-TYC, S. et JANKOWSKA, E. Activités neuroniques somatotopiques et associatives recueillies au niveau de l'aire somatique primaire. *J. Physiol. (Paris)*, **1961,** *53*: 243.

ALBE-FESSARD, D. and FESSARD, A. Thalamic integration and their consequences at the telencephalic level. In G. MORUZZI *et al.* (Eds.), *Progress in brain research. Vol. 1, Brain mechanisms.* Elsevier, Amsterdam, **1963**: 124, Fig. 10.

ALEONARD, P. *Enregistrement et stimulations électriques chez le chat éveillé libre.* Diplôme des hautes études, Paris, **1962,** 55 p.

ANDERSSON, S. A., LANDGREN, S. and WOLSK, D. The thalamic relay and cortical projection of group I muscle afferents from the forelimb of the cat. *J. Physiol. (Lond.)*, **1966,** *183*: 576–591.

BUSER, P. and IMBERT, M. Sensory projections to the motor cortex in cats: a microelectrode study. In W. A. ROSENBLITH (Ed.), *Sensory communications.* Technology Press, Cambridge, Mass., **1961**: 607–626.

BUSER, P. et ROGER, A. Interprétation du conditionnement sur la base des données électroencéphalographiques. *Acta med. belg.*, **1957**: 417–444.

GALAMBOS, R., SHEATZ, G. and VERNIER, V. G. Electrophysiological correlates of conditioned response in cat. *Science*, **1956,** *123*: 367–377.

GRASTYÁN, E., LISSÁK, K., MADARÁSZ, I. and DONHOFFER, H. Hippocampal electrical activity during the development of conditioned reflexes. *Electroenceph. clin. Neurophysiol.*, **1959,** *11*: 409–430.

HEARST, E., BEER, B., SHEATZ, G. and GALAMBOS, R. Some electrophysiological correlates of conditioning in the monkey. *Electroenceph. clin. Neurophysiol.*, **1960,** *12*: 137–152.

JANKOWSKA, E. et ALBE-FESSARD, D. Sur l'origine et l'interprétation de la seconde phase du potentiel évoqué primaire de l'aire somatique. *J. Physiol. (Paris)*, **1961,** *53*: 374–375.

JASPER, H. and AJMONE MARSAN, C. *A stereotaxic atlas of the diencephalon of the cat.* Nat. Res. Council of Canada, Ottawa, **1954**.

JASPER, H., RICCI, G. and DOANE, B. Microelectrode analysis of cortical cell discharge during avoidance conditioning in the monkey. *Electroenceph. clin. Neurophysiol.*, **1960,** *Suppl. 13*: 137–155.

JOHN, E. R. and KILLAM, K. F. Electrophysiological correlates of avoidance conditioning in the cat. *J. Pharmacol. exp. Ther.*, **1959,** *125*: 252–274.

JOHN, E. R., RUCHKIN, D. S. and VILLEGAS, J. Experimental background: signal analysis and behavioral correlates of evoked potential configurations in cats. *Ann. N. Y. Acad. Sci.*, **1964,** *112*: 362–420.

JOUVET, M. et HERNÁNDEZ-PEÓN, R. Mécanismes neurophysiologiques concernant l'habituation, l'attention, et le conditionnement. *Electroenceph. clin. Neurophysiol.*, **1957,** *Suppl. 6*: 39–49.

KONORSKI, J. *Conditioned reflexes and neuron organization.* Cambridge Univ. Press, London, **1948,** 267 p.

KONORSKI, J. The cortical representation of the UC reflexes. *Electroenceph. clin. Neurophysiol.*, **1960,** *Suppl. 13*: 81–90.

KRUGER, L. and ALBE-FESSARD, D. Distribution of responses to somatic afferent stimuli in the diencephalon of the cat under chloralose anaesthesia. *Exp. Neurol.*, **1960,** *2*: 442–467.

LELORD, G. *L'acquisition libre. Aspects neurophysiologiques chez l'animal et chez l'homme.* Thèse Sci. Nat., Paris, **1967,** 199 p.

LELORD, G., MAHO, C. et REYMOND, M. C. Comparaison de l'évolution au cours du conditionnement de réponses obtenues dans diverses aires corticales et structures sous-corticales. *J. Physiol. (Paris)*, **1965,** *57*: 647.

LELORD, G. et KUMMER, J. L. Réponses évoquées au niveau du cortex somatique primaire du chat éveillé libre par des stimulations sonores, alternées avec des stimulations non douloureuses du nerf radial. *J. Physiol. (Paris)*, **1962,** *54*: 368.

LIBOUBAN, S. et ALEONARD, P. Sur un mode d'implantation d'électrodes à demeure chez le rat, permettant l'observation du même animal pendant plusieurs mois. *C. R. Soc. Biol. (Paris)*, **1960,** *154*: 540–543.

LIVANOV, M. N. et POLYAKOV, K. L. Activités électriques dans le cortex cérébral du lapin pendant la formation d'un réflexe conditionné défensif à une stimulation rythmique. *Byull. Acad. Nauk. USSR*, **1945,** *3*: 286–307.

LIVANOV, M. N. et RYABINOVSKAYA, A. M. Le problème de la localisation des modifications électriques dans l'écorce cérébrale du lapin au cours de la formation d'un réflexe conditionné à un stimulus rythmique. *Fiziol. Zh. (Leningr.)*, **1947,** *33*: 523–534.

MAHO, C. *Variations des activités évoquées de diverses structures centrales au cours du conditionnement.* Dipl. Ét. Sup. Sci. Nat. (Paris), **1968,** 63 p.

MALLART, A. Projection des afférences musculaires de la patte antérieure au niveau du thalamus chez le chat. *C.R. Acad. Sci. (Paris)*, **1964,** *259*: 1215–1218.

MALLART, A. *Projection des afférences somatiques vers les structures cérébrales spécifiques et non-spécifiques.* Thèse Sci. (Paris), **1967,** 126 p.

MALLART, A., MARTINOYA, C. et ALBE-FESSARD, D. Comparaison entre les types de stimulations naturelles qui évoquent des réponses dans les relais spécifiques ou les relais associatifs. *J. Physiol. (Paris)*, **1961,** *53*: 421–422.

MASSION, J., LELORD, G. et ANGAUT, P. Étude microphysiologique des projections sensorielles dans la région du noyau ventrolatéral. *J. Physiol. (Paris)*, **1963,** *55*: 166–167.

MORRELL, F. and JASPER, H. Electroencephalographic studies of the formation of temporary connections in the brain. *Electroenceph. clin. Neurophysiol.*, **1956,** *8*: 201–215.

NAUMOVA, T. S., POPOVA, N. S. et ULYANINA, N. N. Évolution de l'amplitude des potentiels évoqués dans les aires de projection visuelle et auditive du chien au cours d'un conditionnement défensif. *Zh. vyssh. nerv. Deyat. Pavlova*, **1966,** *16*: 984–992.

OSCARSSON, O. and ROSEN, I. Short latency projections to the cat's cerebral cortex from skin and muscle afferents in the contralateral forelimb. *J. Physiol. (Lond.)*, **1966,** *182*: 164–184.

PAVLOV, I. P. *Leçons sur l'activité du cortex cérébral.* Legrand, Paris, **1929,** 418 p.

POGGIO, G. F. and MOUNTCASTLE, V. B. A study of the functional contributions of the lemniscal and spinothalamic systems to somatic sensibility. Central nervous mechanisms in pain. *Bull. Johns Hopk. Hosp.*, **1960,** *106*: 266–316.

POPOV, N. A. Études électroencéphalographiques du problème des réflexes conditionnés. *Ann. psychol.*, **1948,** *46*: 132–148.

SALMON-LEGAGNEUR, A. *Comparaison des activités unitaires des cellules du cortex moteur et somatique du singe et du chat.* Dipl. Ét. Sup. Sci. Nat. (Paris), **1966,** 82 p.

STEPIEN, I., STEPIEN, L. and KONORSKI, L. The effect of unilateral and bilateral ablation of sensori-motor cortex on the instrumental (type II) alimentary conditioned reflexes in dogs. *Acta Biol. exp. (Warszawa)*, **1961,** *21*: 121–140.

TARNECKI, R. The formation of instrumental conditioned reflexes by direct stimulation of sensori-motor cortex in cats. *Acta Biol. exp. (Warszawa)*, **1962,** *22*: 35–45.

YOSHII, N. and MAENO, S. An electroencephalographic study of conditioned salivary reflex. *Folia psychiat. neurol. jap.*, **1958,** *12*: 296–316.

YOSHII, N., PRUVOT, P. et GASTAUT, H. À propos d'une activité rythmique transitoirement enregistrée dans la formation réticulée mésencéphalique et susceptible de représenter l'expression EEG de la trace mnémonique. *C.R. Acad. Sci. (Paris)*, **1956,** *242*: 1361–1364.

Référence: LELORD, G. et MAHO, C. Modifications des activités évoquées corticales et thalamiques au cours d'un conditionnement sensoriel. I. Localisation des réponses et variations avec la vigilance. *Electroenceph. clin. Neurophysiol.*, **1969,** *27*: 258-269.

Electroencephalography and Clinical Neurophysiology
Elsevier Publishing Company, Amsterdam – Printed in The Netherlands

MODIFICATIONS DES ACTIVITÉS ÉVOQUÉES CORTICALES ET THALAMIQUES AU COURS D'UN CONDITIONNEMENT SENSORIEL. II. ÉVOLUTION DES RÉPONSES AVEC LES STADES DU CONDITIONNEMENT

G. LELORD[1] ET C. MAHO

Laboratoire de Physiologie des Centres Nerveux, Faculté des Sciences, 4, avenue Gordon-Bennett, Paris 16e (France)

(Accepted for publication: December 30, 1968)

Depuis les travaux classiques de Pavlov (1929) attribuant au cortex cérébral un rôle prédominant dans la formation du réflexe conditionné, différents auteurs, se basant sur des données électrophysiologiques, ont insisté sur le rôle des structures sous-corticales dans le conditionnement (Fessard et Gastaut 1958; Yoshii et Hockaday 1958).

Effectivement des enregistrements explorant des structures sous-corticales associatives, formation réticulée du tronc cérébral (Morrell et Jasper 1956), hippocampe et amygdale (Grastyán *et al.* 1959), hypothalamus (Yoshii et Hockaday 1958) ont montré que les réponses conditionnées y sont observées précocement, avant même l'apparition des modifications corticales. De même, Gastaut *et al.* (1957), étudiant les modifications de la réaction d'arrêt conditionnée sur le cortex, en déduisent que les phénomènes les plus précoces traduisent la mise en jeu de la formation réticulée du tronc cérébral, puis des noyaux intralaminaires du thalamus.

Ces données ne sont pas confirmées par Morrell (1960), Lelord (voir Albe-Fessard et Fessard 1963) et, plus récemment, Kitai *et al.* (1965) qui observent des réponses conditionnées apparaissant en premier lieu sur le cortex et précédant les modifications sous-corticales.

Ayant mis en évidence sur l'aire primaire somatique et dans la région du relais primaire thalamique de la sensibilité des réponses électivement modifiées par un conditionnement couplant un son bref et une stimulation appliquée sur un nerf somatique (Lelord et Maho 1969), nous avons considéré que ces zones se prêtaient tout particulièrement à une étude comparative du conditionnement sur le cortex et dans le sous-cortex (Lelord 1967; Maho 1968).

Désirant en outre préciser l'influence du couplage des stimulations sur la formation des réponses conditionnées, nous avons effectué non seulement des expériences de conditionnement classique comportant des stimulations couplées, mais encore des expériences "d'acquisition libre" (Lelord 1967), où le son et la stimulation du nerf sont appliqués séparément et dans le désordre.

TECHNIQUE

Les principes généraux de la technique d'implantation des électrodes, des enregistrements et du protocole expérimental ont été décrits précédemment (Lelord et Maho 1969).

Les stimulations sont d'intensité faible. Le stimulus conditionnel est un son bref de 5 msec d'une fréquence de 2500 c/sec. Le stimulus inconditionnel est appliqué directement sur une branche cutanée du nerf radial; c'est une impulsion rectangulaire de durée (0,2 msec) et de voltage (0,5 V) peu élevé.

Dans les expériences de conditionnement le son est couplé avec la stimulation du nerf qu'il précède régulièrement, un délai de 300 msec séparant ces deux stimulations.

Dans les expériences d'acquisition libre le son est séparé de la stimulation du nerf, si bien que

[1] Chargé de Recherches au C.N.R.S.

les stimulations sont distribuées dans le désordre, en séries de 1, 2 ou 3 sons succédant à des séries de 1, 2 ou 3 stimulations du nerf. Cette distribution dispersée est répartie de telle sorte qu'elle ne diffère pas de façon significative d'une distribution au hasard.

Dans toutes ces expériences, des intervalles de temps variant entre 15 et 120 sec séparent les stimulations qui se succèdent, qu'il s'agisse des couples de stimuli contigus du conditionnement classique, ou des sons et des stimulations du nerf dispersés des expériences d'acquisition libre. De toute façon, la distribution des stimulations est effectuée de telle sorte qu'il n'y ait pas d'intervalles de temps préférentiels (Lelord 1967).

RÉSULTATS

Évolution des réponses corticales et sous-corticales avec les principaux stades du conditionnement

La comparaison des activités évoquées conditionnées sur le cortex (aire somatique I) et dans le thalamus (zone susjacente au VPL) sera étudiée à titre d'exemple chez le chat Pile (Fig. 1). Avant le conditionnement le son évoque sur le cortex une réponse négative, de 5–10 μV d'amplitude, dont la latence varie entre 20 et 25 msec, et dans le thalamus, une double réponse positive de latence un peu plus longue (30 msec).

Le premier temps du conditionnement (*1*) se déroule au cours des 4 premières séances de

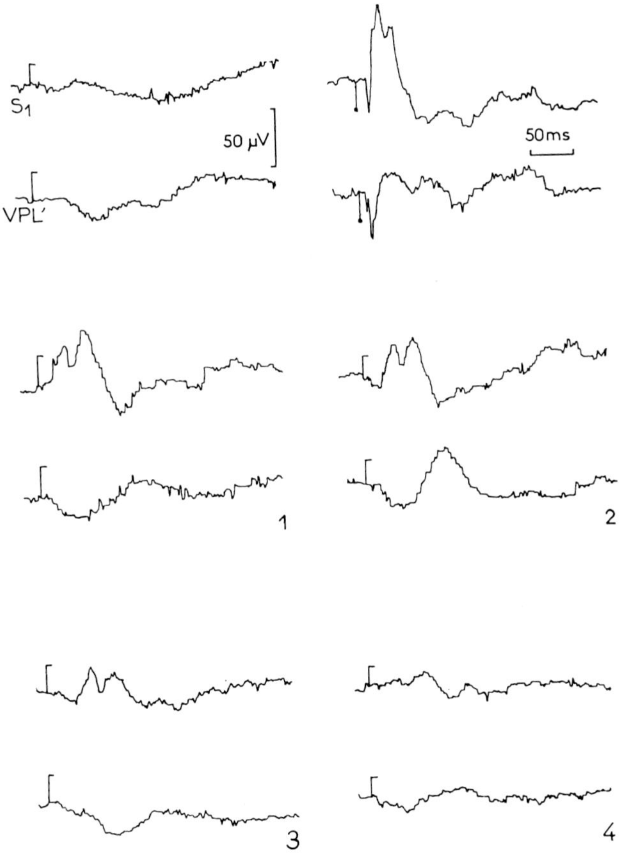

Fig. 1

Comparaison des réponses évoquées par le son sur le cortex et dans le thalamus au cours du conditionnement. Chaque image représente la moyenne des réponses à 25 stimulations. Les signets indiquent les artéfacts des sons, les traits, les artéfacts de la stimulation du nerf. Tracé supérieur: aire primaire somatique (S_1), tracé inférieur: région du noyau VPL. En haut et à gauche: réponses au son avant conditionnement. En haut et à droite: réponses à la stimulation du nerf. *1–3*: différents stades de la formation du conditionnement, *4*: extinction.

couplage des stimulations et se traduit d'abord par l'apparition sur le cortex d'une onde ample, négative et bifide (latence: 20 msec, amplitude: 50 μV, durée: 75 msec). Ce n'est que dans un deuxième temps (*2*) du conditionnement allant de la 4ème à la 8ème séance que la réponse thalamique est profondément modifiée et se caractérise non seulement par un accident positif de latence brève (10 msec), mais par une onde négative ample. Ultérieurement (*3*) les réponses thalamiques et corticales s'atténuent mais leur morphologie, et, pour les réponses thalamiques, leur latence restent différentes de ce qui était observé avant le conditionnement. Enfin, la répétition du son seul au cours des séances dites d'extinction (*4*) amène une réduction importante des deux réponses.

L'apparition des modifications thalamiques à un stade relativement tardif du conditionnement est un fait constant retrouvé chez tous les animaux. Ce phénomène apparaît bien sur la Fig. 2 qui représente les amplitudes moyennes par séance des réponses enregistrées chez le chat C au cours de 25 séances de conditionnement. Les premières séances "d'extinction" du son seul ne provoquent qu'une réduction légère de l'amplitude de la réponse. De même, cette réponse est peu modifiée par les premières séances d'association (expériences 5–10). Par contre des modifications importantes sont observées au cours des 7ème, 8ème et 9ème séance d'association (expériences 11–13). Elles se traduisent d'abord par une diminution puis par une augmentation importante de l'amplitude de la réponse au son qui reste élevée, non seulement au cours des séances suivantes de conditionnement (expériences 14–19) mais encore au cours des premières séances de répétition du son conditionné appliqué seul (expériences 20–23), la diminution d'amplitude n'apparaissant qu'à un stade relativement tardif de l'extinction (expériences 24 et 25).

Ces résultats sont confirmés par l'étude des latences de toutes les réponses représentées sur la Fig. 3. En effet la mesure précise de ces latences montre peu de modifications au cours des premières séances d'association (expériences 5–9). Par contre, à partir de la 6ème séance d'association (expérience 10) apparaît déjà pour certaines

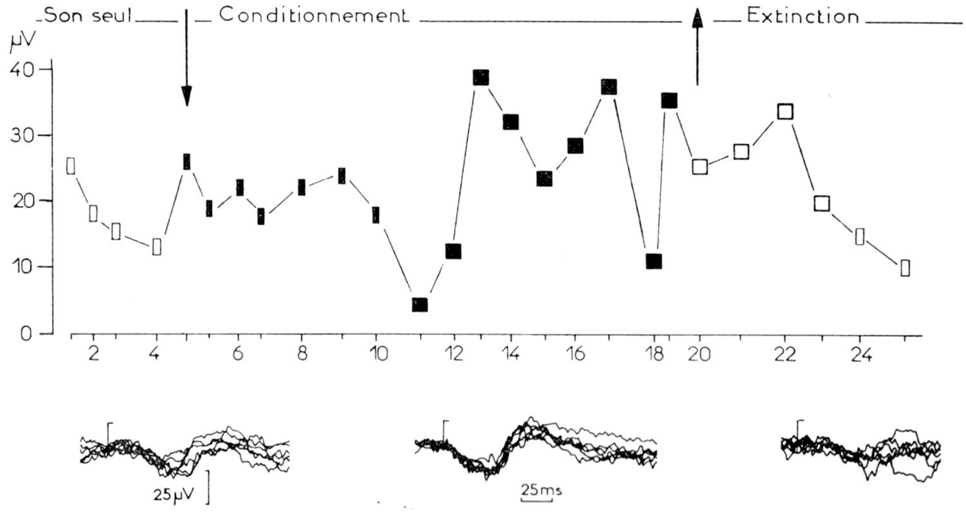

Fig. 2

Amplitude moyenne, par séance, des réponses évoquées par le son. En ordonnées, valeur des amplitudes en microvolts. En abscisses, les séances successives (comportant 6–8 réponses, l'importance des séances correspond au nombre de réponses obtenues). Rectangles blancs: réponses au son seul avant les associations. Rectangles noirs: réponses à longue latence des premières séances d'association. Les carrés noirs correspondent aux réponses à latence brève des séances suivantes. Les carrés blancs, aux réponses à latence brève persistant pendant les premières séances d'extinction. Les images situées sous la courbe montrent l'aspect des réponses correspondantes. Chaque image est constituée par la superposition graphique des 6 potentiels moyens, dont chacun correspond à 25 réponses.

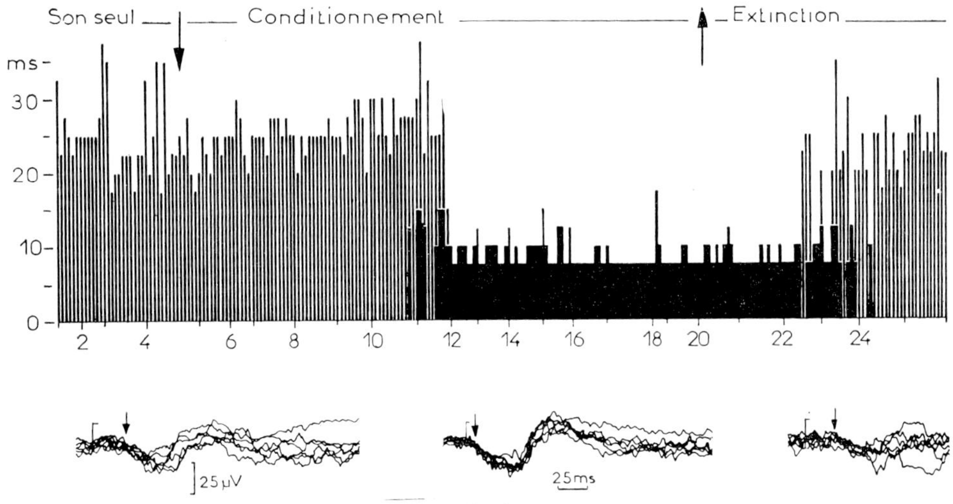

Fig. 3

Latence moyenne des réponses évoquées par le son. En ordonnées, les valeurs des latences en millisecondes. En abscisses, les séances successives (comportant 6–8 réponses). Les images situées sous le schéma montrent l'aspect des réponses. Chaque image est constituée par la superposition graphique des 6 potentiels moyens, dont chacun correspond à 25 réponses.

réponses une réduction marquée des latences. Cette réduction s'étend à toutes les réponses pendant les séances suivantes (expériences 12–19) et persiste au cours des premières séances de répétition du son seul (expériences 20–23). De telles modifications semblent caractéristiques du conditionnement.

Comparaison de l'évolution des réponses corticales et sous-corticales au cours du conditionnement et de l'acquisition libre

Afin de préciser le rôle exact du couplage des stimulations dans la formation du conditionnement, une étude comparative est effectuée de la manière suivante: chez chaque animal sont effectuées 1–3 séances de répétition du son seul, puis 6–9 séances d'acquisition libre (sons et stimulations du nerf étant distribués séparément et dans le désordre) puis 1–3 séances de répétition du son seul, puis 7–11 séances de conditionnement (sons et stimulations du nerf étant appliqués sous forme de couples) suivies de 3–5 séances de répétition du son seul. Les résultats obtenus avec ces deux méthodes d'application des stimulations sont différents sur le cortex et dans le thalamus.

1. *Réponses corticales.* Que la méthode d'association des stimulations soit le conditionnement ou l'acquisition libre, les modifications observées sur le cortex ont sensiblement le même aspect, la même localisation et la même évolution.

Comme les réponses conditionnées, les réponses acquises par la méthode des stimulations dispersées prédominent sur l'aire somatique primaire et présentent le plus souvent un aspect biphasique. C'est ce que montre la Fig. 4 où sont superposées par une méthode graphique des séries de 6 réponses chez trois animaux différents. Avant toute association le son provoque sur l'aire somatique des réponses peu amples et de forme très variable. L'acquisition libre fait apparaître des réponses de morphologie caractéristique qui sont très semblables aux réponses conditionnées et qui diffèrent sensiblement par leur aspect et leur latence des réponses à la stimulation du nerf. L'évolution de ces activités évoquées et plus précisément de leur partie précoce est représentée sur le graphique de la Fig. 5 qui montre les modifications d'amplitude du premier accident négatif de la réponse au son au cours du conditionnement et de l'acquisition libre chez le chat P. Avant toute association le son ne provoque que des réponses de faible amplitude. Les modifications notables qu'entraîne l'acquisition libre ne se manifestent pas immédiatement. Elles sont très inconstantes au début

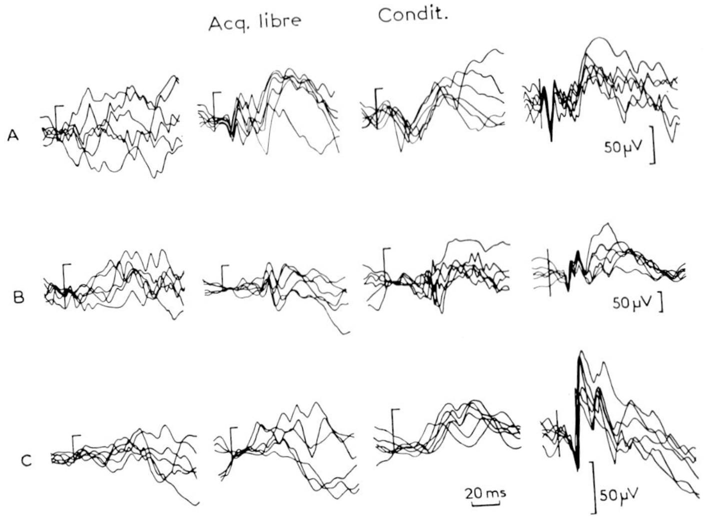

Fig. 4

Acquisition libre et conditionnement des activités évoquées chez trois chats différents. Aire primaire somatique = réponses photographiées une par une et superposées par séries de 6 à l'aide d'une méthode graphique. Chaque ligne *A*, *B*, *C* correspond à un animal différent. Les signets indiquent les artéfacts du son, les traits les artéfacts de la stimulation du nerf. Les trois premières colonnes montrent les réponses au son au cours de moments différents des séries d'experiences. De gauche à droite: extinction du son, puis distribution de la stimulation du nerf suivant la méthode dispersée, puis combinaison du son et de la stimulation du nerf. La colonne de droite montre les potentiels évoqués par la stimulation du nerf.

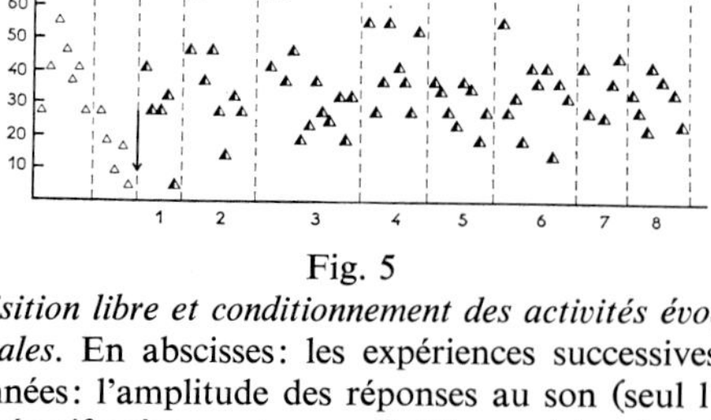

Fig. 5

Acquisition libre et conditionnement des activités évoquées corticales. En abscisses: les expériences successives. En ordonnées: l'amplitude des réponses au son (seul l'accident négatif précoce est mesuré). Chaque triangle indique le chiffre trouvé pour l'amplitude du phénomène évoqué moyen correspondant à 25 réponses. Triangles blancs: avant l'intervention de la stimulation du nerf; triangles noirs: après l'application de cette stimulation sous forme dispersée; triangles noirs et blancs: après couplage des stimulations.

des expériences d'association (II et III), évidentes pendant la IVème expérience, et elles se stabilisent au cours des VIème, VIIème et IXème expériences.

Les phénomènes observés au cours du conditionnement sont comparables. Après "l'extinction" de la réponse au son appliqué seul, le couplage de cette stimulation avec la stimulation du nerf fait apparaître très rapidement (expériences 1 et 2) la réponse conditionnée, qui persiste au cours des expériences suivantes. Cette précocité du conditionnement est liée ici au fait que la réactivité de l'animal a été modifiée par les séries d'expériences d'acquisition libre effectuées auparavant et dont l'effet n'a pas disparu.

2. *Réponses thalamiques.* Alors que des potentiels évoqués conditionnés d'amplitude et de latence caractéristique sont mis en évidence dans le thalamus, les réponses au son recueillies dans cette structure au cours d'expériences distribuant les stimulations sous une forme dispersée sont peu modifiées. Ce contraste entre

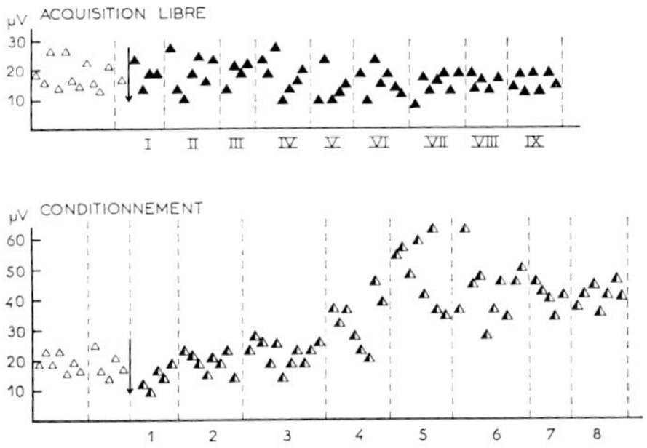

Fig. 6

Réponses thalamiques au cours de l'acquisition libre et du conditionnement. En abscisses: les expériences successives. En ordonnées: l'amplitude des réponses au son (écart entre la pointe de l'accident positif précoce et le sommet de l'onde négative qui lui succède). Chaque triangle indique l'amplitude en microvolts de la réponse. Triangles blancs: avant l'intervention de la stimulation du nerf; triangles noirs: après l'application de cette stimulation sous forme dispersée; triangles noirs et blancs: après couplage des stimulations.

les résultats obtenus avec les deux méthodes est d'autant plus frappant que dans les deux cas les réponses corticales sont semblables.

Un tel contraste apparaît nettement sur la Fig. 6 où sont portées les amplitudes de chaque réponse thalamique au cours d'une série d'expériences de conditionnement et d'une série d'expériences d'acquisition libre.

Ces résultats sont confirmés par le calcul des amplitudes moyennes des réponses corticales et thalamiques chez trois chats différents (Tableau I). Alors que les différences d'amplitude des réponses corticales dans les expériences de conditionnement et d'acquisition libre varient suivant les animaux, l'amplitude des réponses thalamiques est nettement plus élevée chez tous les animaux dans les expériences de conditionnement que dans les expériences d'acquisition libre.

Extinction des réponses

Des différences notables sont également observées entre les réponses acquises par la méthode des stimulations dispersées et les réponses conditionnées au cours des expériences "d'extinction" pendant lesquelles le son est répété seul. En effet, après une série d'expériences d'acquisition libre, une seule séance d'extinction suffit pour faire disparaître les modifications provoquées par l'association du son et de la stimulation du nerf sous forme dispersée (Fig. 7,*3*). Il faut au contraire 3 à 5 séances de répétition du son seul pour obtenir la disparition de réponses conditionnées (Fig. 7,*4*).

La stabilité des réponses électrophysiologiques conditionnées est donc remarquable. Elle s'observe après seulement quelques expériences de conditionnement, que ces expériences aient été ou non précédées par une série de séances de stimulations dispersées. Au contraire, les réponses obtenues au cours de l'acquisition libre sont labiles et leur extinction survient généralement après quelques répétitions du son seul.

DISCUSSION

L'étude comparative des réponses conditionnées corticales et thalamiques confirme tout d'abord certaines observations (Lelord *et al.* 1965) suivant lesquelles le conditionnement apparaît en premier lieu sur le cortex. Chez les animaux examinés ici, les modifications corticales apparaissent dès la 3ème séance d'asso-

TABLEAU I

Comparaison des amplitudes moyennes des réponses corticales et thalamiques chez trois animaux. Les réponses corticales sont plus amples chez le chat Pile au cours de l'acquisition libre et, chez le chat Blanche Neige au cours du conditionnement. Elles sont peu différentes chez le chat Tinto. Les réponses thalamiques sont plus amples au cours du conditionnement chez les trois animaux

	Cortex			Thalamus		
	Acq. libre	Condit.	Seuil prob.	Acq. libre	Condit.	Seuil prob.
Pile	30,2	25,7	$P < 0,01$	18,5	28,5	$P < 0,0002$
Tinto	38,1	40	$P < 0,10$	19,5	25,9	$P < 0,005$
Bl. Neige	26	35,5	$P < 0,005$	16,4	37,1	$P < 0,00003$

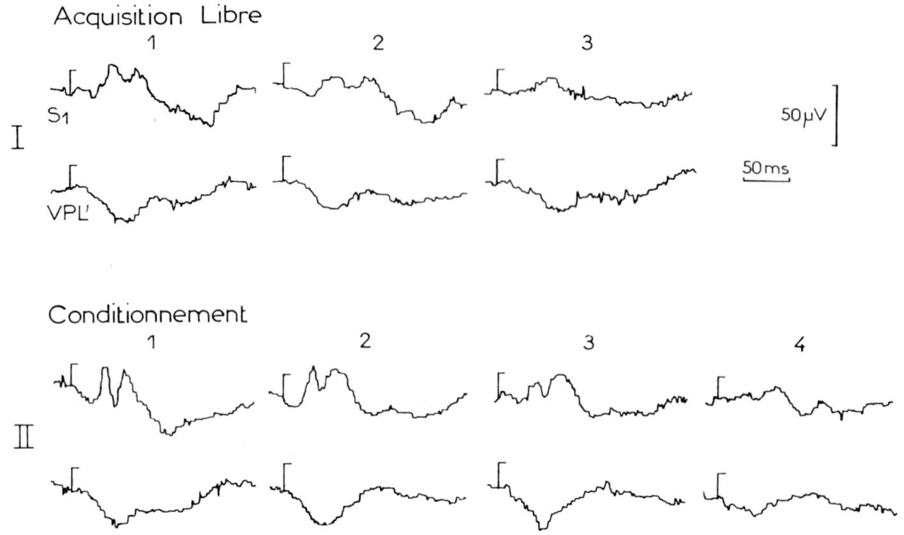

Fig. 7
Extinction des réponses évoquées par le son sur le cortex et dans le thalamus après l'acquisition libre et après le conditionnement. Chaque image représente la moyenne des réponses à 25 stimulations. Tracé supérieur: aire primaire somatique (S_1); tracé inférieur: région du VPL (VPL′). L'artéfact du son est représenté par un signet. En haut: réponses évoquées après acquisition libre (*1*), première (*2*) et deuxième (*3*) séances d'extinction. En bas: réponses évoquées après conditionnement (*1*), première (*2*), troisième (*3*) et cinquième (*4*) séances d'extinction.

ciation tandis que les modifications thalamiques ne surviennent que de la 4ème à la 8ème séance d'association.

Cette précocité d'apparition des réponses corticales est retrouvée aussi bien dans les expériences de stimulations dispersées que dans les expériences de conditionnement. De plus la localisation, la latence et la morphologie de ces réponses est la même dans les deux cas. De telles similitudes confirment les observations déjà effectuées avec la technique EEG (Lelord 1966), montrant que la dispersion des stimulations n'aboutit pas nécessairement à une forme dégradée de conditionnement (pseudoconditionnement) mais peut réaliser une association spécifique, l'acquisition libre.

Cependant l'absence de modifications thalamiques au cours de l'acquisition libre n'en constitue pas moins un résultat inattendu. C'est pourquoi nous envisagerons successivement les mécanismes possibles de formation des réponses thalamiques conditionnées avant d'aborder le problème du "silence" thalamique observé dans l'acquisition libre.

L'apparition de modifications thalamiques à un stade relativement tardif du conditionnement, ne s'accorde pas avec les données électrophysiologiques habituellement admises (Gastaut *et al.* 1957), et paraît peu compréhensible en regard du fait que les convergences observées au niveau de SI sont déjà présentes à proximité du noyau ventral-postéro-latéral (VPL) (Albe-Fessard et Fessard 1963). Il est alors difficile d'imaginer qu'une liaison puisse se produire au niveau du cortex sans affecter d'abord le thalamus.

En fait, ces convergences se manifestent dans le thalamus dès les premières applications du son seul qui provoque à ce moment dans la région du VPL une réponse positive. Cette réponse dont la latence est proche de la latence de la réponse corticale susjacente traduit bien par sa présence l'existence de convergences thalamiques préexistant au conditionnement.

L'apparition retardée, dans un deuxième temps du conditionnement, de modifications thalamiques importantes, permet de penser que ces modifications sont non seulement précédées mais encore facilitées par les modifications corticales. Il est en effet admis que le cortex cérébral exerce un contrôle sur de nombreuses structures sous-corticales (Hugelin et Bonvallet 1957a, b). Ce contrôle s'exerce également sur la partie du noyau ventro-latéral (VL) immédiatement adjacente au VPL (Massion *et al.* 1965) et sur le VPL comme en témoigne la présence de projections corticifuges issues de l'aire somesthésique (Auer 1956) et les observations électrophysiologiques montrant que la stimulation strychnique ou électrique du cortex somatomoteur (Niemer et Jimenez-Castellanos 1950; Stratford 1954) évoque des réponses au niveau de ce noyau.

L'existence de boucles corticales, empruntant les aires primaires et jouant un rôle régulateur sur les structures sous jacentes (Buser et Ascher 1960; Ascher 1965) permet alors de comprendre qu'un "modelage" précoce des réponses évoquées conditionnées sur le cortex SI puisse retentir secondairement sur la formation des activités évoquées conditionnées thalamiques.

Bien plus, l'apparition de ce second temps thalamique, observé dans les expériences de conditionnement, semble traduire la mise en jeu d'un circuit court pouvant échapper au contrôle cortical (Maho 1968). En effet, la latence de la réponse thalamique conditionnée est plus brève que la latence de la réponse corticale et l'influence du niveau de vigilance, très marquée sur cette réponse corticale, reste faible au niveau thalamique. Enfin, chez certains animaux, l'amplitude de la réponse corticale diminue au moment ou le conditionnement se manifeste dans le thalamus.

De telles modifications, caractéristiques du deuxième stade du conditionnement, n'en sont pas moins minimes ou absentes dans l'acquisition libre.

Il faut donc admettre que le couplage des stimulations exerce un effet déterminant sur l'apparition des modifications thalamiques. Mais le mécanisme responsable de cet effet reste à déterminer.

Peut-être faut-il assimiler les stimulations couplées du conditionnement à une stimulation répétitive et considérer que la "coque" du VPL, comme d'autres structures associatives du thalamus (Dempsey et Morison 1942), ne réagit de façon régulière qu'à des trains d'influx?

Peut-être le couplage des stimulations permet-il l'établissement d'effets "en retour" (Dusser de Barenne et McCulloch 1941) entre le cortex et le thalamus pendant l'intervalle de temps de 300 msec qui sépare le stimulus conditionné du stimulus inconditionnel?

Il est possible enfin que les structures sous-corticales soient électivement modifiées par l'application de cycles de stimulations[1] et que ces modifications une fois apparues présentent une stabilité particulière. Cette conservation de traces "cycliques" dans les structures sous-corticales a déjà été signalée sur des préparations décortiquées qui présentent une série d'activités stéréotypées déclenchées à volonté par l'expérimentateur et restent identiques à elles-mêmes aussi longtemps que dure la survie de l'animal (Popov 1950). Plus récemment l'exploration électrophysiologique de ces structures a permis de mettre en évidence soit des reproductions de cycles d'excitation provoquées par le couplage des stimuli conditionnels et inconditionnels (Kitai *et al.* 1965), soit des modifications de cycles d'excitabilité décelées par l'application de deux ou plusieurs stimulations successives (Buser *et al.* 1958).

Ainsi le facteur chronologique liant les stimulations du conditionnement classique et aboutissant à la stabilisation de l'acquisition traduirait une forme d'acquisition apparentée au conditionnement au temps caractérisée par la coexistence de réponses à la fois dans le cortex et le sous-cortex. Au contraire l'indépendance temporelle des stimulations de l'acquisition libre favoriserait la formation d'une association plus labile prédominant au niveau du cortex.

RÉSUMÉ

Cette étude porte sur la comparaison des activités évoquées corticales et thalamiques au

[1] L'existence d'une reproduction par le système nerveux de "cycles d'excitation" a été observée depuis longtemps chez les organismes inférieurs (Pieron 1925) et dans certaines formes dégradées du conditionnement (conditionnement "au temps" de Pavlov). Cette aptitude à reproduire les cycles temporels, appelée "cyclochronie" (Popov 1950), interviendrait également dans le conditionnement classique puisque le stimulus conditionné est capable à lui seul de faire apparaître l'ensemble de phénomènes successifs provoqués habituellement par l'application des couples de stimulations.

cours d'expériences d'association du son et de la stimulation du nerf chez le chat.

Les électrodes sont placées au niveau des voies afférentes correspondant au stimulus inconditionnel, c'est-à-dire sur l'aire corticale primaire somatique (SI) et dans la région du relais thalamique primaire (VPL). Les stimulations sont distribuées différemment dans des expériences de conditionnement où elles sont régulièrement couplées et dans les expériences d'acquisition libre où elles sont appliquées séparément et dans le désordre.

Au cours des expériences de conditionnement les modifications des activités évoquées par le son apparaissent dans un premier temps (1ère–4ème séance) sur le cortex et dans un deuxième temps seulement (4ème–8ème séance), dans le thalamus où elles sont marquées par une réduction importante de la latence de la réponse initiale. Au cours des expériences d'acquisition libre, les réponses corticales provoquées par le son sont très semblables aux activités évoquées conditionnées. Par contre, les modifications thalamiques font défaut en dépit de la répétition des séances d'association. Enfin, les expériences d'extinction par répétition du son seul permettent de distinguer les réponses obtenues par l'acquisition libre, qui sont labiles, des réponses conditionnées qui restent stables.

La précocité d'apparition des réponses corticales confirme ici les théories classiques suivant lesquelles le conditionnement affecte d'abord le cortex. Mais ultérieurement les modifications thalamiques traduisent probablement la mise en jeu d'un circuit court sous-cortical qui semble intervenir dans la stabilisation du conditionnement.

Contrairement aux données généralement admises, il est possible que le facteur chronologique liant les stimulations du conditionnement classique et aboutissant à une acquisition stable traduise une forme particulière d'association apparentée au conditionnement au temps et caractérisée chez le chat par la coexistence de réponses sur le cortex et dans le sous-cortex. Au contraire l'indépendance temporelle des stimulations de l'acquisition libre, bien qu'aboutissant à la formation d'une association tout aussi spécifique est marquée par la prédominance des activités évoquées sur le cortex.

SUMMARY

CHANGES IN CORTICAL AND THALAMIC EVOKED ACTIVITY DURING SENSORY CONDITIONING. II. EVOLUTION OF THE RESPONSES WITH THE STAGES OF CONDITIONING

In a continuation of the preceding study, electrodes were situated in the afferent pathways of the unconditioned stimulus, *i.e.*, on the primary somatic cortex (area S_1) and in the primary thalamic relay (VPL). Stimuli were applied in two different ways: for conditioning they were coupled strictly; for free acquisition they were applied separately and at random.

During conditioning experiments the modifications of activities evoked by an acoustic stimulus appeared earlier in the cortex (1st–4th session) than in the thalamus (4th–8th session), where they were characterized by significant reduction of the initial latency. During free acquisition experiments the cortical responses to acoustic stimulation were similar to conditioned evoked activities. In contrast, thalamic responses were not modified despite repeated associations. Extinction experiments using acoustic stimulation alone gave a further distinction between responses obtained during free acquisition, which were labile, and the conditioned responses, which remained stable.

The early appearance of cortical responses confirms the classical theories; but at a later stage, the thalamic changes probably reflect the activation of a subcortical short-circuit concerned with the consolidation of conditioning. Contrary to generally accepted notions, it seems in these experiments that temporal linking of stimuli leads to a particular case of time-dependent conditioning whereas the temporal independence of stimuli corresponds more closely to the conditions of a more general acquisition.

BIBLIOGRAPHIE

ALBE-FESSARD, D. and FESSARD, A. Thalamic integration and their consequences at the telencephalic level. In G. MORUZZI *et al.* (Eds.), *Progress in brain research. Vol. 1, Brain mechanisms*. Elsevier, Amsterdam, **1963:** 115–148.

ASCHER, P. *La réaction de sursaut du chat anesthésié au chloralose.* Thèse Sci. Nat., Paris, **1965,** 126 p.

AUER, J. Terminal degeneration in the diencephalon after ablation of frontal cortex in the cat. *J. Anat. (Lond.)*, **1956**, *90*: 30–41.

BUSER, P. et ASCHER, P. Mise en jeu réflexe du système pyramidal chez le chat. *Arch. ital. Biol.*, **1960**, *98*: 123–164.

BUSER, P., JOUVET, M. et HERNÁNDEZ-PEÓN, R. Modifications au cours du conditionnement chez le chat du cycle d'excitabilité au niveau de la réticulée mésencéphalique. *Acta neurol. lat.-amer.*, **1958**, *4*: 268–278.

DEMPSEY, E. W. and MORISON, R. S. The production of rhythmically recurrent cortical potentials after localized thalamic stimulation. *Amer. J. Physiol.*, **1942**, *135*: 293–300.

DUSSER DE BARENNE, J. G. and MCCULLOCH, W. S. Suppression of motor response obtained from area 4 by stimulation of area 4s. *J. Neurophysiol.*, **1941**, *4*: 311–323.

FESSARD, A. et GASTAUT, H. Correlations neurophysiologiques de la formation des réflexes conditionnels. In *Le conditionnement et l'apprentissage*. Presses Universitaires de France, Paris, **1958**: 15–106.

GASTAUT, H., JUS, A. et C., MORRELL, F., STORM VAN LEEUWEN, W., DONGIER, S., NAQUET, R., REGIS, H., ROGER, A., BEKKERING, D., KAMP, A. et WERRE, J. Étude topographique des réactions EEG conditionnées chez l'homme. *Electroenceph. clin. Neurophysiol.*, **1957**, *9*: 1–34.

GRASTYÁN, E., LISSÁK, K., MADARÁSZ, I. and DONHOFFER, H. Hippocampal electrical activity during the development of conditioned reflexes. *Electroenceph. clin. Neurophysiol.*, **1959**, *11*: 409–430.

HUGELIN, A. et BONVALLET, M. Tonus cortical et contrôle de la facilitation motrice d'origine réticulaire. *J. Physiol. (Paris)*, **1957**a, *49*: 1171–1200.

HUGELIN, A. et BONVALLET, M. Étude expérimentale des interrelations réticulocorticales. *J. Physiol. (Paris)*, **1957**b, *49*: 1201–1223.

KITAI, S. T., COHEN, B. and MORIN, F. Changes in amplitude of photically evoked potentials by a conditioned stimulus. *Electroenceph. clin. Neurophysiol.*, **1965**, *19*: 344–349.

LELORD, G. Étude EEG chez l'animal et chez l'homme d'un mode d'association spécifique, distinct du conditionnement classique, l'acquisition libre. *Acta Biol. exp. (Warszawa)*, **1966**, *20*: 379–405.

LELORD, G. *L'acquisition libre: Aspects neurophysiologiques chez l'animal et chez l'homme*. Thèse Sci. Nat., Paris, **1967**, 199 p.

LELORD, G. et MAHO, C. Modifications des activités évoquées corticales et thalamiques au cours d'un conditionnement sensoriel. I. Localisation des réponses et variations avec la vigilance. *Electroenceph. clin. Neurophysiol.*, **1969**, *27*: 258–269.

LELORD, G., MAHO, C. et REYMOND, M. C. Comparaison de l'évolution au cours du conditionnement de réponses obtenues dans diverses aires corticales et structures sous-corticales. *J. Physiol. (Paris)*, **1965**, *57*: 647.

MAHO, C. Variations des activités évoquées de diverses structures centrales au cours du conditionnement. Dipl. Ét. Sup. Sci. Nat., Paris, **1968**, 63 p.

MASSION, J., ANGAUT, P. et ALBE-FESSARD, D. Activités évoquées chez le chat dans la région du nucleus ventralis lateralis par diverses stimulations sensorielles. II. Étude microphysiologique. *Electroenceph. clin. Neurophysiol.*, **1965**, *19*: 452–469.

MORRELL, F. Micro-electrode and steady potential studies suggesting a dendritic locus of closure. *Electroenceph. clin. Neurophysiol.*, **1960**, *Suppl. 13*: 65–80.

MORRELL, F. and JASPER, H. Electroencephalographic studies of the formation of temporary connections in the brain. *Electroenceph. clin. Neurophysiol.*, **1956**, *8*: 201–215.

NIEMER, W. T. and JIMENEZ-CASTELLANOS, J. Corticothalamic connections in the cat as revealed by "physiological neuronography". *J. comp. Neurol.*, **1950**, *93*: 101–123.

PAVLOV, I. P. *Leçons sur l'activité du cortex cérébral.* Legrand, Paris, **1929**, 418 p.

PIERON, H. La persistance à l'obscurité du rythme lumineux du lampyre. *Feuille nat.*, **1925**, *21*: 186–188.

POPOV, N. A. Études électroencéphalographiques du problème des réflexes conditionnés. *Ann. psychol.*, **1950**, *49*: 222–250.

STRATFORD, J. Cortico-thalamic connections from gyrus proreus and first and second somatic areas in the cat. *J. comp. Neurol.*, **1954**, *100*: 1–14.

YOSHII, N. and HOCKADAY, W. J. Conditioning of frequency characteristic repetitive EEG response with intermittent photic stimulation. *Electroenceph. clin. Neurophysiol.*, **1958**, *10*: 487–502.

Référence: LELORD, G. et MAHO C. Modifications des activités évoquées corticales et thalamiques au cours d'un conditionnement sensoriel. II. Évolution des réponses avec les stades du conditionnement. *Electroenceph. clin. Neurophysiol.*, **1969**, *27*: 270–279.

Electroencephalography and Clinical Neurophysiology
Elsevier Publishing Company, Amsterdam – Printed in The Netherlands

LONG-TERM EEG CHANGES DURING DIRECT CORTICAL STIMULATION[1]

M. J. O'CONNOR[2], M. ROSENTHAL[3] AND F. F. JÖBSIS

Department of Physiology and Pharmacology, Duke University, Durham, N. C. 27706 (U.S.A.)

(Accepted for publication: December 5, 1968)

INTRODUCTION

Electrophysiological literature has reported many examples of changes in brain potentials associated with conditioning or learning (John 1961; Morrell 1961). These can be broken down into three main classes: (1) classically conditioned changes in the spontaneous brain wave activity (Adrian and Matthews 1934; Jasper and Shagass 1941): (2) changes in responses evoked by peripheral stimulation (Jouvet and Hernández-Peón 1957; Hearst *et al.* 1960): and (3) changes in the response of the brain to direct cortical stimulation (Doty *et al.* 1956). In addition, single cells have demonstrated conditioned activity in response to intracerebral electrical stimulation (Hori *et al.* 1967). In all the experiments that led to the above results, it was stated, assumed or implied that the observed effects were in some manner related to the neurophysiological processes involved in learning.

Recently, Ursin *et al.* (1967) reported that initial presentations of electrical stimulation to the posterior suprasylvian gyrus resulted in low voltage fast EEG activity. Repeated stimulation, however, gradually failed to elicit arousal; *i.e.*, a habituation mechanism came into play. Ursin *et al.* postulated that the cortex is able to treat direct electrical stimulation in the same manner as it treats adequate sensory information.

It seemed possible to us that direct cortical stimulation might elicit changes in the EEG frequency pattern that could be described in terms analogous to those of learning and memory. Although the response to direct cortical stimulation has been extensively studied (see *e.g.*, Adrian 1936; Chang 1951), most studies were concerned with the analysis of the nerve nets involved in its genesis and propagation. In the first experiments reported in this article we answer whether during long lasting continued electrical stimulation of the cerebral cortex in the *cerveau isolé* preparation the frequency distribution of the EEG shows phases similar to those characterizing attention and habituation as seen during the presentation of sensory stimuli. From the later experiments, we describe long lasting effects of stimulation that persist after a rest period of several hours. These later investigations will be referred to as the "memory" experiments. A preliminary report has been published (O'Connor *et al.* 1968).

METHODS

Experiments were carried out on cats weighing between 1.4 and 2.8 kg. All surgery was done under general anesthesia, usually ether followed by i.v. pentothal after cannulation of the trachea and a femoral vein. Occasionally pentobarbital was used alone. The cerebral cortex was exposed bilaterally and an intercollicular brain-stem transection was performed. Anesthesia was then suspended and the cat was allowed to rest for different periods of time (1–27 h). Body temper-

[1] Supported in part by Grant DA-AMC-18 035 085 (A) of the Medical Directorate, Edgewood Arsenal, U. S. Army Chemical Corps and by Grant 5R01 NB06729 of the National Institutes of Health.

[2] Supported in part by the Medical Student Research Training Program of the University of Pennsylvania.

[3] Supported in part by Training Grant 2T01-GM-00929-06 of the National Institutes of Health. This work is part of a dissertation to be submitted to Duke University in partial fulfillment of the requirements for the degree of Doctor of Philosophy.

ature was monitored with a rectal thermocouple and was maintained constant with a heating pad. The cortex was kept moist by irrigation with saline. Experiments were usually concluded within 36 h but occasionally they ran for 4–5 days.

The head of the animal and the electrodes were mounted in a stereotactic apparatus. Two silver-ball recording electrodes of 1 mm diameter with an inter-electrode distance of 2–3 mm were placed on the cortex parallel to a pair of stimulating electrodes which were two tungsten wires of 0.2 mm diameter placed 1–2 mm apart. The stimulus was applied 1 mm below the surface of the cerebral cortex.

In all experiments, the EEG was amplified and recorded by an Offner Type R 8-channel Dynograph. After amplification, the EEG was fed into a filter system and, in many cases, into an Ampex type SP300 4-channel tape recorder. Filter outputs (at 8, 14, 19, 22, 26, 30 and 35 c/sec) were recorded on other channels of the Dynograph.

Each filter channel consisted of two filter sections in series, slightly detuned to achieve a relatively flat, narrow bandpass filter. Each filter section was an operational amplifier with a "parallel-T" null circuit in the feedback loop. Direct current recording of filter output was achieved by peak detection. The recording time constant was essentially that of the filter; *i.e.*, about 1 sec. (Typically in the 22 c/sec filter, for example, the response was down 50% at 21 and 23 c/sec at an input frequency of 22.)

After preliminary explorations, forty-five cats were stimulated mostly at 22 c/sec with 0.5 msec rectangular pulses which were applied for 1 sec out of every 4 sec. The presentation was in "units" of 10 min duration interspersed with 5 min rest periods. Stimulus intensity was at the threshold value (see below) in these initial experiments but was increased to 1.5 times threshold for the second group of experiments. In these later or "memory" experiments, it was decided that the occurrence of a memory mechanism would be indicated if the phases of the tri-phasic pattern which appeared during direct cortical stimulation (*cf.* Results) occurred statistically earlier in subsequent stimulation sessions than in the initial session.

An additional thirty-four cats were used in the "memory" experiments. Two schedules of experimentation were performed. In one group, stimulation was commenced 20 h after the intercollicular brain-stem transection. This initial stimulation session, will be referred to as the "morning session". After the 12th unit of stimulation, no further stimuli were presented for 4 h. Stimulation for 12 units was then presented anew. This session (occurring approximately 27 h after the transection) will be referred to as the "afternoon session". In order to determine whether the delay from the beginning of the afternoon session had any effect on the experiments, a second group of cats was transected at the same time as the first group, but was stimulated in the afternoon without any previous morning session.

In order to systematize the evaluation of records for the "memory" experiments, a set of criteria and contradictions was adopted to determine the time of transition from one phase to another. It was decided that one contradiction would nullify any number of changes that would otherwise be considered valid criteria for the occurrence of a phase change. Changes in the 35 c/sec channel, however, were not taken into account since the responses at this frequency tended to vary randomly. The phases with their criteria and contradictions can be outlined as follows:

Phase I. This is considered to be initiated when the stimulus intensity (progressively increasing) reaches a threshold level. The threshold is defined as that stimulus strength which elicits a response at the frequency of stimulation ("isofrequent response") and at one other frequency. In this phase, one or more non-isofrequent responses sometimes showed some variations in the amount of activity. But the isofrequent response was normally more or less constant or showed a slight decrease with time.

Phase II. This is characterized by a growing enhancement of the isofrequent response in comparison with the non-isofrequent responses. Ideally and most often, the isofrequent response increases and the activity at the other frequencies decreases.

The following criteria were considered acceptable for the transition from phase I to phase II: (1) the isofrequent response stays constant while the responses of at least two nearby frequencies (± 8 c/sec) decrease; (2) the isofrequent response increases considerably while the responses at the other frequencies remain constant.

Contradictions are: (1) any decrease in the isofrequent response, even if much smaller than simultaneous decreases in the non-isofrequent responses; (2) any increase in the response at another frequency, whether the isofrequent response increases or remains constant.

Phase III. This is characterized by a reversal of the changes used for identifying phase II. Ideally and most often, the isofrequent response decreases while the responses at the other frequencies increase.

The following criteria were considered acceptable for the transition from phase II to phase III: (1) the isofrequent response stays constant while the responses of at least two nearby frequencies (± 8 c/sec) increase; (2) the isofrequent response decreases while the responses at other frequencies remain constant.

Contradictions are: (1) any increase in the isofrequent response; (2) any decrease in the response at another frequency when the isofrequent response either decreases or remains constant.

RESULTS

When pairs of stimulating and recording electrodes were placed on the suprasylvian gyrus about 5 mm apart, each supra-threshold train of stimuli would result in a response at the recording electrodes. In Fig. 1, we present the responses of the filter channels as they record the increased activity at 7 frequency bands resulting from a 1 sec train of stimulation. These responses were usually not synchronous with the onset and termination of the 1 sec trains. Some would show a definite delay after the beginning of the stimulation before their output was increased. Others would exhibit continued high activity after stimulation ceased. Generally, the responses to individual trains of stimuli were variable between successive trains. However, on a minute to minute basis, trends could be distinguished as variations of the average response height. This feature was emphasized when the record was compressed by recording at a slow paper speed (*cf.* Fig. 2). These trends could also be brought out by integration of the area under the response curves (*cf.* Fig. 3). With this approach we have investigated the long-term changes in the response patterns over several 10 min "units" of stimulation.

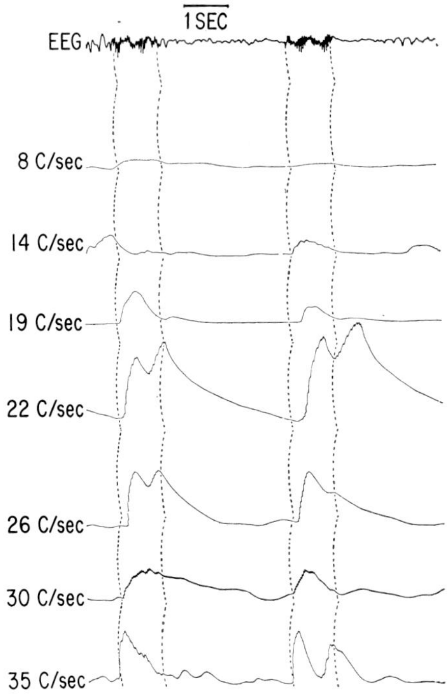

Fig. 1
Changes in activity at a number of frequencies evoked by two 1 sec trains (between dotted lines) of 1.5 times threshold stimulation at 22 c/sec. The figure shows the variability in time course of the responses at different frequencies as well as the variability of responses at a given frequency to successive stimulus trains. Vertical displacement of the traces is directly related to the voltage reached by the active filter and reflects the amount of EEG activity at each of the frequencies. Gains were set to show a significant response at each frequency, however, the gain settings at 8 and 14 c/sec were dictated more by the large but infrequent spontaneous activity at those frequencies than by the response to stimulation.

A tri-phasic pattern to long-term stimulation

In thirteen of the forty-five cats a pattern could be recognized in the distribution of the frequencies when stimulation was close to threshold levels and at a frequency between 19 and 30 c/sec. This response pattern showed three distinct phases which can be presented as follows.

Upon the first presentation of the stimulus at threshold intensity, for example at 22 c/sec, the frequencies present in the response showed a non-specific distribution; *i.e.*, response occurred at all frequencies with the exception of the very low range (less than 10 c/sec). This type of response (phase I) persisted usually for two to four 10 min units of stimulation. As stimulation continued, a new state emerged (phase II) in which the responses became more and more confined to the frequency band most closely matching that of the stimulus frequency. In most records, a definite increase of this "isofrequent" response would be accompanied by a sharp decrease in the output at other frequencies, this decrease being largest at the frequencies close to the isofrequent one (± 8 c/sec). The average value of the isofrequent response during this stimulation period (phase II) was 1.5–2 times greater than the response at that frequency in early phase I and the phase itself lasted usually for 1–5 units. This phase was followed by a third phase in which the disparity between the isofrequent response and the non-isofrequent responses was lost in one of three ways: by a decrease in the isofrequent response: by an increase in one or more of the non-isofrequent responses or, most commonly, by a combination of both.

The tri-phasic response pattern was never observed under the following conditions: (1) when the operation had been performed under pentobarbital anesthesia; (2) when the EEG showed marked spindling activity; (3) when an electrical after-discharge developed; (4) when the brain was extensively swollen; (5) when there were precipitous, temporary depressions of EEG activity or when the latter was permanently depressed; (6) when the intensity of stimulation was inadequate, as a result of a rise in the threshold during the course of the experiment (this was signalled by a gradual decrease of responses at all frequencies without a decrease in the total EEG); (7) when the stimulating and recording electrodes were separated by distances much greater than 5 mm or were separated by a sulcus; (8) when the delay between stimulus trains was greater than 5 sec.

Experiments with twenty-five of the cats exhibited one or more of the above characteristics. Of the remaining twenty cats, thirteen (or 65%) exhibited the tri-phasic pattern.

Stimulation at 1.5 times threshold brought about a much better display of the tri-phasic pattern. The upper strip of Fig. 2 which contains the first 4 stimulation units, shows the transition from phase I to phase II, which was judged to occur in the fourth unit. Activity at 19 and 26 c/sec, *i.e.*, close to the isofrequent response (22 c/sec), increases markedly before it dwindles at the start of the second phase. Note that the responses at 14 and 30 c/sec go through a similar cycle which, in this case, is confined to the first unit. This type of reaction occurred in the majority of the cats showing a three-phase response pattern to 1.5 times threshold stimulus intensity.

In units 5 and 6 (deleted from Fig. 1), the relative intensity of the responses at 19 and 26 c/sec continued to fall whereas the isofrequent response rose markedly. The resulting frequency distribution is depicted in the lower part of the record in Fig. 2 which shows the sequence of units 7, 8 and 9. Transition from phase II to phase III was judged to occur within unit 8 since the isofrequent activity decreases while the activity at the other frequencies remains more or less constant and, since in unit 9, the activity at the frequencies adjacent to the isofrequent ones rises markedly. This trend continues in units 10 and 11 (not shown) within which the responses at 19 and 26 c/sec were greatly increased and at 14 and 30 c/sec were slightly increased. Unit 12 (bottom right in Fig. 2) shows the increased final state of 19 and 26 c/sec and the relatively low response in the isofrequent channel.

In Fig. 3 the results of the same experiment are analyzed by integration of the response at each frequency. These results are presented on a per cent scale with 100% being the mean value of the response throughout the 12 stimulation periods. This method of data analysis shows quite well the transitions between phases but is deficient in showing changes which occur within one unit (such as those which occur at 14 and 30 c/sec in unit I). This figure also shows the events which occur during phase III and in the

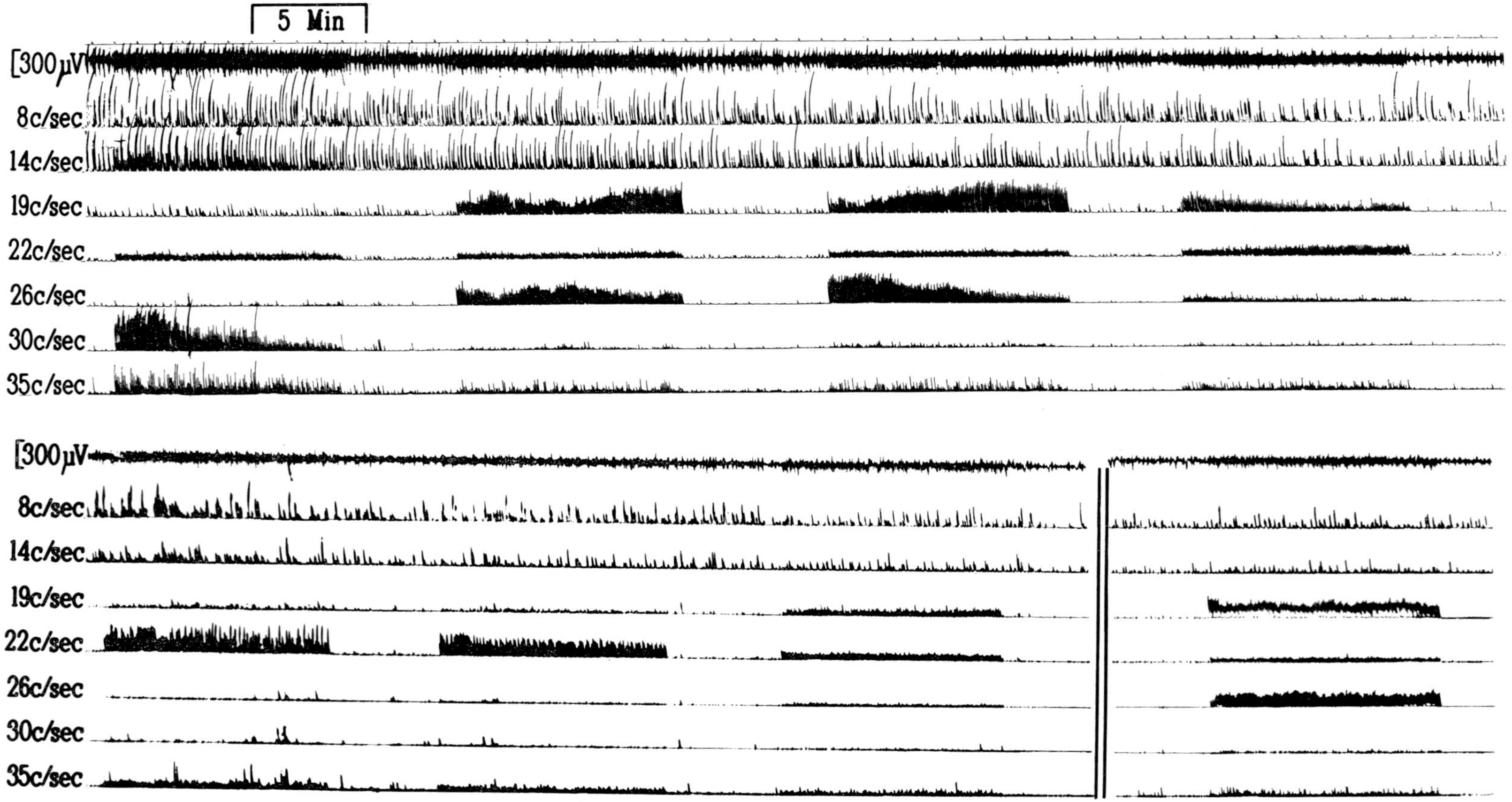

Fig. 2

A long-term record of responses to stimulation showing a triphasic response pattern to 22 c/sec stimulation. The activity at 8, 14, 19, 22, 26, 30 and 35 c/sec (as indicated on the left) is shown together with the total EEG (top channel). Stimulation units 1 through 4 are shown in the top strip. The transition from phase I to phase II was judged to occur in unit 4. In units 5 and 6 (not shown) the activity at 22 c/sec increased further whereas that at 19 and 26 c/sec decreased further. This pattern is continued in unit 7 (beginning of lower strip) until the transition from phase II to phase III occurs towards the end of that unit. In units 8 and 9, the isofrequent activity drops, while the 19 and 22 c/sec channels register gains. This trend continues in units 10 and 11 (not shown) until in unit 12 the isofrequent response is much less prominent than the responses at 19 and 26 c/sec. The EEG was originally recorded on tape. The record shown here was read out with gain settings for the various channels so that maximum activity at each frequency could be accommodated without saturation of the amplifiers.

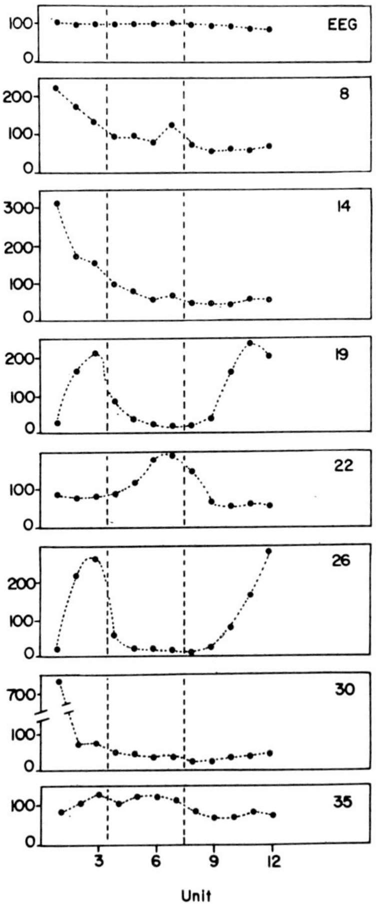

Fig. 3
An integrator analysis of the areas of the response curves of Fig. 2. The mean unit area compiled from the 12 units is the 100% value. The values of the individual unit areas were expressed as percentages of this mean value. Responses at 8, 14, 19, 22, 26, 30 and 35 c/sec were analyzed together with the untreated EEG record. Determination of the moments of phase transitions were made from the original record and are noted by the vertical dashed lines.

8, 14 and 30 c/sec responses. By this treatment it becomes clear that the responses at these three frequencies also tend to rise slightly in the last few units. The integrator analysis confirms that the response at 35 c/sec does not fit the same pattern of those at 14 and 30 c/sec. This has been a recurrent feature in the great majority of our experiments. A limited number of trials has also shown an inability to call forth indications of tri-phasic changes at frequencies higher than 35 c/sec.

In one way, the experiment shown in Fig. 2 is not typical for all preparations in that the depression of the response at 30 c/sec (during the first unit) was generally a much less prominent effect at this frequency.

"Memory" experiments

Of the thirty-four cats used in this study, ten were eliminated from the final tally because they possessed one or more of the 8 characteristics which were found to be incompatible with the occurrence of a three-phase response. An exception was made for the occurrence of spindling in the EEG which apparently was not

TABLE I

Times of phase transitions*

Session	a.m.		p.m.	
Hours after surgery	20		27	
Phase transition	I→II	II→III	I→II	II→III
Cat				
A-1	3.0	7.8	+	+
A-2	3.4	7.5	3.0	7.3
A-3	4.8	7.2	1.8	5.3
A-4	6.3	10.0	—	—
A-5	2.8	11.7	2.0	2.8
A-6	3.2	6.5	0.3	3.8
A-7	6.9	—	2.0	—
A-8	1.9	5.6	+	+
A-9	2.4	3.8	1.8	—
A-10	1.2	—	2.9	—
A-11	5.8	9.7	1.8	7.5
Mean	3.8	7.8	2.0	5.5
B-1			3.5	5.0
B-2			4.0	7.4
B-3			5.3	7.4
B-4			1.5	7.0
B-5			5.9	9.0
B-6			5.2	7.1
B-7			5.0	7.4
B-8			7.5	9.7
Mean			4.9	7.5

* The transition times are given in multiples and one-tenth fractions of the number of 10 min units of stimulation that had been presented when the EEG first exhibited the new frequency response pattern as defined in the text.
\+ = animal dead; — = negative result (*i.e.*, no phase change).

as strict an impediment to a tri-phasic response when stimulation of 1.5 times threshold was used. Of the remaining twenty-four cats, seventeen exhibited an unequivocal tri-phasic response pattern and two cats exhibited a transition from phase I to phase II but did not reach a transition from II to III.

Table I shows a quantitative analysis of the data of the "memory" experiments in terms of the time of occurrence of phase II and III of the two sessions. Group A cats were stimulated in both morning and afternoon sessions. Group B cats were stimulated only in the afternoon. The occurrence of the phase changes was determined independently by the three investigators[1], expressed as multiple and one-tenth fractions of stimulation units and then averaged for each animal.

It is seen that in five out of five Group A cats that exhibited a tri-phasic pattern in both the morning and afternoon session, there is in the second session a decrease in the number of units necessary to undergo the transitions to phases II and III of the tri-phasic response pattern. In only one cat (A 10) is there an increase in the time required for the occurrence of phase II. This cat, however, did not exhibit a phase III response in either stimulation session and is, therefore, atypical.

The fact that there was a decrease in the time required for the occurrence of phase II and phase III in subsequent stimulation sessions, pointed to a possible memory mechanism at work between the two stimulation sessions. However, a time effect on the preparation had not been ruled out. For this reason, the number of units required for the tri-phasic response patterns of the Group A cats in their first stimulation session was compared with those of the Group B cats in their first stimulation session, which occurred at the later time (the time of the second stimulation session of the Group A cats). The Student *t* test (Fisher 1958) was used. It was found that the transition from phase I to phase II was not significantly different between the two groups ($P > 0.2$) and the same was true for the moment of the phase II to III transition ($P > 0.5$). Thus, a difference of approximately 7 h in the post-operative recovery period did not seem to affect the results.

The Student *t* test was also used to determine whether there was a significant difference between the results of the afternoon sessions in the two groups (A, B) of cats. For the transition from phase I to phase II, the probability value was $P < 0.002$. For the II to III transition the difference was not as marked, but probably significant ($P < 0.06$). Since the additional time after the transition has been shown not to influence the results, it should be re-emphasized that all but one of those cats in the Group A that showed phase changes in both the morning and afternoon sessions, went through the tri-phasic pattern more rapidly the second time.

DISCUSSION

In this study, spectral analysis was applied to the EEG during and after intermittent, frequency-specific cortical stimulation. This type of analysis has a distinct advantage over previous methods of interpreting the changes associated with cortical stimulation (Adrian 1936; Ursin *et al.* 1967) in that these long-term changes can be studied more quantitatively.

We have found that the direct cortical stimulation presented in a frequency specific pattern for periods up to 3 h produced a tri-phasic response pattern in the frequency distribution of the EEG. Furthermore, repetition of the stimulation brings about a sizable increase in the speed of the phase transitions after a period of delay sufficient for consolidation.

Measurements of the more rapid electrical events by means of an oscilloscope indicated that, under our conditions, the voltage levels used in the present study are too low to elicit either the negative "spike" or the subsequent positive then negative "wave" of the short-term direct cortical response of Adrian (1936) and Chang (1951). We speculate that subtle changes in the spontaneous EEG are expressed as increased activity

[1] Failure of only one man to recognize the occurrence of a phase change was considered sufficient to invalidate the entire stimulation session. This occurred in only one instance. The average spread between the highest and lowest judgements among the three investigators was 0.24 units for all phase transitions. The largest spread was 0.8 units which occurred in three cases whereas in 11 instances there was no spread; *i.e.*, no disagreement among the investigators larger than ± 0.05 units.

at certain frequencies. When stimuli were used in the voltage range that evokes the "spike" response (*i.e.*, 2.5–5.0 V), the responses were much larger and the individual responses were much more constant; in addition no phase changes were found in the frequency spectrum. The still higher stimulus strengths required to evoke the "wave" (5–25 V) have not been studied since they tend to precipitate spreading depression or after-discharges when continued for extended periods of time. It appears, therefore, that the tri-phasic phenomenon described here is not directly related to either the spike or the wave response. A subthreshold change of excitability and activity is implied as the underlying basis of the frequency changes studied by us.

The long-term changes in frequency distribution often showed a remarkably symmetrical progress from frequencies most removed from the stimulation frequency to an isofrequent response. For example, an early waning at 14 and 30 c/sec would be followed by an increase at the frequencies more closely adjacent to the isofrequent one (19 and 26 c/sec), until they also decreased at the time that the isofrequent response grew; *i.e.*, at the beginning of phase II (*cf.* Fig. 2). Somewhat later, this close synchronization is apparently lost and the response becomes increasingly more generalized in phase III. Further analysis and experimentation, meant to clarify the cause of this pattern, are presently in progress.

The tri-phasic response pattern which we have elicited in the frequency distribution of the EEG exhibits some parallels to the three phases of reactions that occur when an inconsequential stimulus is repeatedly presented to a subject.

In a study on orienting behavior of cats with chronically implanted electrodes, Ursin *et al.* (1967) noted that low voltage fast activity, resulting from direct cortical stimulation, was associated with orienting behavior. Continued cortical stimulation brought about a decrease of the low voltage fast activity and of the orienting behavior indicating a habituation reaction. In our study, a general increase in high frequency response to the stimulation (phase I) was nearly always noted before frequency specific changes were initiated (phase II). This phase II isofrequent activity is followed by a return to a more generalized response with a decrease in the isofrequent activity usually accompanied by an increase in the activity at other frequencies (phase III). This third phase is considered analogous to the habituation phase observed by Ursin *et al.* (1967) although a demonstration of direct relationships with behavioral phenomena could not be attempted.

It is interesting to note that photic driving is readily obtained in the frequency range of 8–12 c/sec (Morrell and Jasper 1956). This has also been demonstrated at 16 c/sec by the use of a spectral analyzer (Trehub 1965). This is the frequency range in which the tri-phasic response pattern is difficult to elicit, whereas it is readily obtained above 20 c/sec. A possible reason for this may have been demonstrated by Scheibel and Scheibel (1965) who showed that only high frequency cortical stimulation results in reticular activation, even though single stimuli may do so via normal sensory paths. This could indicate that reticular activation may be necessary to elicit the changes noted in this study.

The results from the Group B cats which were stimulated in the afternoon after skipping the morning stimulation showed that any effects which might be due to a time-dependent deterioration of the preparation were statistically insignificant. Thus, the occurrence of a memory-like phenomenon appears responsible for the fact that the tri-phasic response pattern is elicited earlier in subsequent stimulation session than in the initial session.

SUMMARY

When repetitive electrical stimuli are directly applied to the cerebral cortex of the *cerveau isolé* preparation of cats, long-term changes can be observed in the relative predominance of certain frequencies in the EEG spectrum. This response to stimuli presented at a constant frequency for several hours exhibits three distinct phases. In the first phase there is an increase in activity at most examined frequencies. The second phase is characterized by an increase in the response at the frequency of stimulation which is usually accompanied by a decrease in the other frequencies. The third phase shows a reversal of the latter pattern; *i.e.*, a relative fall of the activity at the frequency of stimulation. The tri-phasic pattern is reminiscent of the three response phases of organisms to non-reinforced stimulation.

It was also found that the transitions between phases of the tri-phasic response would occur significantly earlier in cats that had been stimulated in a previous session than in cats that had not been previously stimulated. The results indicate that a lasting effect resembling memory of the first stimulation session continues to be present for at least 4 h afterwards.

RÉSUMÉ

MODIFICATIONS EEG À LONG TERME PENDANT LA STIMULATION CORTICALE DIRECTE

Si des stimuli électriques répétitifs sont appliqués directement au cortex cérébral de chats en préparation cerveau isolé, des modifications à long terme peuvent être observées dans la prédominance relative de certaines fréquences du spectre EEG. Cette réponse à des stimuli présentés à une fréquence constante pendant plusieurs heures évolue en 3 phases distinctes. Dans la première phase il y a une augmentation de l'activité dans la plupart des fréquences examinées. La seconde phase est caractérisée par une augmentation de la réponse à la fréquence de stimulation, accompagnée habituellement d'une diminution dans les autres fréquences. La 3ème phase montre une inversion du pattern précédent, c'est-à-dire une chute relative de l'activité à la fréquence de stimulation. Ce pattern tri-phasique rappelle les réponses en 3 phases des organismes à des stimulations non renforcées.

Les auteurs observent également que les transitions entre les phases de la réponse tri-phasique surviennent nettement plus tôt chez des chats qui ont été stimulés dans une session préalable que chez les chats qui n'ont pas été stimulés antérieurement. Ces résultats montrent qu'un effet durable, ressemblant au souvenir de la première session de stimulation, reste présent pendant au moins 4 heures.

REFERENCES

ADRIAN, E. D. The spread of activity in the central cortex. *J. Physiol. (Lond.)*, **1936,** *88*: 127–161.

ADRIAN, E. D. and MATTHEWS, B. H. C. The Berger rhythm: potential changes from the occipital lobe in man. *Brain*, **1934,** *57*: 355–385.

CHANG, H. T. Dendritic potential of cortical neurons produced by direct electrical stimulation of the cerebral cortex. *J. Neurophysiol.*, **1951,** *14*: 1–21.

DOTY, R. W., RUTLEDGE JR., L. T. and LARSEN, R. M. Conditioned reflexes established to electrical stimulation of the cat cerebral cortex. *J. Neurophysiol.*, **1956,** *19*: 401–415.

FISHER, R. A. *Statistical methods for research workers.* Hafner, New York, N.Y., **1958,** 356 p.

HEARST, E., BEER, B., SHEATZ, G. and GALAMBOS, R. Some electrophysiological correlates of conditioning in the monkey. *Electroenceph. clin. Neurophysiol.*, **1960,** *12*: 137–152.

HORI, Y., TOYOHARA, I. and YOSHII, N. Conditioning of unitary activity by intercerebral stimulation in cats. *Physiol. and Behavior*, **1967,** *2*: 255–259.

JASPER, H. H. and SHAGASS, C. Conditioning the occipital alpha rhythm in man. *J. exp. Psychol.*, **1941,** *28*: 373–388.

JOHN, E. R. Brain functions and learning. *Ann. Rev. Physiol.*, **1961,** *23*: 451–484.

JOUVET, M. et HERNÁNDEZ-PEÓN, R. Mécanismes neurophysiologiques concernant l'habituation, l'attention et le conditionnement. *Electroenceph. clin. Neurophysiol.*, **1957,** *Suppl. 6*: 39–49.

MORRELL, F. Electrophysiological contributions to the neural basis of learning. *Physiol. Rev.*, **1961,** *41*: 443–494.

MORRELL, F. and JASPER, H. H. Electrographic studies of the formation of temporary connections in the brain. *Electroenceph. clin. Neurophysiol.*, **1956,** *8*: 201–215.

O'CONNOR, M. J., ROSENTHAL, M. and JÖBSIS, F. F. A tri-phasic EEG response with parallels to learning. *Fed. Proc.*, **1968,** *27*: 388.

SCHEIBEL, M. E. and SCHEIBEL, A. B. The adaptive response of individual reticular units to repeated stimuli. *Recent Advanc. biol. Psychiat.*, **1965,** *7*: 85–96.

TREHUB, A. Spontaneous slow modulation of flicker-evoked response in human brain. *Electroenceph. clin. Neurophysiol.*, **1965,** *19*: 182–184.

URSIN, H., WESTER, K. and URSIN, R. Habituation to electrical stimulation of the brain in unanesthetized cats. *Electroenceph. clin. Neurophysiol.*, **1967,** *23*: 41–49.

Reference: O'CONNOR, M. J., ROSENTHAL, M. and JÖBSIS, F. F. Long-term EEG changes during direct cortical stimulation. *Electroenceph. clin. Neurophysiol.*, **1969,** *27*: 280–288.

Electroencephalography and Clinical Neurophysiology
Elsevier Publishing Company, Amsterdam – Printed in The Netherlands

FUNCTIONAL CHANGES OF SOMATO-SENSORY SYSTEM DURING DEEP SLEEP

CESARE CASATI, NICOLA DAGNINO, EMILIO FAVALE, MARIO MANFREDI, ANDREA SEITUN AND ANTONIO TARTAGLIONE

Clinica delle Malattie Nervose e Mentali dell'Università di Genova, Genoa, and Clinica delle Malattie Nervose e Mentali dell'Università di Sassari, Sassari (Italy)

(Accepted for publication: December 9, 1968)

In experiments directed to investigating the transmission by thalamic synapses during deep sleep and related spells of rapid eye movements (REMs) we observed that REMs coincided with an increase of transmission in the ventro-postero-lateral (VPL) nucleus of the thalamus (Dagnino *et al.* 1965a, 1967), as shown by constant enhancement of VPL responses on stimulation of the medial lemniscus (Dagnino *et al.* 1969).

This finding seemed to lose physiological significance in the light of observations of Carli *et al.* (1967); in fact these authors were able to demonstrate that responses in the medial lemniscus to peripheral inputs show a phasic decrease in amplitude during the bursts of REMs. They postulated therefore that REM spells of deep sleep are associated with "*some kind of physiological isolation of the brain*...*from somatic afferent volleys*" due to "*block of transmission* ...*through the dorsal column system*", thus discounting the importance of VPL transmission changes.

A further reason for caution was that increased thalamic output to direct stimulation of the medial lemniscus could be considered merely artefactual, as an unnaturally synchronized volley of impulses was made to impinge upon the nucleus; as a matter of fact, in a similar experimental situation in the optic system, lateral geniculate output during REMs increased on optic tract stimulation (Dagnino *et al.* 1965a) and decreased on retinal stimulation, no changes being attributable to the retina itself (Mouret *et al.* 1963; Bizzi 1966).

Another possibility, however, is that functional changes of opposite sign are taking place and mutually interacting at the different levels of the somatic path in coincidence with REMs; should this be the case, the effects of somatic afferent volleys impinging upon the cortex after being filtered in relay stations are hardly predictable unless they are compared with the final result, *i.e.*, responses of the cortical population.

When "total patency" of an afferent system is estimated, the modifications taking place in the intracortical neuronal nets themselves must be taken into consideration. In this connection it seems of interest that quite recently Allison and Goff (1968), after investigating, throughout the sleep-wakefulness cycle, somatic cortical responsiveness to stimulation of the somaesthetic radiation, came to the unexpected conclusion that no reliable estimate of cortical excitability can be obtained; in fact, according to these authors, small but significant changes in amplitude of the pre-synaptic component of the radiation-cortical response may occur, thus hindering the achievement of a constant cortical input.

In the present study experiments were directed to this double aim: (1) to assess the relative efficiency of the somatic path, from periphery to cortex, during REMs with respect to non-REM periods; (2) to re-examine the problem of changes of cortical excitability during REMs, Allison and Goff's remarks being taken into consideration.

It will be shown that the occurrence of REMs is associated, at least in the majority of cases, with a final increase of somatic afferent volleys, due to phasic enhancement of either VPL transmission or cortical responsiveness.

MATERIAL AND METHODS

Experiments have been carried out in twenty adult, unanaesthetized cats. In a previous surgical session, under general anaesthesia and in aseptic conditions, electrodes (two stainless steel wires insulated except for their tips, each 0.2 mm in diameter, stuck together with an inter-electrode distance of 0.5 mm) were stereotaxically implanted in the somaesthetic radiation, to be used either for stimulating or for recording. Bipolar recording was generally adopted, but results were similar in control experiments with reference recording against an indifferent lead placed in the bony septum between the frontal sinuses. Also, silver wires were sewn into the skin of the contralateral forepaw; metal screws were fixed into the floor of the frontal sinuses, ipsilateral to the radiation electrodes, to contact the dura covering the posterior sigmoid gyrus, in suitable position for recording responses upon forepaw stimulation. Similar screws were placed over the contralateral sigmoid gyrus and over the lateral gyri for EEG recording, and on the superior orbital wall for monitoring ocular movements. Needles were inserted into the posterior cervical muscles for EMG recording.

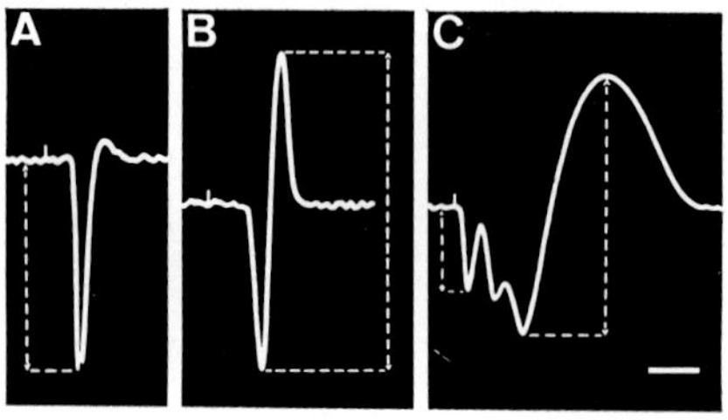

Fig. 1

A: periphero-radiation response; *B*: periphero-cortical response; *C*: radiation-cortical response. Arrows denote measured amplitudes. Time base: 10 msec for *A* and *B*, 2 msec for *C*.

The experimental sessions started 24 h after the operation: the animals were placed in a

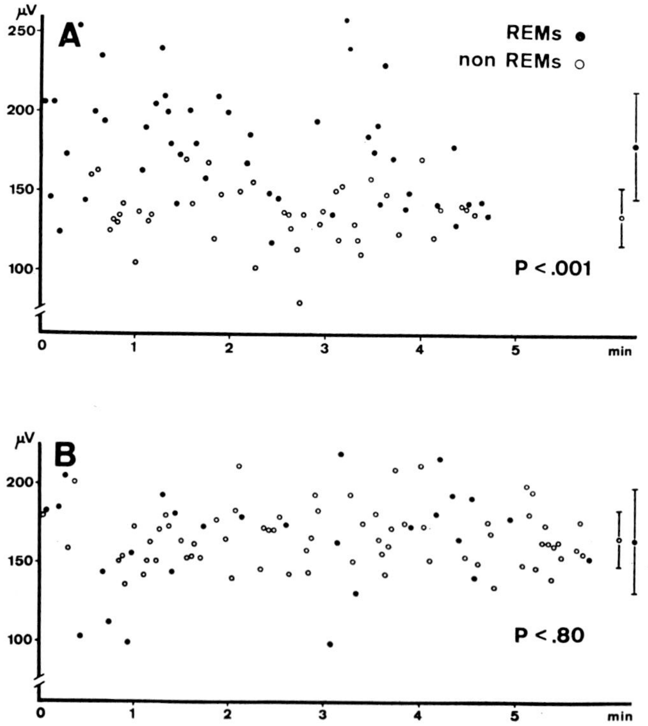

Fig. 2

Behaviour of periphero-cortical responses during two episodes of deep sleep in the same experimental session. During REMs the mean amplitude of responses significantly increases in *A*, remaining unchanged in *B*. In this and the following figure the bars at the right of diagrams indicate the standard deviations of the means.

quasi soundproof cage, where they were able to move freely, EEG, EMG and electro-oculographic activity being continuously monitored. During deep sleep episodes threshold stimuli (square waves of 0.05–0.1 msec, one every 2–3 sec) were delivered to the skin of the forepaw, responses being recorded from the contralateral posterior sigmoid gyrus and corresponding somaesthetic radiation, or to the somaesthetic radiation, the responses being recorded from the ipsilateral posterior sigmoid gyrus. Responses were then divided into two classes: those occurring during rapid eye movements (either single or bursts) and those occurring during ocular quiescence, and the difference between the mean amplitudes of the two classes were statistically evaluated with the Student *t* test. Since there is indirect evidence (*cf.* Sakakura and Iwama 1965) that phasic changes of thalamic transmission may outlast REMs, responses falling within 500 msec from REMs were discarded.

The amplitudes of responses were measured as shown in Fig. 1.

RESULTS

Both the shape and latency of responses evoked at the different levels of the somatic path by peripheral or central stimulation have been extensively described in previous contributions (Favale *et al.* 1965; Dagnino *et al.* 1969); therefore the present results will deal only with changes in amplitude of somatic cortical responses chronologically associated with REMs and their relationships with cortical responsiveness to somatic afferent volleys.

A. *Somatic cortical responses to peripheral (cutaneous) stimulation during REMs*

A significant increase in amplitude of the post-synaptic component (*i.e.*, the positive–negative deflection) of responses evoked in the somatic sensory cortex by cutaneous stimulation (*periphero-cortical*) was observed during REM as compared to non-REM periods in two-thirds of deep sleep episodes, while in the other cases the mean values remained statistically unchanged. Both these possibilities could occur in the same animal and, quite often, even in the same experimental session (Fig. 2). However, *individual* responses during prolonged bursts of REMs could be depressed in spite of a significant increase of the mean amplitude.

B. *Somatic cortical responses to somaesthetic radiation stimulation during REMs*

It has been assumed that changes in amplitude of cortical responses evoked by stimulation of the somaesthetic radiation (*radiation-cortical*) during the sleep-wakefulness cycle concern only the post-synaptic component, the pre-synaptic one being due to the activity of radiation fibres which are directly stimulated at constant pulse strength (Favale *et al.* 1965). Since this assumption has been recently contested by Allison and Goff (1968), the mean values of both pre- and post-synaptic components chronologically related to REMs were considered. In the large majority of deep sleep episodes (about 90%) no statistically significant variations of the pre-synaptic component were observed; the remaining ones showed a slight but significant increase during REMs.

The mean values of the post-synaptic component (*i.e.*, the positive-negative deflection) could be either increased or decreased, but usually (more than 50% of cases) they remained statistically unchanged. All these possibilities could occur in the same animal and sometimes even in the same experimental session (Fig. 3). This holds true even regarding those cases in which the pre-synaptic component increased in coincidence with REMs.

C. *Somatic cortical responsiveness to constant VPL output on peripheral stimulation during REMs*

In order to evaluate possible changes of cortical responsiveness to afferent impulses, a constant input to the cortex is required. This condition was achieved by direct stimulation of thalamo-cortical fibres. However, stimuli to the radiation produce a greater and more synchronized activation of intracortical neuronal nets than peripheral stimuli. In fact, it seems obvious that peripheral receptors bring about, at equal stimulus strengths, much more temporally dispersed volleys than directly activated thalamo-cortical fibres. For this reason it seemed correct to control the behaviour of cortical responsiveness after peripheral stimuli, the corresponding VPL output being concurrently monitored by simulta-

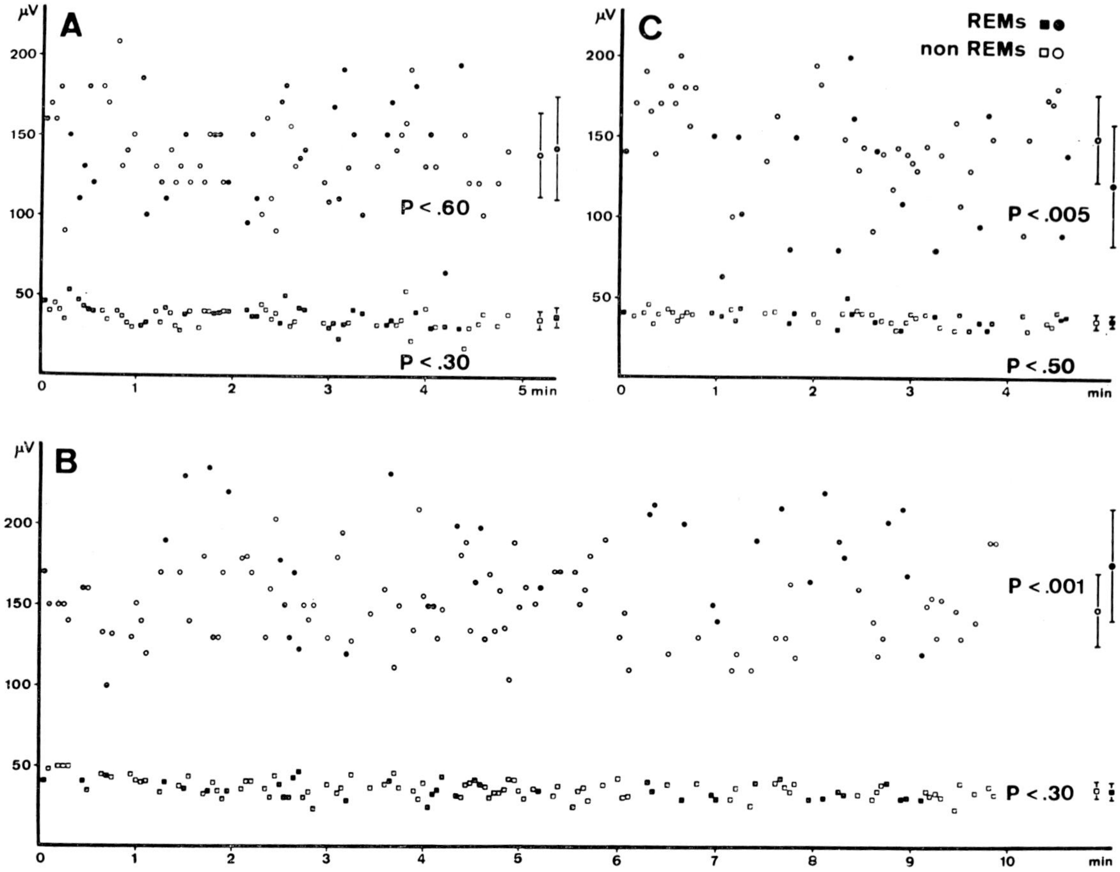

Fig. 3
Variations of cortical responsiveness as expressed by the behaviour of post-synaptic component of radiation-cortical responses during three episodes of deep sleep in the same experimental session. In *A* no significant change, in *B* increase, in *C* decrease in mean amplitude of post-synaptic component (circles) during REMs, the mean amplitude of the pre-synaptic component (squares) being unchanged throughout.

neous recording of the *periphero-radiation* response.

To ensure constant input to the cortex we selected only the cases in which the mean amplitude of periphero-radiation response remained statistically unchanged during REMs. Under these conditions it was observed that, during REMs, the mean amplitude of the post-synaptic component of cortical responses may be either increased or unvaried. Each of these patterns could occur in the same animal and, exceptionally, even in the same experimental session.

DISCUSSION

It has thus been demonstrated that the mean size of responses evoked in the somato-sensory cortex by cutaneous stimulation is significantly increased during REM spells as compared to non-REM periods, at least in the majority of cases. It seems therefore indisputable that, at variance with the assumption of Carli *et al.* (1967), there are no signs of isolation of the brain from somatic inputs during REM periods of deep sleep; on the contrary, somatic input during REMs sets up activity in larger fractions of the cortical cell population.

On the basis of the results herein reported, it seems reasonable to state that the final changes undergone by somatic afferent volleys during REMs represent the result of functional changes of variable sign occurring at the different levels of the lemniscal system; in particular, while the final changes of a somatic afferent volley are relatively constant, the single factors responsible for them are hardly predictable.

(1) Regarding the functional changes occurring at the level of the first station (dorsal column nuclei) the data of Carli *et al.* deserve further consideration. These authors concede that "*not every burst of REMs is associated with a depression of the orthodromic lemniscal response*". In our experience, in a similar experimental situation, the mean amplitude of the orthodromic lemniscal response to peripheral stimulation during REM as compared to non-REM periods remains statistically unchanged in more than 50% of deep sleep episodes (unpublished observations). This striking discrepancy might depend, at least in part, on the different criteria employed to select REM periods. In fact, while Carli *et al.* seem to pay particular attention to "*strong and prolonged bursts*" of REMs, we treated all ocular movements of deep sleep as members of the same class (Dagnino *et al.* 1965a).

It seems thus correct to assume that somatic afferent volleys impinging on VPL neurones are not necessarily reduced during REMs, even because the "patency" of pre-synaptic terminals of medial lemniscus remains usually unchanged under the same experimental conditions (Dagnino *et al.* 1969). Nevertheless a significant reduction of cuneate transfer can occur in a considerable number of cases, thus partially confirming the results of Carli *et al.* This might possibly account for the minority of cases in which the mean amplitude of cortical responses to peripheral stimulation does not show significant changes during REMs.

In any case, however, the modifications of peripheral input taking place in the dorsal column nuclei cannot explain, *per se*, the behaviour of summated responses in somato-sensory cortical areas and further integration of peripheral input must be admitted to take place before the cortex is reached (*i.e.*, at thalamic level), or even in the cortex itself.

(2) As to the second relay station (VPL nucleus) we have previously shown that monosynaptic activation of thalamic neurones is accompanied by a constant increase of VPL output during REMs (Dagnino *et al.* 1965a, 1967, 1969). On the other hand VPL output on cutaneous stimulation can be either increased or remain unchanged during REMs, while a decrease must be considered exceptional (unpublished observations). We feel that the variability of VPL output on cutaneous stimulation is largely due to the irregular changes in synaptic transfer occurring at the first station during REMs.

The modulation that peripheral input has undergone after relaying in the second station, however, cannot always account for the modifications of periphero-cortical responses. In fact, though in many cases an increased thalamic output is probably the main factor accounting for facilitation of cortical responses, the latter may be augmented in face of an unchanged thalamic output, or remain unvaried in spite of a concurrent enhancement of thalamic output. The occurrence of either an increase or a decrease of cortical responsiveness seems therefore required, at least in particular cases.

(3) In order to validate the latter assumption, the mean amplitude changes of cortical responses to a fixed input were investigated during REM and non-REM periods of deep sleep. Apparently, the most reliable method to investigate cortical responsiveness should be direct stimulation of the thalamo-cortical radiation, as intracortical neuronal nets are the only synaptic structure between stimulating and recording electrodes. However, this approach involves some pitfalls. First, it has been shown by Allison and Goff (1968) that the pre-synaptic spike of the radiation-cortical response, which gives an estimate of the input impinging upon the cortex, may increase during REM as compared to non-REM periods of deep sleep. Secondly, there is no proof that the behaviour of cortical responsiveness after direct stimulation of the radiation, *i.e.*, to a heavily synchronized afferent volley, should be really representative of the behaviour after peripheral stimulation, *i.e.*, to a desynchronized and presumably more discrete input.

As to the first problem, a phasic increase during REMs of the pre-synaptic component of the radiation-cortical response has also been observed occasionally in the present study. Factors responsible for this change include: (a) enhanced excitability of the thalamo-cortical fibres due to small changes in impedance of the tissue surrounding the stimulating electrode, affecting the number of afferent fibres stimulated (*cf.* Allison and Goff 1968). We feel, however, that such changes, attributed to variations of cerebral temperature or blood flow, are too sluggish to be limited within periods of time as short as bursts of REMs; (b) changes in the level of polarization of intracortical pre-synaptic endings; however, this possibility has not yet been demonstrated; (c) a concurrent increase of thalamo-cortical background discharge, with consequent enhancement of cortical input; in fact, Belugou (1967) has recently observed a phasic increase of "integrated" VPL activity during REMs; (d) antidromic activation of pyramidal tract cells, whose responsiveness appears to be phasically increased during REMs (Dagnino *et al.* 1965b); it should be pointed out, however, that the latency of the surface correlate of antidromic invasion of pyramidal cells (Humphrey 1968) is well beyond the range of the pre-synaptic component of radiation-cortical response; (e) lastly, and most probably, concurrent stimulation of somata of thalamo-cortical cells, which are admittedly more excitable in coincidence with REMs (Dagnino *et al.* 1969). In fact, VPL (or juxta-VPL) electrical stimulation evokes a cortical response whose pre-synaptic component is made of two spike potentials, respectively due to direct excitation of thalamic relay cells (alpha spike) and to direct excitation of pre-synaptic fibres in the thalamus and subsequent activation of thalamic neurones (beta spike) (Andersen *et al.* 1964). The latter component is often interfered with by the negative deflection of the first one; thus, the pre-synaptic component of thalamo-cortical response may appear as a single spike potential whose initial and peak latencies are very close to those of the pre-synaptic component of the radiation-cortical response, as shown in Fig. 4.

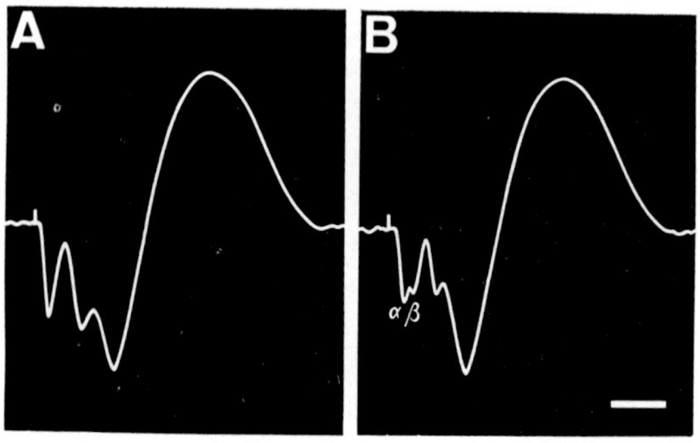

Fig. 4
To show the shape and latency similarities between cortical responses evoked by stimulation of the somaesthetic radiation (*A*) and VPL thalamic nucleus (*B*). The first positive deflection represents in (*A*) the pre-synaptic afferent volley; in (*B*) it is made up of two spike potentials, respectively due to direct (alpha) and synaptic (beta) activation of thalamic relay cells. Time base: 2 msec.

Whichever factor might play a role, to prevent variations of input to the cortex from biasing the results we limited evaluation of cortical responsiveness to those cases (about 90%) in which the pre-synaptic component remained unchanged during REM and non-REM periods of deep sleep. In this regard we observed that cortical excitability can be increased, decreased or remain unvaried during REMs, the latter possibility being the most frequent. In confirmation of this finding we could not establish any relationship between modifications of pre- and post-synaptic components of the radiation-cortical response even in those cases in which an enhancement of pre-synaptic spikes occurred during REMs.

Evaluation of cortical responsiveness after peripheral stimulation was achieved by comparing the mean amplitude changes of cortical responses during REM and non-REM periods in animals in which simultaneous recording of periphero-radiation potentials showed no significant changes of thalamic output during REMs. In fact we can safely assume that this condition ensures a fixed input from periphery to cortex. Even in this case results turned out to be quite variable, as well as those obtained upon direct stimulation of the radiation, thus confirming that the occurrence of REMs may be associated with different patterns of cortical responsiveness.

Summing up, the cortex intervenes in regulating the level of function of the somato-sensory system during REM periods of deep sleep; the cortical outcome of peripheral volleys will represent the interaction of processes of different sign, usually resulting in an increased effectiveness of somatic input during REMs. Quite surprisingly, though combination of modulatory effects gives a chance for such a change, we never observed a decrease of the *mean amplitude* of periphero-cortical responses in coincidence with REMs. *Individual* responses, however, could be reduced during prolonged bursts of eye movements; the latter observation suggests that the hypothesis of Carli *et al.* (1967) cannot be ruled out, at least in principle.

SUMMARY

1. The level of function of the somato-sensory pathway from periphery to cortex was investigated with the evoked potential technique during REM and non-REM periods of deep sleep.

2. The occurrence of REMs is usually associated with an increased effectiveness of afferent volleys, as a greater amount of the cortical cell population is activated during REM periods.

3. This change is due either to a phasic enhancement of transmission through the VPL nucleus of the thalamus or to increased cortical responsiveness.

4. However, cortical responsiveness to a fixed input does not show constant modifications during REM with respect to non-REM periods.

RÉSUMÉ

MODIFICATIONS FONCTIONNELLES DU SYSTÈME SOMATO-SENSITIF AU COURS DU SOMMEIL PROFOND

1. Le niveau fonctionnel de la voie somato-sensitive, de la périphérie au cortex, est exploré par la technique des potentiels évoqués au cours du sommeil profond avec et sans mouvements oculaires rapides.

2. La survenue des mouvements oculaires rapides s'accompagne généralement d'une efficience accrue des vollées afférentes, ce qui ressort du fait qu'une proportion plus grande de la population de cellules corticales est activée pendant les périodes de mouvements oculaires rapides.

3. Cette modification est due soit à une augmentation phasique de la transmission au travers du noyeau VPL du thalamus, soit à un accroissement de la réactivité corticale.

4. Toutefois la réactivité corticale à une efférence donnée ne montre pas de modifications constantes pendant les phases de mouvements oculaires rapides par comparaison aux périodes sans mouvements oculaires rapides.

REFERENCES

ALLISON, T. and GOFF, G. D. Potentials evoked in somatosensory cortex to thalamocortical radiation stimulation during waking, sleep and arousal from sleep. *Arch. ital. Biol.*, **1968,** *106*: 41–60.

ANDERSEN, P., BROOKS, MCC., ECCLES, J. C. and SEARS, T. A. The ventrobasal nucleus of the thalamus: potential fields, synaptic transmission and excitability of both presynaptic and postsynaptic components. *J. Physiol. (Lond.)*, **1964,** *174*: 348–369.

BELUGOU, J. L. *Étude de l'activité électrophysiologique des noyaux de relais somesthésiques pendant le sommeil.* Thèse de Médecine, Paris, **1967,** 72 p.

BIZZI, E. Changes in the orthodromic and antidromic response of optic tract during the eye movements of sleep. *J. Neurophysiol.*, **1966,** *24*: 861–870.

CARLI, G., DIETE-SPIFF, K. and POMPEIANO, O. Transmission of sensory information through the lemniscal pathway during sleep. *Arch. ital. Biol.*, **1967,** *105*: 31–51.

DAGNINO, N., FAVALE, E., LOEB, C. and MANFREDI, M. Thalamic transmission changes during the rapid eye movements of deep sleep. *Arch. int. Physiol.*, **1965**a, *73*: 858–861.

DAGNINO, N., FAVALE, E., LOEB, C., MANFREDI, M. and SEITUN, A. Nervous mechanisms underlying phasic changes in thalamic transmission during deep sleep. *Electroenceph. clin. Neurophysiol.*, **1967,** *Suppl. 26*: 156–163.

DAGNINO, N., FAVALE, E., LOEB, C., MANFREDI, M. and SEITUN, A. Presynaptic and postsynaptic changes in specific thalamic nuclei during deep sleep. *Arch. ital. Biol.*, **1969,** in press.

DAGNINO, N., FAVALE, E. and MANFREDI, M. Cortical activation of pyramidal tract during the sleep-wakefulness cycle. *Arch. int. Physiol.*, **1965**b, *73*: 854–857.

FAVALE, E., LOEB, C., MANFREDI, M. and SACCO, G. Somatic afferent transmission and cortical responsiveness during natural sleep and arousal in the cat. *Electroenceph. clin. Neurophysiol.*, **1965,** *18*: 354–368.

HUMPHREY, D. R. Re-analysis of the antidromic cortical response. I. Potentials evoked by stimulation of the isolated pyramidal tract. *Electroenceph. clin. Neurophysiol.*, **1968,** *24*: 116–129.

MOURET, J., JEANNEROD, M. et JOUVET, M. Activité électrique du système visuel au cours de la phase paradoxale du sommeil chez le chat. *J. Physiol. (Paris)*, **1963,** *55*: 305–306.

SAKAKURA, H. and IWAMA, K. Presynaptic inhibition and postsynaptic facilitation in lateral geniculate body and so-called deep sleep wave activity. *Tohoku J. exp. Med.*, **1965,** *87*: 40–51.

Reference: CASATI, C., DAGNINO, N., FAVALE, E., MANFREDI, M., SEITUN, A. and TARTAGLIONE, A. Functional changes of somato-sensory system during sleep deep. *Electroenceph. clin. Neurophysiol.*, **1969,** *27*: 289–295.

Electroencephalography and Clinical Neurophysiology
Elsevier Publishing Company, Amsterdam – Printed in The Netherlands

ACTION OF DRUGS ON THE ELECTRICAL ACTIVITY OF THE RED NUCLEUS

G. GOGOLÁK, G. LIEBESWAR AND CH. STUMPF

Department of Pharmacology, University of Vienna, Vienna (Austria)

(Accepted for publication: November 28, 1968)

Although a considerable literature exists on the electrophysiology of the red nucleus (*cf.* Massion 1967; Eccles *et al.* 1967), surprisingly little is known about its spontaneous or drug-induced electrical activity as recorded with gross electrodes. The spontaneous activity of the red nucleus in cats under β-erythroidine has been found to be characterized "by 20–30/sec waves, whose amplitude was capable of undergoing great variation" (Starzl *et al.* 1951). A pharmacological study by Schimmerl and Stumpf (1958) revealed that in the rabbit hypnotic barbiturates and meprobamate elicit an exceedingly regular activity in the red nucleus, whereas other central nervous system depressants are ineffective in this respect. Thus, the elicitation of a regular red nucleus rhythm seemed to be a highly specific effect of only a small group of drugs acting on the central nervous system. In the present study a detailed pharmacological analysis of the effect of drugs as well as interactions of drugs on the electrical activity of the red nucleus was carried out. The specificity of the effect of barbiturates and a few other drugs was confirmed, but the study on the interactions of drugs brought some unexpected results, showing that drugs may have antagonistic and synergistic actions simultaneously in different regions of the brain.

METHODS

Forty-five male rabbits weighing between 2.5 and 3 kg were used in this study. Records were taken from the precentral cortex and the red nucleus of one side, and in some experiments also from the dorsal hippocampus. In twelve experiments the electrode position in the red nucleus was verified histologically, but since it turned out that the red nucleus activity produced by barbiturates is restricted to the red nucleus and does not occur in the midbrain around the nucleus, we decided that for this reason histological verification was not necessary for the remaining experiments. The procedure adopted in most experiments was to give a test dose of a short-acting barbiturate (*e.g.*, 20 mg/kg hexobarbital i.v.) and then to insert the electrode in the appropriate stereotaxic coordinates until the barbiturate-induced activity could be recorded.

Two types of preparations were used: rabbits with chronically implanted electrodes and rabbits acutely anaesthetized with the drug under investigation and curarized (gallamine, 3 mg/kg/60 min). Careful local anaesthesia was used prior to any surgery. For acute and chronic experiments the stereotaxic coordinates of Sawyer *et al.* (1954) were used. Conventional bipolar recording of the electrical activity of the appropriate brain areas was carried out, using a Schwarzer electroencephalograph. The acute preparations were used only for exploratory experiments and studies in which the interaction of barbiturates and other drugs were investigated. The other studies were done in chronically prepared rabbits in which barbiturate anaesthesia was used as a localizing technique to implant the red nucleus electrodes. At least one week was allowed to elapse before these animals were used in drug studies. Each drug was tested in three to five animals and some animals were used more than once. If a drug was found not to induce a regular rhythm in the red nucleus, a short-acting barbiturate was given afterwards, and only when the barbiturate produced a regular rhythm was the negative result obtained with the other drug considered conclusive.

All drugs were dissolved in water or saline if not stated otherwise in the text, and were injected i.v. over a time interval of less than one minute.

RESULTS

1. *Spontaneous electrical activity of the red nucleus*

In the normal, alert rabbit the spontaneous electrical activity of the red nucleus consists in a high frequency small amplitude activity which is inconspicuous and hardly distinguishable from that seen in adjacent areas of the brain. For this reason the insertion of recording electrodes was always carried out under the action of barbiturates, as outlined in Methods.

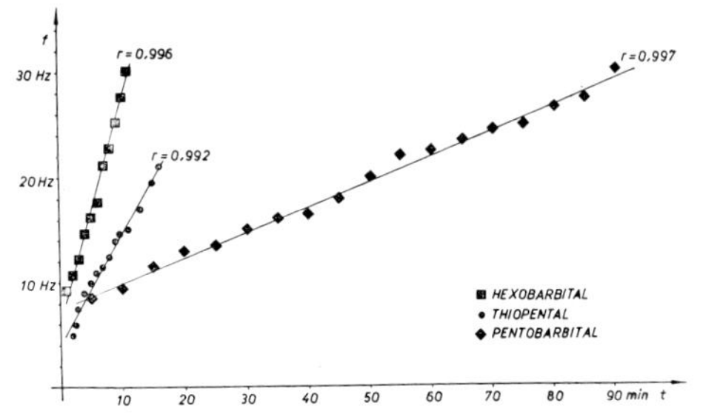

Fig. 2
Correlation between frequency of regular red nucleus activity (ordinate) and time after administration of various barbiturates (abscissa). Doses: 25 mg/kg hexobarbital, 20 mg/kg thiopental, 30 mg/kg pentobarbital.

2. *Action of barbiturates on red nucleus activity*

The following barbiturates were administered: hexobarbital (25–35 mg/kg), pentobarbital (30 mg/kg), phenobarbital (150 mg/kg) and thiopental (15–20 mg/kg). In accordance with the results obtained previously by Schimmerl and Stumpf (1958), it was found that these hypnotic barbiturates elicit in the red nucleus a very regular, quasi-sinusoidal rhythm with a frequency that is related to the depth of anaesthesia (Fig. 1).

Immediately after injection of hexobarbital, pentobarbital or thiopental in the dose ranges mentioned above, regular slow activity at 4–9 c/sec appears in the red nucleus recordings. Apparently a drug-induced red nucleus rhythm with a frequency of less than about 4 c/sec cannot be produced because, after administration of higher doses of barbiturates, regular activity disappears and the first rhythm that appears as the anaesthesia becomes lighter has a frequency of about 4 c/sec. On the other hand, as anaesthesia lightens, a point is reached where regular activity in the red nucleus can no longer be distinguished from the low voltage fast activity seen in the red nucleus which is not under the influence of drugs. The maximal frequency of regular activity which can be clearly distinguished is about 25–30 c/sec. For the short acting barbiturates a positive linear correlation with highly significant correlation coefficients (r = 0.992–0.997) exists, during emergence from anaesthesia, between time (after injection) and frequency of red nucleus rhythm. Fig. 2 shows the results of three experiments of this kind. It may be seen that hexobarbital had the shortest, pentobarbital the longest, and thiopental an intermediate duration of action. It may also be seen in Fig. 2 that each of the short acting barbiturates had a distinct slope of regression line and although this slope varied from animal to animal, in none of our studies did the regression line for one overlap that of another. The lowest frequencies were seen with the higher barbiturate doses.

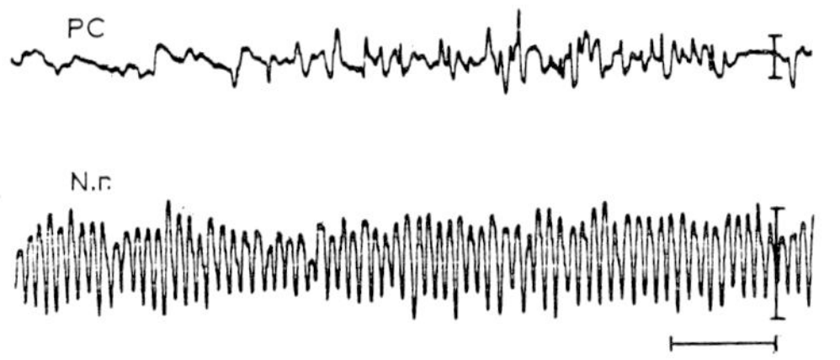

Fig. 1
Regular electrical activity in the red nucleus (N.r.) and slow, irregular spindles in the precentral cortex (PC) 10 min after the administration of 30 mg/kg pentobarbital. Calibrations: 100 μV; 1 sec.

As might be expected from the known slow entrance into and exit from the brain and body, a very different picture was seen with phenobarbital. Following 150 mg/kg phenobarbital, red nucleus frequencies reached their lowest values (12–14 c/sec) 3 h after the injection and increased very slowly afterwards, attaining about 18 c/sec 6 h after the injection. Thus, phenobarbital, unlike the short-acting barbiturates, produced a biphasic action on the red nucleus which was probably related to its slow onset of action.

The apparent depth of anaesthesia may also

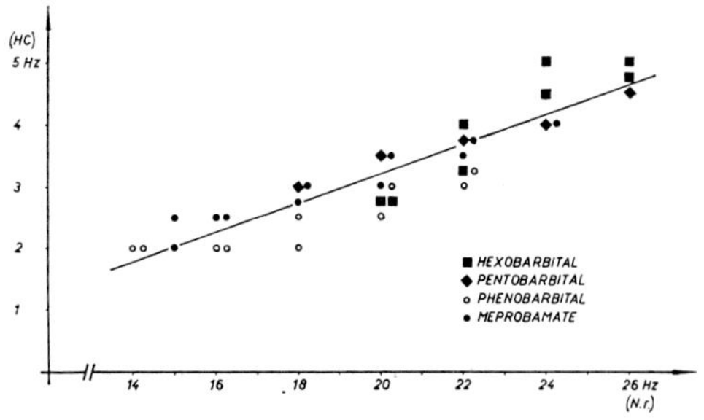

Fig. 3
Correlation between frequency of regular red nucleus activity (abscissa) and frequency of theta rhythm in the hippocampus (ordinate) at various depths of anaesthesia induced by hexobarbital, pentobarbital, phenobarbital and meprobamate.

be estimated from changes of the electrical activity of other brain areas. For comparison we used the activity of the doral hippocampus because it is known (Brücke *et al.* 1957) that the frequency of the theta rhythm elicited in this structure during an arousal reaction decreases with increasing depth of barbiturate anaesthesia. Theta rhythm was elicited by a standard passive movement of one hind leg of the rabbit. In deep anaesthesia such a stimulus is ineffective but, as anaesthesia lightens, a low frequency theta rhythm appears and its frequency increases during emergence from anaesthesia. In Fig. 3 the frequency of the regular red nucleus rhythm is plotted against the frequency of the (evoked) hippocampal theta rhythm during emergence from anaesthesia induced by hexobarbital, pentobarbital, phenobarbital and meprobamate. The meaning of the figure can be understood easily if one imagines that emergence from anaesthesia corresponds to a movement along the regression line from bottom left to top right. It will be seen that, irrespective of the drug used, the frequency of the red nucleus rhythm is related to the frequency of (evoked) hippocampal theta rhythm. Since the red nucleus and the hippocampus are two brain areas without known significant connections with each other, this finding may indicate that the anaesthetic effect of these drugs has to be considered as rather unspecific or that some other system in the brain may affect both red nucleus and hippocampus. Similar correlations seem to exist between the frequency of the red nucleus rhythm and changes of activity in the precentral cortex, but these are more difficult to evaluate quantitatively (see later).

Without any exceptions, whenever the barbiturate-induced red nucleus rhythm could be recorded with large amplitude and free from interference by other activity originating in the surrounding areas of the midbrain, histological examination showed afterwards that the tip of the electrode had been situated near the centre of the magnocellular part of the red nucleus. In experiments in which the electrode had been placed in appropriate stereotaxic coordinates for the red nucleus but in which appropriate red nucleus rhythms could not be recorded, histological examination showed that the electrode tip was in fact not in the red nucleus but in its neighbourhood.

3. *Action of other drugs on red nucleus activity*

Except for the hypnotic barbiturates we have

TABLE I

Doses indicated are ranges or maxima, given intravenously (except ether)

A. Drugs which induce a regular rhythm in the red nucleus:
Barbiturates (given as sodium salts):
  Hexobarbital (25–30 mg/kg)*
  Pentobarbital (30 mg/kg)*
  Phenobarbital (150 mg/kg)
  Thiopental (15–20 mg/kg)*
Propanidid (15 mg/kg)
Meprobamate (100–150 mg/kg)*,**
Benzodiazepine compounds:
  Chlordiazepoxide hydrochloride (50 mg/kg)
  Diazepam (8 mg/kg)**
  Oxazepam hemisuccinate (150 mg/kg)

B. Drugs which do not have such an action on red nucleus activity:
Morphine hydrochloride (30–120 mg/kg)*
Scopolamine hydrobromide (0.25–1 mg/kg)*
Chlorpromazine (10–20 mg/kg)*
Lidocaine hydrochloride (10–20 mg/kg) and
  Procaine hydrochloride (10 mg/kg)*
Mephenesin (150 mg/kg)
Ethyl ether (given as inhalation)
Urethane (1–2 g/kg)*
Ethyl alcohol (30%, 1 g/kg)
Nitrazepam (8 mg/kg)**

* The effects of these drugs on red nucleus activity have already been described by Schimmerl and Stumpf (1958).
** These drugs are dissolved in special organic solvents.

found few other drugs which produce the characteristic changes in red nucleus activity that we have described but we have found many drugs with hypnotic actions which do not have this effect. Table I lists the drugs whose effects on red nucleus activity have been studied.

It can be seen that, in addition to the barbiturates, propanidid and some "minor tranquillizers" (meprobamate and three benzodiazepine compounds) induce a regular rhythm in the red nucleus of the rabbit. The results with propanidid and meprobamate are quite clear. Propanidid induces a rhythm in the red nucleus which in form and frequency is indistinguishable from that which would be induced by a barbiturate and propanidid had a duration of action shorter than that of hexobarbital: at the peak of action, 1 min after injection of 15 mg/kg, there were isoelectric periods in the cortical recording and no regular rhythm was present in the red nucleus, but a few seconds later a 6 c/sec rhythm reappeared and its frequency, increasing linearly with time, reached 20–25 c/sec 4 min after the injection. On the other hand, meprobamate had a longer lasting effect. About 15 min after injection of 150 mg/kg, the frequency of the regular rhythm had decreased to 13–17 c/sec and did not change during the following 3 h. Associated with this red nucleus rhythm was slow wave activity and decreased spindling in the cortical recording, similar to that during the action of barbiturates at a level of anaesthesia characterized by a 13–17 c/sec rhythm in the red nucleus. The correlation with hippocampal activity was mentioned above (see Fig. 3). Unfortunately, the meprobamate dose could not be increased because of its low solubility (80 mg/ml) in relation to the required dose. And though meprobamate was administered in a complex commercial solvent, its effects given i.v. paralelled those produced by it when given orally in earlier experiments (Schimmerl and Stumpf 1958). The effects of chlordiazepoxide and the other benzodiazepine compounds are not as clear cut. When they are injected in the maximal doses that we tested, there appears in the red nucleus a regular rhythm that in form is identical to the barbiturate-induced rhythm (as can be seen for chlordiazepoxide in Fig. 4), but the frequency is never slower than 20–25 c/sec. This might be a quantitative difference

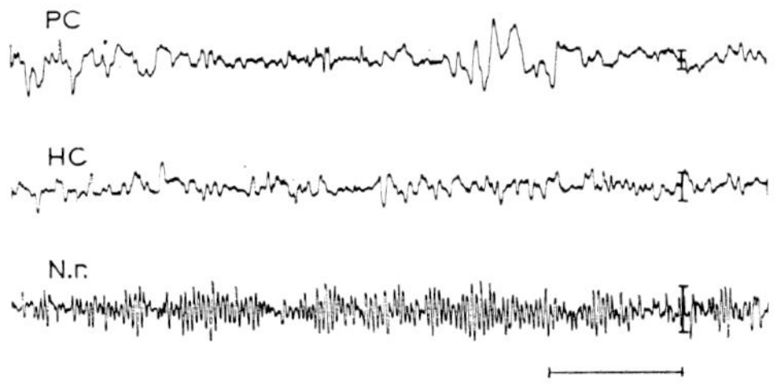

Fig. 4
Effect of 50 mg/kg chlordiazepoxide on the electrical activity of precentral cortex (PC), hippocampus (HC), and red nucleus (N.r.). Calibrations: 100 μV; 1 sec.

which could be solved by the administration of larger doses but experiments with these drugs were complicated by their limited solubility in water. Thus, the aqueous solutions of chlordiazepoxide and oxazepam hemisuccinate were dilute and the need to inject large volumes of solution limited the doses which could be given. We were then not quite sure where we were on the dose effect curve. However, at the upper range of the doses used, the animals appeared deeply narcotized and unresponsive and, as can be seen in Fig. 4, absence of spindling activity in the precentral cortex indicated a fairly deep level of narcosis. In addition, the doses used were much larger than those which block arousal reactions in rabbits by stimulation of the mesencephalic reticular formation (Gogolák and Pillat 1965). The experiments with diazepam and nitrazepam were complicated not only by the amount of the drug which could be administered but by the fact that these drugs were in solution in complex organic vehicles. Surprisingly, nitrazepam did not induce regular rhythm in the red nucleus at the maximal doses used, even though the animal appeared narcotized.

The effects of the vehicles used to dissolve diazepam and nitrazepam were tested in doses comparable to those used for the injection of the drugs and, although the diazepam solvent had no effect on pentobarbital-induced regular rhythms in the red nucleus, the nitrazepam solvent abolished the red nucleus rhythms. Because of this fact we are not completely sure of a lack of interaction in all cases between the vehicle and the drug and we consider our findings with these benzodiazepine compounds as tentative.

In addition to nitrazepam in the form of its commercial preparation several agents with important actions on the central nervous system were tested and found not to induce regular activity in the red nucleus. Morphine, scopolamine, and chlorpromazine, which had already been noted not to induce such rhythms in the red nucleus (Schimmerl and Stumpf 1958), were not retested. Procaine was retested in the present study and again found to have no effect. Lidocaine was injected in doses of 10 and 20 mg/kg and, like procaine, had no effect on red nucleus activity. Mephenesin in doses of 150 mg/kg, which are more than sufficient to produce complete flaccid paralysis in the rabbit, had no visible effect on the red nucleus. Ethyl ether was given by inhalation until deep anaesthesia was reached, with total suppression of cortical electrical activity, and no regular rhythm appeared in the red nucleus during the course of the anaesthesia. It had been shown previously that urethane in anaesthetic doses did not induce synchronous activity in the red nucleus (Schimmerl and Stumpf 1958). We have repeated these studies and in addition we have studied the effects of alcohol which, in doses of 1 g/kg, also induced no regular activity in the red nucleus.

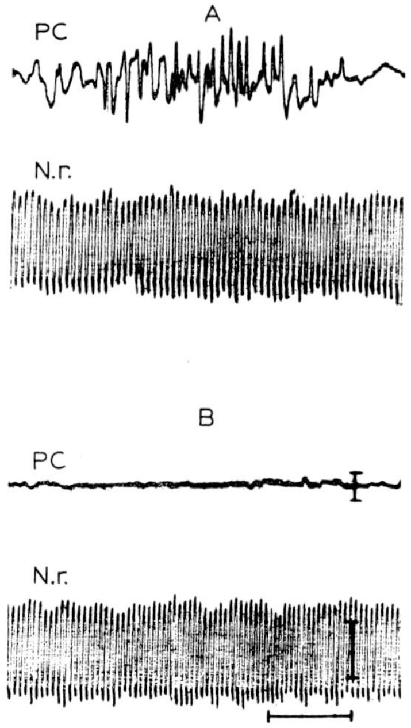

Fig. 5
Effect of urethane (400 mg/kg) on the electrical activity of the precentral cortex (PC) and red nucleus (N.r.) of a rabbit in pentobarbital anaesthesia. *A*: pentobarbital alone; *B*: after administration of urethane in addition to the barbiturate. Calibrations 500 μV (PC) and 100 μV (N.r.); 1 sec.

3. *Interaction of drugs on red nucleus activity*

In an attempt to solve the seeming paradox that alcohol and urethane, both potent central nervous system depressants, did not induce regular rhythms in the red nucleus, we studied the interaction of barbiturates with these agents. These studies were made on acute preparations in which the accurate localization of the electrodes in the red nucleus was done under pentobarbital. When the pentobarbital anaesthesia had lightened to a point where regular rhythms in the red nucleus had a frequency of about 11–18 c/sec, urethane or ethyl alcohol was injected and the effect on the red nucleus rhythm studied. When 0.4 g/kg of urethane was injected in such an animal, it produced the expected cortical signs of deepening depression with suppression of cortical spindling and eventual flattening of the precentral cortical recording to an almost isoelectric state. Unexpectedly, however, the frequency of the red nucleus rhythm was increased (Fig. 5). This increase was not great and never sufficient

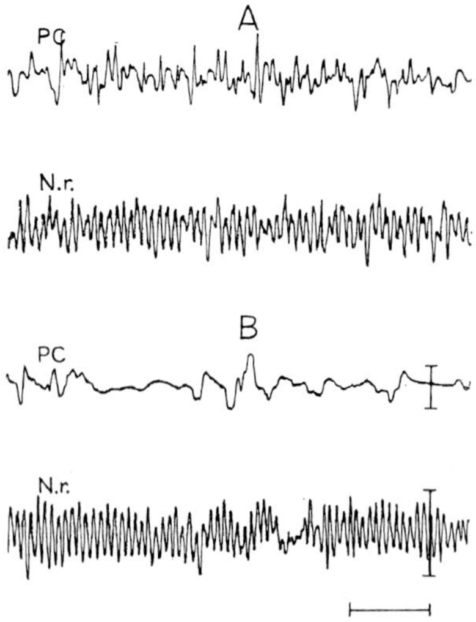

Fig. 6
Effect of ethyl alcohol (1.5 g/kg) on the electrical activity of the precentral cortex (PC) and red nucleus (N.r.) of a rabbit in pentobarbital anaesthesia. *A*: pentobarbital alone; *B*: after administration of alcohol in addition to the barbiturate. Calibrations: 200 μV; 1 sec.

to cause disappearance of regular rhythms. When alcohol was administered to rabbits under pentobarbital, effects similar to those of urethane were seen, that is, deepening depression of the cortex and increase of frequencies in the red nucleus (Fig. 6).

In the interest of completeness, the interaction of pentetrazol, a recognized central nervous system stimulant, and barbiturates was studied. With 8 mg/kg of pentetrazol an antagonistic effect occurred both in the cortex and red nucleus. In a typical experiment, pentetrazol was injected when the frequency of the pentobarbital-induced red nucleus rhythm had reached 14 c/sec. Under pentetrazol the frequency increased temporarily up to 20 c/sec and in the cortex the electrical activity showed changes corresponding to a shift in the direction of lighter anaesthesia.

DISCUSSION

We have shown that not only do the barbiturates reliably induce regular rhythms in the red nucleus but that the frequency of these rhythms is low with deep levels of barbiturate narcosis and increases linearly with time after injection. This effect has not only a linear correlation with time but also a correlation with barbiturate effects on the hippocampus and on the cortex and may be a very useful index of the depth of narcosis, since the red nucleus effects are clearer and more easily measured than barbiturate effects elsewhere in the brain. Of course, we have no evidence at present that the red nucleus is the primary site for the action of barbiturates and similar drugs in inducing the characteristic rhythms in the red nucleus. Such rhythms may well originate in the cerebellum or in the cerebral cortex, areas which are known to send prominent fibre tracts to the red nucleus. We have some preliminary evidence that these rhythms may in fact occur in the cerebellum.

Since barbiturates are eliminated basically according to a first order reaction (Remmer 1963), it is hoped that the frequency of induced red nucleus rhythms will be inversely proportional to the logarithm of the blood or brain barbiturate concentration and these studies are in progress. We have also shown that the slopes of the regression lines for thiopental and hexobarbital are similar and that the lesser slope of the pentobarbital regression line correlates roughly with the expected longer duration of action of pentobarbital in the rabbit. We feel that the data cited by Siegert *et al.* (1964) for the half-life of barbiturates in the rabbit do not apply in our study because their half-life times were calculated on the later part of the blood level curve and do not correlate with the initial time course of anaesthesia with these compounds.

We have also shown that other central nervous system depressants in the general class of "minor tranquillizers" or sedatives can duplicate the effects of barbiturates on the red nucleus. Propanidid and meprobamate appear to have effects qualitatively identical to the barbiturates. The benzodiazepine data are complicated by dose and solvent problems but it is clear that chlordiazepoxide, diazepam and oxazepam hemisuccinate can induce synchronous activity in the red nucleus. The apparent dissociation between cortical and red nucleus effects of the benzodiazepines and the fact that the rhythms induced by large doses of benzodiazepines are never as slow as those induced by barbiturates, need to be further evaluated and may be significant. The fact that one of the benzodiazepine compounds, nitrazepam, did not induce regular rhythms in the red nucleus is complicated by problems with the solvent of this compound. 5 ml of nitrazepam solution ("solution for research purposes only") are prepared by mixing the contents of two ampoules, the first containing 10 mg of nitrazepam, 75 mg of benzyl alcohol and 0.5 ml of ethanol with enough propylene glycol to make 2.5 ml. The second ampoule contains 250 mg of sodium benzoate in 2.5 ml of distilled water. The ethanol concentration by itself is not adequate to account for the possible antagonism of the effects of nitrazepam on the red nucleus and we have not tested the interaction of the drug with the other ingredients in the solvent. Vieth *et al.* (1968) showed that the nitrazepam solvent had effects similar to alcohol on the central nervous system and since alcohol in our hands antagonized the barbiturate effect on the red nucleus, it might be that further study of this compound in different doses might class it with the rest of the benzodiazepines.

At the present time the biological significance

of the red nucleus rhythm induced by the drugs mentioned above remains obscure. Similarly, it is difficult to ascribe one common property to all drugs which elicit a regular red nucleus rhythm that could be responsible for this elicitation. Barbiturates, propanidid, meprobamate and benzodiazepines belong to this group of drugs. Clearly, all of them are central depressants. Propanidid has been shown to cause qualitatively similar EEG changes to barbiturates (Hoffmeister 1965) and to have generally similar pharmacological properties to barbiturates (Wirth and Hoffmeister 1965). The benzodiazepines chlordiazepoxide, diazepam and oxazepam have been used, in the same manner as short-acting barbiturates, for induction of general anaesthesia and it has been said that after i.v. administration of these drugs "a marked hypnotic effect resembling light thiopental anaesthesia is observed" (Dobkin and Po-Giok-Su 1966). In the present study, to elicit a similar effect on red nucleus activity, chlordiazepoxide had to be used in higher doses than diazepam. This accords with the findings of Randall (1962), who also reported that diazepam is more potent than chlordiazepoxide in a variety of tests of central activity. Meprobamate is usually placed, together with the benzodiazepines, in a group of drugs for which, among others, the terms "minor tranquillizers" (Møller 1966; Bowman *et al.* 1968), "drugs for anxiety" (Jarvik 1965) or "euhypnotics" (Muñoz and Levitas 1965) have been used. In many respects, its actions are similar to those of barbiturates, in others different (Domino 1962a, b). Although meprobamate apparently has not been used for induction of anaesthesia, it is highly probable that it could be used for this purpose. Thus, it would appear that elicitation of a regular red nucleus rhythm is a property common to a group of drugs which actually are, or at least theoretically could be, used as hypnotics-narcotics. It is hoped that further experimentation will furnish more information on the significance of this phenomenon.

SUMMARY

The action and interaction of several drugs on the electrical activity of the red nucleus of the rabbit have been investigated. The following results have been obtained:

1. Barbiturates, propanidid, meprobamate and benzodiazepines elicit in the red nucleus an exceedingly regular rhythm in the frequency range between 4 and 30 c/sec.

2. Under barbiturates the frequency increases linearly with time and it is assumed that it is inversely proportional to the logarithm of barbiturate concentration in blood or brain tissue. For this reason the frequency may be used as a highly reliable indicator of the depth of barbiturate anaesthesia.

3. Urethane and ethyl alcohol potentiate the action of barbiturates at cortical levels but antagonize it at the level of the red nucleus. Solvents of some pharmaceutical preparations also interfere with the action of barbiturates on red nucleus activity. Pentetrazol has an antagonistic effect both at the cortical level and at the level of the red nucleus.

4. All drugs thus far studied which elicit a regular red nucleus rhythm belong to a group of hypnotics-narcotics which are, or could be, used for induction of general anaesthesia.

ZUSAMMENFASSUNG

WIRKUNG VON PHARMAKA AUF DIE ELEKTRISCHE TÄTIGKEIT DES NUCLEUS RUBER

An Kaninchen wurden die Wirkungen und Wechselwirkungen verschiedener Substanzen auf die elektrische Tätigkeit des Nucleus ruber untersucht. Diese Untersuchungen lieferten folgende Ergebnisse:

1. Barbiturate, Propanidid, Meprobamat und Benzodiazepin-Derivate lösen im Nucleus ruber einen ausserordentlich regelmässigen Rhythmus mit einem Frequenzbereich von 4 bis 30 c/sec aus.

2. Unter der Wirkung von Barbituraten nimmt die Frequenz linear mit der Zeit zu und es wird daher angenommen, dass sie sich zum Logarithmus der Barbituratkonzentration im Blut oder Gehirn verkehrt proportional verhält.

3. Urethan und Äthylalkohol potenzieren die Wirkung der Barbiturate auf den Cortex, aber antagonisieren deren Wirkung auf den Nucleus ruber. In verschiedenen pharmazeutischen Präparaten enthaltene Lösungsmittel beeinflussen ebenfalls die Barbituratwirkung auf den Nucleus

ruber. Pentetrazol antagonisiert die Wirkung der Barbiturate auf Cortex und Nucleus ruber.

4. Alle bisher untersuchten Substanzen, die einen regelmässigen Rhythmus im Nucleus ruber auslösen, gehören in eine Gruppe der Hypnotica-Narcotica, die für die Narkoseeinleitung verwendet werden oder zumindest dafür verwendet werden könnten.

The authors wish to thank Dr. Harry L. Williams for his valuable criticism and his help in presenting the paper. The authors wish to make the following acknowledgements for the drugs generously supplied for this study: pentobarbital (Nembutal, Abbott Laboratories, North Chicago and Vienna); propanidid (Epontol, Bayer-Pharma G.m.b.H., Vienna); meprobamate (Cyrpon, Tropon-Werke, Köln, and Dr. Kolassa und Co., Vienna); chlordiazepoxide hydrochloride (Librium), diazepam (Valium), and nitrazepam (Mogadon), all supplied by Hoffmann-La Roche, Wien G.m.b.H., Vienna; oxazepam hemisuccinate (hemisuccinate of Adumbran, C. H. Boehringer, Sohn, Ingelheim/Rhein, and Bender und Co., G.m.b.H., Vienna); mephenesin (Reorganin, Frika G.m.b.H., Vienna); gallamine (Flaxedil, C. H. Boehringer Sohn, Ingelheim/Rhein).

REFERENCES

BOWMAN, W. C., RAND, M. J. and WEST, G. B. *Textbook of pharmacology*. Blackwell, Oxford, **1968,** 1025 p.

BRÜCKE, F., SAILER, S. und STUMPF, CH. Pharmakologische Beeinflussung der Frequenz der Hippocampustätigkeit während retikulärer Reizung. *Naunyn-Schmiedeberg's Arch. exp. Path. Pharmak.*, **1957,** *231*: 267–278.

DOBKIN, A. B. and PO-GIOK-SU, J. Newer anaesthetics and their uses. *Clin. Pharmacol. Therap.*, **1966,** *7*: 648–682.

DOMINO, E. F. Site of action of some central nervous system depressants. *Ann. Rev. Pharmacol.*, **1962**a, *2*: 215–250.

DOMINO, E. F. Human pharmacology of tranquilizing drugs. *Clin. Pharmacol. Therap.*, **1962**b, *3*: 599–664.

ECCLES, J. C., ITO, M. and SZENTÁGOTHAI, J. *The cerebellum as a neuronal machine*. Springer, Berlin, **1967,** 335 p.

GOGOLÁK, G. and PILLAT, B. Effect of Mogadon on the arousal reaction in rabbits. In K. AKERT *et al.* (Eds.), *Progress in brain research. Vol. 18. Sleep mechanisms.* Elsevier, Amsterdam, **1965:** 229–230.

HOFFMEISTER, F. Zur Wirkung von Propanidid auf Spontan-EEG und induzierte Potentiale von Katzen und Kaninchen. *Anaesth. Resusc.*, **1965,** *4*: 47–61.

JARVIK, M. E. Drugs used in the treatment of psychiatric disorders. In L. S. GOODMAN and A. GILMAN (Eds.), *The pharmacological basis of therapeutics*. Macmillan, New York, **1965**: 159–214.

MASSION, J. The mammalian red nucleus. *Physiol. Rev.*, **1967,** *47*: 383–436.

MØLLER, K. O. *Pharmakologie als theoretische Grundlage einer rationellen Pharmakotherapie*. Schwabe, Basel, **1966,** 918 p.

MUÑOZ, J. G. und LEVITAS, A. Über den durch Medikamente und Placebo hervorgerufenen Schlaf. *Arzneimittel-Forsch.*, **1965,** *15*: 1118–1125.

RANDALL, L. O. Pharmacodynamics of chlordiazepoxide and other benzodiazepine derivatives. In J. H. NODINE and J. H. MOYER (Eds.), *Psychosomatic medicine*. Lea and Febiger, Philadelphia, **1962:** 476–479.

REMMER, H. Die Ursache der Gewöhnung an oxydable Barbiturate. *Naunyn-Schmiedeberg's Arch. exp. Path. Pharmak.*, **1963,** *244*: 311–333.

SAWYER, CH. H., EVERETT, J. W. and GREEN, J. D. The rabbit diencephalon in stereotaxic coordinates. *J. comp. Neurol.*, **1954,** *101*: 801–824.

SCHIMMERL, G. und STUMPF, CH. Die Tätigkeit des Nucleus ruber nach Verabreichung von Barbituraten und Meprobamat. *Naunyn-Schmiedeberg's Arch. exp. Path. Pharmak.*, **1958,** *235*: 33–40.

SIEGERT, M., ALSLEBEN, B., LIEBENSCHÜTZ, W. und REMMER, H. Unterschiede in der mikrosomalen Oxydation und Acetylierung von Arzneimitteln bei verschiedenen Arten und Rassen. *Naunyn-Schmiedeberg's Arch. exp. Path. Pharmak.*, **1964,** *247*: 509–521.

STARZL, T. E., TAYLOR, C. W. and MAGOUN, H. W. Collateral afferent excitation of reticular formation of brain stem. *J. Neurophysiol.*, **1951,** *14*: 479–496.

VIETH, J. B., HOLM, E. and KNOPP, P. R. Electrophysiological studies on the action of Mogadon on central nervous structures of the cat. A comparison with pentobarbital. *Arch. int. Pharmacodyn.*, **1968,** *171*: 323–338.

WIRTH, W. und HOFFMEISTER, F. Pharmakologische Untersuchungen mit Propanidid. *Anaesth. Resusc.*, **1965,** *4*: 17–47.

Reference: GOGOLÁK, G., LIEBESWAR, G. and STUMPF, CH. Action of drugs on the electrical activity of the red nucleus. *Electroenceph. clin. Neurophysiol.*, **1969,** *27:* 296–303.

Electroencephalography and Clinical Neurophysiology
Elsevier Publishing Company, Amsterdam – Printed in The Netherlands

CLINICAL AND LABORATORY NOTES

THE INFLUENCE OF END-TIDAL CARBON DIOXIDE TENSION ON EEG CHANGES DURING ROUTINE HYPERVENTILATION IN DIFFERENT AGE GROUPS

C. D. Binnie, P. A. Coles and J. H. Margerison

Department of Clinical Neurophysiology, St. Bartholomew's Hospital, London, E.C.1 (Great Britain)

(Accepted for publication: January 10, 1969)

Hypocapnia is an important factor in the development of slow waves in the EEG with overbreathing. Thus Preswick *et al.* (1965) found a greater fall of end-tidal carbon dioxide tension (pCO_2) among the surprisingly small proportion of normal subjects (5%) in their series who developed such slow waves. Most reports stress the failure of slow waves to occur at any constant level of hypocapnia (Davis and Wallace 1942; Blinn and Noell 1949; Morrice 1956; Meyer and Waltz 1960). However, no quantitative information is available concerning the correlation between falls in end-tidal pCO_2 and EEG changes among subjects displaying a wide range of responsiveness to overbreathing. Similarly, little is known of possible relationships between the fall in pCO_2 and other factors, notably age, known to influence the EEG response. The present study concerns the effects both of age and of change in pCO_2 upon the EEG responses in adolescents and in adults undergoing clinical EEG investigation.

MATERIAL AND METHODS

The subjects formed a consecutive series of twenty-four outpatients aged 12–50 years who met the following criteria: (i) a resting EEG classified, for clinical purposes, as normal; (ii) no qualitative EEG abnormality on overbreathing; (iii) no evidence of intracranial pathology and (iv) no systemic condition thought likely either to influence the EEG response or to hinder overbreathing, *e.g.*, spontaneous hypoglycaemia, pulmonary disease etc.

As preliminary observations had suggested that the EEG became more stable to overbreathing during the fourth decade, the patients were divided into categories: Group I, less than 35 years old, comprised thirteen patients with a mean age of 22.3 years; Group II, more than 35 years old, contained eleven patients whose average age was 41.9 years. It was predicted that the younger patients would produce a greater fall in end-tidal pCO_2 and show more marked EEG changes.

Twenty-three chlorided silver stick-on electrodes were applied in a pattern similar to that described by Pampiglione (1956). The EEG was recorded on 12 channels of an Elema-Schönander electroencephalograph. A routine resting record was first obtained and overbreathing was then performed for 3 min. Samples of end-tidal air were taken at the start of recording and immediately before, and immediately after, overbreathing. CO_2 concentrations were measured with a Hartmann and Braun infra-red gas analyser and subsequently converted to partial pressures.

All EEGs were assessed by the same individual. A rating scale was devised to categorize changes from the resting record during overbreathing, ranging from no observable change to a maximal response, in 13 steps each separated by one "just-noticeable-difference". The mid-point of the scale, grade 7, was that at which isolated frontal slow waves appeared. The EEG changes seemed to lie on a continuum and once a few records had been classified the remainder could be graded by interpolation with surprising ease. In order to assess the reliability of the procedure, the EEGs were subsequently regraded at a single session without reference to the previous scores.

RESULTS

The test-retest stability of the EEG assessments was high. In only 3 out of 24 records was there a difference of

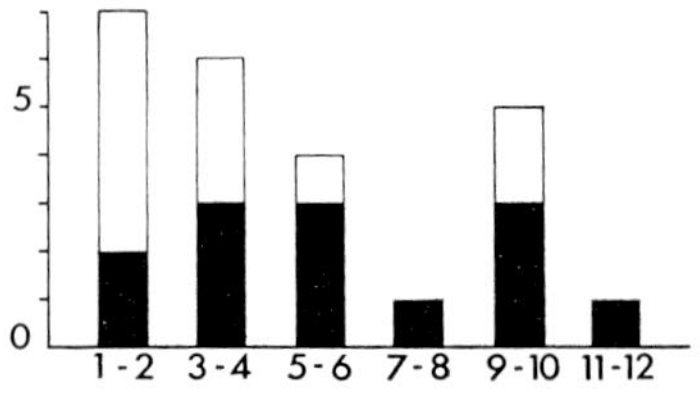

Fig. 1
Grade of EEG change as a function of age: the black areas indicate those subjects less than, and the white areas those more than, 35 years old. Ordinate = number of subjects.

more than one between the first and second scores. The rank orders agreed closely (Spearman's $r = 0.91$, $t = 10.0$, degrees of freedom (d.f.) $= 22$, $P < 0.001$). The results to be presented are based on the second assessment.

EEG ratings for the two age groups are illustrated in Fig. 1. The younger subjects showed greater differences between their EEGs at rest and those taken during hyperventilation. Frontal slow activity occurred in 5 records from Group I but in only 2 from Group II. As predicted, the amount of EEG change was negatively correlated with age ($r = -0.40$, $t = 2.05$, d.f. $= 22$, $P < 0.025$ for a one-tailed test).

As there were no appreciable differences between end-tidal pCO_2 at the start of the resting record and the level immediately before overbreathing, the figures were combined to provide mean values for comparison with the measurements obtained after overbreathing. Marked EEG changes tended to be accompanied by large falls in pCO_2. For example, among patients with EEG ratings of 7 or more (*i.e.*, producing frontal slow activity), the mean fall in pCO_2 was 16.5 mm of Hg (S.D. $= 3.02$) whereas in those with a less marked EEG response, the mean drop was 12.9 mm (S.D. $= 4.49$). The differences between these means is significant at the 5% level ($t = 2.02$, $P < 0.05$ for a one-tailed test).

The changes in end-tidal pCO_2 were smaller in the older patients. Only two patients over 35 years old achieved a fall of pCO_2 exceeding 14 mm (the mean value for the entire sample), whereas a majority of the younger patients did so (Table I).

TABLE I

Change in end-tidal pCO_2 during overbreathing in relation to age

Change in pCO_2	Age (years)	
	12–35	35–50
More than 14 mm	7	2
Less than 14 mm	6	9

$P < 0.05$.

DISCUSSION

The results confirm that EEG changes during overbreathing are influenced both by age and by the magnitude of the fall in end-tidal pCO_2. They indicate further that these two variables are not independent, for the change in pCO_2 itself declines with increasing age. When only those patients showing a drop in pCO_2 between 10 and 20 mm of Hg are considered, thus eliminating that third of the original sample with the more extreme high or low values, no correlation remains between age and EEG rating ($r = -0.16$, $t = 0.605$ with 14 degrees of freedom, $P < 0.5$). Thus the differences in EEG response between younger and older subjects may merely reflect a greater fall of pCO_2 in the former. There is an undoubted need for further studies of factors determining EEG changes during overbreathing, but it is provisionally suggested that, in adolescents and adults, the loss of EEG responsiveness to hyperventilation with increasing years may indicate not so much a change in cerebral physiology as a difference, either in pulmonary function or in the vigour with which overbreathing is performed.

SUMMARY

In twenty-four patients aged 12–50 years a significant positive association was found between the change in end-tidal pCO_2 during 3 min overbreathing and the development of slow activity. There was a significant negative correlation between age and amount of change in the EEG. The fall in pCO_2 grew less with increasing age. It is tentatively suggested that in adolescents and adults the apparent influence of age upon EEG responses to overbreathing may be secondary to a decline in ventilatory performance with increasing years.

RÉSUMÉ

RELATION ENTRE PRESSION PARTIELLE DE GAZ CARBONIQUE DE L'AIR DE RÉSERVE ET MODIFICATIONS EEG PENDANT L'HYPERPNÉE DE ROUTINE DANS DIFFÉRENTS GROUPES D'ÂGE

Chez vingt-quatre malades de 12–50 ans, une relation positive significative s'observe entre les modifications du pCO_2 de l'air de réserve au cours d'une hyperpnée de 3 min et la survenue d'activités lentes à l'EEG. On note une corrélation négative significative entre l'âge et l'importance du changement EEG. La chute du pCO_2 est moindre au-fur-et-à-mesure que l'on augmente en âge. Les auteurs font l'hypothèse que chez l'adolescent et l'adulte, l'influence apparente de l'âge sur la réponse EEG à l'hyperpnée puisse être secondaire à une diminution de l'efficacité de ventilation au-fur-et-à-mesure de l'âge.

It is a pleasure to acknowledge the advice and assistance of Drs. B. W. Watson and D. Bethune (St. Bartholomew's Hospital) and also that of Miss P. A. Ward (Senior EEG Technician) who recorded the EEGs.

REFERENCES

Blinn, K. A. and Noell, W. K. Continuous measurement of alveolar CO_2 tension during the hyperventilation test in routine electroencephalography. *Electroenceph. clin. Neurophysiol.*, **1949**, *1*: 333–342.

Davis, H. and Wallace, W. Factors affecting changes produced in the EEG by standardized hyperventilation. *Arch. Neurol. Psychiat. (Chic.)*, **1942**, *47*: 606–625.

Meyer, J. S. and Waltz, A. G. Arterial oxygen saturation and alveolar carbon dioxide during electroencephalography: I. Comparison of hyperventilation and induced hypoxia in subjects without brain disease. *Arch. Neurol. Psychiat. (Chic.)*, **1960**, *2*: 631–643.

Morrice, J. K. W. Slow wave production in the EEG with reference to hyperpnoea, carbon dioxide and autonomic balance. *Electroenceph. clin. Neurophysiol.*, **1956**, *8*: 49–72.

Electroenceph. clin. Neurophysiol., **1969**, *27*: 304–306

PAMPIGLIONE, G. Some anatomical considerations upon electrode placement in routine EEG. *Proc. electrophysiol. Technol. Ass.*, **1956,** *7*: 20–30.

PRESWICK, G., REIVICH, M. and HILL, I. D. The EEG effects of combined hyperventilation and hypoxia in normal subjects. *Electroenceph. clin. Neurophysiol.*, **1965,** *18*: 56–64.

Reference: BINNIE, C. D., COLES, P. A. and MARGERISON, J. H. The influence of end-tidal carbon dioxide tension on EEG changes during routine hyperventilation in different age groups. *Electroenceph. clin. Neurophysiol.*, **1969,** *27*: 304–306.

BEHAVIOURAL AND EEG AROUSAL INDUCED BY STIMULATION OF UNSPECIFIC PROJECTION SYSTEMS IN A PATIENT WITH POST-TRAUMATIC APALLIC SYNDROME

R. HASSLER, G. DALLE ORE, G. DIECKMANN, A. BRICOLO AND G. DOLCE

Department of Neurosurgery, City Hospital, Verona (Italy) and Department of Neuroanatomy, Max-Planck-Institut für Hirnforschung, Frankfurt/M. (W. Germany)

(Accepted for publication: December 22, 1968)

The increasing number of serious traffic accidents has produced cases of post-traumatic coma that fail to recover even for several months. These patients survive in a state of akinetic mutism with a spontaneous sleep-waking rhythm but without any conscious reaction to sensory stimuli. Why some of these patients spontaneously recover after prolonged periods of deep coma vigil is not understood (Gerstenbrand 1967).

These apallic patients present a remarkably uniform syndrome of akinetic mutism regardless of additional damage to cortical structures, although autopsy findings are by no means uniform. The reason why the mesencephalic reticular formation fails to exert its non-specific action on the cerebral cortex is not known. In the light of the hodological findings, supported by experience with patients during and after stereotaxic surgery, one of us was led to the concept that stimuli from the non-specific activating system might travel through pallidal and thalamic relays (Hassler 1950, 1958). Experimental evidence supporting this concept was provided by Dieckmann (1968).

Pursuant to the idea that pathological changes in this complex neuronal system might account for failure of recovery from prolonged post-traumatic coma, we tried to treat a suitable case of coma vigil by repeated bilateral stimulation of the pallido-thalamic system.

METHOD

In a patient with an apallic syndrome of 5 months' duration we inserted flexible platinum electrodes, 0.5 mm in diameter, with tin-plated tips 6 mm apart, into the basal part of the right pallidum and into the basal portion of the left latero-polar nucleus of the thalamus (VA) (Fig. 1, *A*), *i.e.*, into structures which we believe to represent constituents of the non-specific projection system. The procedure was carried out by the localization method of Hassler and Riechert (1954) and with the stereotaxic apparatus of Riechert and Mundinger (1955). We inserted the flexible electrodes by means of guiding sheaths into the target under control of an X-ray amplifier, withdrew the guiding sheaths and fixed the electrodes to the burr holes with a special dental cement.

After verifying the electrode positions radiologically, we connected them to a Tönnies stimulator providing trapezoid and rectangular pulses with plateaus of 1–3 msec and a frequency range of 1–100 c/sec, voltages being measured within the stimulation circuit. Polygraphic recordings were obtained with a 16-channel electroencephalograph (Galileo) from the scalp, the right pallidum and the left VA, along with the EMG of the neck muscles, ECG and electro-oculogram.

Intensive care of the apallic patient, with high caloric feeding, was continued for the 19 days of stimulation.

RESULTS

1. *Behaviour*

The patient, a male aged 26, was found unconscious in a place in the mountains. He presented a laceration of the scalp in the right parietal region and fracture of the lambdoid suture as evidence of head trauma, though he was also reported to have suffered from occasional generalized seizures since childhood. During the first 20 days of deep coma there were vegetative disorders, but no extension spasms. After 8 weeks the patient opened his eyes spontaneously for the first time; during such waking periods, delta waves (or 6 c/sec waves) were seen in the EEG.

Most of the night he slept, with only short interruptions by opening of the eyes for some minutes. During the day sleeping and waking states of 1–2 h duration alternated. No signs of sensory awareness could be observed, or any

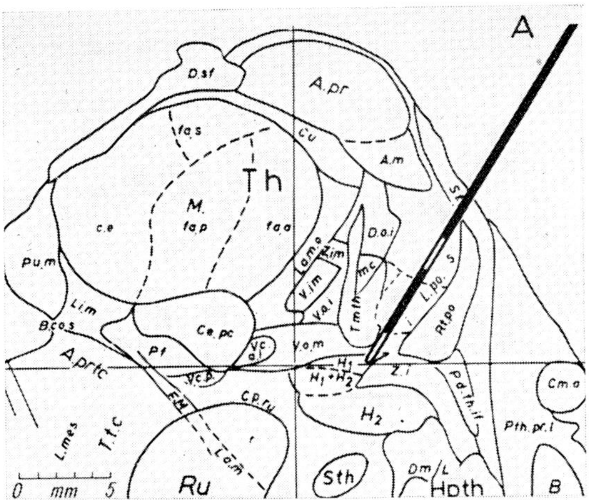

Fig. 1
A: Position of the left stimulating electrode with uninsulated tip in the base of the ventral anterior thalamic nucleus (Lpo. i) and thalamic fascicle (H_1). The other pole is located in the upper part of VA belonging to Lpo. s in the figure. Sagittal diagram of thalamus, 6.5 mm from midline. (According to Hassler 1959).
B: The apallic patient in coma vigil with both flexible electrodes implanted, before stimulation: typical head posture, slightly to the right, with half-closed eyes deviated to the right (unless divergent strabismus predominated).
C: Clinical arousal effect during stimulation of left VA (50 c/sec, 20 V) and right pallidum (8 c/sec, 30 V). The eyes are open, gazing upwards with dilated pupils and gaping eyelids. Pseudo-intentional movements of left arm and hand during stimulation. Disappearance of head posture to the right.

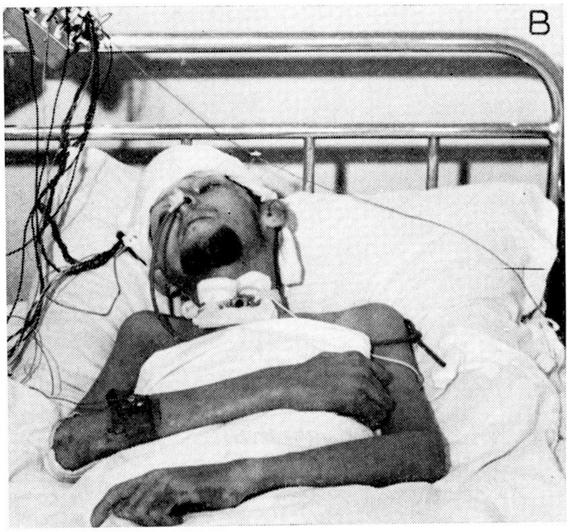

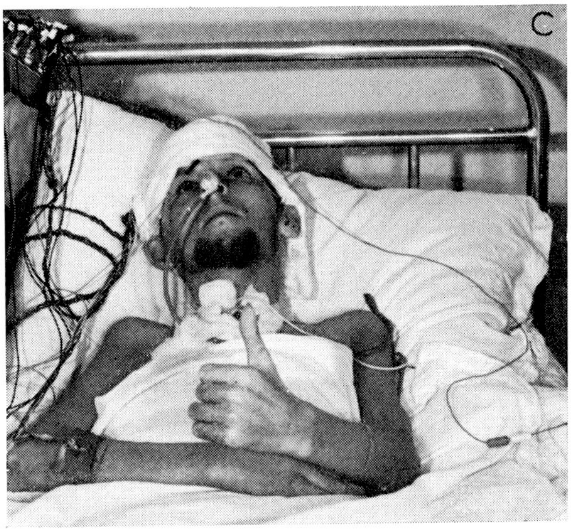

emotional reactions to the nurses or to the visiting parents. He was unable to direct attention to environmental stimuli. During sleep it was always possible to produce behavioural arousal by passive bending of the head against the chest, combined with flexion of the upper and lower extremities.

Stimulation of parts of the non-specific system was started 21 weeks after the head injury. Stimulation of the left VA elicited opening of the eyelids with the eyes in a parallel position, whereas in the absence of stimulation the patient presented a typical divergent strabismus. If the patient was thus stimulated while asleep he would promptly open his eyes (pupils dilated) and direct his gaze to the side opposite stimulation. This behavioural arousal reaction subsided from 10 to 20 sec after the end of stimulation.

Stimulation of the right pallidum and lamella pallidi interna produced sluggish opening of the eyes, even with higher current intensity less pronounced than to stimulation of VA; the eyes took a conjugate position. During stimulation of the pallidum there were sporadic movements of the left arm of greater amplitude than the spontaneous movements which occurred between stimuli. When stimulation was discontinued the left eye was half closed, retracted into the socket, and divergent strabismus was restored.

Simultaneous stimulation of the right pallidum and left VA produced a stronger behavioural arousal (Fig. 1, *B* and *C*) with a shorter latency. Conjugate deviation of the eyes to the left was less than with VA stimulation alone. If one of the stimuli was interrupted its effect subsided. Movements of the left arm were brisk, with a rhythm independent of the frequency of the applied stimuli. During bilateral stimulation the patient sometimes tried to remove his feeding tube. His gaze was wakeful and apparently fixed on some definite object. Sometimes the head was moved slightly to follow eye movements; often, however, the gaze was directed upwards during bilateral stimulation (Fig. 1, *C*).

Higher frequency stimulation of VA (25, 50 and 100 c/sec) occasionally produced a convulsive seizure starting with upward gaze and head raising. Such seizures could always be terminated by passive flexing of the head on the chest.

After 2 days of repeated stimulation (3 or 4 times daily for 15 min each time) with 25 c/sec to the left VA and 8 c/sec to the right pallidum the patient appeared more wakeful and exhibited a purposeful gaze more often between stimuli. Left arm movements also became somewhat more frequent and the left leg was also moved; this had never occurred before stimulation was instituted.

On the fifth day the patient opened his eyes and turned his head toward the left after discontinuation of the stimuli. During his parents' visit he turned spontaneously toward his mother and fixed his gaze on her; his face was flushed and smiling. The parents were sure that the patient recognized them; they were delighted to see that he made apparently coordinated movements with his left arm and

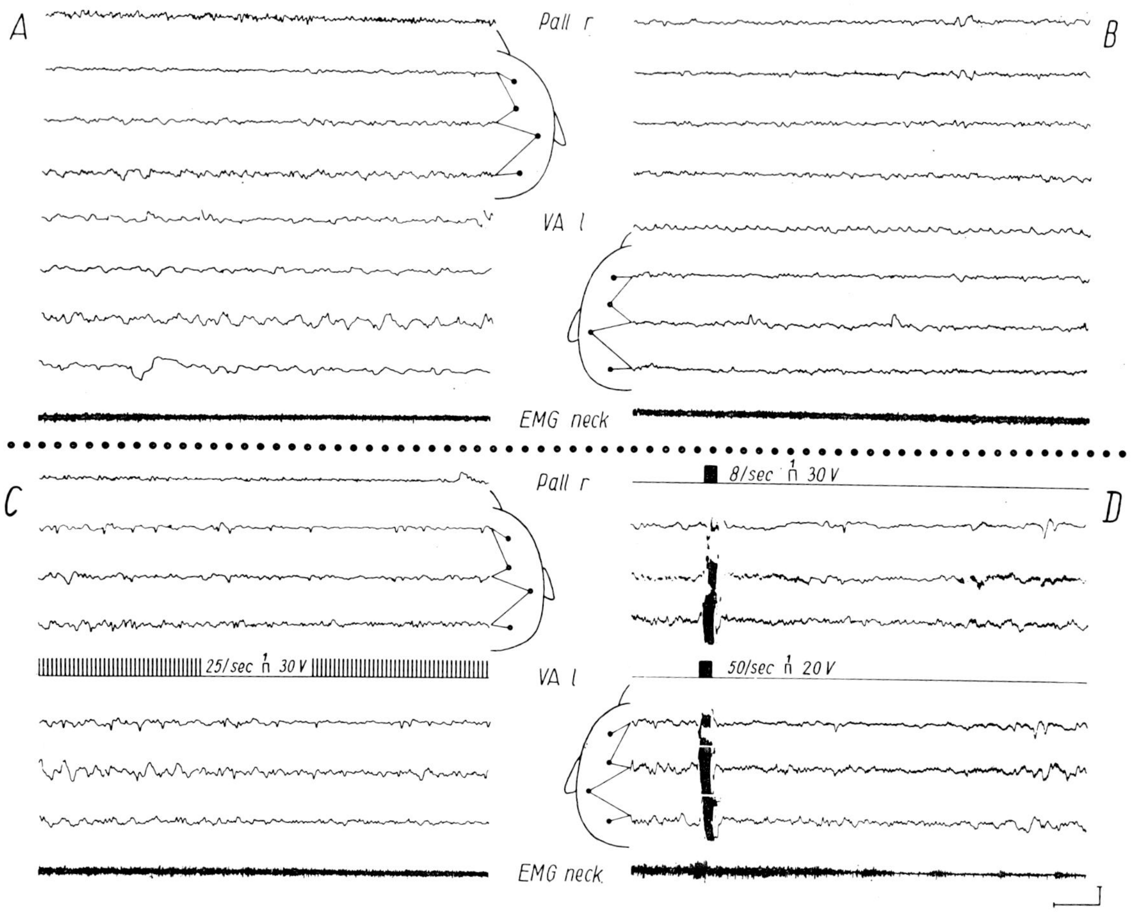

Fig. 2

A: Spontaneous EEG and subcorticogram after implantation of electrodes, before stimulation. Asymmetric background rhythm in the two hemispheres. Activity of left hemisphere is slower and of greater voltage, with left temporal delta activity. Background rhythm on right side consists of faster and lower voltage waves. Pallidum shows mixed activity of 10 c/sec waves with superimposed theta waves. Thalamus (VA l) shows slow waves of various frequencies and small amplitude.

B: EEG and subcorticogram after 2 days of intermittent electrical stimulation of right pallidum and left VA nucleus. Background activity modified to desynchronized pattern. Asymmetry and delta activity have abated. Spontaneous activity in the pallidum has slowed down; in the thalamus, regular 2 c/sec waves appear.

C: EEG and pallidogram during stimulation of left VA with 25 c/sec, 30 V, in rectangular pulses of 1 msec each for 15 min. Desynchronization of slow background rhythm and disappearance of delta activity during stimulation. Alpha frequencies are partially reached in both hemispheres. Pallidal activity is also desynchronized.

D: Simultaneous stimulation of the right pallidum (8 c/sec, 30 V) and left VA (50 c/sec, 20 V) for 0.5 sec results in immediate bilateral desynchronization with blocking of left temporal delta activity. Electrical activity of neck muscles is reduced. Calibration: 2 sec, 100 μV.

hand (*e.g.*, touching his beard and opposite arm), as well as with his left leg. After 8 days of repeated bilateral stimulation (3 or 4 times daily for 15 min each) the tracheotomy cannula could be removed. Thereafter, the patient began to vocalize spontaneously, if unintelligibly, and to turn toward nearby persons.

Continuing stimulation during the following days produced further activation and increase of spontaneous movements of the left hand, with some semblance of purposefulness. When called, the patient would slowly turn his head and gaze toward the voice. At the same time, he was generally more awake and receptive to various sensory stimuli; he moved his left limbs spontaneously. He also tried repeatedly to pull off the stimulating electrodes by elaborate motions of the left arm and hand; thereby the left electrode in the base of VA was broken outside the skull. Because this was the more effective electrode, the stimulation effects became less, and finally perhaps ineffective, while the left electrode could not be replaced. Therefore the electrodes had to be removed on the 19th day.

After 19 days of stimulation the level of consciousness was definitely improved: spontaneous movements of the left limbs were seen both during and between stimuli; unintelligible vocalization occurred and turning reactions to both sides, particularly to the left, were definitely more marked than before treatment. The same was true of spontaneous movements of the left hand toward his own body and immediate surroundings. When the electrodes were withdrawn at 19 days the improvement of the conscious level and spontaneous motility of the left limbs were maintained; however, there was no further gain of either consciousness or vocalization beyond that point.

2. *Electroencephalographic findings*

The spontaneous EEG before stimulation (Fig. 2, *A*) revealed an irregular activity at 6 or 7 c/sec, with overriding slow waves, from the left hemisphere, particularly from the temporal region. There was a left temporal delta focus. During spontaneous movements there was an alteration of the background rhythm toward desynchronization, with an increased frequency reaching into the alpha range. Skin stimulation failed to produce EEG arousal but increased the amplitude of the slower waves. From the pallidum, a low voltage 10 c/sec activity was mixed with theta waves.

Stimulation of VA (25 c/sec, 30 V) produced a desynchronization which included the pallidum. Delta activity was reduced on the left side and alpha frequencies appeared on both sides (Fig. 2, *C*).

Double stimulation of the right pallidum (8 c/sec, 30 V) and left VA (50 c/sec, 20 V) for half a second blocked the delta activity on the left side and immediately desynchronized all tracings bilaterally. The effect was much more marked than with single stimulation. Stimulation reduced electrical activity in the neck muscles (Fig. 2, *D*).

As early as 2 days after the inception of electrical stimulation of the pallidum and of the VA, the background rhythm showed a tendency toward desynchronization, disappearance of delta activity and regression of the asymmetry. Electrical activity in the pallidum was slowed down and regular 2 c/sec waves appeared in the VA (Fig. 2, *B*).

At the end of the 19 day period of stimulation the EEG differences between right and left sides were reduced and the left delta focus was consistently absent.

We have observed comparable results with bilateral stimulation of the pallidal system in another two cases of coma vigil; these will be reported in a separate paper.

DISCUSSION

The apallic syndrome is not due to an anatomical loss of all cortical fields, as suggested by the name, nor is it due to an interruption of all their connections in both directions. It is only a functional loss of cortical activity on account of a loss of the non-specific activation of the cortical fields. This failure of non-specific activation is caused by a lesion in the non-specific projection mechanism, either in the midbrain reticular activating system or in their diencephalic forerunners, including the pallidum. Occasionally such lesions have been found at autopsy (Jellinger 1966). The fact that the EEG, as in the described coma vigil, shows some cortical activity, usually slower than the alpha rhythm, indicates that the action of at least one of the projection systems fails. During the waking state the delta activity of the present case was not altered; on the other hand no EEG or behavioural arousal, or an accelerated activity, was elicited by somato-sensory stimulation, even by a noxious stimulus. The ascending activation of the reticular system failed in coma vigil but the rhythmic descending influence on the eyes and on the autonomic functions was restored after 5 weeks and is still present. The ascending non-specific action on the cortical fields seems to be invariably lost in all apallic syndromes of longer duration.

In many cases a spontaneous recovery from an apallic syndrome with coma vigil occurs after weeks or a few months. This is produced by resumption of the non-specific acitvation of all cortical fields exerted by the diencephalic forerunners of the reticular activating system. The most important of these diencephalic forerunners, perhaps with a spontaneous automatic activity, seems to be the pallidum. Previous experience in stereotaxic operations showed a behavioural and EEG arousal by stimulation of the intralaminar thalamic nuclei and of the pallidum. Both are able to induce non-specific activation of the cortical fields. The pallidal activation includes lateral turning of the eyes and head, awareness and motor activity. The partial functional loss of this non-specific cortical activation after pallidal coagulation for relief of involuntary movements results in slowing down of the alpha rhythm (Ganglberger 1961).

In the apallic patients without spontaneous recovery it was our concept to activate bilaterally the ascending influence of the rostral non-specific thalamic projection nuclei or their pallidal forerunners, to overcome the partial inactivation of electrical cortical activity, which seems to be a precondition of the behavioural recovery from coma vigil. The anatomically undamaged neurones or parts of this non-specific system should be induced to take up again their spontaneous ascending activation of the cortex, necessary for EEG arousal and awareness, by long-term stimulation. This was the hope.

The bilateral repeated stimulation of long duration proved to be effective in respect of behavioural and EEG arousal. Even the electrical activity of pallidum and VA could be excited and accelerated. This stimulus-induced activation of cortical rhythms was connected with motor and psychomotor activities completely independent of the stimulus frequency, such as opening of the eyes, conjugate eye turning to the side opposite to the stimulus, and even spontaneous movements of the left extremities. The long-term stimulation was able to induce even spontaneous activity. Thereby our concept proved to be correct, at least for this behavioural arousal. We failed, however, to induce the return of spontaneous activity in this patient, surviving for more than 5 months after the onset of the apallic syndrome. The same long-term stimulation in apallic syndromes of shorter duration promises the enduring and even progressive therapeutic effect of resuming conscious activity.

SUMMARY

A patient in a state of coma vigil from an apallic syndrome of 5 months' standing was treated by repeated stimulation of the right pallidum and basal portion of the left latero-polar nucleus of the thalamus (VA) by means of flexible electrodes inserted into these structures. Treatment lasted 19 days. Stimulation produced clinical arousal, with spontaneous movements of the left limbs, turning toward nearby persons and affective reactions with unintelligible vocalization, between stimuli. Treatment resulted in a consistently higher level of consciousness, but no further gains were seen after removal of the electrodes at 19 days. EEG monitoring during treatment revealed the disappearance of a left temporal delta focus, reduction of the initial asymmetry and partial restoration of the alpha rhythm. Short bilateral stimuli (pallidum 8 c/sec, VA 50 c/sec) produced immediate desynchronization in all tracings. Stimulation of the left VA (25 c/sec) produced a predominantly ipsilateral acceleration of spontaneous activity with reduced amplitudes.

ZUSAMMENFASSUNG

WECKEFFEKTE IN VERHALTEN UND EEG DURCH REIZUNG DER UNSPEZIFISCHEN PROJEKTIONS-SYSTEME BEI EINEM PATIENTEN MIT POST-TRAUMATISCHEM APPALLISCHEM SYNDROM

Ein Patient mit traumatischem apallischem Syndrom von 5 Monaten Dauer im Stadium des Coma vigile, aber ohne jeden Anhalt für Bewusstseinsvorgänge, wurde durch flexible Elektroden im rechten Pallidum einschliesslich der Lamella pallidi interna (8 oder 25/sec; 30 V) und in der Basis des linken vorderen Thalamuspols (VA) einschliesslich des Bündels H_1 mit 50/sec und 20 V gereizt. Die Doppelreizungen bewirkten klinische Weckeffekte mit Spontanbewegungen der linken Gliedmassen, Spontanzuwendungen zu Personen in der Umgebung und adaequaten affektiven Reaktionen, besonders gegen offenbar erkannte Angehörige; zwischen den Reizungen unverständliche Lautäusserungen. Im EEG hatten die beiderseitigen Reizungen im Pallidum und VA unmittelbar eine Desynchronisation in allen Ableitungen zur Folge. Reizungen des linken VA mit 25/sec bewirkten eine vorwiegend ipsilaterale Beschleunigung der Spontanaktivität mit reduzierten Amplituden.

Als nach 19 Tagen mit täglich 3 Reizperioden von je 15–20 Min. die Reizungen wegen Elektrodenbruchs und verminderter Reaktion der Hirnstrukturen abgebrochen wurden, behielt der Patient die erreichte hellere Bewusstseinslage mit vermehrten Spontanbewegungen der linken Gliedmassen und Zuwendungsreaktionen bei, ohne dass sich eine weitere Besserung anschloss. Der temporale Alpha-Focus links war verschwunden und der Alpha-Rhythmus wiederhergestellt. Durch beiderseitige langdauernde Reizungen der pallidären und der nachgeschalteten thalamischen Strukturen ist es also möglich, beim Coma vigile Weckeffekte nach dem Verhalten und im EEG hervorzurufen. Dabei kann eine anhaltende Besserung der Bewusstseinslage und der Spontanaktivität, aber keine spontan weitergehende Restitution erreicht werden. Die pallidothalamischen Systeme werden als Teile des unspezifischen Aktivierungssystems der Grosshirnrinde angesehen.

REFERENCES

DIECKMANN, G. Cortical synchronized and desynchronized responses evoked by stimulation of the putamen and pallidum in cats. *J. neurol. Sci.*, **1968**, *7*: 385–391.

GANGLBERGER, J. A. Vorübergehende Herdveränderungen im EEG nach stereotaktischen Operationen an den Basalganglien. *Arch. Psychiat. Nervenkr.*, **1961**, *201*: 528–548.

GERSTENBRAND, F. *Das traumatische apallische Syndrom.* Springer, Wien, **1967**, 344 p.

HASSLER, R. Contribution morphologique à la physiologie des lobes frontaux. *C. R. 1st Congr. mond. Psychiat.*, Paris, **1950**, *III*: 118–127.

HASSLER, R. Functional anatomy of the thalamus. *Ann. Vol. Physiol. exp. med. Sci. India*, **1958**, *1*: 56–91.

HASSLER, R. Anatomy of the thalamus. In G. SCHALTENBRAND and P. BAILEY (Eds.), *Introduction to stereotaxis with an atlas of the human brain.* Thieme, Stuttgart, **1959**: 230–290.

HASSLER, R. und RIECHERT, T. Indikationen und Lokalisationsmethode der gezielten Hirnoperationen. *Nervenarzt*, **1954**, *25*: 441–447.

JELLINGER, K. Läsionen des extrapyramidalen Systems bei akuten und prolongierten Komazuständen. *Wien. Z. Nervenheilk.*, **1966**, *23*: 40–73.

RIECHERT, T. und MUNDINGER, F. Beschreibung und Anwendung eines Zielgerätes für stereotaktische Hirnoperationen. (II. Modell). *Acta neurochir. (Wien)*, **1955**, *Suppl. III*: 308–337.

Reference: HASSLER, R., DALLE ORE, G., DIECKMANN, G., BRICOLO, A. and DOLCE, G. Behavioural and EEG arousal induced by stimulation of unspecific projection systems in a patient with post-traumatic apallic syndrome. *Electroenceph. clin. Neurophysiol.*, **1969**, *27*: 306–310.

Electroencephalography and Clinical Neurophysiology
Elsevier Publishing Company, Amsterdam – Printed in The Netherlands

TECHNICAL CONTRIBUTIONS

DISCRIMINANT ANALYSIS IN AVERAGE EVOKED RESPONSE STUDIES: THE STUDY OF SINGLE TRIAL DATA

EMANUEL DONCHIN[1]

Ames Research Center, NASA, Moffett Field, Calif. 94035 (U.S.A.)

(Accepted for publication: January 21, 1969)

An approach to measurement of the similarity of an EEG segment following the onset of a specific stimulus to a given average evoked potential (AEP) is presented. The problem can be stated as follows: given a group of observations on some variable, find a measure of the relative standing of each individual observation in the group with respect to the group mean. This problem is commonly faced by students of psychometrics, and the general approach developed in that field can be usefully applied in evoked response work (Rulon *et al.* 1967).

The basic tool used in specifying the relative standing of a specific individual in a specified group is the "standard score". A standard score is a measure of the deviation of the individual's score from the group mean measured in units of variability. Thus, for example, the mathematics score of an individual might be reported as being one or two standard deviations above or below his peer-group mean score. In addition, when assumptions can be made about the distribution of the variable in question, probability statements can be made about the individual score of the form "the probability that an individual from population X will have a standard score Z is Y".

The following is thus required for a study of individual observations relative to the group mean: (1) a proper estimate of the group mean; (2) a measure of the "distance" between the group mean and the individual observation; (3) a measure of variability in the group in whose units the distance can be expressed. Furthermore, in the case probability statements are sought about the observations, tenable assumptions about the distribution of the data in the parent population must be made. These requirements can be studied in relation to AEPs if one accepts the basic model common to most evoked response studies which leads to conceptualizing each EEG record following the stimulus as a multivariate observation (Donchin 1966), or as a point in an *n*-dimensional space, where *n* is the number of discrete time points at which the EEG is observed following the stimulus.

The basic data in an evoked response experiment are the segments of EEG that follow each stimulus. These segments are digitized at *n* time points; thus, for each stimulus, a vector $X(x_1, x_2, .. x_i, .. x_n)$ is obtained where x_i is the voltage recorded between the electrodes at time point *i*. Each such vector defines a point in an *n*-dimensional space. The collection of vectors obtained for the presentations of each stimulus defines a swarm of points in the space. If we assume that each of the x_i is the sum of the evoked response and normally distributed additive noise, uncorrelated with the evoked response, then the vector has a multivariate normal distribution.

A multivariate normal distribution is completely characterized by two parameters: the mean vector and the variance–covariance matrix. These parameters can be estimated from the data by computing the mean vector $\bar{X}$ with elements $\bar{x}_i$, where each $\bar{x}_i$ is the arithmetic mean of the x_i over the sample. The variance-covariance matrix V is a square symmetric matrix, where v_{ii} is the variance of the x_i, and v_{ij} is the covariance of x_i and x_j.

For a multi-variate distribution of this type, a statistic equivalent to the standard score can be computed. It is defined as

$$(1)\ Z = (X - \bar{X})\, V^{-1}\, (X - \bar{X})'$$

The locus in the space of all the vectors X that yield a specific value for Z is an ellipsoid. The proportion of the distribution that is contained inside the ellipsoid can be computed and thus, in the usual manner, the divergence of any individual observation from the group mean can be specified in terms of the probability that such an observation will be obtained when the distribution is characterized by a specific mean and a variance–covariance matrix.

Thus, the degree to which any individual trial record diverges from a specific average evoked response wave form can be expressed by the probability that such a raw record would be obtained when the evoked response has a specific shape. These probabilities can be obtained through the computation of the appropriate Z scores defined above.

METHODS AND RESULTS

The computations required to obtain these "multivariate standard scores" as well as the calculation of

[1] National Research Council resident research associate on leave from the University of Illinois. This report was presented in a different form before the American EEG Society (*this Journal*, 1968, *24*: 284).

the associated probabilities are performed as part of the computations required in developing a discriminant function. Discriminant analysis is a classification technique that uses the data obtained from members of different groups whose group membership is known to derive criteria for the classification of an observation whose group membership is doubtful. The major outcome of discriminant analysis is a set of discriminant functions which, when applied to the data, can be used to determine in which of a number of groups a new observation should be classified (Rao 1965). It is possible to conceptualize one of the proposed criteria for decision about group membership as a computation of a multivariate standard score for each of the groups in question and the classification of the observation to the group with the smallest score (Rulon *et al.* 1967; for a detailed exposition of the application of discriminant analysis to EEG data, see Walter *et al.* 1967).

The discriminant analysis program I have used is a Step Wise Discriminant Analysis program (SWDA) available as part of the UCLA BMD program package (Dixon 1965, Program 07M). Its use is particularly advantageous in evoked response work because it takes into account the considerable intercorrelation that exists between successive time-points in the AEP. It is common in evoked response research to use digitizing rates of 100–400 samples/sec. However, the evoked responses are usually described by a considerably smaller number of measurements — typically in terms of the peak-to-peak amplitudes and latencies of 6–10 "components". I have shown elsewhere (Donchin 1966) that most of the variance contained in an evoked response data matrix can be accounted for by 6–10 orthogonal components. It is thus clear that it is possible to reduce the dimensionality of the measurement space in which the evoked responses are

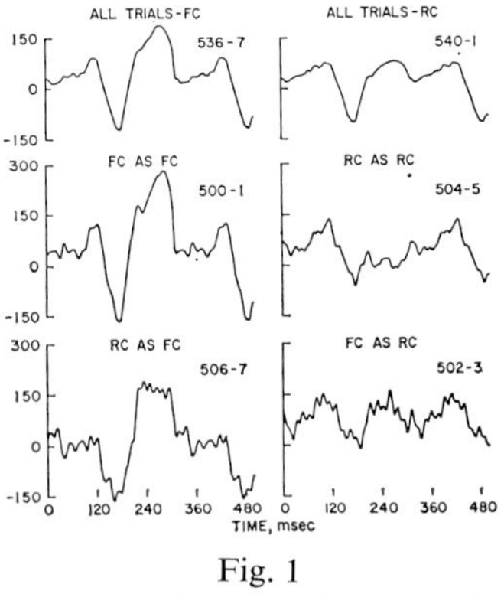

Fig. 1

Visual average evoked potentials recorded between an occipital electrode and an ear reference in two experimental conditions labeled FC and RC. Positivity at the occipital electrode is indicated by an upward deflection. The vertical scale is arbitrary. *Top row*: AEP obtained for all trials in each conditions, $N = 100$. *Other rows*: AEP obtained for different classifications of the trials; *e.g.*, "FC as FC" are those tallied in the last 5 rows of col. 2, Table I, $N = 76$. Note that these are *averages* and thus N does not affect the amplitudes.

TABLE I

Distribution of posterior probabilities for 200 EEG segments

Probability P	Number of FC assigned to FC with P	Number of RC assigned to RC with P
0.001–0.100	1	6
0.101–0.200	4	8
0.201–0.300	6	9
0.301–0.400	7	5
0.401–0.500	6	11
0.501–0.600	5	6
0.601–0.700	14	2
0.701–0.800	14	9
0.801–0.900	24	15
0.901–1.000	19	29
Total	100	100

studied from the 100–400 dimensions represented by the time points to a space of 6–10 dimensions (see Donchin, in press, for a discussion of the dimensionality of the evoked response space). Such a reduction of dimensionality is performed by the SWDA program. The program selects initially that time point which provides the best possible discrimination between the groups in question. After all the information correlated with this point is "removed" from the data, a new point is selected, one that produces the maximal improvement in the discrimination, in combination with the first point. This process continues until there are no points whose inclusion provides a significant improvement in the discrimination. Usually, 6–10 points are sufficient in an evoked response experiment to produce the optimal discrimination between the groups.

To illustrate this technique, I shall present data obtained in a study described in detail by Donchin and Cohen (1967). This study demonstrated a difference in the form of the AEP elicited by the same stimulus as a function of the degree to which that stimulus was task-relevant. The difference can be seen in the two evoked responses in the top row of Fig. 1[1]. Both were elicited by a 50 msec flash of light superimposed on a fluctuating background. The AEP marked FC was obtained when the subject counted the flashes; the one obtained when the subject counted the fluctuations in the background is marked RC. Note, in particular, the difference in the amplitude of the positive-going 300 msec wave (P300). It was precisely at this point that the difference between RC and FC averages was obtained for all subjects in the study.

[1] The digitization rate used in the experiment was 512 points/sec, and all the plots are of 512 point vectors. However, the SWDA program sets a limit of 80 points per input vector; therefore, the input vectors to the program consisted of 80 points per vector evenly spaced at 6 msec per point.

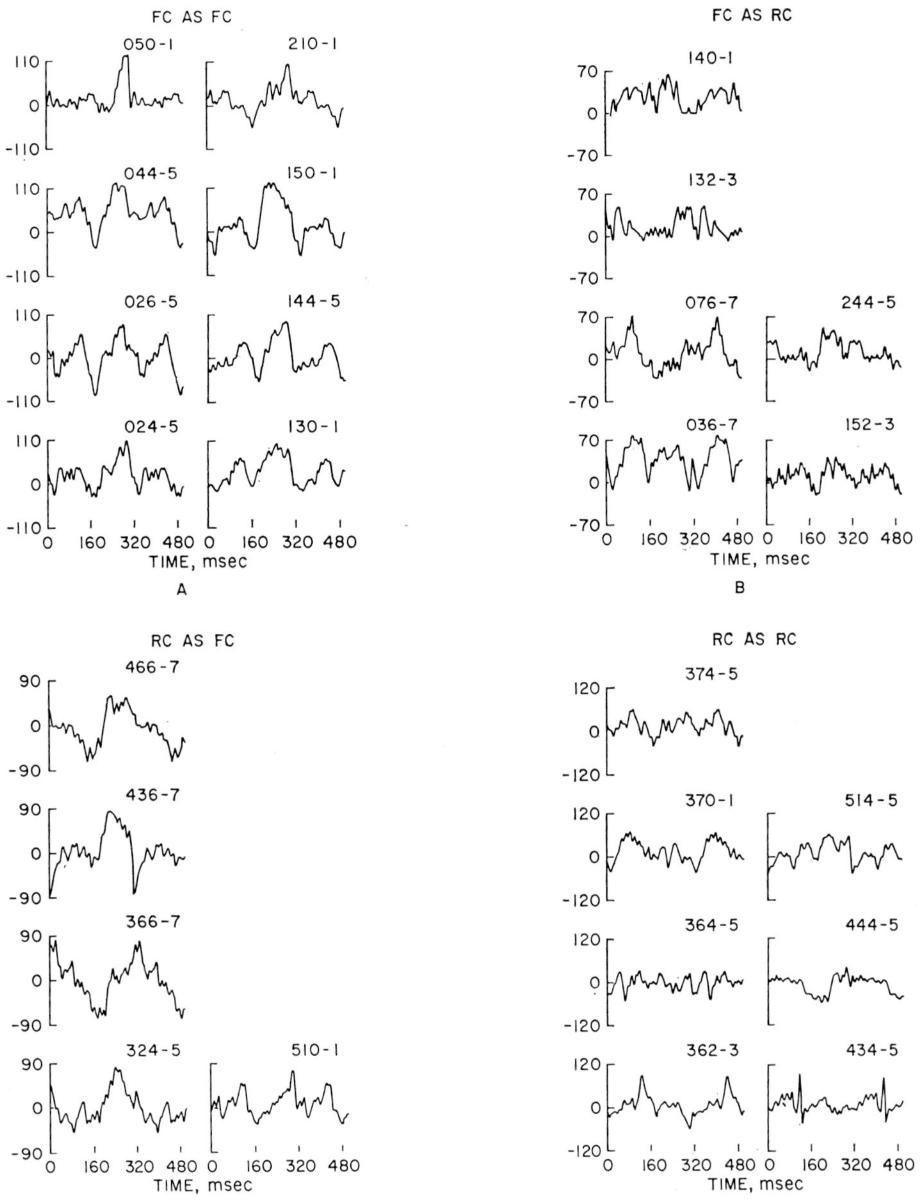

Fig. 2

Some individual segments of EEG used in computing the AEP presented in Fig. 1; the beginning of each segment coincides with stimulus onset. Each segment was assigned with a high probability (greater than 0.80) to the indicated group.

Each of these averages was based on 100 stimulus presentations. The 200 individual EEG segments were used as input to the SWDA program. Only five points were found to be useful by the program; these were (in the order selected) at 330, 360, 420, 162 and 480 msec, respectively. The probability that each observation belongs to each of the two groups was obtained. The probability distribution is presented in Table I, which shows the frequency with which members of each group were assigned to that group with a given probability. Most members of a given group were assigned a high probability of belonging to that group, though some members of each group were assigned a higher probability of belonging to the alternate group. The interpretation of these assignments is shown in Fig. 2 where individual observations with a high and a low probability of belonging to each group are plotted. Interestingly, all the traces classified as belonging with a high probability to group FC show a considerable positive swing with a latency of about 300 msec, whereas all those assigned to group RC are rather flat.

Some indication of the implications of the classification operation can be obtained from rows 2 and 3 of Fig. 1. The four AEP curves were obtained by averaging all observations in one group (FC and RC) that were classified as belonging to a given group. It will be noted that such selective averaging serves to underline the difference between the FC and RC experimental condition: trials classified as FC tend to show a prominent P300 component while in "RC trials" this component is virtually absent. These data have an interesting implication. It appears that during the period in which the stimulus was presumably task-relevant some trials yielded an AEP wave form that is typical of irrelevant stimuli. It is, of course, to be expected that subjects would perform such tasks with a fluctuating degree of zeal, and we might thus be able to detect such trials. However, this cannot be established without access to some independent behavioral measure of trial-to-trial variability in "zeal".

SUMMARY

The data presented suggest that it is possible to make meaningful comparisons between EEG records obtained with a single presentation of the stimulus and the average evoked potential. The technique for measuring evoked response similarity assumes that each record represents a point in a multi-dimensional space, and similarity is defined as the Euclidean distance in this space.

RÉSUMÉ

ANALYSE DISCRIMINATOIRE À L'INTÉRIEUR DES ÉTUDES DE RÉPONSES ÉVOQUÉES MOYENNES: L'ÉTUDE DES DONNÉES PAR STIMULUS UNIQUE

Les faits présentés indiquent qu'il est possible de faire des comparaisons significatives entre les réponses EEG obtenues par présentation unique d'un stimulus et les potentiels évoqués moyens. La technique permettant de mesurer la similarité des réponses évoquées postule que chaque tracé représente un point dans un espace multidimensionnel, et la similarité est définie comme la distance Euclidienne dans cet espace.

REFERENCES

DIXON, W. J. (Ed.). *BMD-biomedical computer programs.* Univ. of California, Los Angeles, **1965,** 620 p.

DONCHIN, E. A multivariate approach to the analysis of average evoked potentials. *IEEE Trans. biomed. Engng.*, **1966,** *BME-13*: 131–139.

DONCHIN, E. Data analysis techniques in evoked potential research. In E. DONCHIN and D. B. LINDSLEY (Eds.), *Average evoked potentials—methods, results, evaluation.* NASA SP-191. Government Printing Office. In press.

DONCHIN, E. and COHEN, L. Average devoked potentials and intramodality selective attention. *Electroenceph. clin. Neurophysiol.*, **1967,** *22*: 537–546.

RAO, C. R. *Linear statistical inference and its applications.* Wiley, New York, **1965,** 522 p.

RULON, P. J., TIEDMAN, D. V., TATSUOKA, M. M. and LANGMUIR, C. R. *Multivariate statistics for personnel classification.* Wiley, New York, **1967,** 406 p.

WALTER, D. O., RHODES, J. M. and ADEY, W. R. Discriminating among states of consciousness by EEG measurements. A study of four subjects. *Electroenceph. clin. Neurophysiol.*, **1967,** *22*: 22–29.

Reference: DONCHIN, E. Discriminant analysis in average evoked response studies: the study of single trial data. *Electroenceph. clin. Neurophysiol.*, **1969,** *27*: 311–314.

ÉTUDE DU BRUIT RÉSIDUEL DES POTENTIELS ÉVOQUÉS MOYENS

D. Arnal[1] et P. Gerin[2]

Laboratoire de Neuroélectrologie, Hôpital Neurologique, 59 Bd. Pinel, 69-Lyon 3 (France)

(Accepted for publication: December 6, 1968)

A la suite de Kitasato et Hatsuda (1965, 1966), nous étudions la contamination des potentiels évoqués moyens (PEM) visuels par du rythme alpha résiduel, mais les notions développées ici et les résultats sont valables pour n'importe quel potentiel évoqué moyen. De nombreux PEM visuels possèdent une réponse oscillante tardive à la fréquence moyenne du rythme alpha du sujet, (Barlow 1960); est-elle du rythme alpha mal éliminé par la sommation ou au contraire une composante significative de la réponse évoquée? L'étude de ce problème nous a conduit: (1) à regarder comment s'élimine le rythme alpha au cours d'une sommation, et (2) à déterminer quelle amplitude doit atteindre un grapho-élément d'un PEM en fin de sommation pour se distinguer significativement du bruit de fond résiduel avec un risque d'erreur donné. Nous appliquons cette méthode pour discuter la nature de la réponse oscillante tardive.

MÉTHODE

Le matériel utilisé a été décrit dans un article précédent (Arnal et Gerin 1969).

L'EEG a été enregistré en montage monopolaire à partir d'un point situé à 3 cm au-dessus de l'inion sur la ligne médiane, la tension de référence étant prise aux lobules des oreilles court-circuités entre eux. Les stimuli lumineux étaient présentés aux deux yeux simultanément soit de façon périodique, soit de façon aléatoire grâce à un générateur produisant une succession d'intervalles de temps aléatoires distribués suivant une probabilité uniforme, la dispersion maximum des stimuli par rapport à la valeur moyenne des intervalles étant de 100 msec.

Nous supposons que les stimuli sont présentés de façon suffisamment espacée pour qu'il n'y ait aucune interférence entre potentiels évoqués successifs, et qu'un potentiel évoqué est un phénomène aléatoire stationnaire du second ordre, c'est-à-dire que la forme moyenne du potentiel évoqué et sa variance sont constantes bien qu'il ne se répète pas toujours de façon identique à lui-même.

Nous avons adopté la définition suivante du rapport (S/b) qui caractérise non pas un potentiel évoqué tout entier mais un élément particulier choisi en fonction du problème étudié.

$$(1) \qquad (S/b)_1 = \frac{E(s)}{\sqrt{p}}$$

le symbole E désignant l'espérance mathématique, p étant la puissance de l'activité électrique cérébrale et s étant l'amplitude de l'élément considéré. Par exemple, si on veut savoir si le système visuel a répondu au stimulus, on prendra pour s l'amplitude maximum du potentiel évoqué. La définition correspondante pour un PEM est,

$$(2) \qquad (S/b)_N = \frac{E(S)}{\sqrt{P}}$$

P étant la puissance transportée par le bruit sommé N fois et S étant l'amplitude correspondant à s. Naturellement $E(S) = N\cdot E(s)$. L'amélioration du rapport (S/b) due à N sommations est donc:

$$(3) \qquad \frac{(S/b)_N}{(S/b)_1} = \frac{E(S)/\sqrt{P}}{E(s)/\sqrt{p}} = N\sqrt{\frac{p}{P}}$$

Remarquons que nous appelons potentiel évoqué "moyen" la somme et non la moyenne de plusieurs potentiels évoqués.

La notion de rapport (S/b) peut être facilement reliée à la notion de variance puisque, pour un bruit de fond, les définitions de la puissance et de la variance coïncident. La variance du bruit de fond est $\sigma_1^2 = p$; celle du bruit sommé N fois est $\sigma_N^2 = P$. Par conséquent, si nous appelons variance normalisée le rapport σ_N^2/σ_1^2 celle-ci est reliée à l'amélioration du rapport (S/b) par la relation (4):

$$(4) \qquad \text{Amélioration de } (S/b) = \frac{N}{\sqrt{\text{variance normalisée}}}$$

Les variances sont estimées de la façon suivante: les enregistrements sur papier de bruit seul ou de bruit sommé sont échantillonnés à 50 c/sec; la variance empirique est calculée par la formule,

$$(5) \qquad \sigma^2 = \frac{1}{r-1} \sum_{i=1}^{r} (x_i - \bar{x})^2$$

[1] Attachée de Recherches à l'I.N.S.E.R.M.
[2] Maître de Recherches à l'I.N.S.E.R.M.

qui donne une estimation sans biais de la variance. r est le nombre d'échantillons et x leur amplitude.

RÉSULTATS

Les résultats expérimentaux présentés donnent: *1ère partie*: l'évolution de la variance et du rapport (S/b) *au cours de la sommation* d'une activité électrique occipitale de repos riche en rythme alpha.

2ème partie: une étude statistique sur 100 sujets de l'amplitude de l'oscillation tardive des PEM par rapport à l'écart-type du bruit résiduel *en fin de sommation*.

1ÈRE PARTIE

A. *Expérience modèle*

Afin de voir schématiquement ce qui se passe nous avons simulé un rythme alpha par une sinusoïde (raie de bruit) de fréquence $f = 10$ c/sec que nous avons sommée:

1. *De façon périodique*

(i) La période de sommation T étant un multiple entier de $1/f$. Dans ce cas, la sinusoïde se retrouve exactement en phase avec elle-même à chaque pas de la sommation et son amplitude croît linéairement en fonction de N (Fig. 1, ligne 1).

(ii) T n'étant pas un multiple entier de $1/f$. Il se produit alors un phénomène de battements; l'amplitude de la sinusoïde sommée croît puis décroît périodiquement en formant une succession de fuseaux dont un seul est représenté sur la figure (Fig. 1, ligne 2).

Calculons l'évolution de la variance et du rapport (S/b). Soit $x(t)$ une fonction aléatoire de moyenne nulle stationnaire du second ordre.

(6) $$\sigma_N^2 = \sum_{u=0}^{N-1}\sum_{v=0}^{N-1} E[X(t+uT)\cdot X(t+vT)]$$

(7) $$\sigma_N^2 = \sum_{u=0}^{N-1}\sum_{v=0}^{N-1} C[(u-v)\,T]$$

$C(\tau)$ représentant la fonction d'autocorrélation de $X(t)$. Si $X(t)$ est une raie de bruit de puissance p, $C(\tau) = p\,e^{2\pi\, \mathrm{i}f\tau}$

(8) d'où

$$\sigma_N^2 = \sum_{u=1}^{N-1}\sum_{v=1}^{N-1} p\,e^{2\pi\, \mathrm{i}f(u-v)T} = p\left(\frac{\sin N\pi Tf}{\sin \pi Tf}\right)^2$$

Or $\sigma_1^2 = p$

(9) d'où la variance normalisée:

$$\frac{\sigma_N^2}{\sigma_1^2} = \left(\frac{\sin N\pi Tf}{\sin \pi Tf}\right)^2$$

D'après la relation (4) l'amélioration du rapport (S/b) due à N sommations est donc:

(10) $$\frac{(S/b)_N}{(S/b)_1} = N\left(\frac{\sin \pi Tf}{\sin N\pi Tf}\right)$$

De ces formules on peut déduire:

(i) si $T = \frac{k}{f}$, k entier, alors:

(11) $$\frac{\sigma_N^2}{\sigma_1^2} = N^2;\ \frac{(S/b)_N}{(S/b)_1} = 1;\ \frac{\sigma N}{\sigma_1} = N$$

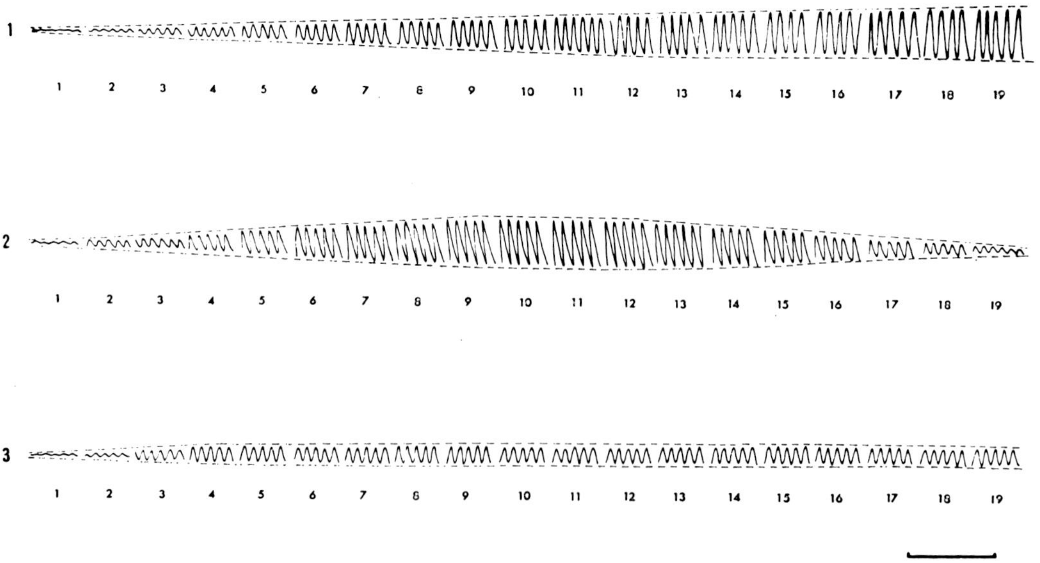

Fig 1

Sommation d'une raie de bruit $f = 10$ c/sec. 1, avec une période $T = 1$ sec. Croissance linéaire du bruit en fonction de N. 2, avec une période T légèrement différente de 1 sec. Phénomène de battements. 3, avec des intervalles aléatoires. Croissance comme $\sqrt{N}$.

Physiquement, l'écart-type σ_N du bruit sommé croît linéairement (donc aussi vite que le signal) (Fig. 1, ligne 1). La variance croît paraboliquement (Fig. 2, courbe C) et le rapport (S/b) ne s'améliore absolument pas (Fig. 2, courbe C′).

(ii) Si le produit $T{\cdot}f$ est différent d'un nombre entier, la variance s'annule chaque fois que $N = k/fT$, k étant un nombre entier. Physiquement, il se produit un phénomène de battements (Fig. 1, ligne 2). L'amélioration du rapport (S/b) se fait en moyenne comme N.

2. *De façon aléatoire*

L'amplitude croît alors comme $\sqrt{N}$ (Fig. 1, ligne 3) ce qui coïncide avec les résultats de Kitasato et Hatsuda (1965, 1966) qui ont démontré que l'amélioration du rapport (S/b) se faisait alors comme $\sqrt{N}$ (Fig. 3, courbe E′) ce qui implique une variance se comportant comme N (Fig. 3, courbe E).

Cette expérience modèle montre que si un bruit est une sinusoïde pure, la sommation peut, soit ne pas l'éliminer du tout (cas i), soit l'éliminer très énergiquement (cas ii), soit l'éliminer comme $\sqrt{N}$.

B. *Évolution du rythme alpha au cours d'une sommation*

Le rythme alpha étant proche d'une sinusoïde, nous avons refait cette même expérience, avec le rythme alpha de vingt sujets laissés au repos les yeux fermés. Nous distinguons l'évolution à court terme (0.5–1 min) de l'évolution à long terme, qui s'avère plus complexe.

(a) *Évolution à court terme*

1. *Sommation périodique à court terme*

(i) Cas $T = k/f$, k entier (Fig. 2). La variance normalisée croît paraboliquement, moins vite que dans le cas de la raie de bruit (courbe C), mais beaucoup plus vite que la variance d'un bruit à large bande qui, d'après un résultat classique, croîtrait comme N (courbe A). L'évolution correspondante du rapport (S/b) déduite de l'évolution de la variance normalisée par la formule (4) se fait suivant une portion de branche d'hyperbole avec une asymptote horizontale. Autrement dit, le rapport (S/b) s'améliore correctement pendant les premières sommations puis il y a tendance à saturation. L'amélioration est beaucoup moins bonne que $\sqrt{N}$.

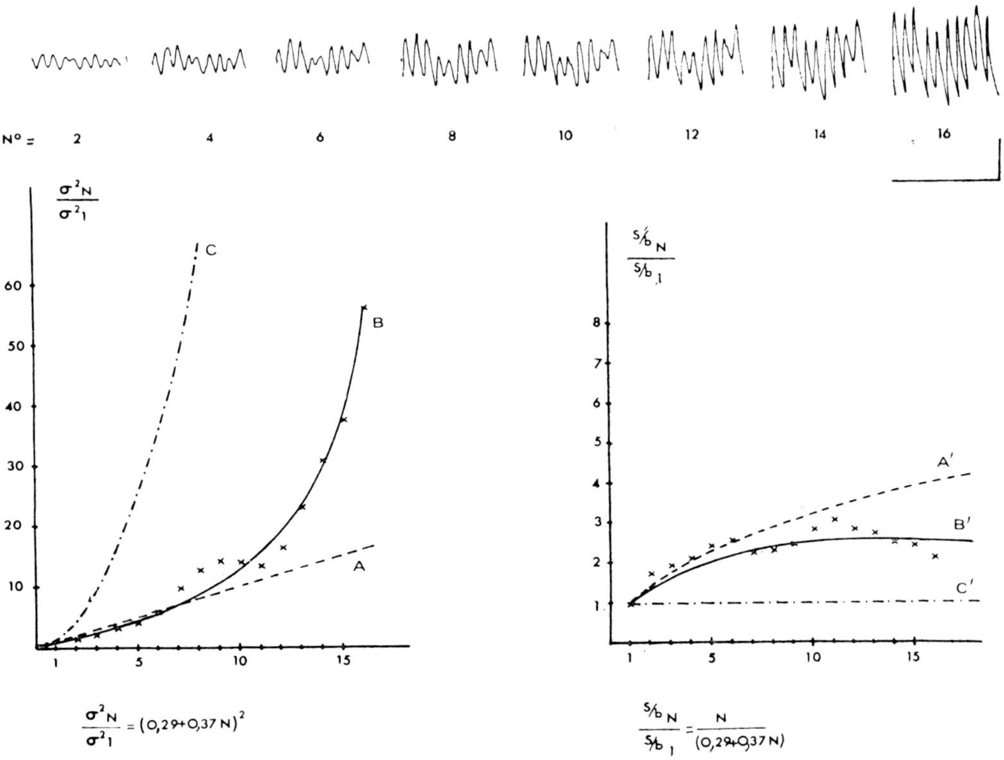

Fig. 2

Évolution de la variance normalisée (à gauche) et de l'amélioration du rapport (S/b) (à droite) dans le cas d'une sommation périodique, la période $T = 1$ sec étant un multiple entier de celle du rythme alpha. Courbes A et A′: bruit à large bande (courbes théoriques), Courbes B et B′: rythme alpha de fréquence moyenne, $f = 10$ c/sec, Courbes C et C′: raie de bruit de fréquence 10 c/sec, (courbes théoriques), Calibration horizontale: 1 sec. Calibration verticale: 0,5 mV. Les chiffres de la 2ème ligne signifient le nombre de sommations.

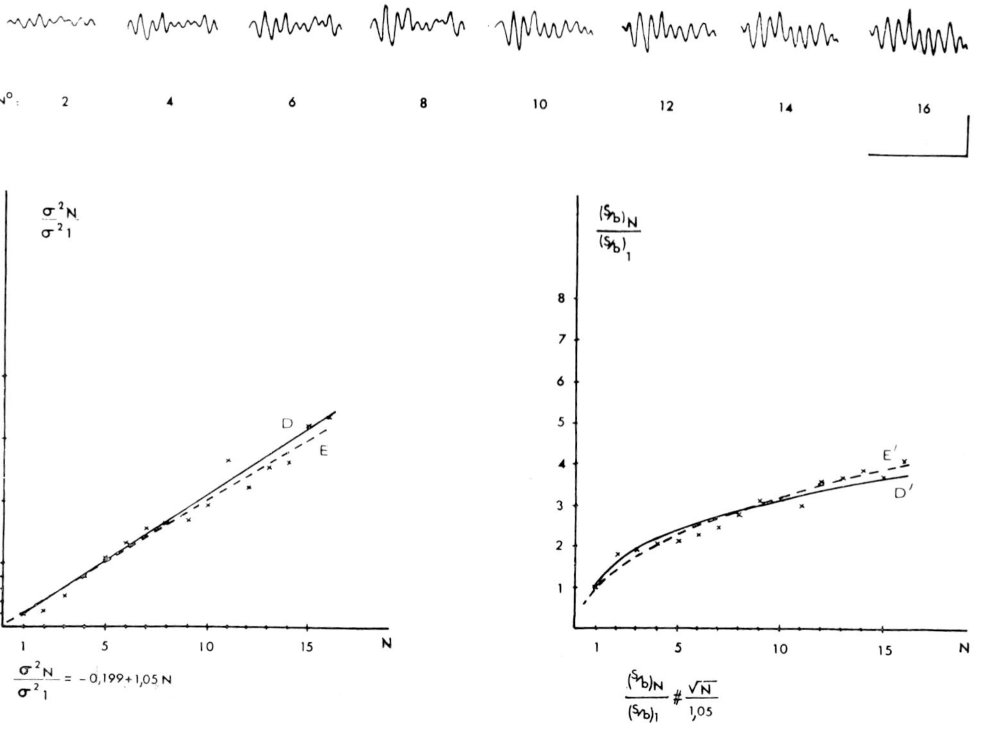

Fig. 3

Évolution de la variance normalisée (à gauche) et de l'amélioration du rapport (S/b) (à droite) dans le cas d'une sommation aléatoire d'un rythme alpha. Courbes D et D′: expérimentales. Courbes E et E′: théoriques. Calibration horizontale: 1 sec. Calibration verticale: 0,5 mV.

(ii) Cas $T \neq k/f$, k entier. Le phénomène de battements peut être observé lorsque le rythme alpha est extrêmement stable et continu. La variance normalisée fluctue autour d'une valeur moyenne constante et l'amélioration du rapport (S/b) se fait en moyenne linéairement donc beaucoup plus vite que $\sqrt{N}$.

Lorsque le rythme alpha est instable, les deux évolutions typiques que nous venons de décrire s'estompent et on observe une évolution intermédiaire, approximativement linéaire pour la variance normalisée et comme $\sqrt{N}$ pour le rapport (S/b).

2. *Sommation aléatoire à court terme*

Ruchkin (1965) a proposé un mode de sommation aléatoire particulier (distribution uniforme des intervalles de temps) devant permettre de ramener le plus possible le comportement d'un bruit à bande étroite à celui d'un bruit à large bande ce qui élimine le cas 1 (i) où l'extraction du signal du bruit est très mauvaise. Nous avons essayé expérimentalement ce mode de sommation et les résultats sont les suivants: la variance normalisée évolue toujours à peu près linéairement et le rapport (S/b) paraboliquement (Fig. 3).

(b) *Évolution à long terme*

1. *Sommation périodique.* A long terme, c'est à-dire lorsque la période de temps analysée dépasse 0.5–1 min, l'évolution du bruit au cours de la sommation est en général moins homogène: les courbes expérimentales ressemblent à une succession de courbes comme celles que nous avons obtenues à court terme. On peut observer de brusques accélérations paraboliques de la variance correspondant à des plateaux dans l'amélioration du rapport (S/b) (Fig. 4, parties 1 et 4), ainsi que des zones où la variance croît linéairement (Fig. 4, partie 2) et des zones où la variance oscille (Fig. 4, partie 4, amorce d'un phénomène de battements). Enfin, l'amélioration finale du rapport (S/b) est en général de l'ordre de $\sqrt{N}$.

2. *Sommation aléatoire*

Les courbes expérimentales à long terme en sommation aléatoire montrent elles-aussi quelques fluctuations mais s'écartent relativement moins d'une évolution comme N pour la variance, comme $\sqrt{N}$ pour le rapport (S/b).

L'évolution expérimentale de l'amélioration du rapport (S/b) est donc fonction de différents facteurs: la stabilité du rythme alpha, le mode de sommation périodique ou aléatoire, la valeur de la fréquence moyenne f du rythme alpha par rapport à la période T de la sommation.

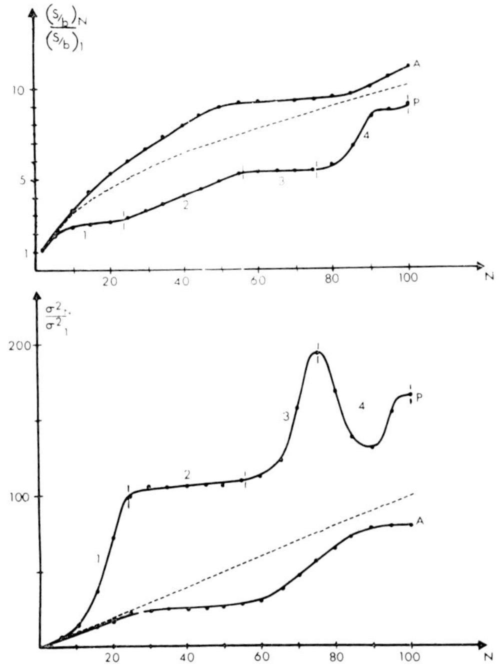

Fig. 4

Évolution à long terme du rapport (S/b) (en haut) et de la variance normalisée (en bas). Courbes A: sommation aléatoire. Courbes P: sommation périodique, $T = 1$ sec.

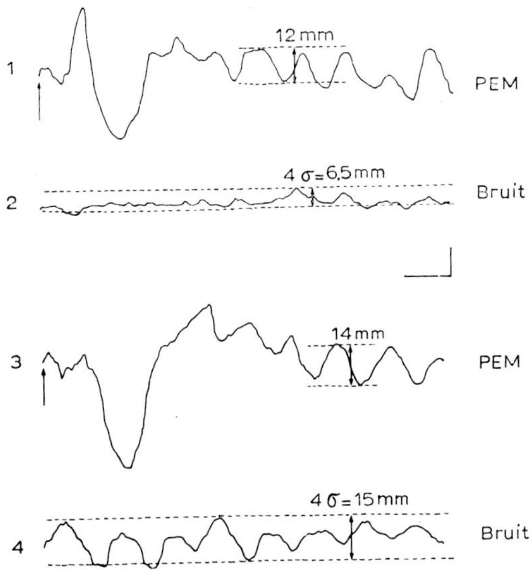

Fig. 5

PEM (ligne 1) et bruit résiduel correspondant (ligne 2). L'oscillation tardive de ce PEM n'est pas du bruit résiduel. PEM (ligne 3) et bruit résiduel correspondant (ligne 4). L'hypothèse que l'oscillation tardive est du bruit résiduel ne peut pas être rejetée. Calibration horizontale: 100 msec. Calibration verticale: 1 mV.

2ÈME PARTIE

Comparaison de l'amplitude de l'oscillation tardive avec l'écart-type du bruit résiduel

L'extraction du signal du bruit ne pouvant être parfaite, il est nécessaire de déterminer en fin de sommation quelle amplitude doit atteindre un grapho-élément d'un PEM pour se distinguer significativement du bruit de fond résiduel.

(a) *Détermination du seuil d'amplitude significative.* Si on admet que le bruit de fond est un processus aléatoire gaussien, ce qui est justifié par les résultats de Saunders (1963), le bruit sommé est encore gaussien et on peut calculer la probabilité pour que son amplitude dépasse un certain seuil. Considérons un tracé résultant de la sommation de N tranches de bruit seul (Fig. 5, ligne 2, par exemple); il peut être échantillonné en r échantillons. Un échantillon quelconque x_i est une variable aléatoire normale dont la variance peut être estimée par:

$$\sigma^2 = \frac{1}{r-1} \sum_{i=1}^{r} (x_i - \bar{x})^2 \tag{12}$$

Donc $t_i = (x_i - \bar{x})/\sigma$ est une variable aléatoire normale centrée réduite. D'après les tables donnant la probabilité pour qu'une telle variable dépasse un certain seuil,

$$\text{Prob}\ [\,|t_i| > 2\,] = \text{Prob}\ [\,|x_i - \bar{x}| > 2\sigma] = 0{,}0456 \tag{13}$$

La probabilité pour que l'amplitude maximum du bruit par rapport à la ligne moyenne dépasse 2σ est donc légèrement inférieure à 5%. Or, sous réserve de stationnarité, l'écart-type σ mesuré sur l'enregistrement du bruit seul est également celui du bruit résiduel contenu dans le PEM obtenu dans les mêmes conditions. Par conséquent, si l'amplitude d'un grapho-élément du PEM par rapport à la ligne de base (ligne moyenne du bruit seul) est supérieure à $2\,\sigma$, on est en droit de conclure avec un risque d'erreur inférieur à 5% que cet élément est significatif; par contre, si son amplitude est inférieure à $2\,\sigma$, on ne peut pas rejeter l'hypothèse que c'est du bruit résiduel. Le critère est naturellement valable pour la réponse évoquée toute entière, des grapho-éléments de la phase précoce à ceux de la phase tardive.

(b) *Solution pratique pour mesurer 4 σ.* La méthode classique d'estimation de σ par échantillonnage et calcul de la somme des carrés des écarts étant très longue, nous proposons une solution pratique pour mesurer $4\,\sigma$ de façon simple et suffisamment précise. La probabilité pour que l'amplitude du bruit par rapport à la ligne de base dépasse $2\,\sigma$ étant environ 5%, le bruit va effectivement dépasser cette limite soit au-dessus soit au-dessous de la ligne de base pendant environ 1/20e du temps analysé; ceci peut être remarqué sur la Fig. 5, tracés 2 et 4. Il suffit donc de tracer deux droites parallèles équidistantes par rapport à la ligne de base de façon que le bruit dépasse cette marge pendant environ 1/20e du temps analysé; la distance entre ces deux droites donne alors une bonne estimation du $4\,\sigma$.

(c) *Application à l'étude de l'oscillation tardive des PEM.* D'après le paragraphe a, si l'amplitude crête à crête de l'oscillation tardive d'un PEM est supérieure à 4 σ on est en droit de conclure avec un risque de 5 % que cette oscillation est une composante significative du PEM; si elle est inférieure ou égale à 4 σ, on ne peut pas rejeter l'hypothèse que c'est du bruit résiduel.

Sur 100 sujets, nous avons systématiquement comparé l'amplitude crête à crête de l'oscillation tardive avec 4 fois l'écart-type σ du bruit résiduel mesuré sur une sommation du bruit seul effectuée dans les mêmes conditions, immédiatement avant ou après la série de stimuli. Lorsque les sujets gardent les yeux fermés, 40 % des PEM présentent une oscillation tardive mais 30 % seulement sont supérieures à 4 σ et 10 % lui sont inférieures. Lorsque les sujets gardent les yeux ouverts, 10 % des enregistrements montrent une oscillation tardive et toutes sont inférieures à 4 σ.

Le critère proposé permet d'interpréter ces résultats de la façon suivante: on observe une réponse oscillante tardive significative chez près d'un tiers des sujets quand on stimule les yeux fermés, mais jamais les yeux ouverts. Ceci confirme les relations étroites entre les générateurs d'alpha et cette oscillation tardive, déjà suggérées par la fréquence de cette dernière.

DISCUSSION

Du point de vue méthodologique, l'estimation de σ^2 gagnerait à être automatisée ainsi que l'enregistrement des courbes d'évolution de la variance.

Un rythme biologique n'étant jamais une sinusoïde pure, son comportement devrait être mieux décrit par un bruit à "bande étroite" que par une raie de bruit. C'est pourquoi nous avons mené une comparaison systématique de nos résultats expérimentaux avec les résultats théoriques de Weiss (1963) et Ruchkin (1965) sur les bruits à "bande étroite", qu'il serait trop long de rappeler ici. A court terme la forme des courbes expérimentales concorde bien avec les courbes théoriques. En particulier la méthode de sommation aléatoire proposée par Ruchkin (1965) apporte effectivement une amélioration comme le montre la comparaison des Fig. 2 et 3 obtenues à partir du même rythme alpha.

A long terme, la divergence entre les résultats expérimentaux et théoriques s'accentue ce qui peut s'expliquer par plusieurs raisons: les fluctuations de la fréquence centrale f de l'alpha qui peuvent faire passer l'évolution du bruit d'un mode à un autre ($f = k/T$ à $f \neq k/T$, par exemple); les changements de phase possibles de l'alpha au début de nouvelles bouffées.

Enfin, après une période de temps assez longue (2 min environ), la fréquence centrale ayant beaucoup fluctué, tout se passe comme si le rythme alpha avait été un bruit à bande beaucoup plus large; il n'est pas étonnant que l'amélioration finale du rapport (S/b) soit alors de l'ordre de $\sqrt{N}$. La méthode de sommation aléatoire proposée par Ruchkin est donc intéressante pour obtenir une meilleure extraction du signal du bruit à court terme mais s'avère inutile à long terme.

Les conclusions de la seconde partie de cette étude confirment partiellement celles de Kitasato et Hatsuda (1965, 1966) qui reconnaissent globalement les ondes oscillantes "alpha like" tardives comme une véritable réponse à la stimulation photique. Mais la méthode présentée ici est beaucoup plus générale puisqu'elle permet d'éviter d'interpréter à tort tous les éléments d'amplitude trop faible des PEM. (Nous pensons en particulier aux éléments précoces qui ont souvent fait l'objet d'interprétations hâtives.) Nous avons choisi le seuil à 5 % car la grandeur 4 σ est très proche de la notion très subjective habituellement utilisée d'amplitude crête à crête du bruit. La comparaison que nous faisons est donc très naturelle puisqu'elle revient à comparer les amplitudes crête à crête de l'oscillation tardive et du bruit résiduel.

Naturellement ce critère repose sur l'hypothèse fragile de la stationnarité du bruit de fond. Il faut donc ajouter au risque de 5 % de conclure à tort qu'un élément de la réponse est significatif, le risque malheureusement non mesurable dû à la non-stationnarité.

RÉSUMÉ

Cet article donne une étude expérimentale de l'évolution réelle du rapport (S/b) au cours d'une sommation et du bruit résiduel en fin de sommation. Il en résulte que:

1. La description du rythme alpha qui concorde le mieux avec les résultats expérimentaux est celle d'un bruit à bande étroite mais dont la fréquence centrale fluctue lentement de façon aléatoire;
2. La méthode de sommation aléatoire proposée par Ruchkin (1965) est intéressante pour obtenir une meilleure extraction du signal du bruit à court terme mais s'avère inutile à long terme;
3. Seuls les grapho-éléments des potentiels évoqués moyens d'amplitude supérieure à 2 fois l'écart-type du bruit résiduel se distinguent significativement du bruit de fond avec un risque d'erreur inférieur à 5 %;
4. En appliquant le critère précédent à une centaine de sujets, des réponses tardives oscillantes significatives ont été observées chez 30 % des sujets gardant les yeux fermés mais chez aucun sujet gardant les yeux ouverts;
5. Une solution pratique simple est proposée pour mesurer 4 fois l'écart-type du bruit résiduel.

SUMMARY

STUDY OF THE RESIDUAL NOISE OF AVERAGE EVOKED POTENTIALS

This paper describes an experimental study of the actual evolution of the signal-noise ratio during summation and of the residual noise at the end of summation. The results were as follows.

1. The description of the alpha rhythm which agreed best with the experimental results was that of narrow band noise in which the central frequency fluctuated slowly in a random fashion;
2. The method of random summation proposed by Ruchkin (1965) was valuable to obtain better extraction of the short term noise but proved useless in the long term;
3. Only the components of the averaged evoked po-

tentials with amplitudes greater than twice the standard deviation of the residual noise were significantly different from the background noise, with a probability of error less than 5%;

4. Applying the above criteria to 100 subjects, significant late oscillatory responses were seen in 30% of the subjects with the eyes closed but in no subject with the eyes open;

5. A simple practical way of measuring 4 times the standard deviation of the residual noise is proposed.

Nous tenons à remercier tout spécialement M. le Professeur R. Arnal (I.N.S.A. Lyon) pour l'aide et les encouragements qu'il nous a sans arrêt prodigués, Mme. David et Mlle. Munier pour l'apport de leur expérience des PEM.

BIBLIOGRAPHIE

ARNAL, D. et GERIN, P. Comparaison des potentiels évoqués moyens à l'aide d'un test T^2 généralisé. Application au problème de l'interférence des réponses évoquées visuelles successives. *Electroenceph. clin. Neurophysiol.*, **1969**, *26*: 325–331.

BARLOW, J. S. Rhythmic activity induced by photic stimulation in relation to intrinsic alpha activity of the brain in man. *Electroenceph. clin. Neurophysiol.*, **1960**, *12*: 317–326.

KITASATO, H. and HATSUDA, T. The degree of contamination of averaged evoked responses with alpha waves and alpha-like waves evoked by photic stimulation. *Jap. J. Physiol.*, **1965**, *15*: 492–504.

KITASATO, H. and HATSUDA, T. The cortical responses evoked by double photic stimuli in various states of man. *Jap. J. Physiol.*, **1966**, *16*: 227–237.

RUCHKIN, D. S. An analysis of average response computations based upon aperiodic stimuli. *IEEE Trans. bio.-med. Engng.*, **1965**, *2*: 87–94.

SAUNDERS, M. G. Amplitude probability density studies on alpha and alpha-like patterns. *Electroenceph. clin. Neurophysiol.*, **1963**, *15*: 761–767.

WEISS, M. S. *An evoked reponse study of a differential conditioned avoidance response utilizing an average response computer*, M.S. Thesis, Univ. of Rochester, Rochester, NY., **1963**.

Référence: ARNAL, D. et GERIN, P. Étude du bruit résiduel des potentiels évoqués moyens. *Electroenceph. clin. Neurophysiol.*, **1969**, *27*: 315–321.

Electroencephalography and Clinical Neurophysiology
Elsevier Publishing Company, Amsterdam – Printed in The Netherlands

SOCIETY PROCEEDINGS

A REVIEW OF SOVIET PAPERS

Published in the first half of 1967

V. A. TCHERNYSHEVA

Institute of Experimental Medicine, Kirovsky 69/71, Leningrad P-22 (U.S.S.R.)

1. [Analysis of the ascending activation of evoked potentials in cerebral cortex to stimulation of urinary bladder receptors.] P. K. Anokhin and G. K. Kadyrov. — Fiziol. Zh. (Leningr.), 1967, 53: 473.

According to the concepts of P. K. Anokhin's laboratory, ascending influences on cortial synaptic organization are of multiple character and interact inevitably either on one and the same neurone or on the synaptic organization of adjacent neurones.

Evoked potentials from the focus of maximum activity of the sciatic nerve projection in the contralateral cortex prior to, against the background of, and after the cessation of urinary bladder stimulation were used as a cortical activity indicator. Two stimuli of different modalities: to the sciatic nerve and by distension of the urinary bladder, one visceral and the other somatic, were sent to the cortical neurones. It was presumed that any variation in the evoked potential would testify to the competition of the two stimuli on the dendrites of the cortical neurones. The experiments were performed under acute conditions on 20 rabbits anaesthetized with urethane. The electrical activity of the reticular formation of the pons, the mesencephalon, the thalamus and the sensori-motor and occipital (bilateral) cortex was recorded from nichrome electrodes, 0.1–0.2 mm in cross-section. Comparative analysis of the EEG of the cortex and subcortical regions with stimulation of the interoceptors showed that the desynchronization of rhythm appeared first in the reticular formation of the brain-stem, the cortical changes being somewhat delayed. Restoration of the background electrical activity developed in the reverse order.

With intensification of the signal from the bladder quite consistent regular adverse changes occurred, first in the components and parameters of the evoked potential, which led to a sharp drop and then to a temporary attenuation, *i.e.*, the so-called masking, of the evoked potential.

In accordance with F. Ata-Muradova's findings (that the negative component of the evoked potential is an expression of post-synaptic potentials at apical dendrites, *i.e.*, in the plexiform layer of the cortex) it is concluded that the masking is associated with desynchronization developing on the same synaptic organizations in the plexiform layer which are activated by the ascending influences from the reticular system of the brain-stem, the latter being activated by afferent signals from the vegetative organs.

This served as a proof of the specific ascending activating influence of the reticular formation of the brain-stem, depending on the character of the afferent impulses transmitted to the cortex (Anokhin *et al.*).

Under the effect of 1% benactyzine no marked changes in the components of the evoked potential were produced by the stimulation of the bladder. Prolongation of the latency of the evoked potential during bladder stimulation and the action of benactyzine might be due to its cholinolytic effect.

It is concluded that interoceptive influences from the bladder on the cortical synaptic organizations in the plexiform layer are of a cholinergic nature.

2. [Ontogenetic study on development of secondary components of evoked response in rabbit.] F. A. Ata-Muradova. — In E. M. Kreps (Ed.), [Evolutionary neurophysiology and neurochemistry]. Leningrad, 1967: 89–98.

The author's earlier works demonstrated the heterochronicity of maturation of the primary response of the sensori-motor region of the rabbit's cortex in the course of ontogenesis. As a result of these investigations a new concept was advanced of the genesis of the primary response, and a concept was evolved of the multiple character of the influences ascending to the cortex, each being expressed by a certain component of the response evoked. The object of the paper is the analysis of the development in ontogenesis of the secondary components of evoked cortical responses.

The paper points out the later maturation of the structure of the secondary negative component. This system is characterized by a considerably lower conduction velocity compared with the conductive structures of the primary negative component. In all its temporal parameters and properties and, consequently, in all its synaptic organization in the cortex the secondary negativity is a superficial axo-dendritic phenomenon.

In the course of the first 3 days after birth, long before the appearance of the positive response component, three channels for the conduction of afferent excitation in the cerebral cortex are maturing in a certain sequence: for the primary negative response of the newborn, for the secondary Forbes' response and for the secondary negative component. Hence, by that time the major non-specific systems of the brain (the hypothalamus and non-specific thalamic nuclei) have already established connections with the cerebral cortex through synapses at the apical dendrites. These earliest maturing ascending influences are referred to the plexiform layer, *i.e.*, the most ancient formation of the cortex. Thus, the first to mature are the working channels of non-specific character, transmitting information from the most important region of the brain, *i.e.*, information of modulating and energetic value (hypothalamus, reticular formation). Several days later channels are formed through which information of discrete character is conveyed from the thalamic relay nuclei.

3. [Peculiarities of electrical activity and steady component of cerebral cortex during sleep and wakefulness in infants between 3 and 12 months of age.] M. N. Akhundi. — Byull. eksp. Biol. Med., 1967, 63 (6): 3.

78 normal, physiologically mature infants were investigated. Bipolar EEGs were taken from the frontal, parietal and occipital lobes. The DC component was recorded by the Monakhov and Loginov technique (1962). Special graphical analysis of the EEG curves was performed to define the peculiarities of the distribution of frequencies in different areas of the cortex by the method of Arshavsky and Gokhblit (1965).

The findings suggest that changes in the EEG in infants from the age of 3 months are characterized by the following features: the formation of the state of drowsiness with a gradual development, at the beginning, of a stage approximating the transitional one (C) and afterwards approximating that of moderately deep sleep (D); the appearance of increasing differences characterizing the EEG at rest, in active wakefulness and sleep, and gradual deepening of the positivity of the DC component in sleep, particularly well pronounced in children over the age of 8 months.

The gradual appearance of these features is correlated with, and possibly depends on, the organization of active wakefulness following the feeding of the infant and its progressive prolongation.

It is suggested that the question of the similarity of slow activity of types Q and delta recorded during sleep in infants below 1 year of age and adults, cannot be regarded as one comprehensively explored, inasmuch as it has been demonstrated by the work of the laboratory that, as distinct from the sleep of adults, sleep in earlier ages is an active state characterized by a higher muscle tone and greater energy reserves per unit of body mass.

4. [Analysis of hypothalamic influences on mono- and polysynaptic potentials of the spinal cord and on the electrocorticogram.] O. G. Baklavadjan and T. K. Kipryan. — Fiziol. Zh. (Leningr.), 1967, 53: 506.

In an effort to analyse further the mechanisms of the descending inhibitory influence of the hypothalamus on somato-motor activity, the sensitivity of the hypothalamo-spinal path to atropine and aminazine was studied in a series of experiments. To define more precisely the site of the drug action, simultaneous recording of EEG, mono- and polysynaptic potentials of the anterior roots of the spinal cord was employed.

Using the method of pharmacological analysis and polygraphic recording of descending and ascending effects of the hypothalamus, an attempt was made to determine whether descending inhibition and ascending activation with stimulation of the same neurones, were associated with dichotomized ascending and descending axons, as described in relation to the reticular formation of the mesencephalon, or whether they resulted from spatial overlapping of two independent structurally differentiated systems at the hypothalamic level. The experiments were performed on cats. The EEG was recorded from needle electrodes. Different structures of the hypothalamus and the reticular formation of the mesencephalon were stimulated with a frequency of 100–200 c/sec. Aminazine, chlorpromazine and atropine were administered i.v. (1–4 mg/kg).

It was found that 2–3 mg/kg atropine i.v. blocked selectively the ascending activating influence of the hypothalamus and the reticular formation without exerting any appreciable effect on the descending inhibition of the activity of the spinal cord motoneurones. Aminazine 1–2 mg/kg i.v. resulted in a noticeable depression of monosynaptic potentials. In such comparatively small doses aminazine, although raising the threshold, did not eliminate the ascending and descending effects of direct stimulation of the hypothalamus and the reticular formation of the mesencephalon.

In doses of 3–4 mg/kg aminazine depressed completely the descending influence of the hypothalamus and the midbrain reticular formation without eliminating the ascending activation of the cortex. Thus, by the administration of aminazine pharmacological dissociation of the descending and ascending effects of the hypothalamus may be achieved.

5. [Physiology and pathological physiology of deep structures of human brain (essays).] N. P. Bechtereva, A. N. Bondarchuk, V. M. Smirnov and A. T. Trokhachev. — Medizina (U.S.S.R.), Leningrad–Moscow, 1967, and People and Health (G.D.R.), Berlin, 1967: 259.

The book is based on some of the results obtained by the application of the method of long-term deep electrodes for treatment and diagnostic purposes. It contains data on the electrical activity of the deep parts of the human brain, on stereotaxic operations, with the introduction of multiple electrodes in the deep cerebral structures, on acute pathophysiological reactions prior to and after the introduction of the electrodes, and on the neurological and neuropsychological studies of the effects of electric stimulation of the deep structures.

Of major importance from the viewpoint of electrophysiology are the studies of the neurophysiological basis of cerebral activity. Investigations of the activity of the human brain were conducted under the following conditions: (1) Observations of psychic, motor and vegetative reactions, as well as local and distant electrical changes following electrical stimulation of different parts of the brain. (2) Studies of the dynamics of different specified activities following electrical stimulation of the brain. Under these conditions changes in an arbitrarily wide range of activities were traced: from more or less elementary neurological symptoms to the very complex forms of psychic activity. (3) Investigations of the dynamics of the physiological indicators of the brain under normal conditions (sleep, wakefulness), with the application of rhythmical and trigger photic stimulation as well as pharmacological agents, while engaged in different activities, etc.

Owing to the fact that, with direct multi-point contacts with the brain, records were analysed not only of the data related to electrical stimulation but also of such phenomena as cellular activity and variations in the DC potential and available oxygen, it was possible to investigate the neurophysiological basis of specifically human activity. The discovery of changing and steadily reproducible patterns of the parameters of the functional state of subcortical structures made it possible to advance a working hypothesis of certain mechanisms underlying psychic activity. Psychic activity is provided by the cortico-subcortical functional system with links characterized by different degrees of rigidity. The system provides the basis for two possible and combining mechanisms which determine comparative rigidity and, at the same time, economy, on the one hand, and flexibility, on the other, in the realization of a particular form of psychic activity.

The "rigid" links of the structuro-functional "skeleton" of the cerebral system, which provide the emotional-psychic reactions, are in all probability those structures the stimulation of which provokes the appearance of, or characteristic changes in, the reactions under study, in which changes in the reproducible indicators of the state of the brain are the most stable. The "flexible" links of the system are those structuro-functional elements which are less constantly involved in the reaction.

6. [Changes in blood serotonin titre in rabbits during sustained stimulation of the anterior segments of the hypothalamus with electric current.] N. L. Vekshina. — Byull. eksp. Biol. Med., 1967, 63 (5): 7.

The study aimed at determining the serotoninergic structures in the hypothalamic region of the rabbit's brain. Investigations were made on 30 unanaesthetized rabbits with electrodes implanted in the brain. Variations in serotonin concentration in central and peripheral blood following electrical stimulation of different regions of the hypothalamus and other structures of the diencephalon (optic tract, caudate nucleus, internal capsule, anterior commissure, septum pellucidum) were studied. EEG and ECG changes were recorded by means of a multi-channel "Galileo" polygraph. Serotonin was assayed in acetone extracts of blood by biological testing. Creatinine sulphate (Lawson Chemicals Co.) was used as the standard solution. Two standard solutions of serotonin were used: 0.1 mg/ml and 1 mg/ml.

Electrical stimulation of the medial pre-optic region, the supra-optic nucleus, the antero-lateral region, the ventro- and dorso-medial nuclei of the hypothalamus gave rise to higher concentration of serotonin in cerebrofugal blood, while in peripheral blood the serotonin content variations were ambiguous. In 6 experiments reserpine was administered intramuscularly as Rausedil (Gedeon Richter Co., Hungary) in a dose of 0.4 mg/kg for 4 days prior to the determination of serotonin; the blood of these rabbits contained no serotonin.

The material testifies to the presence in the anterior regions of the hypothalamus of structures whose stimulation results in a higher serotonin content of cerebrofugal blood. The fact that at the same time the serotonin content of peripheral blood decreased or remained unchanged suggests that higher concentration of the compound in cerebrofugal blood is not associated with its peripheral output by enterochromaffin cells. It is probably the extrusion of serotonin from the serotoninergic structures of the brain under the effect of reserpine, described by several authors, that accounts for the absence of any increase in serotonin in central blood following stimulation of the anterior regions of the hypothalamus in rabbits previously subjected to reserpine treatment.

7. [Extra- and intracellular investigation of neurone responses in the motor cortex of alert rabbits to acoustic and photic stimuli.] L. L. Voronin and V. G. Skrebitsky. — Zh. vyssh. nerv. Deyat. Pavlova, 1967, 17: 523.

The experimental procedure was earlier described by the authors (1965, 1966). The region of representation of one of the extremities was determined by the threshold of the motor reaction to electrical stimulation of the brain through thinned bone near the coronal suture. Extracellular potentials were amplified by UBPl-01 U.S.S.R. apparatus, and intracellular potentials by DC amplifiers of the Cl–4 U.S.S.R. "Diza-indicator" oscillograph. Glass micro-electrodes with a resistance of 5–150 MΩ, filled with 2.5 *M* KCl or (more often) NaCl for extracellular and 2.5 *M* KCl and 2 *M* potassium citrate for intracellular leads, were used.

The results support Buser's conclusion, based on the derivation of evoked potentials, that the motor cortex of the rabbit, like that of the cat, is the centre of polysensory convergence. The findings attest the convergence of signals of different modalities on a considerable part of the neurones of this region. Intracellular records corroborate the assumption that at least a part of the neurones which do not respond to non-specific stimuli by a change in impulse activity can receive only subthreshold synaptic bursts. The same conclusion is suggested by the results of experiments on the application of "non-specific" stimuli against a background of polarization of individual neurones through an extracellular micro-electrode (Voronin 1966). The distribution of neurones according to responses to non-specific stimuli, noted in some experiments, may signify that this type of cortical organization is universal.

8. [Rhythmical oscillations of electrical activity in the vertebrate brain. I. Rhythmical oscillations of electrical activity in the olfactory analyser of vertebrates.] V. I. Gusselnikov, K. G. Gusselnikova and G. S. Voronkov. — Nauch. dorl. Vyssh. Skoly (Biol.), 1967, 4 (40): 45.

A short review of available data on the nature of rhythmical electrical activity of the olfactory analyser, or so-called olfactory waves (Adrian 1950), in vertebrates.

9. [Concerning the relation between the duration of depression of basic cortical rhythms and the latent period of motor reaction in man.] M. P. Ivanova. — Byull. eksp. Biol. Med., 1967, 63 (3): 3.

The aim of the investigation was to correlate changes in the latency of the motor reaction with variations in the duration of the depression of rhythms, not only in the area which was specific for the signal or reaction, but also in one which did not directly participate in the organization of a particular connection. Gripping a hand dynamometer with a force of 14–20 kg was adopted as the motor reaction and sound as the conditioned signal. The EEG was recorded from bipolar derivations from the parieto-occipital and sensori-motor areas of both cerebral hemispheres.

A close relationship between the two indices was not always observed. It manifested itself distinctly only when the latency of motor reaction was correlated with the rhythm variations of the specific area to which the signal or movement was referred. Changes in the spatial distribution of incoming information depended on its distribution in time, the information being transmitted via very complex multi-neurone chains. It was probably this that was reflected in the variations of the latency of motor reaction, on the one hand, and in the duration of the changes in the electrical activity of the brain, on the other.

10. [Influence of the frequency of rhythmic photic stimulation on the harmonic composition of the driving response in the human brain.] V. A. Ilyanok. — Zh. vyssh. nerv. Deyat. Pavlova, 1967, 17: 304–311.

It is generally known that under the action of rhythmic light flashes rhythm "transformation" may occur in the electrical currents of the brain of man and animals, *i.e.*, the appearance of so-called harmonics and subharmonics whose frequencies are multiples of the stimulus frequency.

The purpose was to study the harmonic composition of the reaction of cortical rhythms of the human brain in a wider frequency range than has been done by other authors, primary consideration being given to the relationship between the number and magnitude of harmonics and subharmonics and the frequency of rhythmic light flashes. For quantitative analysis of the EEG Walter's frequency analyser was used, some of the filters being readjusted to the frequencies of two harmonic series ranging from 5 to 160 c/sec (Ilyanok 1960). The frequencies of light flashes varied within the same range. The investigations were carried out on 10 persons from 18 to 30 years of age.

Because the origin of harmonics, as well as the suitability of a frequency analyser for their identification, are open to discussion, the author presents spectograms of different wave forms (sinusoidal, symmetrical triangular, asymmetrical triangular and rectangular) obtained at the same analyser amplification, and considers the possible versions of harmonics and their amplitudes in each particular case.

On the basis of the results the author assumes that the ratio between the magnitude of different harmonic amplitudes according to analyser readings may serve as a rough indication of the form and number of the components of the electrical response of the brain to photic stimulation. Moreover, the harmonics detected by frequency analysis of the EEG during driving are, on the one hand, the result of a complex, real multicomponent composition of the responses to each flash and, on the other, the consequence of expansion into the Fourier series of the non-sinusoidal form of both single- and multi-component responses.

The relationships between the harmonic composition of the driving response and the functional state of the brain, as well as the parameters of rhythmic photic stimuli, testify to the fact that in such cases consistent changes occur in the magnitude and also in the number and form of cerebral potentials following each flash of light.

11. [Changes in electrical and conditioned activity after ablation of the lateral hypothalamus in rabbits.] L. V. Kalyuzhny, L. I. Nekrasova and I. N. Zakharova. — Zh. vyssh. nerv. Deyat. Pavlova, 1967, 17: 1.

The experiments were made on 5 freely moving rabbits. Electrical activity was recorded from the dorsal hippocampus, reticular nucleus of the thalamus, medial reticular formation of the mesencephalon and the lateral and latero-medial regions of the hypothalamus, using implanted electrodes, according to Kotlyar's technique.

Bilateral destruction of the lateral region of the hypothalamus was accomplished by 3–4 mA direct current for 30 sec. It resulted in disappearance of conditioned and unconditioned food reactions without changing the orientation and defensive conditioned reflexes. It was noted that after destruction of the lateral hypothalamus the frequency of potential oscillations diminished only in response to conditioned food signals, while in the case of other stimuli the usual frequency persisted.

The findings support the assumption, to be found in the literature, that synchronized activity with a frequency of 8–10 c/sec (characteristic for freely moving rabbits) is the result of the integration of two flows of excitation: non-specific, reflecting behavioural "attention", and specific, reflecting unconditioned excitation, each being expressed by theta rhythm.

12. [Relation of electrical to metabolic evidence of cell excitation.] A. B. Kogan. — Fiziol. Zh. (Leningr.), 1967, 53: 260.

In present physiological investigations of the activity of excitable tissues practically no use is made of the evidence of cellular metabolism to characterize the working processes of excitation. They are considered only as the consequence of excitation, its "metabolic tail".

On the basis of the author's own investigations and those of his co-workers, facts are presented illustrating the remarkable velocity of development of certain metabolic reactions, possibly even matching that of the electric reactions. Thus, an integrated electrophysiological and cytochemical study of an individual neurone in the extension of the abdominal segment of the crayfish showed that with adequate stimulation the frequency of its pulse activity increased against the background of the increasing disorganization of concentric series of RNA structures in the paranuclear zone, and the general redistribution of RNA in the neurone. The original structure was restored only 30–40 min after the cessation of moderate stimulation.

Metabolic characteristics, including RNA and suxindehydrase dynamics, were correlated with electrical indices to evaluate the topography of the optic projection area of the cortex, to investigate the structure of the "alimentation" centre, in the description of the type of neuronal organization of central mechanisms at different levels of development of the nervous system.

The fact that metabolic reactions reflect minute intracellular changes and the cyclical changes in functional states, and possess universal character as a means of revealing dynamic localization of complex systems, suggests that the deterrents to the use of metabolic evidence in the study of excitation and inhibition are technical and determined by the methodological limitations of present-day cytochemistry.

13. [Electrographic expression of human trace conditioned reflexes to signals of different modalities.] V. F. Konovalov. — Zh. vyssh. nerv. Deyat. Pavlova, 1967, 17: 29.

The experiments were performed on students and schoolchildren 17–24 years of age. Bipolar EEGs from the occipital and Rolandic areas of the cortex, galvanic skin reactions (Tarkhanov), the EMG of hand muscles and oculomotor reactions, were recorded.

It was found that all the stages in the formation of trace conditioned reflexes could be followed by changes in the alpha rhythm, Rolandic rhythm and galvanic skin reflex, with the subject remaining for a long time in the wakeful and drowsy states. Specific features are noted in the formation of trace temporary connections in response to signals of different modalities. Much importance is attached to the time factor, which is an integral part of a trace reflex. Before a temporary connection between a conditioned and an unconditioned stimulus begins to form, the cerebral cortex probably evaluates the given interval by means of some clock mechanism. It is assumed that the counting of time by the nervous system is a result of the activity of the brain as a whole.

14. [EEG study of the effect of vincamine on the central nervous system of rabbits.] A. G. Kurmukov. — Farmakol. i Toksikol., 1967, 30: 286.

The investigation aimed at determining the effect of vincamine (Gedeon Richter Co., "Devincan", for the treatment of cerebral form of hypertension, hypertensive encephalopathy, etc.) on different parts of the brain in rabbits with chronically implanted electrodes. Two phases were found in the effect of the drug, the dose being 1–1.5 mg/kg. Phase I (10–15 min after administration): smaller amplitude and higher frequency in the cortex, regularization of rhythm and larger amplitudes in the hippocampus and mesencephalic reticular formation, regularization of rhythm with no change in the initial amplitude in the medial thalamus. Phase II: the appearance of slow high voltage potentials in the cortex, the return of the electrical activity to the initial level in the hippocampus, the appearance of slow high voltage potentials in the medial thalamus and the mesencephalic reticular formation.

Larger doses of the drug, 5–10 mg/kg i.v., gave rise to aggressive behaviour, sharp waves and spikes appearing in the cortex and the hippocampus and, less frequently, in the medial thalamus and the reticular formation, against a background of low voltage high frequency activity.

15. [Influence exerted on the electrical activity of the brain by benactyzine, apzofenum (α,α-diphenylpropionic acid β-diethylamino-ethyl ester hydrochloride) and corresponding quinuclidine ethers.] M. D. Mashkovsky and L. F. Roschina. — Farmakol. i Toksikol., 1967, 30: 415.

The investigations were carried out on unanaesthetized cats immobilized with suxamethonium (under artificial respiration) with potentials led off from the optic area of the cortex, and on rabbits with electrodes implanted in the optic cortex and the hippocampus. The effects of the drugs on the background activity, on the changes due to photic stimulation and on the activation following electrical stimulation of the sciatic nerve were studied, as well as the effects on EEG changes brought about by an anticholinesterase drug, galanthaminum, and cholinonimetic substances, arecoline and nicotine.

All the cholinolytics under study gave rise to changes in the activity of the cerebral cortex and the hippocampus: slow irregular oscillations with a frequency of 4–6 c/sec and an amplitude of 150–250 μV appeared; they impaired or blocked the response to rhythmic photic stimulation and raised the threshold for activation by electrical stimulation of the sciatic nerve.

Galanthaminum (2 mg/kg), arecoline (0.5 mg/kg) and nicotine (0.4 mg/kg) immediately induced desynchronization in the cerebral cortex in cats and the appearance of a high voltage Q rhythm in the hippocampus of rabbits. The cholinolytics in question prevented and eliminated the activating effect of galanthaminum and arecoline on the cortex and the hippocampus. The cholinolytic substances benactyzine and apzofenum and their quinuclidine analogous were found to exert a marked influence on the electrical activity of the brain and the hippocampus.

These findings make it possible to correlate the effects of the drugs on the cerebral activity with their chemical constitutions. The replacement in the benactyzine molecule of the open alkylamine chain by the bicyclic system of quinuclidine does not affect the extent of its influence upon the EEG, although the duration of the effect increases.

16. [Local pre-potential, spreading impulse and closing of the temporary connection.] R. S. Mnukhina. — Zh. vyssh. nerv. Deyat. Pavlova, 1967, 17: 212.

In earlier experiments performed on dogs and rabbits the author demonstrated that, in the final phase of the formation of a conditioned reflex, the evoked responses (intensification of the process of local excitation) and the negative shift of the cortical steady potential were strongly pronounced. This led to the assumption that the formation of a conditioned reflex was proceeding at a certain limited level of depolarization of the neurones of the corresponding cortical areas of the analysers involved, while the impulse activity arising on its basis was directly responsible for closing the temporary connection.

The purpose of the present investigation was to verify the consistent relationship established earlier with derivations from the deep layers of the cortex. Silver electrodes were implanted in the auditory and motor areas of the cortex of dogs and rabbits, with monopolar derivations. Auditory and defensive conditioned reflexes in response to an acoustic stimulus were elaborated.

The author points out the similarity of the dynamics of impulse activity in the cortical neurones in the course of the elaboration of a conditioned reflex to that observed in the case of electrical stimulation of the sensory thalamic nuclei (Li *et al.*, *J. Neurophysiol.*, 1956, *19*: 11). He presumes that under such circumstances the functional state of the cortex is similar to that resulting from optimal electrical stimulation of the sensory nuclei of the thalamus. With the potential led off from the deep layers of the cortex in the course of conditioned reflex elaboration, the dynamics of the transition of the local deep negative slow pre-potential into extending impulse activity is shown, which promotes contacts between the neurones and thereby brings about the closing of temporary connections. A conditioned reflex is formed according to the mechanism of a polarization-depolarization process and, under the conditions of normal functioning of the cortex, the fact of the closing of temporary connections provides support for the monistic concept of Vvedensky and Oukhtomsky of the unity of local and extending excitation.

17. [Changes of evoked potential duration in the course of defensive conditioning in dogs.] T. S. Naumova and N. S. Popova. — Zh. vyssh. nerv. Deyat. Pavlova, 1967, 17: 442.

Results are reported of studying changes in the duration of three components (1st positive, negative and 2nd positive) of the auditory and optic evoked potential in the primary projection zones in the course of the development and consolidation of defensive conditioned reflexes in dogs. Defensive conditioned reflexes were elaborated by Petropavlovsky's method. Monopolar EEG recording through the thinned cranial bone was used, the electrodes being implanted mainly over the auditory or optic areas of the left hemisphere according to the technique proposed by Lourie and Trofimov.

Five stages were determined in the dynamics of the duration of the components of evoked responses. The distinctness and duration of each stage in the formation of a conditioned reflex were found to depend upon both the modality of the stimulus and the individual peculiarities of the nervous system of the experimental animal. The duration of the 1st positive, negative and 2nd positive components of the evoked response, in the course of the elaboration of the defensive conditioned reflex, changed conjugately, which testifies to the uniform effect of reflex elaboration on both the earlier (primary) and later (secondary) components of evoked response.

18. [Trace phenomena in a dominant state.] R. A. Pavlygina. — Zh. vyssh. nerv. Deyat. Pavlova, 1967, 17: 505.

The work represented an attempt to appraise the significance of the steady potential shift accompanying trace phenomena in a dominant state. The investigations were conducted on 20 rabbits in chronic experiments. Polarization was accomplished by pulsed current. A dominant focus was formed in the cortical area of the left forelimb. Continual photic and acoustic stimuli were used to support the dominant focus. The electrical activity of the motor, optic and auditory areas of the cortex was recorded and, in 5 rabbits, also that of the medial nuclei of the thalamus and of the mesencephalic reticular formation.

Trace phenomena depended wholly upon the dominant state. From this it was inferred that polarization of neurones promoted the preservation of traces (corroborated in the literature). The trace activity was characterized by the maintenance of a certain stimulus model: constant frequency characteristics with a corresponding change in the steady potential level. The sign of the polarization was also important. In these investigations the dominant focus was best formed by anodal polarization.

19. [Development of extinctive inhibition in children in early ontogenesis.] R. I. Polikanina and L. N. Sergeeva. — Zh. vyssh. nerv. Deyat. Pavlova, 1967, 17: 228.

The present work completes a series of investigations conducted by the authors into the elaboration and development of the orienting reflex in newborn infants. A group of healthy mature infants (weighing 2700–4900 g at birth) were observed and the results were compared with those of earlier studies made on premature infants (the conditions of observation were similar).

The results concerning the changes in the EEG and the relation between the vegetative and somatic components during extinction of the orienting reflex to rhythmic acoustic stimuli in mature and premature infants corroborated the differences in functional possibilities of the brains of infants of different degrees of maturity, previously established by the authors.

An assumption is made on the mode of evolution of the inhibitory process in the earliest ontogeny of man. The presence of generalized non-extinctive reactions in foetuses of 5–6 months' antenatal development, resembling the reactions of decorticated animals, attests to an extensive irradiation of the excitation process over the central nervous system, due to the weakness or absence of the inhibitory process.

As the structure and function of the cerebral cortex develop, the character of the reactions changes gradually and their extinction becomes possible, which is associated with differences between the processes of excitation and inhibition.

Thus, the specialized orienting reflex is a comparatively late product of the ontogenetic development in man. Its appearance and, especially, extinction require a certain relation between the processes of excitation and inhibition in the cortex. The differences in the electrical activity of the brain in infants of different degrees of maturity and post-natal age, revealed during extinction of the orienting reflex to rhythmic acoustic stimuli, testify to the relationship between the process of extinction and the degree of maturity of the central cortical part of the auditory analyser in children at the earliest stages of ontogeny. In the present study the dominant role of the cortical part has been revealed.

20. [Organization of cortical mechanisms for closing motor conditioned connections.] M. Ya. Rabinovitch. — Zh. vyssh. nerv. Deyat. Pavlova, 1967, 17: 3.

In research on the major problem of the physiology of the brain, the mechanisms of formation of conditioned connections, the importance is emphasized of further analysis of the significance and role of such morphologically differentiated and complex structures as the cortical layers.

The investigation was conducted on dogs with layer-by-layer implantation of nichrome 30–40 μ electrodes to the specified depth of the cortex of the motor, skin, auditory and optic analysers. EEGs were recorded from monopolar derivations.

Analysis of the EEG activity of individual cortical layers made it possible to distinguish three principal stages in the formation of the motor conditioned reflex. The first comprised higher frequency and amplitudes of waves in the cortex in response to the first application of the conditioned signal and electrodermal support much in advance of the appearance of the motor conditioned reaction. The activation was generalized, and in all layers of the cortex of the analysers of the conditioned and unconditioned stimuli. Against the background of generalized changes, after some 20–30 combinations, local forms of activity could sometimes be distinguished in layers IV and II or in layer IV alone of the analyser to which the conditioned signal was referred.

In the second stage the signal stimulus activated equally the structures of the afferent and efferent cortical links of the conditioned reflex arc, uniting their activities into a single system of conditioned reflex excitation. Local reactions arising primarily in layers IV and II were associated with the structurally determined presence of the two principal systems of cortical specific afferentation (one from the subcortical links of the analyser involved, and the other consisting of the association and commissure fibres from different cortical areas).

In the third stage, when the motor response to the stimulus was sufficiently stable and automatic in the EEG there was a decrease in amplitude or predominance of slow wave activity against the background of activation of layer V of the cortex of the motor analyser and the motor conditioned reaction. At this stage the stimulus did not produce distinct changes in the electrical activity in the cortical layers of the skin analyser.

These observations suggest that in the case of a reinforced conditioned motor reflex the volley of impulses is switched towards the cortical centres of the unconditioned reflex at the subcortical level of the conditioned stimulus analyser, bypassing its cortical structures. At the initial stage of the elaboration of a conditioned reflex its realization is ensured predominantly by transcortical (forward and feedback) connections between the cortical centres of the conditioned and unconditioned stimuli. A moderately reinforced conditioned reaction is induced by signal impulses propagated for the most part subcortically towards the efferent links of the cortical centres of the conditioned connection.

21. [The effect of calcium and magnesium on dendritic potentials.] A. I. Roitbak and T. N. Oniani. — Fiziol. Zh. (Leningr.), 1967, 53: 251.

Upon application to the cerebral cortex of an electrical stimulus of sufficient intensity, a negative potential with a duration of 20–30 msec is recorded at any point within a radius of 6 mm, its latent period increasing with increase in the distance from the stimulating electrode. It is almost universally accepted that this negative potential expresses the response of the apical dendrites of pyramidal neurones.

The authors have demonstrated that a change in the ratio of Ca^{2+} and Mg^{2+} concentrations in the intercellular space of the surface layers of the cortex produces a most profound effect upon the synaptic transmission of excitation on the apical dendrites of the pyramidal neurones. The experiments were performed on 10 cats. Deep Nembutal anaesthesia (75–90 mg/kg) was applied to exclude the influence of the brain-stem reticular formation on the cortex and to depress, as much as possible, the impulse activity of the cortical neurones. The small interpolar distance of the stimulating electrodes and the low intensities of the stimuli assured local stimulation.

The fact that the dendritic potentials rise consistently under the influence of Ca^{2+} ions and drop under the action of Mg^{2+} ions, is conclusive evidence that these potentials are post-synaptic and that axo-dendritic synapses on apical dendrites are synapses with chemical transmission. Synapses on the apical dendrites of the neocortex resemble neuromuscular synapses as well as those on the neurones and ganglia of invertebrates, and on the motoneurones of the spinal cord, in that an increase in $[Ca^{2+}]_n$ is attended by an increase in the amount of transmitter liberated under the effect of the nerve impulse, *i.e.*, the intensity of the exciting post-synaptic current is increased. The absence of any change in latency and in the time of dendritic potential increase under the effect of Ca^{2+} and Mg^{2+} indicates that there is no appreciable change in the rate of transmitter liberation.

The findings explain the second dendritic potential drop in the case of paired stimuli. It is well known that a pre-synaptic impulse results in an enormous increase in the emission of transmitter, *i.e.*, in its production, on the one hand, and in its mobilization, on the other. Thus the principal cause of the second dendritic potential drop in the case of paired stimuli is a decrease within 60 msec of the quantity of transmitter available to the second pre-synaptic impulse.

It is emphasized that $[Ca^{2+}]$ and $[Mg^{2+}]$ are effective in minimum concentrations and that they have a fairly lasting effect (up to tens of minutes). This leads to the assumption that ionic processes in synaptic endings, a change in the $[Ca^{2+}]/[Mg^{2+}]$ ratio in particular, play an important role in the appearance of the "traces" of nervous activity which underlie recent memory.

22. [Modulation of the activity of optic cortex neurones in waking rabbit by different non-visual stimuli.] V. G. Skrebitsky and O. Z. Bomshtein. — Fiziol. Zh. (Leningr.), 1967, 53: 129.

In an earlier investigation (Skrebitsky and Voronin 1965) one of the forms of heteromodal convergence was defined, *viz.*, the inhibition of the evoked activity of the neurones of the rabbit's optic cortex in the course of acoustic stimulation. The present series of experiments was designed to ascertain whether this inhibition was modality specific or not.

The effects of different non-specific stimuli (sound, electrical skin stimulation) on the spontaneous and evoked activity of the optic cortex neurones in a waking rabbit, as well as of stimulation of the brain-stem reticular formation—the structure mediating generalized non-specific reactions—were correlated. The investigations have demonstrated that the direction of change in the spontaneous and evoked activity of the optic cortex neurones in an unanaesthetized rabbit is identical in the case of two different sensory stimuli inadequate for the optic analyser. This shows that the modulation of the activity of the optic cortex neurones by non-visual stimuli is modality non-specific.

It is assumed that a change in the cellular activity due to a non-visual stimulus, which is attended by EEG activation, is a manifestation of the animal's orientating reaction to a new stimulus. This is borne out by the attenuation of the neurone reaction with repeated application of the stimulus. The predominant type of reaction to non-visual stimuli was the inhibition of spontaneous and photically evoked discharges.

One of the most interesting problems arising from these experiments is that of the mechanism of "non-specific inhibition", described by the authors. It may be assumed that in the reticular formation of the mesencephalon or thalamus there are multi-sensory neurones whose activation inhibits the discharges of the optic cortex cells. The results obtained with stimulation of the reticular formation corroborate this assumption.

23. [Steady potentials of the human brain during alertness, anaesthesia and sleep.] M. Kh. Starobinets. — Zh. vyssh. nerv. Deyat. Pavlova, 1967, 17: 2.

Steady brain potential levels were studied in 20 subjects (3–8 times in each, under conditions of complete rest, in semi-darkness) during 20–40 min. A modification of Sorokhtin's technique was used.

The results show that potentials derived from the scalp are steady polarization potentials from the cerebral hemispheres. There is evidence that the galvanic skin reflex does not exert any appreciable influence on the potential curve. The possibility of recording the steady potential of the human brain from the scalp is of interest not only from the theoretical point of view. In some cases, *e.g.*, under anaesthesia, the steady potential reflects more completely than the EEG the functional state of the subject. In the waking state emotion, watchfulness and closer attention to the environment are accompanied by marked depolarization of the brain. The fall in the electropositive potential of the cerebral hemispheres noted by Caspers in animals and by the author in people undergoing investigation for the first time is probably accounted for by the orienting reflex. The change in steady potential in natural and barbiturate-induced sleep consists in a rise of the electropositive potential.

The results of the investigation conform to and corroborate the facts described in literature. If, as established by Berger (1931) and Lennox *et al.* (1936), natural sleep and barbiturate anaesthesia are attended by similar EEG changes, the steady potentials of the brain in these states undergo the same type of alterations. Moreover, injury to the brain-stem reticular formation during inter-collicular transection, resulting in an EEG sleep pattern (Bremer 1936; Lindsley *et al.* 1949), simultaneously produces, according to the author's findings, a rise of the electropositive potential of the cerebral hemispheres in cat. Thus, blockade of the activating ascending reticular formation—anatomical (in an isolated brain preparation), pharmacological (barbiturate-induced sleep and anaesthesia) or physiological (natural sleep)—is attended not only by the well known EEG changes but also by surface hyperpolarization of the cerebral cortex. Inasmuch as this is due to cessation of activating impulses, it may be regarded as passive in its origin. It represents an electrophysiological manifestation of the peculiar state of the cerebral cortex during natural or barbiturate-induced sleep.

24. [Some mechanisms of the rhythmicity of electrical activity of the cerebral cortex.] A. Y. Supin. — Zh. vyssh. nerv. Deyat. Pavlova, 1967, 17: 2.

The aim of this work was to ascertain whether inhibitory processes in the cortex could maintain autonomous activity in it, independent of rhythmic stimuli from the thalamus.

The experiments were performed on unanaesthetized uncurarized rabbits. The electrical activity of the cortex was recorded from the surface by means of silver or nichrome electrodes 0.3–0.4 mm in diameter, and from the deep structures with the help of tungsten electrodes. Unit activity of the cortex was recorded by means of micro-electrodes, as noise generated by the mass of cells adjacent to the electrode tips, and revealed by great amplification and a short time constant of the amplifier. A series of experiments were conducted on an "isolated hemisphere" preparation (transection, with separation of the telencephalon from the diencephalon).

The results make it possible to correlate two types of rhythmic activity of the cerebral cortex of the rabbit: alpha-like after-discharge and convulsive after-discharge. The two types of activity are similar in respect of two characteristics under study, *viz.*, the distribution by layers in the cortex and the interrelation with the impulse activity of neurones. This appears to reflect the synchronous initiation of a prolonged inhibitory post-synaptic potential in a great mass of cortical neurones.

Inasmuch as convulsive after-discharge was recorded from "isolated hemispheres", the possibility that rhythmic activity of the cortex is due to impulses from the thalamus was excluded. This testifies to the possibility of the development of regular rhythm not only in the thalamus but also directly in the cortex, the mechanism of the cortical process in this case being essentially similar to that of rhythmic activity in the thalamus, *viz.*, neurone discharge—prolonged inhibitory post-synaptic potential and inhibition of neurones—again neurone discharge, etc.

25. [On neuronal organization of focal epileptiform discharge.] A. G. Sukhov. — Fiziol. Zh. (Leningr.), 1967, 53: 520.

Simultaneously recorded neuronal activity and ECoG were correlated to determine the form of their interaction. The experiments were made on a white rat immobilized with α-tubocurarine (1.5 mg/kg). Series of rectangular 15–20 V impulses, with a duration of 0.1 msec and a frequency of 10/sec were used for 5–6 sec to evoke focal epileptiform activity. The cortex was stimulated at different levels of the sensori-motor area.

A close relationship was found between the epileptiform reaction of neurones and their usual non-epileptiform reaction to electrical stimulation, which attested to the formation of epileptogenous neurone complexes on the basis of regular synaptic connections between neurones. Consistent changes of the usual and epileptiform types under the varying conditions of stimulation showed the possibility of transformation of the neurone complex in response to external influences.

On the basis of probability calculus theoretical computations were made of the probability of the preservation or alteration of the type of neurone participation in repeated focal discharges evoked from different electrodes. The results corroborate the assumption that for neurones with a readily changing reaction the type of participation in epileptiform discharge is determined by the static relationship between excited and inhibited neurones and the probability connections of an individual neurone with all other neurones, rather than by the properties of the neurone itself.

26. [Neurophysiological characteristics of the cortex isolated from subcortical nervous influences.] M. M. Khananashvili. — Fiziol. Zh. (Leningr.), 1967, 53: 224.

In studying the interaction of individual projection areas of the cerebral cortex during conditioned reflex activity, as well as the mechanisms of closing the temporary connection in animals, use was made of the method developed by the author (1954) to sever all nerve connections between the cortex and subcortex with a view to maximum elimination of the influence of subcortical structures on the cortex (see *Fiziol. Zh. (Leningr.)*, 1961, *47*: 661).

Background activity of isolated cortex is described; account is given of the peculiarities of initiation and propagation of evoked responses in such cortex; convulsive activity of the cortex following stimulation with super-threshold current is discussed, and some problems concerning the mechanisms of generalization of synchronous discharges over the cortex are touched upon. Variation of background activity, from deep depression immediately following the operation to that approximating the normal 4–6 months after, is noted. However, some features peculiar to the ECoG of isolated cortex are still distinguishable, the most characteristic being the alternation of groups of fast waves with periods of their complete absence, possibly indicative of the greater functional exhaustibility of the cells of isolated cortex. A fairly intimate correlation is revealed between the background activity of the majority of investigated neurones of isolated cortex and the ECoG waves. Taking into account the evidence in the literature of closer correlation in lower functional states of the brain and considering the character of the background ECoG, the above assumption appears to be quite plausible. A different interpretation cannot be excluded, bearing in mind that transection of the projection pathways of the cortex results in disconnection of the most important mechanisms of nervous regulation and self-regulation of the cerebral hemispheres.

Changes in the ECoG of neuronally isolated cortex in different functional states (sleep, wakefulness) can be accounted for only by the humoral influence of subcortical structures upon the cortex. As the changes in the ECoG in such cases generally correspond to those observed in normal cortex, it may be assumed that in normal animals ECoG changes occurring in different functional states largely depend upon the humoral influences of subcortical structures.

On stimulation of the suprasylvian convolution the responses were recorded at a distance of 20 mm from the site of stimulation. On stimulation of the ectosylvian convolution the responses did not propagate for more than 14–15 mm. It is concluded that an evoked cortical response propagates over a considerable distance without subcortical structures being involved. However, this does not rule out the possibility of interaction of cortical centres via subcortical structures since such a mechanism not only participates but also plays an important role in the integral activity of the brain. Lowering of the stimulation thresholds for isolated cortex is emphasized as a proof of the general principle of higher sensitivity of denervated structures, which is graphically described in the literature.

27. [Unit activity of the neuronally isolated cortex in a chronic experiment.] M. M. Khananashvili, N. N. Vasilevsky and N. S. Burakova. — Zh. vyssh. nerv. Deyat. Pavlova, 1967, 17: 2.

The purpose of the investigation was to study the background activity of individual neurones of isolated cortex and its relation to general ECoG. The experiments were performed on 4 adult cats with the cortex of one hemisphere isolated. Extracellular spike potentials were derived by means of glass-insulated tungsten micro-electrodes in the middle part of the suprasylvian convolution. In 16 experiments 57 neurones with background activity were discovered. Active neurones could not be found on every micro-electrode track. In frequent cases only punctures of membranes were noted. A conspicuous feature of the background activity of individual neurones of isolated cortex is its close correlation with the waves of the surface and deep ECoG, including individual waves and their phases, as well as periods of increased rhythmical activity.

28. [Propagation of epileptiform activity from neocortex and hippocampus in rabbits and monkeys.] G. A. Khosabov and T. G. Urmancheeva. — In E. M. Kreps (Ed.), [Evolutionary neurophysiology and neurochemistry]. Leningrad, 1967: 76–88.

It has been demonstrated (Rozhansky *et al.* 1953, 1956, 1957) that cortical structures of different evolutionary levels, including the neocortex and the hippocampus, possess a distinct functional community which consists in the ability of these structures to become sources of extensive irradiation of facilitating (excitatory) or inhibitory influences. The aim of the present investigation was to compare the conditions of propagation of epileptiform activity evoked by local electrical stimulation of the hippocampus and neocortex in animals with different morphological predominance of the latter over the hippocampus, using multiple implanted electrodes and 16-channel electroencephalographs.

Two types of propagation of epileptiform activity within the cortex are distinguished. Type I is attended by the development in distant structures of an activity fully correlating with that in the stimulated focus. This correlation may have the character of complete duplication of the epileptiform activity of the primary focus, the cessation of epileptiform activity in the area of stimulation resulting in simultaneous cessation of epileptiform activity in all the structures to which it has been propagated.

Type II is characterized by the development in the secondary focus of an epileptiform activity whose elements have no correlates in that of the primary focus. With this type of propagation the cessation of epileptiform activity in the primary focus does not terminate the activity in the secondary focus. This type of propagation characterizes the formation of a secondary self-supporting independent focus of epileptiform activity, a focus which in some cases may develop from the very beginning, while in others it may gradually replace the dependent activity prevailing in the area.

The material presented indicates that the propagating of epileptiform activity within the cortex system in monkey is considerably impeded as compared to that in rabbit. Particularly conspicuous is the fact that the propagation of epileptiform activity in monkeys is never attended by the development of secondary independent foci.

Electroenceph. clin. Neurophysiol., **1969**, *27*: 322–331

Electroencephalography and Clinical Neurophysiology
Elsevier Publishing Company, Amsterdam – Printed in The Netherlands

THE EEG SOCIETY

London, October 4–5, 1968

Secretary: W. A. Kennedy

Brook General Hospital, London, S.E.18 (Great Britain)

THE EEG IN THE DECLARATION OF DEATH

1. EEG and the declaration of death. — M. V. Driver (London).

This communication comprises a review of EEG studies of coma and their relevance to problems concerning resuscitation following cardiac arrest. Jouvet (*Electroenceph. clin. Neurophysiol.*, 1959, *11*: 805) discussed the electrographic diagnosis of death of the CNS in states of profound coma and most investigations since (*e.g.*, Schwab *et al.*, *Electroenceph. clin. Neurophysiol.*, 1963, *15*: 147) have used similar criteria, though generally without the use of intracerebral electrodes. Rosoff and Schwab (*Electroenceph. clin. Neurophysiol.*, 1968, *24*: 283) introduced a caution to the effect that the electroencephalographer should be sure of his role before making any pronouncement regarding the fact of death. Various studies (*e.g.*, Hockaday *et al.*, *Electroenceph. clin. Neurophysiol.*, 1965, *18*: 575 and Pampiglione and Harden, *Lancet*, 1968, *7555*: 1261) have also been concerned with other than "flat" EEGs (the term "flat" is in need of careful definition if it is to be used at all) but the precise and unique contribution of such records to prognosis remains obscure. The monograph by A. M. Gurvitch (*Electrical activity of the brain during dying and resuscitation*. Moscow, 1966) should be consulted by those able to read Russian.

2. Some aspects of evoked responses to stimulation in cerebral disaster. — E. W. Poole (London).

It would seem prudent to consider evoked and spontaneous EEG activities in the assessment of severe brain disorder, and both might be expected to contribute to intensive care monitoring. This dual approach seems especially important where, for therapeutic and other reasons, it is necessary to define reliably the stages of disorder leading to (and beyond) some certain point of massive irreversibility in relation to present therapy. Responses to stimulation can be of a general arousal character (*e.g.*, EEG, muscle, autonomic activity) or of a restricted particular type (*e.g.*, cerebral sensory, local reflex); it seems important to consider carefully the prognostic implications of such responses and their relevance to criteria for ultimate cessation of cerebral function such as "an absolutely linear electroencephalographic tracing (even with stimulation of the brain) recorded under well defined technical conditions." (C.I.O.M.S. Conference, June 1968).

Arousing stimuli of a vigorous, extensive, varied and prolonged character are a convenient bedside approach but can be difficult to interpret unless the response clearly outlasts stimulation which is accurately monitored. Other stimuli might be considered, *e.g.*, electrical. Stimulation producing specific or non-specific evoked responses appears a promising way to assess some aspects of surviving cerebral function. For long-term monitoring purposes stimulation should be safe, acceptable, simple and readily checkable for adequacy; the response should be slowly habituating, consistent though responsive to changing circumstances, large, artefact-free and should require no special processing. Photic and peripheral nerve electrical stimulation seem the best compromise; the relative persistence of specific responses in coma may well be advantageous. Alterations in form and latency might prove as informative prognostically as the presence/absence of response. ERG potentials, myoclonic jerks and brainstem reflexes have also to be taken into account. Extensive multi-disciplinary studies are needed to establish the place of evoked responses in the socially acceptable definition of cerebral death; it is suggested that, whatever the outcome, such studies can scarcely fail to make an important contribution to the management of severe cerebral disorder and to our understanding of the isoelectric EEG.

3. Serial electrophysiological studies (EEG, EMG, ERG, evoked responses) in a case of 3 months' survival with flat EEG following cardiac arrest. — H. J. Crow and A. Winter (Bristol).

Mr. H. Age: 54. Subject to severe attacks of asthma in one of which, on June 20th 1968, he was found to be in a state of cardiac arrest in Casualty Department. The heart was restarted and the patient put on a respirator. The first record, 4 days later, showed no EEG activity during an hour's examination. The second and third examinations, 24 and 48 h later, also failed to show EEG activity. By the usual EEG criteria he had suffered "brain death", yet he had brisk pupillary reactions to light, thus indicating that his midbrain was "alive". Spontaneous respiration gradually returned and he was taken off the respirator completely about 3 weeks after the cardiac arrest. His condition has been unchanged since then to the present time. He appears to be unconscious. His pupils react to light. He makes uncoordinated muscular responses to noise and flash stimuli. The EEG remains flat. Averaging and computing techniques have been used to supplement the routine EEG information.

4. EEG studies following resuscitation after cardiac arrest in 60 babies. — A. Harden (London).

Between 1957 and 1967, 120 babies and children have had EEG studies within a few hours following resuscitation after a known cardio-circulatory arrest. The criteria for selection of this material, the techniques used and the prognostic value of early EEG findings have been published in a recent paper (Pampiglione and Harden, *Lancet*, 1968, *i*: 1261). In the present report 60 of these patients, aged 1 day to 6 months, are described in relation to the special problems that have been encountered in this young age group.

Normal babies under 6 months of age have EEG features quite different from those of older children and adults and are also said to withstand periods of anoxia better. In the babies resuscitated following cardio-circulatory arrest other pre-existing and concomitant factors are common, not necessarily related to the cardiac arrest. In particular, the occurrence of a variety of congenital anomalies, of rapid metabolic alteration and of the greater possibility of repeated cardio-circulatory troubles, may complicate the evaluation of the EEG features. The natural evolution of each condition may be superimposed upon the effect of transitory cerebral ischaemia and anoxia with a greater variety of resulting EEG patterns in comparison with older patients.

5. EEG findings in dying and resuscitated adult patients. — P. F. Prior (London).

This communication reviews our total experience of 96 adult patients unconscious following technically successful resuscitation from cardio-respiratory arrest. Preliminary studies were reported previously (*Electroenceph. clin. Neurophysiol.*, 1968, *24*: 593). In 73 of the patients there were no pre-existing factors (such as cerebral lesions or severe metabolic disorders) that might have influenced the EEG: in 23 patients such factors were present. No group differences in the accuracy of prediction of a fatal outcome occurred. A simple continuous monitoring device was used in association with intermittent conventional EEG recordings to ensure that the sampling was representative.

Sustained isoelectric EEGs occurred in 25 patients, all of whom died within 10 days without regaining consciousness. All those who survived their arrest by more than one day and whose brains were examined histologically (9 patients) showed extensive anoxic brain damage. Records with bursts of activity separated by isoelectric periods of over 1 sec duration occurred in 26 patients. 24 of these remained in coma and died: anoxic brain damage was found in all 6 who were examined histologically. Two patients recovered fully: one had suffered from respiratory obstruction (mediastinal lymphosarcoma) and the other from a barbiturate overdose.

The 45 patients with milder types of abnormality all recovered to some degree but 31 died later from their original illnesses. Brain histology confirmed absence of anoxic changes in all 5 who were examined.

---

1. The effects of hypoxia on the blood pressure and EEG in newborn babies. — N. R. C. Roberton and J. P. M. Tizard (London).

The effect of acute hypoxia on the EEG and blood pressure was studied during episodes of respiratory insufficiency in newborn babies. The babies were all being artificially ventilated for severe Respiratory Distress Syndrome and at the time of study an attempt was being made to "wean" them off the ventilator. During this period, simultaneous recordings of the blood pressure and EEG were made and the blood gas tensions were measured. Nine babies in whom an unsuccessful attempt was made to wean them off the ventilator became hypoxaemic without gross abnormalities of arterial pH or pCO_2. The hypoxaemia was associated with an initial slowing of the EEG activity, followed in some cases by activity of less than 20 μV amplitude. During this time the blood pressure was sustained. The data presented also suggest that acute changes in paO_2 are more likely to have an effect on the EEG than gradual changes. The significance of these findings in relation to anoxic perinatal brain injury is discussed.

2. Subjective estimates of sleep: an EEG evaluation. — S. A. Lewis (Edinburgh).

Although there has been a considerable amount of research into sleep, using either subjective or objective (EEG) estimates, there has been no attempt to validate the accuracy of the subjective estimates. The present study investigates the relationship between subjective estimates of total sleep time, delay to sleep onset and the number of awakenings in 8 normal subjects over 116 subject-nights. They were studied before taking drugs, during drug administration and in withdrawal. It was found that they under-estimated total sleep time but over-estimated the delay to sleep onset and the number of awakenings. There was a significant withdrawal effect. The implications of this withdrawal effect are discussed in relation to the design of hypnotic drug trials. The reliability of norms for sleep are also discussed.

3. The use of methohexitone in electrocorticography. — R. Harris and R. Paul (London).

It is evident from the literature that methohexitone (Brietal) has been found an increasingly convenient drug to use in EEG investigations. Its speed of action and rapid metabolism as well as its over-all safety make it especially valuable in out-patient use, as indicated by Fenton and Scotton (*Electroenceph. clin. Neurophysiol.*, 1967, *23*: 273). The particular value of methohexitone in paediatric EEG has been stressed by Frank *et al.* (*Electroenceph. clin. Neurophysiol.*, 1966, *23*: 76).

At the National Hospital we have been interested to note how abnormal EEG phenomena, occasionally accompanied by clinical attacks, may be rapidly provoked by small doses of the drug, and these observations are continuing. We particularly wish to draw attention to the use of the drug in corticography (Pampiglione, *Electroenceph. clin. Neurophysiol.*, 1965, *19*: 314P), in which provocation during differing recording positions may need to be repeated several times during the operation.

Two patients suffering from incapacitating and uncontrollable epilepsy have been studied in detail. Pre-operative investigations showed the value of the drug in facilitating spike discharges in both patients. In one patient the effect of i.v. methohexitone was compared with that of thiopentone during corticography. The rapid appearance of spikes with methohexitone contrasted markedly with their absence using thiopentone. The continuing efficacy of methohexitone to evoke spikes with each subsequent injection was noted in both patients. Methohexitone has slight but important structural differences when compared with other commonly used short-acting barbiturates. The mechanism whereby abnormal EEG phenomena are so easily facilitated by it merits further study.

4. Are we Geoffrey Parr's successors? — A. Rémond (Paris, France).

Thirty years ago, when the EEG contribution to neurophysiology and medicine was born, the most "physicist" of the period's pioneers happened to define fairly implicitly the characteristics of the instruments and the techniques which were likely to render the spontaneous rhythms produced by cerebral activity actually observable in a practical way.

These characteristics were defined, taking into account both what was known of the electrical activity of the brain and the technological possibilities of the day. Instrumental specifications have little by little emerged from that effort at precision. They have been adopted gradually by specialists, EEG Societies and manufacturers all over the world. The best of what has come out of EEG has been largely conditioned by the coherence and efficiency of those rules, and by the discipline with which they have been followed. Nobody can say what would have happened if the rules had been much different.

Until a few years ago there had apparently been no pressing need to re-examine these generally accepted specifications and it is within their original framework that the considerable advances in technology carried out on basic components have been introduced into present day apparatus.

The question now arises as to whether they in fact constitute a brake on progress and whether an entirely new set would be offered to us if a group exactly like the one that originally founded those specifications were introduced to EEG for the first time today in the same way that yesterday's pioneers were from 1935 to 1945. The physiology of the nervous system, experimental psychology, cellular and "whole brain" electrophysiology have considerably advanced the understanding of brain function; at the same time technology has been radically transformed and expanded.

The fundamental phenomena behind the EEG remaining the same, could new improvements be investigated which would show up their intrinsic dimensions of time, space and amplitude? Although our classical recordings allow us to appreciate easily events lasting from 0.05 to 20 sec, how many facts are we missing because they are contained in much shorter periods of towards 0.001 sec or, even more so, in longer periods of up to 24 h? What would we learn by relating our evaluations better with events in their temporal context, knowing that it is not easy to see the hundredth of a second within a second, the second in a minute or the minute in an hour etc. In the domain of space, what would we discover with a resolution reduced to 1 cm or 1 mm instead of the present one which still remains of the order of 5 cm? As for the estimation of amplitudes, which is still gross, we know that it could be considerably refined to give very precise measurements.

However, all these improvements would certainly be useless if we were to continue examining EEGs with the naked eye. It is impossible to think of using these refinements if the time allowed for reading EEGs and the problems of their significance are not viewed in terms of "information theory". Before any evolution can take place in this direction the capacities of direct human observation and reasoning must obviously be powerfully amplified by using computers. We are really facing the possibility of a veritable mutation in our techniques and methods and if this takes place it will involve not only a few specialists but the entire body of existing EEGers. In the next few years, data processing will have made so much progress that it will seem positively aberrant if anyone does not use it to the full. It already represents a real challenge to our discipline. But who will be the technical and methodological counsellors and successors of Geoffrey Parr who are going to find a way to domesticate the revolution happening in front of our eyes?

Data acquisition, transmission, processing and exploitation are all sciences which did not exist 30 years ago. It has never been more vital, in our adaptation to the future, to set at the practitioner's side the team of engineers, mathematicians and logicians who will allow him to bring rapidly to the patient's service the fruits of technical and scientific progress of our day.

5. A pseudo-random binary sequence generator: an aid to testing low frequency-wave analysers. — A. C. Davies, D. S. L. Lloyd and C. D. Binnie (London).

Calibration checks have to be repeatedly carried out on most low frequency wave analysers used in EEG. On every occasion each filter has to be tested with signals of at least three different frequencies. The procedure can be greatly simplified by the use of a composite signal having components at a number of selected frequencies, thus allowing a large number of filters to be checked simultaneously.

A device has been constructed in the Department of Electrical and Electronic Engineering at the City University to generate a binary wave form with a periodic length of 127 bits. When the device is driven by an oscillator at a clock frequency of f c/sec its output appears as a signal which is being switched between two voltage levels apparently at random. This signal can be considered to be equivalent to the sum of the series of sinusoids at the frequencies: $f/127, 2f/127, 3f/127, 4f/127, \ldots f$ c/sec, where the relative amplitudes of the components are accurately known. It will be shown that up to 8 filters of a BNI analyser can be simultaneously tested by using the composite signals produced by only three different clock frequencies. The apparatus can be used to test different types of analysers although operational details will necessarily vary

6. EEG changes in Wilson's disease. — P. Hansotia, R. Harris and J. Kennedy (London).

66 EEG records, taken from 28 patients with Wilson's disease, all of whom showed the characteristic abnormalities of copper metabolism, were studied. The patients, 15 male and 13 female, ranged in age from 8 to 35 years. Five families contributed 17 cases. There was no family history of the disease in the remaining 11. The main clinical features were neurological in 13 patients, hepatic in 12 and mixed in 3. Five siblings of clinically affected patients were asymptomatic. The duration of the illness at the time of the first EEG studies ranged from 2 months to 25 years.

Fourteen cases showed mild or moderate bilateral abnormalities consisting in an excess of theta rhythm without any clear localization or paroxysmal features (Heller and Kooi, *Electroenceph. clin. Neurophysiol.*, 1962, *14*: 520). The more severe degrees of abnormality were found in cases with severe liver dysfunction and these recovered with improvement in the clinical condition. Moderate or mild EEG abnormalities appeared to be shown more prominently by members of some families than by others. Among siblings the occurrence of these EEG abnormalities did not appear to be closely related to the severity of the disease.

Seven patients with prominent neurological disturbances had normal EEGs. The remainder showed moderate EEG abnormalities save for one patient who had myoclonic and major seizures, a rare occurrence in this disease. This patient's EEG showed multi-focal and generalized spikes, often in association with the myoclonic jerks. Clinical improvement of the epilepsy and neurological state was accompanied by improvement in the EEG.

Moderate EEG abnormalities were found in several patients with Wilson's disease, severe EEG disturbances being associated only with severe complications of hepatic or neurological involvement.

7. An effect of oral contraceptives on the EEG of normal females. — J. H. Margerison, C. D. Binnie, P. A. Levy, M. J. Lewis and D. S. L. Lloyd (London).

Changes in the electrical activity of the brain during the menstrual cycle have previously been reported and, in particular, correlations between EEG changes and variations in plasma sodium have been demonstrated. During serial weekly studies on normal females, one started and another stopped taking oral contraceptives. Low Frequency Wave Analysis indicated that a change in dominant frequency of 1 c/sec occurred on starting or stopping the "pill", the lower dominant frequency being significantly associated with the taking of oral contraceptives in both subjects. This effect appeared to be confined to records obtained 1, 3 and 4 weeks after the onset of bleeding. It is provisionally suggested that oral contraceptives can cause a change in the electrical activity of the brain, although the sample was small and certainly no implication is intended that the effect is harmful.

8. An electroencephalographic and psychiatric study of 32 insane murderers. — Z. A. Sayed, S. A. Lewis and R. P. Britain (Warrington, Edinburgh and Carstairs).

An EEG and psychiatric study was carried out on 32 murderers classified legally as insane. Their EEGs, which were read "blind", were compared with a control (non-patient) group and it was found that the patients had an incidence of EEG abnormality about 4 times that of the control group. None was found to contain a spike and wave abnormality. The study confirmed the general finding that approximately half the psychopaths had abnormal EEGs but the psychotic group had a much higher incidence. Also, it was found that the severity of the EEG disturbance was related to the degree of psychiatric disturbance. Comment is made on the value of electroencephalography for forensic psychiatry.

Electroenceph. clin. Neurophysiol., **1969,** *27*: 332–335

Electroencephalography and Clinical Neurophysiology
Elsevier Publishing Company, Amsterdam – Printed in The Netherlands

BOOK REVIEW

Edited by H. PETSCHE *and* JOHN R. HUGHES

Neurophysiological basis of normal and abnormal motor activities. — M. D. Yahr and D. P. Purpura (Editors). (Raven Press, Hewlett, N. Y., 1968, 500 p., $ 25.00).

This book contains 17 papers dealing with current experimental knowledge of the neurophysiology of the motor system. They were all presented at the Third Symposium of the Parkinson's Disease Information and Research Center of Columbia University in November of 1966. Actually, at least one and perhaps more of the papers were not presented but replaced informal discussions held at that time.

Although the proceedings of symposia are often of transitory significance, the careful planning of this particular symposium has resulted in a book of significant value which deserves careful attention. The book is divided into four main divisions ranging from an analysis of the smaller units of the motor system to papers offering a broad perspective on motor organization as a whole. The general plan presents one or more review and/or analytic papers summarizing the present state of a major area of investigation, supplemented with a number of smaller reports which deal with specific experiments. It is not to be expected that the brief specific reports will be of as much general interest as the analytic papers. For this reason, the papers to be commented upon here are biased towards the latter group.

Granit and Kellerth have written a long, carefully reasoned and well documented review of the current status of their experimental program dealing with the effects of muscle stretch receptors on motoneurons. It is one of the best papers in the volume. Other papers in this section, "Regulation of motoneuron excitability", include a morphological study of long term changes in muscle status, an analysis of facilitory and inhibitory influences on spinal motoneurons and a systems engineering approach to the analysis of the "proprioceptive length servo" relating to the problem of tremor.

Oscarsson opens the section on "Cerebellar and brain stem mechanisms influencing spinal reflex activities" with a detailed, clear discussion of the spino-cerebellar paths and their role in conveying information from the spinal cord to the cerebellum. Ito's discussion of the cerebellar efferent system is briefer but no less clear. Among the specific reports in this section, the one by Ayala and Poppele is of particular interest in that it combines classical physiological analysis with actual rotatory stimulation to investigate the central action of vestibular input. Their paper demonstrates once again that to observe adequately the effects of sustained sensory stimulation in the central nervous system appropriate DC techniques must be used.

The section entitled "Approaches to the analysis of motor system organization" contains a wealth of provocative papers. Purpura *et al.* pull together a number of observations by a variety of workers on the general problem of the intrinsic synaptic organization within the corpus striatum and conclude that the thalamus exerts a major influence on synaptic activity within the caudate and lenticular nuclei. They postulate that caudate-induced inhibition of lenticular elements is a major mechanism for regulating output of the corpus striatum. The paper by Evarts entitled "Representation of movements and muscles by pyramidal tract neurons of the precentral motor cortex" is one of the most elegant presentations of scientific work this reviewer has ever read. The experimental design is clever, the presentation clear, and the sophistication of analysis of a high order without becoming at all complex or obscure. Vernon Brooks presents some new data and an interesting summary on the relation between sensory input and motor output in the motor-sensory cortex. Pompeiano, in a chapter on sensory inhibition during motor activity and sleep, concentrates on phasic inhibitory events which occur in the sensory system during REM sleep at the same time when extrinsic ocular and spinal motoneurons are excited. He proposes a model of sensory-motor integration for the movements that occur during sleep.

The final section entitled "Principles and perspectives" presents three papers of broad scope by Drs. Eccles, Denny-Brown and Mettler. Eccles' chapter, "The way in which the cerebellum processes sensory information from muscle", typically presents a very tidy picture which can serve the valuable heuristic purpose of stimulating experiments to prove or disprove his points. Unfortunately, Eccles is so convincing that the uninitiated is likely to accept everything he writes as a proven fact. Denny-Brown presents a traditional Sherringtonian approach to dystonia and other disorders of movement. Mettler makes a personal statement in a chapter entitled "Cortical–subcortical relations in abnormal motor functions". Many workers will find this stimulating.

The book is well printed, and the illustrations are fairly clear. Unfortunately, a number of serious (to the individuals involved) typographical errors appear. Ayala's name is consistently spelled Ajala, and Denny-Brown's name is spelled at least three different ways on three consecutive pages. The book is expensive for its size but of sufficient importance that anyone seriously interested in the motor system will undoubtedly refer to it frequently.

ROBERT J. GUMNIT
St. Paul-Ramsey Hospital,
St. Paul, Minn. 55101 (U.S.A.)

Electroencephalography and Clinical Neurophysiology
Elsevier Publishing Company, Amsterdam – Printed in The Netherlands

ELECTROENCEPHALOGRAPHIC FINDINGS IN EXPERIMENTALLY INDUCED INTRACRANIAL HYPERTENSION

S. L. H. NOTERMANS AND S. BOONSTRA

Neurological Department, State University Hospital, Groningen (The Netherlands)

(Accepted for publication: February 13, 1969)

There is no common opinion about the relationship between intracranial hypertension and alterations in the EEG (Walter 1938; Hoagland *et al.* 1939; Cobb 1945; Glaser and Sjaardema 1945; Cairns 1952; Jasper and Van Buren 1953; Sahs and Joynt 1956; Bagchi *et al.* 1961; Small *et al.* 1961; Mani and Townsend 1964; Bakay and Lee 1965; Lundberg 1965). Williams (1939) could not find any definite relationships between EEG patterns and alterations in the cerebro-spinal fluid (CSF) pressure, although he noted that if the CSF pressure was raised, the EEG was altered at the same moment. He proposed that the intracellular hydration of the white matter could be responsible for the EEG abnormality and that cerebral oedema could be the cause of the disturbances in the electrical activity of the cortex.

Forster and Nims (1942) induced intracranial hypertension in cats, which resulted in a reduction of voltage in the EEG and diminution of the higher frequencies in the EEG pattern, especially of beta activity. Stein and Sonnenschein (1953) raised the cisternal CSF pressure in cats by 20–50% of the original level, resulting in a reduction of the beta frequencies. Jasper and Van Buren (1953) suggested that slowing of the EEG, which is often seen with brain-stem tumours, could be caused by an increase in the intracranial pressure.

In our series of experiments we investigated the relationships between CSF pressure changes and the EEG. We induced increased CSF pressure in cats in cooperation with the work group of experimental neurosurgery in Groningen (Head: Prof. J. Beks) which has developed an effective method of inducing cerebral oedema, with subsequent herniation of the brain, by local cooling of the brain surface (Beks *et al.* 1965).

MATERIAL AND METHODS

The subjects were twenty-six adult cats of both sexes, weighing about 3 kg. Each animal was anaesthetized with Pentothal 20 mg/kg body weight, and sodium phenobarbital 50 mg/kg. The narcosis was maintained with a nitrous oxide-oxygen mixture and sometimes with halothane if necessary. The animal was intubated but breathing spontaneously. The femoral artery and vein were cannulated for continuous measurement of the arterial and venous pressures. The cat's head was fixed in a stereotaxic apparatus. During the experiments the CSF pressure was measured with the aid of a Statham physiological pressure transducer, P 23 AA, connected with a special needle inserted stereotaxically into the cella media of the right lateral ventricle, according to Jasper and Ajmone Marsan's coordinates (1955). The body temperature was held constant at normal levels by infra-red radiation.

During the experiments the arterial and venous blood pressures and the CSF pressure were recorded continuously, together with the ECG, respiration and EEG, on an 8-channel Elema polygraph. Bipolar EEGs were obtained from 4 cortical silver electrodes, 2 just in front of the coronal suture and 2 in the occipital region, in the same sagittal plane. The time constant was 1 sec. The polygraphic records were visually analysed and the frequencies and amplitudes were measured by hand. To produce cerebral oedema a cryoprobe was applied directly to the intact dura mater via a 13 mm burr hole in the left frontal region, centred 10 mm behind the coronal suture and 15 mm from the midline.

Before the cooling probe was applied, a 1 h base-

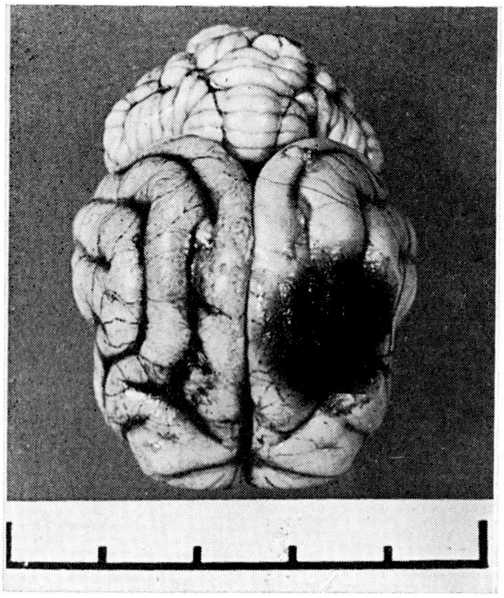

Fig. 1
Photograph of a cat's brain, demonstrating the cortical lesion after cold injury. Calibration in cm.

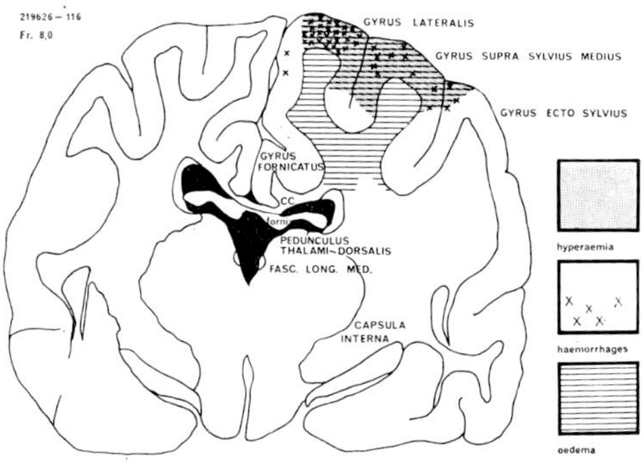

Fig. 2
Schematic drawing of a coronal section of a cat's brain, showing the extent of cerebral oedema and the cortical lesion.

line recording was obtained of the CSF pressure in the ventricular system and of the other parameters, so that every animal could serve as its own control. Then cooled methanol was pumped from a Lauda-ultrakryostat through the thermode. The local temperature obtained was −30°C, maintained for 10 min. The thermode was left *in situ* throughout the experiment to avoid disturbing the intracranial pressure by its removal.

The cortical lesion which resulted from the local cooling was sharply circumscribed, with a diameter of 13–17 mm, and had a slightly swollen region of darker colour compared with the adjacent areas. The cortex immediately around the lesion often seemed a little paler than that of the opposite hemisphere (Fig. 1). The histological features of the cortical lesion resembled those of a recent infarct. Especially in the cortex, and to a lesser degree in the white matter, the chilled area contained lesions of the vascular walls, with leakage of fluid (Fig. 2) (Beks *et al.* 1965; Go *et al.* 1967).

RESULTS

Twenty-six experiments were performed. In twenty-two cats the brains were cooled locally and in sixteen cases this resulted in an increase in the CSF pressure to such a level that herniation of the brain-stem followed. In the other six cats cooling did not produce a very high intraventricular pressure, even if cold was applied twice at the same place. We also did 4 control experiments in order to check the influence of anaesthesia. Table I summarizes the results of these 16 experiments.

The initial intraventricular pressure showed considerable variations, ranging from 50 to 300 mm H_2O. During cooling the CSF pressure usually decreased, in contrast with the findings of Clasen *et al.* (1953, 1962). For about 1–3 h following the cold injury, the intraventricular pressure gradually increased, which led to displacement of the brain mass and compression of the brain-stem. Then changes in the arterial blood pressure, in the ECG and in the type of respiration were noted. Irregular respiration and disturbances in ECG about 10 min before the respiratory arrest were often the initial symptoms of the impending cerebral herniation. Simultaneous with respiratory irregularity the EEG became slower. When the CSF pressure rose to about 1500 mm H_2O the respiration became irregular and often of the Cheyne-Stokes type. About 20 min after the onset of these symptoms of intracranial hypertension and cerebral compression the CSF pressure reached its maximum value. This peak varied considerably, ranging from 1300 to 3000 mm H_2O. When herniation occurred the following symptoms could be noted: the arterial pressure rose sharply, up to 330 mm Hg (normal level ranging about 120–190 mm Hg), the respiration ceased at the highest level of the intraventricular pressure, and piloerection and decerebrate rigidity occurred. Immediately thereafter the ventricular pressure fell below the original level and the arterial pressure rapidly decreased. Unless corrective measures were taken the animal died.

In a number of experiments, 1 min after the onset of respiratory arrest, the cats were infused with hypertonic solutions, urea or mannitol, and artificial respiration was performed. In these cases the spontaneous respiration was re-established after a few minutes (Table I) and the CSF pressure rose again (Beks and ter Weeme 1967). Histological post mortem examination of the brains, fixed in 10% formol solution, showed in most cases herniation of the cerebellar tonsils into the foramen magnum; sometimes herniation of the uncus through the tentorium was seen.

During cooling the following EEG changes were observed (Fig. 3): (1) A diffuse acceleration of cerebral activity, especially an increase of beta and alpha frequencies, were noted. (2) Absolute and relative reductions of the slower frequencies were noted. (3) An amplitude reduction on both sides of about 20–40% of the original level occurred and, in about half of the experiments, this reduction persisted even after cooling was terminated. In the rest of the cases the amplitudes returned to the baseline after a few minutes. (4) Gross asymmetry of voltage developed. The cooled left side had EEG voltages 30–50% lower than the opposite side, which persisted throughout the experiment.

Fig. 4 shows a histogram of the measured voltages of the delta frequencies (less than 3.5 c/sec) in the course of one experiment (EEG No. 65–03, Table I). From this figure it is clear that the first voltage reduction appeared during the cooling period. The second voltage reduction, following cerebral herniation, did not recover unless special measures were taken to prevent the death of the animal. When the CSF pressure increased, for example within 3 min from 700 to 1400 mm H_2O, no gross visible alterations in the EEG occurred during these abrupt rises (EEG No. 65–21, Table I).

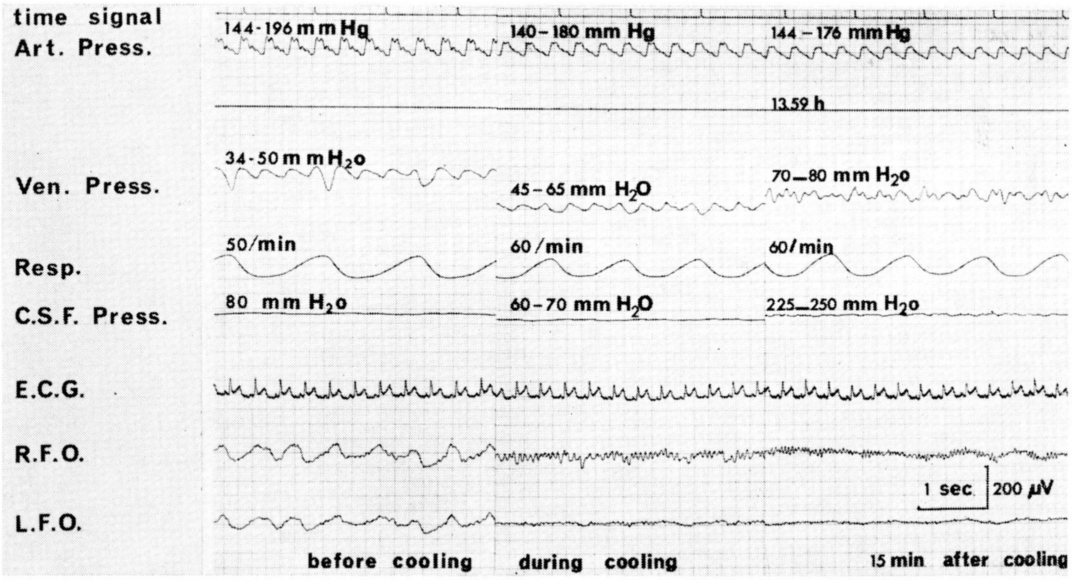

Fig. 3

Polygraphic recording before, during and after cooling. TC 1 sec. Note the increase of beta and alpha frequencies in the EEG during and after cooling, the asymmetry in amplitude between left and right, and the reduction of the amplitude on both sides.

Abbreviations in this and following illustrations: Art. Press.: arterial pressure; Ven. Press.: venous pressure; Resp.: respiration; C.S.F. Press.: cerebro-spinal fluid pressure; E.C.G.: electrocardiogram; R.F.O.: right fronto-occipital EEG; L.F.O.: left fronto-occipital EEG (side of the cerebral cold lesion).

TABLE I

Summary of the most relevant polygraphic values during herniation. CSFP, cerebro-spinal fluid pressure. †, animal died.

EEG No.	First respiration stop after cooling (min)	Maximum CSFP (mm H_2O)	Maximum art. pressure		EEG isoelectrical record		Duration of artificial respiration (min)	Procedure
			(mm Hg)	(mm H_2O)	Time after respiration stop (sec)	Duration (sec)		
65–21	36	1300	230	3128	30	†	No	Blank
–28	139	1350	180	2448	Simultaneously	†	No	Blank
–25	100	2300	240	3264	Simultaneously	†	No	Blank
–02	85	1850	200	2720	No	Only reduction of amplitude of 75%	6	Urea i.v.
–03	63	1720	150	2040	60	45	6	Urea i.v.
–07	42	2800	230	3128	60	4	7	Strophanthin + urea i.v.
–08	73	2000	180	2448	60	4	7	Strophanthin + urea i.v.
–09	46	1400	180	2448	15	75	3	Strophanthin + urea i.v.
–10	62	2600	240	3264	35	50	2.5	Strophanthin + urea i.v.
–05	72	2000	180	2448	No	Only reduction of amplitude of 50%	6	Calcium + urea i.v.
–15	178	1900	200	2720	Simultaneously	5	3.5	Calcium + urea i.v.
–17	58	1900	175	2380	45	90	4	Calcium + urea i.v.
–06	169	2920	254	3454	60	5	8	Mannitol
–14	79	1400	225	3060	Simultaneously	150	8.25	Mannitol
–23	94	2400	250	3400	60	5	45†	Lasix
–24	104	3000	330	4488	30	5	45†	Lasix

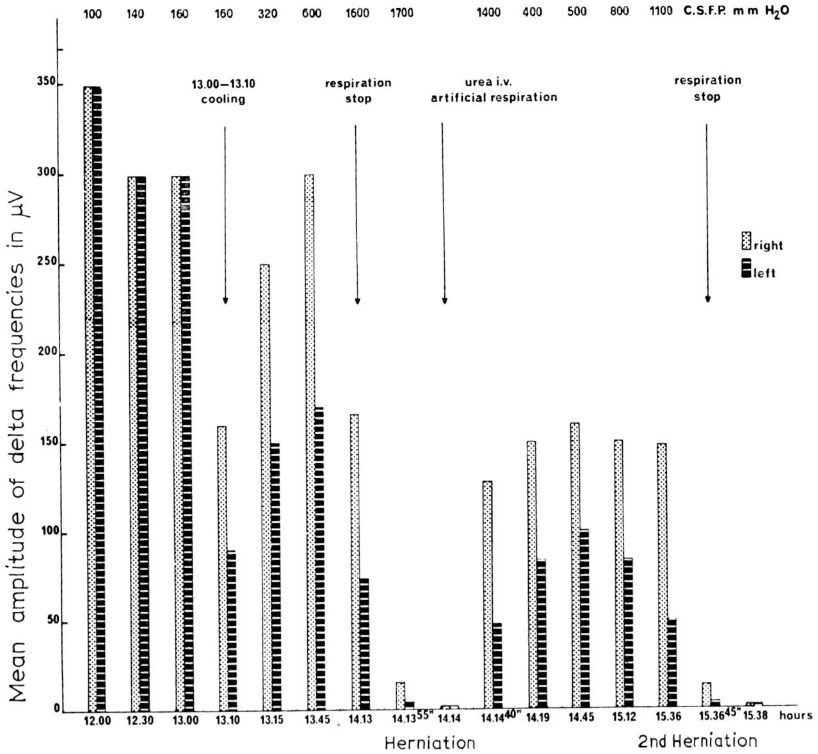

Fig. 4

Histogram of the mean amplitudes of delta activities during an experiment. CSF pressure in mm H_2O above each bar. During herniation the EEG became isoelectric.

EEG disturbances were recognizable in all the 16 records with herniation and may be summarized as follows: about 1 min before the arrest of respiration the EEG became diffusely slower and at the same time voltage reduction occurred (Fig. 5). This reduction in voltage was most evident in the faster frequencies but also appeared in the theta and delta activities. After respiration finally stopped, most of the records showed an isoelectric EEG within 30 sec (Fig. 5, 6), but in two cases the amplitude was reduced only to 50–75% of the level before herniation (EEG No. 65–02, and 65–05, Table I).

In 13 of the experiments (Table I) artificial respiration was started 1 min after breathing stopped (Fig. 6) and the animals were treated intravenously with hypertonic solutions of urea or mannitol to combat the experimentally induced increase in CSF pressure. About 5–25 sec after artificial respiration was begun the EEG activity returned. About 3–9 min (mean 5 min) after the first reappearance of the electrical activity, the EEG was almost comparable to that about 15 min before herniation occurred. In most cases this restoration coincided with the return of spontaneous respiration. Table I shows that we did not administer any medicaments (blank procedure) to three cats; these untreated cats all died immediately as a consequence of the first herniation. In two other animals who received fursemide (Lasix, Hoechst, Germany), instead of urea or mannitol, to correct the cerebral herniation the spontaneous respiration failed to return even after 45 min of artificial respiration.

DISCUSSION

The relationship between the cerebro-spinal fluid pressure and the EEG has been the subject of several investigations (Cobb 1945; Clasen *et al.* 1958; Bagchi *et al.* 1961; Herschkowitz *et al.* 1965; Wilson *et al.* 1965; Langfitt *et al.* 1966).

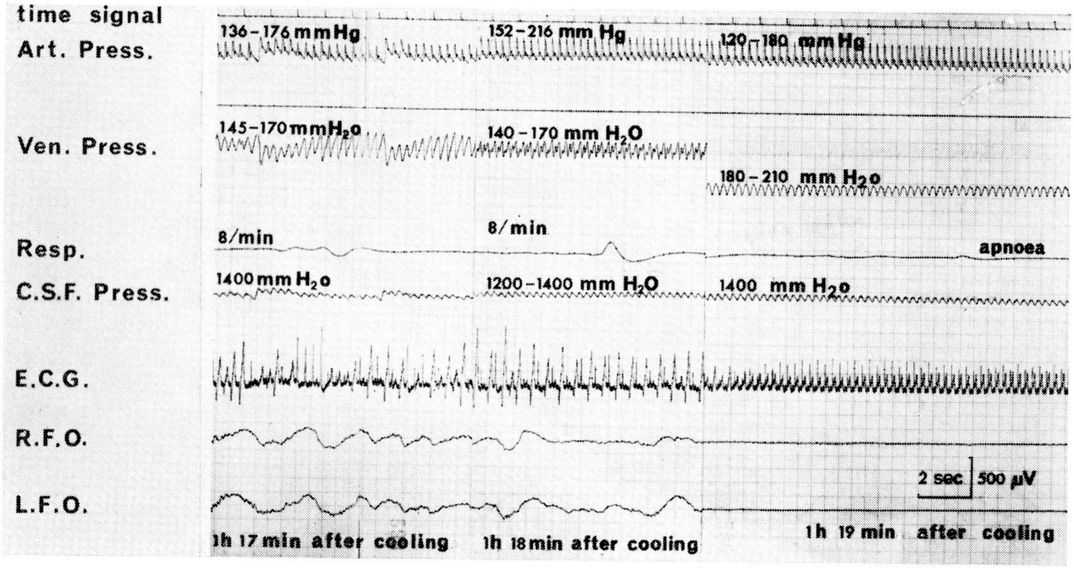

Fig. 5
Polygraphic recording during herniation. Note the irregularity of the ECG and the rapid increase of the CSF pressure. The respiration becomes more and more irregular and slower; after respiration ceases, the EEG becomes slower and finally isoelectric.

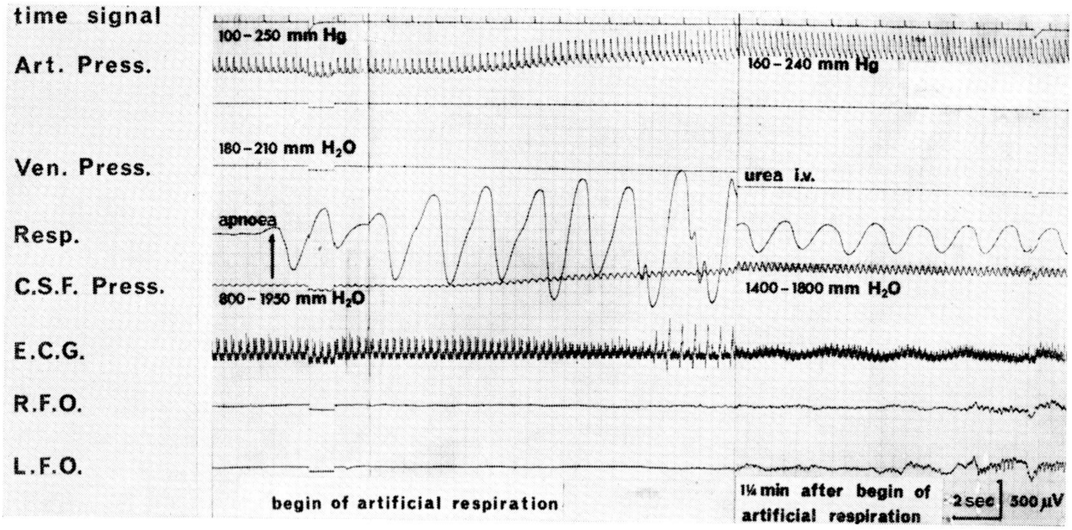

Fig. 6
Polygraphic recording shortly after artificial respiration was started (1 min after respiratory arrest during cerebral herniation). Note that the EEG is gradually restored and that the ECG becomes more regular and faster.

Stewart (1941) emphasized that it was necessary to consider all possible mechanisms which can cause intracranial hypertension. He produced non-communicating hydrocephalus with increased intraventricular pressure in young adult cats, whose EEGs all showed an evident slowing. In a second series of experiments he increased the CSF pressure by raising the hydrostatic pressure in the foramen magnum by means of injections of distilled water, or by ligating the cerebral veins, but these EEGs did not show any specific alterations.

Forster and Nims (1942) and Kramer and Tuynman (1967) found that the EEG became isoelectric when the cisternal CSF pressure rose above the arterial pressure. We did not find this phenomenon in our series of experiments, as shown in Table I. This difference in findings may be due to the different ways of measuring the spinal fluid pressure. Forster and Nims registered the cisternal pressure and we always determined the intraventricular pressure. In most of our experiments, even those in which the arterial pressure was higher than the intraventricular pressure, the EEG became isoelectric as soon as the brain herniated and respiration stopped.

Tiberin *et al.* (1963) also increased the cisternal CSF pressure by intravenous injections of distilled water and did not find significant EEG alterations. They reported some increase in fast EEG activity but only in anaesthetized animals. We could not establish any constant correlation between the EEG patterns and the variations in intraventricular pressure. Gastaut *et al.* (1960) and Cohadon (1964) could not establish any significant changes in the EEG at the time of cerebral oedema and vascular congestion in their series of experiments, in which they evoked encephalomyelitis in monkeys with Japanese B encephalitis virus. We also could not establish any such correlation although cerebral oedema, both cortical and in the white matter, was usually strictly limited to the hemisphere on the side of the cold-induced lesion.

Concerning the EEG asymmetry between sides, appearing during and especially after cooling, we considered the following hypotheses. First, we believe the effect of cooling itself to be responsible for the amplitude reduction in the EEG, secondary to several biochemical alterations in the metabolism of the neurones of the cerebral cortex (Bindman *et al.* 1963; Massopust *et al.* 1964; Pagni and Courjon 1964; Morrell *et al.* 1965). Secondly, the cold lesion of the cerebral cortex in particular showed vascular disorders resembling a recent infarction and to a lesser degree also in the white matter. The chilled area contained lesions of the vascular wall with leakage of fluid (Ebels 1965; Go *et al.* 1967). McGillivray *et al.* (1964) observed that in nearly all their cases of induced cerebral oedema in monkeys a considerable suppression of delta burst activity appeared. It should be noted that they recorded with a TC of 0.1 sec. On the whole it is generally accepted that diffuse cerebral oedema has little effect on the EEG.

There are several clinical studies of the relationship between EEG and cerebro-spinal fluid pressure. Wilson *et al.* (1965) measured the CSF pressure through a lumbar puncture needle inserted into the subarachnoid space at the fourth lumbar interspace in ten patients. Although the maximal measured lumbar pressure was 1175 mm H_2O, they could not establish any EEG abnormality in relation to changes of pressure. Correlations between intracranial hypertension and EEG were not observed, in most cases only minimal EEG changes in relation to CSF pressure being noted (Foley 1955, 1957; Davidoff 1956; Ingvar and Lundberg 1961; Sidell and Daly 1961; Silverman 1964). These clinical findings appear to be in agreement with our experimental results, in which we could not establish a definitive relationship between EEG alterations and CSF pressure changes.

Regarding the EEG changes in our experiments at the moment of the herniation we consider secondary vascular disturbances in the brain-stem as the main cause, in agreement with Le Beau and Dondey (1956) and Langfitt *et al.* (1966). Perhaps the appearance of diffuse slowing of the EEG during herniation is associated with functional disturbances of the upper part of the brain-stem, caused by stretching and compression of the basal arterial rami perforantes. It is important to emphasize that in our animal experiments, even after a totally isoelectric period as the result of cerebral herniation, the EEG activity could return, as an expression of cortical function, if the cerebral anoxia had not been of long duration.

In order to obtain more information about the mechanisms of increased cerebral pressure in relation to the EEG activity it is important to have data on spinal fluid pressures, obtained by cisternal and lumbar measurements, besides the intraventricular pressure values.

SUMMARY

Unilateral cerebral cortical lesions were made in twenty-six cats by the extradural application of a cold probe to produce cerebral oedema, resulting in increased cerebro-spinal fluid pressure. During these experiments the CSF pressure in one of the lateral ventricles, the arterial and venous blood pressures, respiration, ECG and EEG were recorded continuously. Increased CSF pressure was obtained in 16 of 22 experiments to such a degree that herniation of the brain-stem followed. Four control experiments were performed. This study especially concerns the relationship between the EEG and the changes in CSF pressure.

1. There were no obvious correlations between alterations in the intraventricular pressure and the EEG.

2. We did not find a clear relationship between the extent of the cerebral oedema and EEG changes.

3. Cooling caused the following EEG abnormalities: (a) Slow wave activity largely disappeared during local extradural cooling. The faster rhythmic beta and alpha activities increased, especially from 16 to 20 c/sec, relatively as well as absolutely. (b) On both sides, in fronto-occipital derivations, voltage reduction occurred. This was more pronounced on the cooled side, which had a 50% reduction in voltage. This difference continued in most cases after cooling and was probably caused by the local cortical lesion.

4. At the beginning of cerebral herniation the EEG showed gross abnormalities; about 5 min before the respiratory arrest, general slowing of the EEG and reduction of voltage were observed. In most cases the EEG became isoelectric as soon as respiration stopped. After starting artificial respiration electrical activity reappeared after 5–150 sec.

RÉSUMÉ

L'HYPERTENSION INTRA-CRÂNIENNE, PROVOQUÉE EXPÉRIMENTALEMENT, ET L'EEG

Une lésion extradurale par refroidissement a été provoquée dans le cortex cérébral chez vingt-six chats, afin d'obtenir expérimentalement un oedème cérébral et par conséquence une hypertension céphalo-rachidienne. Dans ce but une sonde réfrigérante a été placée sur la dure-mère intacte par une trépanation frontale. Durant ces expériences on a enregistré de manière continue la pression dans les ventricules latéraux, de même que la pression artérielle et veineuse, tandis que la respiration, l'ECG et l'EEG ont été enregistrés polygraphiquement.

Dans ce travail on a obtenu une hypertension ventriculaire dans seize cas sur vingt-deux au moyen de refroidissement local aboutissant à un cône de pression de tronc cérébral. Quatre autres cas ont servi de contrôle.

Le rapport entre l'EEG et les variations de la pression ventriculaire a été spécialement étudié.

Nous voudrions conclure en mentionnant l'influence nette sur l'EEG, exercée par le refroidissement ainsi que par le cône de pression. Par contre il n'y avait pas de rapport evident entre l'augmentation de la pression ventriculaire et l'EEG.

REFERENCES

BAGCHI, B. K., KOOI, K. A., SELVING, B. T. and CALHOUN, H. D. Subtentorial tumors and other lesions: an electroencephalographic study of 121 cases. *Electroenceph. clin. Neurophysiol.*, **1961,** *13*: 180–192.

BAKAY, L. and LEE, J. C. *Cerebral edema.* Thomas, Springfield, Ill., **1965:** 114–120.

BEKS, J. W. F. and TER WEEME, C. A. The influence of urea and mannitol on increased intraventricular pressure in cold-induced cerebral oedema. *Acta Neurochir. (Wien)*, **1967,** *16*: 97–107.

BEKS, J. W. F., TER WEEME, C. A., EBELS, E. J., WALTER, W. G. and WASSENAAR, J. S. Increase in intraventricular pressure in cold induced cerebral oedema. *Acta Physiol. Pharmacol. neerl.*, **1965,** *13*: 317–329.

BINDMAN, L., LIPPOLD, O. C. J. and REDFEARN, J. W. T. Comparison of general body cooling and local cooling of the surface of the brain. *Electroenceph. clin. Neurophysiol.*, **1963,** *15*: 238–245.

CAIRNS, H. Disturbances of consciousness with lesions of the brainstem and diencephalon. *Brain*, **1952,** *75*: 109–146.

CLASEN, R. A., BROWN, O. V. L., LEAVIFF, S. and HASS, G. M. The production by liquid nitrogen of acute closed cerebral lesions. *Surg. Gynec. Obstet.*, **1953,** *96*: 605–616.

CLASEN, R. A., COOKE, P. M., MARTIN, F. A., WILLIAMS, J. R. and HASS, G. M. Cerebral edema and electroencephalographic changes after local acute closed cerebral injury. *Arch. Neurol. Psychiat. (Chic.)*, **1958,** *80*: 696–707.

CLASEN, R. A., COOKE, P. M., PANDOLFI, S., BOYD, D. and RAIMANDI, A. J. Experimental cerebral edema produced by focal freezing. I. An anatomical study utilizing vital dye techniques. *J. Neuropath. exp. Neurol.*, **1962,** *21*: 579–596.

COBB, W. A. Rhythmic slow discharges in the electroencephalogram. *J. Neurol. Neurosurg. Psychiat.*, **1945,** *8*: 65–78.

COHADON, F. EEG and cerebral oedema. An EEG analysis of a series of 30 cases of benign intracranial hypertension. *Electroenceph. clin. Neurophysiol.*, **1964,** *17*: 347P.

DAVIDOFF, L. M. Pseudotumor cerebri. Benign intracranial hypertension. *Neurology (Minneap.)*, **1956,** *6*: 605–615.

EBELS, E. J. Hersenoedeem bij katten door lokale hypothermie. *Ned. T. Geneesk.*, **1965,** *109*: 1226–1227.

FOLEY, J. Benign forms of intracranial hypertension. "Toxic" and "otitic" hydrocephalus. *Brain*, **1955,** *78*: 1–41.

FOLEY, J. Physiology of increased intracranial pressure. In D. WILLIAMS (Ed.), *Modern trends in neurology, 2nd. series*. Butterworth, London, **1957:** 44–65.

FORSTER, F. M. and NIMS, L. F. Electroencephalographic effects of acute increases of intracranial pressure. *Arch. Neurol. Psychiat. (Chic.)*, **1942,** *47*: 449–453.

GASTAUT, H., TOGA, M., BERT, P., PAYAN, H. et NETTER, J. A clinical, EEG and anatomical study of experimental Japanese "B" encephalitis in monkey. *J. nerv. ment. Dis.*, **1960,** *30*: 160.

GLASER, M. A. and SJAARDEMA, H. Effect on the electroencephalogram of localized pressure on the brain. *J. Neurophysiol.*, **1945,** *9*: 63–72.

GO, K. G., EBELS, E. J., BEKS, J. W. F. and TER WEEME, C. A. The spreading of cerebral edema from a cold injury in cats. *Psychiat. Neurol. Neurochir. (Amst.)*, **1967,** *70*: 403–411.

HERSCHKOWITZ, H., MACGILLIVRAY, B. B. and CUMINGS, J. N. Biochemical and electrophysiological studies in experimental cerebral oedema. *Brain*, **1965,** *88*: 557–584.

HOAGLAND, H., HIMWICH, H. E., CAMPBELL, E., FAZEKAS, J. F. and HADIDIAN, Z. Effects of hypoglycemia and pentobarbital sodium on electrical activity of cerebral cortex and hypothalamus (dogs). *J. Neurophysiol.*, **1939,** *2*: 276–288.

INGVAR, D. H. and LUNDBERG, N. Paroxysmal symptoms in intracranial hypertension, studied with ventricular fluid pressure recording and electroencephalography. *Brain*, **1961,** *84*: 446–459.

JASPER, H. H. and AJMONE MARSAN, C. *Stereotaxic atlas of the diencephalon of the cat.* Nat. Res. Council of Canada, Ottawa, **1955.**

JASPER, H. and VAN BUREN, J. Interrelationship between cortex and subcortical structures: clinical electroencephalographic studies. *Electroenceph. clin. Neurophysiol.*, **1953,** *Suppl. 4*: 168–188.

KRAMER, W. and TUYNMAN, J. A. Acute intracranial hypertension and experimental investigation. *Brain Res.*, **1967,** *6*: 686–705.

LANGFITT, T. W., TANNANBAUM, H. M., KASSELL, N. F. and ZAREN, H. Acute intracranial hypertension, cerebral blood flow, and the EEG. *Electroenceph. clin. Neurophysiol.*, **1966,** *20*: 139–148.

LE BEAU, J. and DONDEY, M. EEG studies in some cases of cerebral herniations, some accompanied by brain stem lesions. *Electroenceph. clin. Neurophysiol.*, **1956,** *8*: 173P.

LUNDBERG, N. Continuous recording and control of ventricular fluid pressure in patients with severe acute traumatic brain injury. A preliminary report. *J. Neurosurg.*, **1965,** *22*: 581.

MCGILLIVRAY, B. B., HERSCHKOWITZ, H. et SNOW, E. A. Quelques modifications de l'EEG et de l'impédance dans l'oedème cérébral expérimental. *Rev. neurol.*, **1964,** *111*: 386–391.

MANI, K. S. and TOWNSEND, H. R. A. The electroencephalogram in benign intracranial hypertension. *Electroenceph. clin. Neurophysiol.*, **1964,** *16*: 604–610.

MASSOPUST, L. C., ALBIN, M. S., BARNES, H. W., MEDER, R. and KRETCHMER, H. W. Cortical and subcortical responses to hypothermia. *Exp. Neurol.*, **1964,** *9*: 249–261.

MORRELL, F., PROCTOR, F. and PRINCE, D. A. Epileptogenic properties of subcortical freezing. *Neurology (Minneap.)*, **1965,** *15*: 744–751.

PAGNI, C. A. and COURJON, J. Electroencephalographic modifications induced by moderate and deep hypothermia in man. In P. E. MASPES and B. HUGHES (Eds.), *Hypothermia in neurosurgery. Acta Neurochir. (Wien)*, **1964,** *Suppl. 13*: 35–49.

SAHS, A. L. and JOYNT, R. J. Brain swelling of unknown cause. *Neurology (Minneap.)*, **1956,** *6*: 791–803.

SIDELL, A. D. and DALY, D. D. The electroencephalogram in cases of benign intracranial hypertension. *Neurology (Minneap.)*, **1961,** *11*: 413–417.

SILVERMAN, D. Papilledema and the electroencephalogram. *Neurology (Minneap.)*, **1964,** *14*: 899–907.

SMALL, J. G., BAGCHI, B. K. and KOOI, K. A. Electroclinical profile of 117 deep cerebral tumors. *Electroenceph. clin. Neurophysiol.*, **1961,** *13*: 193–207.

STEIN, S. N. and SONNENSCHEIN, R. R. Some relationships between intracranial pressure and EEG frequencies in cats. *Proc. Soc. exp. Biol. (N. Y.)*, **1953,** *82*: 509–511.

STEWART, A. W. Electroencephalographic changes associated with different forms of experimentally produced increased intracranial pressure. *Bull. Johns Hopk. Hosp.*, **1941,** *69*: 240–265.

TIBERIN, P., PAILLAS, J. et GASTAUT, H. Études cliniques et paracliniques. L'aspect EEG de l'oedème cérébral. In G. LAZORTHES et L. CAMPAN (Eds.), *L'oedème cérébral*. Masson, Paris, **1963:** 66–72.

WALTER, W. G. Critical review. The technique and applications of electroencephalography. *J. Neurol. Psychopath.*, **1938,** *1*: 359–385.

WILLIAMS, D. The abnormal cortical potential associated with high intracranial pressure. *Brain*, **1939,** *62*: 321–334.

WILSON, W. P., TINDALL, G. T. and GREENFIELD, J. C. Effects of an acute increase of intracranial pressure upon the electroencephalogram. *Electroenceph. clin. Neurophysiol.*, **1965,** *19*: 184–186.

Reference: NOTERMANS, S. L. H. and BOONSTRA, S. Electroencephalographic findings in experimentally induced intracranial hypertension. *Electroenceph. clin. Neurophysiol.*, **1969,** *27*: 337–345.

Electroencephalography and Clinical Neurophysiology
Elsevier Publishing Company, Amsterdam – Printed in The Netherlands

HUMAN VIGILANCE AND AUDITORY EVOKED RESPONSES

H. FRUHSTORFER AND R. M. BERGSTRÖM[1]

Institute of Physiology, University of Helsinki, Helsinki (Finland)

(Accepted for publication: January 30, 1969)

Vigilance, as defined by Head (1923), is the dimension of the organizational level of the central nervous functions. Availability, efficiency and integration of sensory, motor and mental processes are determined by the degree of vigilance.

Vigilance is reflected in the electrical activity of the brain. For the spontaneous activity this fact has long been established. The EEG patterns characterizing the vigilance levels between alertness and the onset of real sleep (intermediate stages according to Bente 1964) have, however, been less well described than those occurring in real sleep. This becomes evident in the commonly adopted EEG classifications (Loomis *et al.* 1937 supplemented by the REM stage described by Dement and Kleitman 1957) which distinguish two intermediate stages, A and B, but for sleep stages: C, D, E, REM. As these EEG classifications were usually applied when studying sensory evoked responses at different levels of vigilance, the results naturally do not provide detailed information about the changes occurring within the wide span of wakefulness. And there have been only a few attempts to study evoked responses at the intermediate levels of vigilance, using the spontaneous alpha activity alone as a vigilance indicator (Kooi and Bagchi 1964; Levonian 1966; Artseulova and Ivanitsky 1967).

Much knowledge has been accumulated about changes in the evoked response accompanying fluctuations in the maintenance of an actively raised vigilance level, as judged from discrimination capacity (Haider *et al.* 1964), motor performance (Morrell and Morrell 1966; Donchin and Lindsley 1966; Wilkinson and Morlock 1967) or combinations of these (Näätänen 1967).

The common result emerging from most of these studies is the finding that the evoked response amplitude decreases if vigilance decreases within wakefulness, but, because of different methods, a comparison of the results on the basis of a common vigilance scale is not possible.

This study is an attempt to analyse the auditory evoked response in man quantitatively at several clearly defined levels of intermediate vigilance. The EEG classification of Bente (1964), which is based on Loomis' scheme and uses the subdivision of the B stage proposed by Roth (1961), served as a vigilance indicator. Bente's classification describes seven distinct EEG patterns for the intermediate stages by taking into account the temporo-spatial organization of the alpha activity.

As vigilance fluctuates continuously, its level was determined for every single stimulus response and the responses were summated selectively according to the vigilance levels at which they were evoked. Additionally, care was taken to minimize factors which either are dependent on vigilance and influence the evoked response (*e.g.*, habituation; Marsh and Worden 1964) or which cause vigilance states difficult to assess from the EEG (*e.g.*, directed attention).

METHODS

Subjects and experimental situation

Seven healthy, not sleep-deprived, volunteers (Fig. 1) with good regular alpha activity participated as subjects in the experiments, which took place in a sound-shielded anechoic room (Bergström *et al.* 1969) during day-time. As, in this environment, it proved to be impossible to remain alert with closed eyes for more than a few

[1] R.M.B. was supported by a grant from the Signe and Ane Gyllenberg Foundation.

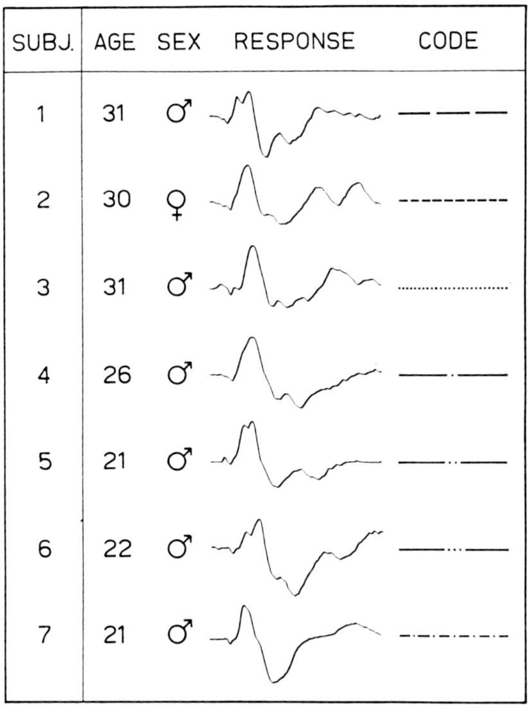

Fig. 1
Age, sex and typical average evoked responses of the subjects together with the codes by which they are represented in the diagrams. (Responses from stage A_4; derivation I; negativity of electrode 2 upward; traces cover the 480 msec following the stimulus onset.)

minutes, two types of experimental situations had to be created:
type 1: for the alert stage the subject was sitting with open eyes in the dimly lit room, receiving 40 stimuli over a period of approximately 8 min;
type 2: for the intermediate stages and sleep the subject was lying on his back with closed eyes in the dark room, receiving about 400 stimuli over a period of approximately 80 min.

In both experimental situations the subject was instructed not to pay attention to the stimulus or react to it. Five experiments of each type were carried out for every subject on different days.

Stimulation

In all experiments a click of about 60 dB above subjective threshold (rectangular pulse, duration 1 msec) served as stimulus. It was presented at intervals of 8–20 sec (mean 12 sec) from a loudspeaker (diameter 210 mm, range 40–18000 c/sec) placed 2 m in front of the subject's head.

Data recording

The EEG was recorded bipolarly from a midsagittal montage which was chosen because it picks up, from only a few derivations, spatial changes in the spontaneous activity as well as the unspecific evoked response at the vertex. Five electrodes (diameter 9 mm) were fixed with collodion along the midline at points equally spaced by 20% of the nasion–inion distance, the first point being 15% of this distance above the nasion. The earth electrode was fixed to the wrist. In the text electrodes and derivations are numbered from frontal to occipital with arabic and roman numerals respectively. The EEG, together with a stimulus mark, was stored on magnetic tape and written on paper. The recording system was set to pass a frequency band between 0.8 c/sec and 50 c/sec (3 dB points).

The level of vigilance was visually determined for every single stimulus response from the 2 sec EEG epoch prior to the stimulus according to the slightly modified classification of Bente (1964) (Table I). The vigilance stages of all responses were then entered into a LINC computer which transferred them in a four bit code to the analog tape just prior to their corresponding stimulus marks. Then, in several runs, the single responses from all four derivations were selectively sampled and summated by the LINC according to the vigilance stages to which they belonged (sampling rate: 500 samples in 60 msec at 8 × recording speed). Single responses which were spoilt by blink, movement or muscle artefacts, or which could not be classified (*e.g.*, occurrence of alpha activity in experiments of type 1), were omitted from summation. The summated responses were stored on digital tape and plotted on paper.

Data processing

Peak amplitudes and latencies of the different components of the summated responses from derivations I and III were measured on the LINC oscilloscope by a cursor program which displayed the coordinate values of any wanted point of the wave form. The latencies were referred to the stimulus onset, the amplitudes to

TABLE I

Criteria according to which EEG samples of 2 sec duration were visually classified. From the classification proposed by Bente (1964) stages B_3 (3–5 c/sec waves > 40 μV), E, and REM were left out because they seldom or never occurred in the experiments of type 2. Stages B_3 and E were covered by C and D respectively. Stage O was added in order to obtain enough data at a high vigilance level. Roman numerals refer to derivations

Stage	Experimental situation	EEG criteria	Comments
O	*Type 1*: Subject sitting, eyes open, relaxed, not attentive; dim light.	Desynchronized low voltage activity over the whole convexity.	Occurrence of only little alpha in one derivation does not belong to this stage.
A_1	*Type 2*: Subject lying on back, eyes closed, relaxed, not attentive; no light.	Continuous monorhythmic occipital alpha with spread to parietal, temporal and central areas.	Continuous regular alpha in IV, moderate in III, little or none in I and II.
A_2		Parietal alpha maximum. Beginning modulation of still continuous regular occipital alpha activity. Beginning slowing.	Continuous regular alpha equal or better in III than in IV.
A_3		Parietal and precentral alpha maximum. Occipital alpha discontinuous. Beginning frequency lability: mainly slower alpha in central and parietal regions.	Maximum as defined rarely seen. Additionally: little or moderate alpha in III and IV; moderate alpha in IV with low and irregular activity in I–III.
A_4		Alpha low and discontinuous. Frequency variations, polyrhythmic activity. Low 16–30 c/sec activity.	Irregular alpha in one of I–IV (mostly III); also: moderate 7–8 c/sec activity in I or II; moderate alpha in IV and III with synchronized 4–7 c/sec activity in I and II.
B_1		Generalized low desynchronized activity. Low 16–30 c/sec activity.	
B_2		Low desynchronized activity with 5–7 c/sec waves < 40 μV mainly in central regions.	Single "spontaneous" V waves without following 12–14 c/sec activity are included.
C		3–7 c/sec activity and 12–14 c/sec activity.	
D		1–3 c/sec activity and 12–14 c/sec activity.	

the mean voltage level during the 38 msec following the stimulus onset. This reference level was close to the components to be measured though it was not influenced by slow evoked activity.

Final reduction and statistical treatment of the data were carried out on a larger general purpose computer.

RESULTS

Changes in vigilance

In all subjects sensory and motor rest in a sound-shielded anechoic environment led to a decrease in vigilance which, in the experiments of type 1, was indicated by the appearance of alpha activity towards the end of the session. In the experiments of type 2 this decrease was rapid and in most cases (30 out of 36 sessions) exceeded the intermediate stages, thus leading to real sleep (Fig. 2, *a–d*). After usually one period of real sleep, which could last from only a few seconds to nearly 1 h, the subjects woke up suddenly, and throughout the rest of the session their vigilance remained with smaller oscillations at a fairly stable level within the intermediate stages. This level was different for the different subjects and could also differ for one subject from session to

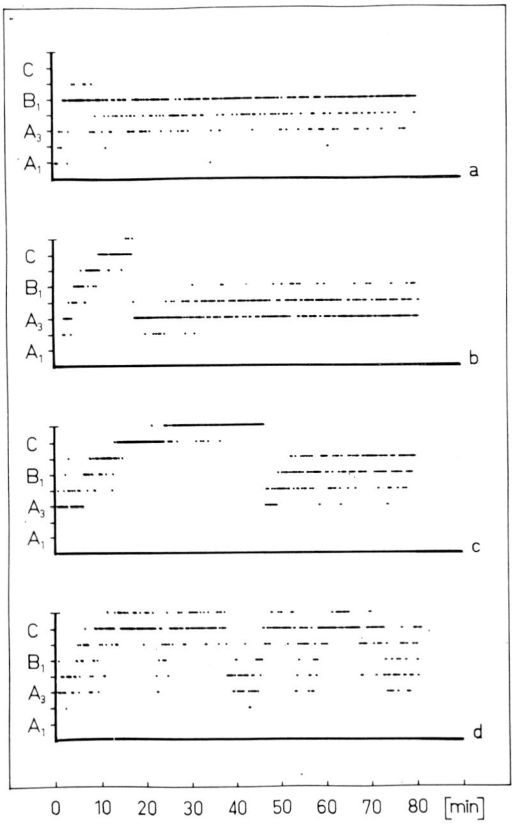

Fig. 2
Vigilance changes in the course of four type 2 experiments. Each point gives the vigilance stage which was determined from a 2 sec EEG epoch sampled at intervals averaging 12 sec. Graph *a* from subject 1, *b* and *c* from 2 and *d* from 6.

session (Fig. 2, *b* and *c*). Less often (in 12 out of 36 sessions) vigilance changed in large oscillations of varying duration throughout the session (Fig. 2, *d*), a phenomenon which was typical for subjects 6 and 7.

14.2% of the 1440 EEG samples obtained from all type 1 experiments and 1.5% of the 14418 samples from all type 2 experiments either could not be classified or contained artefacts. A comprehensive presentation of the frequency with which the different vigilance stages were met in all type 2 experiments is given in Fig. 3.

Changes in the evoked response amplitude

The single unspecific vertex response to a click stimulus was large in wakefulness (stage O) and, because of the small amplitude variation and a favourable signal-to-noise ratio, it could always be seen in the EEG records (Fig. 4, *a*). In sleep the response showed great amplitude variations and was less often seen in the EEG (Fig. 4, *c*). In the intermediate stages single responses were rarely detectable.

In all subjects the summated responses showed the configurations typical for wakefulness and for sleep (Fig. 4, *b* and *d*) with the smoothest and clearest wave form in derivation I. As in most subjects the components N_1 and especially P_2 (nomenclature according to Williams *et al.* 1962) were frequently double-peaked, the individual peaks (N_{1a}, N_{1b}, P_{2a} and P_{2b}) were measured whenever possible. Thc bifid form of N_1 and P_2 which had also been mentioned by Davis *et al.* (1966), was most distinct in the summated responses from intermediate vigilance (Fig. 1),

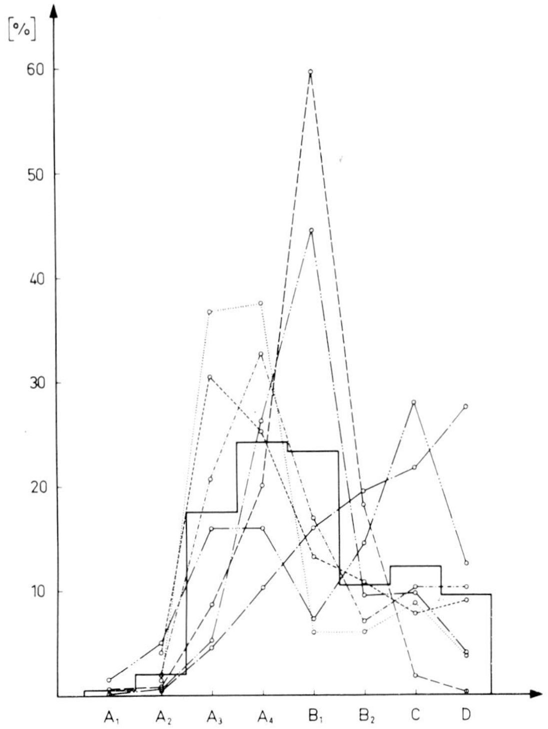

Fig. 3
Frequency distribution of vigilance stages compiled from all type 2 experiments (14205 observations). The data from each subject are given in the form of frequency polygons, the data from all subjects as a histogram.

though in some of the subjects (1, 3, 4 and 6) P_2 was often double-peaked also in the single responses evoked at stage O.

In derivation I all components except P_1 (mean size at stage O: 2 μV) changed in amplitude with declining vigilance. N_{1a} (mean size at stage O: 12 μV), N_{1b} (Fig. 5) and P_{2b} (Fig. 6) were progressively attenuated when vigilance passed the intermediate stages, on the average reaching 46 %, 39 % and 53 % of the original stage O value at A_3, and 32 %, 22 % and 21 % at B_2 (all values significant at $P < 0.1$ %; two-tailed t test). In sleep N_{1a} and N_{1b} were smallest, only one of them being usually demonstrable, whereas P_{2b} was absent. The amplitude of P_{2a} (mean size at stage 0: 8 μV) behaved diversely in the different

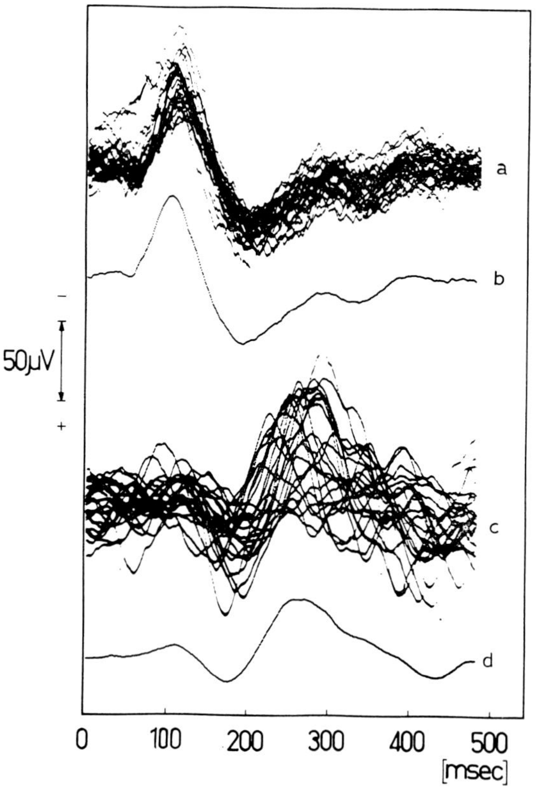

Fig. 4
Twenty photographically superimposed responses to clicks and their computed average, elicited at stage O (graph *a* and *b*) and stage C (graph *c* and *d*). The responses are in succession within the given vigilance stage and are only selected according to the criteria specified in the methods. (Subject 2; derivation I; negativity of electrode 2 upward; stimulus at time O.)

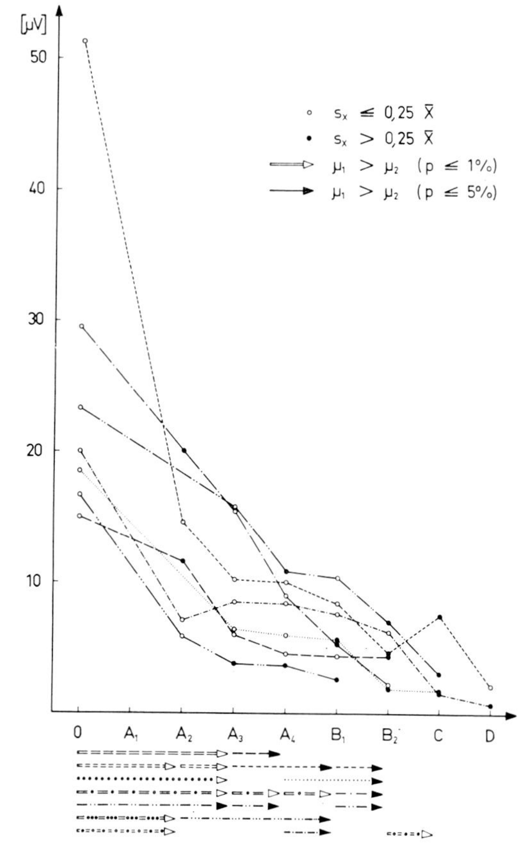

Fig. 5
Amplitude of component N_{1b} in derivation I as a function of vigilance for each subject (see Fig. 1 for codes). Each circle gives the mean of two or more observations. Open circles indicate that the value of the standard deviation is equal to or smaller than a quarter of the mean. Arrows below the diagram indicate the cases in which the amplitude reduction reaches a significant level (one-tailed rank-sum test). The same symbols are used in Fig. 6 and 7.

subjects, the average change being a slight reduction from stage O to B_2 and an increase in sleep. N_2 (Fig. 7) was rarely demonstrable in the intermediate stages and the few measurements indicate that it did not change its amplitude here. However, from stage B_2 to sleep this component showed a clear amplitude increase in all subjects.

Similar amplitude changes occurred in derivation III though all components except P_{2a} had a clear tendency to smaller amplitudes. As a consequence the ratio of amplitude in derivation I/amplitude in derivation III yielded a value usually larger than 1. For component N_{1b} the value of this ratio decreased with falling vigilance

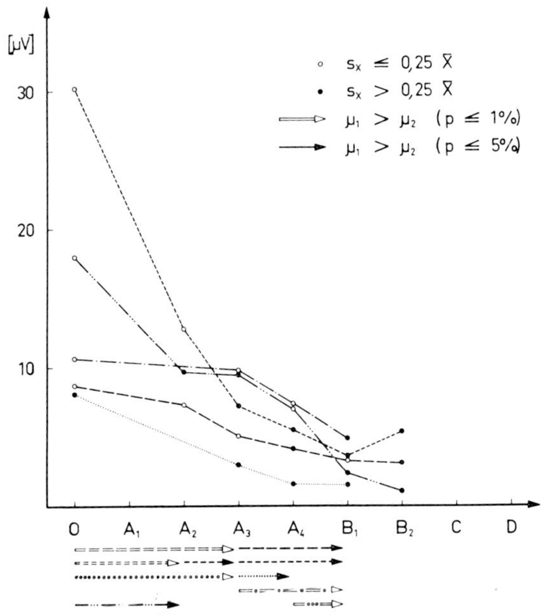

Fig. 6
Amplitude of P_{2b} in derivation I as a function of vigilance for each subject.

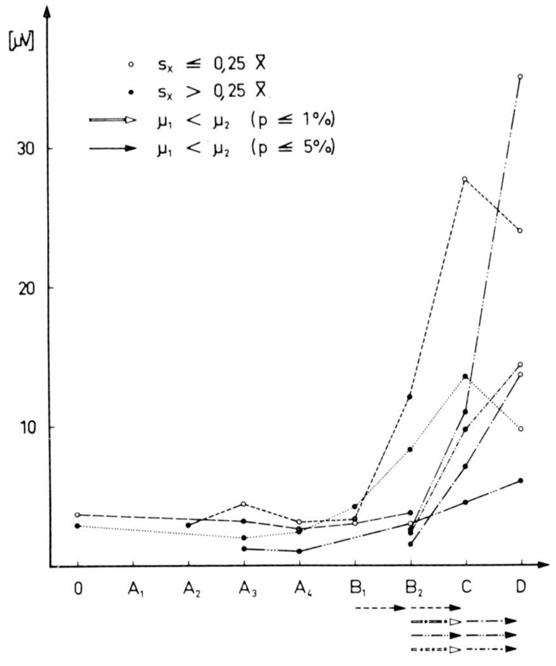

Fig. 7
Amplitude of N_2 in derivation I as a function of vigilance for each subject.

(significant from stage O to stage A_4 and from there to stage D with $P < 1\%$; two-tailed t test).

The voltage maxima (foci) along the midline were estimated for the different evoked response components on the basis of their polarity reversal in the bipolar recordings. It was found that N_{1a} and N_{1b} had their foci near or anterior to electrode 3. The focus of P_{2a} was always near electrode 3, whereas P_{2b} had its focus near electrode 2. All these components showed no shift of their foci along the midline when vigilance changed from alertness to deep sleep. In contrast, the focus of component N_2 abruptly shifted from electrode 2 to electrode 3 when falling vigilance passed stage B_1.

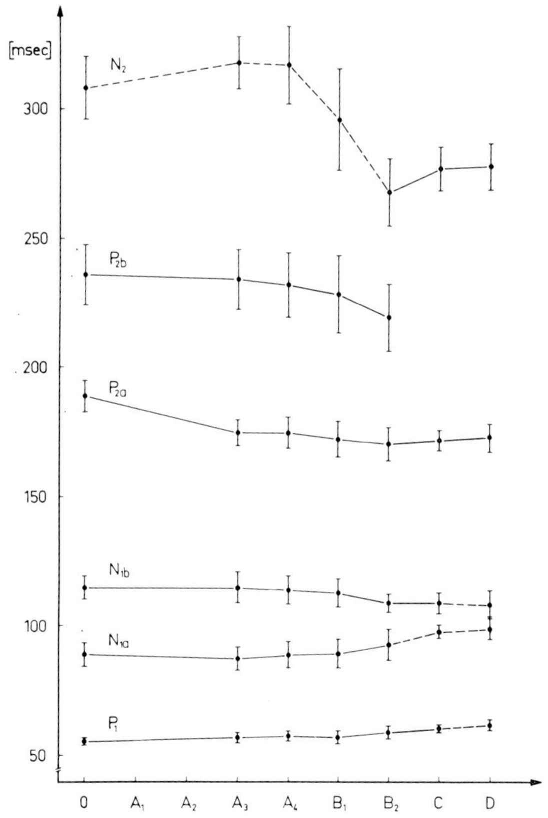

Fig. 8
Latencies of the different components of the evoked response in derivation I as a function of vigilance. Solid lines connect the means of data obtained from four or more subjects, each being represented by a minimum of two observations. The bars give the values of the standard deviations; the intra-individual variation is approximately 1/4 to 3/4 of this value.

Changes in the evoked response latency

The latencies of the different components of the evoked response in derivation I were not markedly affected by vigilance fluctuations (Fig. 8), and only two conspicuous changes could be noted. The latency of P_{2a} decreased on the average by 14 msec when vigilance changed from stage O to stage A_3. This reduction reached a significant level in four subjects ($P < 5\%$; two-tailed rank-sum test). In those three subjects in whom N_2 could be identified over the whole vigilance range, the latency of this component was reduced by approximately 50 msec from stage A_4 to stage B_2 ($P < 5\%$; two-tailed rank-sum test). In derivation III the latencies of all components except N_{1a} were generally somewhat shorter over the whole vigilance range. This difference, however, reached a 5% level of significance only in some subjects (two-tailed sign test). In the four subjects in whom N_{1a} could be measured in both derivations I and III this component had the shorter latency ($P < 5\%$; two-tailed sign test) in derivation I, the average difference being 8 msec.

DISCUSSION

This study has shown that three prominent response components progressively decrease in amplitude when the EEG epochs prior to the stimuli change through a series of typical patterns which presumably reflect successive stages of decreasing vigilance. This progressive amplitude decrease can be interpreted as a decline in the activity of certain brain functions which are essential for the maintenance of an efficient subject–environment relation. In this context it is interesting to note that, like the evoked response, reaction speed (Morrell 1966) and discrimination capacity (Bergström and Häkkinen 1968) decrease as functions of comparable changes in the pre-stimulus EEG.

Although in the present study the variability of the average evoked response was comparatively small, possibly due to the application of a selective rather than a successive summation technique, there was still considerable amplitude variation in the responses elicited at a given EEG activity pattern. An explanation for this phenomenon could be that besides other factors the evoked response is dependent on the degree of interaction ("coupling") between various brain regions occurring just prior to and at the moment of stimulation, as Galbraith (1967) was able to demonstrate for the visual evoked response in the rhesus monkey. Whereas the complex pattern of interaction between the centres processing the sensory information can be only partly reflected in the ongoing activity of the cortex, the EEG is certainly determined by the total pattern of interactions which defines the organizational state of the brain functions.

One of the most important variables which influence the unspecific evoked response is habituation, though its importance is often overlooked. The work of Davis *et al.* (1966) and personal experiments (Fruhstorfer 1966) have shown that only at stimulus presentation rates slower than 1/10 sec is the evoked response not markedly reduced as a function of the number of stimuli. In animal experiments it was found that responses evoked in the auditory cortex at a rate of 1/10 sec were still habituated (Abraham and Marsh 1966) and that habituation at the cortical level was dependent on vigilance (Marsh and Worden 1964).

As a consequence, the results obtained in this study may have been partly influenced by habituation even if the presentation rate was as slow as 1/12 sec. Whereas no habituation was observed in the short experiments of type 1, slight habituation might have occurred in the longer, type 2, experiments. In this case, and provided that habituation does not greatly change within wakefulness as a function of vigilance, the responses during the intermediate stages should have been equally affected by habituation, as these stages were evenly scattered over the whole length of the experiments.

Another factor which might have influenced the results is the different positions of the subjects in the two types of experiment. Nakayama and Hori (1966) have demonstrated that posture has an effect on the evoked response, but the special case of sitting and lying has not been tested. Gross changes in head position with regard to the loudspeaker can be excluded as an error source as they did not occur in wakefulness, and in sleep head position has no noticeable effect on the auditory evoked response (Ornitz *et al.* 1967b).

Finally, the sensitive EEG classification based on visual pattern recognition can be regarded as an error source. For a trained EEG reader the error seems to be mainly a systematic one, as one reader, when analysing 4000 EEG samples twice, classified less than 5% of them differently, whereas two readers, when independently analysing 800 samples, obtained 17% of classifications differing by one stage. Although the error seems to be considerable it certainly does not outweigh the advantages of this classification.

The important finding of this study is the progressive decrease in auditory evoked activity when vigilance falls from alertness to the onset of real sleep. Williams *et al.* (1962) and Weitzman and Kremen (1965), who recorded auditory evoked responses only in "wakefulness" and at one stage of intermediate vigilance (stage 1 according to Dement and Kleitman 1957), report an amplitude decrease which is much less pronounced than that observed by us between stage O and stage B_1. The smaller decrement seems to be mainly due to smaller amplitudes obtained in the waking state. Of the various differences in the methods two points might serve as explanation. First, in both studies cited above the results were obtained in a state of strong habituation (stimuli were presented at rates varying between 1/sec and 1/4 sec). Secondly, the waking state in these studies might in fact have included intermediate stages, as vigilance tends to decrease rapidly when the subject is in a state of sensory and motor relaxation.

This study has not confirmed that auditory evoked activity progressively increases in latency from waking to sleep, as reported for N_2 by Weitzman and Kremen (1965) and for N_1, P_2 and N_2 by Suzuki and Taguchi (1968). On the contrary, for two components the longer latencies were observed during wakefulness, whereas the latencies of the other components did not obviously change. The long latency of P_{2a} at stage O could be explained by the partial neutralization of the early half of this small positive phase caused by the large negative field of N_{1b}, as this masking of P_{2a} is absent whenever N_{1b} is small. N_2 latencies which were also longer in wakefulness cannot be explained by such a mechanism and the question must be raised whether the components observed in wakefulness and in sleep reflect the activity of the same neural processes. For N_2 this is doubtful because simultaneous with the sudden latency change there occurs a posterior movement of the focus and a change in the amplitude behaviour. Goff *et al.* (1966) also question whether the late components of the somato-sensory evoked response in sleep have counterparts in wakefulness.

The great variability of N_2 at a given level of the B and C stages has also been observed by Weitzman and Kremen (1965). Ornitz *et al.* (1967a) have shown that the average amplitude of this component is large only at the onset of sleep. Because of its evident instability it seems to be unsuitable for testing the function of a sensory system. As a consequence of the results obtained in this study the unspecific vertex response would be recorded best in a situation allowing the subject to remain in a state of high vigilance (stage O). At this vigilance level the evoked response is large and stable against a low voltage background, and in most subjects the stability of vigilance can easily be controlled by the EEG. Selection of artefact-free responses (Satterfield 1966) and recording from a derivation distant from neck and masticatory muscles (*e.g.*, Cz–Fpz) would add further precision.

SUMMARY

1. In seven normal subjects vigilance fluctuations and related changes in the auditory evoked response were quantitatively analysed during rest lasting 10 min (eyes open) or 80 min (eyes closed) in a soundproof room. Vigilance was visually determined from the EEG on the basis of a sensitive classification. Responses evoked by slowly repeated clicks were summated selectively according to the vigilance level in the 2 sec immediately prior to each stimulus.

2. During a session vigilance decreased noticeably in all subjects whether the eyes were kept open or closed. With closed eyes the vigilance decrease was rapid and in most cases reached real sleep. After this initial fall vigilance increased again and remained, with smaller oscillations, at a certain level of the intermediate stages.

3. The click-evoked response was large and

stable in the alert state. With decreasing vigilance a progressive amplitude reduction of three prominent response components (N_{1a}, N_{1b}, P_{2b}) was observed. At stage B_2 these components had approximately 25% of their original size at stage O. The transition to real sleep was characterized by a marked increase of N_2 and a slight growth of P_{2a}. P_1 did not change over the whole vigilance range.

4. No progressive changes in latency or shifts in focus were noticed. There was, however, a decrease in latency and a posterior shift in the focus of N_2 at the transition to real sleep.

5. The progressive loss in amplitude is interpreted as a decline in the activity of certain brain functions which are essential for the maintenance of an efficient subject-environment relation.

RÉSUMÉ

VIGILANCE ET RÉPONSES ÉVOQUÉES AUDITIVES CHEZ L'HOMME

1. Chez sept sujets normaux, les fluctuations de la vigilance et les modifications correspondantes des réponses évoquées auditives ont été analysées quantitativement pendant une période de repos de 10 min (yeux ouverts) ou de 80 min (yeux fermés) en chambre insonorisée. Le niveau de vigilance a été déterminé par l'analyse visuelle de l'EEG sur la base d'une classification nuancée. Les réponses évoquées par des clics à fréquences lentes ont été sélectivement sommées en fonction du niveau de vigilance des 2 sec précédant immédiatement chaque stimulus.

2. Pendant l'expérience, la vigilance s'abaisse notablement chez tous les sujets, que les yeux restent ouverts ou fermés. Les yeux fermés, la diminution de la vigilance est rapide et dans la plupart des cas, aboutit au sommeil caractérisé. Après cette chute initiale, la vigilance remonte à nouveau et se maintient, avec des oscillations moindres, à un certain niveau d'état intermédiaire.

3. Les réponses évoquées aux clics sont de grande amplitude et stables pendant l'état vigile. Lors de l'abaissement de la vigilance on observe une réduction progressive de l'amplitude des trois composantes dominantes de la réponse (N_{1a}, N_{1b}, P_{2b}). Au stade B_2, ces composantes ont approximativement 25% de leur taille originelle au stade O. Le passage au sommeil caractérisé se traduit par une augmentation marquée de la composante N_2 et une augmentation légère de P_{2a}. P_1 ne se modifie pas quel que soit le niveau de vigilance.

4. On n'observe aucune modification progressive de latence ni de variation topographique. Une diminution de la latence et un déplacement postérieur du foyer de N_2 surviennent cependant au moment du passage au sommeil caractérisé.

5. La perte progressive d'amplitude est interprétée comme une diminution de l'activité de certaines fonctions cérébrales qui sont essentielles pour le maintien d'une relation efficace sujet-environnement.

REFERENCES

ABRAHAM, F. D. and MARSH, J. T. Amplitude of evoked potentials as a function of slow presenting rates of repetitive auditory stimulation. *Exp. Neurol.*, **1966,** *14*: 187–198.

ARTSEULOVA, O. K. and IVANITSKY, A. M. [Relationship between the components of the evoked potential and background EEG in man] (in Russian). *Zh. vyssh. nerv. Deyat. Pavlova.*, **1967,** *17*: 677–680.

BENTE, D. *Die Insuffizienz des Vigilitätstonus.* Habilitationsschrift, Erlangen, **1964**, 186 p.

BERGSTRÖM, R. M., BLÅFIELD, R., FRUHSTORFER, H., HYTÖNEN, Y. and JAUHIAINEN, T. A sound-attenuating, electrically shielded chamber for experiments in sensory physiology. *Acta physiol. scand.*, **1969,** *75*: 330–332.

BERGSTRÖM, R. M. and HÄKKINEN, V. The effect of vigilance on voluntary motor responses to auditory stimuli. *Scand. J. clin. Lab. Invest.*, **1968,** *21, Suppl. 101*: 60.

DAVIS, H., MAST, T., YOSHIE, N. and ZERLIN, S. The slow response of the human cortex to auditory stimuli: recovery process. *Electroenceph. clin. Neurophysiol.*, **1966,** *21*: 105–113.

DEMENT, W. and KLEITMAN, N. Cyclic variations in EEG during sleep and their relation to eye movements, body motility, and dreaming. *Electroenceph. clin. Neurophysiol.*, **1957,** *9*: 673–690.

DONCHIN, E. and LINDSLEY, D. B. Average evoked potentials and reaction times to visual stimuli. *Electroenceph. clin. Neurophysiol.*, **1966,** *20*: 217–223.

FRUHSTORFER, H. *Der Einfluss von Reizfolgefrequenz, Reizanzahl und Reizort auf die Intensitätsabhängigkeit vibratorisch ausgelöster corticaler Antworten beim Menschen.* Dissertation, Erlangen, **1966,** 90 p.

GALBRAITH, G. C. The effect of prior EEG "coupling" upon the visual evoked response. *IEEE Trans. bio-med. Engng.*, **1967,** *BME-14*: 223–229.

GOFF, W. R., ALLISON, T., SHAPIRO, A. and ROSNER, B. S. Cerebral somato-sensory responses evoked during sleep in man. *Electroenceph. clin. Neurophysiol.*, **1966,** *21*: 1–9.

HAIDER, M., SPONG, P. and LINDSLEY, D. B. Attention, vigilance, and cortical evoked potentials in humans. *Science*, **1964,** *145*: 180–182.

HEAD, H. The conception of nervous and mental energy. II. Vigilance: a physiological state of the nervous system. *Brit. J. Psychol.*, **1923,** *14*: 126–147.

KOOI, K. A. and BAGCHI, B. K. Observations on early components of the visual evoked response and occipital rhythms. *Electroenceph. clin. Neurophysiol.*, **1964,** *17*: 638–643.

LEVONIAN, E. Evoked potential in relation to subsequent alpha frequency. *Science*, **1966,** *152*: 1280–1282.

LOOMIS, A. L., HARVEY, E. N. and HOBART, G. A. Cerebral states during sleep, as studied by human brain potentials. *J. exp. Psychol.*, **1937,** *21*: 127–144.

MARSH, J. T. and WORDEN, F. G. Auditory potentials during acoustic habituation: cochlear nucleus, cerebellum and auditory cortex. *Electroenceph. clin. Neurophysiol.*, **1964,** *17*: 685–692.

MORRELL, L. K. EEG frequency and reaction time—a sequential analysis. *Neuropsychologia*, **1966,** *4*: 41–48.

MORRELL, L. K. and MORRELL, F. Evoked potentials and reaction times: a study of intra-individual variability. *Electroenceph. clin. Neurophysiol.*, **1966,** *20*: 567–575.

NAKAYAMA, T. and HORI, T. Cortical evoked potential and subjective sensation to electric stimulation of the skin: effect of posture and respiratory movement. *Jap. J. Physiol.*, **1966,** *16*: 612–624.

NÄÄTÄNEN, R. Selective attention and evoked potentials. *Ann. Acad. Sci. fenn.*, **1967,** *B 151, 1*.

ORNITZ, E. M., RITVO, E. R., CARR, E. M., LA FRANCHI, S. and WALTER, R. D. The effect of sleep onset on the auditory averaged evoked response. *Electroenceph. clin. Neurophysiol.*, **1967**a, *23*: 335–341.

ORNITZ, E. M., RITVO, E. R., CARR, E. M., PANMAN, L. M. and WALTER, R. D. The variability of the auditory averaged evoked responses during sleep and dreaming in children and adults. *Electroenceph. clin. Neurophysiol.*, **1967**b, *22*: 514–524.

ROTH, B. The clinical and theoretical importance of EEG rhythms corresponding to states of lowered vigilance. *Electroenceph. clin. Neurophysiol.*, **1961,** *13*: 395–399.

SATTERFIELD, J. H. A system for selection of responses for averaging. *Electroenceph. clin. Neurophysiol.*, **1966,** *21*: 86–88.

SUZUKI, T. and TAGUCHI, K. Cerebral evoked response to auditory stimuli in young children during sleep. *Ann. Otol. (St. Louis)*, **1968,** *77*: 102–110.

WEITZMAN, E. D. and KREMEN, H. Auditory evoked responses during different stages of sleep in man. *Electroenceph. clin. Neurophysiol.*, **1965,** *18*: 65–70.

WILKINSON, R. T. and MORLOCK, H. C. Auditory evoked response and reaction time. *Electroenceph. clin. Neurophysiol.*, **1967,** *23*: 50–56.

WILLIAMS, H. L., TEPAS, D. I. and MORLOCK, H. C. Evoked responses to clicks and electroencephalographic stages of sleep in man. *Science*, **1962,** *138*: 685–686.

Reference: FRUHSTORFER, H. and BERGSTRÖM, R. M. Human vigilance and auditory evoked responses. *Electroenceph. clin. Neurophysiol.*, **1969,** *27*: 346–355.

Electroencephalography and Clinical Neurophysiology
Elsevier Publishing Company, Amsterdam – Printed in The Netherlands

EFFECT OF LSD ON VISUALLY EVOKED RESPONSES TO COLOR IN VISUALIZER AND NON-VISUALIZER SUBJECTS

BARBARA B. BROWN, PH.D.

Experiential Physiology, Veterans Administration Hospital, Sepulveda, Calif. 91343, and Department of Psychiatry and Human Behavior, U.C.I. College of Medicine, Orange, Calif. (U.S.A.)

(Accepted for publication: January 13, 1969)

INTRODUCTION

The visually evoked cortical response (VER) in man is reported to differ markedly from subject to subject (Ebe *et al.* 1962; Rietveld 1963; Rietveld and Tordoir 1965) but to remain relatively constant in the same individual over long periods of time (Dustman and Beck 1963; Rietveld 1963). Certain components of the VER reflect visually conducted information as influenced by other neuronal activity related to awareness, attention, perception, and even cognitive ability (Chalke and Ertl 1965; Spehlmann 1965; Callaway 1966; Sutton *et al.* 1967) and may also reflect characteristics of color perception (Monnier *et al.* 1964; Shipley *et al.* 1965). In an earlier study, we related red specific EEG responses to flickering light to degree of visual imagery ability (Brown 1966). The present study was made to determine whether a similar relationship held for VERs to color, and whether LSD-induced enhancement of visual perception could be detected in the VERs to color.

METHOD AND MATERIAL

The data were obtained during experiments from which EEG results have been reported (Brown 1968a). Two groups of subjects were employed. One group of seven was classified as possessing vivid visual imagery ability (claimed "projected" images; *i.e.*, occupied real visual space). A second group of seven was classified as non-visualizers (claimed total absence of visual imagery ability). For other details including those of experimental procedure see the previous papers (Brown 1968a,b).

Fifty flashes were given during the control period for each color condition: white, white while counting the flashes serially, red, blue and green, and were repeated at 40, 80 and 160 min intervals following LSD. Order of the colors was randomized.

Results obtained during the 160 min interval after LSD (0.75–1 μg/kg orally) showed optimal changes and only these are reported.

For analysis the 50 responses for each color condition were summed (CAT 400), using an analysis time of 250 msec. Latencies and peak-to-peak voltages were measured from the responses written out by means of an X–Y plotter.

To analyze these VERs further, all successive, readily identifiable peaks and inflection points were initially measured and grouped. Although a number of trends of cumulative effect were noted, inter-trial variation eliminated all but a few peaks from further consideration. After further analysis of pre- and post-drug VERs, 4 negative peaks were selected. These were peaks which could be identified in both the control and post-LSD responses in all subjects. The criteria required for each of these were: (a) peaks which could be readily identified as dominant peaks in the majority of color VERs and in the majority of subjects both before and after drug; (b) for this majority, a continuing voltage development after change in direction of at least 25% of the largest peak (measured in mm from X–Y plots of the summed responses) occurring in any of the subject's VERs to the 5 color conditions; (c) occurrence within a pre-selected time range, es-

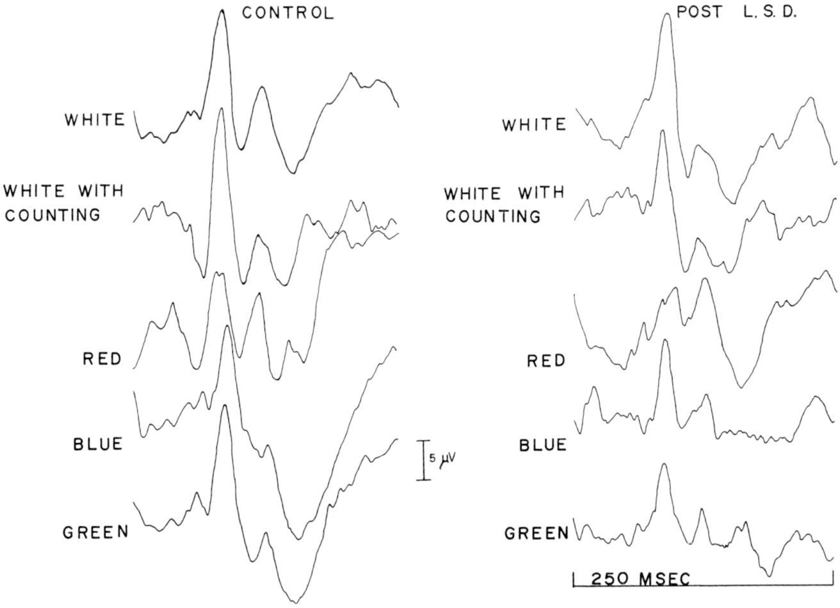

Fig. 1
Examples of VERs to color recorded from right occipital bipolar electrodes in a non-visualizer subject. Each trace is the average of 50 responses (CAT 400).

tablished from the values of times to the highest peaks across all subjects; and (d) by the number of major peaks of similar character which preceded it.

RESULTS

Examples of VERs to color before and after LSD are shown in Fig. 1 for a non-visualizer subject. This is included to indicate the types of differences found among the 5 dimensions of the experiment and the necessity for analyzing the data in terms of patterns.

Average times for the occurrence of each of the selected negative peaks for the two groups of subjects are summarized in Table I. Owing to inter-subject variation, *average* times for individual peaks fell within similar ranges and indicated relatively little change with either change of color or effect of LSD for the majority of responses.

Because of these intra-subject differences as well as the inter-subject differences in pattern, information about the average times for each peak as a function of color did not prove to be a satisfactory index. Further, it was not so much the absolute time of the peak that was important, but (1) the relative times of the same peaks for different colors in an individual subject, and (2) the effect of LSD on these relative times as a function of color.

The difficulties inherent in comparing complex patterns in relation to a variety of variables made it desirable to reduce the quantitative peak times (in msec) to qualitative "ranks" to facilitate these comparisons. The peak patterns were compared along the 5 dimensions of the experiment, namely: (1) visualizers *vs.* non-visualizers; (2) individual subjects within each of these groups; (3) control *vs.* LSD responses; (4) the 5 different colors; and (5) the 4 peaks in the evoked response selected for analysis.

To simplify the comparisons we started with the individual peaks in the evoked response for a single individual. We then scaled the latency times to these peaks in relation to the 5 color situations in the following fashion: for a given peak, for example the second negative peak in a subject's VER, we assigned the number 1 to the *shortest* time for that peak which occurred among

TABLE I

Average times in msec to major VER negative peaks*

Subject group	Color	Control				Post-LSD			
		1	2	3	4	1	2	3	4
Visualizers (7)	White	19	67	103	171	27	52	101	140
	White, counting	25	60	116	165	32	51	100	142
	Red	22	54	109	152	24	59	101	149
	Blue	22	63	107	147	23	59	101	136
	Green	25	63	102	150	27	46	85	129
Non-visualizers (7)	White	35†	67	108	143	32	65	101	140
	White, counting	34	51	96	180	0	57	97	146
	Red	30	57	102	186	35	66	95	163
	Blue	33	62	102	166	32	57	97	156
	Green	31	58	102	173	34	58	97	144

* Standard errors ranged between 9 and 19% of the means for peak 1, between 4 and 14% for peak 2, and 7–10% for peaks 3 and 4.

† All initial negative peaks significantly different between the two subject groups at the 0.02 level (Chi Square Median Test).

the 5 color responses (*e.g.*, this might be for the color red). For the *same* subject and the *same* peak number, the next shortest time was then assigned the number 2 (*e.g.*, the peak in response to white). Times which did not differ by at least 25% were counted as "equal". Thus, if the next shortest time was *not* different by 25%, it also received the rank number 2. Hence for a given subject, if the latencies for each of the 5 color situations differed successively by exactly 25%[1], the resulting "ranks" among the 5 color latencies of a particular peak would be 1, 2, 3, 4, 5.

If some differences for the same peak among the 5 colors were less than 25%, the pattern of "ranks" might be of the following type:

Red	White	White with counting	Blue	Green
1	2	2	2	3

[1] This lower bound of 25% change, required of successive peak times before they were given different "ranks", was assigned on the basis of the standard errors for the averaged peaks given at the bottom of Table I. As an example, if the standard error is 10% of the mean value, and 3 times the standard error is used as the criterion for significance of the differences, then the range of values for any individual peak could contain at least 3 intervals of 25% differences between minimal and maximal values. If, however, the values for the same peak are averaged across *all* colors, the variation is increased, the standard error becomes somewhat larger and 4 intervals of 25% differences are possible.

For some other individual, the pattern of "ranks" for this same peak might be:

Red	White	White with counting	Blue	Green
1	2	1	2	2

After the ranks were assigned in this way for each subject and for each of the 4 peaks, the ranks for a given peak were averaged *across subjects* within the visualizer group. Similar averages were obtained across subjects within the non-visualizer group. These averages were calculated both for the control and for the post-drug conditions.

"Ranks", obtained and averaged in this fashion, are presented in Table II. In this Table, comparisons are meaningful down any column, but not along the rows. Each column should be inspected for its pattern of ranks, and then this *pattern* (not the individual numbers) should be compared between control and post-drug conditions, between visualizers and non-visualizers, and between successive peaks. This makes more apparent the rationale for assigning the ranks. Results in Table II show that an average rank of 3 or more occurred only in 4 instances out of the total of 80 peaks ranked (an incidence of 5%). For a given column within an experimental "block" in this table, the 5 average ranks were inspected for values that deviated significantly

TABLE II

Averaged ordering of VER latencies*

Subject group	Color	Control 1	Control 2	Control 3	Control 4	Post-LSD 1	Post-LSD 2	Post-LSD 3	Post-LSD 4
Visualizers (7)	White	2.0	*1.6*	1.5	1.2	2.0	2.0	1.8	1.2
	White, counting	*3.2*	2.4	1.0	1.0	*1.0**	1.6*	2.2*	1.2
	Red	2.2	*1.4*	1.3	1.5	*1.3**	2.0	1.7	*2.4**
	Blue	2.4	2.4	1.4	1.5	2.0	2.6	2.0	1.2
	Green	2.5	2.4	1.6	1.6	2.2	3.0	1.3	1.0*
Non-visualizers (7)	White	1.8	2.2	1.2	1.6	1.8	2.0	2.2*	1.8
	White, counting	1.8	1.8	1.5	1.6	1.7	1.5	1.7	2.0
	Red	*1.0*	1.6	1.8	*2.4*	*2.6**	*3.0**	1.7	*2.5*
	Blue	1.6	1.8	1.5	2.0	*3.0**	1.7	1.8	1.7
	Green	1.7	2.2	1.6	*1.2*	*2.6**	*2.6*	1.7	*1.0*

* Significant differences (by Student's *t*) are indicated as follows: (a) values in italics are significantly different from those for other color conditions for the same peak number (comparisons down columns); (b) values with asterisks are significantly different from comparable control values.

from the others in that column. Such deviant values are italicized. In each control group (left half of Table II), only 3 rank averages of 20 were significantly different (in italics). Following LSD, the incidence of significant differences increased to six of twenty for visualizers and five of twenty for non-visualizers.

Discussion of the following results was based upon the two criteria[1]: (1) a tendency was assumed when the significance of the difference between any *individual* comparable peaks was at the 1% probability level (Student's *t*), and (2) a real difference between experimental and control data was assumed when at least *two* peaks for any individual VER in one block were significantly different (to the 1% level) from values for comparable peaks in the corresponding VER in the other "block".

A comparison of *column* patterns isolated differences between visualizer and non-visualizer subjects during both experimental conditions.

[1] Since averages of ranks were used to determine significance of differences and since each number represented a 25% difference, the probabilities of extracting significant differences had been reduced. Significance of the results was increased further by requiring that at least 2 peaks of a VER in the experimental "block" (tabulated data for each of the 4 possible combinations of experimental group and conditions) be significantly different from comparable peaks in the corresponding VER in the control block. Such significant differences are marked by asterisks in Table II.

In *visualizers*, averages for ordering of latencies (Table II) revealed no outstanding differences among the color responses except for a tendency for a longer latency for peak 1 for the white while counting reponse and tendencies for shorter latencies for peak 2 in the responses to white and red. A comparison of row patterns within the control block for visualizers indicated that wave form configurations for white and red differed from those for blue and green. After LSD only the VERs to white while counting and to red were significantly changed. The response to white while counting was markedly changed in configuration as indicated by acceleration of peaks 1 and 2 and a slowing of peak 3. The VER to red showed acceleration of peak 1 and slowing of peak 4. A comparison of row patterns indicated that the VERs to white, blue, and green were little changed by LSD in the visualizers.

In *non-visualizers*, differences in VERs for the 5 color conditions in the control block were quite small for peaks 1 and 2 (lower rank averages) as compared to those for the visualizers. The marked differences of peaks 1 and 4 of the VER to red indicate the considerable differences of wave form configuration as compared to that for the other colors. Except for this difference (to red), times for individual peaks were similar for all responses (row patterns) within this block. Following LSD, the latencies for peak 1 showed significant slowing in the VERs to all 3 colors

TABLE III

Average ordering of the largest VER amplitudes

Subject group	Condition	White	White, counting	Red	Blue	Green
Visualizers (7)	Control	2.7	1.6*	2.7	2.0	2.3
	LSD	2.1**	1.6	2.1**	2.4	2.4
Non-visualizers (7)	Control	2.3	1.1	2.2	2.2	1.8
	LSD	1.6	3.0***	2.0	2.1	1.6

* Increase over white and red significant at 1% level (Student's *t*).
** Increase over control significant at 1% level (Student's *t*).
*** Decrease from control significant at 1% level (Student's *t*). Largest of the 4 peaks among the 5 colors was given a value of 1. Values of 2, 3, 4 and 5 were assigned to those peak amplitudes of corresponding latency smaller by successive 25% increments.

but not in the VERs to white or white during counting (comparison of *column* patterns). Comparisons between data blocks for the experimental conditions revealed marked slowing of peaks 1 and 2 in the post-LSD response to red indicating change in wave form configuration. Ranks of latencies of the VER to white while counting were virtually unchanged by LSD.

A position ranking technique was also used to evaluate changes in amplitude of the VERs found for the different conditions of the study. The *largest* of the 4 peaks occurring among the 5 VERs for each subject was assigned a value of 1, and values of 2, 3, 4 and 5 to those peak amplitudes of corresponding latency which were smaller by successive 25% decrements. The remaining 3 selected peaks were not analyzed. The ranks thus obtained for each color VER were then averaged for the subjects of each group and for each experimental condition (Table III). *Visualizers*. Ordering of the amplitudes for the visualizer group showed that the largest amplitudes occurred in the VER to white while counting, and that the corresponding peaks in the VERs to white and red were the smallest. After LSD, amplitudes of the VERs to white and red were reduced in amplitude whereas amplitudes of the other color conditions were relatively unchanged. *Non-visualizers*. As in visualizers, maximal amplitudes also occurred in the VERs to white while counting in spite of the differences in ranks of *latencies* between the two groups. For the non-visualizers, however, no consistent differences among amplitudes of the color VERs were found. Moreover, LSD did not affect amplitudes of any of the color responses. Amplitude of the VER to white was slightly enhanced but the response to white while counting was markedly decreased.

EEG and subjective changes. During both control and post-LSD recording periods, 60% of all subjects retained an alert EEG pattern throughout presentation of the light stimuli. Alpha activity occurred irregularly in the other subjects, but occurred less frequently in the non-visualizers. Following LSD the activation pattern became more intense in the visualizer subjects and less intense in the non-visualizers. Analysis of level of EEG activation for these subjects has been reported (Brown 1968a).

All visualizer subjects reported that the colored light stimuli seemed more intense after LSD and volunteered information as to their beauty, patterns, and interest. In contrast, the non-visualizers expressed little interest in the colors either before or after LSD.

DISCUSSION

The differences in VERs to different color conditions found between visualizer and non-visualizer subjects demonstrate differences in central data processing between the two subject groups. The VERs of visualizer subjects evidenced a tendency for color specificity indicated by differences in both latency and amplitude values when responses to white and to red were compared to those to blue and to green. The VERs in non-visualizer subjects were remarkably like each other except for the VER to red. Ranking of latency and amplitude values revealed that the response configurations for all VERs differed between the two groups. The color responses of the two groups were, moreover, affected differently by LSD.

The differences in VERs to color and their differing changes after LSD between the two subject groups are similar to those reported using colored flickering light and EEG photic following responses (Brown 1968a).

The different configurations found for the VER to red is similar to the result obtained by Monnier *et al.* (1964) and by Shipley *et al.* (1965), both of whom found the VER to red different from that to blue. Monnier *et al.* (1964) also reported VER wave forms to red to be independent of events at the retina. The present report supplies additional information about the peculiarities of the VER to red by the finding that among color VERs, that to red was the most susceptible to effect of LSD and was different for the two subject groups.

The tendency for visualizer subjects to exhibit different wave form characteristics for different sets of colors (red, white *vs.* blue, green) may be a correlate of visual imagery ability. The VER wave forms for blue and green were not significantly changed by LSD and, with the exception of red, relationships among the color responses (both row and column patterns) were not changed. As contrasted to the changes seen for the non-visualizer group, this evidence could suggest the visualizers discriminated and perceived the colors similarly both before and after LSD. The failure of non-visualizer subjects to show significant central color discrimination, except to red, *before* LSD and to show only suggestive evidence of a change in latency but not amplitude of the color VERs *after* LSD parallels the subjective reports that non-visualizers not only lack visual imagery ability, but experienced no conscious change in visual perception after LSD. Employing a somewhat similar technique of analysis, Begleiter *et al.* (1967) found that change in affective meaning of the stimulus significantly altered configuration of the VER. This suggests that colored stimuli may contain greater affective significance for visualizers than for non-visualizers, and indirectly relates such differences in visual perception to the differences in visual imagery ability of the two groups.

An additional indication of difference in perceptual activity was that latter components of the VER to red in visualizers after LSD and in non-visualizers both before and after LSD were significantly different than for the other color conditions. Latter components of the VER as indicators of perceptual activity has been demonstrated by Sutton *et al.* (1967) and John *et al.* (1967).

It has been reported (Eason 1964; García-Austt *et al.* 1964; Donchin and Lindsley 1966) that VERs are enhanced during attentional states accompanied by activated EEGs. In the present study EEG activation levels were higher in non-visualizers during the control periods but were lower than those of the visualizers following LSD; however, these changes were not paralleled by absolute changes in VER amplitudes. Recent studies have shown, however, that selective attention, rather than non-specific attention or vigilance, yields VERs of enhanced amplitude (Haider *et al.* 1964; Spong *et al* .1965). The VER to white while the subject counted the flashes was used as a rough index of effect of increased level of attention. The two subject groups differed significantly in their VERs to this condition both before and after LSD. In the visualizer group this response resembled more closely the VERs to blue and green in both latencies and amplitude, and after LSD not only continued to be maximal in amplitude but also showed accelerated early peak times. Such evidence of an enhanced response may relate to the reported increase in visual interest of the visualizers.

In sharp contrast, in the non-visualizer group the VER to white while counting the flashes was virtually identical to the other VERs (except red) in latencies and these were completely unaffected by LSD. The amplitude of this response was markedly suppressed after LSD and may relate to the lack of change in visual perception reported by this group, and in fact, suggests a loss of externally or perceptually directed attention.

SUMMARY

1. The visually evoked responses (VERs) to color of visualizer subjects evidenced a signifi-

cant degree of color specific characteristics and selective alteration in color specificity after LSD. The changes were somewhat more pronounced in the amplitude domain. Configuration of the VER to white and red were consistently different from those to blue or green. Visualizers also reported enhanced visual perception after LSD.

2. In non-visualizer subjects the VERs to all color conditions except to red were virtually identical. Following LSD, early components of all 3 color VERs, most noticeably for red and green, were changed in configuration, all changes being in the latency domain.

3. Maximal amplitudes occurred in the VERs to white while counting the flashes in both subject groups. After LSD this was unchanged in visualizers but was markedly attenuated in responses of the non-visualizers.

4. A technique for ranking components of a complexly organized set of responses was used which permitted extraction of critical data from a complex of intercurrent intra- and inter-subject variation. The technique isolated patterns of response by which changes over time could be conveniently compared within and between subject groups, and as these were affected by the experimental condition. This proved useful in isolating significant differences in a multi-dimensional system in which the external stimuli, light and LSD, were both contained within reasonable physiologic and pharmacologic limits.

RÉSUMÉ

EFFET DU LSD SUR LES RÉPONSES ÉVOQUÉES À LA COULEUR CHEZ DES SUJETS AVEC ET SANS IMAGERIE MENTALE

1. Les réponses évoquées visuelles à la couleur chez les sujets avec imagerie mentale montrent un degré significatif de caractéristiques spécifiques à la couleur et une altération sélective dans la spécificité des couleurs après LSD. Ces changements concernent surtout l'amplitude. La configuration de la réponse évoquée visuelle au blanc et au rouge est nettement différente de celle au bleu et au vert. Les sujets avec imagerie mentale rapportent également un accroissement de la perception visuelle après LSD.

2. Chez les sujets sans imagerie mentale, les réponses évoquées visuelles à toutes les conditions de couleur, excepté le rouge, sont virtuellement identiques. Après LSD, des composantes précoces des réponses évoquées visuelles aux trois couleurs, et plus particulièrement au rouge et au vert, sont changées dans leur configuration, ces changements affectant les latences.

3. Les amplitudes maximales s'observent pour des réponses évoquées visuelles au blanc lorsque les sujets des deux groupes comptent les éclairs. Après LSD ceci est inchangé chez les sujets avec imagerie mentale, mais est nettement atténué pour les réponses des sujets sans imagerie mentale.

4. Une technique de rangement des composantes d'un jeu de réponses à organisation complexe est utilisée pour permettre l'extraction des données saillantes d'un ensemble de variations intercurrentes intra- et inter-individuelles. Cette technique isole des patterns de réponses au moyen desquels des changements dans le temps peuvent être convenablement comparés à l'intérieur des groupes et entre les groupes, et leur sensibilité à la condition expérimentale mesurée. Cette technique s'est révélée utile pour isoler des différences significatives dans un système multidimensionnel dans lequel les stimuli externes, la lumière et le LSD, étaient contenus à l'intérieur de limites à la fois physiologiques et pharmacologiques raisonnables.

The author gratefully acknowledges the technical assistance of J. E. Shryne, Jr. and particularly the cooperation of J. RB Whittlesey in conceptualizing the scaling procedures used in the multi-dimensional analysis.

REFERENCES

BEGLEITER, H., GROSS, M. M. and KISSIN, B. Evoked cortical responses to affective visual stimuli. *Psychophysiology*, **1967**, *3*: 336–344.

BROWN, B. B. Specificity of EEG photic flicker responses to color as related to visual imagery ability. *Psychophysiology*, **1966**, *2*: 197–207.

BROWN, B. B. Subjective and EEG responses to LSD in visualizer and non-visualizer subjects. *Electroenceph. clin. Neurophysiol.*, **1968**a, *25*: 372–379.

BROWN, B. B. Visual recall ability and eye movements. *Psychophysiology*, **1968**b, *4*: 300–306.

CALLAWAY, E. Averaged evoked responses in psychiatry. *J. nerv. ment. Dis.*, **1966**, *143*: 80–94.

CHALKE, F. C. R. and ERTL, J. Evoked potentials and intelligence. *Life Sci.*, **1965**, *4*: 1319–1322.

DONCHIN, E. and LINDSLEY, D. B. Average evoked potentials and reaction times to visual stimuli. *Electroenceph. clin. Neurophysiol.*, **1966,** *20*: 217–223.

DUSTMAN, R. and BECK, E. C. Long-term stability of visually evoked potentials in man. *Science*, **1963,** *142*: 1480–1481.

EASON, R. G. Activation and behavior: II. Visually evoked cortical potentials in man as indicants of activation level. *Percept. mot. Skills*, **1964,** *19*: 875–895.

EBE, M., MIKAMI, T., AKI, M. and MIYAZAKI, M. Electrical responses evoked by photic stimulation in human cerebral cortex. *Tohoku J. exp. Med.*, **1962,** *77*: 352–372.

GARCÍA-AUSTT, E., BOGACZ, J. and VANZULLI, A. Effects of attention and inattention upon visual evoked response. *Electroenceph. clin. Neurophysiol.*, **1964,** *17*: 136–143.

HAIDER, M., SPONG, P. and LINDSLEY, D. B. Attention, vigilance, and cortical evoked-potentials in humans. *Science*, **1964,** *145*: 180–182.

JOHN, E. R., HERRINGTON, R. N. and SUTTON, S. Effects of visual form on the evoked response. *Science*, **1967,** *155*: 1439–1442.

MONNIER, M., VATTER, O. and HOSLI, L. Action of colour flicker stimuli on the electrical responses of retina and optic cortex in man. *Docum. ophthal. (Den Haag)*, **1964,** *18*: 207–220.

RIETVELD, W. J. The occipitocortical response to light-flashes in man. *Acta physiol. pharmacol. neerl.*, **1963,** *12*: 373–407.

RIETVELD, W. J. and TORDOIR, W. E. M. The influence of flash intensity upon the visual evoked response in the human cortex. *Acta physiol. pharmacol. neerl.*, **1965,** *13*: 160–170.

SHIPLEY, T., JONES, R. W. and FRY, A. Evoked visual potentials and human color vision. *Science*, **1965,** *150*: 1162–1164.

SPEHLMANN, R. The averaged electrical responses to diffuse and to patterned light in the human. *Electroenceph. clin. Neurophysiol.*, **1965,** *19*: 560–569.

SPONG, P., HAIDER, M. and LINDSLEY, D. B. Selective attentiveness and cortical evoked responses to visual and auditory stimuli. *Science*, **1965,** *148*: 395–397.

SUTTON, S., TUETING, P., ZUBIN, J and JOHN E. R. Information delivery and the sensory evoked potential. *Science*, **1967,** *155*: 1436–1439.

Reference: BROWN, B. B. Effect of LSD on visually evoked responses to color in visualizer and non-visualizer subjects. *Electroenceph. clin. Neurophysiol.*, **1969,** *27*: 356–363.

Electroencephalography and Clinical Neurophysiology
Elsevier Publishing Company, Amsterdam – Printed in The Netherlands

THE VISUAL EVOKED RESPONSE: A COMPARISON OF BRIGHT AND DULL CHILDREN[1]

L. E. RHODES[2], R. E. DUSTMAN AND E. C. BECK

Veterans Administration Hospital and University of Utah, Salt Lake City, Utah 84113 (U.S.A.)

(Accepted for publication: February 14, 1969)

A relationship between brain wave patterns and level of intelligence has been sought since the beginning of electroencephalography (Berger 1933). As it has long been known that development of intellectual abilities relates directly to chronological age, as does the emergence of different wave forms, patterns, and frequency of EEG activity, a correlation of level of intelligence with certain EEG parameters has been a reasonable expectation. Indeed, a number of investigators have reported correlations between various parameters of the EEG trace and test scores of intelligence (Kreezer 1936, 1937, 1940; Bernhard and Skoglund 1939; Knott *et al.* 1942; Henry 1944; Kreezer and Smith 1950; Mundy-Castle 1958; Netchine and Lairy 1960). Others have found no relationship (Lindsley 1938, 1944; Shagass 1946; Ostow 1950; Biesheuvel and Pitt 1955; Ellingson 1956; Gastaut 1960; Berkson *et al.* 1961; Hill 1963).

Recently these opposing views have been interestingly summarized and debated by Vogel and Broverman (1964, 1966) and Ellingson (1966). According to Ellingson, evidence concerning the relationship between brain waves and intelligence is contradictory and inconclusive, whereas Vogel and Broverman support the existence of a reliable relationship between EEG and test intelligence. They state that whereas such relationships are not so clear in the normal adult, they are evident in studies of subjects who have either relatively undeveloped intellectual function, such as children and feeble-minded individuals, or those with deteriorating intellectual function, such as geriatric subjects.

Beyond criticisms of technique of the various studies, ranging from EEG recording methods to the types of intelligence tests used, there has been the suggestion that other measures of electrocortical activity should be used (Ellingson 1966). The conflicting findings may be attributable, in part, to the nature of the resting EEG which makes reliable quantification difficult.

The average or summed evoked response has a number of characteristics that suggest it as a promising approach to the problem. It is under stimulus control, thereby providing additional information beyond that which may be derived from resting electrocortical activity. The evoked response pattern reflects individual differences (Dustman and Beck 1963; Uttal and Cook 1964) that are more easily seen and measured than those of the EEG trace. The intra-subject changes in the wave form of the evoked response have been proved to be stable over short and long periods of time, thus providing a reliable measure (Shagass and Schwartz 1961; Dustman and Beck 1963). Finally, amplitude changes in the visually evoked response, particularly in the late wave components, have been reported to change with chronological age (Dustman and Beck 1966, 1969). In view of these findings, we attempted to determine whether evoked response amplitude or the latency of wave components of the evoked response would be significantly related to the mental age of children. We now report the results of studies on forty subjects,

[1] Supported in part by National Institute of Child Health and Human Development, PH-43-67-1451.

[2] Present address: Veterans Administration Hospital, Phoenix, Ariz. 84012. Data in this paper are from a thesis submitted to the faculty of the University of Utah in partial fulfillment of the requirements for the Ph.D. degree in Psychology.

twenty dull and twenty bright children, selected from a sample of several hundred school children.

METHOD

Apparatus

A Grass photo stimulator (PS2B) was employed to evoke cortical responses to a light pulse. Brain electrical activity was amplified, with amplifier frequency response limits of ± 3 dB, 0.8–50 c/sec, and stored on a 7-channel Sanborn-Ampex magnetic data recorder. A Mnemotron Computer of Average Transients (CAT) was used to sum and extract the visual evoked response (VER) from the ongoing EEG. An inked record of each summed response was plotted on 25×38 cm graph paper by a Moseley X–Y Plotter. Latencies, amplitudes, and other pertinent measures of the evoked responses were coded on IBM cards for later analysis by a Control Data 3200 Computer.

Procedure

Subjects. Two experimental groups of 10- and 11-year-old children equated for age and matched for sex were studied: (1) a group of twenty bright children who had a full scale WISC IQ score that ranged from 120 to 140 (mean = 130); and (2) a group of twenty dull children who had a full scale WISC score that ranged from 70 to 90 (mean = 79). Approximately 800 children were initially screened on the basis of school records, previously administered intelligence tests, and physical and mental health summaries. Only those children with group IQ scores below 90 and above 120, who had no record of brain damage or emotional disturbance, and who were adapting satisfactorily to school were considered for further testing. Final selection of subjects for the two groups was made on the basis of WISC IQ score, a biographical inventory, and health status. Although EEG recordings of the usual clinical type were not made, tracings from the central and occipital areas were examined by the authors and later evaluated by an electroencephalographer. Several children with borderline or abnormal EEG patterns were excluded from the study, as were a number of others because of biographical information inplying possible brain injury.

Each child participated in two experimental recording sessions separated by approximately 2 months. Subjects were seated in a padded chair while solder pellet electrodes were applied to the scalp over the central (C_3 and C_4) and occipital (O_1 and O_2) scalp, according to the "10–20" International System. Recording was unipolar against reference electrodes attached to the ear lobes. Two additional electrodes were applied approximately one inch apart on the subject's right thumb, over the opponens pollicis. Muscle discharges from the thumb electrodes served to monitor a mental task used as a gross control for variations in attention. The children were asked to respond by pushing a button with their right thumbs after the 4th and 6th flashes in each sequence of 10 flashes. If during the 100 flashes, a child was "asleep at the switch" or his reaction time was excessive, these responses were excluded. As recording sessions were short, generally 5 min or less, maintaining attention did not appear to be a serious problem.

The child faced a white reflecting hemisphere 70 cm in diameter which was positioned so that its center was 40 cm from his eyes. The photo lamp was located immediately behind and above the child's head, and was aimed at the hemisphere's center which reflected a uniform flash enveloping the child's face. The luminance of the flash reflected from the hemisphere was measured, at the same distance as the child's face (40 cm), in lumens/cm^2 or phots. At the intensities used in the experiments, PS-1 with filter, PS-2, and PS-8, phots were $0.65 \times 10^{+2}$, $1.15 \times 10^{+2}$, and $2.05 \times 10^{+2}$, respectively.

After several practice flashes, two sets of 100 flashes at intensity PS-2 were presented to each child. The two sets of flashes, separated by approximately 5 min, comprised the first session. In the second session (2 months later) 100 flashes at PS-2 were repeated. Two additional series of 100 flashes were included in this session, one at intensity PS-1 plus a filter, and one at PS-8. Thus the two sessions provided measures of reliability of VERs separated by 5 min and by 2 months. Also a comparison of the two groups was possible at three levels of flash intensity. The hemisphere was used in all instances, and inter-flash intervals were never less than 2 sec.

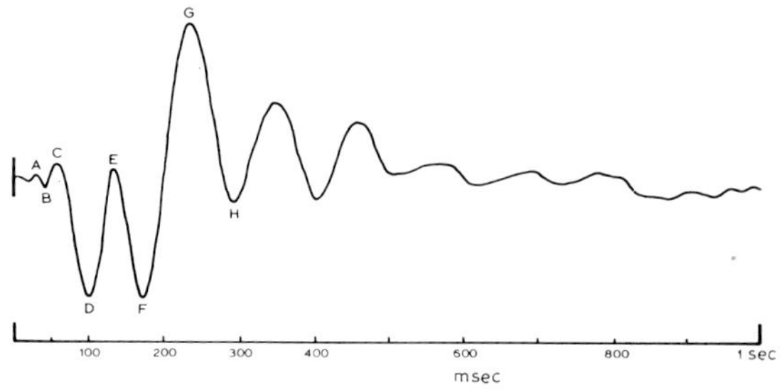

Fig. 1
A typical VER with 8 waves, labeled A to H. In this and subsequent figures, an upward deflection is negative.

Methods of measurement

VERs from each scalp area were plotted for each set of 100 flashes. The typical response (Fig. 1) included eight recurring peaks (waves A–H). Latencies were computed by converting the distance between flash onset and each peak into msec. Amplitude was determined by measuring the vertical distance from the trough or peak of the preceding component to the peak or trough of the component in question. Excursion measures were also used in the present study. Measuring was done by tracing, with a map-reading wheel, the response pattern scribed by the recording pen. By such a method the total excursion of two or more waves occurring during a certain epoch of the evoked response could be measured and compared with others similarly measured (see Dustman and Beck 1969). By this method the following measurements were made: (1) a total excursion obtained by rolling the map-reading wheel from onset of the response to 250 msec; (2) excursions of early components determined by measuring from onset to the peak of the D wave, generally about 100 msec; and (3) excursions of later components defined as the excursion from the peak of the D wave to 250 msec.

Wave form stability was determined by correlating the 100 amplitude measures obtained from one VER with those obtained from another. This method has been previously described (Dustman and Beck 1963, 1966, 1969; Callaway and Layne 1965). The reliability of evoked responses from each recording site was determined by correlating each subject's response from a particular site with his responses recorded from the same site approximately 5 min and 2 months later. Inter-subject correlations were computed for each group; as for example, the right central response of each bright child was correlated with the right central responses of each of the other bright children. This allowed for a comparison of group homogeneity of the VER wave form.

Statistical analysis

A three-factor (intelligence, sex, hemisphere) analysis of variance completely fixed model, with repeated measures on the third factor, was employed. Separate analyses were computed for VER measures from the occipital and the central scalp. An analysis of variance was computed on each excursion measure and latency of each peak. The same basic statistical design was employed to analyze wave form stability; however, since

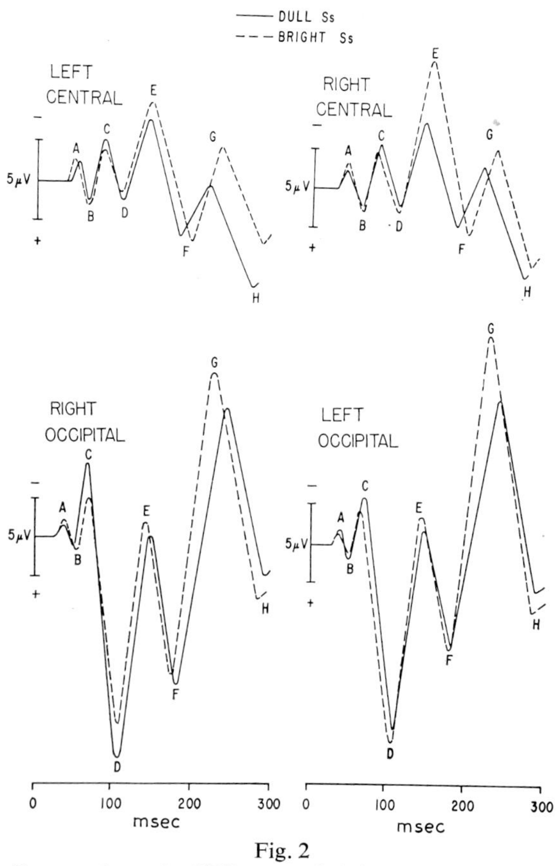

Fig. 2
Group schematic VERs recorded from left and right central and occipital scalp of twenty bright and twenty dull children illustrating amplitude differences between the groups.

correlations above 0.50 do not distribute normally, the Fisher Z Transformation was made on all correlations prior to the analyses of variance.

RESULTS

Group schematic VERs recorded from central and occipital scalp of bright and dull children are illustrated in Fig. 2. These schematic responses were constructed by plotting the mean latencies and amplitudes of the various wave components for each group of subjects. Numerical values for mean peak to trough amplitudes and latencies are presented in Tables I and II.

The excursion measures of the later components (100–250 msec) of both the occipital and central VERs were found to be reliably larger for the bright children ($P < 0.01$ occipital; $P < 0.05$ central). Much of the excursion difference of the central responses could be attributed to the amplitude of the D, E and F waves, especially the D–E deflection (see Fig. 2). Each of these measures differentiated the groups significantly ($P < 0.05$).

TABLE I

Mean peak to trough amplitudes (μV) of VER components recorded from bright and dull children

Groups by area	Components						
	A–B	B–C	C–D	D–E	E–F	F–G	G–H
Left occipital							
Bright children	2.0	3.5	14.5	13.3	10.0	19.7	14.6
Dull children	1.6	5.4	18.9	14.4	9.5	17.9	10.7
Right occipital							
Bright children	1.7	2.8	16.0	15.4	8.6	20.1	16.8
Dull children	1.8	4.0	15.4	13.3	7.6	16.1	12.5
Left central							
Bright children	3.1	3.5	2.9	5.9	8.9	6.0	6.1
Dull children	2.5	4.0	3.8	5.2	7.6	4.8	6.6
Right central							
Bright children	3.0	3.7	4.1	9.8	11.0	5.7	6.7
Dull children	2.6	4.1	4.5	5.6	6.7	4.0	8.0

TABLE II

Mean latencies (msec) of VER recorded from bright and dull children

Groups by area	Peaks							
	A	B	C	D	E	F	G	H
Left occipital								
Bright children	38	52	67	105	140	172	226	281
Dull children	36	48	66	106	146	180	244	291
Right occipital								
Bright children	37	50	65	106	143	176	227	284
Dull children	38	50	67	109	146	182	243	290
Left central								
Bright children	44	63	81	105	146	196	234	284
Dull children	46	63	84	109	142	182	220	269
Right central								
Bright children	44	63	81	106	148	198	232	280
Dull children	44	63	84	110	142	183	216	270

The bright group also differed from the dull group with respect to hemispheric asymmetry. A different hemispheric relationship of the peak to trough amplitudes of waves D–E and E–F recorded from right and left central scalp was attested by significant hemisphere × intelligence interactions ($P < 0.01$ and < 0.05). This difference between groups is best illustrated by the DEF excursion measures. The mean DEF excursions of the right and left central responses of the bright children were 14.5 cm and 11.5 cm, respectively, or a mean amplitude difference of 2.9 cm. For the dull children, the amplitude of the right hemisphere (10.3 cm) exceeded that of the left (9.7 cm) by only 0.6 cm. Thus, while there was essentially no amplitude difference between the right and left central responses of the dull children, the right central responses of bright children were significantly larger than their left central responses.

Fig. 3 graphically illustrates the mean excursion measures of the late central components (waves D through H) recorded from the bright and dull children as a function of stimulus intensity. Consistent with the above findings, the evoked responses of bright children were found to be larger than those of dull children across all three intensity levels ($F = 7.30$, $df = 1/32$, $P < 0.05$).

The latency of wave G (see Table II) recorded from occipital leads was significantly earlier for the bright children, as indicated by an F ratio of 12.19 ($df = 1/36$, $P < 0.01$). Interestingly, this

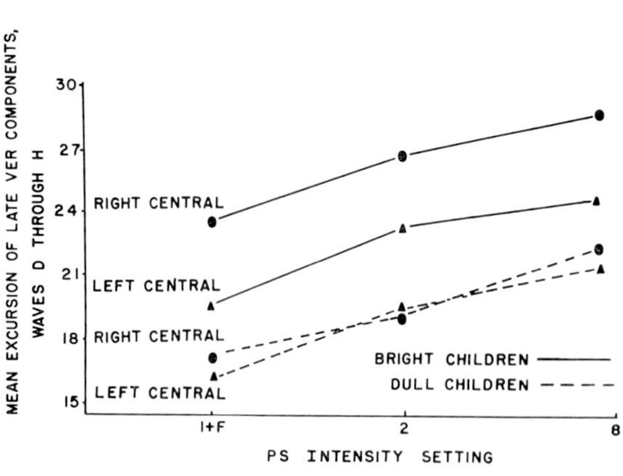

Fig. 3

Mean hemispheric amplitudes in bright children and dull children at various levels of light intensity, showing inter-hemispheric asymmetry for the bright children only.

TABLE III

Mean intra-subject correlations between VERs as a function of time

Area	Bright children		Dull children	
	5 min	2 mo.	5 min	2 mo.
Left central	0.91	0.84	0.87	0.80
Right central	0.94	0.87	0.92	0.84
Left occipital	0.96	0.92	0.96	0.92
Right occipital	0.97	0.92	0.96	0.90

same component, when recorded from central leads, arrived later in the bright children, but this difference was not statistically significant. There were no other reliable latency differences.

The amplitude of late components, *i.e.*, the excursion of waves D–G, of the boys' VERs was greater than that found in the girls on both the occipital and central responses ($P < 0.05$) for both bright and dull children.

The mean intra-subject correlations (*i.e.*, right central response of each subject correlated with another of his own right central responses, left occipital with left occipital, etc.) between VERs recorded 5 min and 2 months apart are given in Table III. Here it may be seen that the response for both groups was stable even for long periods of time.

Since amplitude differences related to intelligence, sex, and hemisphere were found predominantly in the later components, correlations between wave forms of later components (100–250 msec) of the VERs were computed and analyzed. The wave form similarity between later components of the central response was significantly higher among the bright children than among the dull ones, as indicated by the F ratio of 4.32 ($df = 1/36$, $P < 0.05$), indicating that the bright group was more homogeneous. The frequency of alpha and the evoked response after-discharge were found to correlate 0.64 for bright children and 0.79 for dull children. However, non-reliable correlations of −0.18 for bright children and −0.30 for dull ones was found between alpha frequency and the frequency of late wave components; *i.e.*, waves F, G, H. This suggests that alpha frequency is related to after-discharge activity but that the last triphasic component of the VER (FGH) is time-locked to the light flash and is not the result of ongoing alpha rhythm. No reliable differences related to intelligence were found for alpha amplitude ($t=0.83$, $df=32$) or alpha frequency ($t=0.38$, $df=32$). This finding does not support the notion that VER amplitude differences between bright and dull children can be attributed to background alpha activity.

DISCUSSION

The evoked response differentiated bright from dull children in three ways: (1) The bright children had reliably larger amplitudes in the late components of their evoked responses in both central and occipital recordings. (2) Dull children did not demonstrate hemispheric asymmetry in response amplitude as did bright children. The evoked responses of the bright children were consistently of larger amplitude over the right than over the left hemisphere. (3) The late components of VERs of bright children were more similar or homogeneous than those of the dull children.

It may be that the organization of the central nervous system in dull children is less mature than that of intellectually superior children. If this is so, this difference may be reflected in wave form or amplitude of the evoked response. Based on this proposition, the concept of mental age, and the recent maturational data on the VER provided by Dustman and Beck (1966, 1969), we compared the evoked responses of bright 10-year-old children with those of several other age groups. The large late components from the bright children's occipital responses were more similar to the 13- and 14-year-old group than to any of the groups above the age of 10 years. The responses of the dull children, however, were unlike the normative data. The later occipital components were smaller than those recorded from the normal children between the ages of 5 and 10 years. From these observations, we speculate that bright children may exhibit evoked responses similar to those recorded from older subjects. In contrast, responses from dull children are peculiar in that they are of smaller magnitude than responses from normal children of their own age level and below. From this it appears that the differences in VERs between bright and dull children represent something more than a maturational difference.

It should be stressed that while group differences were modestly significant, the possibility of discriminating bright and dull individuals by amplitude of late VER components is limited because of the extreme variability of the response. For example, a seemingly large group difference may be found in the amplitude of the D–E component recorded from the right central scalp (Table I). The mean amplitude of the bright children was 9.8 μV, that of the dull children 5.6, but as the standard deviation for the groups approached 4 μV, overlap of individuals from each group is apparent.

The most interesting characteristic differentiating bright and dull children was that the dull children demonstrated no amplitude differences between the late components of right and left central responses. This peculiarity was a general phenomenon occurring throughout the dull group, not just a function of two or three extreme cases. The bright children consistently exhibited larger amplitudes with right central responses. The amplitude of the VERs recorded from right central scalp was greater in nineteen of the twenty bright subjects. Later components of VERs recorded from the right hemisphere have been reported to be larger than those recorded from the left scalp in normal adults (Cohn 1963, 1964; Kooi *et al.* 1965), left- and right-handed college students (Groberg 1967), and children whose intellectual functioning was in the normal range (Bigum 1969).

Several proposals have been made to explain the asymmetry of amplitude of VERs. Cohn (1964) reported that alpha amplitude may be related to the amplitude differences which are found in later components of the VER. If either alpha amplitude or alpha frequency had a significant effect on evoked response amplitude in the present study, the right hemisphere alpha amplitude of the bright children should be greater than that found with the dull children. Contrary to expectation, we found no reliable differences for either alpha amplitude or alpha frequency between bright and dull children.

As the bright children's responses were larger than the dull children's, the possibility of differences in level of attention cannot be ignored. It has been repeatedly demonstrated that with increased attention there is an enhancement of late components of the evoked response (Haider *et al.* 1964; Spong *et al.* 1965; Sakai *et al.* 1966). Having the children perform a mental task by counting the flashes and pressing a key at certain intervals does not necessarily indicate that a certain level of attention was maintained for all subjects. Bright youngsters may generally operate at a higher level of attention. Or it may be, as Lindsley (1957) speculated, that the dull child's lowered responsiveness, compared to normal and bright subjects, indicates a dysfunctioning reticular activating system. As it is generally accepted that late components of the evoked response derive from extralemniscal pathways passing through the reticular formation, the decreased amplitude of late components of the evoked response in dull children is consonant with Lindsley's hypothesis.

That latency differences between the VERs of bright and dull children did not reach significance is inconsistent with the findings of Chalke and Ertl (1965). They reported a mean difference of 63 msec on a third positive peak, probably our wave F, between responses from thirty-three bright and four mentally retarded subjects. Similarly, bright post-graduate students and eleven Army Cadets who had IQs in the "low normal range" gave means of 142 msec and 175 msec, respectively, for the same peak. We found no such large latency differences, although there was a trend in that direction, particularly in components arriving after 200 msec.

SUMMARY

Visual evoked responses were recorded from central and occipital scalp of twenty bright children (Full Scale WISC scores ranging from 120 to 140, $\bar{X}=130$) and twenty dull children (Full Scale WISC scores ranging from 70 to 90, $\bar{X}=79$). All subjects were 10 or 11 years old and each group was composed of ten boys and ten girls. Results were: (1) The late components (100–250 msec) of responses recorded from both occipital and central scalp were reliably larger for the bright children. (2) Dull children demonstrated essentially no hemispheric differences between the amplitudes of the right and left central responses. The bright subjects had right central responses which were consistently larger than responses from the late components of the left scalp. This finding was consistent at several stimulus intensities.

Differences between the bright and dull children did not appear to be simply a function of the maturational process. The bright children's VER amplitudes were similar to normal 13- and 14-year-old children's; however, the dull children's VER amplitudes were smaller than those of either younger children or normal children their own age.

RÉSUMÉ

LA RÉPONSE ÉVOQUÉE VISUELLE: COMPARAISON ENTRE DES SUJETS D'INTELLIGENCE SUPÉRIEURE ET DES SUJETS D'INTELLIGENCE MÉDIOCRE

Les réponses évoquées visuelles ont été enregistrées au niveau du scalp dans les régions centrales et occipitales chez vingt enfants très intelligents (score à l'échelle globale du WISC allant de 120 à 140, $\bar{X}=130$), et vingt enfants d'intelligence médiocre (score à l'échelle globale du WISC allant de 70 à 90, $\bar{X}=79$). Tous les sujets étaient âgés de 10 à 11 ans et chaque groupe comportait dix garçons et dix filles. Les résultats sont les suivants: (1) les composantes tardives (100–250 msec) des réponses enregistrées au niveau du scalp occipital et central sont nettement plus grandes chez les enfants très intelligents; (2) les enfants d'intelligence médiocre montrent essentiellement une absence de différence hémisphérique entre les amplitudes des réponses centrales droite et gauche. Les sujets intelligents montrent des réponses centrales droites qui sont de façon constante plus grandes que les réponses du scalp gauche en ce qui concerne les composantes tardives. Cette donnée est constante pour plusieurs intensités de stimulation.

Des différences entre enfants très intelligents et enfants d'intelligence médiocre n'apparaissent pas être simplement fonction du processus maturatif. Les amplitudes des réponses évoquées visuelles des enfants très intelligents sont semblables à celles d'enfants normaux âgés de 13 à 14 ans; toutefois, les amplitudes des réponses évoquées visuelles des enfants d'intelligence médiocre sont moindres que celles soit d'enfants plus jeunes, soit d'enfants normaux de leur âge chronologique.

We wish to express our gratitude to Dr. H. Mavor, Director of EEG Laboratories, V.A. Hospital, Salt Lake City, for his valuable help and advice.

REFERENCES

BERGER, H. Über das Elektrenkephalogramm des Menschen. V. *Arch. Psychiat. Nervenkr.*, **1933**, *98*: 231–254.

BERKSON, G., HERMELIN, B. and O'CONNOR, N. Physiological responses of normals and institutionalized mental defectives to repeated stimuli. *J. ment. Defic. Res.*, **1961**, *5*: 30–39.

BERNHARD, C. G. et SKOGLUND, C. R. Recherches sur la fréquence alpha de l'électro-encéphalogramme chez l'enfant. *Acta psychiat. scand.*, **1939**, *14*: 223–231.

BIESHEUVEL, S. and PITT, D. R. Some tests of speed and tempo of behavior as predictors of the primary-secondary function temperament variable. *J. nat. Inst. Personnel Res.*, **1955**, *6*: 87–94.

BIGUM, H. *Visual and somatosensory evoked responses from mongoloid and normal children.* Unpublished doctoral dissertation, University of Utah, **1969**, 77 p.

CALLAWAY, E. and LAYNE, R. S. Evoked responses and segmental set of schizophrenia. *Arch. gen. Psychiat.*, **1965**, *112*: 83–89.

CHALKE, F. C. and ERTL, J. Evoked potentials and intelligence. *Life Sci.*, **1965**, *4*: 1319–1322.

COHN, R. Average evoked cortical response from visual stimulation. *Electroenceph. clin. Neurophysiol.*, **1963**, *15*: 156P.

COHN, R. Rhythmic after-activity in visual evoked responses. *Ann. N.Y. Acad. Sci.*, **1964**, 112: 281–291.

DUSTMAN, R. E. and BECK, E. C. Long term stability of visually evoked potentials in man. *Science*, **1963**, *142*: 1480–1481.

DUSTMAN, R. E. and BECK, E. C. Visually evoked potentials: Amplitude changes with age. *Science*, **1966**, *151*: 1013–1015.

DUSTMAN, R. E. and BECK, E. C. The effects of maturation and aging on the wave form of visually evoked potentials. *Electroenceph. clin. Neurophysiol.*, **1969**, *26*: 2–11.

ELLINGSON, R. J. Brain waves and problems of psychology. *Psychol. Bull.*, **1956**, *53*: 1–34.

ELLINGSON, R. J. Relationship between EEG and test intelligence: a commentary. *Psychol. Bull.*, **1966**, *65*: 91–98.

GASTAUT, H. Correlations between the electroencephalographic and the psychometric variables (M.M.P.I., Rosenzweig, intelligence tests). *Electroenceph. clin. Neurophysiol.*, **1960**, *12*: 226–227.

GROBERG, D. H. *Handedness and late components of visual and somatosensory cerebral evoked responses.* Unpublished doctoral dissertation, University of Utah, **1967**, 73 p.

HAIDER, M., SPONG, P. and LINDSLEY, D. B. Attention, vigilance, and cortical evoked potentials in human. *Science*, **1964**, *145*: 180–182.

HENRY, C. E. Electroencephalograms of normal children. *Monogr. Soc. Res. Child Devel.*, **1944**, *9* (Serial No. 39): 3–66.

HILL, D. The E.E.G. in psychiatry. In D. HILL and G. PARR (Eds.), *Electroencephalography. A symposium on its various aspects.* Macmillan, New York, **1963**: 368–428.

KNOTT, J. R., FRIEDMAN, H. and BARDSLEY, R. Some electroencephalographic correlations of intelligence in eight-year and twelve-year-old children. *J. exp. Psychol.*, **1942**, *30*: 380–391.

KOOI, K. A., GUVENER, A. M. and BAGCHI, B. K. Visual evoked responses in lesions of the optic pathways. *Electroenceph. clin. Neurophysiol.*, **1965**, *18*: 524.

KREEZER, G. Electrical potentials of the brain in certain types of mental deficiency. *Arch. Neurol. Psychiat. (Chic.)*, **1936**, *36*: 1206–1213.

KREEZER, G. The dependence of the electroencephalogram upon intelligence level. *Psychol. Bull.*, **1937**, *34*: 769–770.

KREEZER, G. The relation of intelligence level and the electroencephalogram. *Yearbook nat. Soc. Study of Education*, **1940**, *39 (Part I)*: 130–133.

KREEZER, G. and SMITH, F. W. The relation of the alpha rhythm of the electroencephalogram and intelligence level in the nondifferentiated familial type of mental deficiency. *J. Psychol.*, **1950**, *29*: 47–51.

LINDSLEY, D. B. Electrical potentials of the brain in children and adults. *J. gen. Psychol.*, **1938**, *19*: 285–306.

LINDSLEY, D. B. Electroencephalography. In J. McV. HUNT (Ed.), *Personality and the behavior disorders, Vol. 2.* Ronald Press, New York, **1944**: 1033–1103.

LINDSLEY, D. B. Psychophysiology and motivation. *Nebraska Symposium on Motivation*, **1957**: 44–106.

MUNDY-CASTLE, A. C. Electrophysiological correlates of intelligence. *J. Personality*, **1958**, *26*: 184–199.

NETCHINE, S. et LAIRY, C. Ondes cérébrales et niveau mental: Quelques aspects de l'évolution génétique du tracé EEG suivant le niveau mental. *Enfance*, **1960**, *No. 4–5*: 427–439.

OSTOW, M. Psychic function and the electroencephalogram. *Arch. Neurol. Psychiat. (Chic.)*, **1950**, *64*: 385–400.

SAKAI, M., GINDY, K. and DUSTMAN, R. E. Amplitude changes of components of the visually evoked response as related to mental states. *Proc. Amer. psychol. Ass.*, **1966**, *2*: 139–140.

SHAGASS, C. An attempt to correlate the occipital alpha frequency of the electroencephalogram with performance on a mental ability test. *J. exp. Psychol.*, **1946**, *36*: 88–92.

SHAGASS, C. and SCHWARTZ, M. Reactivity cycle of somatosensory cortex in humans with and without psychosis. *Science*, **1961**, *134*: 1757–1759.

SPONG, P., HAIDER, M. and LINDSLEY, D. B. Selective attentiveness and cortical evoked responses to visual and auditory stimuli. *Science*, **1965**, *148*: 395–397.

UTTAL, W. R. and COOK, L. Systematics of the evoked somatosensory cortical potential: A psychophysical-electrophysiological comparison. *Ann. N. Y. Acad. Sci.*, **1964,** *112*: 60–79.

VOGEL, W. and BROVERMAN, D. M. Relationship between EEG and test intelligence: A critical review. *Psychol. Bull.*, **1964,** *62*: 132–144.

VOGEL, W. and BROVERMAN, D. M. A reply to "Relationship between EEG and test intelligence: A commentary". *Psychol. Bull.*, **1966,** *65*: 99–109.

Reference: RHODES, L. E., DUSTMAN, R. E. and BECK, E. C. The visual evoked response: a comparison of bright and dull children. *Electroenceph. clin. Neurophysiol.*, **1969,** *27*: 364–372.

EVOKED VISUAL, SOMATO-SENSORY AND RETINAL POTENTIALS IN PHOTOSENSITIVE EPILEPSY[1]

ROGER BROUGHTON[2], KARL-HEINZ MEIER-EWERT[3] AND MITURU EBE[4]

Department of Neurology and Neurosurgery, McGill University and the Montreal Neurological Institute and Hospital, Montreal, Quebec (Canada)

(Accepted for publication: January 17, 1969)

In approximately 1% of epileptic subjects, seizures are regularly provoked by sensory triggering factors (Gastaut and Tassinari 1966). By far the majority of these cases of "reflex epilepsy" involve visual stimuli, usually in the form of intermittent photic stimulation (IPS). The seizures consist mainly of bilateral massive myoclonus, absences (often myoclonic), generalized tonic-clonic attacks and seizures with ictal EEG discharges localized to the parieto-occipital regions (Naquet *et al.* 1960; Gastaut and Tassinari 1966).

In subjects with photosensitive epilepsy, IPS delivered by a stroboscope usually elicits abnormal responses of cerebral, muscular, ocular, autonomic and other origin. At present most authors employ the terms "photoconvulsive response" (PCR) for the paroxysmal cerebral potentials and "photomyoclonic response" (PMR) for the muscular potentials (Bickford *et al.* 1952). Investigations of the PMR using the technique of summated evoked potentials (Meier-Ewert and Broughton 1967) indicated that this response is often an abnormal enhancement of the "photomotor response" of Bickford (1964).

The present paper deals with the cerebral evoked potentials of patients with photosensitive epilepsy, a PCR and a PMR. Comparisons have been made between the spatial, temporal and amplitude characteristics of the waking visual and somato-sensory evoked potentials (VEPs and SEPs) and the ERG of these patients and age and sex-matched controls. Scalp recorded potentials of non-cerebral origin, particularly muscular and ocular, have been assessed: and the evolution of the VEP has been studied during different stages of sleep and arousal, as these affect photosensitivity (Rodin *et al.* 1955; Meier-Ewert and Broughton 1967).

METHODS

Subjects

Ten epileptic subjects and ten matched control subjects, aged 14–34 years (average 23.4), have been investigated. Since all patients but one (an 18-year-old girl with an Unverricht-Lundborg syndrome) participated in a study of the PMR (Meier-Ewert and Broughton 1967), the latter article is referred to for details of their clinical features. The recording and visual stimulation techniques and the equipment are also described in the same study.

In the waking studies of evoked potentials, the subjects were asked to relax all head, neck and jaw muscles as completely as possible, in any case until no EMG potentials were evident in the monitor oscilloscopic tracings. If EMG potentials persisted, intense teeth clenching for 1–2 min was almost always followed by a lack of spontaneous myogenic potentials for several minutes. Stimuli were delivered only under such optimal conditions of relaxation.

The VEP was studied 2–6 times in each

[1] Supported in its early stages by a Fellowship of the Medical Research Council of Canada (Dr. Broughton). Presented in part at meetings of the Eastern Society of Electroencephalographers (see Broughton *et al.* 1967; Ebe *et al.* 1967).

[2] Present address: Department of Medicine, University of Ottawa, Ottawa, Ontario (Canada).

[3] Fellow of the German Academic Exchange Service; presently Scientific Assistant, Neurologische Klinik mit Abteilung für klinische Neurophysiologie der Universität, Freiberg/Br., West Germany.

[4] Visiting Scientist; presently Chief, Department of Physiology, Toranomon General Hospital, Tokyo, Japan.

photosensitive epileptic subject and 1–3 times in each normal subject following 20–30 min of dark adaptation. Controls were unpaid colleagues, medical students and the investigators. The VEP was sampled at standard "10–20 international" midline and lateral electrode sites, using both referential (to ipsilateral ear) and bipolar montages. Supra-orbital and infra-orbital electrodes recorded vertical eye movements. To further monitor possible myogenic contamination, the electrical activity of temporal and occipital muscles was recorded either by closely spaced (1.5–2.0 cm) routine EEG electrodes, so that cerebral activity was essentially equipotential despite the possible presence of background EMG activity, or by a pair of subcutaneous wire electrodes (see Hishikawa *et al.* 1965) separated by 0.5–1.0 cm. A commercial low vacuum corneal electrode referred to the ipsilateral ear was used for recording the ERG.

The eyes were closed in all runs, except a single one which included the ERG. Single flashes were delivered manually in random fashion every 1.0–2.5 sec to minimize possible effects of habituation or anticipation and to avoid stimulation during the occasional spontaneous blink, head movement, EMG or other observable and monitored artifacts. In some studies, pairs of flashes were delivered separated by intervals equivalent to the rate of trains of flashes which was most effective in producing a PCR. Flash-trains themselves were not employed for summation.

The VEP to single flashes was studied during sleep in nine of the epileptic subjects (6 with petit mal and 3 with Unverricht-Lundborg syndrome). The sleep classification used is that of Dement and Kleitman (1957); but stage 1 REM is referred to as REM sleep, and the other stages (I–IV) as non-REM or NREM sleep.

In eight of the epileptic subjects, the SEP was also investigated and compared to that of twelve normal controls. Percutaneous stimulation of the median nerve at the wrist was performed by a Grass S4 stimulator, through an isolation unit, using a cathodal electrode positioned over the nerve and with the anodal electrode 3 cm away in a distal and lateral direction. The stimulus was a square wave of 0.1 (occasionally 0.5) msec duration just sufficiently intense (42–90 V) to produce clonic movement of the thumb. A ground electrode was wrapped more proximally around the forearm.

For all studies, the patients' medications were either unchanged or had been diminished 2–3 days before the recording to heighten photosensitivity. The degree of photosensitivity was assessed before and at the termination of each recording system using flash-trains at the most effective frequencies.

Statistical comparisons[1] were performed between epileptic subjects and normal controls for the VEP, SEP and ERG.

[1] With multi-phasic responses such as evoked potentials the technique of quantifying them is very important, although rarely discussed. The features of interest are the onset and offset latencies and the amplitude of each consistent deflection or "component". Whether a polarity reversal is active and so represents a new physiological phenomenon or is passive in the sense of representing waning of a phenomenon, or whether activities of different origin are overlapping (Rosenzweig and Rosenblith 1953) and so partially mask each other, does not alter the desirability of such quantification. Interpretation is a later stage.

The latencies and amplitudes of such deflections can be measured by either baseline-to-peak or peak-to-peak measurements. Some authors have mixed both types of measurements according to unproven preconceptions of underlying physiological mechanisms (Goff *et al.* 1962) or have even required arbitrarily that a component must cross the baseline to be measured at all (Domino *et al.* 1964), thereby potentially disregarding consistent and apparently relevant events.

Baseline-to-peak measures present the problem of accurately establishing a baseline, several more or less approximate techniques being available. More seriously, a deflection with a given polarity (*e.g.*, positive to preceding activity), consistent latencies for its onset and termination and a constant over-all amplitude can give rise to numerical data very different from peak-to-peak measures. Such a potentially unitary phenomenon may even be considered as of either positive or negative polarity, depending upon its position relative to the baseline, and therefore upon the just preceding potential level of the evoked response. Thus, if an ongoing positivity begins negative relative to the baseline and fails to reach the latter, it will still be considered as a negative measurement: and if it does cross the baseline, the component will be considered positive.

Peak-to-peak measurements, by contrast, are purely descriptive of the multi-phasic curve and do not have the above serious inconveniences. In particular, the point of onset of components as determined by preceding evoked activity, does not influence measurements of their amplitude or decision of their polarity. Rather, it is the polarity direction, magnitude and onset and offset latencies of the change which are scored.

TABLE I

Visual evoked potentials at occipital electrode: comparison between normal and photosensitive epileptic subjects

Component	Polarity	Normals M	Normals S.D.	Epileptics M	Epileptics S.D.	Student test	MWU test
Latencies (msec)							
I	+	28.25	4.18	32.56	4.64	—	—
II	—	40.21	6.36	42.20	7.33	—	—
III	+	52.50	8.94	57.80	12.32	—	—
IV	—	74.65	15.48	78.47	19.51	—	—
V	+	123.59	15.15	123.12	35.37	—	—
VI	—	142.33	10.44	179.00	40.28	0.05 (NH)	0.025
VII	+	194.00	18.26	218.00	29.96	—	—
Amplitudes (μV)							
I	+	2.33	0.58	3.56	1.59	—	—
II	—	3.31	0.95	6.11	3.10	—	0.01
III	+	5.54	2.90	17.07	18.31	—	0.01
IV	—	11.59	7.74	26.40	31.57	—	—
V	+	21.53	12.08	34.24	28.63	—	—
VI	—	7.50	4.97	43.80	26.88	0.01	0.001
VII	+	10.80	3.49	24.67	15.17	—	0.03

Abbreviations used in this and subsequent tables: M, mean value; S.D., standard deviation; NH, non-homogeneous; MWU, Mann-Whitney U test.
Probabilities given where $P \leqslant 0.05$.

TABLE II

Visual evoked potentials at C_z electrode: comparison between normal and photosensitive epileptic subjects

Component	Polarity	Normals M	Normals S.D.	Epileptics M	Epileptics S.D.	Student test	MWU test
Latencies (msec)							
A	—	47.38	7.96	55.40	13.89	—	0.025
B	+	84.50	15.22	76.71	31.15	—	—
C	—	119.50	16.66	106.67	51.95	—	—
D	+	196.00	12.95	139.80	40.23	0.01 (NH)	0.005
Amplitudes (μV)							
A	—	6.00	2.33	13.80	3.27	0.001	0.005
B	+	8.14	3.34	24.71	12.27	0.01 (NH)	0.001
C	—	11.88	4.42	34.83	15.46	0.005 (NH)	0.05
D	+	20.75	6.11	40.00	19.69	0.05	0.01

Probabilities given where $P \leqslant 0.05$.

Peak latencies and peak-to-peak amplitudes of all stable deflections (components) of the evoked potentials were measured manually in referential montages at the O_1 or O_2 and C_z electrodes for the VEP, at the C_3 or C_4 electrode for the SEP, and at the corneal electrode for the ERG. Some 1200 curves were available for such measurements. The data were then fed into an IBM 7044 general purpose computer (McGill University) programmed to compare the indexes of each event (*e.g.*, peak latency of a given component of the occipital VEP) for the Student test and for the non-parametric Mann-Whitney U test. Data concerning the anterior diffusion of occipital VEP components were compared by the Chi-square test.

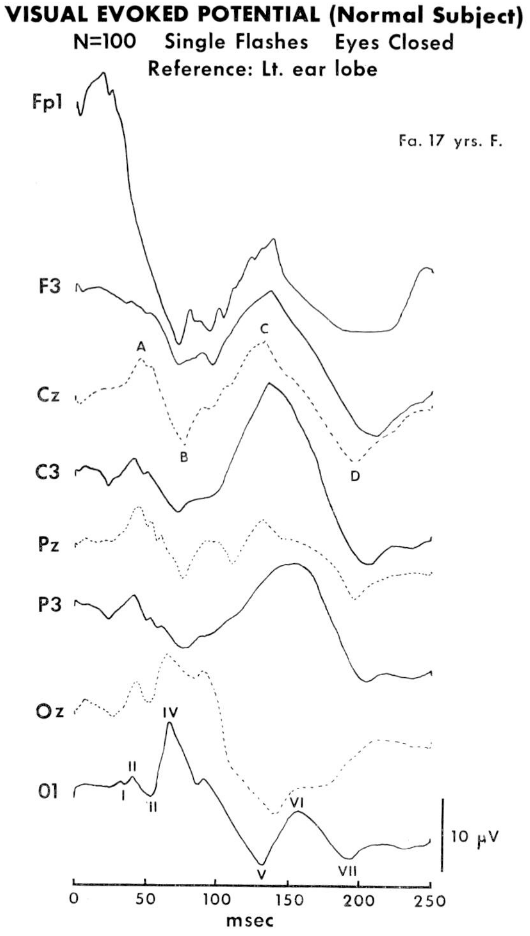

Fig. 1
Spatial distribution of the VEP of a normal subject. Midline responses are in dotted lines. In all referential recordings, surface positivity at the active electrode is down.

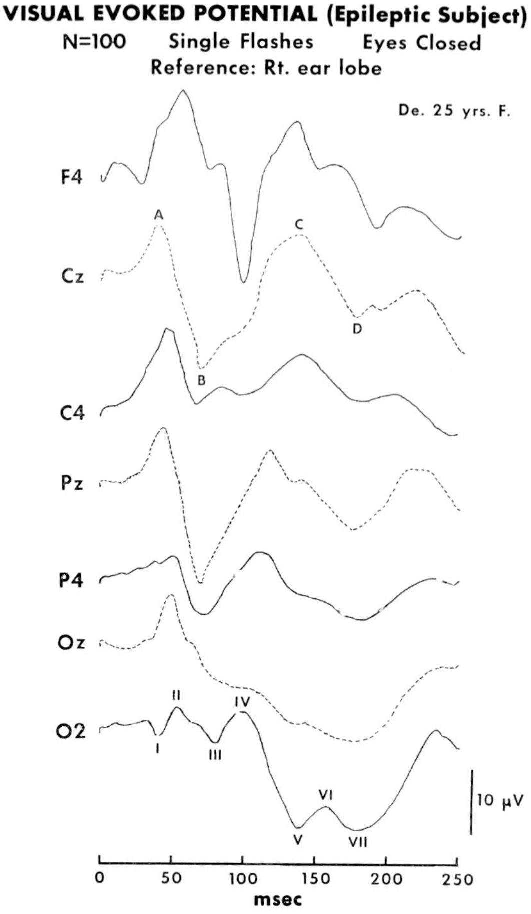

Fig. 2
Spatial distribution of the VEP of a photosensitive epileptic subject. Marked C_z and P_z responses are present in a subject showing little anterior spread of occipital components.

RESULTS

The occipital VEP of normal control subjects (Table I, Fig. 1) was comparable to that described by others (Cobb and Dawson 1960; Cigánek 1961; Ebe *et al.* 1962; Kooi and Bagchi 1964; Gastaut and Régis 1965). VEP components, designated sequentially with Roman numerals, consisted of: an initial surface positivity (component I) at approximately 28±4 msec peak latency, followed by a negativity (component II) at 40±6, a positivity (III) at 52±9 and a negativity (IV) at 75±15, sometimes notched by a small positive wave. These were succeeded by a large positivity (component V) at 140±15, which frequently became split by an intermediate negativity producing a triphasic positive-negative-positive complex (V, VI, VII) with peak latencies of 124±15, 140±16 and 194±18 msec. The potential was completed by a final negativity (component VIII) and an after-rhythm whose frequency approximated that of the parieto-occipital alpha rhythm.

Component I was observed in five of the ten controls, II in eight, III in nine and components V (or the V–VI–VII complex) and VIII in all. Components I, II and III were generally restricted to the parieto-occipital regions, whereas the later components were present more anteriorly at the C_3 or C_4 electrode in about one-third of the subjects.

The C_z electrode (Table II, Fig. 1) generally showed a somewhat different wave form consisting of a negativity (A) at 47 ± 8 msec, positivity (B) at 85 ± 15, negativity (C) at 120 ± 17 and positivity (D) at 196 ± 13. These deflections could be distinguished readily from ERG and ocular potentials evident more anteriorly. Usually this central response was distinctly different from the occipital response (Fig. 1, 2), whereas at other times (about 35% of the potentials) the C_z and occipital electrodes had fairly similar wave forms (Fig. 3).

The photosensitive epileptic subjects had an occipital VEP of wave form comparable to that of normals. But it showed significant differences for a number of components (see Table I). Component VI had both a greater amplitude and latency, and components II, III and VII had greater amplitudes. Statistical analysis (Chi-

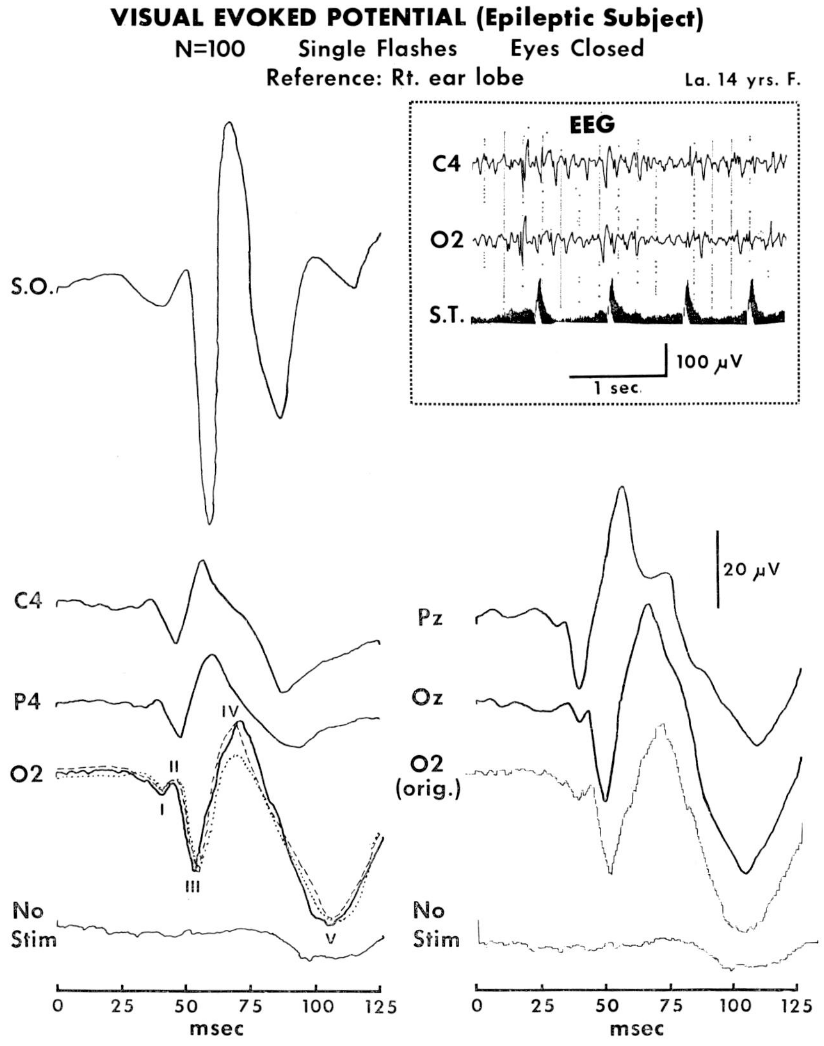

Fig. 3

Spatial distribution of the VEP of a photosensitive epileptic subject. A widespread similar wave form is present. A sample of the background EEG is included. Patient had an Unverricht-Lundborg syndrome. S.O., supra-orbital electrode; S.T., stimulus artifact.

TABLE III

Spatial distribution of visual evoked potentials at the lateral central electrode: comparison between normal and photosensitive epileptic subjects*

Component	Polarity	Normals		Epileptics		Probability
		NonC	C	NonC	C	
I	+	3	2	5	2	—
II	—	10	1	4	3	0.05
III	+	13	1	5	9	0.01
IV	—	14	3	9	7	—
V (V–VI–VII)	+ (+, —, +)	17	0	7	10	0.001
VIII	—	9	8	5	12	—

* Each identified VEP component was scored for its presence or absence at the C_3, C_4 electrode. Component V and the complex V–VI–VII had similar distributions. Seventeen studies compared in each group.
Abbreviations: NonC, number of responses in which component is not present at central electrode (*i.e.*, present only in parieto-occipital region); C, component present at central electrode.
Probabilities from Chi square test, given where $P \geqslant 0.05$.

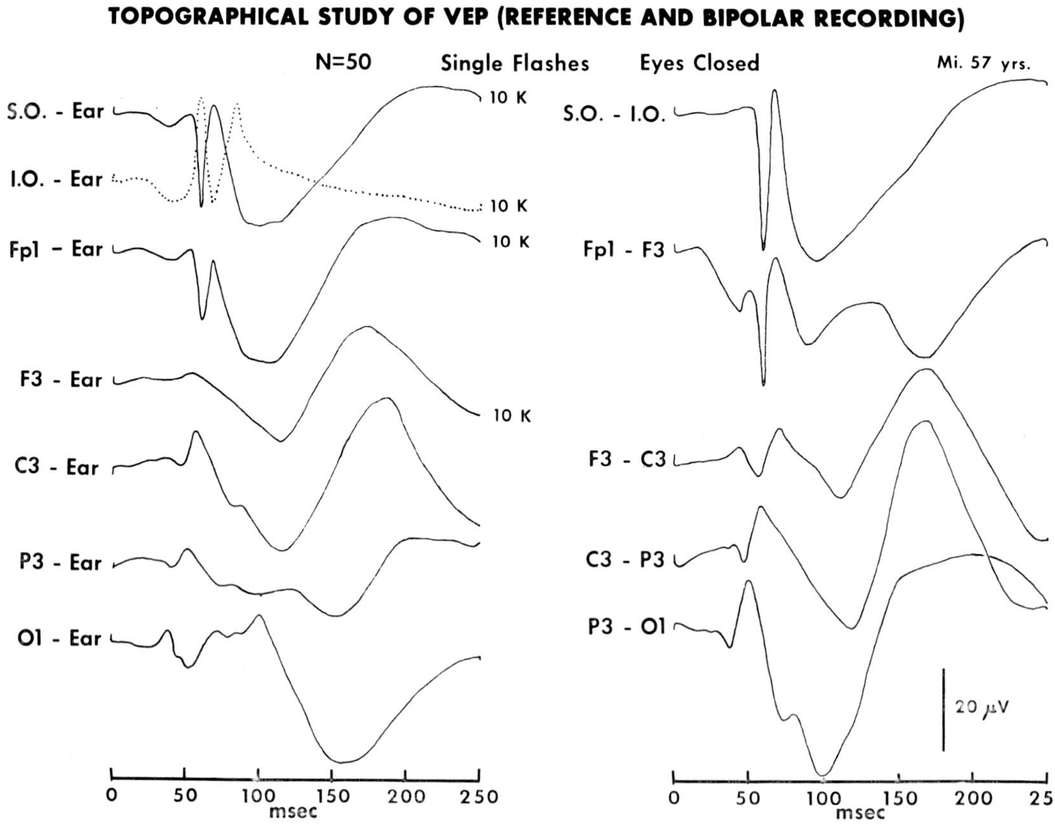

Fig. 4

Comparison of referential and bipolar VEP recording in a photosensitive epileptic subject. The two recording techniques indicate that the potential fields of the occipital VEP and central VEP are quite distinct and that there is a lack of any appreciable oculogenic artifacts posterior to the mid-frontal electrode. S.O., supra-orbital electrode; I.O., infra-orbital electrode.

square test; Table III) indicated that only components II, III and V (or the triphasic V–VI–VII complex) of the VEP of photosensitive epileptics spread significantly anteriorly to the C_3 or C_4 electrodes.

The C_z responses in the epileptic group (Fig. 2) exhibited even more striking differences (Table II). The amplitude of all four components A, B, C and D was significantly greater in photosensitive epileptics: and component A occurred later and component D earlier.

As mentioned, multiple recordings were performed in all subjects. The variability of the VEP, both in multiple determinations in a single session or from session to session (*cf.*, O_2 in Fig. 3), was quite low.

In direct write-out by the UV recorder of taped responses to pairs or series of flashes, the responses to the second or later stimuli could either show simultaneous increases in the occipital and C_z evoked potentials, or the occipital response would increase one or two stimuli before the central region. A proportionately greater increase in amplitude was always observed, however, at the central electrode.

The ERG of normals showed group mean peak latencies of 17.6 ± 1.9 msec for the negative *a* wave and 50.0 ± 9.5 msec for the positive *b* wave. The ERG of epileptic subjects was of identical wave form and distribution, but showed a significantly earlier peak latency of the *a* wave (14.0 ± 1 msec $P < 0.001$). No amplitude differences were present. The potential field in both groups fell off very quickly at the supra-orbital and frontopolar

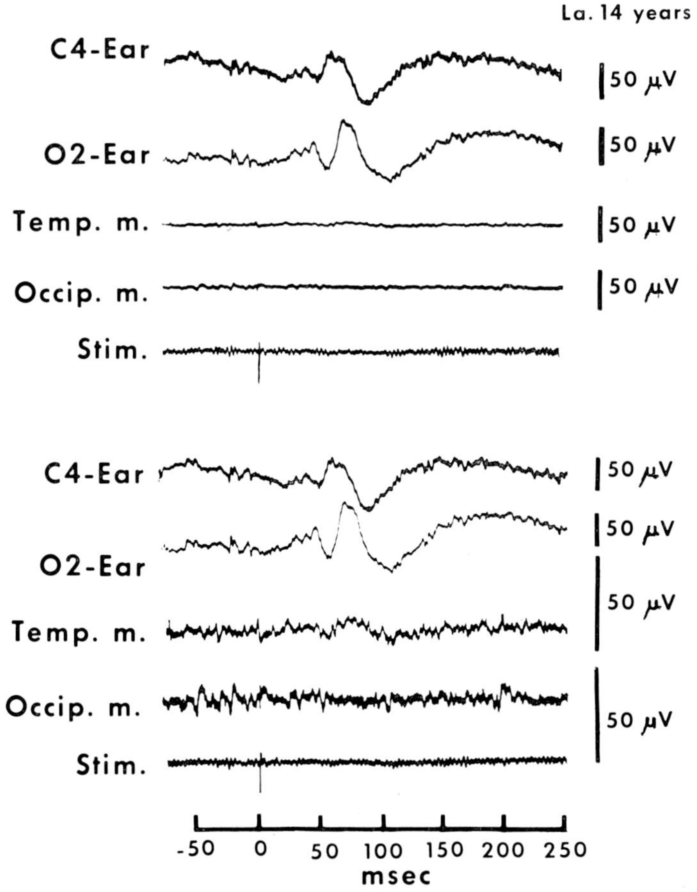

Fig. 5
VEP and subcutaneous EMG (see Hishikawa *et al.* 1965) in an epileptic subject with a marked PMR. Single responses are shown.

electrodes, and usually was indiscernible at the frontal electrode (Fig. 4).

All statistical analyses were performed on potentials believed to be uncontaminated by either oculomotor or muscular activity.

The oculomotor potentials in photosensitive epileptic patients, especially prominent when an "oculoclonic response" was present, were easily identifiable by their inversion of polarity (whereas the ERG had the same polarity) in the supra-orbital and infra-orbital electrodes (Fig. 4). The early reflex ocular movement was quite stable and had fairly constant latencies: frontal positive (*i.e.*, upward movement) at 58 ± 4 msec; negative, 68 ± 6; and positive, 82 ± 8. It was usually followed, at the supra-orbital electrode alone, by inconstant potentials, not related to more posterior activity and probably of palpebral origin. These ocular movement potentials generally were negligible posterior to the F_3–F_4 electrodes (Fig. 4), although at times they would affect the reference ear electrode or, rarely, could even be recorded as a separate potential field of identical polarity in the occipital regions.

Closely spaced scalp electrodes similar to those used to record the peripheral PMR (Meier-Ewert and Broughton 1967) indicated that no muscular contamination was present in the VEP to single flashes. Subcutaneous wire electrodes showed background EMG activity but did not record time-locked synchronous muscle potentials in either averaged or in single (Fig. 5) responses. Finally, the VEPs recorded in two epileptic subjects at corresponding cortical and scalp electrodes (bone reference) during diagnostic cerebral biopsy procedures were similar in the sequence and number of components and in wave form (Fig. 6). It therefore appears that muscular contamination in the VEP was minimal, if not absent.

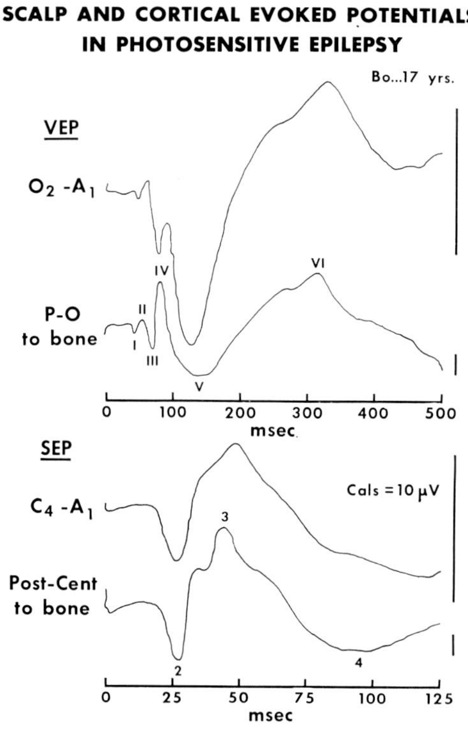

Fig. 6
Cortical and scalp VEP and SEP recordings of a photosensitive epileptic subject. The parieto-occipital cortical VEP and post-central gyrus SEP show the same sequence of components on the cortex compared to scalp, although their relative amplitudes obviously vary.

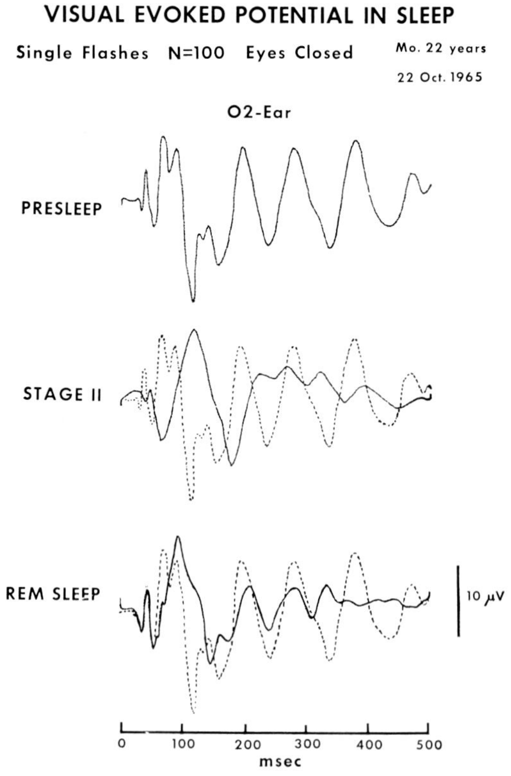

Fig. 7
VEP of a photosensitive epileptic subject during dark adapted pre-sleep wakefulness, NREM sleep (stage II) and REM sleep.

Sleep had marked effects upon cerebral discharges and the VEP. In NREM sleep, spontaneous paroxysmal bursts of poly-spike or poly-spike and wave discharges were recorded in the epileptic group which at times appeared to grow out of the sleep spindles: the PCR, however, was reduced. The VEP (Fig. 7) underwent similar changes in both groups. Components I and II, when identifiable, had slightly increased latencies and occasionally decreased amplitudes. Components III–V were replaced by a widespread triphasic wave, often maximal at C_z, consisting of a positivity peaking at 70–80 msec, a large negativity at 100–200 msec and a positivity at 180–260 msec. The after-rhythm of the VEP disappeared and was sometimes replaced by rhythmic activity of spindle frequency (12–15 c/sec). In REM sleep, no spontaneous discharges occurred in the epileptic subjects and photosensitivity was low. At the occipital electrode, components I and II returned to latencies and amplitudes similar to those of wakefulness, components III, IV and V reappeared with somewhat greater latencies, and no after-rhythm was present (Fig. 7). Moreover, the late C_z responses were greatly diminished in amplitude or were absent.

Following forced arousal from slow wave sleep, the VEP regularly showed increased latencies and amplitudes of later components and sometimes even contained transitory carry-over of components typical of slow wave sleep, as has already been reported for normal subjects

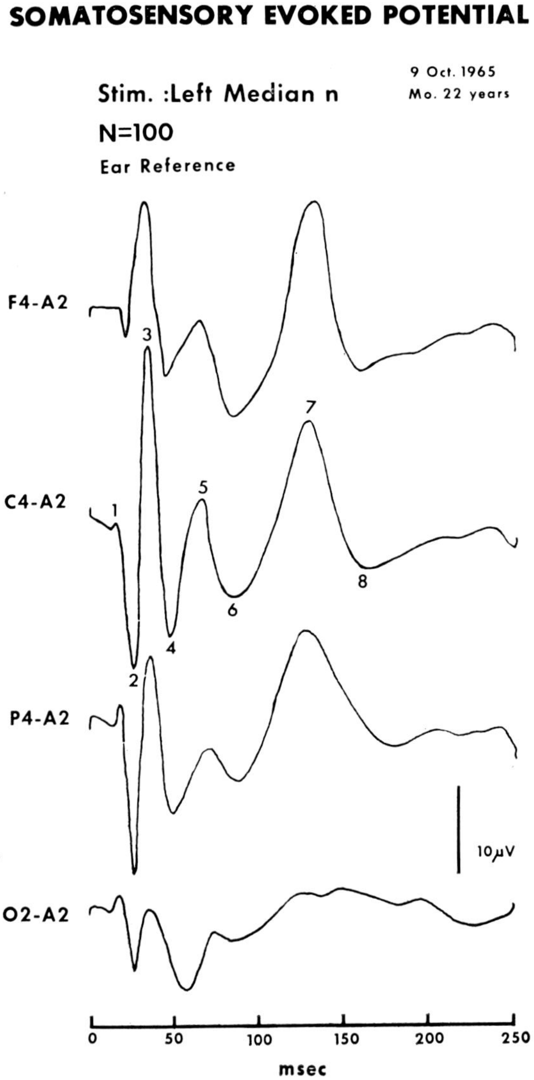

Fig. 8
SEP of a subject with photosensitive epilepsy.

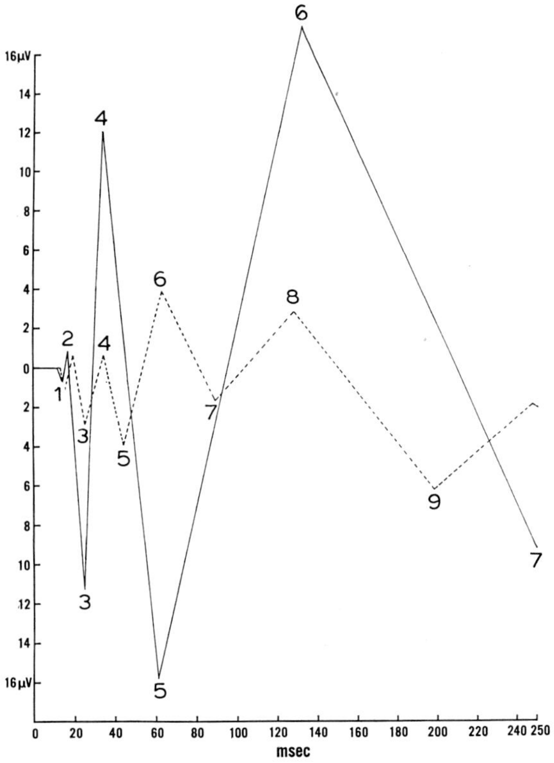

Fig. 9
Group mean SEPs of photosensitive epileptic subjects (——) and normals (- - -). In the epileptic subjects, component 6 and later deflections are of greater latency than 250 msec and are not included in the graph.

TABLE IV

Somato-sensory evoked potential at the central (C_3, C_4) electrode: comparison between normal and photosensitive epileptic subjects

Component	Polarity	Normals		Epileptics		Student test	MWU test
		M	S.D.	M	S.D.		
Latencies (msec)							
0	+	15.00	1.18	14.03	1.75	—	—
1	—	19.14	1.46	17.00	1.15	0.01	0.001
2	+	25.62	4.44	25.43	1.62	—	—
3	—	34.46	4.12	34.74	2.80	—	—
4	+	44.21	2.64	61.14	14.94	0.001 (NH)	0.001
5	—	63.50	7.12	134.43	56.92	0.001 (NH)	0.001
6	+	89.07	10.51	278.29	126.14	0.001 (NH)	0.001
7	—	128.43	14.94	401.43	182.87	0.001 (NH)	0.001
8	+	198.57	30.13	517.83	262.78	0.001 (NH)	0.01
Amplitude (μV)							
0	+	1.15	0.48	0.77	0.28	—	0.05
1	—	1.76	0.57	1.53	1.46	—	—
2	+	3.46	2.01	12.10	9.46	0.01 (NH)	0.001
3	—	3.39	1.79	23.33	10.63	0.001 (NH)	0.001
4	+	4.46	1.93	27.80	14.46	0.001 (NH)	0.001
5	—	7.74	3.05	32.26	33.65	0.01 (NH)	0.001
6	+	5.52	1.91	30.51	25.96	0.01 (NH)	0.001
7	—	4.49	2.64	18.19	13.54	0.01 (NH)	0.001
8	+	9.05	6.82	13.33	7.79	—	—

Probabilities given where $P \leqslant 0.05$.

(Broughton 1968). With arousal from REM sleep, the VEP pattern reverted more or less directly to that of wakefulness although its amplitude remained smaller for a considerable period of time.

The SEP to single stimuli of the median nerve was similar in wave form in the photosensitive epileptic subjects and in normals, having the same sequence of components. However, later components of the epileptic subjects' SEP had greatly increased latencies[1]. The basic wave form of both was similar to that previously described for normal subjects (Dawson 1954; Goff *et al.* 1962; Giblin 1964; Broughton 1967), to that recorded on the apparently normal somato-sensory exposed cortex (bone reference) of patients undergoing surgery for temporal lobe epilepsy (Broughton 1967), and to scalp recorded cerebral potentials uninfluenced by regional changes in muscle tension, as defined by Cracco and Bickford (1968). Subcutaneous EMG recordings (which in our experience provide a more useful technique to assess participation of myogenic potentials than does forced muscle tension) did not contain a somato-motor response in these relaxed subjects. Finally, one subject had a cortical SEP, as well as a VEP, recorded during a procedure for cerebral biopsy, and it was similar in wave form to the scalp response (Fig. 6). It therefore appears that potentials from muscle or scalp movement were negligible or absent.

The waking SEP of the photosensitive epileptic subjects did show quantitative differences from the normal SEP which were at least as significant as those of the visual potentials. All SEP components (designated sequentially by Arabic numbers) were very widespread (Fig. 8) on the scalp as compared to normals. The C_3 or C_4 component 1 was significantly earlier, 4–8 were later and components 2–7 were much larger than in normals (Table IV, Fig. 9). Component 3, for example, was 8 times larger in amplitude in the epileptic subjects, whereas the greatest difference in the VEP concerned components B and C the C_z electrode which were 3 times larger in the epileptic group.

[1] The reason for this difference was not investigated systematically. It is possible that medication and/or cerebral pathology might be responsible in some cases.

DISCUSSION

Photosensitive epilepsy is accompanied by a number of modifications of the VEP. Component VI at the occipital regions shows significant increases of *both* latency and amplitude. This negative component appears to be homologous to V^b of Gastaut and Régis (1965), who also noted that its amplitude increased during photosensitivity, and to component V of Černáček and Cigánek (1962) who reported that it was increased in all epileptic subjects, photosensitive or not. We cannot support their statement that earlier components are all of smaller amplitude in epileptic subjects: at least in photosensitive epileptic patients, some components are significantly increased. Nor do the findings support those of Ebe *et al.* (1963) or Morocutti *et al.* (1964) who state that *all* components are increased in amplitude in *all* epileptic subjects no matter what type or frequency of seizures is present. Only four components were significantly larger in the photosensitive epileptics.

The spread of certain components of the VEP, especially II and V (or the V–VI–VII complex) to the central region is in keeping with previous clinical (Gastaut 1949; Naquet *et al.* 1960) and experimental (Gastaut and Hunter 1950; Hunter and Ingvar 1955) reports indicating a role for irradiation of the response from the occipital to central motor cortex in the genesis of the photic induced convulsion. The finding that components were sometimes recorded earlier in the central than in the occipital regions (*cf.*, Fig. 3) suggests, but in no way proves, that this irradiation might be occurring also, or even primarily, at subcortical levels.

The VEP differences showing greatest statistical significance between the normal and photosensitive epileptic subjects were, however, found in the midline central region, where the potential was much larger in the latter subjects. The visual system appears to have a separate projection to this area, as is suggested by the different VEP wave form frequently recorded there and by its persistence following abolition of the occipital VEP in cortical blindness (Kooi and Sharbrough 1966). This vertex potential is of similar wave form (at least insofar as components over 100 msec peak latency are concerned) for both somato-sensory and visual stimulation in our own studies and, on the basis of other studies (Susuki and Taguchi 1965; Weitzman and Kremen 1965), possibly also for auditory stimulation. The vertex therefore appears to represent an important area of sensory convergence, perhaps mediated through a human equivalent of the diffuse thalamic projection system described in animal experimentation (Dempsey *et al.* 1941; Morison *et al.* 1941a,b; Jasper 1949).

The threefold amplitude increase in the visual vertex potential might indicate participation of such a multi-modal projection system in photosensitivity. But it might also be explained by a local increase in excitability (responsiveness) of the fronto-central cortex.

The diffuse projection system hypothesis, however, is perhaps further supported by the effects of sleep upon the VEP which were most marked at the C_z electrode. In NREM sleep, photosensitivity diminished and the wave form of the C_z VEP radically altered, suggesting suppression of systems related to this potential and therefore to waking photosensitivity. In REM sleep photosensitivity was minimal and the vertex response was virtually abolished, although the occipital VEP was fairly similar to that of wakefulness.

The finding of ERG *a* wave changes suggests retinal involvement as part of the mechanism of photosensitivity. These changes, however, could simply reflect a secondary phenomenon due to alterations in cen[illegible]fugal retinal control from higher centers.

Thus, multiple levels of "primary" and "unspecific" visual systems appear to be affected. The relative predominance of anterior spread *versus* vertex accentuation (whether related to a diffuse projection system or local cortical changes) in individual VEPs may suggest a differential involvement or a combination of these mechanisms in a single subject which is lost in over-all population statistics. These findings, therefore, indicate the possibility of eventually separating photosensitive epileptic subjects into subgroups.

The studies indicate that, at least for potentials evoked by single stimuli, the main sources of non-cerebral potentials may be estimated, even in photosensitive epileptic subjects with a clinical PMR.

After the preliminary reports (Broughton *et al.* 1966, Ebe *et al.* 1967) of these results, Hishikawa *et al.* (1967) have published a study on the VEP in patients with photosensitive epilepsy. They offer no statistical comparisons with controls, nor do they appear to have attempted to assess non-cerebral potentials or to have examined other sensory modalities. On the whole, however, the two studies are in agreement in regards to the VEP changes.

The finding that the SEP is very markedly altered, even more so than the VEP, suggests that the basic defect of photosensitive epileptic patients is multi-modal (auditory stimulation has not yet been tested in this regard). Such SEP changes are not observed in patients with temporal lobe epilepsy (Broughton 1967), but perhaps are in patients with other forms of epilepsy (Dawson 1947; Halliday 1965).

These multi-modal changes affecting early and later components in man may be compared to fairly similar findings in Metrazol induced photosensitivity in the cat (Gastaut and Hunter 1950; Hunter and Ingvar 1955) or, more recently, in a naturally photosensitive Senegalese baboon, *Papio papio* (Killam *et al.* 1967). The latter, in particular, shows a marked local accentuation of excitability in the fronto-central cortex, a situation which may, as mentioned, also hold true in man.

It is suggested that "photosensitivity" in epileptic patients is usually a diffuse and generalized state of cerebral neuronal hyperexcitability, perhaps based upon a fundamental metabolic (?enzymatic) defect.

SUMMARY

A comparison of the group mean visual evoked potential (VEP), somato-sensory evoked potential (SEP) and electroretinographic (ERG) response was made between photosensitive epileptic subjects and age and sex-matched normal controls.

The VEP of epileptic subjects was similar in wave form but differed significantly in a number of other features from that of normals. In the occipital region, components II, III, VI and VII were of larger amplitude, component VI showed a longer latency; and there was a tendency for the response to spread anteriorly to the central electrode. Midline central (vertex) responses were generally dissimilar in wave form from occipital responses and showed greater differences than did occipital potentials between the two groups, all components being of larger amplitude in photosensitive epileptic subjects. There was evidence also for alteration of the ERG in the form of an earlier *a* wave. The changes indicate participation in photosensitivity of: the retina; visual pathways probably of primary, secondary and associative type; unspecific diffuse projection systems projecting maximally to the vertex; or perhaps local changes of the central cortex.

The possibility of contamination of cerebral responses by ERG, eye and muscle potentials was assessed by various recording techniques and, in two cases, by comparing cortex and scalp responses during diagnostic cerebral biopsy. Differential stages of sleep and states of arousal produced quite stereotyped changes of the VEP.

The SEP was altered even more than the VEP. Individual components showed marked changes in amplitude, latency and distribution, some having mean amplitudes of up to 8 times normal.

It is suggested that "photosensitivity", at least in epilepsy, represents a diffuse multi-modal alteration in cerebral excitability affecting various levels of different sensory systems.

RÉSUMÉ

POTENTIELS ÉVOQUÉS VISUELS, SOMATO-SENSITIFS ET RÉTINIENS DANS L'ÉPILEPSIE PHOTOSENSIBLE

Une comparaison des potentiels évoqués visuels moyens des potentiels évoqués somato-sensitifs et des réponses électrorétinographiques est faite entre des groupes de sujets épileptiques photosensibles et de sujets normaux de contrôle appariés quant à l'âge et au sexe.

La forme des potentiels évoqués visuels des sujets épileptiques est identique à celle des sujets normaux, mais un grand nombre d'autres variables diffèrent de façon significative. Dans la région occipitale, les composantes II, III, VI et VII sont plus amples, la composante VI montre une latence plus grande; la réponse a aussi une tendance à diffuser en avant vers l'électrode centrale. Les réponses centrales au niveau de la ligne médiane (vertex) ont en général une forme différente des réponses occipitales et montrent des variations entre les deux groupes plus grandes que les potentiels occipitaux, toutes les composantes étant de plus grande amplitude chez les sujets épileptiques photosensibles. On note également des signes d'altération de la forme de l'onde *a* précoce de l'électrorétinogramme. Ces modifications indiquent la participation dans la photosensibilité: de la rétine, des voies visuelles probablement de type primaire, secondaire et associatif, des systèmes de projection diffuse non spécifiques projetant au maximum vers le vertex, ou peut-être même des modifications locales du cortex central.

La possibilité de contamination des réponses cérébrales par l'électrorétinogramme, les potentiels oculaires et musculaires, a été vérifiée par différentes techniques d'enregistrement au niveau du scalp et, dans deux cas, en comparant les réponses receuilies au niveau du scalp et du cortex au cours d'une biopsie cérébrale diagnostique. Les différents stades du sommeil et les stades d'éveil produisent des modifications tout à fait stéréotypées des potentiels évoqués visuels.

Les potentiels évoqués somato-sensitifs sont encore plus altérés que les potentiels évoqués visuels. Des composantes individuelles montrent des modifications marquées d'amplitude, de latence et de distribution, certaines ayant des amplitudes moyennes atteignant jusqu'à 8 fois l'amplitude normale.

Les auteurs concluent que la "photosensibilité", au moins dans l'épilepsie, représente une altération diffuse multimodale de l'excitabilité cérébrale affectant à différents niveaux différents systèmes sensoriels.

The patients were kindly referred by Drs. F. Andermann, D. Lloyd-Smith, F. McNaughton and P. Robb. Mr. W. Gibson provided technical assistance and Mr. C. Hodge photographed the illustrations.

REFERENCES

BICKFORD, R. G. Properties of the photomotor response system. *Electroenceph. clin. Neurophysiol.*, **1964**, *17*: 456.

BICKFORD, R. G., SEM-JACOBSEN, C. W., WHITE, P. T. and DALY, D. Some observations on the mechanisms of photic and photometrazol activation. *Electroenceph. clin. Neurophysiol.*, **1952**, *4*: 275–282.

BROUGHTON, R. *Somatosensory evoked potentials in man.* Ph.D. thesis, McGill University, Montreal, **1967**, 302 p.

BROUGHTON, R. Sleep disorders: disorders of arousal? *Science*, **1968**, *159*: 1070–1078.

BROUGHTON, R., MEIER-EWERT, K. and EBE, M. Visual and somato-sensory evoked potentials of photosensitive epileptic subjects during wakefulness, sleep and following i.v. diazepam (Valium). *Electroenceph. clin. Neurophysiol.*, **1966**, *21*: 622.

BROUGHTON, R., MEIER-EWERT, K. and EBE, M. Evoked visual, somatosensory, myogenic, oculogenic and electroretinographic potentials of photosensitive epileptic patients and normal control subjects. *Electroenceph. clin. Neurophysiol.*, **1967**, *23*: 492.

ČERNÁČEK, J. and CIGÁNEK, L. The cortical electroencephalographic response to light stimulation in epilepsy. *Epilepsia (Amst.)*, **1962**, *3*: 303–314.

CIGÁNEK, L. The EEG response (evoked potential) to light stimulus in man. *Electroenceph. clin. Neurophysiol.*, **1961**, *13*: 165–172.

COBB, W. A. and DAWSON, G. D. The latency and form in man of the occipital potentials evoked by bright flashes. *J. Physioi. (Lond.)*, **1960**, *152*: 108–121.

CRACCO, R. Q. and BICKFORD, R. G. Somatomotor and somatosensory evoked responses: median nerve stimulation in man. *Arch. Neurol. (Chic.)*, **1968**, *18*: 52–68.

DAWSON, G. D. Investigations on a patient subject to myoclonic seizures after sensory stimulation. *J. Neurol. Neurosurg. Psychiat.*, **1947**, *10*: 141–162.

DAWSON, G. D. Auto-correlation and automatic integration. *Electroenceph. clin. Neurophysiol.*, **1954**, *Suppl. 4*: 26–37.

DEMENT, W. and KLEITMAN, N. Cyclic variations in EEG during sleep and their relation to eye movements, body motility and dreaming. *Electroenceph. clin. Neurophysiol.*, **1957**, *9*: 673–690.

DEMPSEY, E. W., MORISON, R. S. and MORISON, B. R. Some afferent diencephalic pathways related to cortical potentials in the cat. *Amer. J. Physiol.*, **1941**, *131*: 718–731.

DOMINO, E. F., MATSUOKA, S., WALTZ, J. and COOPER, I. S. Simultaneous recordings of scalp and epidural somatosensory evoked responses in man. *Science*, **1964**, *145*: 1199–1200.

EBE, M., MEIER-EWERT, K. and BROUGHTON, R. Further studies of i.v. diazepam (Valium) and evoked potentials of photosensitive epileptic subjects and normal subjects. *Electroenceph. clin. Neurophysiol.*, **1967**, *23*: 492–493.

EBE, M., MIKAMI, T., AKI, M. and MIYAZAKI, M. Electrical responses evoked by photic stimulation in human cerebral cortex. *Tohoku J. exp. Med.*, **1962**, *77*: 352–372.

EBE, M., MIKAMI, T., ITO, H., AKI, M. and MIYAZAKI, M. Photically evoked potentials (PEPs) in brain disorders. *Tohoku J. exp. Med.*, **1963**, *80*: 323–328.

GASTAUT, H. Effets des stimulations physiques sur l'EEG

de l'homme. *Electroenceph. clin. Neurophysiol.*, **1949,** *Suppl. 2*: 69–82.

GASTAUT, H. and HUNTER, J. An experimental study of the mechanism of photic activation in idiopathic epilepsy. *Electroenceph. clin. Neurophysiol.*, **1950,** *2*: 263–287.

GASTAUT, H. and RÉGIS, H. The visually-evoked potentials recorded transcranially in man. In L. D. PROCTOR and W. R. ADEY (Eds.), *Symposium on the analysis of central nervous system and cardiovascular data using computer methods.* NASA, Washington, D.C., **1965,** *Spec. Publ. 72*: 7–34.

GASTAUT, H. and TASSINARI, C. A. Triggering mechanisms in epilepsy. *Epilepsia (Amst.)*, **1966,** *7*: 85–138.

GIBLIN, D. R. Somatosensory evoked potentials in healthy subjects and in patients with lesions of the nervous system. *Ann. N.Y. Acad. Sci.*, **1964,** *112*: 93–142.

GOFF, W. R., ROSNER, B. S. and ALLISON, T. Distribution of cerebral somatosensory evoked responses in normal man. *Electroenceph. clin. Neurophysiol.*, **1962,** *14*: 697–713.

HALLIDAY, A. M. The incidence of large cerebral evoked responses in myoclonic epilepsy. *Electroenceph. clin. Neurophysiol.*, **1965,** *19*: 102P.

HISHIKAWA, Y., SUMITSUJI, N., MATSUMOTO, K. and KANEKO, Z. H-reflex and EMG of the mental and hyoid muscles during sleep, with special reference to narcolepsy. *Electroenceph. clin. Neurophysiol.*, **1965,** *18*: 487–492.

HISHIKAWA, Y., YAMOMOTO, J., FURUYA, E., YAMADA, Y., MIYAZAKI, K. and KANEKO, Z. Photosensitive epilepsy: relationships between the visual evoked responses and the epileptiform discharges induced by intermittent photic stimulation. *Electroenceph. clin. Neurophysiol.*, **1967,** *23*: 320–334.

HUNTER, J. and INGVAR, D. H. Pathways mediating Metrazol induced irradiation of visual impulses. An experimental study in the cat. *Electroenceph. clin. Neurophysiol.*, **1955,** *7*: 39–60.

JASPER, H. Diffuse projection systems: the integrative action of the thalamic reticular system. *Electroenceph. clin. Neurophysiol.*, **1949,** *1*: 405–420.

KILLAM, K. F., KILLAM, E. K. and NAQUET, R. An animal model of light sensitive epilepsy. *Electroenceph. clin. Neurophysiol.*, **1967,** *22*: 497–513.

KOOI, K. A. and BAGCHI, B. K. Visual evoked responses in man: normative data. *Ann. N.Y. Acad. Sci.*, **1964,** *112*: 254–269.

KOOI, K. A. and SHARBROUGH, III, F. W. Electrophysiological findings in cortical blindness. Report of a case. *Electroenceph. clin. Neurophysiol.*, **1966,** *20*: 260–263.

MEIER-EWERT, K. and BROUGHTON, R. J. Photomyoclonic response of epileptic and non-epileptic subjects during wakefulness, sleep and arousal. *Electroenceph. clin. Neurophysiol.*, **1967,** *23*: 142–151.

MORISON, R. S., DEMPSEY, E. W. and MORISON, B. R. Cortical responses from electrical stimulation of the brain stem. *Amer. J. Physiol.*, **1941**a, *131*: 732–743.

MORISON, R. S., DEMPSEY, E. W. and MORISON, B. R. On the propagation of certain cortical potentials. *Amer. J. Physiol.*, **1941**b, *131*: 744–751.

MOROCUTTI, C., SOMMER-SMITH, J. A. e CREUTZFELDT, O. Studio dei potenziali evocati visivi in soggetti normali ed in soggetti affetti da malattie cerebrali. *Riv. Neurol.*, **1964,** *34*: 57–71.

NAQUET, R., FEGERSTEN, L. and BERT, J. Seizure discharges localized to the posterior cerebral regions in man, provoked by intermittent photic stimulation. *Electroenceph. clin. Neurophysiol.*, **1960,** *12*: 305–316.

RODIN, E. A., DALY, D. D. and BICKFORD, R. G. Effects of photic stimulation during sleep: study of normal subjects and epileptic patients. *Neurology (Minneap.)*, **1955,** *5*: 149–159.

ROSENZWEIG, M. R. and ROSENBLITH, W. A. Responses to auditory stimuli at the cochlea and the auditory cortex. *Psychol. Monogr.*, **1953,** *67*: 1–26.

SUSUKI, T. and TAGUCHI, K. Cerebral evoked response to auditory stimuli in waking man. *Ann. Otol. Rhinol. Laryngol. (St. Louis)*, **1965,** *74*: 128–140.

WEITZMAN, E. D. and KREMEN, H. Auditory evoked responses during different stages of sleep in man. *Electroenceph. clin. Neurophysiol.*, **1965,** *18*: 65–70.

Reference: BROUGHTON, R., MEIER-EWERT, K.-H. and EBE, M. Evoked visual, somato-sensory and retinal potentials in photosensitive epilepsy. *Electroenceph. clin. Neurophysiol.*, **1969,** *27*: 373–386.

EEG SPIKES AND THE AVERAGED EVOKED RESPONSE TO CLICKS AND FLASHES[1]

EDWARD M. ORNITZ, M.D., EDWARD R. RITVO, M.D., PETER E. TANGUAY, M.D. AND RICHARD D. WALTER, M.D.

The Neuropsychiatric Institute, U.C.L.A. Center for the Health Sciences, Los Angeles, Calif. 90024 (U.S.A.)

(Accepted for publication: January 22, 1969)

INTRODUCTION

During the course of studies of the averaged auditory evoked response (AER) during sleep (Ornitz *et al.* 1967a,b; 1968) we have recorded from five children with persistent spontaneous spike activity during their sleep EEGs. One of these children showed an unusual tendency to time-lock the spike discharges to both repetitive clicks and flashes. It is the purpose of this report to present data on the relationship of this spontaneous EEG spike discharge and the averaged evoked response to both auditory and visual stimuli during sleep.

METHODS

Subject. The subject was a 53-month-old boy with moderate mental retardation and a severe developmental delay in speech acquisition. There was a history of dystocia. There was no history of clinical seizures. He received no medication and was studied on 3 nights over a 6 week period.

Stimulation. Single clicks or pairs of clicks were generated by a Grass S4 stimulator using a 1.0 msec pulse duration and were delivered after amplification by a speaker 5 ft above the head of the bed at 80–90 dB above normal adult hearing threshold. Single clicks were presented every 2.2 sec. Pairs of clicks were presented every 2.0 sec with intervals of 500, 400, 320, 250, 200 and 80 msec within each pair. Flashes were generated by a Grass PS-2 Photo-Stimulator and were presented 3 ft from the subject's face.

[1] Supported by Grant No. USPHS-MH-13517, Grant No. USPHS-NB-02808, and the McGregor Fund.

Recording. Auditory and visual evoked responses were recorded from C_z–O_1 and C_z–O_2 on a Grass 16-channel electroencephalograph with filters set at 1–35 c/sec. Additional channels recorded EEG and eye movements for sleep staging.

Data sampling and analysis. There were 477 min of sleep including 5 rapid eye movement (REM) sleep periods recorded on the first night and 190 min and 180 min of sleep on 2 additional nights. Fifty or 100 responses to clicks or flashes were summed with an Enhancetron Model 800 and transcribed on a Mosley XY plotter, using a 2 sec time base. Latencies of waves comprising the response were measured to the peak of the wave and amplitudes were measured from the peak of the preceding wave of opposite polarity.

RESULTS

Spikes occurred bilaterally and synchronously throughout frontal, temporal and central derivations. They did not occur in the waking record, appeared only with drowsiness, persisted only during Stage 2 and 3–4 sleep, and almost completely disappeared during REM sleep. They almost invariably became time-locked to ongoing repetitive single and paired clicks and to flashes (Fig. 1–3). However, flashes or clicks presented at 10 to 20 per sec did not induce seizure discharge activity in the EEG.

When the responses to clicks and flashes were summated, both the averaged auditory evoked response (AER) and visual evoked response (VER) reflected precisely the latency and wave form characteristics of the EEG spike and showed it to be temporally associated with a wave which is identical to wave N_2 of the AER (Fig. 3) (com-

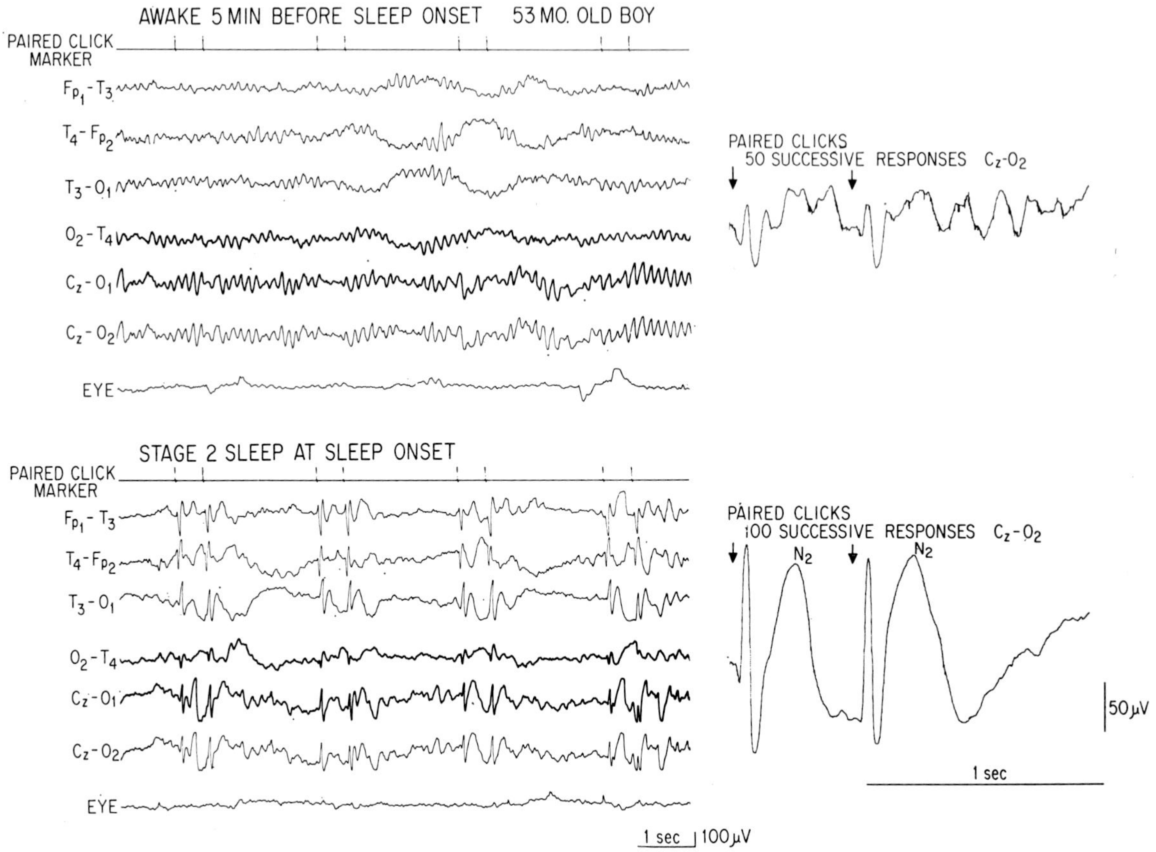

Fig. 1

In the upper left tracing, no random or time-locked spike activity can be seen to occur in the waking EEG. However, the averaged response to the paired clicks (upper right tracing) reveals small peaks (summated spikes) 70 msec after each click. With the onset of sleep, large spikes appear in synchrony with the clicks in the EEG (lower left tracing) and as part of the auditory AER (lower right tracing). In this and subsequent figures, negativity at the vertex is indicated by an upward deflection. The arrows indicate the time that clicks occur.

pare Williams *et al.* 1962; Weitzman and Kremen 1965; Ornitz *et al.* 1967a). The mean latencies of this wave N_2 during Stage 2 sleep (245 msec in response to the first, and 271 msec in response to the second of the paired clicks) were significantly longer than during REM sleep (196 msec and 210 msec) ($P = 0.002$, Mann-Whitney, two-tailed test). The mean amplitudes of wave N_2 during Stage 2 sleep in response to both the first click and the second click were significantly greater than during REM sleep ($P = 0.002$, Mann-Whitney, two-tailed test). There was also a *phasic* inhibition of wave N_2 during the eye movement bursts of REM sleep (Ornitz *et al.* 1967b). Finally, wave N_2 was enhanced at sleep onset (Ornitz *et al.* 1967a).

During Stage 2 sleep, the summated spikes appeared as a sharp wave with a prominent negative peak occurring at about 76 msec in the averaged AER and 78 msec in the averaged VER. This peak virtually disappeared during REM sleep (Fig. 2). In those plots in which small residuals could be measured during REM sleep, the latencies were shorter than during Stage 2. During Stage 3–4 sleep, the paired click interval was reduced by steps from 500 msec to 80 msec and the paired clicks were alternated with single clicks. Spikes were almost always present and

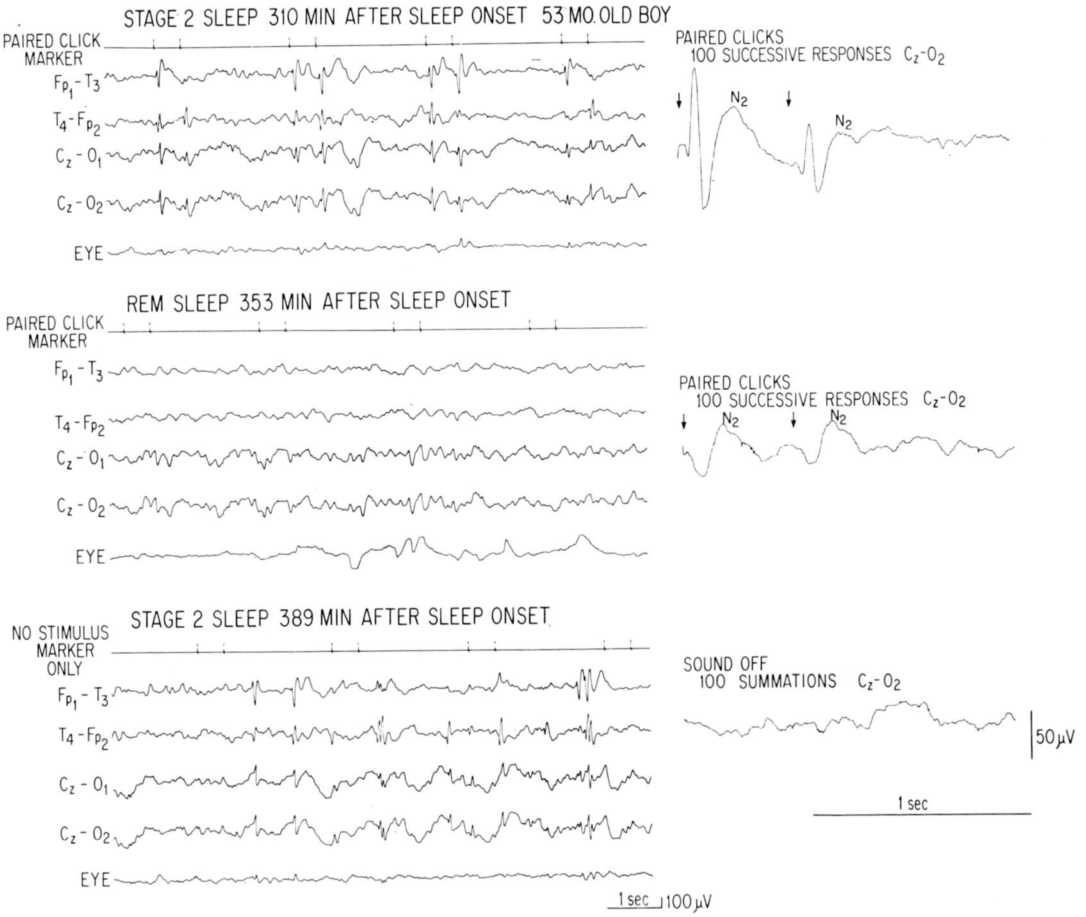

Fig. 2

Spikes time-locked to clicks during Stage 2 sleep (upper left tracing) disappear during REM sleep (middle left tracing) and occur randomly and in short bursts in the EEG when sound is turned off during Stage 2 sleep (lower left tracing). These events are reflected in the averaged AERs which also show the depression of wave N_2 during REM sleep in this case (right middle tracing).

time-locked in the EEG to both clicks of the pair at 500 msec and 400 msec intra-pair intervals. At 320 msec, a spike only occasionally occurred in the EEG in response to the second click. At 250 msec, EEG spikes never occurred in response to the second click. These findings were paralleled by the recovery cycle of the summated spike in the averaged AER. At 500 msec and 400 msec, a summated spike was always present in response to the second click. At 320 msec, it could only be demonstrated by subtraction of the averaged response to the single click from the response to the paired click. At 250 msec, there was no response at the latency of the summated spike to the second click. It was also observed that wave N_2 in the averaged AER had the identical recovery cycle to that of the summated spike; *i.e.*, it did not occur in response to the second click at intra-pair intervals less than 320 msec.

Thus, the latency characteristics of these summated spikes, their recovery cycle and their temporal association with wave N_2 of both the averaged AER and VER suggest that they are the equivalent of wave N_1 of the AER as seen in adults. While wave N_1 is not commonly observed in younger children (Ornitz *et al.* 1967b), Fig. 4 illustrates the presence of this wave in

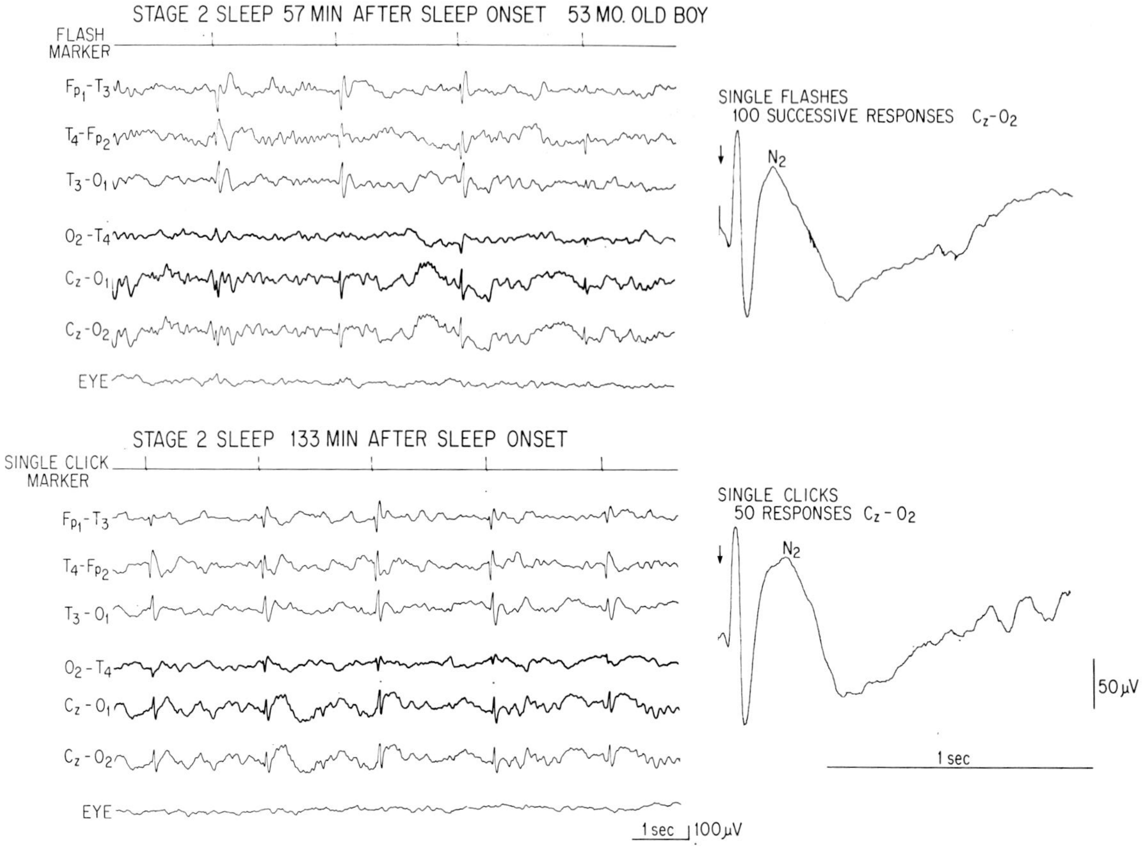

Fig. 3

Spikes in EEG occur synchronously with either flashes (upper left tracing) or clicks (lower left tracing). Averaged VER and AER on right reveal almost identical spike summations at 70 msec latency in association with wave N_2 which occurs earlier in response to flashes than to clicks.

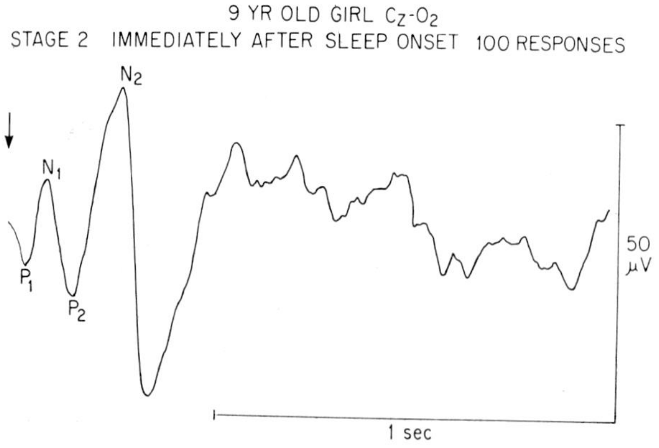

Fig. 4

Averaged AER in an older normal child. Compare latency and wave form characteristics of wave N_1 to summated time-locked spike activity in averaged AERs from subject in Fig. 1–3.

an older child to demonstrate the similarity of wave N_1 to the summated spikes.

DISCUSSION

The observations in this unusual subject demonstrate striking similarities between the spontaneously appearing spiking activity during sleep and the N_1 wave of the averaged AER as seen in older subjects. These similarities include latency, wave form, recovery cycle, alterations induced by the level of sleep, and association with wave N_2. At least in this case then, it could be assumed that the same physiological pathway responsible for an evoked response was also participating in the bilaterally synchronous spike discharge. This abnormality showed a remarkable response to afferent stimulation over both the auditory and visual pathway, yet the patient did not exhibit the classical photoconvulsive response in the waking state.

Though it would appear that in this case a common mechanism exists between the AER and the spontaneous spike, there are no data that might be used to explain the apparent spontaneously occurring nature of the spiking discharge without the presence of external stimuli. It is tempting, however, to view this phenomenon as a special example of the type of recruiting response mediated by multiple sensory modalities.

We are not aware of any previous report of a case in which spontaneously occurring spikes have become time-locked to auditory stimuli and participated in averaged AER formation. Morocutti *et al.* (1966) have reported this phenomenon in response to visual stimuli.

SUMMARY

Spontaneous bilaterally and synchronously occurring spike activity was activated by sleep in a young child and showed the unusual tendency to become time-locked to both clicks and flashes. Averaging of the auditory and visual evoked responses demonstrated that the summated spikes were equivalent to wave N_1 of the averaged evoked response. This finding is tentatively interpreted as a type of recruiting response mediated by sensory modalities that utilize mechanisms common to that of this type of spike discharge.

RÉSUMÉ

POINTES EEG ET RÉPONSES ÉVOQUÉES MOYENNES AUX CLICKS ET AUX ÉCLAIRS

Une activité de pointes survenant spontanément de façon symétrique, bilatérale et synchrone est activée par le sommeil chez un jeune enfant et montre une tendance inhabituelle à l'accrochage temporel avec à la fois les clicks et les éclairs. Le moyennage des réponses évoquées auditives et visuelles montre que les pointes sommées correspondent à l'onde N_1 de la réponse évoquée moyenne. Cette donnée est interprétée à titre d'hypothèse comme un type de réponse par recrutement, induit par les modalités sensorielles qui utilisent des mécanismes communs à ceux de ce type de décharge de pointe.

The authors are grateful for the technical assistance of Miss A. Mason and Mr. G. Low. H. Okada and R. Hicks developed the stimulator control unit.

REFERENCES

MOROCUTTI, C., SOMMER-SMITH, J. A. und CREUTZFELDT, O. Das visuelle Reaktionspotential bei normalen Versuchspersonen und charakteristische Veränderungen bei Epileptikern. *Arch. Psychiat. Nervenkr.*, **1966**, *208*: 234–254.

ORNITZ, E. M., RITVO, E. R., CARR, E. M., LAFRANCHI, S. and WALTER, R. D. The effect of sleep onset on the auditory averaged evoked response. *Electroenceph. clin. Neurophysiol.*, **1967a**, *23*: 335–341.

ORNITZ, E. M., RITVO, E. R., CARR, E. M., PANMAN, L. M. and WALTER, R. D. The variability of the auditory averaged evoked response during sleep and dreaming in children and adults. *Electroenceph. clin. Neurophysiol.*, **1967b**, *22*: 514–524.

ORNITZ, E. M., RITVO, E. R., PANMAN, L. M., LEE, Y. H., CARR, E. M. and WALTER, R. D. The auditory evoked response in normal and autistic children during sleep. *Electroenceph. clin. Neurophysiol.*, **1968**, *25*: 221–230.

WEITZMAN, E. D. and KREMEN, H. Auditory evoked responses during different stages of sleep in man. *Electroenceph. clin. Neurophysiol.*, **1965**, *18*: 65–70.

WILLIAMS, H. L., TEPAS, D. I. and MORLOCK, H. C. Evoked responses to clicks and electroencephalographic stages of sleep in man. *Science*, **1962**, *138*: 685–686.

Reference: ORNITZ, E. M., RITVO, E. R., TANGUAY, P. E. and WALTER, R. D. EEG spikes and the averaged evoked response to clicks and flashes. *Electroenceph. clin. Neurophysiol.*, **1969**, *27*: 387–391.

Electroencephalography and Clinical Neurophysiology
Elsevier Publishing Company, Amsterdam – Printed in The Netherlands

AN ANALYSIS OF THE EFFECT OF 1,2-DIHYDROXYBENZENE ON TRANSMISSION THROUGH THE DORSAL COLUMN SENSORY PATHWAY

A. ANGEL[1]

Department of Physiology, University College London, and the Department of Experimental Neurology, Institute of Psychiatry, London, S.E. 5 (Great Britain)

(Accepted for publication: January 24, 1969)

During his studies of the effects of polyhydroxylic phenols on the nictitating membrane of the cat Bacq (1936) noted that some of these chemicals would cause convulsions. One of the chemicals used by Bacq, 1,2-dihydroxybenzene (catechol), has been injected into anaesthetized rats, rabbits, cats and monkeys. In all these animals two effects have been observed. With small doses, or before the full effect of a larger dose had developed, the animals would give a single brief jerk, or a short group of brief jerks, in response to a sensory stimulus. The type of stimulus used was not critical, it could be a tap on the table on which the animal was resting, or a short electrical stimulus to a limb. When larger doses of catechol were given the animal passed through a phase of convulsive jerking which lasted for several minutes. In this state the jerks occurred without any added sensory stimulation.

One component of the complex muscular response to a sensory stimulus has been shown to be dependent on the integrity of the sensorimotor cortex (Angel *et al.* 1969). It was decided, therefore, to see whether catechol had any effect on the centripetal sensory volley conducted through the dorsal column sensory pathway.

The investigations in this paper, which have been reported in abstract elsewhere (Angel and Dawson 1964), show that, during the jerky state produced by catechol, the cortical responses to sensory stimulation are enlarged and that this enlargement is associated with increased transmission in the sensory pathway through the thalamus.

[1] M.R.C. Research Assistant. Present address: Department of Physiology, The University, Sheffield 10.

METHODS

Preparation

The majority of these experiments were made on albino rats, although rabbits (10), monkeys (4) and cats (4) have also been used. The animals were anaesthetized with urethane administered intraperitoneally, with the exception of the cats which were anaesthetized with Nembutal (Abbott). No premedication was used. The depth of anaesthesia was adjusted so as just to abolish reflex withdrawal of a hind leg when it was pinched firmly. This level was reached with a dose of urethane of 1.3–1.5 g/kg of body weight. Access to the primary cortical receiving area and the ventro-basal thalamus was allowed by an extensive craniotomy, usually on the left side. The dura was reflected. The animal was then mounted in a specially constructed stand. The head was held by a plug in each auditory meatus and by a bar underneath the hard palate behind the incisor teeth. The borders of the skin incision over the cranium were gripped between an inner perspex ring and an outer metal clip; the pool so formed over the cerebral cortex was filled with liquid paraffin (equilibrated with physiological saline) at a temperature of 37° C. To expose the cuneate nucleus the neck muscles were reflected and the arch of the atlas and the posterior margin of the skull overlying the cerebellum were removed. The cerebellum was always left intact. A steel pin was placed transversely deep to the attachment of the back muscles and the dorsal part of the sacrum. The animal was then stretched between the ear plugs and the steel pin, with its body suspended in the air. This arrangement was found to reduce considerably movement of the medulla caused by the animal's respiration, and also by the jerkings.

Recording

Recordings from the ventro-basal thalamus and medulla, of the electrical responses to a peripheral stimulus, were made with a glass micro-pipette, having an outside diameter at the tip of 2–5 μ, filled with a 3 *M* sodium chloride solution with a resistance between 1 and 4 MΩ. It was connected to a cathode follower and through an RC amplifier to a cathode ray oscillograph. The frequency response characteristic of the system was flat from 50 c/sec to 3 kc/sec, falling by 5 dB at 10 c/sec and 9 dB at 10 kc/sec. Records from the cerebral cortex were made through fine silver wires, fused at their tips into small balls, and connected to a similar RC amplifier.

The electrical stimuli applied to the limbs were rectangular pulses of 0.1 msec duration. They were applied through a 1:1 isolating transformer to small strips of lint soaked in 3 *M* NaCl solution, one wrapped round the wrist (−ve) and the other round a digit (+ve). To stimulate the white matter underneath the primary cortical receiving area a micro-pipette was used, having a tip diameter of 2–5 μ and filled with 3 *M* NaCl. The pipette was made the negative electrode, the positive one being a lint pad soaked in concentrated NaCl solution and wrapped round the left wrist. Timing of the stimuli was controlled from a digital timing device (Pitman 1958).

Catechol was dissolved in saline (10 mg/ml) at 37° C, stored under oil to prevent oxidation and administered intravenously via a polythene cannula inserted into the left saphenous vein, or the left short saphenous vein. Averaged responses were obtained in either of two ways: (a) in a number of separate records of responses three ordinates per msec were measured and the average obtained by hand, or (b) the sum of a number of responses was obtained from a

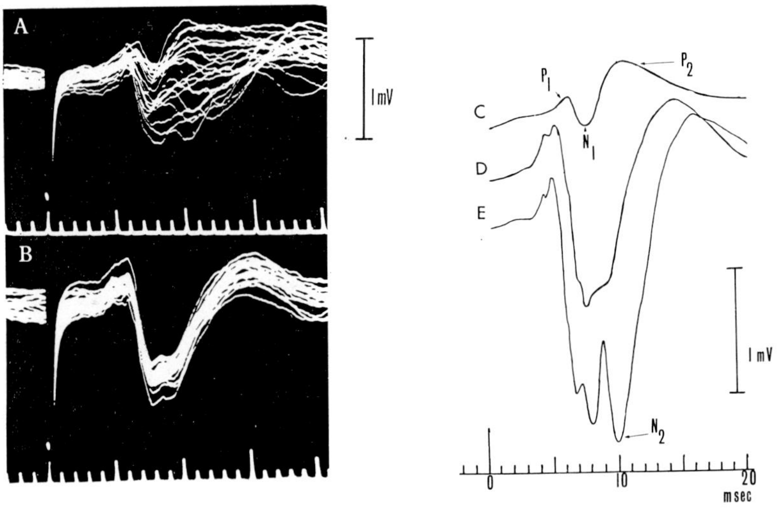

Fig. 1

Responses from the left somato-sensory cortex to stimulation of the right forepaw at a rate of 2/sec in a rat anaesthetized with urethane. Twenty superimposed responses before (*A*) and 55–65 sec after (*B*) i.v. injection of 4 mg/kg of catechol. Time scale 1 and 5 msec intervals. Twenty responses averaged before (*C*) and 1 min after (*D*) the injection of catechol. *E*: The forepaw stimulus was applied 500 msec after the start of a train of shocks (34 in number, with a 3 msec separation) had been applied to the left hind leg before catechol. The averages were obtained by measuring individual records. P_1 and P_2 = first and second positive waves. N_1 and N_2 = first and second negative waves. Stimulus at 0 msec. Positivity under the active electrodes is shown as an upward deflexion in this and subsequent figures.

Mnemotron computer of average transients type CAT 400B.

RESULTS

Cortical responses

All records from the cortex in response to electrical stimulation of the forefoot were made from an area which gave the shortest latency responses (Angel 1962, 1967). At the depth of anaesthesia used the potentials recorded from the primary somatic cortical receiving area were not constant in size, shape and latency but varied considerably (Fig. 1, *A*). For descriptive purposes the cortical potential can be divided into three components, a first positive wave (P_1, Fig. 1, *C*), a second positive wave (P_2, Fig. 1, *C*) and between these two a first negative wave (N_1, Fig. 1, *C*). Fig. 1, *C* shows the average of 20 responses recorded from the cortex in a rat, after stimulation of the forefoot. It can be seen that the latency to the start of the first positive wave (P_1) was 4.9 msec and that it reached its peak 6.5 msec after the stimulus. After this peak there was a small negative wave (N_1) followed by a second positive wave (P_2) with a latency to its peak of 11 msec. A small amount of catechol, injected intravenously, increased the sizes and rates of change of the first positive and first negative waves of the cortical response to a subsequently applied test stimulus (Fig. 1, *D*), decreased their latencies and also made the responses more stereotyped (Fig. 1, *B*).

The duration of the effect of a single injection of catechol depended both upon the amount given and the route of administration. With the intravenous route and using small doses (4–8 mg/kg) the effect lasted for approximately 10 min, whereas with intraperitoneal injection much larger doses were necessary (20–100 mg/kg) and the effect lasted for a much longer time; 20–60 min. With small intravenous doses the first sign of an alteration of the cortical response to peripheral stimulation was seen 5–10 sec (Fig. 8) after the start of the injection. The peak effect was seen 30–45 sec after the beginning of an injection. From 1 to 5 min there was a rather rapid decline towards the resting level after which, from 5 to 10 min, the responses slowly returned to the pre-injection level. Fig. 2,*b* shows the effects on the size of the first negative wave

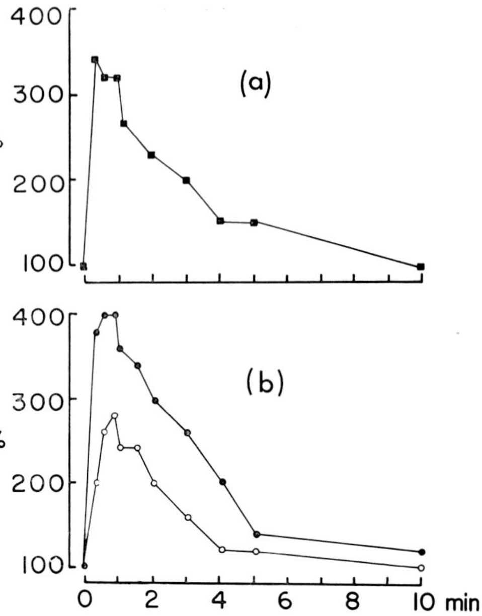

Fig. 2

Shows the mean percentage change in respiratory rate (*a*) and percentage size of the first negative wave of 20 consecutive cortical responses to forepaw stimulation (*b*) at various times after the i.v. injection of catechol in a rat deeply anaesthetized with urethane. (*a*) 4 mg/kg, (*b*) 4 mg/kg (○—— ○) and 8 mg/kg (●—— ●) of catechol.

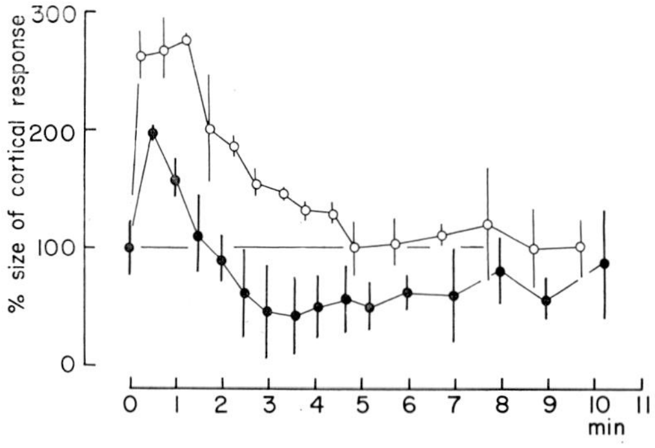

Fig. 3

The effect on the percentage size of the first negative wave of the cortical response to peripheral stimulation (○—— ○) and to stimulation of the white matter underlying the primary somatic receiving area (●—— ●) at various times after the i.v. injection of 4 mg/kg of catechol. The stimuli were adjusted so that the mean sizes of the cortical responses were the same before the injection. The stimuli were alternated during the experiment and each point is the mean response to 20 consecutive stimuli. The vertical bar through each point indicates the scatter of the responses.

of the cortical potential of two different doses of catechol, administered intravenously. Since the responses to peripheral stimulation were not usually stable, to obtain meaningful results it was necessary to superimpose a number of responses. The rate of stimulation was 2/sec; it has been shown that the short latency components of the cortical response will follow this rate (Angel 1963, 1967) without alteration. Each record consisted of 20 superimposed traces, and therefore showed the evoked responses sampled over a 10 sec period. Hence the points of the graphs in Fig. 2, *b* represent not only the average size of the first negative wave of the cortical response but also the average time at which the observation was made.

The change seen in the evoked cortical potential after catechol was very similar to that seen when a testing stimulus was applied after a train of stimuli had been applied to any part of the body surface (Angel and Dawson 1963) in

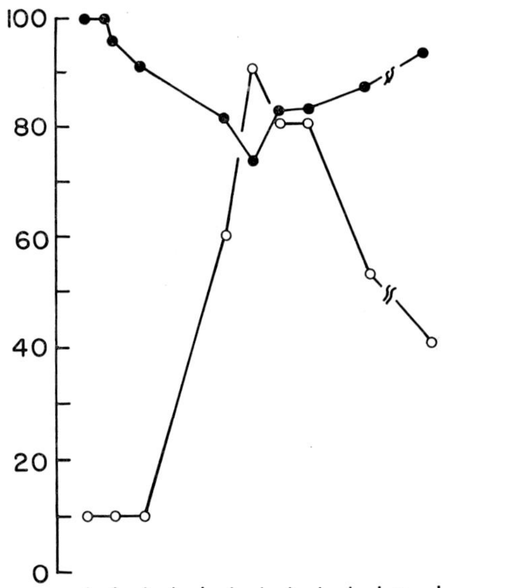

Fig. 4

The effect of an intraperitoneal injection of 20 mg/kg of catechol on the sizes of the post-synaptic cuneate response (●——●) and the first negative wave of the cortical response (○——○) in a rat deeply anaesthetized with urethane. The ordinate shows the percentage size of the cuneate response, and the relative size of the cortical response, at various times after the injection (abscissa). Each point is the mean of 20 responses.

that the first negative wave increased in size. One major difference, however, was that the later negative wave (N_2, Fig. 1, *E*), usually seen after strong peripheral stimulation, appeared to be absent from the responses after catechol. The same effect was seen when rabbits, cats or monkeys were used.

The increase in the size of the cortical response after catechol could be due either to an increased responsiveness of the cortex to an unchanged afferent volley or to an increase, somewhere along the dorsal column sensory pathway, in the size of the corticopetal volley.

Cortical responsiveness

The cortical responses to stimulation of the periphery and to stimulation of the white matter underlying the cortex have been compared. This procedure has been shown to produce responses closely similar in shape and timing of their various components (Angel 1967). These comparisons have been made at various times after the intravenous administration of catechol. In these experiments the stimulus intensity was adjusted so that the amplitude of the first negative wave was equal to that produced by peripheral stimulation. The cortical responses to stimulation of the white matter were enhanced for the first 1–1.5 min after an injection of catechol and were thereafter unaffected or reduced in size for 10 min or more, depending upon the given dose. Fig. 3 is a graphical illustration of one such experiment in which peripheral and white matter stimulation were alternately applied. The responses to peripheral stimulation showed, on the other hand, an increase in the size of the response for 4–5 min after the injection.

Therefore, an increase in the cortical responsiveness alone will only account for the initial effect of catechol. If the later effect is due to an increase in the size of the corticopetal volley then the question arises of where in the dorsal column sensory pathway any modification of responsiveness occurs.

Responses from peripheral nerves

Records were made from the sciatic trunk in response to stimulation of the hind foot and from the medial, ulnar and radial nerves in response to stimulation of the forelimb. No change at all could be detected in the size and synchrony of the ascending volley after a peripheral stimulus when catechol was injected intravenously in a dose sufficient to cause a large increase in the cortical response recorded at the same time.

Responses from the cuneate nucleus

When the responses from the cuneate nucleus were compared before and after the administration of catechol it was found that, in the majority of experiments, the size of the mass response to a peripheral test stimulus was unaffected by the injection of catechol. In a few experiments, however, the injection of catechol caused a decrease in this response, although at the same time the cortical response was increased in size. Fig. 4 shows, in graphical form, the size of the cuneate post-synaptic mass response and the size of the first negative wave of the cortical response after the intraperitoneal injection of catechol (20 mg/kg). Six minutes after the injection the first negative wave of the cortical response was increased to 9 times its pre-injection amplitude and the cuneate response was reduced to 73% of its pre-injection level. No change in the synchrony or latency of the post-synaptic cuneate response was seen.

Ventro-basal thalamic responses

The part of the thalamus from which short

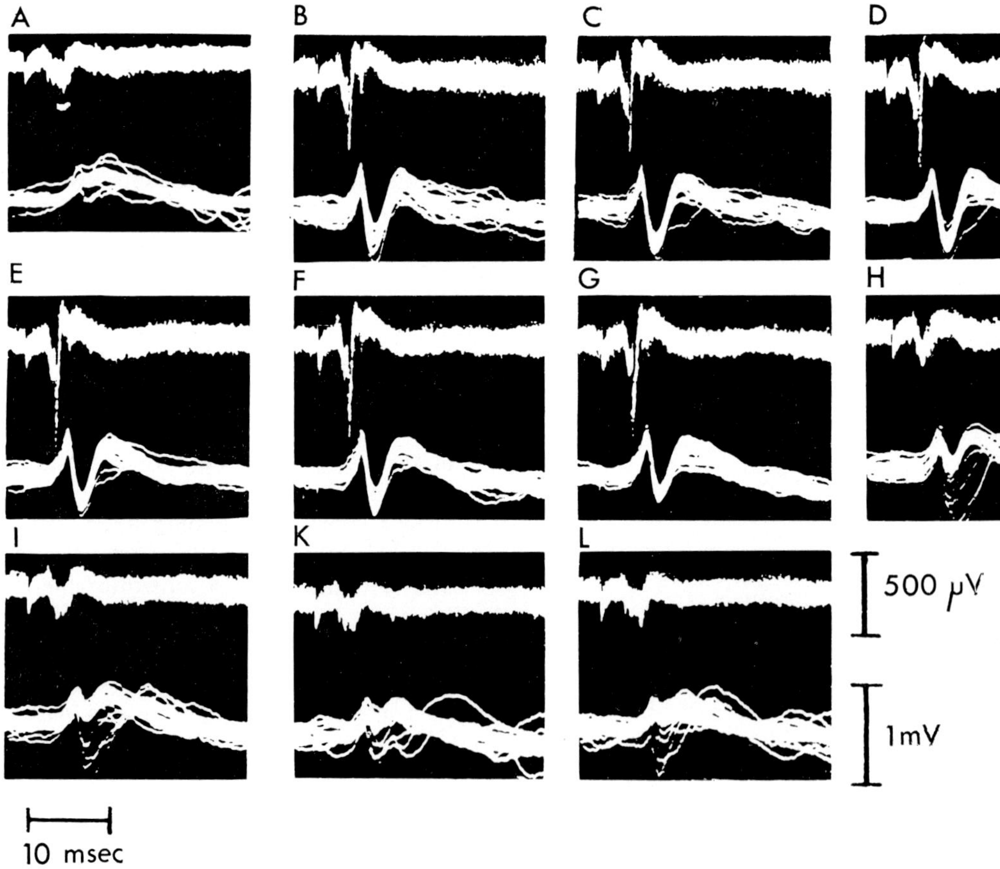

Fig. 5

Each record shows 20 superimposed responses from the left thalamus (top) and left cortex (bottom) to stimulation of the right forepaw at a rate of 2/sec in a rat deeply anaesthetized with urethane, before and at various mean times after an i.v. injection of 4 mg/kg of catechol. *A*: before; *B*: 15 sec; *C*: 30 sec; *D*: 45 sec; *E*: 60 sec; *F*: 90 sec; *G*: 2 min; *H*: 3 min; *I*: 4 min; *K*: 5 min; *L*: 10 min.

latency responses are obtained to stimulation of localized portions of the contralateral body surface has been shown to be the *nucleus ventralis thalami* (Angel and Dawson 1963) (terminology from de Groot 1959) which is analogous in its anatomical location and physiological properties to that region in the rabbit and cat called the ventro-basal thalamus by Rose and Mountcastle (1952). The effect of catechol in the rat was always to increase the size of the thalamic mass response to stimulation of the periphery, and to decrease the latency of the thalamic and cortical responses. Fig. 5 shows the records from one experiment illustrating the changes in the thalamic mass response to peripheral stimuli at various times after the intravenous administration of catechol. Each record is the response to 20 successive stimuli with the individual responses superimposed. The increase in the thalamic mass response lags slightly behind that of the cortical response.

This lag is clearly shown in Fig. 6, in which the percentage sizes of the thalamic mass response and the first negative wave of the cortical response have been plotted at various times after the intravenous injection of an 8 mg/kg dose of catechol. When the response to peripheral stimulation of individual thalamic neurones was studied it was seen that after the administration of catechol the probability of the unit responding was increased and the earliest latency of discharge together with its scatter were decreased. For example, one unit discharged from 5.7 to 8.3 msec after a peripheral stimulus, firing 7 times out of 20 trials in the resting state. One minute after the intravenous injection of catechol (4 mg/kg) the neurone responded 15 times in 20 trials and the latency of discharge was from 4.8 to 6.3 msec.

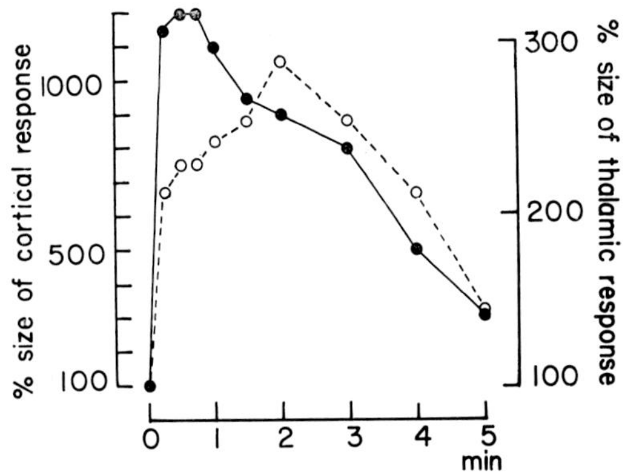

Fig. 6

The sizes, expressed as percentages of the control values, of the thalamic (○--- ○) and cortical (●——●) responses in a rat at various times after the i.v. injection of 8 mg/kg of catechol. Each point is the mean of 20 consecutive responses obtained over a 10 sec period.

Spontaneous cortical activity

The effect of catechol on the spontaneous cortical activity was to change it from a pattern of high voltage low frequency waves to low voltage high frequency waves. An example is shown in Fig. 7. The records were taken from a cat moderately deeply anaesthetized with Nembutal. The EEG (recorded from brass screw electrodes in the skull, one over the sensory cortex the other further back over the occipital cortex) was showing frequent spindle bursts before the injection of catechol. Six to 7 sec after the start of the intravenous injection of catechol (10 mg/kg) very fast waves with a low voltage appeared in the EEG. These fast waves were fully developed 12–15 sec after the start of the injection (Fig. 7, *d*), at which time the animal started to jerk spontaneously as well as to applied tactile stimuli. Three minutes after the injection (Fig. 7, *e*) small spindle bursts began to appear and occasionally could develop into larger spindles. Thirteen minutes (Fig. 7, *f*) after this injection the EEG showed spindling activity at intervals approximately the same as those seen before the injection (Fig. 7, *a* and *f*).

In rats anaesthetized with urethane so that a small reflex withdrawal of the hind paw was just obtainable to a strong pinch, the animals showed signs of behavioural arousal, *i.e.*, feeble movements of the head and trunk after catechol.

Thus far it has been shown that catechol exerts its effect by initially increasing the responsiveness of the sensory cortex to ascending volleys. This is immediately followed by a phase of increased responsiveness of cells in the ventro-basal thalamus. How these two effects are brought about remains to be answered.

Effects of catechol on the thalamic reticular nuclei

An attempt has been made to determine how

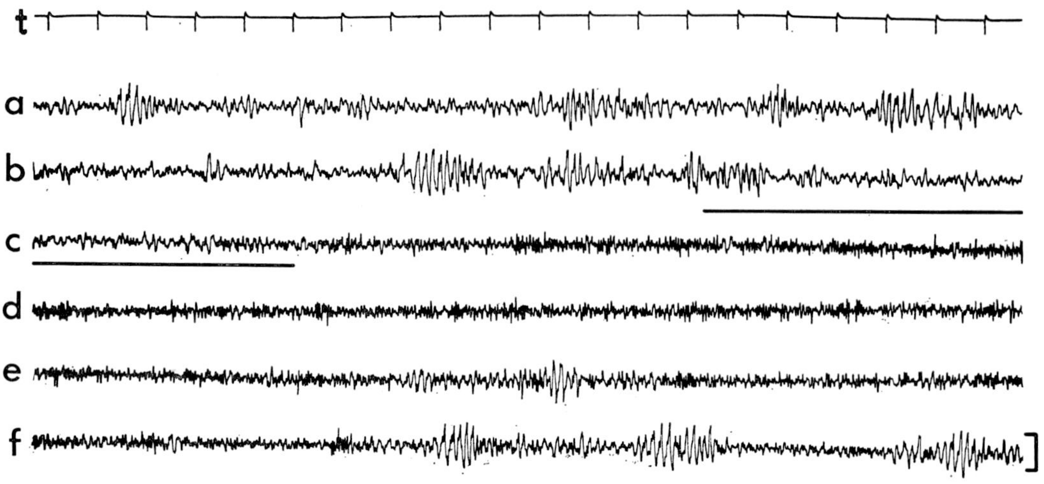

Fig. 7
Records of the spontaneous cortical activity recorded from bipolar sensory-occipital leads in a cat deeply anaesthetized with sodium hexobarbitone, (*a*) before, (*b* and *c*) during, (*d*) immediately after (records *a–d* are consecutive), (*e*) 3 min after and (*f*) 13 min after the i.v. injection of 10 mg/kg of catechol. The horizontal line indicates the duration of the injection. Calibrations: 100 μV and 1 sec (*t*).

an intravenous injection of catechol can increase the responsiveness of cells in the ventro-basal thalamus. It has been reported (Angel 1964) that there is a direct relationship between the discharge frequency of cells situated in the nucleus ventralis pars dorsomedialis and the nucleus reticularis thalami (terminology from de Groot 1959), and the responsiveness of the ventro-basal thalamus. Therefore, records were made from these thalamic reticular cells to determine whether their discharge frequency showed the same changes after an injection of catechol as they do to strong peripheral stimulation. This latter procedure has been shown to increase the responsiveness of the ventro-basal thalamus to an ascending volley (Angel and Dawson 1963). Qualitatively, catechol was found to have the same effect on the discharge frequency of the thalamic reticular cells as strong peripheral stimuli, *i.e.*, cells which in the absence of any intentional stimulus had a low "resting" discharge frequency showed an increase in frequency, and those having a high "resting" discharge showed a decrease in frequency. Difficulty was experienced in keeping the cells under observation for long periods of time since the concomitant incraese in the animal's respiratory effort after the injection of catechol caused movement of the brain and usually the cell became damaged. In two experiments, however, one cell of each type was studied for periods of 10–20 min. Records were obtained of the discharge before, during and after an injection of catechol and the discharge was correlated with the change in the cortical responses seen at the same time. These results have been plotted in Fig. 8 and 9. It can be seen from the graphs that the change in frequency of discharge and the increase in the size of the cortical potentials ran very similar time courses.

In these experiments no change in the amplitude of either the cortical, thalamic or cuneate responses or in the frequency of discharge of the reticular cells was observed after the injection of saline alone.

Effect of catechol on respiration

Catechol was also found to increase the respiratory rate and this change showed the same time course as that of the cortical responses (Fig. 2, *a*). Three groups of experiments were performed to determine whether the cortical changes could be consequent on either: (i) the increased sensory inflow; (ii) any change in the alveolar pCO_2 due to the increased respiratory

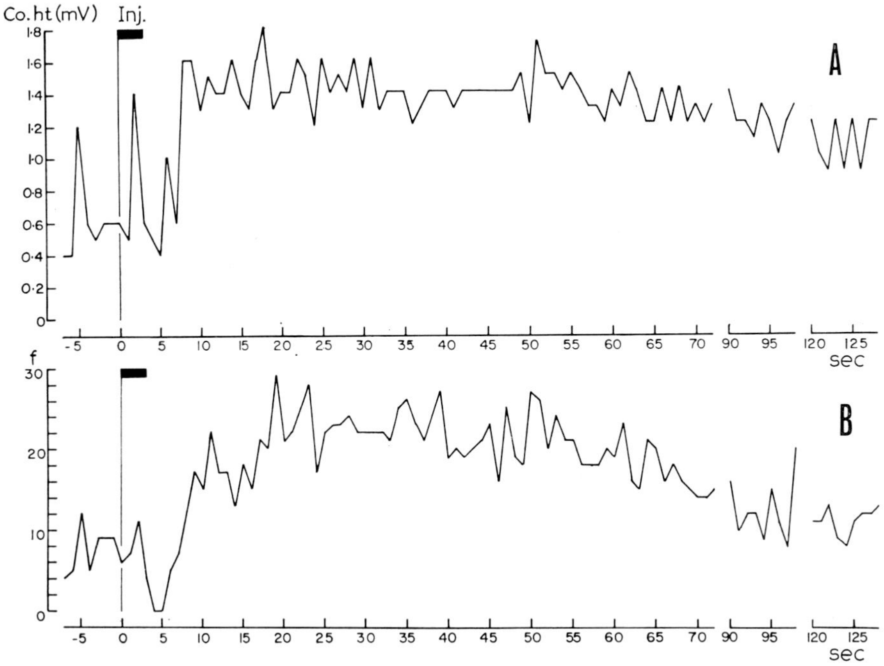

Fig. 8
The size of the cortical response to each peripheral stimulus (*A*) and the frequency of discharge of a cell from the nucleus reticularis thalami (*B*) after an i.v. injection of 4 mg/kg of catechol in a rat deeply anaesthetized with urethane. The horizontal bar indicates the duration of the injection.

effort; or (iii) any change in the oxygen carrying capacity of the blood, since polyhydroxyphenols such as catechol are reducing agents. (i) In the first group of experiments animals breathing room air were suddenly switched onto a 95% O_2, 5% CO_2 gas mixture to stimulate respiration. No maintained changes in the cortical response to a peripheral stimulus were seen as a consequence of this manoeuvre. (ii) The effect of an intravenous injection of catechol was then examined in animals first breathing room air and then the gas mixture. The effect of catechol was found to be similar in the two cases, with the exception that in animals breathing increased CO_2 the initial effect of catechol on the cortical responses was even slightly increased, certainly not diminished. (iii) The slight increase in the effect of catechol in animals breathing the gas mixture may perhaps indicate that sufficient oxygen is carried in solution in the plasma to counteract any loss of O_2 carrying capacity. These experiments showed that if the alveolar pCO_2 was artificially kept high then the effect

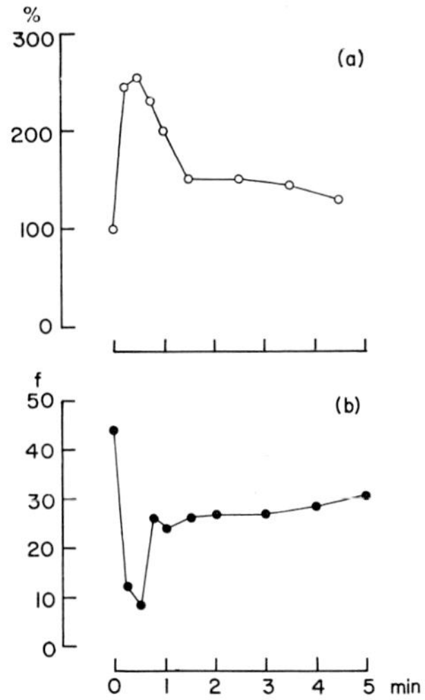

Fig. 9
The mean percentage size of the first negative wave of the cortical response to 20 consecutive stimuli (*a*) and the mean frequency of discharge (obtained during the stimulation period) of another cell from the nucleus reticularis thalami (*b*), in an animal anaesthetized with urethane after an i.v. injection of 4 mg/kg of catechol.

of catechol was unaltered. This indicates that any reduction in the alveolar pCO_2 due to hyperventilation caused by catechol would be ineffective in causing the increase in the cortical response to peripheral stimulation. To confirm this point, experiments were performed on rabbits to see if hyperpnoea, and hence a decrease in the alveolar pCO_2, had any effect on the cortical potentials evoked by a peripheral stimulus. The results shown in Fig. 10 are from one such experiment. Each trace is the sum of the cortical responses to 20 peripheral stimuli at various times before (Fig. 10, *A*) and during (Fig. 10, *B*) a period of artificial overventilation with a pump, sufficient to cause apnoea for 1–1.5 min when the animal was suddenly switched from the pump to its normal respiration. It was found that after an initial increase in the slope of the first positive and first negative waves of the cortical response, with a slight reduction in the latency, there was a gradual decrease in size of the early components and increase in the response latency. The first negative wave was reduced relatively much more than the first positive wave. This decrease in the size of the early components was maintained during the period the animal was overventilated and persisted during the period of apnoea. The size returned to normal when the animal's respiratory efforts returned to normal. In this experiment a transistory increase in the first positive wave of the average cortical response was seen when the animal was made to hyperventilate by increasing its dead space (Fig. 10, *C*). The response returned to normal within 40–60 sec after the dead space was increased and remained at its normal level.

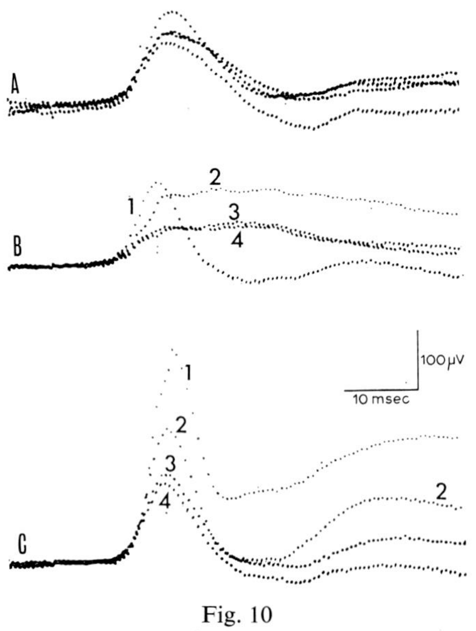

Fig. 10
The summed responses (CAT 400B computer) of 4 groups of 20 consecutive cortical responses to forepaw stimulation at a rate of 1/sec (in a rabbit deeply anaesthetized with urethane). *A*: The "normal" animal. *B*: At various times after the commencement of forced hyperventilation: (1) 0–20 sec; (2) 20–40 sec; (3) 40–60 sec; (4) 60–80 sec. *C*: At various times after increasing the animal's dead space by approximately 4 ml: (1) 0–20 sec; (2) 20–40 sec; (3) 40–60 sec; (4) 60–80 sec.

DISCUSSION

In anaesthetized animals, the increase in the cortical response is due to two factors; there is a small short lasting increase in the cortical responsiveness itself, and a large, long lasting increase in the responsiveness of the ventrobasal thalamus. Two lines of evidence are available from the present experiments to support this. First, the increase in the size of the thalamic responses lags slightly behind that of the cortical response (Fig. 6). Second, if the cortical responsiveness was tested directly by stimulating the underlying white matter, a transient increase in the responsiveness was seen (Fig. 3).

This transitory increase in the cortical responsiveness appears to occur as a consequence of the hyperpnoea produced by the injection of catechol, since in rabbits it was found that the initial effect of hyperventilation was an increase in the size of the early components of the cortical response (Fig. 10, *B*) to peripheral stimulation. The prolonged decrease in cortical responsiveness after the injection of catechol would appear to be due to the same cause since this transient increase was followed by a period of decreased responses (Fig. 10, *B*). This phase of reduction persisted for as long as hyperventilation was continued and during any period of apnoea at the cessation of hyperventilation. The cortical responses only recovered at the same time as the animal's respiratory effort returned to normal.

The increased thalamic responses after catechol were not due to any increase in the volley arriving at the thalamus since the responses from the cuneate nucleus were either unchanged (in the majority of experiments), or were decreased in amplitude. The temporal pattern of the cuneate response was never altered. Therefore, catechol has the property of increasing transmission through the thalamus. It was shown previously (Angel 1964) that the increased thalamic responses after a strong peripheral stimulus were accompanied by changes in the frequency of discharge of cells located in the nucleus ventralis thalami pars dorsomedialis and in the nucleus reticularis thalami; indeed the relation between the change in discharge frequency of these cells and the increased thalamic responsiveness was almost linear. It is of interest, therefore, to find that catechol also influences the discharge frequency of cells in these nuclei (Fig. 8 and 9). The temporal course of the change in frequency of discharge and the increased responsiveness of cells in the ventro-basal thalamus are again very similar and an almost linear relation exists between the two phenomena. Further, the change in the discharge frequency of the cells lying outside the ventro-basal thalamus lags slightly behind the increase in size of the cortical responses after the injection of catechol. It was proposed (Angel 1964) that the cells with a high "resting" frequency of discharge might exert an inhibitory action on ventro-basal thalamic cells and that those cells with a low "resting" discharge frequency might exert an excitatory action. Thus the effect of catechol on the cells located outside the ventro-basal thalamus may cause a decreased inhibitory inflow and an increased excitatory inflow to the ventro-basal thalamus, giving rise to a large increase in the excitability of cells in this nucleus. It has been shown recently in the cat that the cells in the nucleus reticularis thalami send their axons caudad into the thalamus, where they form synapses with neurones in the ventro-basal thalamus (Scheibel and Scheibel 1966). Thus there is both anatomical and physiological evidence that these thalamic reticular cells may be capable of exerting a modulatory influence upon thalamic transmission.

Catechol has also been found to change the discharge frequency of cells in the pontine reticular formation (Yoshii *et al.* 1960), stimulation of which region has been shown to give an EEG "arousal" reaction (Moruzzi and Magoun 1949). Catechol also produces a change in spontaneous electrocortical activity, in animals lightly anaesthetized with barbiturates, from a pattern of high voltage slow waves to low voltage high frequency waves (Fig. 7, see also Bacq *et al.* 1959).

Theoretically catechol may exert its effect in either of three ways. First, it is an inhibitor of catechol-O-methyl transferase (COMT) and may act by means of a central adrenergic mechanism (Bacq *et al.* 1959). However, Angel and Rogers (1968) found that the convulsant action of polyphenols was unrelated to their relative activities as COMT inhibitors, and no change in cerebral 5-hydroxytryptamine, noradrenaline or dopamine was found after catechol administration (Rogers *et al.* 1968). Secondly, catechol inhibits glycolysis in brain cells (Hochstein and Cohen 1960) and thus reduces cerebral ATP supplies. This might then be expected to produce a state analogous to cerebral anoxia. Angel *et al.* (1969) have shown that the action of catechol cannot be related to its effect on glycolysis since the fall in brain ATP concentration bears no relation to the intensity of the convulsions produced by polyphenols. For example, 3 min after an intraperitoneal injection of catechol (60 mg/kg) the cerebral ATP levels in animals breathing room air fell by 28.4% whereas, if the animals were breathing a 95% O_2 5% CO_2 gas mixture, the fall was only 6.5%.

Finally Rothberger (1902) showed that polyhydroxy phenols antagonize the neuromuscular blocking action of curare and recently Otsuka and Nonomura (1963) have shown that catechol increases the amount of acetylcholine liberated by a single nerve impulse at the neuromuscular junction. Preliminary experiments (Angel, unpublished) indicate that the effect of catechol is potentiated by eserine and partially blocked by atropine sulphate but not by atropine methyl nitrate, which latter does not penetrate the blood-brain barrier. Thus a central cholinergic action for catechol cannot be ruled out as yet, although that it acts *per se* without any intermediary is also possible.

SUMMARY

1. Intravenous or intraperitoneal injection of 1,2-dihydroxybenzene in deeply anaesthetized

animals produces a net increase in the excitability of the dorsal column sensory pathway. The effect lasts for 10 min or more, depending upon the dose administered and the route of administration.

2. Responses recorded from the primary somatic cortical receiving area and ventro-basal thalamus, to peripheral stimulation, increase in size and show a reduction in the scatter of both size and latency of the individual responses.

3. Responses recorded from the cuneate nucleus show either no change in their size or temporal pattern or, in some cases, a size reduction.

4. These changes are accompanied by generalized EEG "arousal", increased respiratory effort and changes in the discharge frequencies of cells located in the thalamus outside the dorsal column sensory pathway: in the nucleus reticularis thalami and the nucleus ventralis pars dorsomedialis.

5. It is proposed that the initial increase in excitability is due to an increased responsiveness of the cerebral cortex to a thalamo-cortical volley consequent upon the hyperpnoea produced by the 1,2-dihydroxybenzene. The continuing increase is due to an increased responsiveness of the ventro-basal thalamus brought about by the modulatory influence of the thalamic reticular nuclei. During this latter period the cortical responsiveness to electrical stimulation of the thalamo-cortical fibres is unaltered or decreased.

RÉSUMÉ

ANALYSE DE L'EFFET DE 1,2-DIHYDROXYBENZÈNE SUR LA TRANSMISSION AU TRAVERS DE LA VOIE SENSITIVE DE LA COLONNE DORSALE

1. L'injection intraveineuse ou intrapéritonéale de 1,2-dihydroxybenzène chez des animaux sous anesthésie profonde provoque une nette augmentation de l'excitabilité de la voie sensitive de la colonne dorsale. Cet effet dure 10 min ou davantage, suivant la dose administrée et la voie d'administration.

2. Les réponses à la stimulation périphérique enregistrées au niveau de l'aire corticale somatosensitive primaire et au niveau du thalamus ventro-basal augmentent de taille et montrent une réduction de la dispersion des tailles et des latences des réponses individuelles.

3. Les réponses enregistrées au niveau du noyau cunéiforme montrent soit aucun changement de leur amplitude ou de leur pattern temporel, soit dans quelques cas une réduction d'amplitude.

4. Ces modifications sont accompagnées d'un arousal électroencéphalographique généralisé, d'un effort respiratoire accru, et de modifications des fréquences de décharge des cellules localisées dans le thalamus en dehors de la voie sensorielle de la colonne dorsale: dans le noyau réticulaire thalamique et le noyau ventral dorsomédian.

5. L'auteur fait l'hypothèse que l'augmentation initiale de l'excitabilité est due à une réactivité accrue du cortex cérébral à la volée thalamo-corticale consécutive à l'hyperpnée produite par 1,2-dihydroxybenzène. L'augmentation subséquente est due à une réactivité accrue du thalamus ventro-basal liée à l'influence modulatrice des noyaux thalamiques réticulaires. Pendant cette dernière période, la réactivité corticale à la stimulation électrique des fibres thalamo-corticales est inchangée ou diminuée.

I should like to express my sincere thanks to Prof. G. D. Dawson for his advice and many helpful discussions during the course of this work.

REFERENCES

ANGEL, A. *Investigations into the control of transmission in the direct sensory pathway of the rat.* Ph.D. Thesis, Univ. of London, **1962**.

ANGEL, A. The level of failure of transmission in the sensory pathway to closely spaced stimuli. *J. Physiol. (Lond.)*, **1963**, *169*: 32–33P.

ANGEL, A. The effect of peripheral stimulation on units located in the thalamic reticular nuclei. *J. Physiol. (Lond.)*, **1964**, *171*: 42–60.

ANGEL, A. Cortical responses to paired stimuli applied peripherally and at sites along the somato-sensory pathway. *J. Physiol. (Lond.)*, **1967**, *191*: 427–448.

ANGEL, A. and DAWSON, G. D. The facilitation of thalamic and cortical responses in the dorsal column sensory pathway by strong peripheral stimulation. *J. Physiol. (Lond.)*, **1963**, *166*: 587–604.

ANGEL, A. and DAWSON, G. D. The effect of 1,2-dihydroxybenzene on transmission in the sensory pathway of the rat. *Electroenceph. clin. Neurophysiol*, **1964**, *16*: 312.

Electroenceph. clin. Neurophysiol., **1969**, *27*: 392–403

ANGEL, A., LEMON, R. N., ROGERS, K. J. and BANKS, P. The effect of polyhydroxyphenols on brain ATP in the mouse. *Exp. Brain Res.*, **1969,** *7*: 250–257.

ANGEL, A. and ROGERS, J. K. Convulsant action of polyphenols. *Nature (Lond.)*, **1968,** *217*: 84–85.

BACQ, Z. M. Sensitization to adrenaline and to adrenergic nerve excitation by antioxidants. *Arch. int. Physiol.*, **1936,** *42*: 340–366.

BACQ, Z. M., SCHLAG, J., FAIDHERBE, J. et CHAILLET, F. Étude de l'action excitatrice centrale du catéchol. *C. R. Acad. Sci. (Paris)*, **1959,** *249*: 2839–2841.

GROOT, J. DE. The rat forebrain in stereotaxic co-ordinates. *Proc. kon. ned. Akad. Wet., Natuurk., 2nd Ser., Pt. LII*, **1959,** *4*: 4–10.

HOCHSTEIN, P. and COHEN, G. The inhibitory effects of quinones and dihydric phenols on glucose metabolism in sub-cellular systems of brain. *J. Neurochem.*, **1960,** *5*: 370–378.

MORUZZI, G. and MAGOUN, H. W. Brain stem reticular formation and activation of the EEG. *Electroenceph. clin. Neurophysiol.*, **1949,** *1*: 455–473.

OTSUKA, M. and NONOMURA, Y. The action of phenolic substances on motor nerve endings. *J. Pharmacol. exp. Ther.*, **1963,** *140*: 41–45.

PITMAN, J. R. A digital delay and time scale generator *J. Physiol. (Lond.)*, **1958,** *142*: 3P.

ROGERS, K. J., ANGEL, A. and BUTTERFIELD, L. The penetration of catechol and pyrogallol into mouse brain and the effect on cerebral monoamine levels. *J. Pharm. Pharmacol.*, **1968,** *20*: 727–729.

ROSE, J. E. and MOUNTCASTLE, V. B. The thalamic tactile region in the rabbit and cat. *J. comp. Neurol.*, **1952,** *96*: 441–490.

ROTHBERGER, C. J. Weitere Mittheilungen über Antagonisten des Curarins. *Pflügers Arch. ges. Physiol.*, **1902,** *92*: 398–450.

SCHEIBEL, M. E. and SCHEIBEL, A. B. The organization of the nucleus reticularis thalami: a Golgi study. *Brain Res.*, **1966,** *1*: 43–62.

YOSHII, N., MATSUMOTO, J. and OGURA, H. Studies on the unit discharge of brainstem reticular formation in the cat. II. Effects of catechol, amphetamine, nembutal and megimide. *Med. J. Osaka. Univ.*, **1960,** *11*: 19–33.

Reference: ANGEL, A. An analysis of the effect of 1,2-dihydroxybenzene on transmission through the dorsal column sensory pathway. *Electroenceph. clin. Neurophysiol.*, **1969,** *27*: 392–403.

Electroencephalography and Clinical Neurophysiology
Elsevier Publishing Company, Amsterdam – Printed in The Netherlands

EFFECT OF BRAIN-STEM LESIONS ON METRAZOL-INDUCED SEIZURES IN CATS[1]

Dennosuke Jinnai, M.D., Heitaro Mogami, M.D., Jiro Mukawa, M.D., Yoshikazu Iwata, M.D. and Kiyofumi Kobayashi, M.D.

Department of Neurological Surgery, Osaka University Medical School, Osaka (Japan)

(Accepted for publication: January 22, 1969)

INTRODUCTION

Emphasis has been placed on the intracerebral physiological mechanism of maintaining the epileptic excitability or of generalization of seizure activity since Jung and Tönnies (1949, 1950) proposed the caudate inhibitory theory. The interaction of striatum and cerebellum and its possible role in the control of epileptiform activity have also been considered (Snider and Cooke 1953; Cooke and Snider 1955; Dow 1961). The important concepts of the activating or integrating function of the brain-stem (Jasper 1949; Moruzzi and Magoun 1949) and hypothalamus have recently been re-emphasized in relation to seizure activity (Freedman and Moossy 1953; Starzl *et al.* 1953; Gastaut 1954; Fernández-Guardiola *et al.* 1956; Freedman and Ferris 1956; Caspers 1957; Gellhorn *et al.* 1959; Miyasaka 1960; Sano 1960; Walker and Serrano 1963; Milhorat *et al.* 1966).

In this experimental work, the effect of brain-stem lesions on the Metrazol (pentetrazol)-induced major seizure was studied from the standpoint of threshold changes, and the intracerebral mechanism for the maintenance of epileptic excitability is discussed.

METHOD

Eighty-six adult cats were utilized: twenty-six as controls and sixty as the experimental animals. After the tracheotomy, done under light ether anesthesia, the animal was placed in a stereotaxic apparatus. Intramuscular injection of succinylcholine chloride was intermittently given with local anesthesia of the wound and artificial respiration was maintained for the following experiment.

EEG was recorded with a San'ei electroencephalograph through four or five pairs of bipolar concentric stainless steel needle electrodes which were stereotaxically inserted into both sides of the anterior sigmoid gyrus, various nuclei of the thalamus, lenticular nucleus, substantia nigra, mesencephalic reticular formation and limbic structures. These electrodes were 0.8 mm in the outer diameter and insulated except for the tip.

In the experimental group, a pair of anodal electrolytic lesions were made bilaterally in the brain-stem by passing 4 mA of D.C. for 50–60 sec through a stereotaxically placed stainless-steel needle. The lesion was of oval shape and 2–2.5 mm in its maximum diameter. The cats were all allowed to recover for more than 2 weeks (average 19.5 days) after the lesions were made before the Metrazol seizure was induced.

Metrazol (10 mg diluted by 1 ml of 0.5% saline solution) was injected i.v. every 30 sec until generalized seizure discharges were elicited. Such seizure was induced only once in each cat in both the control or experimental groups. At the end of experiment, the brains were perfused through the carotid arteries with isotonic saline solution, followed by potassium ferrocyanide formalin solution in order to mark the needle point. The recording points and lesions were histologically verified after hematoxylin-eosin staining.

RESULTS

1. *Electrographic findings of Metrazol seizure discharges*

In the controls, the Metrazol spike discharges

[1] Presented at the 25th Meeting of the Japan Neurosurgical Society at Tokyo in 1966.

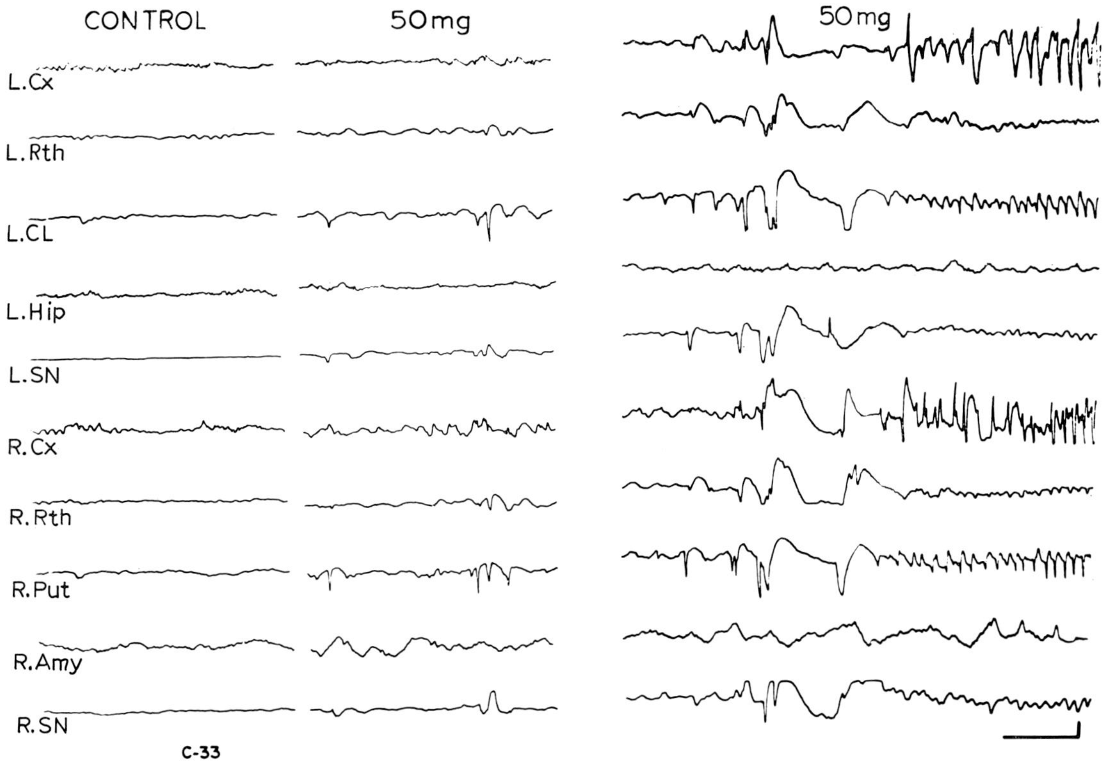

Fig. 1
Metrazol seizure discharges. L. or R.: left or right side of the brain; Cx: anterior sigmoid gyrus; Rth: N. reticularis thalami; CL: claustrum; Hip: hippocampus; SN: substantia nigra; Put: putamen; Amy: N. amygdalae. (Calibration: 100 μV, 1 sec).

appeared to "originate" in various subcortical structures such as claustrum, globus pallidus, putamen, substantia nigra and subthalamic region including the mesencephalic reticular formation in twenty-two out of twenty-six cats. A pure cortical "origin" could not be observed in any of the cases, although a simultaneous "origin" both in the motor cortex and these subcortical structures occurred in the other four cases. The seizure activity did not "originate" in the thalamus or limbic structures in any case. A typical example is shown in Fig. 1. After the injection of 50 mg of Metrazol, spikes were noted at first in the left claustrum and right putamen before seizure discharges became generalized. Limbic structures such as the hippocampus and amygdala were notably silent. These findings suggest that the Metrazol-induced seizure activity "originates" subcortically within the motor system.

2. *Average threshold for Metrazol seizure*

Average or mean value (M) threshold dosage of Metrazol to induce a generalized seizure in the control group was 70 mg (standard deviation, $s = 20.5$) or 23.6 mg/kg ($s = 4.4$). The smaller s of the latter supports the well known fact that the body weight is a significant factor for threshold determination.

3. *Brain-stem lesion and alteration of the threshold*

The threshold (in mg/kg) of the experimental group was compared with that of the control group. The lesions were plotted at various planes from A14.0 to P9.0 as illustrated in Fig. 2 (Snider and Niemer 1961). The lesions which resulted in an increase of the threshold dosage over 28.0 mg/kg ($M+s$) are cross-lined and those which reduced it below 19.2 mg/kg ($M-s$) are dotted. These two groups of lesions are not randomly distributed but appear to be or-

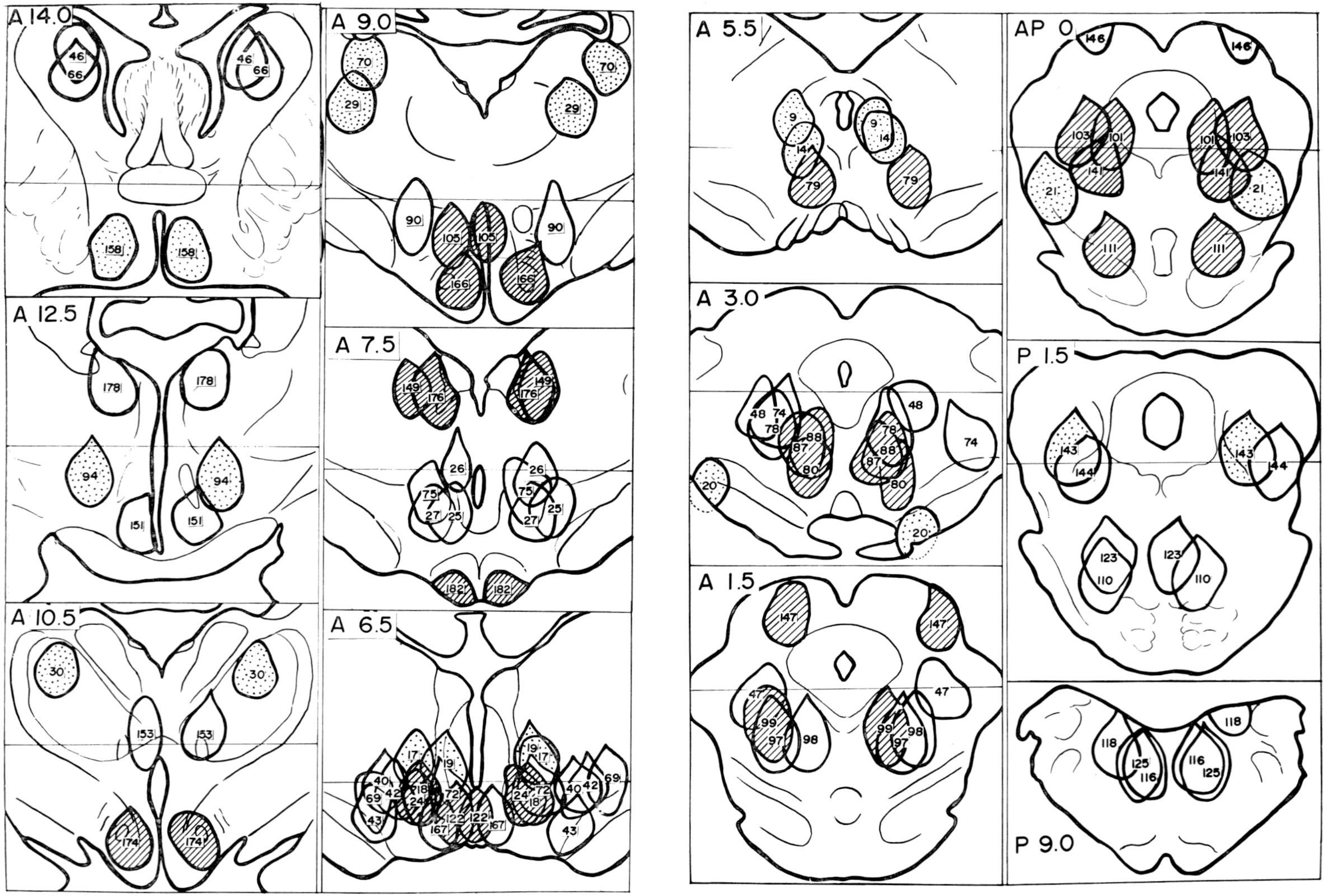

Fig. 2

Brain-stem lesion and threshold change in Metrazol-induced major seizure. Hatched areas: threshold increment; dotted areas: threshold decrement; other areas: no threshold change.

Paired lesions are plotted at each side and the cat numbers are indicated. The horizontal line in the plane 10 mm dorsal to the interaural line, and the numbers following A or P are mm in distance anterior or posterior to the interaural vertical plane (APO). A14.0–A6.5: diencephalon; A5.5–APO: mesencephalon; P1.5: representative of pons; P9.0: representative of medulla.

ganized in a certain meaningful anatomical fashion as suggested by the following analyses.

The numerical threshold dosage of each animal is given in Table I for each of the anatomical regions in which the lesion was performed. The threshold change was statistically more significant when it was over 2*s* in comparison with *s* (see Table II). The former was, therefore, interpreted to indicate a definite threshold change whereas the latter was considered to indicate simply a tendency of the threshold change.

(a) In the hypothalamus, there was a contrast in the threshold change between the anterior and posterior parts. The anterior lesions definitely reduced the threshold in two out of three

TABLE I

Metrazol threshold dosage, and changes for each animal and in relation to different anatomical lesions

Part or Nucleus	Cat number	Metrazol dosage (mg/kg)	Threshold change
(a) Hypothalamic region (A14.0–6.5)			
Anterior	C–151	21.9	
	C–158	13.8	⇓
	C– 94	12.5	⇓
Posterior	C–174	28.2	↑
	C–166	28.4	↑
	C–105	38.0	⇑
	C–182	42.6	⇑
	C–122	36.4	⇑
(b) Thalamic region			
Anterior	C–178	21.1	
Ventro-lateral	C– 30	18.4	↓
	C– 29	17.2	↓
	C– 70	15.8	↓
Ventro-medial	C–153	25.3	
Centre median	C– 17	9.8	⇓
	C– 19	14.9	↓
Dorso-medial	C–149	29.0	↑
	C–176	30.5	↑
(c) Caudate nucleus			
Head	C– 46	25.1	
	C– 66	19.4	
(d) Subthalamic region			
Anterior	C– 90	23.8	
	C– 25	19.8	
	C– 26	22.1	
	C– 27	26.9	
	C– 75	21.1	
Posterior (lateral)	C– 40	27.7	
	C– 42	27.5	
	C– 43	20.8	
	C– 69	22.2	
Posterior (medial)	C– 24	30.6	↑
	C– 18	35.5	⇑
	C– 72	21.8	
	C–167	21.0	
(e) Midbrain			
Rostral (dorso-medial)	C– 48	24.5	
	C– 74	20.0	
	C– 78	20.5	
	C– 9	17.2	↓
	C– 14	21.1	⇓
Rostral (ventro-medial)	C– 79	35.3	⇑
	C– 80	33.3	⇑
	C– 88	33.3	⇑
	C– 87	30.5	↑
Rostral (ventro-lateral)	C– 20	17.5	↓
Caudal	C– 47	22.9	
	C– 97	22.3	
	C– 98	21.6	
	C– 99	37.0	⇑
	C–147	34.2	⇑
	C–101	45.7	⇑
	C–103	34.0	⇑
	C–141	36.1	⇑
	C–111	35.8	⇑
	C– 21	14.5	⇓
	C–146	26.3	
(f) Pons and medulla (P1.5–9.0)			
Pons	C–143	16.7	↓
	C–144	22.7	
	C–110	27.8	
	C–123	26.6	
Medulla	C–118	21.6	
	C–125	22.5	
	C–116	27.9	

⇑ : definite increment, ↑: tendency to increment, ⇓ : definite decrement and ↓: tendency to decrement in threshold.

TABLE II

Statistical analysis of the threshold changes

Threshold changes	Control group 26 cats	Experimental group 60 cats	χ^2
Over s	7	31	4.50 $0.05 > P > 0.025$
Over $2s$	1	18	7.21 $0.01 > P > 0.005$

s: standard deviation. Note the statistical significance of changes in over $2s$; this represents "definite" threshold change.

cats: the posterior lesions did not cause any threshold reduction in all of five cats (rather, the threshold tended to rise in 2 and definitely rised in 3 cats).

(b) In the thalamus, the lesions in the anterior and ventro-medial nuclear group did not change the threshold. The lesions in the ventro-lateral nucleus tended to reduce the threshold in all of three cats. The lesions in the centre median of the medial group resulted in threshold reduction in two cats. The lesions in the dorso-medial nucleus of the medial group tended to produce a threshold rise in two cats.

(c) Lesions in the anterior and postero-lateral subthalamus did not change the threshold, but lesions in the medial part of the posterior subthalamus resulted in a threshold elevation in two out of four cats. These two cats had the lesions in the prerubral Forel's H field bilaterally.

(d) The lesions of the dorso-medial part of the rostral midbrain did not produce a change in threshold or did decrease it when the lesions were bilaterally located at the Forel's tractus fasciculorum. The ventro-medial lesions strongly resulted in threshold elevation in all of four cats.

The lesions at the most caudal level also induced remarkable threshold rise as found in APO of Fig. 2.

(e) No lesions in the pons and medulla caused an elevation of threshold in seven cats. Other effects are indicated in Table I.

In our series of experiments, the maximum increment of the threshold was 93%, and the maximum decrement 57%. The EEG patterns of the Metrazol-induced generalized discharges were not varied by the lesions. It should be noted that there was no evidence that any lesion could prevent the development of the seizure discharges.

DISCUSSION

A threshold decrease can be interpreted as increased intracerebral susceptibility to Metrazol either due to the elimination of the inhibitory function in the destroyed structure *per se*, or to the intercepting of inhibitory influences passing through the destroyed structure, or both. Threshold increase would be the expression of opposite mechanisms. On the basis of such an interpretation the anatomical distribution of facilitatory and inhibitory functions in the brain-stem will be suggested.

In the hypothalamus, there was a functional differentiation, the anterior portion exerting inhibitory and the posterior portion facilitatory influences on Metrazol-induced seizure activity (see also Gellhorn *et al.* 1959). Murphy and Gellhorn (1945) and Miyasaka (1960) observed respectively the facilitation of cortical strychnine discharges and of the neocortical after-discharges, by stimulation of the hypothalamus. There is, however, no report directly concerned with functional differences between the anterior and posterior hypothalamus.

There have been a number of investigations correlating the Metrazol seizure susceptibility and the brain-stem activating system. Fernández-Guardiola *et al.* (1956) demonstrated an active inhibitory process in the mesencephalic reticular formation; Okuma *et al.* (1961) and Milhorat *et al.* (1966) also found that the threshold of the Metrazol seizure was reduced by a lesion of the midbrain reticular formation, and noted that this structure is a powerful inhibitory system. Freedman and Ferris (1956) and Gellhorn *et al.* (1959), on the other hand, pointed out the facilitatory influence of the midbrain reticular formation upon the Metrazol-induced hypersynchronous activity.

In review of other types of investigations using various experimental models of focal seizure activity, Freedman and Moossy (1953) and Miyasaka (1960) pointed out the facilitatory function of the midbrain reticular formation upon the neocortical after-discharges. However, Martin *et al.* (1953) and Sano (1960) could not find any influence of the reticular activating system on the neocortical seizures whereas Caspers (1957) and Andy and Mukawa (1959) demonstrated an inhibitory influence of the midbrain upon the cortical and other forebrain structures. There have been, thus, a variety of opinions on the role of the brain-stem reticular formation in the development and control of seizure activity, and no detailed anatomical correlations have been provided.

Functional differentiations in the midbrain (inhibitory effects from the dorso-rostral part, facilitatory elsewhere) have been found in the present experiments in relation to Metrazol-induced seizures. It should also be noted that no effects could be detected from either the pons or the medulla.

In the thalamus, only the dorso-medial nucleus was found to be facilitatory in our Metrazol experiments. There are several clinical reports of dorso-medial thalamotomy (Spiegel *et al.* 1949; Wada 1952; Handa *et al.* 1961) for the treatment of epilepsy, but none of them clearly gives the physiological explanation of seizure inhibition. According to the anatomical hypothesis of Murphy and Gellhorn (1945), the pathways responsible for hypothalamo-cortical facilitation consist of the primary neuron in the posterior hypothalamus and the secondary neuron in the dorso-medial thalamic nucleus. It is interesting to note that both of these structures were facilitatory in our Metrazol experiment.

On the other hand, the non-specific thalamic projection system (such as VA and CM) was found to have inhibitory influences in our experiment. Starzl *et al.* (1953) were unable to find evidence that the diffuse thalamic projection system plays a prominent role in seizure induction by Metrazol. This system was considered inhibitory as a functional entity with the rostral reticular formation by Caspers (1957) and Milhorat *et al.* (1966).

In the subthalamus, the medio-dorsal part of the caudal level corresponding to the prerubral Forel's H field was facilitatory in this experiment. In our laboratory, Funaki (1959), Kambayashi (1959), Jinnai and Nishimoto (1963) and Jinnai (1966) have found that the existing corticogenic convulsion could be abruptly interrupted by cutting the field bilaterally before the self-sustained discharges propagated from the lenticular nucleus to the substantia nigra and concluded that the conduction pathway for seizure activity was located in the H field. Mukawa (1964a) and Iwata (1967) recently demonstrated the facilitatory function of the H field upon seizure activity in the motor cortex and lenticular nucleus. Mukawa (1964b) stressed the anatomical relations between the H field and the mesencephalic and pontine reticular formations for the seizure inhibitory process.

Lesions of the head of the caudate nucleus in our experimental series were partial and were present in only two cats. The results do not support the hypothesis of Jung and Tönnies (1949, 1950).

In conclusion, a functional differentiation appears to exist in relation to the Metrazol-induced seizure activity in the brain-stem rostral to the pons. A primarily facilitatory system would consist of the caudal mesencephalon extending rostrally to the posterior hypothalamus through the ventral part of the rostral mesencephalon and posterior subthalamus, and also of the medio-dorsal nucleus of the thalamus. An inhibitory system would include the dorsal part of the rostral mesencephalon extending rostrally

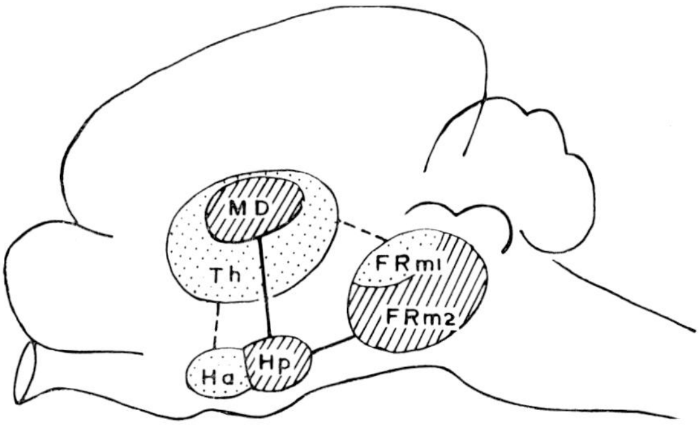

Fig. 3
Schema of cat brain showing the brain-stem systems which are facilitatory (cross-lining) and inhibitory (dotted) for the Metrazol seizure activity and the hypothesized relationship to each other. FRm 1: dorsal part of the rostral level of the mesencephalic reticular formation; FRm 2: the rest of the mesencephalic reticular formation; MD: the medio-dorsal nucleus of the thalamus; Th: the rest of the thalamus; Ha: anterior hypothalamus; Hp: posterior hypothalamus.

to the thalamus and also of the anterior hypothalamus (see Fig. 3).

It may be suggested that the facilitatory system plays a role in the onset and generalization of the Metrazol seizure (see also Gastaut 1954).

SUMMARY

1. The chronic effect of bilaterally paired lesions in the cat's brain-stem on Metrazol-induced seizures was studied in order to clarify the intracerebral mechanism for the maintenance of epileptic excitability.

2. The results seem to indicate that there are two systems of facilitatory and inhibitory functions in the brain-stem rostral to the pons as far as Metrazol-induced seizure activity is concerned. The facilitatory system consists of the caudal mesencephalon extending rostrally to the posterior hypothalamus through the ventral part of the rostral mesencephalon and posterior subthalamus, and also of the medio-dorsal nucleus of the thalamus. The inhibitory system consists of the dorsal part of the rostral mesencephalon extending rostrally to the thalamus and also of the anterior hypothalamus.

3. It may be suggested that this facilitatory system plays a significant role in the onset and generalization of the Metrazol seizure.

RÉSUMÉ

EFFET DES LÉSIONS DU TRONC CÉRÉBRAL SUR LES CRISES INDUITES PAR MÉTRAZOL CHEZ LE CHAT

1. Les auteurs étudient l'effet chronique de lésions bilatérales couplées du tronc cérébral du chat sur les crises induites par Métrazol, afin d'éclaircir le mécanisme intracérébral de maintien de l'excitabilité épileptique.

2. Les résultats paraissent indiquer qu'il existe, en ce qui concerne l'activité critique induite par Métrazol, deux systèmes fonctionnels, facilitateur et inhibiteur, situés dans le tronc cérébral en avant du pont. Le système facilitateur comprend le mésencéphale caudal, s'étendant en avant à l'hypothalamus postérieur au travers de la partie ventrale du mésencéphale rostral et du subthalamus postérieur, et le noyau dorso-médian du thalamus. Le système inhibiteur comporte la partie dorsale du mésencéphale rostral s'étendant en avant au thalamus, et l'hypothalamus antérieur.

3. Les auteurs émettent l'hypothèse que ce système facilitateur joue un rôle important dans le déclenchement et la généralisation de la crise par Métrazol.

REFERENCES

ANDY, O. J. and MUKAWA, J. Brainstem lesion effects on electrically induced seizures (electroencephalographic and behavioral study). *Electroenceph. clin. Neurophysiol.*, **1959,** *11*: 397.

CASPERS, H. Die Beeinflussung der corticalen Krampferregbarkeit durch das aufsteigende Reticulärsystem des Hirnstammes. *Z. ges. exp. Med.*, **1957,** *129*: 128–144.

COOKE, P. M. and SNIDER, R. S. Some cerebellar influences on electrically induced cerebral seizures. *Epilepsia (Amst.)*, **1955,** *4*: 19–28.

DOW, R. S. Some aspects of cerebellar physiology. *J. Neurosurg.*, **1961,** *18*: 512–530.

FERNÁNDEZ-GUARDIOLA, A., ALCARAZ, V. M. y GUZMAN, F. C. Modificación de la descarga convulsiva cortical por estimulación mesencefálica. *Bol. Inst. Estud. méd. biol. (Méx.)*, **1956,** *14*: 15–21.

FREEDMAN, D. A. and FERRIS, G. S. Effect of mesencephalic lesion on Metrazol-induced cortical activity. *Neurology (Minneap.)*, **1956,** *6*: 173–178.

FREEDMAN, D. A. and MOOSSY, J. Effect of mesencephalic lesion on the cortical electroconvulsant threshold. *Neurology (Minneap.)*, **1953,** *3*: 714–720.

FUNAKI, N. [On the propagation mechanism of the epileptic convulsion and its blocking.] (in Japanese). *Okayama Igakkai Zasshi*, **1959,** *71*: 4451–4459.

GASTAUT, H. *The epilepsies. Electro-clinical correlations.* Thomas, Springfield, Ill., **1954,** 149 p.

GELLHORN, E., BALLIN, H. M. and KAWAKAMI, M. Studies on experimental convulsions with emphasis on the role of the hypothalamus and the reticular formation. *Epilepsia (Amst.)*, **1959,** *1*: 233–254.

HANDA, H., MORI, K. and YOSHIDA, K. [Stereotaxic surgery of aggressive idiocy.] (in Japanese). *J. Japan Surg. Soc.*, **1961,** *62*: 1276–1377.

HAYASHI, T. *Neurophysiology and neurochemistry of convulsion.* Dai-Nihon-Tosho, Tokyo, **1959:** 5–136.

IWATA, Y. [Experimental study of epileptic excitability. Its intracerebral facilitation and inhibition.] (in Japanese). *Osaka Daigaku Igaku Zasshi*, **1967,** *19*: 303–312.

JASPER, H. Diffuse projection system. The integrative action of the thalamic reticular system. *Electroenceph. clin. Neurophysiol.*, **1949,** *1*: 405–420.

JINNAI, D. Clinical results and the significance of Forel-H-tomy in the treatment of epilepsy. *Confin. neurol. (Basel)*, **1966,** *27*: 129–136.

JINNAI, D. and NISHIMOTO, A. Stereotaxic destruction of Forel-H for the treatment of epilepsy. *Neurochirurgia (Stuttg.)*, **1963,** *6*: 164–176.

JUNG, R. und TÖNNIES, J. F. Hirnelektrische Untersuchungen über den Elektrokrampf: die Erregungsabläufe in corticalen und subcorticalen Hirnregionen bei Katze und Hund. *Arch. Psychiat. Nervenkr.*, **1949,** *183*: 206–244.

JUNG, R. und TÖNNIES, J. F. Hirnelektrische Untersuchungen über Entstehung und Erhaltung von Krampfentladungen: Die Vorgänge am Reizort und die Bremsfähigkeit des Gehirns. *Arch. Psychiat. Nervenkr.*, **1950,** *185*: 701–735.

KAMBAYASHI, T. [Studies on the interception of the pathways of epileptic convulsion.] (in Japanese). *Okayama Igakkai Zasshi*, **1959,** *71*, 4429–4443.

MARTIN, W. R., VERNIER, V. G. and UNNA, K. R. Effect of stimulation of the reticular activating system of electrically induced cortical after-discharge. *Epilepsia (Amst.)*, **1953,** *3rd Ser.*, *2*: 145.

MILHORAT, T. H., BALDWIN, M. and HANTMAN, D. A. Experimental epilepsy after rostral reticular formation excision. *J. Neurosurg.*, **1966,** *24*: 595–611.

MIYASAKA, M. [Electrophysiological study of seizure discharges in neo-, paleo-, and archicortical system.] (in Japanese). *Recent Advance Res. nerv. Syst. (Tokyo)*, **1960,** *5*: 227–251.

MORUZZI, G. and MAGOUN, H. W. Brainstem reticular formation. *Electroenceph. clin. Neurophysiol.*, **1949,** *1*: 455–473.

MUKAWA, J. Effect of brainstem and subcortical lesions on corticogenic epileptic convulsion with special reference to Forel-H field. *Acta Med. Okayama*, **1964**a, *18*: 153–171.

MUKAWA, J. Fiber connections of the Forel-H field as seen in Marchi preparations. *Acta Med. Okayama*, **1964**b, *18*: 207–220.

MURPHY, J. P. and GELLHORN, E. The influence of hypothalamic stimulations on cortically induced movements and on action potentials of the cortex. *J. Neurophysiol.*, **1945,** *8*: 341–364.

OKUMA, T., LLINAS, R. and ERVIN, F. R. Effect of mesencephalic reticular formation lesion on epileptic seizure threshold in cats. *Electroenceph. clin. Neurophysiol.*, **1961,** *13*: 304–305.

SANO, K. Upper mesencephalic reticulotomy in epilepsy and behavior disorders. *Neurol. med. chir. (Tokyo)*, **1960,** *2*: 138–146.

SNIDER, R. S. and COOKE, P. M. Cerebellar activity in relation to the electrocorticogram before, during and after seizure states. *Electroenceph. clin. Neurophysiol.*, **1953,** *Suppl. 3*, 78 p.

SNIDER, R. S. and NIEMER, W. T. *A stereotaxic atlas of the cat brain.* Univ. of Chicago Press, Chicago, **1961.**

SPIEGEL, E. A., WYCIS, H. T. and FREED, H. Thalamotomy: neuropsychiatric aspects. *N.Y. J. Med.*, **1949,** *49*: 2273–2274.

STARZL, T. E., NIEMER, W. T. and FORGRAVE, P. R. Cortical and subcortical electrical activity in experimental seizures induced by Metrazol. *J. Neuropath. exp. Neurol.*, **1953,** *12*: 262–276.

WADA, T. [Dorsomedial thalamotomy for the treatment of epilepsy.] In Y. UCHIMURA (Ed.), [*Study of epilepsy*]. Igaku-Shoin, Tokyo, **1952**: 192–202. (in Japanese)

WALKER, A. E. and SERRANO, H. R. Brainstem reticular formation influence on convulsions in monkey. *Arch. Neurol. (Chic.)*, **1963,** *8*: 248–256.

Reference: JINNAI, D., MOGAMI, H., MUKAWA, J., IWATA, Y. and KOBAYASHI, K. Effect of brain-stem lesions on Metrazol-induced seizures in cats. *Electroenceph. clin. Neurophysiol.*, **1969,** *27*: 404–411.

Electroencephalography and Clinical Neurophysiology
Elsevier Publishing Company, Amsterdam – Printed in The Netherlands

THALAMO-CORTICAL RECRUITING RESPONSES DURING SLEEP CHARACTERIZED BY A LOW VOLTAGE FAST EEG[1]

I. LEHTINEN AND P. VALLEALA

Department of Physiology, University of Turku, Turku (Finland)

(Accepted for publication: January 3, 1969)

Low frequency repetitive electrical stimulation of "non-specific" thalamus can in certain circumstances elicit so-called recruiting responses in wide areas of the cerebral cortex. This finding, first described in anaesthetized preparations (Dempsey and Morison 1942a; Jasper 1949), could also be found in unrestrained animals during quiet wakefulness (Evarts and Magoun 1957) and during sleep characterized by EEG slow waves (Yamaguchi *et al.* 1963, 1964). By using a threshold intensity for recruiting responses, these responses decreased or were abolished when the mesencephalic reticular formation of the brainstem was simultaneously stimulated (Moruzzi and Magoun 1949). Recruiting responses were also decreased or absent when the animal was attentively awake (Evarts and Magoun 1957; Weinberger *et al.* 1968) or in sleep characterized by a low voltage fast EEG (Rossi *et al.* 1961; Yamaguchi *et al.* 1963, 1964; Allison 1965).

In anaesthetized preparations and during slow wave sleep repetitive stimulation of "non-specific" thalamus elicits recruiting responses at the threshold level as intermittently occurring groups which build up from the level of spontaneous activity, *i.e.*, there are no distinct evoked potentials to be found in the electrocorticogram between successive recruiting response groups. On the other hand, during low voltage fast sleep (Yamaguchi *et al.* 1963) and alert wakefulness (Wells and Sutin 1964) the same type of repetitive thalamic stimulation evokes a cortical potential with every pulse and these potentials do not exhibit typical waxing and waning.

The different types of evoked reactivity to repetitive stimulation of "non-specific" thalamus will here be denominated as follows: *recruiting response* will mean a series of evoked potentials in which the amplitude varies in the manner of spindling. To elicit such responses during low voltage fast sleep the intensity of repetitive thalamic stimulation has to be at a higher level than is needed to elicit recruiting responses during slow wave sleep. *Recruiting wave* will signify a single evoked potential of a recruiting response. *Sustained waves* refer to successive evoked potentials not showing waxing and waning.

The general characteristics of the thalamo-cortical recruiting response during low voltage fast sleep and the relation of such a response to the occurrence of rapid eye movements (REMs) is the main theme of the present study. Furthermore, recruiting responses are related to the electrical activity of levator palpebrae superioris in that stage of sleep.

METHODS

The experiments were performed on six adult, unanaesthetized, freely moving cats, carrying teflon-coated stainless steel electrodes previously implanted under barbiturate anaesthesia. Stimulating electrodes consisted of two wires, each 0.25 mm in diameter. They were insulated to their obliquely cut ends, cemented side by side and their tips were separated vertically by 1 mm. The stimulating electrodes were inserted at coordinates F 8.5–11.0, L 0–1.0, V 0 to +1, according to Snider and Niemer's atlas (1961), but the precise final localization was based on the observation of cortical recruiting responses to thalamic stimulation. The stimuli consisted in rectangular pulses

[1] Aided by a grant from the Juselius Foundation, Finland.

of 0.4–1.0 msec duration at 8/sec and the peak current varied from 0.15 to 0.50 mA, except in one cat in which it amounted to 1.3 mA. The current was monitored on a CRO by measuring the voltage drop over a 0.5 kΩ resistor in series with the electrodes. Stimulation was provided by a Grass S-4 stimulator and an RF isolation unit. For recording of REMs and the movements of the upper eyelids, two wires 0.13 mm in diameter were inserted through the roof of each orbit into the levator palpebrae superioris muscles. The ends of the wires lying inside the muscles were denuded of insulation for a length of about 5 mm. These wires were used for recording the EMG and electro-oculogram (EOG). In the latter case the electrode pair consisted of one lead from each levator muscle. In a control animal a more conventional way of recording the EOG was used by placing the electrodes at the inner canthus of each eye. There were, however, no consistent differences in the temporal distribution of the EOG during low voltage fast sleep when recorded in these two ways.

Cortical electrodes were placed on the dura within 0.5–2.0 mm lateral to the midline for recording electrical activity from both anterior sigmoid gyri. A reference electrode was cemented in the frontal bone. All recording electrodes were fixed according to the technique of Sheatz (1961). Activity led off from the cortex and levator muscles was amplified by conventional techniques, displayed on a CRO and fed to magnetic tape. Concurrent tracings of EEG and EOG were recorded with an ink-writing oscillograph.

To facilitate sleep the animal was kept on a slowly revolving drum during the night before the recording day. During experiments the animal was kept in a shielded sound-attenuated cage provided with a window. During sleep recordings the cage was completely dark. Wakefulness in this study means quiet wakefulness, *i.e.*, the animal sat or was in the "sphinx" position, looking through the window of the cage.

During low voltage fast sleep stimulation was performed as follows: in one part of the experiments the duration of stimulation and the interval between successive stimuli were varied, but an attempt was made to start the stimulation period either during strong REMs or absence of REMs. In another part a systematic scheme was used in three animals; stimulation periods of 10 sec were continually alternated with pauses of the same duration. In this material the recordings obtained with an ink-writing oscillograph were divided into 200 msec parts. With respect to every 200 msec division a judgement was made as to which of the following three categories it belonged: "Only recruiting responses", "Only REM" or "REM and recruiting responses simultaneously". The total numbers of 200 msec periods in these three groups were then determined. In each animal such analyses comprised measurements from several low voltage fast sleep periods.

After experimental series which could last several weeks the positions of the stimulating electrodes were marked by electrolytic deposits of iron. The points were then checked histologically in serial sections which were stained with cresyl violet (Nissl). The marked sites of the electrode tips were found in all cases to be in the general region of n. centralis medialis, within 1.0 mm from the midline.

RESULTS

Recruiting responses during low voltage fast sleep compared with their occurrence during slow wave sleep and wakefulness

When the intensity of repetitive stimulation of "non-specific" thalamus was gradually raised

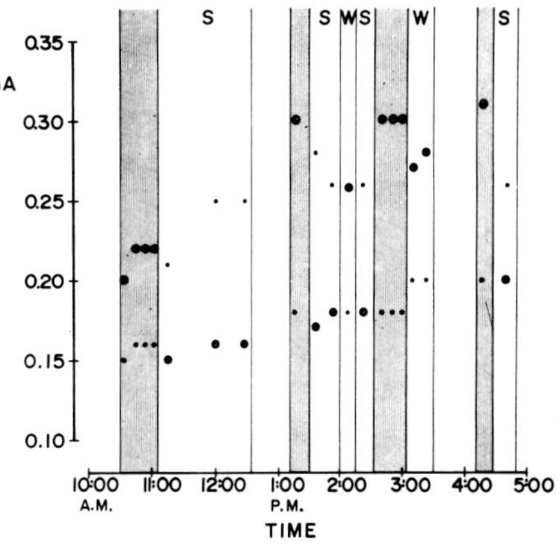

Fig. 1

Thresholds for recruiting responses (large circles) and sustained waves (small circles). Measurements were made from one animal during the same recording session, including the stages of low voltage fast sleep (shaded columns), slow wave sleep (S) and wakefulness (W). Stimulation of "non-specific" thalamus: 8/sec, 1 msec. Ordinate: stimulation current (mA). Abscissa: time (hours).

during low voltage fast sleep, the sustained waves represented the first noticeable reaction in the electrocorticogram. The amplitude of the first wave at the start of stimulation was usually smaller than that of the following waves. When stimulus strength was raised still further, recruiting responses started to appear as intermittent groups, and both recruiting responses and sus-

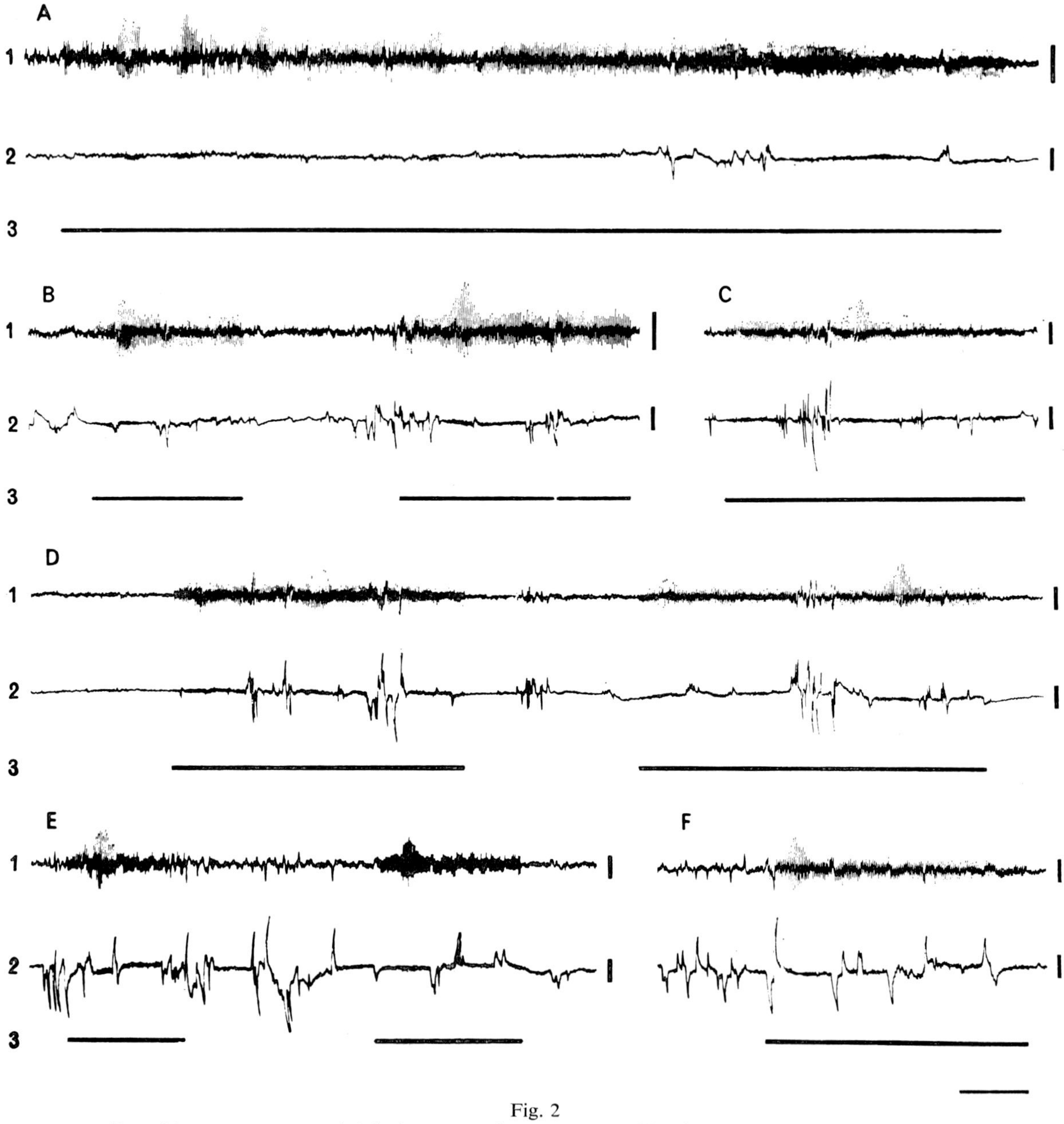

Fig. 2

Recruiting responses recorded during one session. In *A* a transition from slow wave sleep to low voltage fast sleep. Stimulus strength was liminal for recruiting responses during slow wave sleep. In the other samples stimulus strength was raised in order to provoke recruiting responses during low voltage fast sleep (*B*, *C* and *D*) and during wakefulness (*D* and *F*). 1: ECoG of anterior sigmoid gyrus; 2: EOG; 3: stimulus marker. Calibrations: 50 μV, 5 sec. Note the gradual appearance of sustained waves at the beginning of low voltage fast sleep (*A*).

tained waves were seen in the same record (*e.g.*, Fig. 4). There was no considerable difference between the latencies of sustained and recruiting waves. In different animals these latencies varied from 12 to 20 msec, and the difference between their thresholds from 0.05 to 0.15 mA.

Fig. 1 shows the threshold values corresponding to the first appearance of sustained waves (small circles) and of recruiting responses (large circles). Measurements were made during low voltage fast sleep (shaded columns in Fig. 1) and, for comparison, also during slow wave sleep and wakefulness. All the data shown in Fig. 1 were sampled from one animal in the course of one recording day, but the same general type of relationship between threshold levels was found in every animal. The thresholds in Fig. 1 are roughly grouped into two zones, upper and lower. In this figure all thresholds show a gradual rise as a function of time, and this change is about equivalent in the two zones. This kind of gradual rise of threshold was not a consistent finding in all animals and on all recording days and was not further investigated in this study.

It can be seen in Fig. 1 that within the lower zone the threshold values for sustained waves during low voltage fast sleep and wakefulness and, on the other hand, for recruiting responses during slow wave sleep are about the same. These facts with respect to low voltage fast sleep and slow wave sleep can also be found in Fig. 2, *A*, but from another point of view. The figure shows a gradual transition from the latter to the former during the course of the same thalamic stimulation. The stimulus strength was chosen to be liminal for the appearance of recruiting responses. In the beginning of this recording the ongoing cortical activity is interrupted by recruiting response groups. Later the recruiting tendency decreases while the sustained waves start to appear. Eye movements typical of low voltage fast sleep emerge with these events.

The threshold values composing the upper zone in Fig. 1 show more dispersion than in the lower one. It has to be remembered that in the present study we are dealing with quiet wakefulness; if the animal was restless the threshold for recruiting responses was much higher, or these phenomena could not be elicited at all.

Measurements made during slow wave sleep have been indicated in Fig. 1 with the same symbols as for other stages, although the meaning of the symbols is somewhat different: the large circles in Fig. 1 within S columns represent thresholds for eliciting recruiting responses without concomitant sustained waves and, on the other hand, the small circles in S columns indicate the first appearance of sustained waves in the intervening periods of successive recruiting response groups. Thus slow wave sleep with respect to the background of recruiting responses is clearly different from both low voltage fast sleep and wakefulness, which in this respect are quite similar. During the latter the recruiting responses never develop from a background of mere spontaneous cortical activity, as is the case when the animal is drowsy, in slow wave sleep or under barbiturate anaesthesia, but they are always connected with sustained waves coming up during the periods between successive recruiting responses. In addition, during the course of continuous repetitive stimulation the frequency of intermittent recruiting response groups during slow wave sleep is higher and their temporal distribution more regular than in low voltage fast sleep and wakefulness.

The relationship between recruiting responses and rapid eye movements

The investigation of the relationship between recruiting responses and REMs was always started by choosing the lowest intensity of repetitive thalamic stimulation which provoked intermittent recruiting responses, *i. e.*, the level which within the shaded columns in Fig. 1 is indicated by large circles. For example, in Fig. 2, *A* the stimulus intensity was below the threshold level and was therefore raised until recruiting responses started (Fig. 2, *B–D*). This type of thalamic stimulation did not cause any clear temporary cessation of ongoing motor activity in awake animals and never produced any kind of repetitive twitching or obvious autonomic reactions. It has to be emphasized that, when long lasting, it did not prevent shifts from low voltage fast to slow wave sleep or *vice versa*, nor did it clearly activate such transitions.

Fig. 2, *B–D* give examples of cases in which the stimulation periods were varied and attempts were made to start the stimulus either during

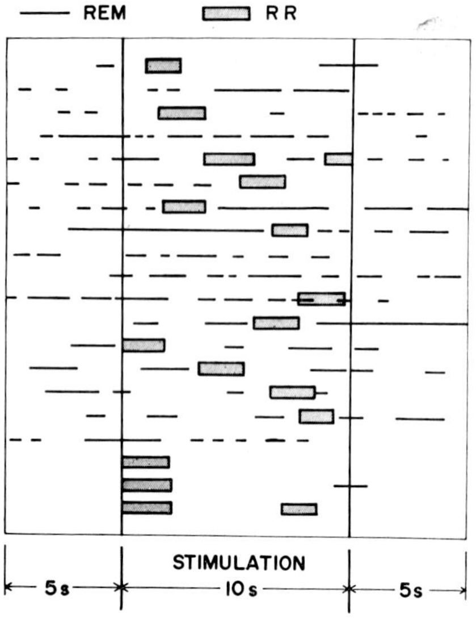

Fig. 3
Temporal distribution of recruiting responses (RR) and rapid eye movements (REM) during one low voltage fast sleep period lasting about 3 min. The continuous recording should be read from left to right and from top to bottom. Stimulation periods of 10 sec alternated with pauses of the same duration. In only one case did recruiting responses and REMs overlap in this recording.

strong REMs or absence of REMs. Fig. 3 shows results from one low voltage fast sleep period during which a systematic stimulation schedule was used (see Methods). The data of Fig. 2 and 3 are from the same animal (Cat 1). In these figures, which are representative of all experiments of this kind, it can be seen that recruiting responses and REMs did not usually occur simultaneously. This was most consistent during the period corresponding to the culmination of recruiting spindling. As shown in Table I the simultaneous occurrence of recruiting responses and REMs in a group of three animals was only of the order of 1%, whereas "Only RR" and "Only REM" classes combined varied from 32.7% to 42.4% of the total stimulation time. On the other hand, the cortical evoked potentials not contributing to intermittent recruiting phenomena, *i.e.*, sustained waves, could occur regularly with REMs.

One low voltage fast sleep period lasting about 3 min is schematically shown in Fig. 3. In the final phase of this period the EEG is actually changing to that of slow wave sleep. This change is indicated by the paucity of REMs and the tendency for recruiting responses to occur with the start of stimulation, while their number during a 10 sec stimulation period tends to increase. In fact, the first spindles characteristic of slow wave sleep started immediately after the last recruiting response group depicted in the lowermost line of Fig. 3.

In those exceptional cases in which recruiting response and REMs occurred simultaneously the waxing of the former was slower and their culmination in spindling was of smaller amplitude as compared with recruiting responses occurring without concurrent REMs. On the other hand, it was also very uncommon that EOG bursts of large amplitude occurred during such overlapping periods.

Fig. 2, *E* and *F* represent experiments from the same recording session as that illustrated in Fig. 2, *A–D*, but in this case the animal was awake. The cat sat still and looked through the window of the cage, which was now partly illuminated. One can observe the same type of

TABLE I

Occurrence of recruiting responses (RR) and rapid eye movements (REM) during low voltage fast sleep in three animals. For analysis see Methods.

Cat (No.)	Number of 200 msec periods	Stimulation				No stimulation
		Only REM %	Only RR %	REM and RR simultaneously %	Total REM %	Total REM %
1	7639	25.5	12.8	0.93	26.5	32.8
2	3050	27.5	14.9	1.15	28.7	30.2
3	2600	20.0	12.7	0.62	20.6	28.3

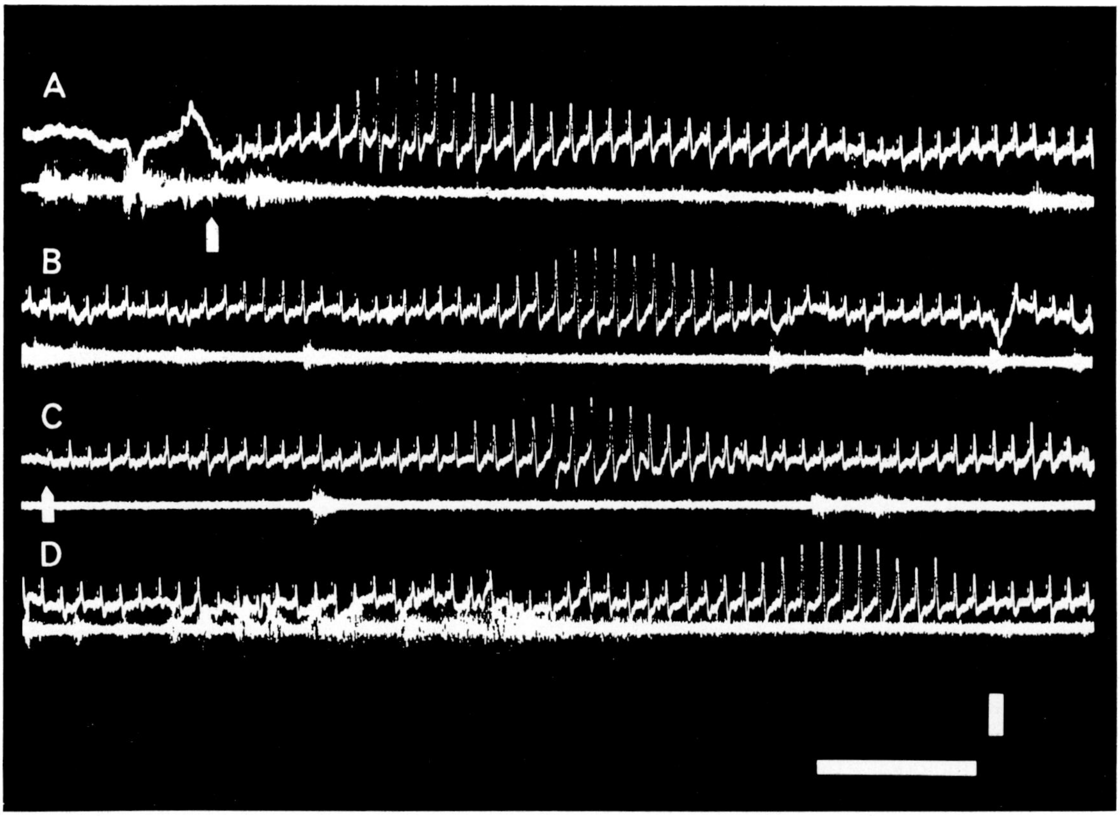

Fig. 4
Relation of recruiting responses to the electrical activity of left levator palpebrae superioris muscle during low voltage fast sleep (4 samples). Upper traces: ECoG of left anterior sigmoid gyrus. Lower traces: EMG of levator muscle. Stimulation is continuous in the second and fourth samples and its start in the first and third samples is indicated by an arrow. Calibrations: 50 μV (ECoG), 1 sec.

relationship between recruiting responses and the eye movements of visual inspection as that encountered in the same animal during low voltage fast sleep.

Finally, the relation of recruiting responses to the electrical activity of levator palpebrae superioris was similar to that to REMs. Thus they did not usually occur concurrently during low voltage fast sleep (Fig. 4). It was sometimes found that the tonic component of the EMG burst which just preceded the recruiting response decreased in parallel with the waxing phase of recruitment (Fig. 4, *A*).

DISCUSSION

In the present study recruiting responses during slow wave sleep and sustained waves during low voltage fast sleep represented the first reactions in records from the anterior sigmoid gyrus when the strength of repetitive stimuli to "non-specific" thalamus was gradually raised. With further increase of stimulus strength during low voltage fast sleep, recruiting responses started as intermittent groups; in this situation the recruiting and sustained waves thus occurred in the same recording and were apparently quite closely related.

Among the similarities between recruiting and sustained waves in this stage of sleep are the relatively long equal latencies, the similar type of minimal or absent initial positivity and the same general wave forms. On the other hand, such characteristics of sustained waves as the increase of the surface-negative component following the second thalamic stimulus as compared to that following the first stimulus (*e.g.*, Fig. 4,*C*), and the lack of the typical spindling to continuous repetitive stimulation are reminiscent of the augmenting response (Dempsey and Morison 1942b; Brookhart and Zanchetti 1956). In the present study the intermingling of sustained waves, *i.e.*, the "augmenting-like" component and the recruiting response varies essentially according to the state of the animal. It has to be remembered that in this study the thresholds for recruiting responses during slow wave sleep and for sustained waves during low voltage fast sleep were about the same, so that the appearance of sustained waves cannot be explained by the spread of stimulating current but rather by a change in transmission circumstances.

It seems obvious that repetitive stimulation of "non-specific" thalamus will uncover one kind of periodic tendency which essentially would determine the frequency of recruiting response groups both during slow wave sleep and low voltage fast sleep. During slow wave sleep these groups often appear with rather regular intervals and at relatively high frequency. During low voltage fast sleep, on the other hand, their occurrence is lower and the intervening intervals between successive groups are irregular. It seems probable that during low voltage fast sleep there are some factors which can modulate and also totally inhibit the periodic tendency. A later discussion will indicate that the factors which are effective during low voltage fast sleep, and possibly strongly modify the influence of this kind of periodic tendency, are the phasic events concurrent with REMs. A tendency to sustained waves during slow wave sleep (Fig. 2, *A*) and that to recruiting responses during low voltage fast sleep would be a sensitive indication of an alteration in the actual sleep stage. Sensitivity of recruiting responses to reveal slight changes in arousal level has been emphasized by Weinberger *et al.* (1968).

When stimulating "non-specific" thalamus during low voltage fast sleep at threshold intensity for recruiting responses, it was highly uncommon for the latter and REMs to occur concurrently. This finding, which confirms and extends the results obtained by Allison (1965), may be explained in two ways. First, the low voltage fast sleep mechanism itself and its phasic accentuations, being temporarily related to REMs, may depress the so-called synchronizing thalamocortical system and thus prevent the appearance of recruiting responses during thalamic stimulation (Rossi *et al.* 1961; Yamaguchi *et al.* 1964; Allison 1965). Supporting this possibility is the higher threshold for recruiting responses during low voltage fast sleep than during slow wave sleep. Moreover, during low voltage fast sleep there is a varying delay to the first recruiting response from the start of stimulation, as can be seen in Fig. 3. During slow wave sleep, on the contrary, the first recruiting response tends to build up soon after the start of stimulation (See transition to slow wave sleep in lower part of Fig. 3). It is possible that REMs which sometimes filled up such a delay were also a causal factor for it, by preventing the appearance of recruiting responses.

Secondly, the repetitive stimulation of "non-specific" thalamus itself, and especially the events relating to recruiting responses during this kind of stimulation, might inhibit the mechanism responsible for REMs. A background to this assumption are the findings concerning the induction of recruiting responses in the mesencephalic and bulbar reticular formation (Schlag and Faidherbe 1961), as well as the changes in motor behaviour, *e.g.*, in the form of an "arrest reaction" (Hunter and Jasper 1949) and the cessation of conditioned movement (Rougeul *et al.* 1967). The finding that recruiting responses and REMs usually did not occur concurrently could be stated in another way: it was highly uncommon for REMs to start during recruiting responses. This point of view indicates that the events caused by thalamic stimulation, being concurrent with recruiting responses, could inhibit the mechanism producing REMs. It is unlikely, however, that this kind of thalamic stimulation, in the present study, exerted any marked effect on the causal mechanism of REMs because of the small difference to be found in cats 1 and 2 in Table I between Total REM (Stimulation) and Total REM (No stimulation). It has to be remembered that the intensity of thalamic stimulation was no higher than was necessary to elicit recruiting responses. Naturally one can not exclude the possibility that such a stimulus could influence some other qualities of REMs than merely the temporal occurrence which was analysed in this study.

When dealing with the relationship between recruiting responses and REMs it thus seems probable that both factors, low voltage fast sleep with REMs and thalamic stimulation with recruiting responses, must be taken into account, although the influence of the former factor is assumed to be the more important and will be further discussed below.

During low voltage fast sleep the generalized thalamo-cortical system can be inhibited by the descending influence mediated by the somatosensory and motor cortex (Krauthamer *et al.* 1968). This influence could explain findings made in the present study providing that its timing corresponds to that of REMs. Some studies could point to such a possibility, because during low voltage fast sleep phasic enhancements in the pyramidal discharge are often related in time with the bursts of REMs and originate from motor (Marchiafava and Pompeiano 1964) as well as from somato-sensory cortex (Morrison and Pompeiano 1965).

Recent evidence suggests that the mechanism causing the spontaneous spindle burst probably is a necessary prerequisite for the presence of the recruiting response (Lehtinen and Valleala 1968). The so-called "spindle-tripping" (Jasper and Droogleever-Fortuyn 1947) can sometimes be demonstrated during the intervals of the REM bursts, thus indicating an increased susceptibility to spindle activity during these periods (Lehtinen and Valleala, in preparation).

In the light of the present study and the findings mentioned above it seems that during low voltage fast sleep in the course of continual repetitive thalamic stimulation the occurrence of the recruiting response indicates a tendency to slow wave sleep. By stimulating the "non-specific" thalamus during this stage of sleep, and thus creating the possibility of the presence of recruiting responses, we are actually measuring the intensity of the mechanism maintaining the state of electrocortical desynchronization. Occasional decrease in this intensity, *i.e.*, a tendency to spindle activity, will then afford the necessary prerequisite for the appearance of the recruiting response.

SUMMARY

1. During sleep characterized by a low voltage fast EEG, recruiting responses could be elicited in cats in the course of repetitive stimulation of "non-specific" thalamus by using a stimulus strength slightly supraliminal for recruiting responses during sleep characterized by EEG slow waves.

2. The occurrence of recruiting responses and "sustained waves" depended on the stimulus strength and the actual state of the animal.

3. In the same animal the thresholds for eliciting recruiting responses during slow wave sleep and "sustained waves" during low voltage fast sleep and quiet wakefulness were about the same. There was no remarkable difference between the latencies of the "sustained" and recruiting waves during low voltage fast sleep.

4. During low voltage fast sleep, recruiting responses and rapid eye movements (REMs) usually did not appear simultaneously; *i.e.*, if stimulation was started during REMs the first recruiting response was often delayed. From another point of view, REMs did not usually start during recruiting responses. A similar relationship was found between recruiting responses and the electrical activity of the levator palpebrae superioris muscles. The decrease of the tonic component of the levator EMG was often parallel with the waxing phase of the recruiting response. In the waking state also the searching eye movements and recruiting responses did not usually occur concurrently.

5. It can be assumed that during low voltage fast sleep in the course of continual repetitive stimulation, the temporal distribution of recruiting response groups corresponds to fluctuations of the low voltage fast sleep level. These fluctuations might indicate an occasional tendency to slow wave sleep.

RÉSUMÉ

RÉPONSES PAR RECRUTEMENT THALAMO-CORTICALES PENDANT LE SOMMEIL CARACTÉRISÉ PAR UN EEG RAPIDE DE BAS VOLTAGE

1. Pendant le sommeil caractérisé par un EEG rapide de bas voltage, des réponses par recrutement ont été obtenues chez des chats au cours de stimulations répétitives du thalamus "non spécifique", en utilisant une intensité de stimulation légèrement supraliminaire à l'intensité nécessaire

pour obtenir des réponses par recrutement pendant le sommeil caractérisé par des ondes EEG lentes.

2. La survenue de réponses par recrutement et d'"ondes entretenues" dépend de l'intensité du stimulus et de l'état actuel de l'animal.

3. Chez le même animal, le seuil nécessaire à l'apparition de réponses par recrutement pendant le sommeil lent et d'ondes entretenues pendant le sommeil rapide et pendant l'état de veille tranquille, est sensiblement le même. Il n'y a pas de différence notable entre les latences des ondes entretenues et des ondes par recrutement pendant le sommeil rapide.

4. Pendant le sommeil rapide, les réponses par recrutement et les mouvements oculaires rapides n'apparaissent pas habituellement de façon simultanée, c'est-à-dire que si la stimulation débute pendant les mouvements oculaires rapides, les premières réponses par recrutement sont souvent retardées. D'autre part, les mouvements oculaires rapides ne débutent pas habituellement pendant les réponses par recrutement. Une relation similaire s'observe entre réponses par recrutement et activité électrique des muscles palpébraux élévateurs supérieurs. La diminution de la composante tonique de l'EMG du muscle élévateur est souvent parallèle à la phase ascendante de la réponse par recrutement. A l'état de veille également, les mouvements oculaires d'exploration et les réponses par recrutement ne surviennent habituellement pas de façon concomitante.

5. On peut donc postuler que pendant le sommeil rapide, au cours d'une stimulation répétitive continue, la distribution temporelle des groupes de réponses par recrutement correspond aux fluctuations du niveau de sommeil rapide. Ces fluctuations pourraient indiquer une tendance occasionnelle au sommeil lent.

REFERENCES

ALLISON, T. Cortical and subcortical evoked responses to central stimuli during wakefulness and sleep. *Electroenceph. clin. Neurophysiol.*, **1965,** *18*: 131–139.

BROOKHART, J. M. AND ZANCHETTI, A. The relation between electrocortical waves and responsiveness of the cortico-spinal system. *Electroenceph. clin. Neurophysiol.*, **1956,** *8*: 427–444.

DEMPSEY, E. W. AND MORISON, R. S. The production of rhythmically recurrent cortical potentials after localized thalamic stimulation. *Amer. J. Physiol.*, **1942a,** *135*: 293–300.

DEMPSEY, E. W. and MORISON, R. S. Activity of a thalamo-cortical relay system. *Amer. J. Physiol.*, **1942b,** *138*: 283–296.

EVARTS, E. V. and MAGOUN, H. W. Some characteristics of cortical recruiting responses in unanesthetized cats. *Science*, **1957,** *125*: 1147–1148.

HUNTER, J. and JASPER, H. H. Effects of thalamic stimulation in unanaesthetised animals. The arrest reaction and petit mal-like seizures, activation patterns and generalized convulsions. *Electroenceph. clin. Neurophysiol.*, **1949,** *1*: 305–324.

JASPER, H. H. Diffuse projection systems: the integrative action of the thalamic reticular system. *Electroenceph. clin. Neurophysiol.*, **1949,** *1*: 405–420.

JASPER, H. H. and DROOGLEEVER-FORTUYN, J. Experimental studies of the functional anatomy of petit mal epilepsy. *Ass. Res. nerv. ment. Dis. Proc.*, **1947,** *26*: 272–298.

KRAUTHAMER, G., BESSON, J. M., GUILBAUD, G., ABDELMOUMENE, M. and LIM, R. K. S. Descending control systems. *Proc. 24th int. Congr. physiol. Sci. (Washington, D. C.)*, **1968,** *6*: 239–240.

LEHTINEN, I. and VALLEALA, P. Spontaneous spindle activity as a gating mechanism for recruiting responses in an unanesthetized cat. *Acta physiol. scand.*, **1968,** *74*: 24A–25A.

MARCHIAFAVA, P. L. and POMPEIANO, O. Pyramidal influences on spinal cord during desynchronized sleep. *Arch. ital. Biol.*, **1964,** *102*: 500–529.

MORRISON, A. R. and POMPEIANO, O. Pyramidal discharge from somatosensory cortex and cortical control of primary afferents during sleep. *Arch. ital. Biol.*, **1965,** *103*: 538–568.

MORUZZI, G. and MAGOUN, H. W. Brain stem reticular formation and activation of the EEG. *Electroenceph. clin. Neurophysiol.*, **1949,** *1*: 455–473.

ROSSI, G. F., FAVALE, E., HARA, T., GIUSSANI, A. and SACCO, G. Researches on the nervous mechanisms underlying deep sleep in the cat. *Arch. ital. Biol.*, **1961,** *99*: 270–292.

ROUGEUL, A., PERRET, C. et BUSER, P. Effets comportementaux et électrographiques de stimulations électriques du thalamus chez le chat libre. *Electroenceph. clin. Neurophysiol.*, **1967,** *23*: 410–428.

SCHLAG, J. and FAIDHERBE, J. Recruiting responses in the brain stem reticular formation. *Arch. ital. Biol.*, **1961,** *99*: 135–162.

SHEATZ, G. C. Electrode holders in chronic preparations. A. Multilead techniques for large and small animals. In D. E. SHEER (Ed.), *Electrical stimulation of the brain.* Univ. Texas Press, Austin, **1961:** 45–50.

SNIDER, R. S. and NIEMER, W. T. *A stereotaxic atlas of the cat brain.* Chicago University Press, Chicago, Ill., **1961.**

WEINBERGER, N. M., NAKAYAMA, K. and LINDSLEY, D. B. Electrocortical recruiting responses during classical conditioning. *Electroenceph. clin. Neurophysiol.*, **1968,** *24*: 16–24.

WELLS, J. and SUTIN, J. Sustained response of the diffuse

thalamic projection system. *Proc. Soc. exp. Biol. (N. Y.)*, **1964**, *116*: 235–237.
YAMAGUCHI, N., LING, G. M. and MARCZYNSKI, T. J. Differences between cortical recruiting responses observed during wakefulness and natural sleep. *Nature (Lond.)*, **1963**, *199*: 186–187.
YAMAGUCHI, N., LING, G. M. and MARCZYNSKI, T. J. Recruiting responses observed during wakefulness and sleep in unanesthetized chronic cats. *Electroenceph. clin. Neurophysiol.*, **1964**, *17*: 246–254.

Reference: LEHTINEN, I. and VALLEALA, P. Thalamo-cortical recruiting responses during sleep characterized by a low voltage fast EEG. *Electroenceph. clin. Neurophysiol.*, **1969**, *27*: 412–421.

ANNOUNCEMENTS

THE SOCIETY OF BIOLOGICAL PSYCHIATRY

The Society of Biological Psychiatry announces two awards to be given in May, 1970. The first is the Gold Medal Award to a distinguished senior scientist in the field of Biological Psychiatry. The second are two $750 awards: one for clinical research and one for basic research in the fields related to Biological Psychiatry. These latter two awards are to be given to young men under 35 years of age.

The deadlines for entries are February 1, 1970.

For details please contact Williamina A. Himwich, Ph.D., Chairman, Committee on Research Awards, Society of Biological Psychiatry, Galesburg State Research Hospital, Galesburg, Illinois 61401, U.S.A.

Electroenceph. clin. Neurophysiol., **1969**, *27*: 421

THE SOCIETY FOR NEUROSCIENCE

Following discussions and assessment of the response by interested scientists throughout the United States, a new society has been formed to promote better understanding of the functioning of nervous systems including the part they play in determining behavior. A steering group was organized by the Committee on Brain Sciences of the National Research Council, culminating in the formation of the Society for Neuroscience. The new group will foster interdisciplinary communication and investigation among scientists from the many fields involved and at all levels of biologic organization. It will also seek to attract potential investigators, to advance their education, and to inform the general public of current research in this area and its implications.

Specific activities envisioned for the society, in addition to national meetings, include sponsorship of local chapters to arrange meetings of scientists of differing backgrounds interested in nervous systems, and establishment of a central source of information on interdisciplinary curricula and training programs in neuroscience. The society will also produce nontechnical reports on new information in this broad area, underlining its relevance to the human condition.

Inquiries should be addressed to the Society for Neuroscience, c/o Dr. Louise H. Marshall, 2101 Constitution Avenue, N.W., Washington, D.C. 20418, U.S.A.

Electroenceph. clin. Neurophysiol., **1969**, *27*: 421

Electroencephalography and Clinical Neurophysiology
Elsevier Publishing Company, Amsterdam – Printed in The Netherlands

CLINICAL AND LABORATORY NOTES

SPONTANEOUS SLEEP IN HEALTHY SUBJECTS IN LONG-TERM SERIAL ELECTROENCEPHALOGRAPHIC RECORDINGS

PAMELA F. PRIOR AND PATRICIA A. DEACON

The London Hospital, London E.1. and Shell Research Limited, Tunstall Laboratory, Sittingbourne, Kent (Great Britain)

(Accepted for publication: February 13, 1969)

Spontaneous drowsiness and light sleep with concomitant changes in the EEG activity are often observed during routine recordings. This was particularly so in a group of subjects taking part in a double blind pharmacological study (described in detail elsewhere, Hunter and Robinson 1967) who had monthly EEGs performed over a 3 year period. These male volunteer subjects received for 2 of the 3 years either a placebo or small daily oral doses of the chlorinated hydrocarbon insecticide dieldrin (this substance contains 85% of the compound 1,2,3,4,10,10-hexachloro-6,7-epoxy-1,4,4a,5,6,7,8,8a-octahydro-1,4-endo-exo-5,8-dimethanonaphthalene (HEOD) and 15% related compounds). The dosage of dieldrin was so arranged that it would produce blood and fat HEOD concentrations greater than those of the normal population (Hunter *et al.* 1963) but less than those known to produce clinical and EEG changes associated with intoxication (Kazantzis *et al.* 1964). The subjects did not at any time complain of any alteration in sleep habit or indeed of any other physiological effect and no laboratory or clinical test showed any change except for an increased concentration of HEOD in those receiving the active capsules.

The purpose of the EEG recordings was to ascertain the continuing normality of the recorded cerebral activity in these subjects: they did, however, afford an opportunity to study in more detail the occurrence of EEG activity concomitant with spontaneous drowsiness and light sleep in a long series of recordings. It is the results of these findings that we report here.

MATERIAL AND METHODS

The EEG records were taken under standard conditions by the same technician, using an Elema Schonander EEG machine located in a quiet but not soundproofed laboratory. The subjects were required to attend at the same time of day after a normal night's sleep and at a constant time after food. Nineteen pad electrodes arranged according to the 10–20 system were used for bipolar recording. In the present study the first 10 min of resting EEG were assessed. Two-thirds were recorded with an antero-posterior montage and one-third with a transverse montage which did not include the occipital electrodes. There were fairly frequent commands to open and close the eyes and small taps or noises at irregular intervals during the test.

The 420 records obtained were assessed independently by the two authors: (a) for the depth and duration of drowsiness and sleep, and (b) for the time taken for the subject to fall asleep.

(a) Eight epochs (every fifth 10 sec epoch) were rated in each EEG according to the method of Tizard (1966). In this method a numerical value is given to each epoch according to the main type of activity present; the 8 figures so obtained were then summed to give a total score for each record. The EEG stages A–D from wakefulness to light sleep designated by Loomis *et al.* (1937) were used, and allocated numbers 0–3: the higher the total score for a record the greater amount or depth of drowsi-

TABLE I

Sleep in serial EEGs over a 3 year period (13 subjects)

	First 3 months	Middle 3 months	Final 3 months
Mean sleep score (total possible 16)*	0.51 (S.E. 0.19)	3.20 (S.E. 0.61)	3.31 (S.E. 0.54)
Percentage incidence of sleep**	23% (S.E. 6.8)	51% (S.E. 8.0)	58% (S.E. 8.2)
Time taken to fall asleep (mean of those sleeping)***	470 sec (S.E. 72)	319 sec (S.E. 49)	281 sec (S.E. 47)

* Means for middle and final months both significantly greater than for first 2 months ($P < 0.1\%$).
** Percentages for middle and final months both significantly greater than for first months ($P < 1\%$).
*** Time for final months significantly less than for first ($P < 5\%$).
The 3-monthly periods selected for the comparisons in this table show the various results in: (a) the first 3 months of the trial, that is, before any capsules were administered; (b) at the midpoint of the trial (when all subjects had received a placebo or one of 3 doses of dieldrin for just over one of the 2 years that they were exhibited); and (c) during the final period of the trial when all capsules had been withdrawn for 9 months.

ness and sleep. We extended Loomis' stage C (spindles on a low voltage fast background) to include epochs which contained any of the paroxysmal features that may occur on a low voltage background in light sleep (vertex waves, K complexes and the occipital positive sharp or "lambdoid" waves of sleep) even if sigma spindles did not occur in the particular epoch. In epochs containing two levels of activity we rated the one that occupied the major portion of the time or the pre-stimulus portion if any stimulus had occurred. There were inter-rater disagreements in the rating of only 2.5 % of the epochs.

(b) The time to onset of sleep was measured from the beginning of recording to the first undoubted paroxysmal feature of light sleep: the order of appearance of these various features was noted and particular attention was paid to the characteristics of the occipital "lambdoid" waves of sleep.

RESULTS

The mean sleep scores of the whole group of thirteen subjects for 3 different periods during the study are compared in Table I. Also shown are the percentage incidences of actual sleep and the average time taken for subjects to fall asleep compared for the same 3 periods. The monthly scores for three individuals (each representing a certain characteristic type of pattern) are detailed in Fig. 1.

Of the 175 records that showed plentiful light sleep almost all (91 %) contained vertex waves, just over half (58 %) also showed sigma activity and in just under half (49 %) occipital "lambdoid" waves were present. K complexes occurred in 22 % of the records. The occurrence of "lambdoid" waves was probably an underestimate because of the use of the transverse montage. The order of appearance of these paroxysmal features was variable even in the same individual on different occasions. The most common paroxysmal feature to herald sleep was a vertex wave in 68 % and a run of "lambdoid" waves in 26 % of the records. Sigma activity appeared first in only 4 % and K complexes were even less common.

Of the ten subjects who slept regularly seven exhibited occipital "lambdoid" waves and, of these, four also had lambda waves when awake with the eyes open. The waves were almost identical, showing a positive, basically triangular, wave form, but minor differences were apparent. The "lambdoid" waves in the four subjects showed more

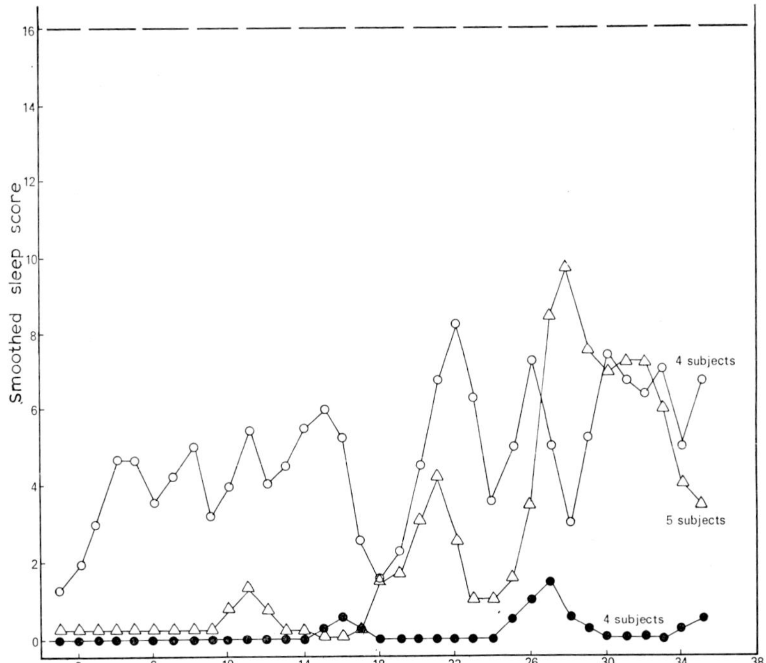

Fig. 1

Individual sleep scores in monthly EEG records from three subjects. The 3 types of curve were characteristic of the group as a whole who, whilst all showing a tendency to increasingly high scores over the 3 year period, showed 3 typical patterns: (a) rare drowsiness or sleep (4 men), illustrated by ●—●, subject 9; (b) sleep prominent mainly in the second half of the trial period (5 men), illustrated by △——△, subject 10; (c) sleep prominent from the first record onwards (4 men), illustrated by ○——○, subject 1. The actual proportion of time spent asleep can be approximated by subtracting the level of the sleep score curve from the horizontal line at the top of the graph which represents the total score possible if the subject was deeply asleep throughout the recording.

variability of form, being often di- or triphasic (the former more commonly in the parieto-occipital and the latter in the temporo-occipital derivations) and tending to appear in clusters. The "lambdoid" waves were of longer duration (120–260 msec) than lambda waves (80–120 msec) and of greater amplitude (50–100 μV) than the lambda waves (rarely reaching 50 μV).

DISCUSSION

Our aim in making the original recordings was to assess each EEG for normality and to exclude specifically those changes which might be due to dieldrin. No changes of the type recorded by Hoogendam *et al.* (1962) or others occurred and none of the EEGs showed any great change from the pre-exposure patterns characteristic of the individual, as assessed in 3 pre-exposure EEGs. We therefore felt justified in considering this to be a sample of normal people who had been studied in considerable detail.

One of our problems in assessing continuing normality was the occurrence of drowsiness and sleep. Indeed we noted that the subjects tended to be alert for only brief portions of the recording and our detailed results confirmed these clinical impressions. The subjects exposed to dieldrin (3 dose-level groups) and the placebo group did not show statistically significant group differences in mean sleep scores, individual curves or percentage incidences of sleep.

The qualitative EEG patterns of sleep recorded were different from those found in the clinical department where sleep is often induced by drugs and the patient is relatively undisturbed. In our subjects sigma spindles were somewhat uncommon. K complexes were likewise infrequent although irregularly occurring stimuli were often used: this may have been due to an adaptation phenomenon to small stimuli (Pampiglione and Ackner 1958).

The comparison of the "lambdoid" waves of sleep and waking lambda waves, in spite of showing certain minor differences, confirmed many of the original observations of Roth and Green (1953) regarding their basic similarities. It was noted that lambdoid waves occurred during sleep and not when the subjects were merely drowsy. We believe that this triangular, positive wave form is a particular characteristic of the occipital region itself rather than that the cause of these two types of wave is necessarily the same. For we have seen morphologically similar waves occurring in the occipital regions in a variety of other states, both pathological (*e.g.*, in localized epilepsies and in some blind children) and physiological (*e.g.*, the responses to single flash stimuli).

SUMMARY

Visual rating scales were used to assess the depth and duration of drowsiness in sleep in the EEGs of thirteen normal subjects taken at monthly intervals over 3 years. There was no evidence that the EEGs or the subjects' physiological state was influenced by exposure to a placebo or to small doses of the insecticide dieldrin administered for 2 out of the 3 years. However, the subjects slept more frequently, more speedily and for more of the recording time as the 3 year period progressed. Certain characteristics of the EEG phenomena of the sleep that occurred are noted and, in particular, comparison of the basically similar wave forms of occipital "lambdoid" waves of sleep and waking lambda waves in the same individual is made.

RÉSUMÉ

LE SOMMEIL SPONTANÉ CHEZ LES SUJETS SAINS D'APRÈS LES TRACÉS ÉLECTROENCÉPHALOGRAPHIQUES EN SÉRIE SUR UNE LONGUE PÉRIODE DE TEMPS

Un système de graduation visuelle a été utilisé pour évaluer la profondeur et la durée de la somnolence et du sommeil dans les tracés de treize sujets normaux relevés à intervalles d'un mois sur une période de 3 ans. Rien ne paraît indiquer que les tracés ou l'état physiologique des sujets aient été affectés soit par un médicament de contrôle soit par l'administration de faibles doses de l'insecticide dieldrin pendant 2 ans sur 3. Toutefois, à mesure que progressait la période de 3 ans, le sommeil des sujets devenait plus fréquent, plus rapide, et couvrait une proportion plus importante du temps d'enregistrement du tracé. Certaines caractéristiques des phénomènes EEG du sommeil relevés sont indiquées, et en particulier la similitude foncière entre les ondes "lambdoïdes" du sommeil dans le tracé occipital et les ondes lambda de la veille chez le même individu.

We wish to thank Dr. C. G. Hunter of Tunstall Laboratory for permission to publish these EEG details from his broad survey of the effects of dieldrin and also for help and encouragement. We also wish to express our thanks for their assistance to Dr. D. F. Scott of the London Hospital, to Dr. J. Volavka of the Psychiatric Research Institute, Prague, and to Mr. M. Roberts of the Statistics Unit of Woodstock Agricultural Research Centre, Sittingbourne.

REFERENCES

Hoogendam, I., Versteeg, J. P. J. and de Vlieger, M. Electroencephalograms in insecticide toxicity. *Arch. environm. Hlth*, **1962,** *4*: 86–94.

Hunter, C. G. and Robinson, J. Pharmacodynamics of Dieldrin (HEOD): 1. Ingestion by human subjects for 18 months. *Arch. environm. Hlth*, **1967,** *15*: 614–626.

Hunter, C. G., Robinson, J. and Richardson, A. Chlorinated insecticide content of human body fat in Southern England. *Brit. med. J.*, **1963,** *1*: 221–224.

Kazantzis, G., McLaughlin, A. I. G. and Prior, P. F. Poisoning in industrial workers by the insecticide Aldrin. *Brit. J. industr. Med.*, **1964,** *21*: 46–51.

Loomis, A. L., Harvey, E. N. and Hobart, G. A. Cerebral states during sleep, as studied by human brain potentials. *J. exp. Psychol.*, **1937,** *21*: 127–144.

Pampiglione, G. and Ackner, B. The effects of repeated stimuli upon EEG and vasomotor activity during sleep in man. *Brain*, **1958,** *81*: 64–74.

Roth, M. and Green, J. The lambda wave as a normal physiological phenomenon in the human electroencephalogram. *Nature (Lond.)*, **1953,** *172*: 864–866.

Tizard, B. Repetitive auditory stimuli and the development of sleep. *Electroenceph. clin. Neurophysiol.*, **1966,** *20*: 112–121.

Reference: Prior, P. F. and Deacon, P. A. Spontaneous sleep in healthy subjects in long-term serial electroencephalographic recordings. *Electroenceph. clin. Neurophysiol.*, **1969,** *27*: 422–424

Electroencephalography and Clinical Neurophysiology
Elsevier Publishing Company, Amsterdam – Printed in The Netherlands

CORTICAL EVOKED POTENTIALS IN HEPATOLENTICULAR DEGENERATION

HANS LÜDERS, MOTOHIRO KATO AND YOSHIGORO KUROIWA

Department of Neurology, Kyushu University, Fukuoka (Japan)

(Accepted for publication: January 14, 1969)

Although electrophysiological changes in patients with hepatolenticular degeneration are not rare, only a few systematic studies are available.

Reported herein are cortical evoked potential changes observed in three patients with this condition. No previous similar reports are known to the authors.

MATERIAL AND METHOD

The patients studied were three men aged 31, 20 and 22 years and with a history of hepatolenticular degeneration for approximately 3, 2.5 and 1.5 years, respectively. The clinical diagnoses were corroborated by low levels of ceruloplasmin and serum copper. Results of routine liver function tests, including BSP (bromsulphthalein), were normal. One patient had borderline abnormal (some slow irregularities) and two had normal EEG. A control group of seventeen normal men, aged 19–29 years, were included in the study.

Electrical somato-sensory stimuli were applied to the median nerve using disc electrodes. The stimulus was a 0.1 msec square pulse of 10 V above the motor threshold for the thenar muscles. For photic stimulation a photic stimulator enclosed in a sound attenuating device was placed about 20 cm in front of the patient's eyes. Both types of stimuli were given at 1.25 sec intervals.

Needle scalp electrodes were fixed one on each side over the post-Rolandic areas, corresponding approximately to the cortical sensory hand area (Shagass and Schwartz 1964), and over the occipital regions according to the 10–20 system.

Recording was referential to the ipsilateral ear, upward deflections denoting negativity at the active electrodes. The time constant of the recording equipment was 0.1 sec.

The potentials from the scalp were recorded by an EEG apparatus and by a 4-channel magnetic tape recorder (TEAC,R-100). The read-out from the tape recorder went to a ATAC-401 digital computer (100 sample points available on each sweep), which was employed to obtain the summation of sequences of 100 stimulations, using analysis times of 62.5, 125, 250, 500 and 1000 msec. The evoked potentials corresponding to each kind of stimulation were recorded at least twice, using sequences of 100 stimulations.

The subject was placed in a supine position, in a semi-

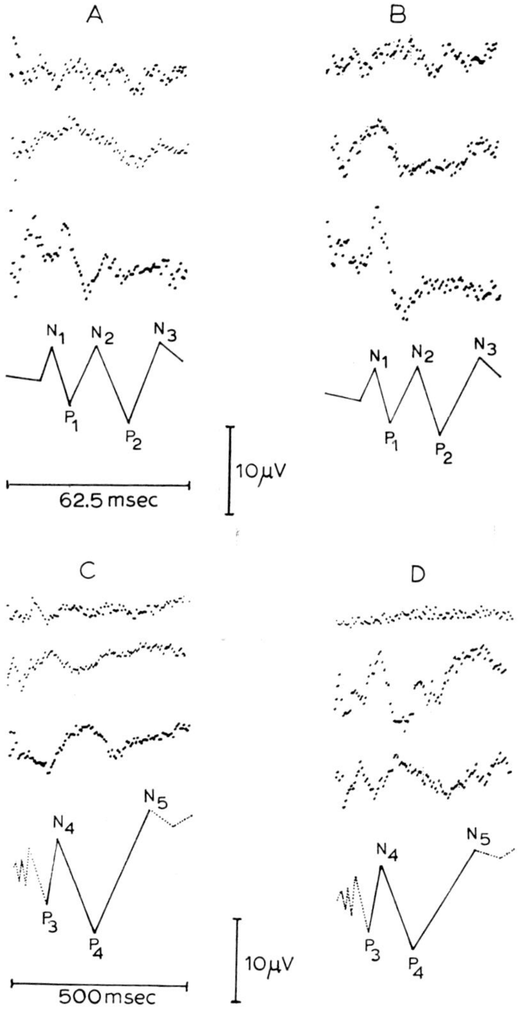

Fig. 1
Somato-sensory evoked potentials. In descending order are shown readings for patients 1, 2 and 3, and the average of the control group. *A*, *C*: Stimulation, right median nerve. Record, left post-Rolandic area. *B*, *D*: Stimulation, left median nerve. Record, right post-Rolandic area.

TABLE I

Somato-sensory evoked potentials. Latencies and amplitudes (62.5 msec analysis time)

	Latencies (msec)					Amplitudes (μV)			
	N_1	P_1	N_2	P_2	N_3	N_1–P_1	P_1–N_2	N_2–P_2	P_2–N_3
1. Stimulation, right median nerve. Record, left post-Rolandic area									
Patient 1	—	—	—	—	—	—	—	—	—
Patient 2	19.4	—	—	—	—	—	—	—	—
Patient 3	19.4	27.3	33.5	39.6	—	8.4	5.3	3.4	—
Normal group									
Mean value	18.3±0.9	24.3±1.5	32.5±2.4	43.5±2.7	54.7±3.8	6.8±2.3	6.7±2.5	8.8±2.2	9.3±4.2
Minimum and maximum value	16.7–19.4	22.0–26.9	30.4–37.8	38.5–49.5	48.8–61.7	3.9–11.3	3.9–12.4	3.9–12.4	3.6–16.8
2. Stimulation, left median nerve. Record, right post-Rolandic area									
Patient 1	—	—	—	—	—	—	—	—	—
Patient 2	19.4	26.4	—	—	—	6.3	—	—	—
Patient 3	19.4	28.2	35.2	—	—	14.4	4.7	—	—
Normal group									
Mean value	17.7±1.1	23.8±1.5	32.7±2.0	42.3±1.4	54.5±3.4	6.3±2.4	6.8±2.5	7.6±2.6	9.5±3.5
Minimum and maximum value	16.5–19.4	21.7–26.4	28.6–36.5	39.6–44.6	49.1–59.9	3.2–9.5	2.6–10.5	3.9–12.9	4.3–16.1

TABLE II

Somato-sensory evoked potentials. Latencies and amplitudes (500 msec analysis time)

	Latencies (msec)				Amplitudes (μV)		
	P_3	N_4	P_4	N_4	P_3–N_4	N_4–P_4	P_4–N_5
A. Stimulation, right median nerve. Record, left post-Rolandic area							
Patient 1	—	—	—	—	—	—	—
Patient 2	86	126	204	—	2.6	3.2	—
Patient 3	105	226	303	—	9.0	5.8	—
Normal group							
Mean value	93±11	131±15	225±40	388±35	7.8±3.0	11.2±3.7	13.5±3.5
Minimum and maximum value	70–116	114–183	162–274	332–436	3.9–15.8	6.8–17.7	6.5–18.4
B. Stimulation, left median nerve. Record, right post-Rolandic area							
Patient 1	—	—	—	—	—	—	—
Patient 2	86	134	204	423	8.7	10.6	11.2
Patient 3	105	169	317	465	6.4	6.4	5.8
Normal group							
Mean value	87±12	127±12	213±40	386±39	7.9±4.0	10.3±4.4	11.8±3.4
Minimum and maximum value	70–112	98–149	155–289	330–458	3.5–18.7	5.5–19.7	8.1–19.0

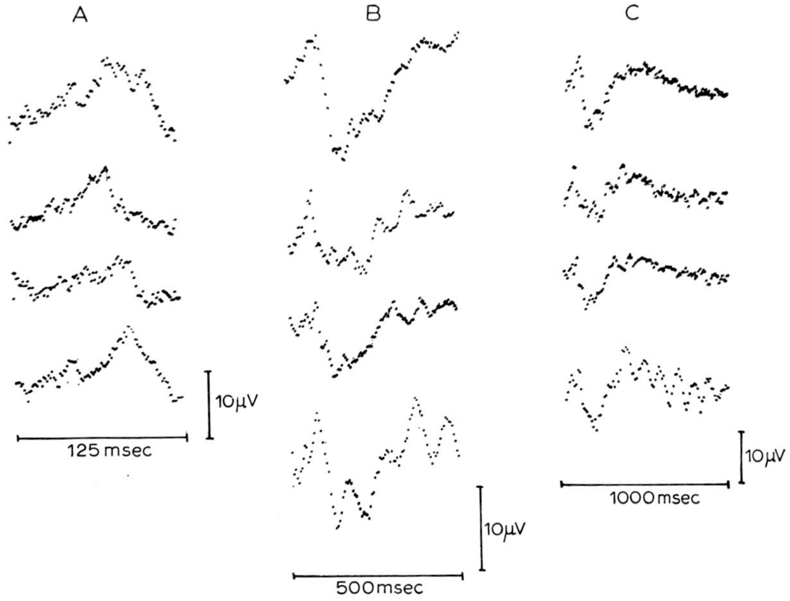

Fig. 2

Photically evoked potentials. Stimulation, flash. Record, occipital region. In descending order are shown readings for patients 1, 2 and 3, and a typical response of the control group. Note different analysis time in *A*, *B* and *C*.

dark room, with closed eyes. The alertness of the subject was assessed by means of the routine EEG.

RESULTS

1. Somato-sensory evoked potentials

These are shown in Fig. 1, using an analysis time of 62.5 msec (*A*, *B*) and of 500 msec (*C*, *D*). The corresponding latency and amplitude of each peak are tabulated in Tables I and II.

Patient 1 presented an extremely abnormal somatosensory evoked potential. It was impossible to differentiate from the background oscillation any one of the 9 peaks which were evident in the normal control group. The evoked responses in patients 2 and 3 showed a more or less well differentiated N_1 and P_1; it was even possible to distinguish N_2 in patient 3. N_3, which was usually the greatest negative peak when using an analysis time of 62.5 msec, could not be differentiated from the background oscillation in any of the patients.

In patient 2, the later components of the evoked response were of normal shape on both sides with P_3, N_4, P_4 and N_5. The response was of normal amplitude on the right side, but was of small amplitude on the left side (smaller than the smallest amplitude recognizable in the normal group). Patient 3 showed an abnormal variability of the later components of the evoked potentials, none of the responses falling within the normal range.

2. Photically evoked potentials

These are shown in Fig. 2 with analysis times of 125 (*A*), 500 (*B*) and 1000 msec (*C*). Taking in consideration the remarkable inter-individual variation of the visual potentials of our normal group the evoked potentials of the patients were within normal limits. Patient 1, in spite of the almost total absence of a somato-sensory evoked potential, showed visual evoked potentials of normal amplitudes.

Rhythmic after-discharges were not differentiated in the three patients whereas they were present in eleven of our seventeen normal subjects. (Since the summation of the routine EEG without any stimulation frequently reveals some rhythmic ondulations, we consider as after-discharges only periodic waves which appear after 200 msec, with a duration of about 100 msec, an amplitude of more than 7 μV and which are more than 2 times greater than the background oscillations measured by summation of the routine EEG using no stimulation.)

SUMMARY

1. Somato-sensory and visual evoked potentials have been studied in three patients with hepatolenticular degeneration.

2. In one patient all of the components of the somatosensory evoked potential were absent. In the other two patients prominent alterations of N_2, P_2 and N_3 were observed.

3. The visual evoked potentials were within normal limits in all patients, except for the absence of rhythmic after-discharges.

4. Our findings suggest that somato-sensory evoked potentials are a more sensitive test than EEG in hepatolenticular degeneration.

RÉSUMÉ

POTENTIELS ÉVOQUÉS CORTICAUX DANS LA DÉGÉNÉRESCENCE HÉPATOLENTICULAIRE

1. Les potentiels évoqués somato-sensitifs et visuels ont été étudiés chez trois malades atteints de dégénérescence hépatolenticulaire.

2. Chez un malade, toutes les composantes du potentiel évoqué somato-sensitif manquaient. Chez les deux autres on observait des altérations prévalentes de N_2, P_2 et N_3.

3. Les potentiels évoqués visuels étaient dans les limites du normal chez tous les malades, excepté en ce qui concerne l'absence de post-décharge rythmique.

4. Ces données suggèrent que les potentiels évoqués somato-sensitifs sont un test plus sensible que l'EEG dans la dégénérescence hépatolenticulaire.

REFERENCE

SHAGASS, C. and SCHWARTZ, M. Recovery functions of somatosensory peripheral nerve and cerebral evoked responses in man. *Electroenceph. clin. Neurophysiol.*, **1964,** *17*: 126–135.

Reference: LÜDERS, H., KATO, M. and KUROIWA, Y. Cortical evoked potentials in hepatolenticular degeneration. *Electroenceph. clin. Neurophysiol.*, **1969,** *27*: 425–428.

EFFECTS OF INTRAVENOUS DIAZEPAM (VALIUM) UPON EVOKED POTENTIALS OF PHOTOSENSITIVE EPILEPTIC AND NORMAL SUBJECTS[1]

MITURU EBE[2], KARL-HEINZ MEIER-EWERT[3] AND ROGER BROUGHTON[4]

Department of Neurology and Neurosurgery, McGill University and the Montreal Neurological Institute, Montreal, Quebec (Canada)

(Accepted for publication: January 17, 1969)

Diazepam (Valium) has been reported to have beneficial effects upon a number of neurological conditions including states of abnormally increased muscle tone (Katz *et al.* 1962; Fowlks *et al.* 1965; Symposia 1963, 1964) and recurrent epileptic seizures especially of petit mal absence, myoclonic or temporal lobe "psychomotor" type (Brock and Dyken 1963; Gastaut *et al.* 1965; Naquet *et al.* 1965; Trolle 1965; Weinberg and Harwell 1965; Muller *et al.* 1966).

Because of the remarkable responsiveness of components of the photosensitive state to diazepam (see Poiré *et al.* 1963, 1964), it was decided to investigate the drug's influence upon the visual and somato-sensory evoked potentials (VEP and SEP), the photomyoclonic response (PMR), the electroretinogram (ERG) and electro-oculographic (EOG) potentials in a number of patients with photosensitive epilepsy reported in a preceding paper (Broughton *et al.* 1969). Preliminary findings have been presented (Broughton *et al.* 1966; Ebe *et al.* 1967).

METHODS

The effects of i.v. diazepam were investigated in seven of the ten subjects with photosensitive epilepsy described in the preceding paper. Four had petit mal absences, two an Unverricht-Lundborg syndrome and one a Ramsay Hunt syndrome (average age 28.1 years). They were compared to nine control subjects consisting of non-paid students, colleagues and investigators, aged 18–44 years (average 29.2).

A polygraphic recording (EEG, EMG, EOG, EKG, respirogram, electrodermogram) was first performed to assess the nature and degree of photosensitivity and the effect of diazepam upon the photoconvulsive response (PCR) and PMR. Photic stimulation was given before, during and after the injection of diazepam at various flash frequencies with the eyes open and closed.

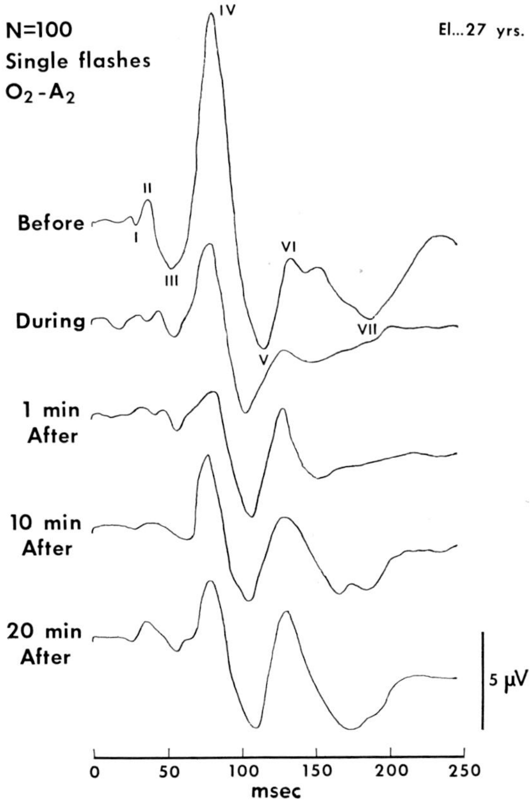

Fig. 1
Effects of diazepam upon the occipital VEP of a normal subject. Scalp positivity is recorded downwards in this and in all other records of cerebral evoked potentials.

[1] Supported in its early stages by a Fellowship of the Medical Research Council of Canada (Dr. Broughton).

[2] Visiting Scientist; presently Chief, Department of Physiology, Toranomon General Hospital, Tokyo, Japan.

[3] Fellow of the German Academic Exchange Service; presently Scientific Assistant, Neurologische Klinik mit Abteilung für klinische Neurophysiologie der Universität, Freiburg/Br., West Germany.

[4] Present address: Department of Medicine (Neurology), University of Ottawa, Ottawa, Ontario (Canada).

At least 4 days later, the evoked potentials were studied (see Broughton *et al.* 1969). These included a VEP, an SEP, an ERG and a peripheral EMG (to summate the PMR). Stimuli were delivered randomly every 1.5–2 sec. The EEG and peripheral EMGs were monitored by an Offner T apparatus. The degree of photosensitivity the day of the evoked potentials was assessed by using flash-trains before and after the administration of diazepam.

Diazepam was injected slowly (10 mg in 2 min) into the antecubital vein of thirteen subjects. In three others, the injection was stopped because of drowsiness or dizziness. The epileptic patients showed no such adverse effects. Evoked potentials were studied before, during and at various intervals up to 4 h after the injection. Subjects were requested to indicate any subjective change in the nature of the stimulus. The monitor EEG, as well as repeated clinical checks, allowed continuous assessment of the level of vigilance. Individual investigations lasted 3.5–5 h.

RESULTS

EEG, polygraphic studies and clinical effects

In all epileptic subjects, i.v. diazepam produced suppression and usually abolition of the photic induced cerebral and muscular responses (PCR and PMR). This effect was almost immediate and often became evident after administration of only 5–6 mg of the drug. The oculoclonic and frontal muscle responses, when present, were similarly quickly abolished, the autonomic effects of flicker (tachycardia, tachypnea, electrodermal responses) became minimal, and the muscle tone decreased. Spontaneous generalized spike and wave or poly-spike and wave discharges and myoclonus (bilateral and associated with spontaneous and evoked EEG discharges in two patients, disseminated and fragmentary in two patients, and action myoclonus in one patient) were also suppressed.

The EEG of both normal and epileptic subjects quickly showed 18–22 c/sec beta activity first over the fronto-central regions then diffusely also over the parieto-occipital areas.

No epileptic patients experienced side effects. Most subjects described a decrease in subjective intensity of the flash allowing them to look more easily at the stroboscope. Some subjects also mentioned that the visual after-image was weaker and of shorter duration. Feelings of bodily relaxation and mental calm were described.

In epileptic subjects the injection was frequently followed by a diminution in seizure frequency for at least 2–3 days.

Visual evoked potentials

The effects of i.v. diazepam upon the VEP (see Broughton *et al.* 1969) were similar in both groups (Fig. 1 and 2). Over the occipital region, components I, II and III, when clearly recognizable, usually exhibited a decrease in amplitude, with or without an increase in latency, and in three cases disappeared completely. In others, however, they appeared little changed. Component

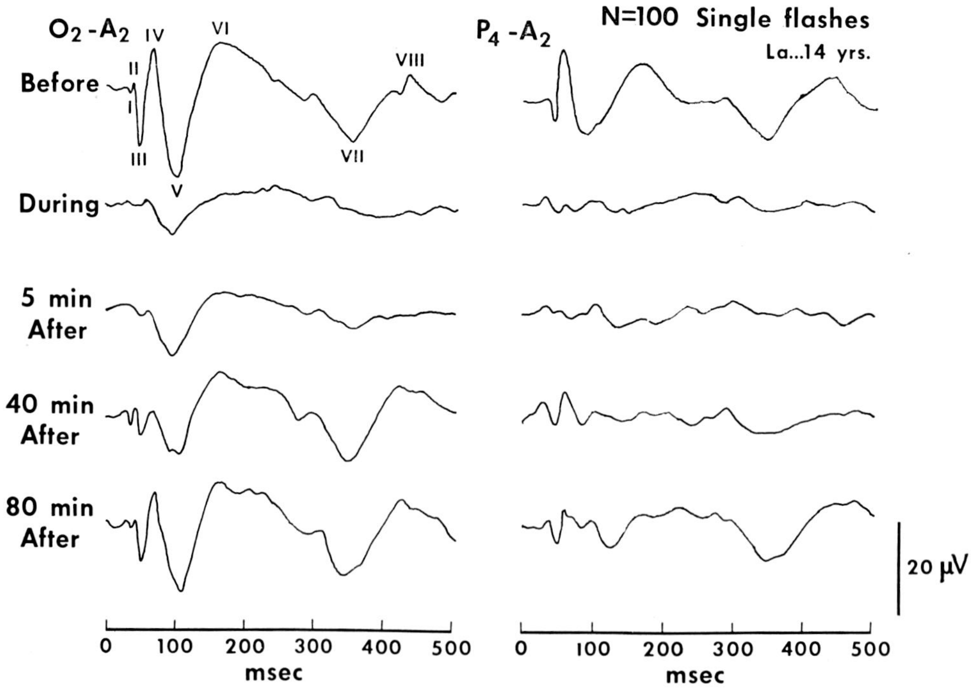

Fig. 2
Effect of i.v. diazepam upon the VEP in photosensitive epilepsy.

IV showed a consistent and marked decrease in amplitude, often associated with decrease or increase in latency. Sometimes this negative component disappeared completely and was replaced by a positivity of similar latency which eventually could either become confluent with component III thereby reducing its peak latency or, occasionally, with component V, leading to an increase in its peak latency. The positive component V was consistently more resistant than component IV to diazepam injections but did decrease in peak amplitude and showed variable changes in latency. Negativity VI by comparison was very sensitive, usually disappearing completely and sometimes producing an apparent broadening of component V (Fig. 2) or even apparently being replaced by a large positivity. Components VII and VIII were usually suppressed. In two cases a monophasic component V was changed to a triphasic complex V–VI–VII. The after-rhythm was regularly abolished.

The summation of smaller samples ($N = 25$ or 10) indicated that diazepam also considerably reduced the variability of the VEP.

The spatial distribution of the VEP was strikingly affected. In four of the seven epileptic subjects in which components I–V (or the complex V–VI–VII) were present at the C_3, C_4 electrodes, such components usually became localized to the occipital electrode after diazepam. The VEP of those rare normal subjects in whom components V, IV or even III were recorded at the C_3, C_4 electrodes underwent a similar reduction in anterior spread.

In those subjects whose C_3, C_4 electrodes exhibited a VEP with a wave form similar to that often recorded maximal at the C_z area (see Broughton *et al.* 1969), identifiable components A, B, C, D (differing from the occipital response) were markedly reduced in amplitude.

The VEP to single flashes gradually reverted to their pre-injection features over a period of 1.5–4 h (*cf.* Fig. 2).

When the two normal subjects passed into light sleep, the monitor EEG contained central 12–14 c/sec spindle activity which was easily distinguishable from the more rapid 18–22 c/sec drug induced beta activity. The occipital VEP then showed the positivity at 60–80 msec followed by a large amplitude negativity peaking at 120–200 msec.

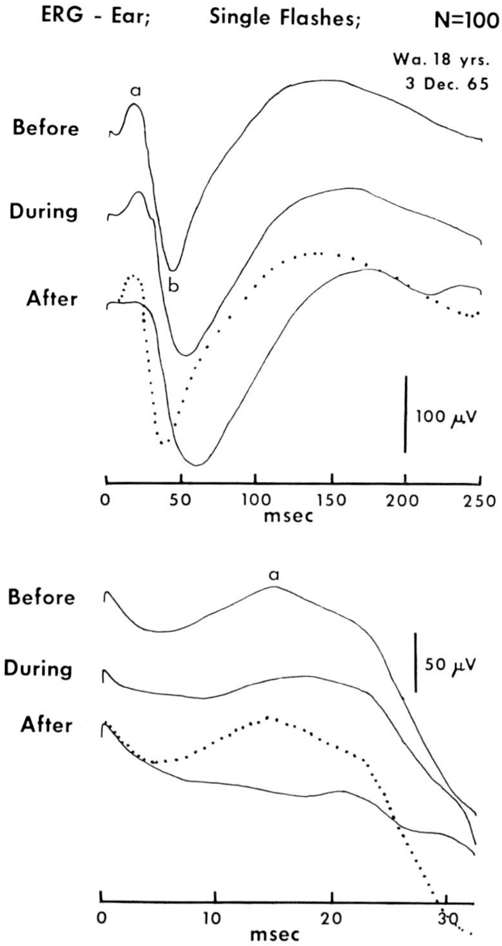

Fig. 3

Effects of diazepam upon the ERG at different post-stimulus analysis times. In this and in subsequent illustrations downward-directed deflections indicate positivity at the corneal electrode. Dotted curves are superimposed pre-injection responses.

Electroretinogram

The modification of the ERG was very stereotyped (Fig. 3, 4) in all (epileptic or normal) subjects. The corneal negative *a* wave showed a consistent decrease in amplitude (mean of 65 to 35 μV) and an increase in latency (17 to 19 msec). The *b* wave (corneal positivity) underwent an increase both in mean peak latency (50 to 65 msec) and in duration, the wave becoming broader. Changes in amplitude of the *b* wave, however, were variable and slight. Perusal of individual ERG responses suggested that some retinal light adaptation took place initially in the series, as was indicated by a tendency for a decrease in amplitude of the *b* wave (Fig. 4). This effect was not sufficiently marked to influence the reliability of changes attributable directly to the drug.

Electro-oculogram

EOG (monitored by supra- and infra-orbital electrodes) contained potentials due mainly to vertical eye movements but also apparently to palpebral movement (slow potentials seen only at the supra-orbital electrode) and to contraction of frontal and facial muscles. The initial EOG changes (frontal positive at 58 ± 4 msec, negative at 68 ± 6 msec, positive at 82 ± 8 msec), which were due to reflex movements of the eyeball, decreased in amplitude and increased in latency following diazepam. The later potentials at the supra-orbital electrode, presumably of palpebral origin, were usually reduced considerably, or even disappeared (the subjects were also observed to blink less frequently).

Somato-sensory evoked potentials

I.v. diazepam (Fig. 5) reduced by about 30–40% the

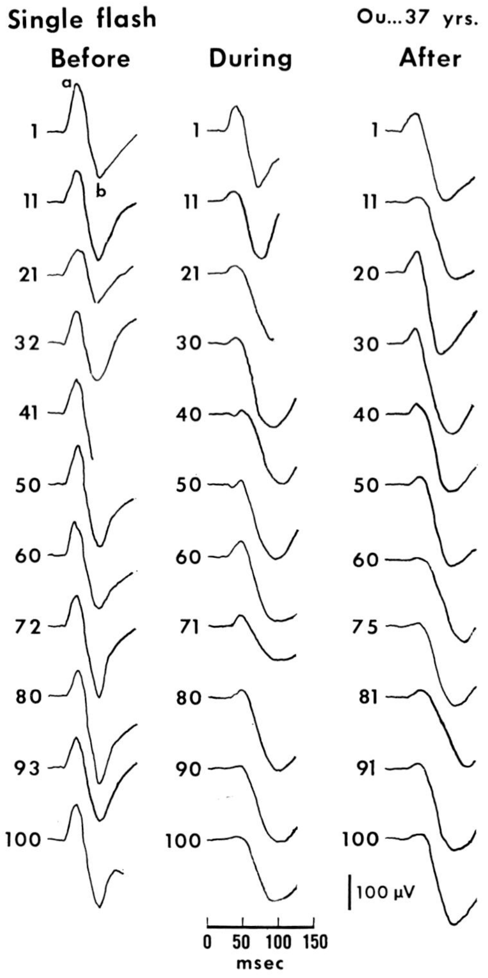

Fig. 4
Effects of diazepam upon single ERG responses in a photosensitive epileptic subject. Approximately every tenth response has been selected. The individual responses were chosen for lack of eye movement or other artifact. Two curves are incomplete, as they were deformed by artifacts during their later parts.

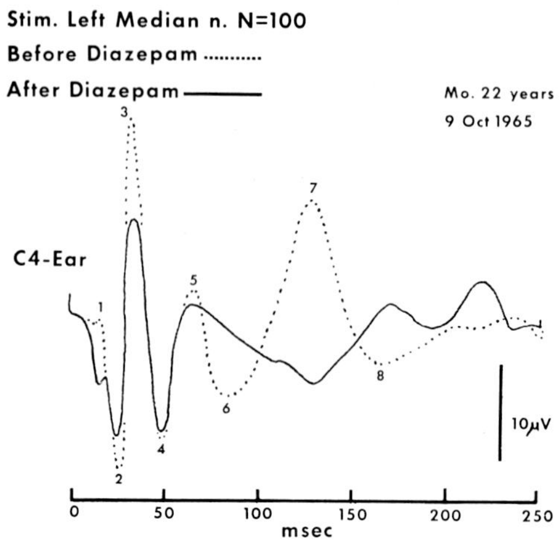

Fig. 5
Effects of diazepam upon the SEP of a photosensitive epileptic subject.

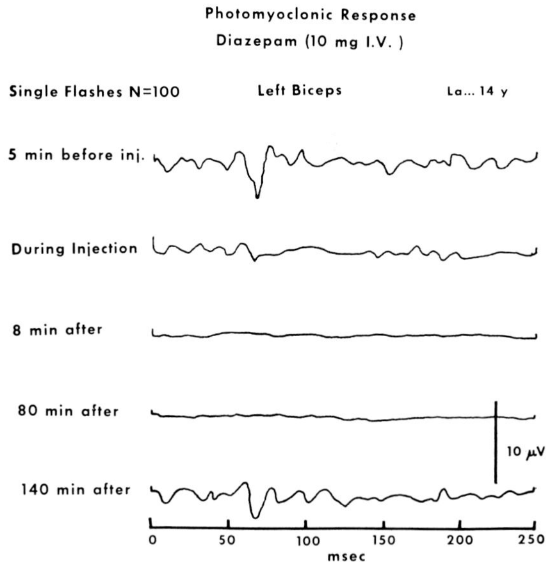

Fig. 6
Effects of diazepam upon the summated photomyoclonic response of a photosensitive epileptic patient.

amplitude of early SEP components 2 and 3 which also became more localized to the central region. Components 5 and perhaps 6 were less affected, and the late negative component 7 disappeared completely or was even replaced by a positivity (Fig. 5). The results were qualitatively similar for all four epileptic subjects in whom the effects of diazepam on the SEP were studied.

Photomyoclonic response

Computer summation of the peripheral muscle jerk (Fig. 6), which is believed to be usually an abnormal enhancement of the normal subclinical photomotor response of Bickford (Meier-Ewert and Broughton 1967), confirmed that such a response is abolished by diazepam. The PMR usually returned after 80–160 min.

DISCUSSION

Our results confirm the earlier clinical studies of Poiré *et al.* (1963, 1964) and the experimental work in the photosensitive baboon of Killam *et al.* (1967) of the effects of diazepam upon the PCR, PMR and autonomic responses.

The ERG effects, inasmuch as they were not similar to those described for a number of physiologic conditions (such as variations of light adaptation, stimulus intensity, stimulus duration or area of retina stimulated—Jacobson 1961), appear to reflect direct drug effects. A similar decrease in total ERG amplitude has been described following administration of diazepam in the cat by Lanoir *et al.* (1965). Since the *a* wave amplitude and *b* wave latency (but not *b* wave amplitude) are believed to reflect photo-chemical events, diazepam probably affects these photo-chemical mechanisms (although changes in centrifugal retinal control—Jacobson 1961—cannot be excluded).

The tendency for decreased amplitudes and increased latencies of VEP components I–III can be compared to similar effects in the cat upon the evoked positive–negative potential recorded at the chiasma (indicating that the retinal efferent discharges in fact do diminish), lateral geniculate body and striate cortex (Requin *et al.* 1963; Lanoir *et al.* 1965). Moreover these animal experiments showed that the negative components of the cortical responses were more affected than positive ones. This also holds true in man, where negative component IV and VI are most sensitive, sometimes being replaced by positivities, and where positive V is altered least. The anterior spread of the VEP in photosensitive epileptic subjects was abolished by diazepam, and apparent vertex-type responses picked up at the lateral central electrode were markedly diminished. A similar suppression of fronto-central responses has been reported for the naturally photosensitive baboon *Papio papio* (Killam *et al.* 1967). This is perhaps the most important single change in reducing photosensitivity, as evoked potentials in the photosensitive group are altered most markedly in this region, suggesting participation of a subcortico-cortical and perhaps a localized fronto-central cortical mechanism (Broughton *et al.* 1969).

The effects of diazepam in photosensitive epileptic subjects are only *quantitatively* different from those in non-epileptic normal subjects and represent a tendency to normalization of the VEP. The VEP effects, like those of the ERG, are not similar to those described for variations of stimulus characteristics, light–dark adaptation, level of vigilance or other physiological changes (Gastaut and Régis 1965), and therefore appear to be directly related to effects of the drugs.

The suppression of later midline components of apparent unspecific origin in both the VEP and SEP are of interest, both because of their possible relevance to the genesis of photosensitivity and because of the experimental evidence of decrease following diazepam of the evoked potentials recorded in the mesencephalic reticular formation (Requin *et al.* 1963; Hernández-Peón *et al.* 1964; Lanoir *et al.* 1965). The reduced autonomic reactivity may be related to such a brain-stem action, or may be due to the known inhibitory influence of the drug upon rhinencephalic structures, especially the amygdala (Requin *et al.* 1963; Hernández-Peón *et al.* 1964; Schallek *et al.* 1964; Schallek and Kuehn 1965).

The effects of diazepam upon motor systems were also very striking. It reduced or abolished the PMR and the oculoclonic response, as well as markedly decreasing background muscle tone. These changes may be attributed to decreased excitability of spinal motoneurones, as evidenced by the inhibition of the H reflex following i.v. diazepam in man (Broughton *et al.* 1968). The precise site of drug action is undetermined, but might either be directly upon the anterior horn cells or upon brain-stem structures modulating their excitability. It is so powerful that in certain circumstances it may lead to apparent cessation of the motor expression of clinical seizures without affecting the cerebral discharge, as reflected in scalp recordings. This dissociation is commonly observed in the case of the periodic myoclonus of subacute inclusion body encephalitis (Broughton *et al.* 1968). It can also occur in temporal lobe seizures with ipsiversion or contraversion (unpublished observations). EEG control is therefore essential for full assessment of the effects of i.v. diazepam.

SUMMARY

The effects of 7.5–10.0 mg of i.v. diazepam were studied in seven patients with photo-sensitive epilepsy and in nine normal controls. Minimal side effects (drowsiness, dizziness and slurred speech) occurred in three controls, but not in the epileptic subjects.

Diazepam very rapidly blocked the photoconvulsive and photomyoclonic responses of epileptic subjects, as well as reducing the blinking and autonomic or vegetative changes induced by photic stimulation. Spontaneous epileptic discharges were also abolished. In both epileptic and normal subjects, beta activity appeared in the EEG maximally in anterior head regions, and marked hypotonia and subjective relaxation were induced.

Visual and somato-sensory evoked potentials (VEP and SEP) and the electroretinogram (ERG) were modified. In epileptics, early occipital VEP components were somewhat decreased in amplitude and increased in latency, and later components underwent variable effects, the most consistent being reduction in amplitude of negative components IV and VI. The VEP after-rhythm was abolished; and apparent midline central responses were greatly attenuated, as was the anterior spread of occipital components. Similar but less marked effects were observed in controls. The SEP in epileptics underwent a consistent reduction in amplitude and became more localized to the central region. The ERG *a* wave decreased in amplitude and *b* wave increased in peak latency and duration. All evoked potential changes appeared to be directly related to the action of the drug.

The effects of i.v. diazepam on the evoked potentials of photosensitive epileptics in large part appeared to represent a normalization of cerebral reactivity.

RÉSUMÉ

EFFETS DU DIAZEPAM (VALIUM) INTRAVEINEUX SUR LES POTENTIELS ÉVOQUÉS DES ÉPILEPTIQUES PHOTOSENSIBLES ET DES SUJETS NORMAUX

L'effet de 7.5 à 10.0 mg de diazepam intraveineux a été étudié chez sept malades atteints d'épilepsie photosensible et chez neuf sujets normaux. Des effets secondaires minimes (somnolence, vertiges et bagouillement) ont été observés chez trois sujets de contrôles, mais chez aucun sujet épileptique.

Le diazepam bloque très rapidement les réponses photoconvulsives et photomyocloniques des sujets épileptiques, de même qu'il réduit le clignement et les modifications autonomes ou végétatives induites par la stimulation photique. Les décharges épileptiques spontanées sont également abolies. Chez les sujets normaux et chez les épileptiques, une activité beta apparaît à l'EEG, maximum dans les régions antérieures, et une hypotonie marquée est induite avec sensation subjective de détente.

Les potentiels évoqués visuels et somato-sensitifs et l'électrorétinogramme sont modifiés. Chez les épileptiques, les composantes précoces du potentiel évoqué visuel occipital sont quelque peu diminuées en amplitude et augmentées en latence, et les composantes plus tardives subissent des effets variables, dont le plus constant est la réduction d'amplitude des composantes négatives IV et VI. La post-décharge du potentiel évoqué visuel est abolie. Les réponses centrales apparaissant au niveau de la ligne médiane sont nettement atténuées, de même que la diffusion antérieure des composantes occipitales. Des effets similaires mais moins marqués sont observés chez les sujets de contrôle. Les potentiels évoqués somatosensitifs des épileptiques subissent une réduction nette d'amplitude et deviennent plus localisés à la région centrale. L'onde *a* de l'électrorétinogramme diminue d'amplitude et la latence du pic et la durée de l'onde *b* augmentent. Toutes les modifications des potentiels évoqués paraissent être directement liées à l'action de la drogue.

Les effets du diazepam intraveineux sur les potentiels évoqués des épileptiques photosensibles paraissent représenter en grande partie une normalisation de la réactivité cérébrale.

The patients were kindly referred by Drs. F. Andermann, D. Lloyd-Smith, F. McNaughton and P. Robb. Mr. W. Gibson provided technical assistance and Mr. C. Hodge photographed the illustrations.

Injectable diazepam (Valium) was supplied for the investigations by the generosity of Hoffman-La Roche, Montreal, Quebec (Canada).

REFERENCES

BROCK, J. T. and DYKEN, M. The anticonvulsant activity of chlordiazepoxide and Re 5-2807. *Neurology (Minneap.)*, **1963,** *13*: 59–65.

BROUGHTON, R., MEIER-EWERT, K. and EBE, M. Visual and somato-sensory evoked potentials of photosensitive epileptic subjects during wakefulness, sleep and following i.v. diazepam (Valium). *Electroenceph. clin. Neurophysiol.*, **1966,** *21*: 622.

BROUGHTON, R. J., MEIER-EWERT, K.-H. and EBE, M. Evoked visual, somato-sensory and retinal potentials in photosensitive epilepsy. *Electroenceph. clin. Neurophysiol.*, **1969,** *27*: 373–386.

BROUGHTON, R., VERA, C., MEIER-EWERT, K., EBE, M. and ANDERMANN, F. H-reflex studies and the effects of i.v. diazepam (Valium) in subacute sclerosing leucoencephalitis. *Electroenceph. clin. Neurophysiol.*, **1968,** *24*: 288.

EBE, M., MEIER-EWERT, K. and BROUGHTON, R. Further studies of i.v. diazepam (Valium) and evoked potentials of photosensitive epileptic subjects and normal controls. *Electroenceph. clin. Neurophysiol.*, **1967,** *23*: 492–493.

FOWLKS, E. W., STRICKLAND, D. A. and PEIRSON, G. A. Control of spastic states in neurological patients with diazepam. *Amer. J. phys. Med.*, **1965,** *44*: 9–19.

GASTAUT, H. and RÉGIS, H. Visually-evoked potentials recorded transcranially in man. In L. D. PROCTOR and W. R. ADEY (Eds.), *Symposium on the analysis of central nervous system and cardiovascular data using computer methods.* NASA, Washington, D.C., **1965,** *Spec. Publ. 72*: 7–34.

GASTAUT, H., RÉGIS, J., SOULAYROL, R., LOB, H. et TASSINARI, C. A. L'action du diazepam (Valium) dans le traitement de formes non-convulsives de l'épilepsie généralisée. *Rev. neurol.*, **1965,** *112*: 99–118.

HERNÁNDEZ-PEÓN, R., ROJAS-TAMIREZ, J. A., O'FLAHERTY, J. J. and MAZZUCHELLI-O'FLAHERTY, A. L. The experimental study of the anticonvulsive and relaxant actions of Valium. *Int. J. Neuropharmacol.*, **1964,** *3*: 405–412.

JACOBSON, J. H. *Clinical electroretionography.* Thomas, Sprinfield, Ill., **1961,** 167 p.

KATZ, R. A., ALDES, J. H. and RECTOR, M. A new drug approach to muscle relaxation. *J. Neuropsychiat.*, **1962,** *3, Suppl. 1*: 91–95.

KILLAM, K. F., KILLAM, E. K. and NAQUET, R. An animal model of light sensitive epilepsy. *Electroenceph. clin. Neurophysiol.*, **1967,** *22*: 497–513.

LANOIR, J., REQUIN, S., DOLCE, G. et CHIRINOS, E. Étude neurophysiologique comparative de deux drogues anticonvulsantes: le Valium et le Mogadon. *(Congress of Electroencephalography and Clinical Neurophysiology), Excerpta med. (Amst.)*, **1965**: 49.

MEIER-EWERT, K. and BROUGHTON, R. J. Photomyoclonic response of epileptic and non-epileptic subjects during wakefulness, sleep and arousal. *Electroenceph. clin. Neurophysiol.*, **1967,** *23*: 142–151.

MULLER, H. R. VON, KLINGLES, M., KAESER, H. E. und HIRT, H. R. Zur Behandlung des Status epilepticus, mit Diazepam (Valium). Erfahrungen in 12 Fallen. *Schweiz. med. Wschr.*, **1966,** *96*: 121–127.

NAQUET, R., SOULAYROL, R., DOLCE, G., TASSINARI, C., BROUGHTON, R. and LOB, H. First attempts at treatment of experimental status epilepticus in man with diazepam (Valium). *Electroenceph. clin. Neurophysiol.*, **1965,** *18*: 427.

POIRÉ, R., DEGRAEVE, M. et BECK, L. Comparaison des propriétés anticonvulsantes du chlordiazepoxide (Librium) et du diazepam (Valium) par l'étude électroclinique de l'inhibition des réponses paroxystiques à la stimulation photique intermittante. *C. R. Congr. Psych. Neurol.*, **1963,** *61*: 570–582.

POIRÉ, R., DEGRAEVE, M. et BECK, L. Étude électrographique comparative de l'action inhibitrice de certaines drogues (trimethadione, acetazolamide, dichlorphenamide, chlordiazepoxide, diazepam) sur les photomyoclonies de l'homme. *Rev. neurol.*, **1964,** *110*: 270–290.

REQUIN, S., LANOIR, J., PLAS, R. et NAQUET, R. Étude comparative des effets neurophysiologiques du "Librium" et du "Valium". *C. R. Soc. Biol. (Paris)*, **1963,** *157*: 2015–2019.

SCHALLEK, W. and KUEHN, A. An action of Mogadon on the amygdala of the cat. *Med. Pharmacol. exp.*, **1965,** *12*: 204–208.

SCHALLEK, W., ZABRANSKY, F. and KUEHN, A. Effects of benzodiazepines on central nervous system of cat. *Arch. int. Pharmacodyn.*, **1964,** *145*: 467–483.

Symposium on Diazepam. *West. Medicine.*, **1963,** *4*, *Suppl. 1*: 1–64.

Symposium of Diazepam ("Valium"). *Ann. phys. Med.*, **1964,** *June Suppl.*

TROLLE, E. Diazepam (Valium) in the treatment of epilepsy. *Acta neurol. scand.*, **1965,** *41*, *Suppl. 13*: 535–539.

WEINBERG, W. A. and HARWELL, J. L. Diazepam (Valium) in myoclonic seizures. Favourable response during infancy and childhood. *Amer. J. Dis. Child.*, **1965,** *109*: 123–127.

Reference: EBE, M., MEIER-EWERT, K.-H. and BROUGHTON, R. Effects of intravenous diazepam (Valium) upon evoked potentials of photosensitive epileptic and normal subjects. *Electroenceph. clin. Neurophysiol.*, **1969,** *27*: 429–435.

ANNOUNCEMENT

AMERICAN BOARD OF QUALIFICATION IN ELECTROENCEPHALOGRAPHY

The Board of Qualification of the American Electroencephalographic Society has been reorganized by agreement among the American EEG Society, the American Academy of Neurology, and the American Neurological Association, and has been incorporated under the name American Board of Qualification in Electroencephalography, Inc. The new Board has been expanded to seven members, including one each nominated by the AAN and ANA.

The present Board is as follows:

Chairman:
Daniel Silverman, M.D., Philadelphia, Pa.
Secretary-Treasurer:
Robert J. Ellingson, Ph.D., M.D., Omaha, Neb.
Robert J. Joynt, M.D., Rochester, N.Y. (ANA Member)
Kenneth A. Kooi, M.D., Ann Arbor, Mich.
Richard P. Schmidt, M.D., Gainsville, Fla. (AAN Member)
Jolyon S. Tucker, M.D., Hartford, Conn.
Richard D. Walter, M.D., Los Angeles, Calif.

The American Board of Qualification in Electroencephalography, Inc., held oral examinations in Omaha, Nebraska, April 9 and 10, 1969. The following candidates were qualified:

James Battershill, M.D., Winnipeg, Man.
James C. Daniels, M.D., Maywood, Ill.
Stephen J. Dutch, M.D., Omaha, Neb.
Andrija Lauber, M.D., Iowa City, Iowa
William S. Masland, M.D., Philadelphia, Pa.
Peter Morgan, M.D., Iowa City, Iowa
Richard R. North, M.D., Dallas, Texas
Sandra Forbes Olson, M.D., Chicago, Ill.
Lorenzo G. Runk, M.D., Montgomery, Ala.
Barry R. Tharp, M.D., Palo Alto, Calif.

Diplomates of the former Board of Qualification of the American EEG Society are eligible to receive the certificate of the new Board on application and payment of a nominal fee. They will be notified individually.

The next written examination will be given on January 10, 1970. The next oral examination will be given at Duke University, Durham, North Carolina in March 1970. Completed applications for examination must be submitted by November 15, 1969. Information and application forms may be obtained from the Secretary, Nebraska Psychiatric Institute, 602 South 44th Avenue, Omaha, Nebraska 68105.

Electroencephalography and Clinical Neurophysiology
Elsevier Publishing Company, Amsterdam – Printed in The Netherlands

TECHNICAL CONTRIBUTIONS

A METHOD FOR DETECTING CHANGE IN A TIME SERIES APPLIED TO NEWBORN EEG[1]

RICHARD H. JONES[2], DAVID H. CROWELL[3] AND LINDA E. KAPUNIAI[3]

University of Hawaii, Honolulu, Hawaii 96822 (U.S.A.)

(Accepted for publication: January 30, 1969)

The advent of analog to digital converters has provided a source of precisely recorded accurate digital representation of the EEG which in turn has permitted processing large samples of the EEG by means of computer techniques (see Brazier, 1961). A critical problem, however, has been the lack of a technique for determining whether a change has occurred in the EEG and the statistical significance of such changes. The model described herein was developed to enable the researcher to make objective evaluations of possible changes in the EEG of a single subject during and after stimulation. No attempt is made, however, to interpret the statistical changes in terms of specific neurophysiological mechanisms.

METHOD

A series of 10 stimuli designed for the purpose of examining sensory reactivity and arousal within the visual, auditory, tactile and olfactory modalities was presented to a 2-day-old male neonate who was in a quiescent state. The stimuli were as follows:

1. A 40 W incandescent light directed toward the subject's eyes for 3 sec from a distance of 61 cm (L_1).
2. A 60 dB modulated pure tone at 1000 c/sec with a duration of 4 sec, emanating from a speaker placed 17.8 cm from the subject's ear. This tone was produced by a Beltone audiometer, Model 10A, sound reference level, 0.0002 dynes/cm^2, and modulated at 5% of the basic frequency at a rate of 6 c/sec by an Allison Warble Tone Adapter, Model 101 ($S_1$60 dB 1000 c/sec).
3. A second 60 dB pure tone equivalent to stimulus 2 but at 8000 c/sec ($S_1$60 dB 8000 c/sec).
4. A second light like the first, but using a 75 W lamp (L_2).
5. An 80 dB 1000 c/sec tone presented as in item 2 ($S_2$80 dB 1000 c/sec).
6. An 80 dB 8000 c/sec tone as in item 2 ($S_2$80 dB 8000 c/sec).
7. A puff of nitrogen having a pressure of 1.68 atm, 10 lb/sq. in., delivered through a vented plastic cone placed on the infant's abdomen above the umbilicus for 0.5 sec (N_2).
8. A series of 5/sec 60 dB auditory clicks produced by a Grass PS-2 Photic Stimulator synchronization circuit for a period of 2 sec (AC).
9. Full-strength glacial acetic acid on a Q-tip, held 5 mm from the subject's nose for 2 sec (O).
10. Repetitive photic stimulation at a rate of 5/sec for 6 sec from a Grass PS-2 Photic Stimulator, intensity "8", with the lamp 25 cm from the subject's eyes (Photic).

The EEG recordings were obtained from Grass silver disc electrodes approximating C_3 linked to C_4, referred to A_1. EEGs were recorded on an Offner Type R dynograph at a sensitivity setting of 50 μV/cm with a paper speed of 10 mm/sec.

The EEG signals were digitized by an Electronic Engineering Company of California Model 762 analog to digital converter and recorded on a Precision Instrument Model 1167F incremental digital tape recorder. The sampling rate for the digital tape recorder was 72 samples/sec. Every 4th sample was the EEG, and every 20th was the stimulus event channel; the stimulus channel was one sample-interval before the EEG. Other physiological data were recorded on the intervening channels, but are not reported here.

The sampling rate was, therefore, 18 samples/sec on the EEG and 3.6 samples/sec for the stimulus event marker. The digitized EEG was converted to μV at the University of Hawaii Statistical and Computing Center on an IBM 360/50 computer. For each stimulus, 196 pre-stimulus data points (approximately 10.8 sec) and 200 post-stimulus onset data points (approximately 11 sec) constituted the basic data used in the analysis.

Change detection model

A digitized EEG signal is a time series; that is, it

[1] Preparation of this manuscript was supported in part by Research Grant HD00869-06 and Training Grant HD00079-04 from the National Institute of Child Health and Human Development, and in part by the Pacific Biomedical Research Center (DHC), and by the Air Force Office of Scientific Research under Contract No. F 44620-69-C-0035 (RHJ). Assistance of the University of Hawaii Statistical and Computing Center is also acknowledged.

[2] Information Sciences Program.

[3] Newborn Psychological Research Laboratory. Department of Psychology and Pacific Biomedical Research Center.

possesses some randomness or lack of complete predictability. Because the data are collected in time, the usual assumption of statistical independence which is necessary for standard statistical tests is violated. Therefore, it is necessary to attempt to remove the statistical dependence. The technique used herein for removing this statistical dependence is auto-regression; that is, predicting each observation using past observations. If this prediction is carried out correctly, the difference between the predicted and actual observation represents the random input (sometimes called innovation) to the time series. This random input or innovation represents the unpredictable component of the observation at a given time. Statistical tests can be performed on these random differences. If the structure or underlying parameters of the process do not vary with time, these differences will have a variability which can be estimated; however, if a change occurs, such as an evoked response, much larger differences would be observed. This is the basis for the proposed method of change detection.

The model considered here is an auto-regression of order p,

$$x_t = \mu + \alpha_1 (x_{t-1} - \mu) + \alpha_2 (x_{t-2} - \mu) + \ldots + \alpha_p (x_{t-p} - \mu) + \varepsilon_t \quad (1)$$

where μ is the process mean and $\alpha_1, \ldots, \alpha_p$ are the auto-regressive parameters to be estimated. Under certain assumptions (Jones 1964), Equation 1 is a stationary model. It is, therefore, appropriate during pre-stimulus intervals since the subject is in a quiescent state. If the data are truly a pth order auto-regression, the errors, ε_t, are uncorrelated in time (Quenouille 1949) with variance, σ^2. These errors represent the random inputs to the time series. This means that all information which can be extracted from the past by linear methods has, in fact, been extracted, and that deviations of the one-step predicted values from observed values are uncorrelated. Based on this, statistical tests for change can be designed. If ε_t are correlated in time, the order of the auto-regression should be increased in an attempt to remove this correlation. Therefore, a major task is to determine the correct order auto-regression to remove serial correlation.

Durbin (1960) has developed a step-wise method for estimating the auto-regressive parameters of a time series. The equations are similar to the usual step-wise techniques in ordinary regression (Efroymsen 1960), except that Durbin's (1960) equations are simpler, making use of the symmetries of stationary process covariance matrices. Jones (1964) used the latter technique on meteorological data and included a test of significance at each step in order to indicate when the correct order auto-regression has been fit to the data.

Testing for change

After selection of the appropriate order auto-regression, one-step predictions are made using the following equation:

$$\hat{x}_t = \hat{\mu} + \hat{a}_1 (x_{t-1} - \hat{\mu}) + \hat{a}_2 (x_{t-2} - \hat{\mu}) + \ldots + \hat{a}_p (x_{t-p} - \hat{\mu}). \quad (2)$$

Let $\hat{\sigma}$ be the estimated variance of the one-step prediction error. For a Gaussian process the prediction error squared divided by this estimated variance is approximately distributed as chi-square with one degree of freedom (d.f.). These predictions are made by starting at the beginning at time $p + 1$ and moving forward point by point to the end of the data. A large chi-square is obtained when the predicted value is far from the observed value, indicating that a change has occurred. A change in the form of an evoked response or increase in variance would give large values of chi-square. There is also the possibility that the predictions will be extremely close to the observed value. This would give a low chi-square, which is likewise significant and indicative of change. Therefore, a two-tailed test of change is possible which uses both low values of chi-square (close to zero) and large values of chi-square. A simple decrease in the variance of the process without a change in the shape of the spectrum would tend to show up as a low chi-square. Based on these two approaches, change can be detected at any point in the time series.

If no change occurs, the sequence of chi-squares will be essentially independent. In order to test for change in an interval, the chi-squares can be summed over the interval, giving a new chi-square with the appropriate d.f. The smoothing procedure is more likely to detect a change that persists in the interval being tested. This smoothing was done here using a moving sum, summing the chi-squares over a time interval, shifting one point forward and summing again until all the data points were used. The summed chi-squares now have d.f. equal to the number of points entering into the sum. Only the summed chi-squares from non-overlapping intervals are independent. The 1 d.f. chi-squares are used for temporal resolution and the summed chi-squares increase the power of the statistical test over an interval. A Fortran IV program has been developed to implement the above analysis.

RESULTS

The pre-stimulus EEG for all 10 stimuli was scanned to determine if any artifact was present that would invalidate the stationary assumption. On this basis, the $S_2$80 dB 1000 c/sec stimulus was not included in the statistical analysis. Using the step-wise procedure, auto-regressions of increasing order were fit to the pre-stimulus data of the 9 stimuli. A 9th or 10th order auto-regression was appropriate. Proceeding to the test for change, one-step predictions were made using the 10th order auto-regression. The difference between the predicted and observed values squared was divided by the one-step prediction variance, giving the chi-square test for change. The moving sum over 9 time points gave tests for change over 0.5 sec intervals.

Analysis of the 9 stimuli showed that there was a clear response to the photic, $S_1$60 dB 8000 c/sec and olfactory stimuli. Plots of 3 of the 9 stimuli (Fig. 1–3) are presented to illustrate examples of response and no response to the stimuli. In each figure the stimulus event channel shows the duration of the pre-stimulus, stimulus and post-stimulus periods. The EEG is plotted from the digitized data. The horizontal lines through the EEG tracings are

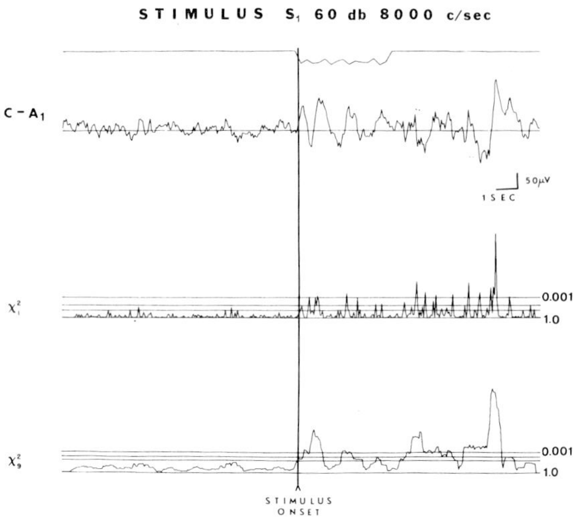

Fig. 1
Example of significant response to an $S_1$60 dB 8000 c/sec tone in the EEG of a 2-day-old male neonate. Monopolar recordings were obtained from electrodes placed approximately at C_3 linked to C_4 referred to A_1 ($C–A_1$). The chi-square test with 1 d.f. is indicated by χ_1^2. The chi-square test with 9 d.f. with the chi-squares smoothed over 0.5 sec intervals is noted by χ_9^2. Significance levels of 0.05, 0.01, 0.001 are shown to the right of the chi-square curves.

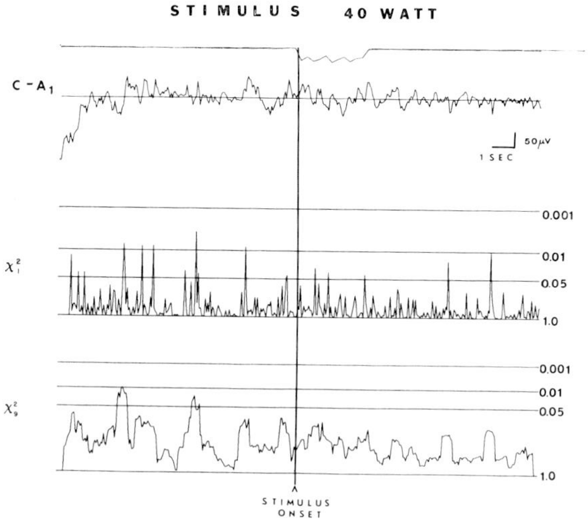

Fig. 2
No significant response to a 40 W flash in the EEG of a 2-day-old male neonate (see Fig. 1).

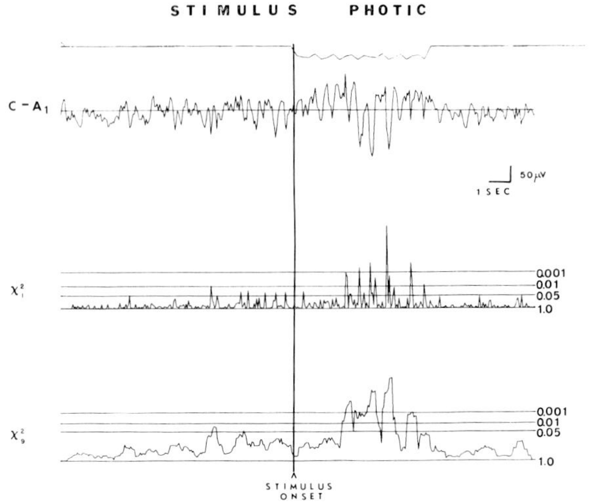

Fig. 3
Significant response to a repetitive photic (5/sec for 6 sec) stimulus in the EEG of a 2-day-old male neonate (see Fig. 1).

the pre-stimulus sample means ($\hat{\mu}$) estimated from all the pre-stimulus data. The chi-squares are obtained from the deviations from the one-step predictions, not from the deviations from this line. The chi-squares are shown starting from time point $p + 1$ near the beginning of the tracing, since the first p time points must be used as predictors. The chi-squares are shown in the pre-stimulus periods as an indication of possible artifacts or non-stationarities which may temporarily affect the EEG prior to stimulus onset. Fig. 1–3 present the results of the one-tailed chi-square tests with 1 and 9 d.f. The vertical scale for each tracing was set by the range of the chi-squares. For significance level p, the curve would be expected to spend $100p$ per cent of its time above the level with no response to the stimulus. For the data shown, each stimulus has 200 post-stimulus onset points. Therefore, on the average, two points would be expected to appear above the 0.01 level.

There is clear evidence of change in Fig. 1 to the $S_1$60 dB 8000 c/sec stimulus because of the number of points above the 0.001 level. The 1 d.f. curve gives the resolution necessary for determining when the change occurs. For a change which persists for 0.5 sec or longer, the 9 d.f. curve would be much more powerful for detecting this change. The latency can be determined by a print-out of the data or from measurements on the plotted curve. At approximately 0.42 and 0.81 sec after the stimulus onset, two peaks of the 1 d.f. curve touched the 0.001 line. Lack of precision in the stimulus onset is ± 0.18 sec. From this curve there may still be some doubt of response directly after the stimulus onset; however, the chi-square with 9 d.f. curve increases confidence in the response.

Fig. 2 is an example of no response to a 40 W light stimulus because the number of peaks above any given significance level could be attributed to chance.

In Fig. 3 there is a clear response to repetitive photic stimulation, since five peaks are above the 0.001 level in a portion of the post-stimulus region. Again, the first peak in the chi-square with 1 d.f. indicates the response onset. There is the possibility that the peaks in the chi-squares are related to the frequency of the photic stimulation.

DISCUSSION

A workable auto-regression model has been developed which objectively evaluates change. The application of this technique is appropriate for experimental designs where a stationary model can be assumed for all pre-stimulus data and through the post-stimulus regions if there is no response to the stimulus. The stationary assumption is obviously an approximation. Data collected under steady state conditions justify making this assumption. Even though the model detects non-stationarity as change, one must be aware that non-stationarity can be introduced by spurious factors.

Any attempt to define individual differences in autonomic function should ultimately focus on response patterns of the individual to extract neurophysiological parameters for inter-individual comparisons. The model which has been developed facilitates making such comparisons. The determination of whether a response has been made to stimulation can be objectively defined in terms of levels of statistical significance. The neurophysiological meaning of the change is in part a function of the experimental design and inferences which can be deduced or inferred from the biological functions being measured. It is in this sense that statistics is most contributory and becomes a functional tool for assessing underlying neurological activity.

The single subject model developed here is a practical technique for resolving some of the complexities of the time-varying EEG signal for interpretation relative to other neurophysiological facts. Thus, in the single subject design analyzed by the current change detection model, definite evidence is shown for selective responsivity within several sensory modalities. The latency as well as duration of the response is fairly accurately established. In the light of current theories concerning the orienting reflex (Moruzzi and Magoun 1949; Lindsley 1960; Sokolov 1960), a reasonable interpretation suggests evidence of an arousal reaction. To determine whether the EEG changes are in the classical adult pattern of low voltage fast activity would require further spectral analysis or further analysis in the frequency domain. The suggestive evidence of reactivity to photic stimulation is in line with earlier data on rhythmic fluctuations (Ellingson 1960; Glaser and Levy 1965) which have, as in this case, been observed outside the occipital region (Ellingson 1967). That responsivity can be related to a 60 dB 8000 c/sec modulated tone provides a foundation for more definitive audiometric plotting in newborn humans without the necessity for signal averaging techniques. Although this EEG change can be viewed only as a non-specific response to auditory stimulation, it becomes a first approximation to auditory sensitivity. The effects of the olfactory stimulus are probably complex and reasonably interpreted as relating to stimulation of the trigeminal as well as the first cranial nerves.

Further application of the technique can be visualized for precise study of cortical and subcortical activity. In combination with analysis of changes in autonomic variables, such as heart rate, respiration volume, and electrodermal shifts, the temporal course of responses may provide a base for exploring whether stimulus analysis occurs first in the cortex and is secondarily followed by the orientation reaction (Sokolov 1960).

SUMMARY

An auto-regression model using a step-wise procedure for estimating the parameters has been developed to test for change in the post-stimulus onset EEG of a single subject. A stationary process is assumed for the pre-stimulus data and if there is no significant change, for the post-stimulus region. Change can be detected at any point in the time series giving a measure of response latency and duration.

This analysis was performed utilizing the responses of a human newborn to sensory stimulation to demonstrate the applicability of the model for detecting changes in digitized EEG data and relating these to underlying neurophysiological activity.

RÉSUMÉ

MÉTHODE DE DÉTECTION DE MODIFICATIONS DANS UNE SÉRIE TEMPORELLE APPLIQUÉE À L'EEG DU NOUVEAU-NÉ

Un modèle d'auto-régression utilisant un déroulement par étapes pour l'estimation des paramètres a été mis au point afin de tester tout changement dans les parties de l'EEG immédiatement consécutives à un stimulus sur un sujet isolé. Les données pré-stimulus sont considérées comme un processus stationnaire et, s'il n'y a pas de modification significative, il en est de même de la période post-stimulus. Une modification peut être décelée à tout point de la série temporelle qui donne une mesure de latence et de durée de la réponse.

Cette analyse a été réalisée en utilisant les réponses d'un nouveau-né humain à la stimulation sensorielle pour démontrer l'applicabilité du modèle à la détection de changements dans les données EEG quantifiées et à leur mise en relation avec l'activité neurophysiologique sousjacente.

REFERENCES

BRAZIER, M. A. B. Computer techniques in EEG analysis. *Electroenceph. clin. Neurophysiol.*, **1961**, *Suppl. 20*, 98 p.

DURBIN, J. The fitting of time series models. *Rev. int. statist. Inst.*, **1960**, *28*: 233–244.

EFROYMSEN, M. A. Multiple regression analysis. In A. RALSTON and H. S. WILF (Eds.), *Mathematical methods for digital computers*, Part V (17). Wiley, New York, **1960**: 191–203.

ELLINGSON, R. J. Cortical electrical responses to visual stimulation in the human infant. *Electroenceph. clin. Neurophysiol.*, **1960**, *12*: 663–677.

ELLINGSON, R. J. The study of brain electrical activity in infants. In L. P. LIPSITT and C. C. SPIKER (Eds.), *Advances in child development and behavior*, Vol. 3. Academic Press, New York, **1967**: 53–97.

GLASER, G. H. and LEVY, L. L. Photic following in the EEG of the newborn. *Amer. J. Dis. Child.*, **1965**, *109*: 333–337.

JONES, R. H. Prediction of multivariate time series. *J. appl. Meteorol.*, **1964**, *3*: 285–289.

LINDSLEY, D. B. Attention, consciousness, sleep and wakefulness. In J. FIELD *et al.* (Ed.), *Handbook of physiology*, *Sect. I*. Amer. Physiol. Soc., Washington, **1960**, *3*: 1553–1593.

MORUZZI, G. and MAGOUN, H. W. Brain stem reticular formation and activation of the EEG. *Electroenceph. clin. Neurophysiol.*, **1949**, *1*: 455–473.

QUENOUILLE, M. H. Approximate tests of correlation in time series. *J. roy. statist. Soc.*, *B* (Methodological), **1949**, *11 (1)*: 68–84.

SOKOLOV, E. N. Neuronal models and the orienting reflex. In M. A. BRAZIER (Ed.), *The central nervous system and behavior*. Macy, New York, **1960**: 187–276.

Reference: JONES, R. H., CROWELL, D. H. and KAPUNIAI, L. E. A method for detecting change in a time series applied to newborn EEG. *Electroenceph. clin. Neurophysiol.*, **1969**, *27*: 436–440.

AN ELECTRODE FOR THE STUDY OF LINGUAL SENSITIVITY

D. A. MAJEAU AND A. K. PLEASONTON

Department of Otorhinolaryngology and Biocommunication, Louisiana State University Medical Center, New Orleans, La. 70112 (U.S.A.)

(Accepted for publication: February 26, 1969)

The study of lingual sensitivity has been hampered by the lack of suitable surface electrodes capable of adequate contact with a surface as moist as that of the lingual mucosa. Two types of electrodes used in the oral cavity have been described: suction electrodes (Harris *et al.* 1964; Cooper 1965) and probe-like electrodes (Krarup 1958; Harbert *et al.* 1962; Pulec *et al.* 1963; Bekesy 1964; Jauhiainen *et al.* 1967). Suction electrodes are used for recording muscle potentials, but are not appropriate as stimulating electrodes for the following reasons: (1) They can alter the normal physiological state of the recording site by causing an increase in evaporation of water from the tissue surface and an abnormal blood flow through the region. (2) The mechanical deformation resulting from the suction may stimulate the receptors under study and induce a state of adaptation and decreased responsiveness. The probe-like electrodes described by Bekesy for taste studies require immobilization of the tongue and constant visual monitoring to make sure contact is unbroken. They are thus inadequate for studies of larger groups of normal subjects. The hand-held probe electrodes described by the other investigators cited exert a variable pressure and are thus inappropriate for touch studies.

METHODS

Electrodes avoiding these difficulties were designed by Majeau and used for a study of thresholds of lingual tactile sensitivity by Pleasonton (1968). These electrodes are shown in Fig. 1. They consist of a silver foil point of approximately 1 mm² surface area embedded in a thin plastic disc 1 cm in diameter cut from commercially available plastic sheets (0.0075″ [0.188 mm] is found to be a suitable thickness as it is neither too heavy nor too flexible). The foil is wrapped around a copper wire 0.11 mm in diameter and inserted into a hole made in the center of the plastic disc by a 22-gauge hypodermic needle. The protruding part is pressed into a 1 mm² area. This holds the electrode firmly and produces only minimal protrusion. Aluminum foil may be substituted for silver if the electrodes are to be used solely for short duration stimulation. Aluminum is polarizable and can react with body fluids to produce junctional potentials of a magnitude as high as 40 mV, in contrast to silver which rapidly

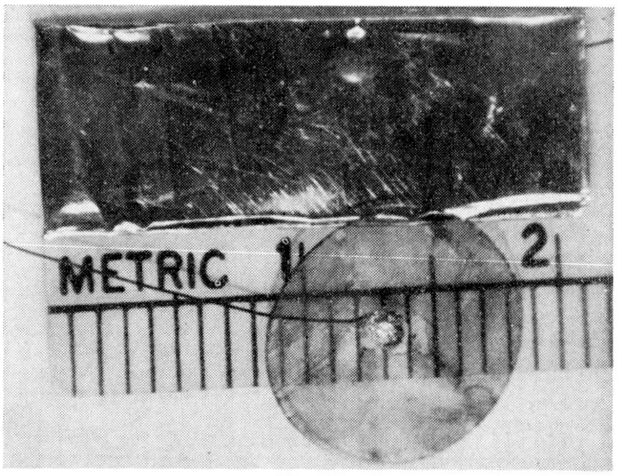

Fig. 1
Electrodes.

forms a chloride coating and produces potentials which do not exceed 1 μV.

The indifferent electrode consists of a foil strip 2 cm long and 0.7 cm wide. It is placed under the tongue so that its long axis is perpendicular to the tongue's. This allows maximum stability for the electrode against lingual movements and permits collection of the stimulus current by a broad area.

The electrodes are connected to the output of an electronic laboratory stimulator by insulated copper wires.

RESULTS

These electrodes adhere to the lingual mucosa by surface tension. Pressure, if any, is minimal, and remains constant during the duration of the experiment. Retention at the precise area under investigation is monitored visually by the experimenter and kinesthetically by the subject. Small lingual movements, as during swallowing, do not interfere with retention and accuracy of placement. In subjects unable to avoid gross lingual movements, replacement between threshold determinations may occasionally be necessary.

DISCUSSION

These electrodes are appropriate for the measurement of lingual tactile sensitivity in normal and clinical populations because they fulfil the following requirements: (1) Their application is painless. (2) They are capable of retention in one area without immobilizing the tongue, and without suction. (3) They do not produce lingual deformation, and the pressure they exert remains minimal and constant to avoid stimulation of receptors sensitive to deformation. (4) They are very small in area, to provide highly localized current density and avoid stimulation of too large a receptor population.

SUMMARY

Simple electrodes are described which can be made inexpensively and with a minimal time expenditure after a short period of practice. They are used as disposable electrodes.

RÉSUMÉ

ÉLECTRODE POUR L'ÉTUDE DE LA SENSIBILITÉ LINGUALE

L'auteur décrit des électrodes simples qui peuvent être réalisées de façon économique et dans un minimum de temps après une courte période d'entraînement. Ces électrodes peuvent être jetées après usage.

Support is acknowledged from NIH NB-07005, U.S. Public Health Service.

REFERENCES

BEKESY, G. VON. Sweetness produced electrically on the tongue and its relation to taste theories. *J. appl. Physiol.*, **1964,** *19*: 1105–1113.

COOPER, F. S. Research techniques and instrumentation: EMG. *ASHA Reports*, **1965,** *1*: 153–168.

HARBERT, F., WAGNER, S. and YOUNG, I. M. The quantitative measurement of taste function. *Arch. Otolaryng.*, **1962,** *75*: 138–143.

HARRIS, K. S., ROSOV, R., COOPER, F. S. and LYSAUGHT, G. F. A multiple suction electrode system. *Electroenceph. clin. Neurophysiol.*, **1964,** *17*: 698–700.

JAUHIAINEN, T., ALLAS, Y. and AHO, J. Subjective scale of electric taste. *Acta Otolaryng.*, **1967,** *63*: 462–466.

KRARUP, B. On the technique of gustatory examinations. *Acta Otolaryng.*, **1958,** *Suppl. 140*: 195–200.

PLEASONTON, A. K. *Sensitivity to and temporal resolution of electrical stimuli to the tongue.* Unpublished Ph.D. Diss., Louisiana State Univ., **1968.**

PULEC, J. L., URBAN, J. and HOUSE, W. F. *A new taste tester.* Presented as a New Instrument at the Amer. Acad. Ophthal. and Otolaryngol., October 24, **1963.**

Reference: MAJEAU, D. A. and PLEASONTON, A. K. An electrode for the study of lingual sensitivity. *Electroenceph. clin. Neurophysiol.*, **1969,** *27*: 440–441.

Electroencephalography and Clinical Neurophysiology
Elsevier Publishing Company, Amsterdam – Printed in The Netherlands

IMPLANTATION OF STERILE ELECTRODES IN CHRONIC ANIMALS[1]

VICTOR MILSTEIN

Division of Neurology, University of Oregon Medical School, Portland, Ore. 97201 (U.S.A.)

(Accepted for publication: February 25, 1969)

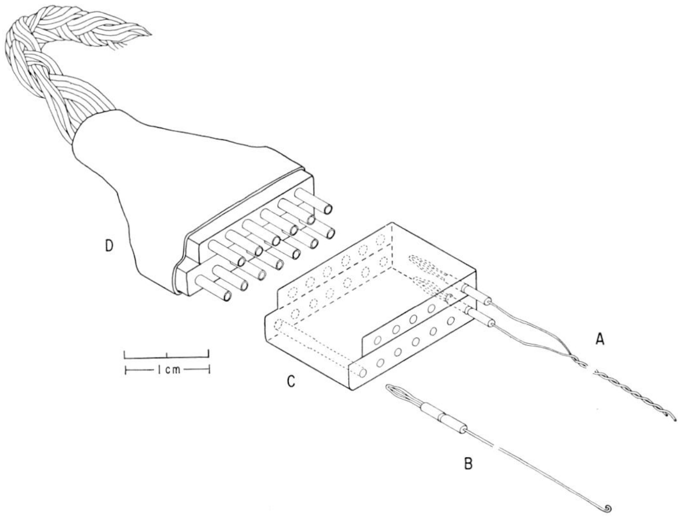

Fig. 1
Schematic representation of the electrodes, connector, and cable. *A*: Bipolar depth electrode partially inserted into connector. *B*: Surface electrode. Not indicated is the fact that the insulation has been removed from the 5 mm comprising the curved portion. *C*: The 13-hole connector formed by cementing together two strips of Micro-Rac. *D*: The matching cable.

Many techniques for the implantation of chronic electrodes unfortunately involve soldering over the surgically exposed preparation (McAdam *et al.* 1961; Jimenez and Escobar 1963; Ray 1965; Yules *et al.* 1966; Reeves and Hagamen 1968). Alternatives to this procedure have been the use of conductive paint and cement (Spooner 1965), crimping (Retzlaff and Fontaine 1964) and screw attachment (Sutton 1962). When electrodes are simply to be slipped through burr holes by hand onto or under the dura, they can be soldered to the connector prior to implantation, that is, a pre-fabricated electrode can be employed (Lagerwerff and Smith 1961; Roth *et al.* 1966). However, this is rarely possible for depth electrodes which must be inserted stereotaxically with an electrode holder. Unless a single depth implant only is to be made, or some sort of break-away extension employed, such electrodes are usually inserted, cemented to the calvarium, removed from the electrode holder, cut to length, and soldered to the connector. The connector is then attached to the animal's skull.

A simple procedure for avoiding the need to solder during the implantation procedure is described herein. Commercially available components are used which result in a small, neat connector attached to the animal with sterile technique.

Amphenol "Wire-Form" 220 series contacts and 220 series Micro-Rac connectors are employed. (Both Nadler (1965) and Rose (1966) have employed Amphenol No. 221 series connectors in implant procedures.) The depth electrodes are prepared by twisting together two lengths of 0.01 in. enamel-coated stainless steel wire (Driver Harris Type 316). These are then given an additional coat of Formvar insulation and cut to approximate length.

[1] Supported in part by Grant No. 687 of the Medical Research Foundation of Oregon.

The connector ends of the electrode are scraped free of insulation and soldered to male Wire-Form contacts (Fig. 1, *A*). These are sterilized by soaking in a germicidal solution or by autoclaving, whichever is more convenient. Our surface electrodes (Fig. 1, *B*) consist of single strands of insulated wire with 5 mm of the tip scraped bare and twisted into a tight circle. As with the depth electrode, the connector end is scraped and soldered to a male Wire-Form contact. This technique can also be used for electrodes that are glued with epoxy cement to the outside of insulated stainless steel cannulae through which materials are injected into the brain substance or ventricular system of the animal.

At the time of surgery the surface electrodes are inserted through burr holes in the skull and placed on the dura. The hole is filled with dental acrylic, and a small mound of this material is built up around the electrode. The depth electrodes are implanted at the desired locations with the needle carriers of the stereotaxic instrument. They are then cemented to the skull in the same way that the surface electrodes were. The cannulae with attached electrodes are inserted in identical fashion, very carefully cemented to the skull, and a larger mound of cement built up around them. Employing a high-speed air drill, the cannula is then cut off approximately 5 mm above the top of the mound of dental acrylic. A stainless steel stylet, with an L-shaped bend at the top is cut to the exact length of the cannula to maintain patency of the distal end. The electrodes that are now firmly cemented to the calvarium are simply inserted into the appropriately formed, sterile Micro-Rac connector (Fig. 1, *C*) using a sterilized Amphenol Insertion Tool (No. 294-123). The extra lengths of wires that may be present are simply pushed down against the skull and the Micro-Rac connector is cemented in place with dental acrylic. Two tantalum or stainless steel screws are ordinarily inserted into the calvarium to serve as anchors for the mound of dental cement that holds the Micro-Rac connector.

Because at times there is sufficient seepage from the wound to fill the holes of the connector, we have routinely capped it with a matching plug. This plug has the same conformation as the connector which will be used to attach the animal to the recording apparatus (Fig. 1, *D*).

SUMMARY

A simple and rapid technique which obviates the need for soldering over a surgically exposed preparation is described.

RÉSUMÉ

IMPLANTATION D'ÉLECTRODES STÉRILES CHEZ DES ANIMAUX CHRONIQUES

L'auteur décrit une technique simple et rapide qui évite la nécessité de soudure sur une préparation à cerveau ouvert.

REFERENCES

JIMENEZ, J. I. and ESCOBAR, I. A simple method of securing connectors to the heads of animals for EEG recordings. *Electroenceph. clin. Neurophysiol.*, **1963,** *15*: 123–124.

LAGERWERFF, J. M. and SMITH, M. H. Completely prefabricated chronic cortical electrode units. *Electroenceph. clin. Neurophysiol.*, **1961,** *13*: 643–644.

MCADAM, D., SNODGRASS, L. and KNOTT, J. R. A prewired circuit board for use in chronic electrode implantations. *Electroenceph. clin. Neurophysiol.*, **1961,** *13*: 798–799.

NADLER, R. D. A simplified cannula system for implanting and injecting chemicals into the brains of small animals. *Electroenceph. clin. Neurophysiol.*, **1965,** *19*: 312–313.

RAY, C. D. Multiple electrode implantation in animals. A simplified plastic cap technique. *Electroenceph. clin. Neurophysiol.*, **1965,** *19*: 529–530.

REEVES, A. G. and HAGAMEN, W. D. A re-usable nylon socket holder for use with chronically embedded electrodes in the cat. *Electroenceph. clin. Neurophysiol.*, **1968,** *25*: 185–186.

RETZLAFF, E. and FONTAINE, J. Chronic cortical electrodes for small animal studies. *Electroenceph. clin. Neurophysiol.*, **1964,** *17*: 700–701.

ROSE, G. H. Permanently implanted recording electrodes for immature animals. *Electroenceph. clin. Neurophysiol.*, **1966,** *21*: 395–396.

ROTH, J. G., MACPHERSON, C. H. and MILSTEIN, V. The use of carbon electrodes for chronic cortical recording. *Electroenceph. clin. Neurophysiol.*, **1966,** *21*: 611–615.

SPOONER, C. E. Preparation and implantation of brain electrodes in the young chick. *Electroenceph. clin. Neurophysiol.*, **1965,** *18*: 419–421.

SUTTON, D. A multiple electrode appliance for chronic recording from small animals. *Electroenceph. clin. Neurophysiol.*, **1962,** *14*: 772–773.

YULES, R. B., OGDEN, J. A., GAULT, F. P. and FREEDMAN, D. X. An implanted electrode for recording both rapid eye movements and muscle tone during sleep. *Electroenceph. clin. Neurophysiol.*, **1966,** *20*: 410–411.

Reference: MILSTEIN, V. Implantation of sterile electrodes in chronic animals. *Electroenceph. clin. Neurophysiol.*, **1969**, *27*: 442–443.

Electroencephalography and Clinical Neurophysiology
Elsevier Publishing Company, Amsterdam – Printed in The Netherlands

SOCIETY PROCEEDINGS

BULGARIAN SOCIETY OF NEUROLOGY, PSYCHIATRY AND NEUROSURGERY

SECTION OF EEG AND CLINICAL NEUROPHYSIOLOGY

Fourth Annual Session

Sofia, February 26, 1968

Secretary: DR. D. B. TCHAVDAROV

V.M.I., Sofia 31 (Bulgaria)

1. On the mechanisms of picrotoxin epileptic seizure (macro- and micro-electrode investigations). — G. Usunoff, E. Atsev and D. Tchavdarov (Sofia).

The investigations dealt with ECoG changes in the somato-sensory cortex of 34 cats after i.v. injection of picrotoxin 0.5–1 mg/kg body weight. Simultaneous micro-electrode recordings of the action potentials of cortical neurones were also made from 18 of the cats. After the injection a desynchronization, lasting 1–2 min, of the ECoG was witnessed, followed by a progressive increase in background amplitude and slowing. Spikes and sharp waves appeared during the 3rd min, which quickly increased in number so that from the 4th to 6th min they grew into an ECoG attack of a tonic-clonic kind. After the picrotoxin injection the potentials evoked by single somato-sensory stimuli increased progressively in amplitude, turning into evoked epileptic spikes. Later on single stimuli might even provoke epileptic attacks. When the action potentials of one and the same neurone were continuously recorded, their increase in frequency was often seen after the picrotoxin injection. Neuronal discharges grouped themselves in high frequency volleys at the time of the spikes. Just before the tonic-clonic seizure some neurones gave a rather prolonged volley of action potentials accompanied by a gradual decrease in amplitude, resulting in their complete disappearance in the tonic phase, and followed by volleys of neuronal discharge during the clonic attacks. Under the influence of picrotoxin single somato-sensory stimuli evoke volleys of discharge even in neurones which have never before reacted to such stimuli.

The investigations provide grounds to assume that after injection of picrotoxin a progressive accumulation of excitation takes place in cortical neurones, growing at a certain level into an abnormal epileptic excitation. The character of the changes in spontaneous and evoked global and unit activity occurring under picrotoxin indicates rather a primary influence on the deep subcortical structures.

2. Changes in evoked perifocal electrical activity with an acute epileptogenic focus in cat's cortex. — E. Atsev and T. Yosiphov (Sofia).

ECoG investigations on the changes in focal and perifocal structures with a strychnine epileptogenic focus in the visual or somato-sensory cortex were carried out on 20 cats. The changes in evoked potentials under a local application at the focus of maximum activity (FMA) were especially studied. It was found that at the time of increase in the positive, and especially the negative, phase of the primary response in FMA and during the subsequent appearance of "triggered" spikes, characteristic changes in the evoked activity of perifocal structures take place. These changes depend on the importance of epileptic manifestations at the focus, on the distance between the region in question and the FMA, on the strength and frequency of the specific stimulation, etc. With constant conditions a gradual change in the amplitude and configuration of the evoked potentials was observed on departing from the FMA. At a distance of 5–8 mm from the FMA an inversion of phase of the evoked potentials took place. The triggered spikes remained, however, with a primary negative phase, which came later than the one in FMA.

The authors discussed the roles: (1) of perifocal specific afferentation; (2) of cortico-cortical associative connections and (3) of the electrotonic effect.

3. On the mechanisms of "triggering" epileptic manifestations (macro- and micro-electrode investigations). — E. Atsev (Sofia).

Experiments were performed on 49 cats and 6 rabbits. In 43 of the cats strychnine epileptogenic foci were created (33 in primary somato-sensory cortex and 10 in visual cortex). A cobalt focus in the somato-sensory cortex was created in 6 cats and 6 rabbits. A great number of leads were taken from the focal region and from extrafocal structures. In 28 of the experiments simultaneous micro-electrode investigations were also carried out. Peripheral and electrical stimuli of relay, associative and non-specific subcortical structures, as well as some direct cortical stimulation of the focus, were used.

It was found that in certain conditions the various stimuli might provoke epileptic manifestations. The effectiveness of "triggering" depended mainly on the character and location of the focus, on the type, strength and frequency of the stimulus and on the functional condition of extrafocal brain structures. In equivalent conditions the evoked epileptic manifestations were always more vivid with a strychnine focus than with a cobalt one.

Of first importance to "triggering" is specific afferent stimulation directed to the focus. With single stimuli of this kind, various time ratios between primary evoked responses and evoked epileptic spikes were seen, depending on their strength and frequency (from complete coincidence of the spike with the negative phase of the primary response, to their appearance some hundreds of milliseconds later). In the cobalt focus the "triggered" spike had a comparatively more constant shape and latency (usually some milliseconds after the peak of the negative phase of the primary response). Peripheral stimulation of a modality "unspecific" for the epileptogenic focus, as well as electrical stimulation of associative or non-specific thalamic nuclei, had a rather weaker triggering effect but could, in certain conditions (greater intensity and frequency), provoke even fully developed epileptic crises.

The micro-electrode investigations showed that, coinciding with the "triggered" spikes, a far greater number of neurones fired than at the time of evoked potentials. Often there were neurones in the focus which fired simultaneously with the "triggered" and "spontaneous" spikes but not at the time of normally evoked potentials. Neuronal discharges with triggered spikes were longer and of higher frequency than those with evoked responses. Intracellular investigations revealed neurones reacting only at the time of "triggered" spikes, with an abnormally strong depolarizing shift and without any action potentials.

An attempt to shed more light on the nature of "triggered" epileptic manifestations is based on these investigations. It is assumed that neuronal mechanisms at the time of "triggering" the epileptic manifestations are similar to, but not identical with, those of normal evoked potentials. There is a suggestion that "triggering" of the epileptogenic focus might be reached only when the afferent volleys coming into the epileptogenic focus cause a definite critical rise in the excitation process, leading to an abnormally strong paroxysmal depolarization in a huge number of the neurones.

4. Spatio-temporal study of the average somaesthetic potential evoked on the scalp in man by stimulation of the median nerve. — I. Mezan (Sofia), A. Rémond and N. Lesèvre (Paris, France).

See "Société d'Électroencéphalographie et de Neurophysiologie clinique de Langue Française", meeting of 6 March 1968 (*This Journal*, 1969, *26*: 637).

5. Modifications of the EEG and of cerebral vascular resistance (CVR) during hyperventilation. — D. Tchavdarov (Sofia).

The close correlation between the EEG and the variations of cerebral irrigation, as induced by hyperventilation, are well known. The injection of non-diffusible radio-indicators into the blood stream offers the possibility of investigating variations in the cerebral blood volume, which is a direct function of the cerebral blood flow and of the CVR, simultaneously with the EEG. When the cerebral vascular reactions are tested by hyperventilation lasting 3–5 min, the results obtained can be loosely classified into two groups: patients with fair mobility of the cerebro-vascular reactions and adequate EEG responses and cases with abnormal changes in the cerebral blood volume, exhibiting various EEG symptoms. The simultaneous application of these two methods of investigation could help to achieve a better physio-pathological interpretation of EEG data and a better differentiation between the vascular and the neural backgrounds of some cerebral affections. Progress in therapy could also be better followed and documented.

6. EEG and cerebral blood flow following cortical application of strychnine and mescaline. — D. Tchavdarov (Sofia).

The mechanisms of changes in the regional cerebral blood flow (rCBF) induced by an experimental epileptogenic focus are still not elucidated. The heat clearance principle was employed in an investigation with this in view. The experiments were carried out on anaesthetized cats. A high correlation was found between the local ECoG and the rCBF. At first the rCBF increased in proportion to the desynchronization. With the appearance of spikes this increase became nearly stepwise. Then the rCBF remained unchanged though the number and the amplitude of the spikes increased, but was again augmented with the appearance of polyphasic spikes. Besides this general type of evolution, there were also some specific differences between the effects of the two epileptogenic agents.

These data seem to indicate that the modifications of the rCBF are due to an increase of the neuronal metabolism caused by the epileptogenic irritation, while the differences between the effects of the two agents could be attributed to their specific vascular actions.

7. Electrocorticographic modifications induced by stimulation of the ventral amygdaloid complex. — R. Tzicalova (Sofia).

Experiments have been carried out on 20 phenobarbital-anaesthetized cats (50 mg/kg). Stimulation of the ventral amygdala produced ipsilateral changes in cortical activity. In 14 cases an acceleration of the background rhythm was observed, in 6 cases slower (6–8 c/sec) rhythms appeared. The changes in the ECoG were correlated with the parameters of stimulation. With 5 V only local effects were observed. An optimal cortical effect was obtained by stimulation with 15–20 V and 100–150 c/sec. This effect did not vary in the different cortical regions and no after-discharge was produced once the stimulation was arrested. Modifications of respiration, muscular activity and pupillary size were also observed during stimulation.

8. Modifications of the electrocorticogram, the vegetative and the motor functions after suboccipital injection of noradrenalin and serotonin in rabbits. — A. Tzenov, C. Merdjanov and R. Harizanov (Sofia).

Noradrenalin was injected into the cisterna magna of rabbits in doses of 50–100 μg. This caused an arousal reaction (high frequency, low voltage activity in the sensori-motor area, theta activity in the occipital region) whose duration was related to the dose. The respiration became deeper and faster, the cardiac activity was slower. The maximum of these vegetative phenomena was observed between 5 and 10 min after the injection. The motor reactions became slower, with increasing hypotonia, to a full arrest of motor initiative followed by muscular twitches and disturbances of coordination (3–5 h).

Serotonin was introduced suboccipitally in 100–1500 μg doses. Moderate doses (250–500 μg) induced phasic (in Pavlovian terminology) modifications of the electrical activity (see K.R. Iliutchenu): the initial EEG activation was followed by a period of relative slowing and amplitude increase, then by another activation beginning 30–40 min after the injection and lasting even after the third hour. The vegetative phenomena were in general milder than those induced by noradrenalin but the bradycardia was sensibly stronger. The muscular hypotonia which gradually immobilized the animals was accompanied by frequent scratching movements, nods and tremor of the masticatory muscles. The EEG modifications did not always evolve in parallel with the vegetative and with the motor phenomena and this was equally true for both drugs.

9. Effect of intravenous infusion of D-cycloserine on the EEG of the rabbit. — B. Vassileva and M. Staneva (Sofia).

It is known that i.v. injected L-cycloserine produces in the experimental animal a sedative behavioural effect and a synchronization of the EEG. We have attempted to analyse and compare the effects of D-cycloserine on the waking, non-restrained rabbit. The effect of the drug, administered in a large range of doses (0.05–1.0 g/kg), is expressed in relaxation, motor inhibition, atonia and akinesia. The EEG is markedly hypersynchronized, the amplitude of the background activity increases by several hundred microvolts, its frequency is slowed to 2–3 c/sec. This hypersynchronization is maintained for more than 2 h and is even more accentuated by rhythmic photic stimulation. Low and medium doses of D-cycloserine increase the frequency range of photic driving.

10. The effect of local or suboccipital application of D-cycloserine on the cortical activity of the rabbit. — B. Vassileva (Sofia).

A local application of D-cycloserine (1–3% solution or crystals) to the visual cortex of rabbits does not produce any epileptic phenomena. It is known that L-cycloserine behaves in the same manner. On the other hand suboccipital administration of D-cycloserine (0.01–1.0 g/kg) produces a severe intoxication with atonic stupor and repeated clonic jerks or tonic contractions of all the muscles. The intensity and the duration of the tonic contractions are dose related. The EEG is desynchronized with a background of low voltage slow waves. Slow waves of large amplitude, groups of high voltage sharp waves, occasionally even spike and wave complexes, appear during the convulsive manifestations. These peculiar convulsive phenomena could be tentatively interpreted as a particular form of subcortical or brain-stem epilepsy.

11. An EEG study of healthy premature babies. — G. Vladimirova (Sofia).

A study is made of 100 EEGs recorded from 52 healthy premature babies aged 5–65 days. Their average post-conceptional age was 34 weeks. The EEGs were recorded during diurnal sleep. Two problems are considered:

1. The correlation between the amplitude of the background activity and its frequency. A log frequency/amplitude relation was found ($P < 0.001$) with a negative correlation between the two parameters ($r = -0.9916$). The magnitude of the amplitude is defined by $\lg A_{\mu V} = 1.704 - 0.53759 \lg F_{c/sec}$ (So = 0.02398, Sb = 0.02104). The confidence interval of the amplitude was computed.

2. The ratio between the mean amplitude of the background activity and the mean amplitude of the activity following exteroceptive stimulation (flicker, clicks and temperature skin stimulation). It was found that when the background amplitude was small exteroceptive stimulation caused a relative increase ($P < 0.001$). It is defined by $\overline{A}_{response} = 10.026 + 0.5497\ \overline{A}_{backgr}$ (So = 3.277, Sb = 0.0124). Thus, in theory, for an average background amplitude of 22.3 μV, the response to stimulation would not be significantly higher.

12. Primary hypothyreosis and EEG. — G. Vladimirova, L. Peneva and R. Slavova (Sofia).

Nine children, aged 9 months to 14 years, with primary hypothyreosis (congenital in 8, acquired in one) have been followed for 2–14 months. EEGs were recorded before the treatment, at the end of the first and of the second week and then monthly. The patients were treated with dry thyroid extract. Before the treatment the EEG was as a rule slow and of low voltage, particularly in nursing infants. It was also hyporeactive to flicker and hyperventilation. In the course of treatment the clinical improvement went in parallel with an increase of frequency (by 1–3 c/sec) and amplitude (up to 100%). These modifications did not appear before the second week of treatment and manifested a tendency to reversal after its cessation. The gain in amplitude was considered abnormally high in 5 children and its peak corresponded to the maximum dosage of the thyroid hormone.

13. The EEG in vibration sickness. — P. Petrov (Sofia).

An EEG study has been carried out on 120 workers exposed to local or general vibration, compared with 40 healthy controls without any professional contact with vibrations. The EEG of the professionally exposed patients differed from the controls in a great number of cases. Low voltage records, marked or predominant theta activity and poor reaction to flicker were often observed, sometimes even diffuse sharp waves and a few spikes were seen. The proportions of abnormal records were 61.66% in the vibration group and 7.5% in the controls. An abnormal EEG was more frequent in workers with clinically proved vibration sickness. The physiopathology of vibration sickness and the practical usefulness of EEG examination in this disease were discussed.

14. EEG findings in Alzheimer's disease. — D. Dascalov (Sofia).

EEG records were taken in 20 patients (18 female and 2 male) with Alzheimer's disease. Nearly all of them showed diffuse abnormalities without asymmetry or topical predilection. The background activity consisted of polymorphous theta and delta waves of small and medium amplitude. Overbreathing increased moderately the slow wave activity. An attempt at activation with chlorpromazine in 3 patients did not produce significant results. One of the patients who had epileptic seizures displayed diffuse sharp waves and spikes. The EEG abnormalities in Alzheimer's disease are characteristic enough to serve as additional evidence for the diagnosis.

Electroenceph. clin. Neurophysiol., **1969**, *27*: 444–447

PAVLOV'S PHYSIOLOGICAL SOCIETY OF THE U.S.S.R. MOSCOW AND LENINGRAD BRANCHES

September, 1967–March, 1968

EEG reports selected by D. K. KAMBAROVA

Institute for Experimental Medicine, Academy of Medical Sciences of the U.S.S.R., Leningrad (U.S.S.R.)

1. Correlations between membrane potential and inhibitory post-synaptic potential in spinal motor neurones. — Zh. G. Alexandrova, G. A. Vartanian, Yu. Ya. Zakher and N. M. Yakovlev (Leningrad).

Mono- and poly-synaptic post-synaptic potentials (PSP) in response to orthodromic or antidromic 0.5 c/sec stimulation were recorded, with intracellular microelectrodes filled with 0.6 M K_2O_4 solution, from 30 spinal motor neurones in 12 adult cats. The membrane potentials (MP) fluctuated about -60 to -70 mV during a few minutes or hours. In the end depolarization developed because of the damaging effect of the micro-electrode. Correlation between MP value and evoked post-synaptic potential (EPSP) amplitude was usual: the EPSP increased during hyperpolarization and decreased during depolarization. Various correlations between inhibitory post-synaptic potential (IPSP) amplitude and MP were observed: (1) a stable IPSP value during depolarization and hyperpolarization; (2) decreasing IPSP at the same MP value; (3) increase of the IPSP (up to a certain level) during depolarization; (4) steady IPSP decrease with short periods of increase during depolarization. The latter happened rather often. In some cases the depolarization not only entailed decrease of the IPSP to zero, but even its reversal, *i.e.*, its transformation into an EPSP. The time parameters of the PSP did not essentially alter, although sometimes elongation of the falling phase of the IPSP was observed during depolarization.

Depolarization of a neurone caused by damage by a micro-electrode is mainly due to an inflow of sodium ions into the cell. This entails an IPSP shift to depolarization (Eccles *et al.* 1964) which evokes decrease of the IPSP amplitude at an unaltered MP. The various IPSP amplitude changes accompanying the MP shifts are probably due to discrepancy between rates of shifts of the equilibrium potential of IPSP and MP.

2. Neuronal mechanisms of the temporary connexion. — N. N. Vassilevsky and V. V. Trubatchev (Leningrad).

Neuronal activity in the somato-sensory I cortical area was studied in rabbits under curare during orienting responses and elaboration of the temporary connexion. Sound, light or tactile stimulation (during 1.6 sec) served as the conditioned stimulus, and electrical skin stimulation of a receptive field (0.3–0.5 sec duration) as the unconditioned one. Spikes were recorded extracellularly for 2–6 h. Functional properties of type I neurones (with local receptive fields), type II (with diffuse receptive fields) and type III (with no distinct receptive fields) have been described elsewhere (Vassilevsky 1965, 1966). According to Vassilevsky's method of a double experiment, the same neurone could be studied either in a focus of conditioned or unconditioned stimulation.

Two forms of conditioned response were revealed for types I and II neurones. First, after 2–30 pairings, conditioned changes occurred as a diffuse increase of the

Electroenceph. clin. Neurophysiol., **1969**, *27*: 447–451

firing rate during the whole period of isolated action of the conditioned stimulus with 0.1–0.3 sec latency. Further, in some neurones, after formation of the diffuse response, a so-called specialized response appeared as a high frequency train after 5–50 pairings during the second half of the conditioned stimulus action, with 0.5–1.3 sec latency. The level of the response fluctuated from 40 to 90%. On stimulation of skin areas ajacent to the receptive field, exerting an inhibitory influence, an inhibitory form of the conditioned response could be observed in the focus of the reinforcing stimulus.

No conditioned responses could be obtained for type III neurones.

A stable specific evoked response remained in the conditioned stimulus focus when the receptive field of the neurones was activated with a conditioned tactile stimulus.

Neurones with conditioned responses had, on average, almost twice as high a background firing rate as the neurones with no conditioned responses. In some neurones there had been initially a high background level, in others the background activity increased on reinforcement. However, in 3 neurones elaboration of the above response forms was observed with a background frequency lower than 10/sec.

After the end of reinforcement the conditioned responses disappeared after 4–20 conditioned stimuli. With prolonged training conditioned responses remained after scores of non-reinforcements.

It should also be noted that the formation of a conditioned neuronal response not only depends on the orientation of the reinforcing stimulus to the receptive field of a neurone and to the level of its excitability, but also on the ecological-biological characteristics of the conditioned stimulus. Thus, for instance, for elaboration of responses of the neurones representing the forelimbs, tactile conditioned stimulation of the skin of the body and hind limbs proved to be the most effective, and stimulation of the skin of the head the least effective.

The authors suggest that the basis of the mechanisms for alerting response extinction and conditioned reflex elaboration consists in the control of excitability and transfer of functions in associative structures which, in the authors' opinion, are represented in the cerebral cortex by type II neurones.

3. Trace effects of stimulation of single neurones. — L. L. Voronin (Moscow).

Recovery of the background neuronal activity in the sensory-motor cortex of an unanaesthetized rabbit was studied during the seconds or scores of seconds after the current passed through a recording micro-electrode had been switched off. Extracellularly observed trace effects after an exciting (outgoing) current could be excitatory or inhibitory and their sign was contrary to the trace effect in the same neurones after switching off an inhibitory (entering) current. Intracellular recording only revealed trace decrease after depolarizing current and trace increase of the firing rate after hyperpolarizing current. A series of data obtained with intracellular recording (slow adaptation of the firing rate during the passage of current, no essential change in the average membrane potential or of the synaptic inflow during after-discharge, changes in threshold of some neurones etc.) testifies that the above trace effects are not related to the prolonged circulation of impulses in the neuronal network, but to adaptation of the excitable membranes. Comparative study of the similar effects on an isolated stretch-receptor neurone of a crawfish confirms the possibility of prolonged after-discharge in the absence of synaptic influences from other neurones. After switching off the current in either direction the trace effects of opposite sign, in different neurones during extracellular recording, are probably due to the current exerting a depolarizing influence on some membrane areas and hyperpolarizing on others.

4. Oxygen availability in human deep cerebral structures and its behaviour during some functional tests. — V. B. Gretchin (Leningrad).

Oxygen availability (O_2a) in human deep cerebral structures was studied by the polarographic oxygen cathode method in 6 hyperkinetic patients treated with implanted electrodes. Pre-operative testing of the electrodes made it possible to show the specific structural distribution of levels and the patterns of O_2a fluctuations in various subcortical structures and their individual variability, accounted for by the character of the neurological disease and, apparently, by the patient's age.

Oxygen availability is a highly sensitive parameter characterizing the functional state of a given brain area. After inhalation of oxygen, or overbreathing, diffuse O_2a changes occur as a result of systemic changes in the processes of oxygen supply. In both cases, the O_2a changes develop as a multi-stage process, separate links of which could reveal certain peculiarities in some structures. If the inhalation of oxygen entails widespread hyperoxia, differently expressed in different structures, overbreathing leads to a pronounced mixed brain hypoxia.

For theoretical purposes the O_2a data were interesting for investigation of the functional–anatomical organization of the subcortical structures. Thus, investigation of the O_2a dynamics during motor tests made it possible to divide all structures under study into three groups: (1) structures with no reproducible O_2a pattern in successive tests; (2) structures with reproducible O_2a patterns only in response to motor tests of the contralateral limbs; (3) structures with reproducible O_2a patterns in response to motor tests both of contralateral and ipsilateral limbs.

In the O_2a dynamics of ventro-lateral and central thalamic nuclei and of the pallidum, the role of alertness was noted. In some subcortical structures (thalamic nuclei, pallidum, hippocampus, amygdala and caudate nucleus) reproducible O_2a patterns occurred in successive tests of mental activity of the operative memory type. In them, the patterns had different time and amplitude characteristics, and in some structures could be related to correct completion of the tests. "Artificial noise" (triggered photic stimulation) caused changes in the distribution of the reproducible O_2a pattern: it disappeared or was suppressed in some structures and appeared in others.

Investigation of the O_2a pattern is of great practical importance: ascertainment of "significant" intracerebral vessels close to the electrodes; making the identification of electrode placement more exact; checking the state of the brain tissue during all stages of therapeutic and diagnostic electrical procedures; evaluating duration and intensity of the effect of threshold and supra-threshold electrical stimulation; determining the spread and degree of brain tissue alterations caused by therapeutic procedures.

5. On the possibilities of using for EEG analysis the method of fields of average velocities of change in brain activity. — V. V. Dubikaitis (Leningrad).

In physiology the rate of change of some process often has more importance than its amplitude characteristics. Therefore, investigation of the cerebral electric fields was carried out by studying the fields of average velocity of potential change. The velocities were determined for every 12.5 or 25 sec at 20 points all over the head. EEG epochs of about 5 sec duration were analysed. It has been asserted that there are only two areas of homogenous electric sign at any moment: one of increase (positive velocities) and one of decrease (negative velocities) of potentials. The area of increasing potentials coincides with the projection of the area of excited cortical dendrites to the scalp. The form, period and amplitude of EEG waves are shown to depend on the character of alteration in the trajectory of the excited area. For instance, if excitation passes over minor circuits of the brain, the EEG amplitude is small; with passage of the excitation to larger circuits, the amplitude increases; if the excitation passes over the same pathway for some time, no modification of the potential amplitude is observed. The data on excitation spreading in different directions testify to the existence of a scanning mechanism with circular spatial development, sudden alteration of which entails transformation of the EEG waves.

Investigation of the spatial distribution of the absolute average velocities of potential change showed the highest velocities in the parieto-occipital areas of healthy subjects, somewhat less in the anterior parts of the frontal lobes and least in the posterior frontal and temporal areas. Analysis of the velocity fields in 126 patients with various local brain pathologies shows that they differ from those of healthy man. At a superficial focus the configuration of the field starts to change. In different patients with similar foci and stages of the developing pathology the velocity fields are identical. With spreading of the pathology towards midline structures disturbances of the spatial distribution of velocities of potential change become more and more pronounced.

6. Alterations of evoked potentials in psychotic patients under the influence of chlorpromazine and trifluoperazine. — T. V. Kopylova (Leningrad).

Evoked potentials (EP) in response to rhythmic photic stimulation (from 1 to 70/sec) and the spontaneous EEG were studied in 90 patients with schizophrenia, epilepsy and various organic brain diseases, in 4 series of trials.

1. The partial range of the EP (especially the upper limit) EP index and EP irradiation over the brain decreased 1.0–1.5 h after chlorpromazine 25–150 mg i.m. The above EP parameters increased 18 h after the drug in patients with a positive therapeutic effect.

2. The range, amplitude, EP index and EP irradiation over the brain increased 2 h after administration of trifluoperazine 5–15 mg per os.

3. In the course of long-term therapy with chlorpromazine (from 4 to 48 months) clinical improvement of 12 out of 22 patients corresponded to increase of the range, upper limit and EP index. In 9 patients out of 22, in whom no clinical improvement was achieved, the EP changes were insignificant. If the clinical condition got worse, the frequency range and EP index decreased.

4. In 16 out of 21 patients in the course of trifluoperazine therapy a positive clinical effect was observed, accompanied by increase of the frequency range and upper limit of the EP. In 2 patients who got worse the range and EP index decreased. In 3 patients with neither effect no EP changes were observed.

In all 4 series of trials the spontaneous EEG showed no significant alterations, while the EP changes were statistically reliable.

The alterations in the functional state by drugs, revealed by EP, permit assessment of the lability, reactivity and excitability of specific and non-specific brain systems, and greatly aid in the selection and determination of individual doses of a drug.

7. Clinico-electroencephalographic correlations in patients with cerebral arachnoiditis. — S. A. Movsisiants (Leningrad).

Clinical and EEG examinations were made of 70 patients with cerebral arachnoiditis, diagnosed by detailed neurological examination and pneumoencephalography. The EEGs were analysed both visually and by statistical processing of data according to Moiseeva and Orlov's method for the "Minsk-1" computer.

The following reliable EEG differences were noted for any focus of arachnoiditis: (a) increased fast and sharp waves, both diffuse and in bursts, mainly with arachnoiditis of the convexity; (b) increased slow (mainly theta) activity, diffuse and in bursts, mainly with basal arachnoiditis; (c) regular spindles of alpha rhythm with grossly disturbed spatial distribution, often alternating with theta rhythm, with diffuse basal-convexity arachnoiditis.

Particularly marked pathological EEG components were observed in patients in whom the arachnoiditis led to pronounced signs of diencephalic dysfunction.

Continuous examination of the patients in many cases showed correlations between the development of the disease and the EEG changes. Functional tests showed almost half of the patients to have a significant lowering of reactivity. In some cases, overbreathing and trigger stimulation helped to reveal a pathological focus.

In general, the EEG changes in patients with cerebral

arachnoiditis, *i.e.*, altered spatial distribution of the alpha rhythm, presence of hypersynchronous low frequency beta rhythm and sharp waves anteriorly and centrally, frequent paroxysmal bursts of bilaterally synchronous activity, apparently indicate involvement of non-specific structures in the upper brain-stem and diencephalon in the pathological process, and suggest two mechanisms of the pathological electrical activity: (1) changes in neuronal activity because of the altered ascending reticular influence; (2) alteration of conditions in the same structures because of the atrophy and metabolic disturbances in the cerebral cortex.

8. Evaluation of working ability of man under normal conditions and in neurotic states by prevalence of slow EEG potentials during movement. — E. B. Sologub and T. P. Fanagorskaya (Leningrad).

Complex clinical, neurological and EEG examinations were carried out in sportsmen with neurotic disturbances consequent on overtraining. To evaluate physical working ability, functional tests were used (running on the spot for 10 sec at 4–5 steps/sec). The EEG was recorded with reference leads from frontal, pre-central, inferior parietal and occipital areas at rest and during muscular work. In overtrained sportsmen disturbances of brain function mainly appeared as astheno-neurotic syndromes and vegetative disturbances (chiefly of the cardio-vascular system). In the EEG of the overtrained sportsmen at rest, a low alpha index, small amplitude, fast background activity up to 13–14/sec, sometimes up to 17/sec, were found in cases with prevailing excitation and sympathetic tone, or low voltage and frequency of the alpha rhythm with a high alpha index in depressive states. During running tests the EEG of the overtrained sportsmen showed the following phenomena: the index of the working form of electrical activity (slow waves related to rate of movement) was halved as compared with that of healthy sportsmen; this working activity prevailed in the right hemisphere and, particularly, it disappeared during repeated tests, which indicates low working ability, quick fatigue and unsatisfactory restoration of the cortex, as well as disturbance of cortico-subcortical interrelations in the process of controlling motor activity.

9. EEG data on relation of the brain association areas to the organization of complex voluntary activity in children from 1 to 4 years of age. — T. P. Khrizman (Leningrad).

The EEG was recorded with reference leads from 10 points in the frontal, motor, parietal, occipital and temporal areas of children from 1 to 4 years of age, under conditions of relative rest and during play. The data were subjected to correlation analysis with constructing of maximal correlation columns and selection of correlation rows. Mutual inter-central correlations (from +1.0 to −1.0) of potential oscillations between these areas were considered. Functional connexions between various cortical structures were judged by the amount and degree of the correlation.

Anterior parts of the right frontal lobe were shown to have the maximal correlation with the electrical activity of other areas, with the right lower parietal area in second place. There were no functional structures with a clear interrelation

During play the maximal correlation was noted in the motor cortex, the frontal area was in second place and the lower parietal area third. The amount of distinct connexion between anterior association and motor structures was increased by 60% as compared with that between motor and posterior associative areas. Apparently the roles of the frontal and lower parietal areas in the organization of voluntary activity are not functionally identical.

In children, along with the ontogenetic development of the ability to attach a concrete meaning to voluntary activity, the anterior and posterior associative structures, with the motor centres, unite in a single correlation row.

In children the finding of significant correlations between potential changes in association areas and other centres, primarily the motor, during voluntary activity confirms the theoretical suggestion that human voluntary motor activity is organized and accomplished by a complex functional system, in which the associative structures have, apparently, an important controlling role.

10. Clinical-electroencephalographic comparisons in patients with aphasic and anosognosic syndromes. — A. N. Shandurina (Leningrad).

The results of EEG, psychological and neurological examinations were compared for 50 patients, from 19 to 82 years of age, with syndromes of aphasia (33 subjects) and anosognosia (17 subjects), mainly of vascular origin. The patients were watched from the first days of the disease and for a period from 2–3 months to 2 years. Bipolar EEGs were recorded with 16- and 8-channel machines. All EEG records were analysed visually, and some of them were subjected to statistical processing with a computer by Moiseeva and Orlov's method (1965, 1967).

In patients with different types of aphasia, reliable differences in distribution of the slow waves over brain areas were revealed. In general, our data corresponded with contemporary views on the localization of pathological foci with certain forms of speech disorders. Differences in the prominence of pathological activity in patients with different degrees of aphasia were also statistically reliable.

The EEGs of patients with anosognosia and hemisomatognosia had some peculiarities: (1) diffuse changes were more pronounced and prevailed in the right hemisphere, especially in the fronto-temporo-parietal area; (2) in numerous records paroxysmal bursts of activity were rather diffuse and mainly right-sided; (3) distinct inter-hemisphere asymmetry was often observed, due to prevailing slow waves on the right and beta waves on the left.

In most cases repeated EEGs corresponded to the clinical development of aphasia and anosognosia. In some patients diminished EEG pathological signs preceded the regression of the psychopathological disorders, which permitted the use of EEG data for prognosis in some cases.

In some patients during rhythmic and trigger photic stimulation and overbreathing, asymmetry was noted, due to decreased alpha suppression and driving in the diseased hemisphere, especially in the area of a pathological focus.

The clinical-EEG correlations permit discussion of some neurophysiological mechanisms underlying aphasia and anosognosia. Apparently, development of these syndromes is not only related to a pathological focus with a certain localization in a hemisphere, but also to alteration of the functional state of other brain structures, to disorder of cortico-subcortical interrelations and to dissociation in the activity of the hemispheres. Depending on which prevails, the clinical and EEG patterns of disturbances of the higher mental functions may change.

11. Using clipped electroencephalograms for sleep studies. — A. N. Shepovalnikov and V. S. Shneiderov (Leningrad).

The search for sufficiently simple methods of processing prolonged electrograms, measured in hours, compels restricting analysis to the most informative parameter, frequency for instance.

In consequence of peak amplitude restriction (clipping) the EEG acquires two significances: $+1$ and -1. To reveal the information contained in the intervals between base-line crossings, each interval is recorded as a point on the X axis, which is the greater according to the greater distance between two consecutive zeros. Thus intervals related to delta activity were noted in the upper parts of a frame, while those related to fast activity occurred in the lower parts. After constructing a scale corresponding to delta, theta, alpha and beta activities, the number of points for each frequency band was counted and histograms of interval distributions were constructed characterizing certain EEG sleep stages.

The interval distribution was found to correspond more exactly than the spectral density with changes in the EEG parameters. Also the mean number of EEG base-line crossings was determined by histograms which reflected EEG behaviour in different sleep stages and within one stage. Spectral densities of clipped and initial EEGs were investigated. The results of periodograms and spectral analysis of the clipped EEG of a sleeping man are quite comparable with the usual methods of EEG data processing. This provides the possibility of significantly simplifying EEG magnetic recording and the subsequent processing of data with analysing devices using the binary system.

Electroenceph. clin. Neurophysiol., **1969,** *27*: 447–451

GROUPEMENT BELGE D'ÉTUDES EEG

Brussels, November 23, 1968

Secretary: J. Titeca

11 rue de la Luzerne, Brussels 3 (Belgium)

1. Spectral analysis of EEG in the monkey *Papio papio*. Effects of anoxia. — F. Bostem, R. Naquet, C. Vuillon-Cacciuttolo and J. Bimar (Liège and Marseille, France).

The EEG modifications provoked by anoxia in animals and man have been studied for a long time. However, it seemed interesting to take advantage of the modern methods of information to analyse the spectral content and to study these modifications in a primate, *Papio papio*, which has the characteristic of often presenting electro-clinical epileptic manifestations, electively provoked by intermittent light stimulation.

These animals were subjected to hypoxia, obtained only by lowering the relative quantity of oxygen in the ventilated gas mixture. The EEG data were amplified and stored on magnetic tape. These records were first analysed visually, then adequate epochs were chosen and submitted to analysis.

The following facts were observed: (a) The stage of pre-anoxic "desynchronization", observed by spectral repartition in asymptotic exponential decrements, is rarely present in this animal. This stage is observed in cats, but the observation must be compared with that in man, in whom the stage of pre-anoxic "desynchronization" is lacking. (b) At the stage of anoxic slow waves in the animals which demonstrate spike and wave discharges during intermittent light stimulation, paroxysmal discharges of spikes and waves and of multiple spikes and waves appear. The latter are observed in the frontal areas and are demonstrated in the power spectral density curve by a bimodal distribution of energy, a maximum around 8 c/sec corresponding to the spikes. It is interesting to note that, at this stage, intermittent light stimulation becomes unable to provoke spike and wave discharges. (c) During the whole anoxic period, a progressive change of energy towards the low frequencies is noted. A reverse change is observed during the stage of recovery. (d)

Electroenceph. clin. Neurophysiol., **1969,** *27*: 451–452

During the period of recovery a particular stage is observed which suggests the EEG stage of "desynchronization". However, spectral analysis shows that this activity is different, at least in the fronto-Rolandic area, where a bimodal distribution of energy is encountered, with one peak around 6 c/sec and the other, intense, around 20 c/sec; this rather transitory pattern lasts for about 20 sec, then completely disappears. Instead of considering the records as "desynchronized", one must invoke a facilitation of the rhythmic fast activities characteristic of the fronto-Rolandic areas This observation can be compared with the activity observed during anaesthesia with halothane, which is similar in location and spectrally identical. (e) Although the records show an apparently precocious recovery after re-oxygenation, it is interesting to observe that the power spectral density curves remain abnormal for a much longer period, approximately 5 min.

2. Perpendicular referential montages in EEG. — M. L. Sorel (Louvain).

Classical bipolar recording cannot accurately establish the localization and potential gradient of an extensive activity or determine the exact polarity of a paroxysm. As perfect unipolar recording cannot be realized, a possible method to decrease the difficulties would consist of using a reference electrode which would have little activity; such activity, however, could be easily and always detected.

The new technique uses two connected reference electrodes, situated on each side at the base of the neck; this "reference" montage is called the "perpendicular referential montage". The use of 24 EEG channels enables the simultaneous recording of classical longitudinal or transverse bipolar montages and perpendicular referential montages. The combined study of these and of the phase reversals enables one to determine the activity of the reference electrode at any given moment. This technique makes it possible to establish: (a) the existence of spikes, either only negative or simultaneously negative and positive in different parts of the scalp; (b) a precise potential gradient for activities such as waves and spikes; (c) a great variety of temporal paroxysms, depending on whether the reference electrode is affected or not; (d) the electrical field of the basic rhythm in man. This does not seem to be an activity with a posterior predominance, as appears from the bipolar montage, but a cap located predominantly in the occipital and neck areas in some people, in the central or anterior areas in others.

From the electro-clinical correlations of these data, important information can be obtained to dissociate the different forms of epilepsy. In addition, it was observed that the alpha rhythm in the normal adult is usually situated in the parieto-Rolandic areas and an anterior shift is frequent in organic and psychological troubles.

3. First clinical result with Depakine. Study of 30 cases. — M. D. de Biolley and L. Sorel (Louvain).

Dinitropropylacetate of sodium or Depakine is a new anti-epileptic drug; its chemical formula is entirely different from the other anti-epileptic drugs used. It was studied in 30 cases and gave good results, mainly in grand mal, symptomatic petit mal and in certain forms of psychomotor epilepsy. It seems ineffective in the sequelae of myoclonic encephalopathy with hypsarrhythmia as well as in cases of startle epilepsy. In cases of Lennox syndrome, the results are average. Though the drug is usually well tolerated, digestive troubles and sleepiness, usually temporary, can be observed.

4. Results obtained with Depakine in cases of epilepsy resistant to other treatment. — Mme. M. Dumon-Radermecker (Antwerp).

The author presents her own results with a new anti-epileptic drug, Depakine, in 38 proved cases of epilepsy which did not respond to any classical drug treatment, even in diverse combinations. The most important group consisted of 25 cases of absence with atypical spikes and waves and multiple spikes and waves; in 17 of these there were also attacks of grand mal. The other observations consist of 7 cases of temporal lobe epilepsy, 3 cases of myoclonus epilepsy, 2 cases of Jacksonian epilepsy and one case of hyperthermic convulsions. The most spectacular and interesting results have been obtained in cases of absence of the "Lennox disease" type. Depakine has, however, been used with phenobarbital or with Mysoline, the dose of which was progressively reduced.

Electroenceph. clin. Neurophysiol., **1969**, *27*: 451–452

BOOK REVIEWS

Edited by H. Petsche *and* John R. Hughes

Klinische Elektroenzephalographie. Lehrbuch und Atlas. — W. Christian. (Thieme, Stuttgart, 1968, 336 p., 226 Fig., DM 98.00).

This new textbook and atlas was compiled by an expert who, because of his broad experience in both EEG and clinical neurology, is most capable of undertaking such a task. Accordingly, the main purpose of this book has been to discuss EEGs from the clinical point of view. It is surprising, however, that in spite of this intentional limitation, several physiological features are well outlined, as for instance the origin of the EEG. Nevertheless, so many EEG textbooks have been published in recent times that the reviewer has to put to himself the question whether or not publishing this particular volume was a pressing necessity, a question forcing the reviewer to judge books of this kind by severe standards.

First of all, the 226 figures, almost exclusively samples of EEG records, are excellent, though considerably reduced in size. One main drawback is the high degree of redundancy of most of these figures, because the greater part of the records were obtained referentially with the ipsilateral ear as reference. What makes the matter still worse: in many cases only paramedian electrodes were recorded from, temporal records being lacking. This is particularly regrettable in the recording of psychomotor seizures when the legend says "steep theta rhythms are present, synchronously over all brain regions" (Fig. 107). On the other hand, Fig. 28 represents "bilateral temporal delta wave groups", a conclusion simply drawn from bipolar records. But in this case, the potentials being bilateral, fronto-parietal delta waves cannot be excluded. An additional reference recording would have resolved this question.

That the author does not seem to be too familiar with the physical bases of bipolar and reference methods and their ranges of application, follows from the montages he prefers and also from sentences such as "laboratories working exclusively with bipolar technique have to use more electrodes". One wonders why? And if he claims to obtain with his type of montages "results not essentially poorer than those obtained with more electrodes", then this is only a confirmation of the fact that it depends not so much on the number of electrodes used as on their montage whether or not an optimum of results is attained.

Rather sparse is the chapter on nomenclature. Instead of taking over the concepts of the Terminology Committee of IFSECN, at least as far as those terms were generally accepted, the author creates, in different fields, his own nomenclature, without giving sufficiently clear criteria for definition in each case. Thus, for instance, the concept of "dysrhythmia", insufficient as it may be, is described not less than three times under different names: the record of Fig. 44 is considered as dysrhythmia, the one of Fig. 16 is described as "irregular EEG". In the text is written: "In adults, dysrhythmia occurs in about 10%" and on page 43: "In 10–15% of healthy persons EEGs are recorded that can be considered to be slightly and generally altered." And page 21 says: "Irregular EEG...as a constant finding in about 15% of healthy persons". Other new concepts, which the reviewer considers to be unnecessary, are "focal dysrhythmia" and "focal paroxysmal potentials". On the other hand, the concept "sharp waves and spikes" is used, indeed, but no definition is given. One main criticism concerns the frequent mention of "typically (or: specific) epileptic potentials". There is complete agreement among scientists since Lennox' days that no such potentials exist. Besides, some formulations are not quite clear: what are, for instance, "temporal foci without focal discharges" (page 183) and "temporal foci without epileptic potentials" (Table 1)? Moreover, several other inconsistencies ought to be avoided in a further edition.

It may seem unfair to enumerate the pitfalls of the book instead of emphasizing its good features. There are many. One of them is the good presentation of EEG changes in sleep, especially with respect to the epileptic patient. Particularly to be appreciated is the critical position the author takes with regard to the evaluation of the EEG in cases of epilepsy, which is also reflected in his consideration of epileptic equivalents. Regarding location of tumours, the reviewer is convinced that a better exploitation of the recording facilities might have supplied, in some cases, still more impressive pictures, giving more details for location. The chapters on vascular diseases, encephalitides, metabolic diseases and brain trauma are well written and give evidence of the author's wide experience in these fields.

As a whole, after having read this book, the reviewer regrets not having to deal with its second edition (which will probably be written soon) from which, it is hoped, many of the inconsistencies contained in the first edition will be eliminated.

H. Petsche
Neurological Institute,
University of Vienna (Austria)

Electroenceph. clin. Neurophysiol., **1969**, *27*: 453

Elektricheskie reakcii mozga na tormoznye signaly [Electrical reactions of the brain to inhibitory signals]. — J. G. Kratin. (Publishing House "NAUKA", Leningrad, 1967, 258 p., lr. 70k.).

The first four chapters (78 pages) of this monograph represent an extensive introduction to the following problems: reaction of excitation and inhibition from the standpoint of the Russian physiological school (Pavlov, Wedensky, Ukhtomsky), electrogenesis and subcortical structures, electrophysiology of the cerebral cortex, EEG and the highest nervous activity. This review, very informative mainly for a beginner, tries to confront orthodox Russian concepts with the results of the Western electrophysiological schools.

The author's own results were obtained on man, cat and rabbit. In human subjects a rather permanent state of drowsiness or light sleep (stage A to B) was introduced by the monotony of the experimental conditions. Persistence of this EEG stage in spite of applied stimulation was interpreted as the presence of inhibition, alpha rebound (paradoxical Berger's reaction) as a sign of excitation. In animals desynchronization and a resting record or spindle stage (cats) were looked for as correlates of excitation and inhibition respectively. The situations most frequently tested for the presence of EEG signs of inhibition thus defined were: inhibition of the orienting reaction to repeated irrelevant stimuli, differentiation of conditioning and test stimuli with verbal instruction (unconditioning stimulus) to perform voluntary movement (unconditioned reaction) in man, and alimentary or defensive reactions in animals, conditioned reactions with delayed unconditioning stimuli, extinction of conditioned reactions etc. The reported EEG signs of inhibition were nearly always found where they were expected. The EEG signs of excitation persisted, however, much longer than the inhibited reactions. The author interprets this as the persistence of excitation in the analysing branch of the system while the effectors are already fully inhibited. In some of the reported experimental situations, reactions of primary and secondary evoked potentials are described, without very persuasive correlations with the other events discussed. The monograph is closed by some rather speculative concepts exceeding the boundaries of the presented experimental data.

Excepting some summarizing graphs there is no endeavour to make a statistical evaluation of the results. Numerous figures of good quality are illustrative rather than documentary. As can be seen from this short review no new EEG signs of excitation and inhibition are presented. The contribution to the problem consists in showing systematically situations in which the well known signs of alertness occur. The question remains open of whether the reported EEG signs are specific for the different kinds of inhibitory processes described, evidently taking place in definite cerebral structures, or if they represent signs of different general states of alertness.

L. Ciganek
Institute of Normal and Pathological Physiology, Slovak Academy of Sciences, Bratislava (Czechoslovakia)

Electroenceph. clin. Neurophysiol., **1969**, *27*: 453–454

Progress in brain research. Vol. 30. Cerebral circulation. — W. Luyendijk (Editor). (Elsevier, Amsterdam, 1968, 511 p., Dfl. 95.00).

The volume contains 70 of the papers given at the Third European Neurosurgical Congress. The authors are eminent investigators of cerebral circulation. The volume is divided into nine sections and begins with the new results in the fields of basic research — anatomy, physiology and pathology.

The first three papers deal with the anatomy of the arteries of the brain. Van den Bergh and Vander Eecken describe two arterial systems in the cerebrum and cerebellum, two patterns of centrifugal and centripetal arteries. Lazorthes *et al.* emphasize that the blood flow of the cortex is not uniform, either from the point of view of anatomy or of haemodynamics. Not only do the archicortex, the paleocortex and the neocortex differ from each other, but even in the same parts of the neocortex conditions are different. Salamon *et al.* describe their results from examining cerebral arteries with a micro-radiographic technique.

In Section II there are 18 papers. Capon *et al.* survey, briefly but clearly, the methods used in the study of cerebral circulation. They summarize the procedures applicable to animals and man separately and discuss their theoretical basis. Jennett and Harper emphasize that in the course of neurosurgical interventions the technique which is best suited to the special circumstances of the case, and which may be expected to yield the data required, should be used. On the basis of his investigations with the isotope clearance method, using 8 or 16 detectors, Ingvar distinguishes 3 kinds of cerebrovascular disturbance, the focal hyperaemic, the ischaemic and the non-focal low rCBF type, which represents the "chronic brain syndrome". Symon describes a method for the study of traumatic cerebral vasospasm in experimental animals. It is the intima and internal elastic lamina of the traumatized artery that are damaged; it may be assumed that vasoactive substances, liberated intra-murally in the artery, are implicated in the production of spasm. Lundberg *et al.* deal with a special form of intracranial pressure variations called "plateau waves", their mechanism of development and their effect on cerebral haemodynamics. Hulme and Cooper call attention to the fact that in the "paradoxical" stage of sleep intracranial pressure may increase, possibly as a result of vasodilatation due to increased metabolism. According to McDowall *et al.* halothane and trichloroethylene cause cerebral vasodilatation, which increases blood flow and at the same time reduces cerebral O_2 uptake, and cerebrospinal fluid pressure rises. The increase in pCSF may be so great as to reduce CBF. The papers of Zwetnow *et al.*, Siesjö *et al.* and Betz, completing and confirming each other, emphasize the role of extracellular pH in the regulation of CBF and present data to support their opinion. On the basis of their animal experiments Shalit *et al.* support former data in the literature by assuming a neural reflex mechanism in the vasodilatation produced by CO_2. Lesions in the pons and mesencephalon reduce or abolish the vasodilating effect of CO_2. According to the observations of Waltz and Sundt the auto-regula-

Electroenceph. clin. Neurophysiol., **1969**, *27*: 454–456

tion of CBF fails to come into play in the territory of an occluded middle cerebral artery. Observations by Raudam *et al.* show that during transitory ischaemic attacks the O_2 demand and supply remain in equilibrium as a result of the increased O_2 consumption. The equilibrium is disturbed when infarction develops. If the upper brain-stem is involved, hyperventilation and hypocapnia develop and the patients "breathe themselves to death". Lassen deals with the mechanism of the "luxury perfusion syndrome" described by him. He calls attention to the fact that mild local compression of the cortex might bring about hyperaemia, which is documented also by the experiments of Brock. Jenkner expounds modifications and the theoretical basis of the rheoencephalographic technique. Himwich and Clark describe the results of their model experiments clarifying the haemodynamics of occlusive vascular processes. Heck deals with vascular pulsatile phenomena in the cortex and their changes in the case of an open rather than a closed calvarium and in increased intracranial pressure.

In Section III Zülch discusses separately the roles of the local and of the extracranial factors in the mechanism of intracranial haemorrhage. Yates makes a brief survey of occlusive cerebrovascular disease, mentioning occlusion of the intracranial vessels caused by thrombi and emboli, stenosis of extracranial vessels, disturbance of the blood flow in the internal carotid and vertebral arteries when the neck is turned, and the subclavian steal syndrome.

In Section IV Fischgold *et al.* expound the possibilities and advantages of cerebral angiography in neurosurgical cases. According to them, in atherosclerosis the isotope clearance technique is to be preferred. Ziedses des Plantes supports the significance of the subtraction method of cerebral angiography with excellent figures.

In Section V the use, in cerebrovascular disease, of EEG is dealt with by Carvalho, that of gammaencephalography by Oeconomos, that of echoencephalography by De Vlieger, that of pallencephalography by Barcia-Goyanes and Barcia-Salorio, and that of thermography by Wackenheim, in each case with the authors' experience reported. Perria *et al.* give their opinion on the diagnostic value of the intracarotid and intravertebral injection of amobarbital sodium.

In Section VI David *et al.* describe the symptomatology, pathology, aetiology and therapy of vertebro-basilar stenoses and thromboses on the basis of their experience, documented with excellent roentgenograms. Tolosa demonstrates the role of the middle meningeal artery in collateral circulation in cases of occlusion of the internal carotid and middle cerebral arteries. Vink and Dicke shortly summarize symptomatology, operative indications and techniques, and the possibilities of operative anaesthesia, in extracranial occlusive lesions. Hejhal and Firt deal with reconstructive surgery on the branches of the aortic arch. Donaghy and Yasargil describe a surgical technique for vessels less than 4 mm in outside diameter.

Section VII deals with intracranial aneurysms. Richardson reports his experience with aneurysms treated by strict bed rest, which experience is of great importance for practice. Sachs *et al.* present their observations on 126 intracranial aneurysms dissected macroscopically and point out that angiograms do not always give the precise information about the anatomy of aneurysms which is important for the surgeon. Govaert and Walker deal with the pathological anatomy of intracranial aneurysms and the mechanisms of their development. In the opinion of Taylor and Kak studies of cerebral circulation time may be of great help in the management of subarachnoid haemorrhage. Norlén reports his experience with the surgery of aneurysms of the anterior communicating artery and points out the importance of arterial spasm as an unfavourable prognostic sign. Guidetti also discusses the problems of surgery of the anterior communicating artery, timing of the operation, the use of hypothermia and operative techniques. Kunc emphasizes that in aneurysm of the carotid and the posterior communicating artery the patient's somatic condition and conscious state greatly influence the outcome of an operation. According to Maspes and Marini, in unfavourable risk patients mortality is almost equal between operated and non-operated groups; in favourable risk patients, however, prognosis is much better for the operation. It is only in cases of irrecoverable patients with vertebro-basilar aneurysms in catastrophic condition that Laine does not operate. Morello compares the results of operations performed under three kinds of condition: (1) normothermia and hypotension; (2) hypothermia and controlled respiration and (3) normothermia and mild hypotension. Mortality is smallest in the third group. Zoltán prefers surgical treatment of the saccular aneurysm to its conservative therapy. Björkesten and Troupp, comparing the results of surgical and conservative treatment of intracranial aneurysms, do not find a significant difference. Taptas and Katsiotis call attention to arterial embolism as a possible cause of hemiplegia after subarachnoid haemorrhage from aneurysm. Stepien deals with the technique of reinforcement of aneurysms with adherent plastics. Gillingham describes his experience with the cardiac pacemaker. Kristiansen deals with the cardiac pacemaker and the method of extracorporeal circulation.

Section VIII discusses some of the problems of arterio-venous aneurysms. Verbiest surveys the localization, types, symptoms and techniques of surgical treatment of arterio-venous aneurysms of the posterior fossa. Kunicki deals with micro-angiomas and angiomas of the central area, which is followed by an article by Zoltán on the operability of centrally located arterio-venous angiomas. Kostić presents some observations on the surgical treatment of cerebrovascular diseases. Wappenschmidt *et al.* point out the significance of vertebral angiography in the diagnosis of arterio-venous malformations. Examining arterio-venous angiomas microscopically, Paillas *et al.* have nearly always found sclerosis of the vascular walls and, in one third of the cases, also more special lesions: conglomerates of histiocytes, calcification and iron deposits in the walls of blood vessels. The incidence of migraine and that of epileptic manifestations are high in such cases. In Ameli's opinion the prognosis of arterio-venous malformations may be complicated by intracerebral haemorrhage, for which he suggests surgical treatment. Carrea and Girado deal with arterio-venous fistulous and angiomatous aneurysms in children and with their surgical treatment. Arutiunov *et al.* describe techniques for the surgical treatment of carotico-cavernous fistulae on the basis of their own experience. Riechert presents a case of pulsating exophthalmus and its surgical management, compression of the cavernous sinus with a tantalum plate. According to Röttgen in the treatment of aneurysms the method of choice is occlusion of the aneurysm without injuring the artery.

Dealing with the pathogenesis of hypertensive intracerebral haemorrhage on the basis of their experimental experience in Section IX, Margolis *et al.* draw the conclusion that it is not the elevated blood pressure *per se*, but the tonic reaction of cerebral vessels, and their structural and functional properties, which play the primary role. Pia emphasizes the significance of surgical treatment in intraventricular haemorrhage. Feindel *et al.* describe their experience with fluorescein angiography during craniotomy. According to Hollin *et al.* hyperbaric oxygenation reduces the mortality of experimentally produced cerebral oedema and compression.

In this volume all those who are interested in the results of the basic sciences bearing on cerebral circulation, and also neurosurgeons, can find such information as is indispensable to their further activities.

L. Molnár
Psychiatric-Neurologic Clinic,
University of Pécs, Pécs (Hungary)

Electroenceph. clin. Neurophysiol., **1969**, *27*: 454–456

Hepatocerebral degeneration. — H. Asao and K. Oji. (C. C. Thomas, Springfield, Ill., 1968, 83 p., $7.50).

This short monograph is written in an English that would have benefited from considerable editing. Representative of the authors' style, this sentence was taken from the Introduction:

"A disease described as *Hepatocerebral Degeneration* is defined to be a hepatogenic encephalopathy, of which the influence upon neurologic manifestations is different according to the nature and severity of the liver dysfunction."

and another from the Summary:

"Hepatocerebral Degeneration is the name of a disease based on the pathoanatomical standpoint. However, the clinical and pathological findings of this disease in general resemble in various points the so-called hepatic coma. From these facts, hepatic coma due to liver failure and the specific forms (Inose type and pseudoulegyria type) are classified as a sub-form of hepatocerebral degeneration in a wide sense."

Unfortunately, the style between the Introduction and the Summary is of about the same standard; this unintelligible sentence is from the section on Treatment:

"In hypopotassemia caused by removal of a large amount of ascites, ammonia more easily entering into the cells, because of the deficiency of potassium or magnesium caused by vomiting and diarrhea, is often noted in coma."

The numerous syntactical, grammatical, and constructional deficiencies are detracting.

The book has been written for neurologists, internists, and investigators interested in the biochemical and physiologic aspects of hepato-cerebral syndromes. An abundant literature—to which the authors have contributed—has appeared over the years on this complex subject. To have condensed it effectively to 24 pages would have been a remarkable achievement if the authors had succeeded.

Two chapters are devoted to a review of the clinical and pathologic features of the "specific" forms of hepatocerebral degeneration described by Inose and Shiraki; those not familiar with these syndromes, or who do not regularly peruse the Japanese and the German literature, will find them worth reading.

The EEG aspects of hepatic encephalopathy are alluded to very briefly: EEG findings in the "specific" types of hepato-cerebral degeneration resemble those seen in the more usual forms of hepatic coma; they also correlate better with the degree of disturbance of consciousness than with any other single parameter, including blood concentration of ammonia, short-chain fatty acids, nucleic acid derivatives, and so forth.

In the last chapter, conventional and less conventional means of correcting the metabolic derangements of hepatic encephalopathy are presented, however, without a critical evaluation of their therapeutic efficacy.

Hepatocerebral Degeneration is a poorly edited book of limited interest.

Jean Reiher
Mayo Clinic and Mayo Foundation,
Rochester, Minn. 55901 (U.S.A.)

Electroenceph. clin. Neurophysiol., **1969**, *27*: 456

ALTERATIONS OF THE HUMAN ELECTROENCEPHALOGRAM INDUCED BY STRESSFUL VERBAL ACTIVITY[1]

JAN BERKHOUT, DONALD O. WALTER AND W. ROSS ADEY

Space Biology Laboratory, Brain Research Institute, University of California, Los Angeles, Calif. 90024 (U.S.A.)

(Accepted for publication: March 24, 1969)

The EEG has been proved an efficient and sensitive indicator of CNS reactivity in several distinct areas of laboratory stress evaluation. One such area includes the presentation of symbolic or verbal stimuli of a potentially stressful nature, the affective value of these stimuli being assessed under conditions of passive perception. Under such conditions the phase relationships of dominant rhythmic segments of the EEG, measured between opposite sides and poles of the head, have proved to be valuable parameters for discerning and quantifying human reactions. Darrow and Converse (1950), Darrow and Hicks (1965) and Darrow (1967) have published a series of papers describing the changing of such lead and lag indices as functions of the emotional significance or information content of discrete symbolic or verbal stimuli. These phase shifts were apparently proportional to the stress value of particular words, and were also sensitive to the appearance of "anticipation" stress in the period of apprehension preceding the presentation of stimuli.

Grey Walter (1965) has also reported a scalable EEG response to such forms of stimuli, the responses consisting of relatively long-term anterior lobe negative base-line shifts or depolarizations. Black and Walter (1965) state that under certain circumstances the extent of this depolarization is a function of the probability of association between information-bearing stimuli in other sensory modes. These responses are both complementary to and compatible with the phase shift phenomena described by Darrow and his co-workers.

Several other facets of the EEG have been associated with the perception of discrete verbal stimuli since the earliest observations on the relationship of the EEG and behavior. Travis and Egan (1938) reported an increase in the frequency of the alpha rhythm following verbal stimulation, which appeared to be consistent over several subjects, despite very crude control over the stimuli used and the method of frequency analysis employed. Hoagland *et al.* (1938) made use of an EEG delta index in an experiment on emotion in humans involving hostile personal and sexual comments in a confrontation situation. Both the quantity of sub-alpha frequency material and its pharyngeal (hypothalamic)-cortical phase lag were good indicators of the subjective annoyance and rage evoked by the stimuli, as confirmed by simultaneous autonomic activity and subsequent interviews.

We have substantially confirmed the existence and direction of such transient changes in the EEG during a variety of both simulated and genuinely stressful circumstances (Adey *et al.* 1967; Walter *et al.* 1967b). We have also noted a similar range and variety of EEG responses to be closely associated with potentially stressful presentations of semantic stimuli, including phase shifts, changes in spectral intensity and spindling (Walter *et al.* 1967a; Adey 1969).

The present study of the relationship of the EEG to verbal behavior was directed at two specific aspects of this problem: (1) the extent to which the EEG is altered across the definable

[1] This study was aided by Contract NONR 233 (91) between the Office of Naval Research, Department of the Navy and the Brain Research Institute of the University of California, Los Angeles. The computer analysis was done in the Data Processing Laboratory of the Brain Research Institute supported by U.S. Public Health Service Grant NB 02501, and in the Health Sciences Computing Facility supported by National Institutes of Health Grant FR-3.

stages of a verbal exchange, independent of content; and (2) the extent to which the EEG is altered by the specific information content of given verbal stimuli, or by the different alerting or stress values of a series of such stimuli.

METHODS

A. *Data collection*

The definable stages of our formalized verbal exchange may be tentatively described as perception, decision and anticipation epochs, as these are delimited by the question duration, the question–answer interval, and the answer–next comment interval (Fig. 1). These three epochs were considered integral in this study although the question–duration interval might be further divisible according to the grammar of the verbal stimulus.

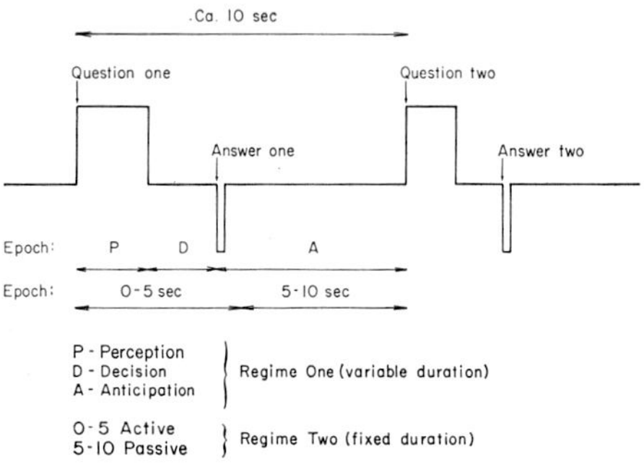

Fig. 1
Schematic representation of epoch definitions.

Our subjects for this study consisted of fourteen paid male student volunteers, ranging in age from 18 to 22. They were isolated in a soundproof room and presented with identical tape-recorded sequences of 20 questions covering a variety of personal and ethical topics, and ranging from embarrassing or offensive to innocuous in their subjective effect. Simultaneous monitoring of autonomic activity (heart rate pulse volume and galvanic skin potential) served to confirm the affective value of the questions asked. The questions varied in duration from 1.0 to 3.5 sec and occurred at 10 sec intervals, the entire session lasting 200 sec. The subjects were instructed to reply only "yes" or "no" to each question. A voice-operated relay coded the times during which questions were asked and answers produced with $\pm$ 50 msec accuracy.

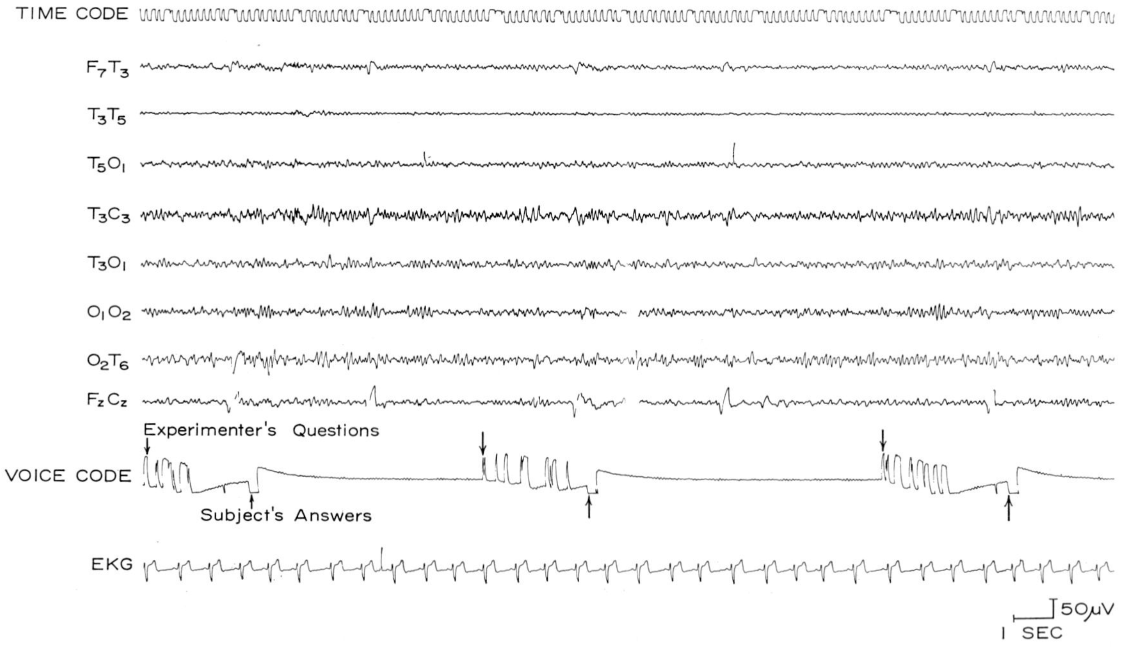

Fig. 2
EEG activity during questioning of a non-reactive subject (No. 48). Note the absence of any EEG activity regularly altered by the occurrence of questions or answers.

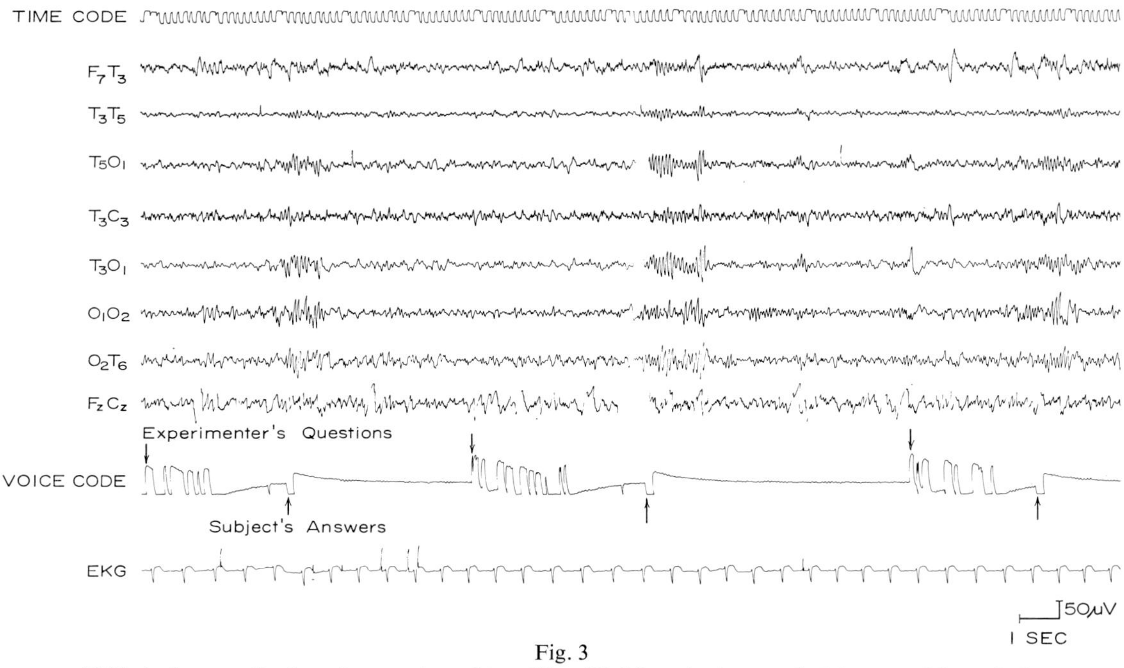

Fig. 3
EEG during questioning of a reactive subject (No. 42). Note the bursts of alpha material regularly following this subject's answers.

Nine channels of EEG were recorded on an analog instrumentation tape recorder during the question session and for the 1.0 min preceding and following. Bipolar derivatives were used exclusively in the recording montage.

The paper tracings were screened for muscle and eye movement artifacts and classified as reactive or non-reactive according to whether alpha spindling or alpha attenuation accompanied the presentation of the question stimuli. Fig. 2 and 3 illustrate excerpts of reactive and non-reactive EEG tracings obtained during the experimental question sessions.

The EEG records of each subject were divided into short epochs with reference to the voice-code mentioned above. For those subjects who generally delayed answering for more than 1.5 sec past the termination of each question, the three epochs defined in Fig. 1, Regime 1, were constructed. These epochs were necessarily of varying length. For those subjects whose answers followed questions very closely, only two epochs were defined: active and passive (Fig. 1, Regime 2). The active (0–5) epoch consisted of the 5.0 sec immediately following question onset, and contained both the question and answer; the passive (5–10) epoch consisted of the subsequent 5.0 sec of empty time. Thus 40 or 60 epochs were defined for each subject.

The questions asked were classified as highly stressful, moderately stressful or not stressful on the basis of the autonomic responses of a group of sixty-five subjects previously studied (Berkhout *et al.* in preparation). The separation of the questions into three autonomic response classes was based on the criteria listed in Table I. The standard deviations referred to in that table were obtained by pooling responses from all subjects across all questions.

Variability within the three classes was not great, as many questions were excluded to obtain a tri-modal distribution. As our intention was to isolate tentatively homogeneous sets of verbal stimuli rather than homogeneous sets of autonomic responses, the high-stress and low-stress classes of stimuli were further divided into groups differing only in verbal content; a division eventually supported by the analyses applied to the concomitant EEG activity.

Autonomic activity of subjects contributing to the present study was monitored for unusual or extreme responses. The stressful character of

TABLE I

Description of question sets. Autonomic criteria are based on evoked circulatory responses to each item, averaged across an independent group of sixty-five subjects

Question set	Autonomic criteria	Typical verbal content
High stress I (Sex)	Severe (± 2 S.D.) fluctuations of heart rate and pulse volume coincident with question presentation	"Do you masturbate?" "Do you have homosexual urges?" (4 items)
High stress II (Lie)	As above	"Have you lied answering those questions?" (repeated 3 times)
Low stress I (Read)	Mild (less than 1 S.D.) fluctuations of heart rate and pulse volume coincident with question presentation	"Do you approve of the material you have just read?" (3 items)
Low stress II (Query)	As above	"Does anyone know you are here?" (repeated 2 times)
Non-stress	No fluctuations of heart rate or pulse volume noted	"Do you believe in capital punishment?" (2 items)

our question stimuli was generally confirmed in our present experimental group. The lengths of the epochs used in this EEG study were too short to permit a statistically valid evaluation of autonomic activity occurring during individual epochs.

B. *Data reduction*

The EEG activity accompanying the various epochs defined above was subjected to a procedure of spectral analysis (Walter 1963). The auto-spectral derivatives generated by this procedure included intensity and bandwidth. These parameters were defined for each of the six frequency bands specified between 1 and 30 c/sec.

Intensity was defined in units of $\log_{10} \mu V^2/c/sec$ summed over each specific band. Bandwidth was defined in c/sec for each band, that value being the bandwidth of an ideally filtered noise function with the same maximum spectral intensity and same total intensity as the EEG segment analyzed. Bandwidth is interpreted as an estimator of "peakedness" in the spectral distribution; where strongly rhythmic activity or spindling is present bandwidth will be small, where such activity is lacking, bandwidth will be large. Cross-spectral derivatives included phase and coherence. Phase was defined as the sine of the angle by which the first channel of each pair led or lagged the second in a given frequency band. The coherence function provides a measure of linear relationship between pairs of EEG channels. Coherence was defined in non-physical units as the difference between an observed value and the calculated 95% confidence level for non-random occurrence of that value, taking epoch length and spectral resolution into account.

This coding of coherence was used to compensate for unequal bias of the coherence estimator as a function of epoch length; hence all coherence values listed in the tables for all regimes are directly comparable.

Five channels of EEG (F_7T_3, T_3T_5, T_5O_1, O_1O_2 and O_2T_6) were excerpted for spectral analysis of this type. Thus, with 6-band resolution of the frequency spectrum, 60 auto-spectral parameters were defined for each epoch. With 10 channel-pairs analyzed, 120 cross-spectral parameters were also defined. This produced 7,200 data values per subject under the 40-epoch regime; under the 60-epoch regime 10,800 data values per subject were generated. Consequently, a further step of data reduction was considered necessary. For this purpose, we employed the stepwise discriminant analysis program DISCAN (Dixon 1967; Walter *et al.* 1967c). This program has as one of its capabilities the generation of a multi-dimensional canonical variable which maximizes the differences between distinct and non-overlapping families of epochs for which comparable parameters are available. Such families of epochs must be initially segregated and defined. Sufficient parameters to achieve 100% separation of these families are then introduced step by step, compensating those remaining unselected at each step for variance common to previously selected items. Thus each parameter eventually included represents a group of variables of common tendency among which it is the most efficient discriminator. The parameters selected are consequently relatively independent of each other.

The percentage separation achieved by a given number of discriminators is a good index of the true distinctiveness of the families of data tentatively set apart when the program was initiated. The nature and dimensions of such distinctiveness and the internal consistency and anomalies inherent in the experimental data must be deduced from the tactical developments appearing at each step of the discriminant analysis. Basically, the program is used to identify a small number of relevant index parameters from a large mass of data.

Fiducial confidence limits or significance levels are generated as part of the DISCAN computation procedure. This calculation takes into account the number of parameters originally available for selection; if this number is very large the confidence limits are adjusted to compensate for the increased likelihood of a random agreement between some variable and the desired categorization.

Interpretation of the discriminant analysis output required an evaluation of the increment of classification successes with the addition of each step. Physiological interpretation of a parameter chosen by the program at a given step was based on detailed study of the distribution of its values for the initially defined groups, and on a study of the changes in patterns of classification between steps, assessing the distribution of values for those groups from which the previously misclassified cases were retrieved.

RESULTS

A. *Identification of spectral parameters best correlated with perception, decision and anticipation*

The stimulus conditions of a verbal interchange appeared to impose a set of response characteristics on the EEG which were rapidly established and rapidly replaced, being expressed in epochs 3–5 sec long, and yet reliably consistent, being uniformly repeated over 20 cycles of verbal interchange elapsing within 4 min.

1. *Individual characteristics of perception–decision–anticipation cycles.* The first evaluation of our data was directed at distinguishing between the perception, decision and anticipation epochs of Regime 1, apart from the specific content and stress value of the questions asked. We applied our discriminant analysis procedure to data from those four subjects whose question–answer delay times were sufficiently long to permit a valid estimate of spectral characteristics for all three types of epochs. The computation

TABLE II

Summary of a stepwise discriminant analysis. Data for a single subject were evaluated by epoch type, 60 epochs contributing. Values of Intensity are given in $\log_{10} \mu V^2$/c/sec. Values of Phase and Coherence are in coded units (see text). The parameters are weighted differently as selection steps proceed

Step	Parameter (3 c/sec bandwidths)	Percent correct after step	Average values over 20 epochs		
			Perception epochs	Decision epochs	Anticipation epochs
Subject 8:					
1.	$T_5O_1 \times O_1O_2$ Coherence, 6 c/sec	54%	−0.34	−0.12	−0.23
2.	T_5O_1 Intensity, 12 c/sec	62%	2.40	2.52	2.60
3.	$O_1O_2 \times O_2T_6$ Coherence, 6 c/sec	79%	−0.23	−0.10	−0.33
4.	$O_1O_2 \times O_2T_6$ Coherence, 18 c/sec	83%	−0.26	−0.18	−0.33
		97% correct attained at Step 15			

procedure was designed to select those parameters which most consistently identified the epochs in question. These parameters were then combined into a multi-dimensional index variable and cut-off points were established which allowed a tentative identification of each of the 60 epochs in question as being one of the three types defined.

The four subjects compatible with Regime 1 had individually distinctive EEGs, and a discriminating canon applicable to the entire group of individuals was highly unsuccessful. Considering each subject separately, we were able to achieve over 90% correct identification of the 60 epochs in each case. In this particular analysis both auto- and cross-spectral derivatives were evaluated simultaneously, competing with each other for admission to the discriminating canon. We will describe one case in detail to give an example of the procedure, and summarize the similarities and contrasts with the other individuals tested. Table II contains a detailed listing of the initial parameters selected for subject 8, in their order of selection.

Fifty-eight out of 60 epochs were correctly identified for subject 8, with 15 parameters contributing. The initial parameter selected was a cross-spectral derivative, coherence between T_5O_1, and O_1O_2 at 6 c/sec. Coherence was lowest during the perception epoch and highest during the decision epoch between question and answer. Using that parameter as a sole criterion for identifying epochs, over 50% were correctly attributed. The correct attributions were primarily drawn from the perception and decision categories, which averaged the lowest and highest coherence, respectively. Values of coherence for the anticipation epochs fell, on the average, between values for the other two groups. This particular coherence parameter was the best discriminator among several coherence parameters similarly distributed over the three epochs; these included $T_5O_1 \times O_1O_2$ at 9 c/sec, and $O_1O_2 \times O_2T_6$ at 12 c/sec. In the succeeding steps of the analysis the remaining available parameters were corrected for variance common to items already chosen, so that such covarying families of parameters, as the family of coherences mentioned above, would be represented by their best member. Each increment of correctly classified epochs was usually drawn from the extreme tails of the distribution of the particular parameter added at each step.

Upon the selection of T_5O_1 intensity as the second step in Table II, five additional epochs were correctly identified. All were anticipation epochs for which average alpha intensity was high. The symmetrical channel (O_2T_6) displayed a similar pattern of alpha intensities: low during question presentation, slightly higher before the answer, and highest while attending the subsequent question.

Using such EEG criteria exclusively, no more than 5 of the 60 epochs were misclassified for each individual with 15 parameters contributing; with only 5 parameters contributing, no more than 15 of the 60 epochs were misclassified.

For all four subjects, perception epochs were characterized by an attenuation of parietal-occipital alpha compatible with an alert state, decision epochs were characterized by over-all increases in coherence in the theta and beta bands compatible with a state of increased stress, and anticipation epochs were characterized by low coherences and generally high alpha intensities.

These characteristics differed in detail from subject to subject, and an individual-specific calibration was necessary to identify the various epochs. An attempted discrimination across the four subjects simultaneously failed, not reaching 40% correct identifications in 15 steps. Fiducial confidence limits for the individual-specific discriminations exceeded 99% levels in every case.

2. *Individual characteristics of active–passive cycles.* The remaining ten subjects were not suitable for the detailed epochal analysis of Regime 1 and were subjected to the fixed-epoch-length analysis of Regime 2 (Fig. 1). Under the latter regime the initial epoch contained both the question and answer and was considered "active", the subsequent epoch being "passive". A combined spectral and discriminant analysis procedure similar to that reported above was applied to these subjects to determine those EEG parameters most consistently discriminating between the active and passive states. The stepwise analysis procedure for four selected subjects is summarized in Table III. As with the previous cases, auto- and cross-spectral parameters were competing together for admission to the discriminating canon. Only 40 epochs of two types

TABLE III

Summary of four stepwise discriminant analyses. Data for single subjects were evaluated by epoch type, 40 epochs contributing for each subject

Step	Parameter	Percent correct after step	Average values: Active epochs	Average values: Passive epochs
Subject 39:	(Reactive)			
1.	F_7T_3 Intensity 8–12 c/sec	77%	4.6	4.8
2.	$F_7T_3 \times O_1O_2$ Phase 8–12 c/sec	87%	0.53	0.07
3.	$T_5O_1 \times O_2T_6$ Phase 0–2 c/sec	90%	−0.16	0.15
	100% correct attained at Step 7			
Subject 48:	(Non-Reactive)			
1.	$F_7T_3 \times T_3T_5$ Phase 8–12 c/sec	70%	0.11	−0.13
2.	T_3T_5 Intensity 3–7 c/sec	77%	2.64	2.56
3.	$T_5O_1 \times O_1O_2$ Phase 8–12 c/sec	85%	−0.18	0.00
4.	$F_7T_3 \times O_2T_6$ Coherence 8–12 c/sec	95%	−0.36	−0.28
	98% correct at Step 6 100% correct at Step 15			
Subject 46:	(Reactive)			
1.	O_1O_2 Intensity 8–12 c/sec	77%	4.06	4.37
2.	$F_7T_3 \times T_5O_1$ Coherence 20–30 c/sec	90%	−0.34	−0.45
3.	T_3T_5 Bandwidth 13–20 c/sec	95%	2.15 c/sec	2.00 c/sec
	100% correct attained at Step 10			
Subject 23:	(Reactive)			
1.	O_1O_2 Bandwidth 20–30 c/sec	62%	1.97 c/sec	2.15 c/sec
2.	O_2T_6 Intensity 20–30 c/sec	82%	2.56	2.45
3.	$F_7T_3 \times T_5O_1$ Coherence 0–2 c/sec	87%	−0.48	−0.38
	92% correct at Step 5—100% correct at Step 10			

were involved for each subject and 100% correct identifications were obtained in every case. A survey of the parameters selected for the various subjects in Table III will illustrate the great variety between individuals in the manner in which they most consistently reacted to the two epoch conditions defined.

Subject 39 consistently demonstrated lower

alpha intensity in the F_7T_3 derivation during the active epochs, and alpha material from the frontal-temporal area led occipital alpha in phase by 30°. During the passive epochs this phase difference disappeared.

Subject 48 displayed a similar phase shift in alpha material along the anterior-posterior axis, the anterior leading during the active epochs, posterior leading during the passive epochs. This parameter was selected as the first step in the discriminating canon. However, alterations in alpha intensity between the two kinds of epoch were not a consistent feature of this subject. Theta intensity appeared slightly but consistently higher in the temporal area during the active epoch.

This subject illustrates one of the limitations of the discriminant analysis procedure. With six parameters contributing, all epochs but one were correctly identified. Seven further items had to be entered before the single anomalous case was assigned to its proper category. Obviously, such recalcitrant epochs are distinct from the others (though perhaps only because of sampling variance in the measurements), hence the parameters utilized in such a forced distinction are likely to generalize poorly.

Subject 46 displayed the usual alpha attenuation pattern during the active epochs, but other parameters chosen were unique for this subject. Subject 23 did not present a consistent alpha attenuation pattern during the active epochs, but rather a more intense narrow band occipital high beta (20–30 c/sec) activity, along with ambiguous coherence shifts in the delta band. Nevertheless, 100% correct identification of the 40 epochs was achieved for this subject.

Parameters reflecting the alpha spindling following answers which characterized the "reactive" EEG records of some of these subjects were not always chosen to enter the discriminating canon. The DISCAN procedure is biased to select small but consistent differences between groups over large but erratic differences. Thus, for subject 46 in Table III, who generated a reactive EEG (similar to Fig. 3), alpha intensity in the occipital area, obviously related to the observed alpha spindling, was selected as the best discriminating parameter. However, for subject 23 in Table III, notwithstanding an apparently similar pattern of EEG reactivity, beta activity characteristics not notable in the raw paper tracings proved a more consistent discriminator of sequential active and passive epochs than the

TABLE IV

Summary of a stepwise discriminant analysis. Data for five subjects were evaluated by stress level. One "active" epoch was included for each subject and question, providing 140 epochs for the analysis

Step	Parameter	Percent correct after step	Average values	
			Stress epochs	Non-stress epochs
Group A: *Non-reactive EEG*				
1.	$F_7T_3 \times T_5O_1$ Coherence 0–2 c/sec	67%	−0.48	−0.38
2.	T_3T_5 Bandwidth 3–7 c/sec	68%	2.2 c/sec	2.4 c/sec
3.	$O_1O_2 \times O_2T_6$ Coherence 8–12 c/sec	70%	0.01	−0.32
4.	O_2T_6 Bandwidth 8–12 c/sec	74%	1.77 c/sec	1.9 c/sec
5.	F_7T_3 Intensity 20–30 c/sec	75%	3.00	2.80
6.	T_3T_5 Phase 13–19 c/sec	84%	−0.12	0.02
		92% correct at Step 12		

more obvious, but apparently less consistent, changes in alpha activity.

Whatever the parameters eventually selected for the various subjects, the differences between active and passive epochs were compatible with greater emotional significance and heightened alertness being associated with the active state. Active states were characterized by attenuated alpha and phase shifts of alpha material along the frontal-temporal-occipital axis.

B. *Application of discriminant analysis to high and low stress questions*

EEG changes associated with strings of alternating active and passive epochs were individual-specific. However, when the active epochs alone were excerpted, EEG characteristics associated with question stress values and with the verbal content of the questions themselves were determined to be similar, within strict numerical limits, over many subjects simultaneously.

Such epochs were excerpted from five subjects with non-reactive type EEGs. All high-stress category questions were combined in one set, and the innocuous and low stress questions in another. By restricting the discriminating procedure to these two classes, the parameters chosen as the basis of separation could be related to the differential autonomic response characteristics used to define the two sets. This procedure was definitely not equivalent to a linear correlation of EEG and autonomic activity, since the criteria for designating a given question as stressful included contradictory patterns of autonomic arousal and widely varying baselines. Table IV lists the characteristics of high and low stress which emerged from this analysis. Over 90% of the epochs tested were correctly identified.

The parameters listed in Table IV may be interpreted as defining a tentative EEG stress index. Our high stress epochs were characterized by a distinct narrowing of the temporal-parietal theta bandwidth, a similar narrowing of the occipital alpha bandwidth, and a 70% increase in frontal-temporal beta intensity. Cross-spectral discriminators included a slight but consistent decrease in delta band coherence between the left frontal and left temporal channels during stress, and a major increase in alpha band coherence between the right occipital and right parietal channels during the same epochs. There was an average 10° phase lag of beta material between the left temporal and left occipital areas during the stress epochs which was not noted at other times.

Over-all, 92% of the epochs tested were correctly identified as stress or non-stress events by means of their associated EEG characteristics. The residual 8% (6 epochs) may well represent accurate evaluations of truly anomalous responses rather than mistaken evaluations of true stress or non-stress EEG patterns.

C. *Effect of subjective content on EEG changes*

Our final step in evaluating this material was directed at determining the extent to which the EEG was altered by the subjective content, or differential stress value, of the various questions asked. By treating sets of questions according to content we discovered several EEG parameters which differentiated among the sets across groups of five subjects simultaneously.

Fourteen of our verbal stimuli were divided into five sets of homogeneous subject matter, as listed in Table I. We are not at all confident of the true independence of subjective affect between these five sets, and they may well overlap to some extent. Since we were able to derive a relatively good discriminating EEG index for each set, the uncertainty of our initial stress evaluation could not have been particularly severe.

A discriminant analysis procedure similar to that described above was applied to spectral parameters derived from the active type of 5 sec epochs, incorporating one epoch per question for two groups of five subjects each. The groups were separated by reactive and non-reactive EEGs; this separation was necessary for the success of the discriminations.

It was not our intention to demonstrate an EEG signature for each of the verbal circumstances defined by our question sets, but rather to show that their differential operational value, insofar as it was distinct for each set, was reflected in the spectral characteristics of the contributing EEG in a manner both fairly consistent within subjects, and substantially similar across subjects. Over 80% of the epochs tested were correctly identified in association with one of the five types

TABLE V

Summary of two stepwise discriminant analyses. Data for two groups of five subjects each were evaluated by question content. Each analysis included 140 "active" epochs

Step	Parameter	Average values				
		High stress epochs		Low stress epochs		Non-stress epochs
		"Sex" content	"Lie" content	"Read" content	"Query" content	
Group A: *Non-reactive EEG*						
1.	$T_3T_5 \times O_1O_2$ Phase 0–2 c/sec	0.22	−0.26	−0.54	−0.05	−0.35
2.	$T_5O_1 \times O_1O_2$ Phase 8–12 c/sec	0.34	0.15	0.05	−0.27	0.07
3.	$F_7T_3 \times O_1O_2$ Coherence 0–2 c/sec	−0.43	−0.45	−0.53	−0.41	−0.41
4.	$T_3T_5 \times O_1O_2$ Coherence 8–12 c/sec	−0.54	−0.50	−0.48	−0.52	−0.50
5.	$F_7T_3 \times O_2T_6$ Coherence 13–19 c/sec	−0.41	−0.46	−0.39	−0.48	−0.34
		58% correct at Step 5 84% correct at Step 15				
Group B: *Reactive EEG*						
1.	$T_5O_1 \times O_2T_6$ Phase 13–20 c/sec	0.19	0.19	0.20	0.55	0.28
2.	$T_3T_5 \times T_5O_1$ Coherence 8–12 c/sec	−0.11	−0.27	−0.16	−0.33	−0.28
3.	$T_3T_5 \times O_2T_6$ Phase 3–7 c/sec	0.14	0.43	0.00	0.19	−0.11
4.	$F_7T_3 \times T_5O_1$ Phase 3–7 c/sec	0.46	0.13	0.16	0.26	−0.18
		54% correct at Step 4 81% correct at Step 15				

of verbal content. The identifying characteristics are listed in Table V.

Because the analysis reported in Table V was required to establish a discrimination between some sets of questions with equivalent stress value and differing only in verbal content, it was not possible to interpret these particular results as expressing a stress "signature" of the EEG. The parameters selected did not exhibit low values with low stress, and high values with high; nor *vice versa*. Indeed, the parameters listed in Tables IV and V (A) do not overlap to any considerable extent. The procedure generating Table V was constrained to distinguish groups of epochs similar in stress value and differing only in verbal content; procedures for Table IV were constrained to separate epochs by their subjective stress concomitants only. It is quite predictable that two independent sets of parameters should have emerged from these procedures.

The elements of the EEG that appeared to be sensitive to the verbal aspects of our experimental presentation (in ways which generalized adequately across subjects) were almost completely restricted to the cross-spectral derivatives of coherence and phase. This was true of both the reactive and non-reactive types of EEG. For the non-reactive group, these phase and coherence differences appeared in all four frequency bands, always involving the bioccipital channel. The phase lead or lag of this area with the left frontal-temporal region was the most powerful parameter in the discriminating canon for this group. No auto-spectral derivatives were selected at all. For the reactive EEG group a different mix of contributing parameters and channels was noted, and an occasional auto-spectral derivative, for example parietal theta bandwidth, was incorporated into the discrimination.

The distribution of incorrect attributions among subjects was uniform: no one subject generated more than 3 incorrect attributions for the 14 epochs evaluated per subject, and no one question generated more than 2 incorrect attributions for the 5 epochs evaluated per question. Confidence levels associated with these discriminant procedures exceeded 99% levels in both cases. It would appear that there are indeed some alterations in the EEG reflecting differences in content of spoken stimuli which are consistent across small groups of individuals.

DISCUSSION

Spontaneous changes of intensity occurring in the resting EEG appear to differ greatly between individuals. These differences are stable so long as the resting condition is maintained, but tend to be obliterated during conditions of arousal, sensory perception or sleep (Henry 1941; Berkhout and Walter 1968). Many auto-spectral parameters reflecting such individual-specific EEG activity in the passive state were incorporated in the computation differentiating active *vs.* passive epochs. It is thus not surprising that this discrimination could not be extended across individuals. Within individuals, the sequence of 40 interleaved active and passive epochs provoked generally coincident changes in auto-spectral values which were consistent throughout the 20 cycles of active–passive alternation.

In the discrimination of high stress *vs.* low stress events several auto-spectral responses associated with active epochs were consistent enough across subjects to contribute to the discrimination.

These responses, including decreases in theta- and beta-frequency bandwidth, are not usually observed in the resting EEG, and seem to be typical of EEG responses to external events. They are more stereotyped across a large population than is spontaneous, resting, or passive EEG activity. The stress index values derived from such bandwidth characteristics were valid for five subjects simultaneously, with no recalibration needed for given individuals.

In the discriminations of semantic content presented during active epochs, auto-spectral parameters were almost completely excluded from the discriminating canons in favor of cross-spectral derivatives. Phase shifts between frontal and occipital alpha material following emotionally significant stimuli, as reported by Hoagland *et al.* (1938) and Darrow and Hicks (1965), were confirmed to be consistent changes in about half of our subjects. The phase shifts derived from our particular mode of cross-spectral analysis are defined for each frequency band evaluated and as such are quite distinct from the wave comparator data of Darrow. Nevertheless, our measurements did indicate a shift in relative latency in the dominant alpha band during some stress epochs, with the frontal regions lagging at those times. The stress signature indicated in Table IV contains elements analogous to both the antero-posterior phase shifts of dominant wave activity reported by Darrow for similar types of stressor stimuli, and to the increased coherences and theta band intensity reported by Adey *et al.* (1967) in an entirely different stressor situation involving orbital space flight.

The computation of cross-spectral measurements, including phase angles, would seem to be essential in evaluating EEG responses to this type of situation. Boyle *et al.* (1965) reported no correlation between resting and mildly stressed situations and EEG frequency components. Their frequency analysis was based on single channel wave counts, a mode of analysis which we too have found to be most insensitive under such conditions.

The relationships of coherence and phase values over the various areas of the head are not known to be particularly characteristic of individuals, and in this study these parameters seemed to reflect those complex mental processes associated with assimilating and evaluating our different species of verbal stimuli, processes common across this series of subjects. A unique, physiologically interpretable description of these coherence and phase relationships, as they were associated with the different kinds of questions, is not possible at this time. We have found evidence in the chimpanzee (Hanley *et al.* 1968) and in the monkey (Berkhout *et al.* 1969) that physiologically meaningful descriptions of the correlates of symbolic mental processes require data from allocortical, thalamic and midbrain structures.

We have previously reported a study on the automatic classification of states of consciousness using a similar discriminant analysis data reduction technique (Walter *et al.* 1967c). In that study, the classes of epochs to be discriminated were defined by stimulus conditions directly related to states of consciousness, and with known EEG correlates (*e.g.*, eyes open, eyes closed, responding to tone). That such states could be discriminated on the basis of rigidly specified EEG criteria is encouraging but not unexpected. In the present study, several of the conditions discriminated were defined by their verbal content only. The EEG criteria evolved to discriminate them are thus implicated among phenomena associated with subjective perception of meaning, and with verbal stress. The application of EEG analysis in this area has hitherto been based on largely non-numerical evaluation of tracings from single subjects.

In the 1967 study, it was not found possible to establish discriminating criteria for four subjects simultaneously, although within single subjects a completely effective index of consciousness could be derived. The current study reports three independent discriminations valid across five subjects simultaneously, with two non-overlapping sets of subjects. This illustration of the possibility of using EEG criteria to separate epochs differing only in verbal activity content, valid over five subjects simultaneously is to our knowledge unique.

SUMMARY

Certain auto- and cross-spectral components of the EEG appear to be characteristic of responses to verbal stimuli. Employing a discriminant-analysis procedure applied to spectral parameters, it proved possible to separate subjectively stressful from non-stressful verbal stimuli, and to determine distinctive EEG responses to verbal stimuli of similar stress value differing only in semantic content. The EEG components characteristic of these response states were consistent over small populations, and the criteria developed for their identification proved valid over several different subjects without requiring individual calibration.

Other, individual-specific characteristics of the EEG were observed consistently to parallel the cyclical occurrence of several constituent epochs in a twenty-item question–answer sequence.

RÉSUMÉ

MODIFICATIONS DE L'ÉLECTROENCÉPHALOGRAMME HUMAIN PROVOQUÉES PAR UNE ACTIVITÉ VERBALE STRESSANTE

Certaines composantes auto et cross-spectrales de l'EEG paraissent caractéristiques des réponses aux stimuli verbaux. En utilisant un procédé d'analyse discriminative appliqué aux paramètres du spectre, il s'est révélé possible de séparer les stimuli verbaux subjectivement stressants des stimuli non stressants, et de déterminer des réponses EEG distinctes aux stimuli verbaux de valeur similaire de stress, ne diffèrant que par leur contenu sémantique. Les composantes EEG caractéristiques de ces réponses sont constantes sur de petites populations et les critères développés pour leur identification se sont montrés valables pour plusieurs sujets différents sans nécessiter de calibration individuelle.

Par ailleurs, des caractéristiques EEG spécifiques d'un individu sont observées de façon constante parallèlement à la survenue cyclique de plusieurs époques constituantes d'une séquence de 20 items question–réponse.

REFERENCES

ADEY, W. R. Spectral analysis of EEG data from animals and man during alerting, orienting and discriminating responses. In T. MULHOLLAND and C. EVANS (Eds.), *Conference on neurophysiology and attention.* Butterworth, London, **1969** (in press).

ADEY, W. R., KADO, R. T. and WALTER, D. O. Computer analysis of EEG data from Gemini flight GT-7. *Aerospace Med.*, **1967**, *38*: 345–359.

BERKHOUT, J., ADEY, W. R. and CAMPEAU, E. Simian EEG activity related to problem solving during a simulated space flight. *Brain Res.*, **1969**, *13*: 140–145.

BERKHOUT, J. and WALTER, D. O. Temporal stability and individual differences in the human EEG. *IEEE Trans. bio-med. Engng.*, **1968**, *BME-15*: 165–168.

BLACK, S. and WALTER, W. G. Effects on anterior brain

responses of variation in the probability of association between stimuli. *J. psychosom. Res.*, **1965**, *9*: 33–43.

BOYLE, R. H., DYKMAN, R. and ACKERMAN, P. T. Relationships of resting autonomic activity, motor impulsivity, and EEG tracings in children. *Arch. gen. Psychiat.*, **1965**, *12*: 314–323.

DARROW, C. W. Problems in the use of the galvanic skin response as an index of cerebral function: implications of the latent period. *Psychophysiology*, **1967**, *3*: 389–396.

DARROW, C. W. and CONVERSE, M. EEG phase and autonomic function. *Electroenceph. clin. Neurophysiol.*, **1950**, *2*: 225.

DARROW, C. W. and HICKS, R. G. Interarea EEG phase relationships following sensory and ideational stimuli. *Psychophysiology*, **1965**, *1*: 337–346.

DIXON, W. J. (Ed.), *BMD biomedical computer programs (2nd ed.)*. University of California Press, Los Angeles, **1967**: 214A–214H.

HANLEY, J., WALTER, D. O., RHODES, J. R. and ADEY, W. R. Chimpanzee performance data: computer analysis of electroencephalograms. *Nature (Lond.)*, **1968**, *220*: 879–881.

HENRY, C. Electroencephalographic individual differences and their constancy. I. During sleep. II. During waking. *J. exp. Psychol.*, **1941**, *29*: 117–132; 236–246.

HOAGLAND, H., CAMERON, D. E., RUBIN, M. A. and TEGELBERG, J. J. Emotion in man as tested by the delta index of the EEG. II: Simultaneous records from cortex and from a region near the hypothalamus. *J. gen. Psychol.*, **1938**, *19*: 247–261.

TRAVIS, L. E. and EGAN, J. P. Increase in frequency of the alpha rhythm by verbal stimulation. *J. exp. Psychol.*, **1938**, *23*: 385–393.

WALTER, D. O. Spectral analysis for electroencephalograms: mathematical determination of physiological relationships from records of limited duration. *Exp. Neurol.*, **1963**, *8*: 155–181.

WALTER, D. O., BERKHOUT, J. and ADEY, W. R. Patterns of EEG and autonomic reactivity to laboratory stress. In L. FOGEL and E. GEORGE (Eds.), *Progress in biomedical engineering*. Spartan, New York, **1967a**: 125–130.

WALTER, D. O., KADO, R. T., RHODES, J. and ADEY, W. R. EEG baselines in astronaut candidates estimated by computation and pattern recognition techniques. *Aerospace Med.*, **1967b**, *38*: 371–379.

WALTER, D. O., RHODES, J. and ADEY, W. R. Discriminating among states of consciousness by EEG measurements. *Electroenceph. clin. Neurophysiol.*, **1967c**, *22*: 22–29.

WALTER, W. G. Brain responses to semantic stimuli. *J. psychosom. Res.*, **1965**, *9*: 51–61.

Reference: BERKHOUT, J., WALTER, D. O. and ADEY, W. R. Alterations of the human electroencephalogram induced by stressful verbal activity. *Electroenceph. clin. Neurophysiol.*, **1969**, *27*: 457–469.

Electroencephalography and Clinical Neurophysiology
Elsevier Publishing Company, Amsterdam – Printed in The Netherlands

EEG CHANGES DURING PERFORMANCE OF VARIOUS TASKS UNDER OPEN- AND CLOSED-EYED CONDITIONS[1]

H. LEGEWIE, O. SIMONOVA AND O. D. CREUTZFELDT

Abteilung für Neurophysiologie, Max-Planck-Institut für Psychiatrie, Munich (West Germany)

(Accepted for publication: March 11, 1969)

Ever since the classical studies of Berger (1931) and of Adrian and Matthews (1934) the general viewpoint has prevailed that alpha activity is characteristic of the relaxed waking state with eyes closed, whereas during mental activity, especially when the eyes are open, alpha activity decreases. This basic view has been maintained up to the present, although some authors have reported an increase in alpha activity during a state of attention when the eyes are open (*e.g.*, Mundy-Castle 1957; Mulholland and Runnals 1962; Kreitman and Shaw 1965; Mulholland 1969).

The particular questions posed in the present study developed from an earlier investigation of the EEG activity in sixteen normal subjects during performance of 8 different tasks with the eyes open (Grünewald *et al.* 1968; Simonova *et al.* 1968; Creutzfeldt *et al.* 1969).

Those results pertinent to the discussion of this paper are presented here briefly:

1. With eyes open the marked reduction in alpha activity, such as is frequently described in the literature, occurred. During longer recording periods, however, a considerable number of alpha waves remained (actual number of waves 80–300/min). The effect upon alpha activity of opening the eyes (blocking) was considerably stronger than the effect of individual tasks upon the already reduced level of alpha activity present when the eyes were open.

2. Subjects differed from one another in their temporo-occipital alpha reaction: one-third showed a consistent increase during performance as opposed to rest; one-third showed a consistent decrease; the remaining subjects showed an increase with some tasks and a decrease with others.

3. During performance fronto-central activity within the alpha frequency range (mu rhythm) decreased consistently (see Discussion).

4. No clear change in the means of wave frequencies could be shown between rest and performance.

5. During performance beta activity tended to increase temporo-occipitally but not fronto-centrally; theta activity did not change significantly in either the temporo-occipital or the fronto-central records.

6. Although the tasks which were studied differed considerably in the degree of mental effort involved, no clear relationship between this variable and EEG activity could be shown. However, various differences between cognitive and visuo-motor tasks were found (see Grünewald *et al.* 1968).

These results were the basis for the following questions considered in the present study:

1. Can the temporo-occipital increase and the fronto-central decrease in "alpha" activity, shown during task performance when the eyes were open, be substantiated in another group?

2. Will changes in alpha activity during task performance when eyes are closed be similar to those found when eyes are open?

3. Can a systematic difference between tasks with and without full visual control be demonstrated under open-eyed conditions?

METHOD

The investigation was conducted on eight healthy 20–27-year-old male students possessing

[1] This study was partially supported by the Deutsche Forschungsgemeinschaft (Grant Cr 30).

normal EEGs with a clear alpha rhythm. The EEGs were recorded with bipolar electrodes located fronto-centrally (F_3–C_3) and temporo-occipitally (T_5–O_1) on the left side (10–20 system). Also, heart rate and breathing were recorded. Telemetric recording was used since this allowed the subjects to move during the long experimental sessions. This resulted in better relaxation.

Experimental design

The questions being investigated required tasks which could be performed under otherwise identical conditions with eyes open and eyes closed. On the basis of preliminary studies the following tasks were chosen:

Task 1: Drawing a wavy line in a writing manner;

Task 2: Writing a complicated test word ("Dampfschiffahrtsgesellschaft");

(In 1 and 2 under the open-eyed conditions the subject's view of the writing hand was obstructed.);

Task 3: Repeated mental arithmetic (multiplication);

Task 4: Acoustic tracking: a 50 dB tone oscillated periodically (sine waves of 0.1 c/sec) between 600 and 1000 c/sec. The subject had to attempt to maintain the tone at a steady level through compensatory regulation;

Task 5: Optical tracking: the vertically deflected beam of an oscilloscope was moved back and forth along the x axis by a slow sine wave generator (±3 cm; 0.25 c/sec). The subject had to attempt to hold the beam on a marker in the middle of the screen by means of compensatory adjustments with a potentiometer. In 4 and 5 the error was recorded simultaneously with the EEG. This error was the potential difference between the input sine wave and the subject-adjusted potentiometer output. In case of perfect performance the error record would be a straight line.

Tasks 1–4 were conducted both with eyes open and eyes closed; task 5 was only performed with the eyes open.

In order to ensure that the instructions had been understood properly and that the particularly strong individual differences evident in the first attempt were balanced out somewhat, the

TABLE I

Stability of EEG measures (Rank-correlations (Spearman) of the relative numbers of waves, see text)

Experimental conditions correlated	Temporo-occipital						Fronto-central					
	Theta		Alpha		Beta		Theta		Alpha		Beta	
Eyes	closed	open	closed	open	closed	open	closed	open	closed	open	closed	open
Rest before/during tasks 1–4	*0.75*	*0.76*	*0.76*	0.29	*0.83*	0.55	*0.64*	**0.91**	0.45	*0.72*	−0.42	−0.60
Average correlation of resting condition before tasks 1–4	**0.82**	**0.72**	**0.78**	**0.62**	**0.65**	*0.42*	**0.77**	**0.80**	**0.96**	**0.87**	0.17	*0.41*
Rest before tasks 1–4/tasks 1–4	**0.95**	*0.81*	*0.75*	0.55	**0.84**	0.59	0.51	0.36	*0.67*	**0.90**	0.07	0.05
Average correlation tasks 1–4	**0.80**	**0.66**	**0.76**	**0.74**	**0.57**	0.26	*0.52*	**0.66**	**0.60**	**0.61**	*0.41*	*0.47*

Significance limits ($N = 8$): $P < 5\%$ $< 1\%$
Rank correlation *0.64* **0.83**
Average rank correlation *0.34* **0.55**

subject had the opportunity to practise each task before the start of the actual experiment.

Prior to each task a 60 sec rest period was given, announced by a tone of 0.5 sec duration. A second tone sounded 10 sec before the start of the task and a third served as start signal. After 2 min a final tone signalled the end of the task.

Before the start of the actual experiment the resting EEG was recorded with eyes closed and eyes open. Half of the subjects received the tasks with eyes closed first and then with eyes open, the other half in the opposite order. Within these conditions the order of the tasks was varied systematically.

Apparatus

The taped time signals were presented to the subject by loudspeaker. The tapes also regulated the oscillations of the tone in task 4 and of the line in task 5.

After telemetric transmission from an Alvar transmitter to a receiver developed in our laboratory the EEG was fed to both an EEG amplifier and an 8-channel storage tape (Honeywell). Also recorded with the EEG were the EKG,

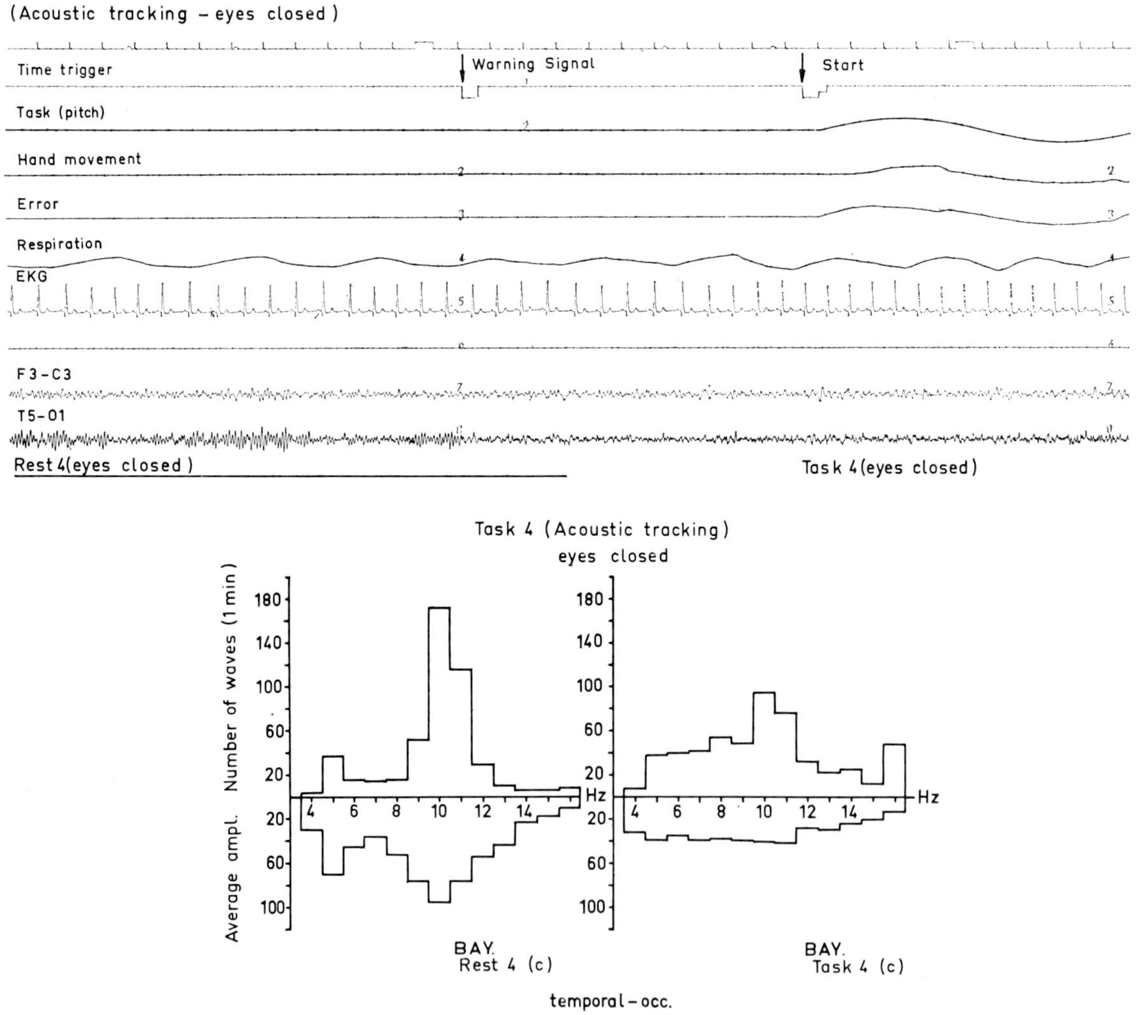

Fig. 1

Record during rest and start of task with eyes closed. Below: frequency distribution based on period analysis, and average amplitudes of the different frequencies. Analysis time 1 min during rest (left) and during task (right).

respiration and, for tasks 4–5, the errors as an indication of performance.

For illustrative purposes Fig. 1 and 2 present original protocols showing records during rest and performance with eyes closed and eyes open.

Analysis of data

Before automatic analysis was begun, all curves were subjected to a thorough visual inspection, being checked for possible artefacts. Muscle artefacts (causing slight distortions in the beta range) and artefacts in the fronto-central leads as a result of eye movements (affecting the theta range in particular) could not be eliminated entirely. The automatic period and amplitude analysis (zero-crossing method) which followed was performed by a digital computer, IBM 1130, equipped with an interface developed in our laboratory (Färber and Probst 1968).

For each 1 min time segment the computer yielded the following parameters for temporo-occipital and fronto-central EEG activity (Legewie and Probst 1969):

1. Histogram of the numbers and average amplitudes of the various wave frequencies (4–16 c/sec), tabulated in steps of 1 c/sec.

2. Numbers and average amplitudes of waves in the following frequency ranges: theta 5–7.9 c/sec; alpha 8–12.9 c/sec; beta over 12.9 c/sec.

3. Average wave frequency (and variance) within the total filter range as a measure of the relative weight of the different sub-frequencies.

To eliminate slow base line shifts the records were passed through a broad-band filter (4–16 c/sec, 12 dB/oct., Schwarzer) prior to automatic analysis. This left activity undistorted in the alpha range, which was of particular interest here, whereas waves of adjoining frequency ranges were slightly attenuated. This may have eliminated from the analysis some smaller waves mainly in the theta range.

To answer the questions we had raised, the

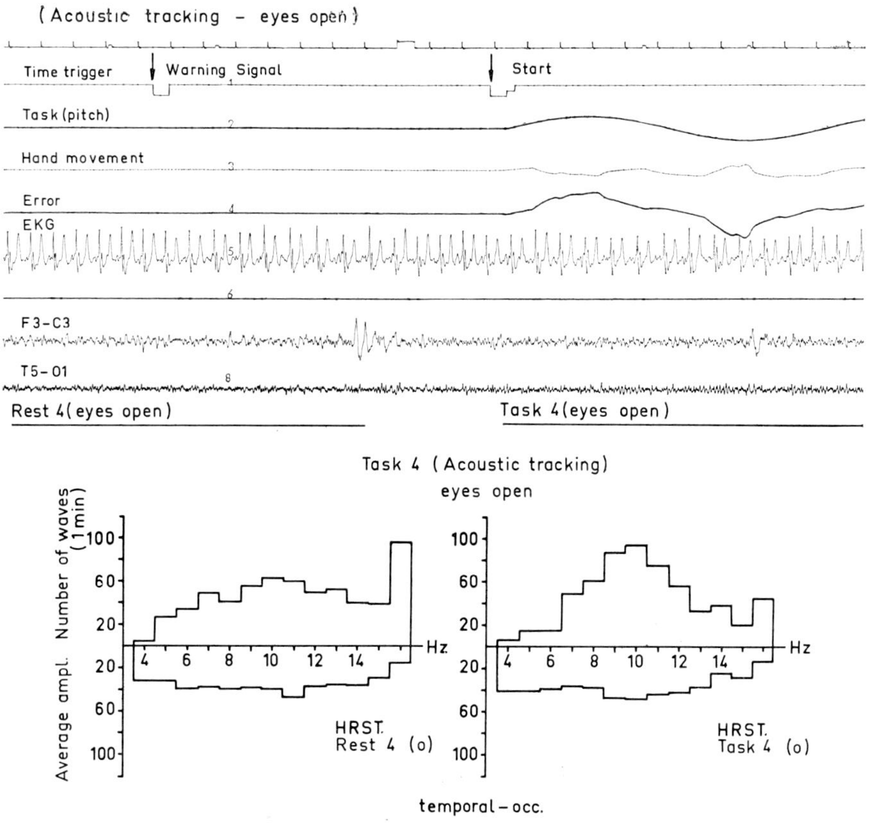

Fig. 2
Record during rest and start of task with eyes open. For explanation see Fig. 1.

number of alpha, theta and beta waves seemed particularly suitable for statistical analysis. In order to assess the stability or reliability of these EEG measures under varying conditions, rank correlation coefficients (according to Spearman, see Siegel 1956, p. 202) of the relative numbers of theta, alpha and beta waves with eyes open and eyes closed (temporo-occipital and fronto-central) were computed over 4 combinations of conditions. As can be seen in Table I, the reliability coefficients were generally large, being significant ($P \leq 0.05$) or highly significant ($P \leq 0.01$). This means that subjects with a high value in a particular measure in one situation tend to have a high value in the same measure in another situation.

RESULTS

1. *Differences between open- and closed-eyed conditions*

Temporo-occipital recordings. Fig. 3,*a* provides an impression of the absolute numbers of theta, alpha and beta waves during rest with eyes open and eyes closed. The differences between the open- and closed-eyed conditions are highly significant for all three frequency ranges (Wilcoxon Matched Pairs Signed-Ranks Test, see Siegel 1956, p. 75). The number of alpha waves is reduced to about half when the eyes are open. In none of the 1 min periods investigated (these involved for every subject 13 experimental conditions, 5 resting periods and 4×2 min under task) was the number of alpha waves as great when the eyes were open as when they were closed.

In contrast, the numbers of theta and beta waves were approximately doubled when the eyes were closed ($P \leq 0.05$ in each case).

Use of the broad-band filter permitted only limited conclusions regarding changes in beta frequency, since beta waves of low voltage were not recorded.

Fronto-central recordings. Fronto-centrally smaller amounts of alpha and beta activities, as well as a greater amount of theta activity, were found than in the temporo-occipital records (Fig. 3, *b*).

Eyes being open produced almost as great a reduction in the number of alpha waves here as it did temporo-occipitally. However, no significant differences were found in the theta and beta activities between when the eyes were open or closed.

2. *Differences between the various tasks*

Significant differences between the various tasks were only found within the theta range, while all differences were insignificant in the alpha and beta ranges, both temporo-occipitally and fronto-centrally.

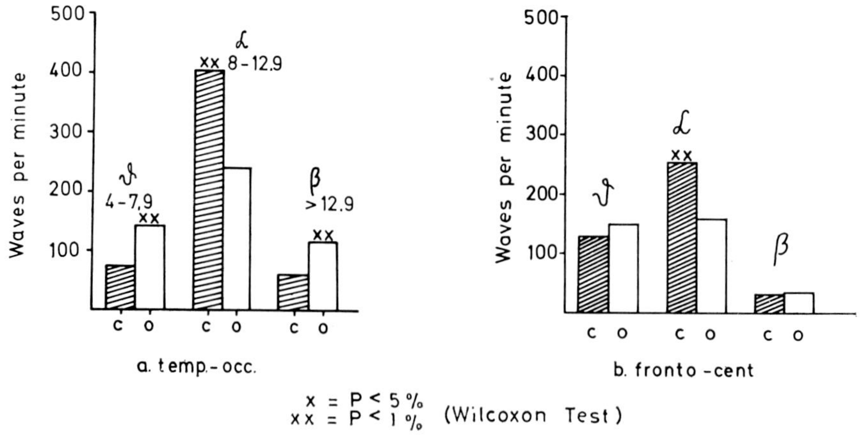

Fig. 3

Average number of waves (8 subjects) of different frequencies during rest with eyes closed (c) and eyes open (o) (mean values for 4 resting periods of 1 min each).

3. *Differences between rest and performance*

No significant differences were found between the first and second minutes of performing a given task (Wilcoxon Test). Thus, in the discussion which follows we shall deal only with the first minute.

In evaluating the differences between resting and the first minute of a given task, we computed for each subject the percentage of change in comparison with the immediately preceding rest period. Fig. 4 indicates the corresponding percentage changes for each of the three frequency ranges (black columns) and for the respective averages in amplitude (white columns).

(a) *Alpha range*

Temporo-occipital recordings. When the eyes were closed tasks 1–3 brought a decrease in both the number and the average amplitude of alpha waves. The decrease was relatively small in percentage (5–10% on the average), but occurred consistently, so that it was clearly significant. When the eyes were open a greater change occurred, but in the opposite direction: for all tasks (1–5) the number and amplitude of the alpha waves increased. This increase in alpha activity was found consistently in seven out of eight subjects. Noteworthy is the fact that the same increase occurred in task 5 (in which visual control was involved).

Fronto-central recordings. Fronto-centrally, in contrast to temporo-occipitally, task performance led to a reduction in "alpha" activity (number and amplitude of waves), both with eyes open and eyes closed (Fig. 4, *b*).

(b) *Theta range*

Temporo-occipital recordings. When the eyes were closed tasks 1–3 produced a definite increase in theta activity. This was statistically significant for tasks 1 and 3, but was not evident at all in task 4. When the eyes were open, task performance produced a slight and non-significant reduction in theta activity. Changes in average amplitude within the theta range (clear columns) were not of a consistent nature.

Fronto-central recordings. When the eyes were closed task performance led to an increase in theta waves. This increase was more marked fronto-centrally than temporo-occipitally, being significant for all tasks. An accompanying decrease in amplitude was present; this was greater than chance for two of the tasks. When the eyes were open the effect of task performance upon theta activity was less uniform. Nevertheless, 3 of the tasks produced a significant increase in theta activity.

(c) *Beta range*

Temporo-occipital recordings. When the eyes were open task performance generally produced an increase of 45–90% in the number of beta waves; this occurred during all tasks. Changes in amplitude were not evident. The high percentage change obtained in task 1 did not reach significance, since in the beta range a high degree of individual variation was present. When the eyes were open task performance led to a slight and non-significant increase in beta activity.

Fronto-central recordings. Fronto-centrally as opposed to temporo-occipitally, task performance when the eyes were closed produced no clear increase in beta activity. When the eyes were open a reduction in beta activity (in the number and amplitude of waves) occurred, achieving significance in a portion of the cases.

4. *Mean and variability of the various wave frequencies*

Temporo-occipital recordings. During task performance a slight increase of the mean frequency occurred (0.2–0.5 c/sec) indicating an increase in beta activity, as mentioned above. When the eyes were closed task performance appeared to increase the variability of wave frequencies; when the eyes were open some tasks produced an increase, others a decrease in variability.

Fronto-central recordings. Fronto-centrally, in contrast to temporo-occipitally, task performance produced a slight decrease in average wave frequency (up to 0.5 c/sec), both with the eyes open and closed. This corresponded to the increase in theta activity mentioned above.

When the eyes were closed task performance resulted in a significant increase in the variability of wave frequencies; when the eyes were open it had no apparent effect.

DISCUSSION

The most marked experimental effect found was that the alpha activity was only about half

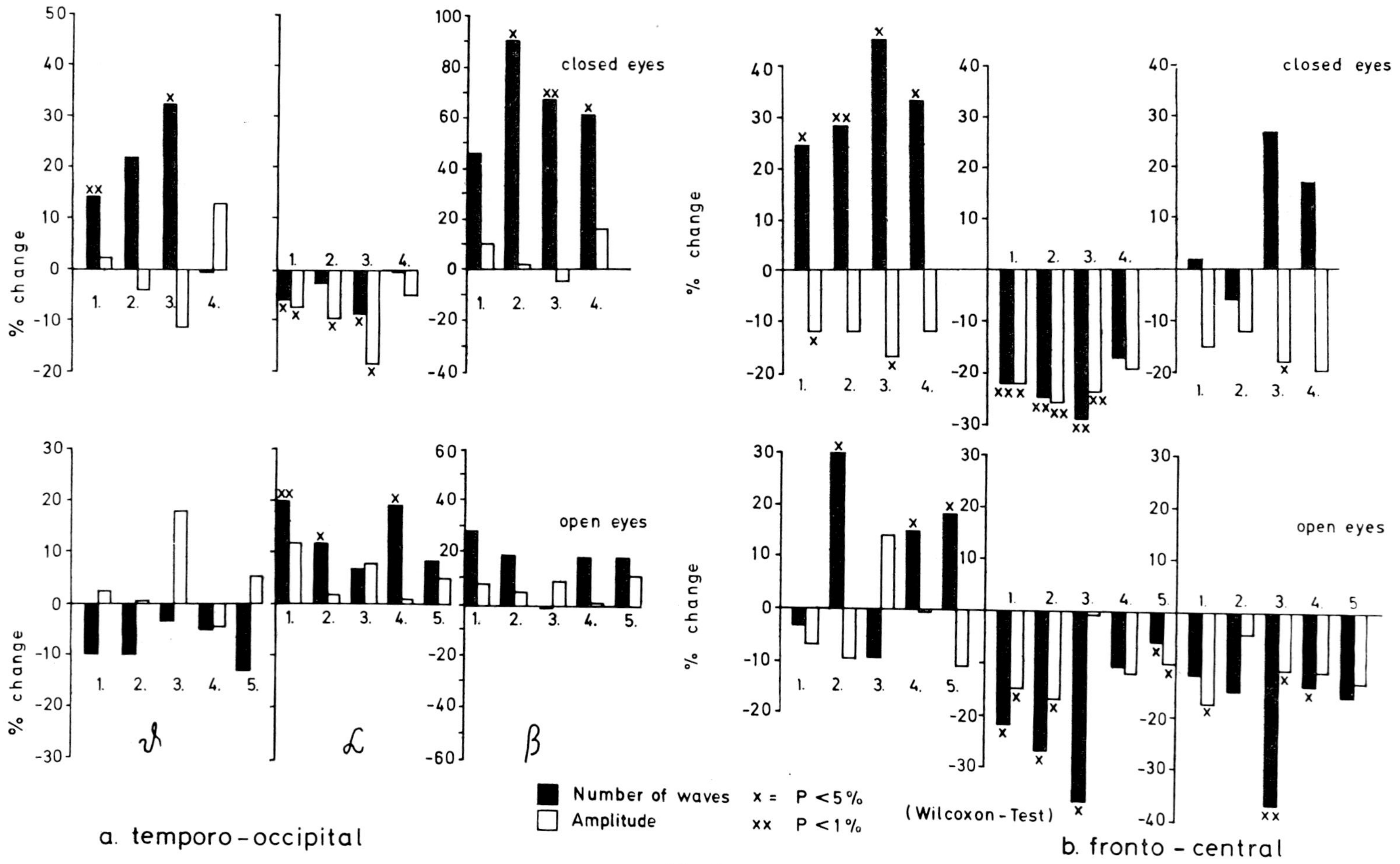

Fig. 4

Percentage changes in numbers of waves and amplitudes (average of 8 subjects) during performance compared to rest. Tasks 1–4 (eyes closed) above, tasks 1–5 (eyes open) below. (Enhancement during performance shown by positive % change on the ordinate, reduction by negative change.)

as great when the eyes were open as when they were closed. This occurred without exception both temporo-occipitally and fronto-centrally.

These differences between the open- and closed-eyed conditions were greater than those between rest and performance. This finding concurs with classical results (Cobb 1963). Temporo-occipitally the decrease in alpha activity when the eyes were open was accompanied by an increase in the number of waves in the adjoining ranges of frequency.

The differences between the results obtained in the individual tasks were slight in comparison with the differences between rest and performance. A finer differentiation between the various tasks would require more tasks and a larger number of subjects (Grünewald *et al.* 1968).

Let us now consider the questions raised at the start:

1. The increase in temporo-occipital alpha activity between rest and performance when the eyes are open, reported in the earlier study (Creutzfeldt *et al.* 1969), was fully substantiated in the present investigation: this was shown in most of the tasks in seven of the eight subjects. The fact that in only one subject did the alpha activity decrease does not contradict the earlier finding of a decrease in one-third of the subjects; such discrepancies are attributable to the random differences in samples of small size. The important point is that the earlier results were corroborated with an independent sample and with partially different tasks.

The findings of the first study that fronto-central activity in the alpha frequency range (mu rhythm) is consistently decreased during performance when the eyes are open also gained full support. In contrast to the temporo-occipital results, the fronto-central mu reduction occurred under open- and closed-eyed conditions alike. The differences between the fronto-central and the temporo-occipital changes in the alpha band underline the independence of the various central mechanisms contributing to alpha activity, which various authors have reported (*e.g.*, Gastaut 1952; Mundy-Castle 1957).

2. The findings relative to EEG activity during rest and performance with eyes open (previous investigation) were supplemented by the following: when the eyes are closed performance produces, not the increase in alpha activity noted when eyes are open, but rather (under otherwise identical conditions) a reduction in the number of alpha waves, both temporo-occipitally and fronto-centrally. These results are more in harmony with the classical desynchronization theory of mental performance than are those pertaining to the open-eyed conditions (Lindsley 1960).

3. In assessing the influence of the visual system upon alpha activity it should be borne in mind that the major effect found was the reduction in alpha activity from closed- to open-eyed conditions. This implies that the decisive element determining alpha activity is the presence or absence of visual input. Since alpha activity increased during a task involving visual control it appears that, under the conditions present here, the active participation of the visual system was of lesser importance.

The tendency for performance to produce a reduction in alpha activity when the eyes are closed and an increase when the eyes are open can be interpreted as the result of synchronizing and desynchronizing mechanisms reacting to both individual and situational factors.

Fig. 5 summarizes our results and suggests an interpretation of them: performance appears

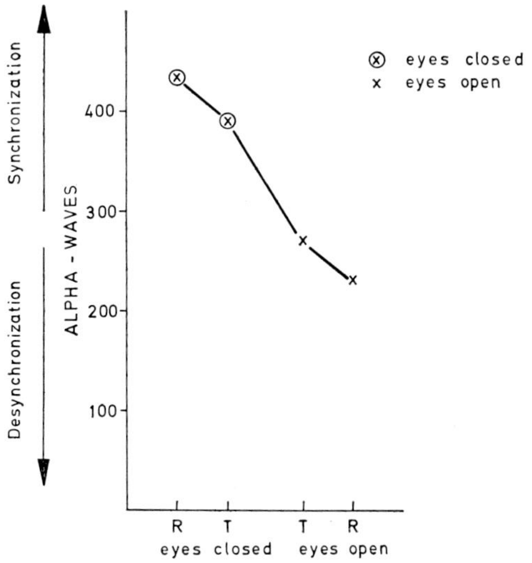

Fig. 5

Average number of alpha waves in 1 min (8 subjects) during rest (R) and task (T) with eyes closed and eyes open (mean values for 4 conditions).

to produce desynchronization only when synchronizing elements are initially predominating (eyes closed). When desynchronization is clearly present from the start, however, as under open-eyed conditions, performance tends to produce no further increase in desynchronization, but rather a decrease.

SUMMARY

Telemetric EEG recordings of eight healthy persons were obtained during rest and during performance of 4 different tasks with eyes closed and of 5 tasks with eyes open. Automatic analysis of temporo-occipital and fronto-central EEG (period–amplitude analysis) yielded the following results:

1. When the eyes were open, temporo-occipital and fronto-central alpha activity were in all cases less than when the eyes were closed (on average approx. 50%).

2. Fronto-central "alpha" activity, both with eyes open and closed, was decreased during performance.

3. Performance produced a significant trend toward intermediate degrees of temporo-occipital alpha activity. With eyes closed a decrease in the number of alpha waves (desynchronization) and with eyes open an increase (synchronization) was observed.

4. The increase in synchronization with eyes open appeared largely independent of whether visual components were directly involved in the task.

ZUSAMMENFASSUNG

EEG-VERÄNDERUNGEN IN VERSCHIEDENEN LEISTUNGSSITUATIONEN BEI OFFENEN UND GESCHLOSSENEN AUGEN

Bei acht Versuchspersonen wurde telemetrisch das EEG unter Ruhe und unter 4 verschiedenen Tätigkeiten mit geschlossenen Augen und 5 Tätigkeiten mit offenen Augen registriert. Die automatische Analyse der temporo-occipitalen und der fronto-centralen EEG-Aktivität (aperiodische Intervall–Amplituden-Analyse) zeigte folgende Ergebnisse:

1. Bei offenen Augen fand sich temporo-occipital und fronto-central ohne Ausnahme eine annähernd 50% geringere Aktivität im Alphafrequenzbereich als bei geschlossenen Augen.

2. Die Aktivität im Alphafrequenzbereich zeigte fronto-central bei geschlossenen und offenen Augen eine Verminderung unter Tätigkeitsbedingungen gegenüber Ruhe.

3. Die Veränderungen bei psychischen Tätigkeiten zeigten temporo-occipital eine überzufällige Tendenz zum Erreichen einer Mittellage der Alpha-Aktivität. Bei geschlossenen Augen wurde diese Mittellage erreicht durch Abnahme der Ruhe-Häufigkeit (Desynchronisation); bei offenen Augen durch Zunahme (Synchronisation).

4. Die Zunahme der Synchronisation bei offenen Augen schien weitgehend unabhängig davon zu sein, ob bei der Leistung visuelle Komponenten unmittelbar beteiligt waren.

We gratefully acknowledge the help of Dr. Hansert in consulting the statistical evaluation of the data and of Dr. Goldsmith in preparing the English manuscript.

REFERENCES

ADRIAN, E. D. and MATTHEWS, B. H. C. The Berger rhythm: Potential changes from the occipital lobes in man. *Brain*, **1934**, *57*: 355–385.

BERGER, H. Über das Elektrenkephalogramm des Menschen. III. *Arch. Psychiat. Nervenkr.*, **1931**, *94*: 16–60.

COBB, W. A. The normal adult EEG. In D. HILL and G. PARR (Eds.), *Electroencephalography*. Macmillan, New York, **1963**: 232–249.

CREUTZFELDT, O., GRÜNEWALD, G., SIMONOVA, O. and SCHMITZ, H. Changes of the basic rhythms of the EEG during performance of mental and visuomotor tasks. In C. EVANS and T. MULHOLLAND (Eds.), *The concept of attention in neurophysiology*, Butterworth, Oxford, **1969** (in press).

FÄRBER, G. und PROBST, W. Automatische Versuchssteuerung und Versuchsauswertung mit dem IBM System 1133, dargestellt an einem Beispiel aus der Medizin. *IBM Nachrichten*, **1968**, *188*: 126–131.

GASTAUT, H. Étude électroencéphalographique de la réactivité des rythmes rolandiques. *Rev. neurol.*, **1952**, *87*: 176–182.

GRÜNEWALD, G., SIMONOVA, O. und CREUTZFELDT, O. Differentielle EEG-Veränderungen bei visuomotorischen und kognitiven Tätigkeiten. *Arch. Psychiat. Nervenkr.*, **1968**, *212*: 46–69.

KREITMAN, N. and SHAW, J. C. Experimental enhancement of alpha activity. *Electroenceph. clin. Neurophysiol.*, **1965**, *18*: 147–155.

LEGEWIE, H. and PROBST, W. On-line analysis of EEG with a small computer (period–amplitude analysis). *Electroenceph. clin. Neurophysiol.*, **1969**, *27*: 533–535.

LINDSLEY, D. B. Attention, consciousness, sleep and wakefulness. In J. FIELD *et al.* (Eds.), *Handbook of physiology, Sect. 1.* Amer. Physiol. Soc., Washington, **1960,** *III*: 1553–1593.

MULHOLLAND, T. The concept of attention and the electroencephalographic alpha rhythm. In C. EVANS and T. MULHOLLAND (Eds.), *The concept of attention in neurophysiology*, Butterworth, Oxford, **1969** (in press).

MULHOLLAND, T. and RUNNALS, S. Increased occurrence of EEG alpha during increased attention. *J. Psychol.*, **1962,** *54*: 317–330.

MUNDY-CASTLE, A. C. The electroencephalogram and mental activity. *Electroenceph. clin. Neurophysiol.*, **1957,** *9*: 643–655.

SIEGEL, S. *Nonparametric methods for the behavioral sciences.* MaGraw-Hill, New York, **1956,** 312 p.

SIMONOVA, O., GRÜNEWALD, G., CREUTZFELDT, O. und SCHMITZ, H. Über Zuordnung von EEG-Kriterien und Aufmerksamkeitsverhalten. *Zbl. ges. Neurol. Psychiat.*, **1968,** *191*: 166.

Reference: LEGEWIE, H., SIMONOVA, O. and CREUTZFELDT, O. D. EEG changes during performance of various tasks under open- and closed-eyed conditions. *Electroenceph. clin. Neurophysiol.*, **1969,** *27*: 470–479.

Electroencephalography and Clinical Neurophysiology
Elsevier Publishing Company, Amsterdam – Printed in The Netherlands

EEG AVERAGE FREQUENCY AND INTELLIGENCE

DUILIO GIANNITRAPANI

Institute for Psychosomatic and Psychiatric Research and Training, Michael Reese Hospital, Chicago, Ill. 60616 (U. S. A.)

(Accepted for publication: February 25, 1969)

The purpose of this study is to investigate the relationships between EEG average frequency and intelligence. Most experiments studying EEG activity and intellectual functioning have focussed on the mentally retarded (*e.g.*, Kreezer and Smith 1950; Netchine *et al.* 1959; Gibbs *et al.* 1960) or on the mentally ill (Liberson 1951). The few investigators who have addressed themselves to the study of EEG and a broader range of intelligence have failed to find any relationship between intelligence and alpha amplitude; on the other hand, the studies of the relationships between intelligence and either alpha index or alpha frequency have produced inconsistent results.

Alpha index showed no significant correlations with intelligence in the children's groups studied by Knott *et al.* (1942) and Lindsley (1938), but in adults Mundy-Castle (1958) found alpha index correlating 0.33 with Verbal I.Q. and 0.48 with the Arithmetic subtest of the South African Version of the Wechsler-Bellevue Intelligence Scale.

Occipital alpha frequency did not correlate with various intelligence scores in the studies by Lindsley (1938), Henry (1944) and Shagass (1946). Knott *et al.* (1942) found a correlation of 0.50 in their sample of 8 year olds but only 0.12 in their sample of 12 year olds. Netchine and Lairy (1960) found differing correlations depending on the age groups (the sample included children 5–12 years old), the highest being 0.38 in the 11–12 year olds.

Later, Netchine and Lairy (1962) developed an index that included a measure of amplitude differential between the occipital, parietal and Rolandic leads. This index, in conjunction with an occipital alpha frequency score, showed a strong relationship with I.Q. in their sample of 128 5–9 year olds.

Working with adults Mundy-Castle (1958) found the highest correlation (0.51) between alpha frequency and total I.Q. (South African WBI Scale). Saunders (1961) found a low but significant correlation between Digit Span of the WBI and alpha frequency. He stated that the correlation would have been higher had he used dominant frequency rather than alpha frequency.

Frequency changes occurring in the EEG during mental activity have also been observed. Berger (1929) first noted reduction of alpha concurrent with attention. Travis and Egan (1938) noted an increase in alpha frequency in subjects listening to verbal material. Knott (1938) found similar increases in alpha frequency during silent and oral reading. His scores were mean wave/sec not restricted to alpha activity. Strong beta activity must have been included in the scores to obtain his averages.

Hadley (1941) used a similar wave-counting procedure to show an increase in average frequency (up to 14 c/sec) with mental multiplication. Mundy-Castle (1951) demonstrated an increase in beta activity with mental arithmetic and (1957) attributed this increase to a correlate of mediation of information in the brain. Similar observations were made more recently with electronic scoring methods by Chapman *et al.* (1962) and Glanzer *et al.* (1964).

In conclusion, increase of alpha frequency seems to correlate weakly with intelligence. With some form of attention or mental work there has been observed an increase not only of alpha frequency but of dominant frequency (which may enter the low beta range) and of beta frequency proper.

Another factor to be considered is that the EEG activity in homologous brain areas is not as symmetrical as generally believed (Strauss *et al.*

1943), and there is some evidence that this asymmetry increases with mental work (Giannitrapani 1966a).

From the foregoing analysis, three sets of tentative correlations can be abstracted: (a) greater alpha frequency with intelligence; (b) greater EEG frequency during mental work; and (c) greater EEG frequency differential between the hemispheres during mental work. The alleged increase of alpha frequency with intelligence might very well be produced by the same processes responsible for the increase in frequency during mental activity in a given subject. To study this, I.Q. scores should be correlated with EEG scores which involve differentials between resting and thinking and differentials between the two hemispheres.

For this purpose subjects were administered an intelligence test and the average EEG frequency of eight brain areas (4 left and 4 homologous right) was obtained under two conditions: while the subjects were resting (control) and while the subjects were performing mental multiplication problems. A measure of incidence of occipital alpha rhythm (alpha index) was also obtained to make possible the evaluation of the relationship between this rhythm and I.Q.

METHOD

The sample was constituted by eighteen volunteer subjects (ages 21–45; 11 males and 7 females) without EEG abnormalities, as determined by a standard clinical EEG examination. They were selected on the basis of their WAIS I.Q. and divided into two groups: Middle (I.Q. 93–118) and High (I.Q. 119–143). The I.Q. scores were evenly distributed throughout the range.

The equipment consisted of an 8-channel Grass Polygraph. Recordings were made from eight scalp electrodes (left and right frontal, temporal, parietal and occipital) with reference to both ears. No filtering was used. Standard electrodes (with electrolite jelly) were held in place with collodion.

The subject, with eyes closed, lay on a bed in a dimly lit room. The recording was obtained during a "resting" condition and while "thinking" (*i.e.*, when the subject was requested to perform a mental multiplication and prior to his answering aloud). To obtain uninterrupted 5 sec periods for the Thinking condition, the difficulty of the problem was adjusted for each individual. The record then contained at least six problems for which the subject required more than 5 sec for the solution. Sample problems were 3 × 7, 7 × 9, 13 × 3, 12 × 8, 17 × 12.

Six 5 sec periods of record for a total of 30 sec were analyzed for each of the two conditions, Resting and Thinking, and for each of the eight electrode placements. The periods chosen did not contain obvious muscle artifacts. To obtain the average frequency scores the changes in pen deflection were totaled for each of these 30 sec periods. Such scoring included frequencies from 6 to 50 c/sec. To include activity in the beta range (15–50 c/sec) each visually detectable change in pen deflection, regardless of amplitude, was counted, thus including signals of 1–3 μV.

A group of assistants, unaware of the purpose and of the conditions of the experiment, were instructed in scoring; each record was scored independently by two of them. To determine the reliability of the scores, a Pearson correlation was performed for the pairs of scores for each of the twenty subjects. The distribution of these correlations had a range of 0.48 to 0.99, a mean of 0.81, and a mode between 0.90 and 1.00.

The average of the two scores for each period was used as the raw score in this study. There was a total of 96 scores per subject for a grand total of 1,728 scores.

An alpha index was also derived from the data. Scores for the alpha index were obtained by visually inspecting every one-fifth of a second of the left and right occipital tracings for presence (score = 1) or absence (score = 0) of alpha activity. The summation of these scores for the 30 sec of each of the two conditions constituted the alpha scores used in this experiment.

Thus the variables in this study were: Conditions (Resting, Thinking); Areas (left and right frontal, temporal, parietal and occipital); Periods (six 5 sec periods) and I.Q. groups (Middle and High I.Q.).

Several repeated measurement analyses of variance were performed via computer program (Sorkin *et al.* 1964) with the following variables: Conditions, Periods, Areas and two I.Q. groups as a nested subject category. Following this,

Spearman Rho correlations of pertinent EEG variables with the three I.Q. scores (*i.e.*, Verbal I.Q., Performance I.Q. and Full I.Q.) were computed.

RESULTS

An analysis of variance shows, in Fig. 1, a significant decrease ($P < 0.01$) in average frequency between the first and the second time periods of the Thinking condition. There were no other significant differences between any other periods within either the Thinking or the Resting conditions.

The interaction which tested the differences between the two conditions (Thinking minus Resting) for the two I.Q. groups was insignificant.

The interaction between the two sides of the brain was significant ($P < 0.05$); the histograms

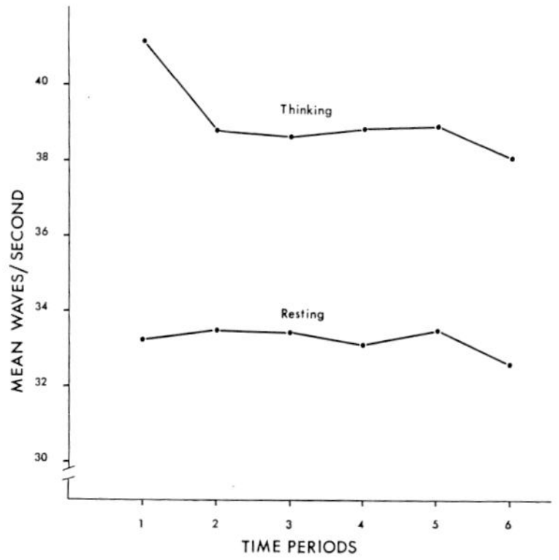

Fig. 1
Mean waves/sec for the two conditions: Thinking (multiplication task) and Resting for each of the six 5 sec periods.

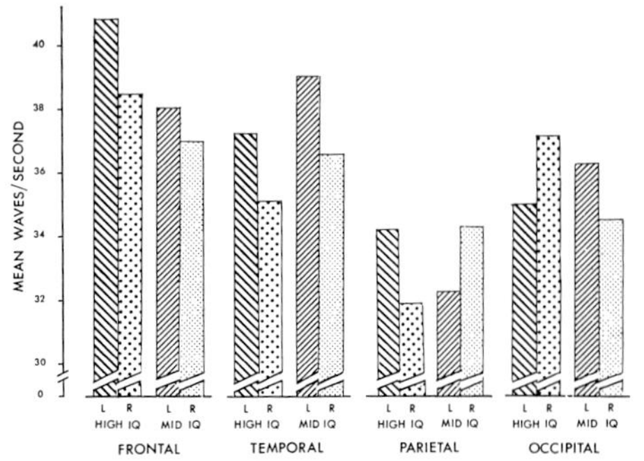

Fig. 2
Mean waves/sec of the left and right side of the four brain areas (frontal, temporal, parietal and occipital) for each I.Q. group (Middle 93–118, High 119–143).

in Fig. 2 show that there was, in general, greater average frequency on the left side except in the parietal areas of the Middle I.Q. group and the occipital areas of the High I.Q. group.

To test the significance of the distribution of activity of the left and right parietal and occipital areas an analysis of variance with difference scores (Left minus Right) was performed for all areas. The interaction of Areas and Groups was significant ($P < 0.01$) and is presented in Fig. 3. The parietal as well as the occipital differences in mean frequency between the High and Middle I.Q. groups were also significant ($P < 0.05$).

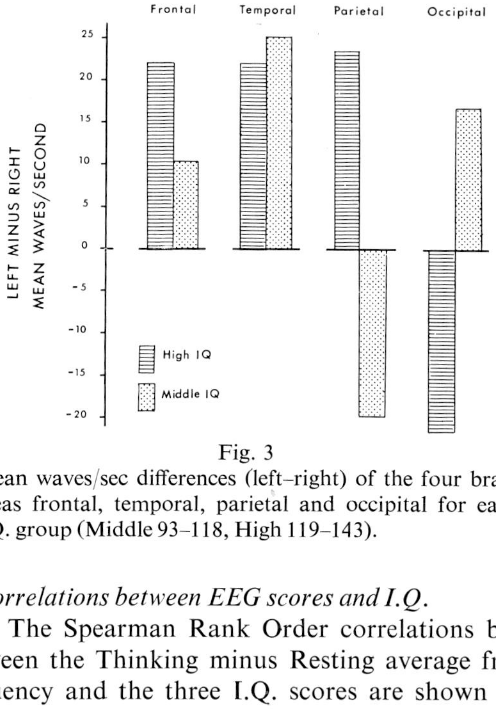

Fig. 3
Mean waves/sec differences (left–right) of the four brain areas frontal, temporal, parietal and occipital for each I.Q. group (Middle 93–118, High 119–143).

Correlations between EEG scores and I.Q.

The Spearman Rank Order correlations between the Thinking minus Resting average frequency and the three I.Q. scores are shown in Table I, *A*. The highest correlations were obtained between the left parietal area and Performance I.Q. The correlations were predominantly negative, indicating that the higher the I.Q., the lower the difference in average frequency between Thinking and Resting.

The correlations between the Left minus Right average frequency and the three I.Q. scores for each of the four areas separately are given in Table I, *B*. This shows that: (1) the Left minus Right EEG scores of the frontal areas correlate highest (even though not significantly) with Verbal I.Q. while thinking; (2) temporal activity shows

TABLE I

Spearman rank order correlations

A. EEG average frequency (Thinking minus Resting) *vs*. WAIS I.Q. scores

I.Q. scores	Frontal		Temporal		Parietal		Occipital	
	Left	Right	Left	Right	Left	Right	Left	Right
Verbal I.Q.	0.18	0.02	0.07	−0.05	−0.37	−0.08	0.09	−0.15
Performance I.Q.	−0.25	−0.27	−0.03	−0.43	−0.54*	−0.40	−0.11	−0.38
Full I.Q.	−0.06	−0.16	−0.01	−0.23	−0.48*	−0.23	−0.05	−0.22

B. EEG average frequency (Left minus Right) *vs*. WAIS I.Q. scores

I.Q. scores	Frontal		Temporal		Parietal		Occipital		F + T + P − O	
	Thinking	Resting	Thinking	Resting	Thinking	Resting	Thinking	Resting	Thinking	Resting
Verbal I.Q.	0.37	0.19	0.21	0.10	0.19	0.30	−0.22	−0.33	0.59*	0.41
Performance I.Q.	0.10	0.10	0.09	−0.17	0.54*	0.57*	−0.44	−0.54*	0.78**	0.39
Full I.Q.	0.26	0.14	0.13	0.00	0.39	0.49*	−0.38	−0.48*	0.72**	0.46

C. Alpha index *vs*. WAIS I.Q. scores

I.Q. scores	Left occipital		Right occipital		Left + Right occipital	
	Thinking	Resting	Thinking	Resting	Thinking	Resting
Verbal I.Q.	0.46	0.56*	0.54*	0.64**	0.52*	0.48*
Performance I.Q.	0.65**	0.38	0.67**	0.40	0.67**	0.31
Full I.Q.	0.58*	0.51*	0.64**	0.57*	0.62**	0.43

* $P < 0.05$.
** $P < 0.01$.

low correlations throughout; (3) the parietal areas show the highest correlations of any single area with Performance and Full I.Q.; and (4) the occipital areas show high negative correlations.

To maximize the findings by decreasing the between groups variance, correlations between the I.Q. scores and a composite EEG average frequency score were computed. The composite score was obtained by adding the scores used for the frontal, temporal and parietal, and subtracting the occipital because of its negative correlations. The composite score of the Thinking condition (frontal + temporal + parietal − occipital) showed by far the highest correlation with Performance I.Q.

The correlations between alpha index in the occipital areas and the three I.Q. scores are given in Table I, *C*. Relatively higher correlations are shown with Performance I.Q. and during the Thinking condition.

DISCUSSION

Resting minus Thinking

The first set of correlations, dealing with I.Q. and the average frequency difference between Resting and Thinking, were not as high as expected.

The hypothesis tested the possibility that the degree of change in activity in a given brain might be related to diversity of intellectual functioning which could be assumed to be a necessary correlate of high intellectual ability. It is quite possible that one reason for the low correlation is the notorious unhomogeneity of the Resting condition.

Left minus Right

Previous studies on behavioral laterality preference in the phase analysis of the EEG showed patterns of asymmetry in selected left–right homologous areas (Giannitrapani 1965, 1966b; Giannitrapani *et al.* 1966). While current research investigated average frequency, homologous areas asymmetries were also present. In the frontal areas significantly higher frequency on the left side was found in the High I.Q. group. By far the most interesting finding occurred in the parietal areas where a unique mirror image distribution of scores, relatively constant for both conditions, was present.

The frontal asymmetries correlated highest with Verbal I.Q. while thinking. The earlier experiment (Giannitrapani 1966a) had demonstrated that when comparing all areas, the greatest changes in average frequency between Resting and Thinking was in effect in the frontal areas, mental multiplications being considered to be a verbal task.

In contrast with the frontal areas, the parietal and occipital areas showed greater correlation with Performance I.Q. Clinical studies seem to indicate greater parietal and/or occipital involvement with Performance I.Q. functions, but there are no EEG studies to support these findings. The individuality of asymmetries in different areas is in support of historical findings and previous work with phase analysis of the EEG (Giannitrapani *et al.* 1964; Giannitrapani 1967). These studies demonstrated a variety of patterns inconsistent with a simple hemispheric dominance notion.

The composite score involving all areas tested showed the highest correlation between the Thinking condition and Performance I.Q. The differential treatment afforded the occipital scores is *ex-post-facto*, and the only defense for its use is as a preliminary finding, the validity of which remains to be tested in the future.

This method of average frequency scoring is not related to frequency of alpha activity, since the alpha rhythm, when present, constitutes a small percentage of the frequency counted. There is the danger that some muscle artifact of small amplitude may have been included in the scores, but it is difficult to theorize how the left–right differential of the potentials might correlate with I.Q.

Alpha index

The positive correlations between alpha index and I.Q. during the Resting condition were in general agreement with, but higher than, those obtained by Mundy-Castle (1958). In addition to this corroborated finding in the Resting condition, the present experiment showed a consistently higher correlation in the Thinking condition (not studied by Mundy-Castle), performance I.Q. showing the highest relationship with alpha index. This finding indicated a negative relationship between I.Q. and alpha activity desynchronization in general, a relationship that is enhanced during mental activity.

Each subject was given a mental multiplication problem designed to be subjectively equal; *i.e.*, that required a little over 5 sec to solve, 5 sec being the unit time for scoring purposes. Even though the tasks were objectively more difficult for the higher I.Q. subjects, mental multiplication produced less desynchronization of the alpha rhythm in the individuals of higher I.Q. While the smaller-degree-of-desynchronization-while-thinking-in-High-I.Q.-subjects rationale is intriguing, one cannot be but skeptical of a strong relationship between alpha index and I.Q.

Changes through time

The significant drop in average frequency between the first and second mental multiplication problems is of great interest here. Is the additional fast activity which occurs during the first time period unrelated to the performance of mental multiplication as such? Is it perhaps a consequence of other activities concurrent with the novelty of the situation such as an orienting reflex, or is it a by-product of a process which could be subsumed under the general label of anxiety such as muscle artifacts?

Considering the variances introduced by the hand counting of the data, EEG amplitude recording levels, and the variances connected with individual administration of I.Q. tests, the resulting correlations are very high indeed. It is because of these and similar difficulties which hamper research in this area that Ellingson (1966) had to conclude that the weight of available evidence suggested no relationship between normal brain wave phenomena and intelligence in normal adults.

In conclusion, the greatest shortcoming of the method used is the difficulty in obtaining additional data. Instead of the hand counting of average frequency, future work will have to rely on some automated method of data reduction such as digitizing the EEG tracings, performing a Fourier analysis in a computer and obtaining the output of the power spectra for further analysis. Such a new method, currently being developed at this laboratory, permits the analysis of separate frequency components and their relative contribution to the observed average frequency scores of the present experiment.

SUMMARY

An investigation of the relationship between the average frequency of the EEG and WAIS I.Q. scores indicated a strong relationship between I.Q. and average frequency asymmetries in left and right homologous areas. The correlations were higher in the posterior areas and for Performance I.Q. A composite score of all EEG areas tested, which took into account the negative correlations of the occipital areas (frontal + temporal + parietal − occipital), showed for the Thinking condition a Spearman Rho with Verbal I.Q. of 0.59, with Performance I.Q. of 0.78, and with Full I.Q. of 0.72. Alpha index correlations were also higher during the Thinking conditions and Performance I.Q.

RÉSUMÉ

FRÉQUENCE EEG MOYENNE ET INTELLIGENCE

Une recherche sur les relations entre la fréquence moyenne de l'EEG et les scores du quotient intellectuel aux tests de WAIS indique une forte relation entre le quotient intellectuel et l'asymétrie de fréquence moyenne sur les aires homologues droite et gauche. Les corrélations sont plus élevées au niveau des régions postérieures, et pour les scores performance du WAIS. Une quantification combinée de toutes les aires EEG explorées, tenant compte des corrélations négatives des aires occipitales (frontal + temporal + pariétal − occipital) montrent en condition d'activité mentale un Rho de Spearman de 0.59 avec le quotient verbal, de 0.78 avec le quotient performance, et de 0.72 avec le score global. Les corrélations de l'index alpha sont également plus élevées en conditions d'activité mentale et avec le quotient performance.

The data were collected at the VA Consolidated Center, Wadsworth, Kansas, and the study was supported in part by the VA Grant P9-60. The concluding and most important phase of this experiment which included theoretical development and computer analysis of these data was performed at the Michael Reese Psychiatric and Psychosomatic Institute and was supported in part by U.S. Public Health Service Grant No. 5519.

REFERENCES

Berger, H. Über das Elektrenkephalogramm des Menschen. *Arch. Psychiat. Nervenkr.*, **1929,** *87*: 527–570.

Chapman, R. M., Armington, J. C. and Bragdon, H. R. A quantitative survey of kappa and alpha EEG activity. *Electroenceph. clin. Neurophysiol.*, **1962,** *14*: 858–868.

Ellingson, R. J. Relationship between EEG and test intelligence: a commentary. *Psychol. Bull.*, **1966,** *65*: 91–98.

Giannitrapani, D. EEG phase asymmetries and laterality preference. *Clinical Neurophysiology EEG–EMG, 6th int. Congr. Electroenceph. clin. Neurophysiol.*, Vienna, **1965:** 301–305.

Giannitrapani, D. EEG differences between resting and mental multiplication. *Percept. mot. Skills*, **1966**a, *22*: 399–405.

Giannitrapani, D. Attenuation of the EEG in left- and right-preferent subjects. *Proc. 74th Ann. Convention*, APA, Washington, D. C., **1966**b: 127–128.

Giannitrapani, D. Developing concepts of lateralization of cerebral functions. *Cortex*, **1967,** *3*: 353–370.

Giannitrapani, D., Darrow, C. W. and Sorkin, A. Asleep and awake interhemispheric EEG phase relationships in left- and right-handed subjects. *Amer. J. Psychol.*, **1964,** *19*: 480–481.

Giannitrapani, D., Sorkin, A. I. and Enenstein, J. Laterality preference of children and adults as related to interhemispheric EEG phase activity. *J. neurol. Sci.*, **1966,** *3*: 139–150.

Gibbs, E. L., Rich, C. L., Fois, A. and Gibbs, F. A. Electroencephalographic study of mentally retarded persons. *Amer. J. ment. Defic.*, **1960,** *65*: 236–247.

Glanzer, M., Chapman, R. M., Clark, W. H. and Bragdon, H. R. Changes in two EEG rhythms during mental activity. *J. exp. Psychol.*, **1964,** *68*: 273–283.

Hadley, J. M. Some relationships between electrical signs of central and peripheral activity: II. During "mental work". *J. exp. Psychol.*, **1941,** *28*: 53–62.

Henry, C. E. Electroencephalograms of normal children. *Soc. Res. Child. Devel. Monogr.*, **1944,** *9*: 1–71.

Knott, J. R. Brain potentials during silent and oral reading. *J. gen. Psychol.*, **1938,** *18*: 57–62.

Knott, J. R., Friedman, H. and Bardsley, R. Some electroencephalographic correlates of intelligence in eight-year- and twelve-year-old children. *J. exp. Psychol.*, **1942,** *30*: 380–391.

Kreezer, G. L. and Smith, F. W. The relation of the alpha rhythm of the electroencephalogram and intelligence level in the non-differentiated familial type of mental deficiency. *J. Psychol.*, **1950,** *29*: 47–51.

Liberson, W. T. Ondes électriques du cerveau et intelligence chez les malades mentaux. *Ann. psychol.*, **1951,** *5*: 678–703.

LINDSLEY, D. B. Electrical potentials of the brain in children and adults. *J. gen. Psychol.*, **1938,** *19*: 285–306.

MUNDY-CASTLE, A. C. Theta and beta rhythm in the EEG grams of normal adults. *Electroenceph. clin. Neurophysiol.*, **1951,** *3*: 477–486.

MUNDY-CASTLE, A. C. The electroencephalogram and mental activity. *Electroenceph. clin. Neurophysiol.*, **1957,** *9*: 643–655.

MUNDY-CASTLE, A. C. Electrophysiological correlations of intelligence. *J. Personality*, **1958,** *26*: 184–199.

NETCHINE, S. et LAIRY, G. C. Ondes cérébrales et niveau mental: quelques aspects de l'évolution génétique du tracé EEG suivant le niveau mental. *Enfance*, **1960,** *No. 4–5*: 427–439.

NETCHINE, S. and LAIRY, G. C. Comparison of EEG data and intelligence level in children. *Proc. London Conf. Sci. Study ment. Defic.* (May and Baker, Dagenham), **1962,** *2*: 378–383.

NETCHINE, S., TALAN, I., LAIRY, G. et ZAZZO, R. EEG et niveau mental. *Ann. psychol.*, **1959,** *59*: 356–372.

SAUNDERS, D. R. Digit span and alpha frequency: a cross validation. *J. clin. Psychol.*, **1961,** *17*: 165–167.

SHAGASS, C. An attempt to correlate the occipital alpha frequency of the electroencephalogram with performance on a mental ability test. *J. exp. Psychol.*, **1946,** *36*: 88–92.

SORKIN, A., ENENSTEIN, J., GIANNITRAPANI, D. and DARROW, C. W. An IBM 7090 FORTRAN Program for 1-through 4-way analysis of variance. *Behav. Sci.*, **1964,** *9*: 377–378.

STRAUSS, H., LIBERSON, W. T. and MELTZER, T. Electroencephalographic studies: bilateral differences in alpha activity in cases with and without cerebral pathology. *J. Mt. Sinai Hosp.*, **1943,** *9*: 957–962.

TRAVIS, L. E. and EGAN, J. P. Increase in frequency of the alpha rhythm by verbal stimulation. *J. exp. Psychol.*, **1938,** *23*: 384–393.

Reference: GIANNITRAPANI, D. EEG average frequency and intelligence. *Electroenceph. clin. Neurophysiol.*, **1969,** *27*: 480–486.

Electroencephalography and Clinical Neurophysiology
Elsevier Publishing Company, Amsterdam – Printed in The Netherlands

ELECTROPHYSIOLOGICAL AND BEHAVIOURAL CHANGES OWING TO SPLITTING OF THE BRAIN-STEM IN CATS

MAURO MANCIA

Laboratorio di Fisiologia Umana dell'Università di Milano and Laboratorio di Biologia Spaziale del C.N.R., Milan (Italy)

(Accepted for publication: February 14, 1969)

It has been recently shown (Michel and Roffwarg 1967) that a longitudinal midline section through the brain-stem from the mesencephalon to the bulb can induce in cats a persistent increase in wakefulness with reduction of both synchronized and desynchronized sleep. A marked reduction in sleep and an increase in wakefulness with concomitant behavioural alterations has been reported in monkeys (Mancia *et al.* 1967, 1968) following a midline split limited to the medio-rostral part of the pontine tegmentum (almost at the level of n.reticularis pontis oralis).

The purpose of this investigation was to study the modifications of the sleep-wakefulness cycle and the parallel electrophysiological and behavioural changes chronically induced in cats by splitting the brain-stem at the pontine, bulbar or mesencephalic level.

A histological study was performed during this research in order to investigate any retrograde changes which might occur in the median and paramedian aspecific structures of the brain-stem from bulb to mesencephalon following the splitting procedures.

Some of the results have been presented as preliminary notes (Mancia 1968a, b; Mancia and Rustioni 1968).

METHODS AND MATERIAL

The experiments were carried out on thirty cats. All the animals, anaesthetized by intraperitoneal injection of sodium pentobarbital (30 mg/kg), were placed in a stereotaxic apparatus.

Pontine split. A hole was trephined in the occipital bone in order to expose the surface of the cerebellum. After the dura had been cut, a thin spatula (10 mm wide on the cutting edge), inclined at 30° to the vertical, mounted on an electrode holder and calibrated, was introduced at the midline through the cerebellum and progressively lowered into the brain-stem at the pontine level until the base was reached. The same technique was used for bilateral pontine splits. In this case the spatula was inserted at 3 mm from the midline on both sides.

Bulbar split. A tracheal cannula was introduced through the mouth under local anaesthesia. An inclined (30° to vertical) spatula, the same as the one used for the pontine split, was stereotaxically inserted through the posterior part of the corpus cerebelli and medulla oblongata till the base was reached. Artificial respiration was generally started as the spatula approached the brain-stem and maintained for 6–12 h, until the anaesthesia ceased and the animal could breathe spontaneously.

Mesencephalic split. The occipital lobe on the left was widely exposed, the dura cut, the occipital lobe lifted by means of a spatula and the tentorium cerebelli removed in order to open a passage to the mesencephalon. A straight spatula, the same size as above, was inserted between the two hemispheres and lowered through the midbrain till it reached a position from 1 to 2 mm above the base. When both midbrain and bulbar splitting was performed, both operations were carried out during the same session.

In all animals, after the split had been made, a thin polythene sheet was placed over the opening, to prevent adhesion, and fixed with dental cement. Two screw electrodes were implanted over the frontal and parieto-occipital cortex of each side for EEG recording. The eye movements (EOG) were recorded from two screws fixed in the superior wall of the orbital cavity on each side. Stainless steel wire electrodes were introduced into the posterior cervical muscles for EMG recording. The terminals of all electrodes were soldered to a 9-way plug which was fixed to the bone with dental cement. The cats were left to recover for about 48 h in a thermostatic cage, then placed in a soundproof and shielded cage and connected to an 8-channel ECEM inkwriting electroencephalograph. The EEG, EMG and EOG were recorded for 2–5 weeks, continuously day and night, except for 30 min every 6 h so that the animal could be fed and studied neurologically. A dim light was placed in the cage so that the behaviour of the animals could be observed at any time through a one-way glass window placed on the top of the cage. Intramuscular penicillin was daily injected for a week after the operation. The cats were always weighed before receiving through a cannula their daily diet of 100 g of homogenized baby food diluted in 200 ml of milk. The percentages of wakefulness, synchronous sleep and desynchronized sleep were calculated on the basis of the EEG, EMG and EOG components of each record.

In one animal the split of the pons was not complete and in another a split of the bulb and mesencephalon was carried out.

As a control a series of normal cats, with electrodes implanted under Nembutal anaesthesia, were recorded from uninterruptedly for 15 days, starting 48 h after the operation, in the same cages and under the same experimental conditions as for the animals with split brain-stems. In one cat the cerebellum was divided at the midline, leaving the brain-stem intact.

Histological controls. At the end of the experiment the cat was anaesthetized and perfused through the aorta with 10% formalin in physiological solution. 30 μ thick serial sections of the brain-stem from bulb to mesencephalon were stained, using the Nissl method. Thus the extent of the splitting lesion was determined and the retrograde changes observed in the aspecific median and paramedian nuclei of the brain-stem were studied in order to draw a complete map of degeneration of the reticular nuclei from bulb to mesencephalon.

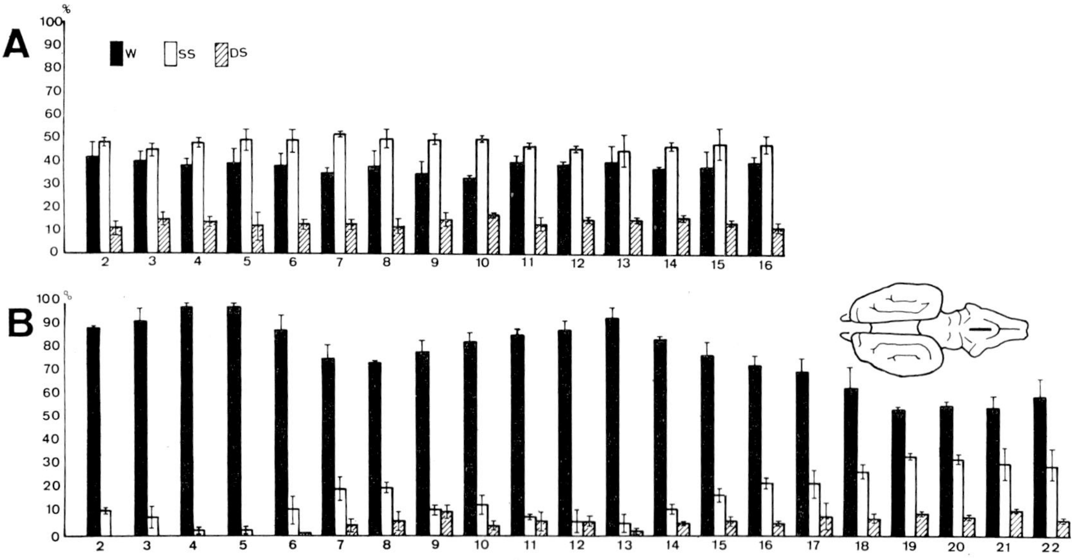

Fig. 1

Histogram showing average percentage values and standard deviations of wakefulness (W), synchronized sleep (SS) and desynchronized sleep (DS) for each day after operation (abscissa) during 22 h recording in four normal (*A*) and five midline-pontine-split cats (*B*). Drawing on right in *B* shows position and extent of pontine cut (heavy line). In *B* note total disappearance of DS during first 5 days after the split, the constant increase of W and its tendency to stabilize at higher values than normal even 20 days after operation.

RESULTS

1. *Electrophysiological, behavioural and neurological changes induced by pontine splitting*

a. *Midline pontine split*. All cats with a midline pontine longitudinal section showed a significant alteration of the sleep-wakefulness cycle. Some of the physiological data relative to their percentages of wakefulness, synchronized and desynchronized sleep are presented in Fig. 1, *B*. Table I shows the mean percentage values of sleep and wakefulness under different experimental conditions. Soon after recovering from anaesthesia the split-pons cats presented an intense bilateral desynchronization, high nuchal tone and some vertical eye movements. This alert pattern could be observed day and night for several days after operation, as can be seen in Fig. 1, *B*. Wakefulness, calculated from data obtained during the first 2 weeks following the operation, reached an average of 78.9%. Synchronized sleep was drastically reduced and its percentage remained very low for at least 2 weeks after operation (Fig. 1, *B*). Both values were significantly different from normal (Table I). High voltage slow waves typical of the synchronized phase of sleep were persistently much reduced and this phase was mainly characterized by the presence of short lasting spindles followed by long interspindle lulls. As can be seen in Fig. 1, *A* and *B*, desynchronized sleep normally disappeared during the first week and reappeared only 6 or 7 days after the operation, always remaining at very reduced levels (Table I; Fig. 1, *B*). An analysis of the sleep-wakefulness cycle of normal and midline-pontine-split cats is presented in Fig. 2, *A* and *B*. Here it can be seen that, during a continuous 22 h recording, long periods of EEG desynchronization and alertness replace the prevalent synchronized pattern of a normal cat. Synchronized episodes are rare and very short lasting.

Desynchronized sleep also appeared in rare, brief episodes which directly followed a state of intense wakefulness, without passing through synchronization. This latter phenomenon is also clearly visible in the continuous records shown in Fig. 3, *A* and *B*. Eye movements during desynchronized sleep were frequently absent or very rare and of low voltage (Fig. 3, *A* and *B*) for 10 or 15 days after the operation. Subsequently more complex eye movement patterns could be observed which, however, were never comparable to the bursts of rapid eye movement typical of the paradoxical phase of sleep in a normal cat.

Fig. 3, *C* illustrates some peculiar electrophysiological aspects of sleep after pontine splitting. During this stage the EEG was synchronized with very low muscular tone and eye movements resembling those of desynchronized sleep. Generally the EEG was not asymmetric during the whole recording time; however, in one cat a

TABLE I

Mean percentages of wakefulness (W), synchronized sleep (SS) and desynchronized sleep (DS), and standard deviations calculated from data obtained during the first 2 weeks following operation in day-and-night recording. Pooled data from four cats (normal), five cats (midline pontine split), two cats (bilateral pontine split), four cats (midline bulbar split) and five cats (midline mesencephalic split). Note the highly significant changes in all three stages after midline and bilateral pontine split, whilst no changes are observed after bulbar and mesencephalic split except for the reduction of desynchronized sleep in the latter experimental condition

Stage	Normal cats %	Midline pontine split %	Bilateral pontine split %	Midline bulbar split %	Midline mesencephalic split %
W	37.8 (±5)	78.9 (±8) $P < 0.01$	78.6 (±8) $P < 0.05$	47.8 (±8) n.s.	50.8 (±8) n.s.
SS	48.1 (±3)	16.7 (±8) $P < 0.05$	19.7 (±7) $P < 0.05$	42.5 (±8) n.s.	43.2 (±9) n.s.
DS	14.1 (±2)	4.4 (±3) $P < 0.05$	1.7 (±1) $P < 0.05$	9.7 (±3) n.s.	6 (±3) $P < 0.05$

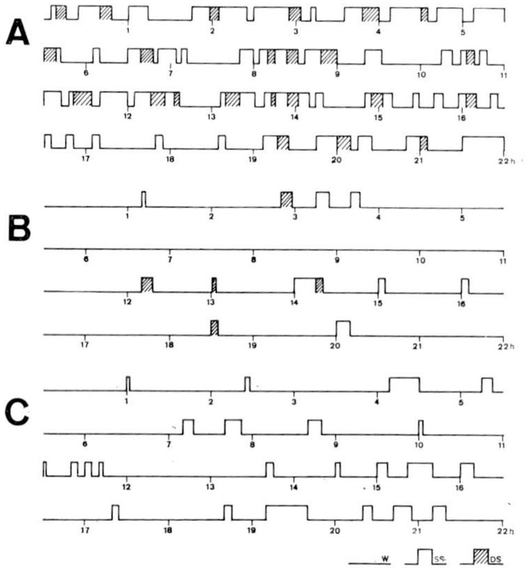

Fig. 2
Schematic representation of typical sleep-wakefulness rhythms of normal (*A*), midline-pontine-split (*B*) and bilateral-pontine-split (*C*) cats. Diagram indicates for each animal the periods of wakefulness (W), synchronized sleep (SS) and desynchronized (DS) recorded on the sixth day after operation for 22 h. Stages represented as indicated at bottom of figure. Time in hours. Note lengthening of straight lines in *B* and *C*, indicating increased wakefulness, and the few episodes of desynchronized sleep in *B*, which follow directly an alert state. In *C* no desynchronized sleep is present.

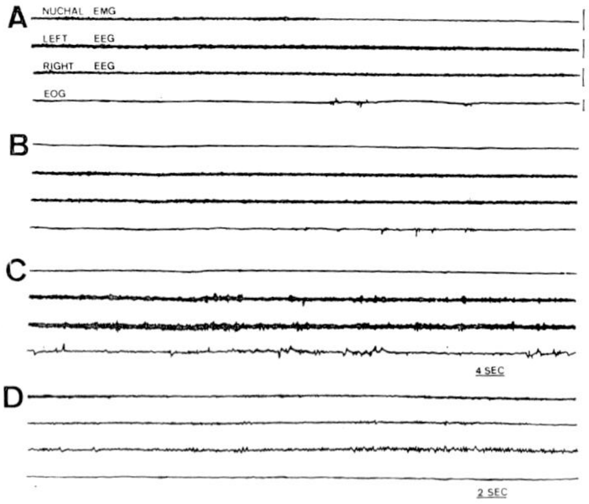

Fig. 3
Examples of EEG, EMG and eye movements (EOG) of three different midline-pontine-split cats. *A* and *B*: continuous records taken a week after operation, showing an episode of desynchronized sleep directly following wakefulness. Note rareness of eye movements during this stage of sleep. *C*: another cat showing a mixed pattern with very low nuchal EMG and eye movements, whilst EEG is synchronized. *D*: another cat with slight EEG asymmetry during synchronization. Calibration 200 μV.

slight asymmetry was found during spontaneous synchronization (Fig. 3, *D*). This asymmetry faded away a few days after the operation.

Three to 5 weeks after operation most pontine-split cats regained some synchronized and desynchronized sleep. However, the sleep-wakefulness cycle showed a tendency to stabilize at much higher values of wakefulness than in normal cats (Fig. 1, *A* and *B*). No strict relationship was found between synchronized and desynchronized sleep episodes. The appearance of desynchronized sleep was more predictable and more easily observable when the sleep-wakefulness rhythms were becoming more stable and slightly closer to normal, as can be observed in the histograms of Fig. 1, *B*.

From the behavioural point of view the cats which had lost their normal cycle after pontine splitting underwent marked changes which consisted in restlessness, aggressivity towards the experimenter, high irritability. No sign of hypervoracity similar to that reported in split-pons monkeys (Mancia *et al.* 1967, 1968) could be found. The symptoms reported were strictly related to the loss of sleep since they were not present in other split-brain-stem or control animals (see below) and they disappeared after the midline-pontine-split cat regained some sleep (40% of synchronized and 10% of desynchronized sleep). A dramatic reduction in body weight (up to 30–40 g /day) was also observed, parallel to the consistent changes in sleep and wakefulness brought about by the midline pontine split. This sign was also strictly related to the loss of sleep since the pontine-split cats regained their normal weight as their insomnia diminished and no weight loss was found in those brain-stem-split animals whose sleep-wakefulness cycles were not modified.

The neurological symptoms produced by the midline pontine split consisted in a complete loss of normal posture: the cat lay on one side for some days after the operation. In this position the cat made frequent pedalling movements which increased when it was stimulated by the presence of the experimenter. When helped to stand the animal showed a marked increase of postural tone, which was more evident in both forelimbs, wide oscillations of the body and a tendency to opisthotonus. A few days after the splitting procedure a marked incoordination, ataxia and dysmetria resulted when the cat was helped to walk. Some of these motor symptoms were less evident after the first week and had a tendency to recede as time passed. The pontine-split animal had an expressionless face because of bilateral facial paralysis and could not eat spontaneously. Pupils tended to be mydriatic, isocoric and reactive to light. Isolated and conjugate lateral eye movements were permanently abolished. The cats showed spontaneous vertical eye movements which occurred more frequently as the time from operation increased. No nystagmus was ever observed. The corneal reflexes, which were normally present, became more prompt a few days after the operation. A slight bilateral deficit of trigeminal sensitivity was seen in some cats. No gross sensory disturbance was found when the body was stimulated.

In one cat the midline pontine split was not complete and reached the dorsal half of the pontine tegmentum. Under these conditions the cat showed an alteration of the sleep-wakefulness cycle with reduction of sleep (synchronized and desynchronized) and increase of wakefulness. The mean percentage values obtained from data recorded during the first 2 weeks after operation were as follows: wakefulness 54.5% (±2), synchronized sleep 36.2% (±1.5), desynchronized sleep 9.2% (±0.7). These values were significantly different from the ones obtained after complete pontine splitting. The insomnia and behavioural alterations which followed the incomplete pontine split were very slight and not comparable with those induced by complete section of the brain-stem at the same level.

b. *Bilateral pontine split*. In order to ascertain whether the important changes in sleep and wakefulness in all animals after complete pontine midline split were due to section of crossing fibres or to damage to pontine raphe nuclei (Brodal *et al.* 1960a, b; Taber 1961), two experiments were performed in which bilateral longitudinal sections were made at the pontine level about 3 mm from the midline, so that the raphe cells remained intact while the fibres were cut. After this procedure the cats had a pattern of intense electrophysiological and behavioural wakefulness

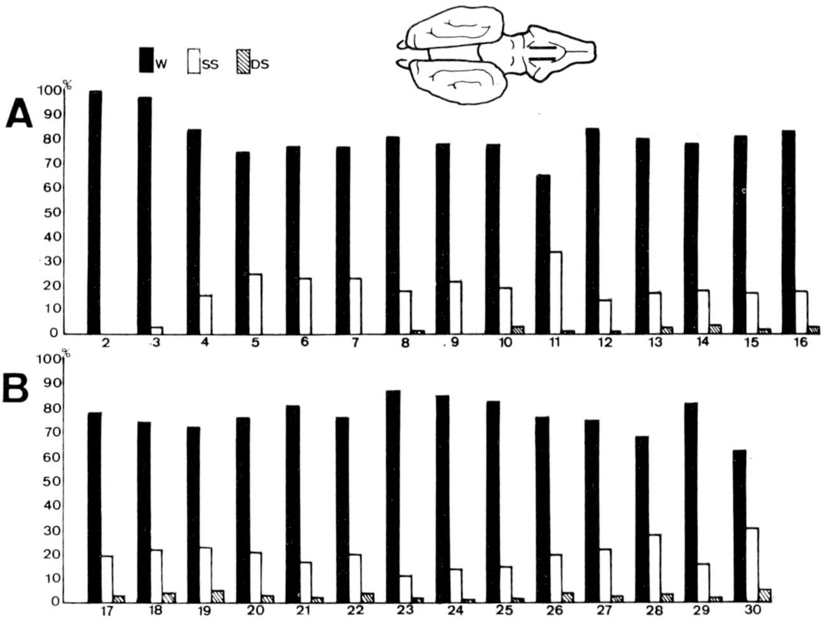

Fig. 4

A and *B*: continuous histogram showing average percentage values of wakefulness (W), synchronized sleep (SS) and desynchronized sleep (DS) for each day (22 h recording) in two cats with bilateral pontine split as shown in the drawing (heavy lines). Abscissa: days after operation. Note disappearance of DS for entire first week after operation and increase of W, which remains very high for following 23 days.

comparable to that seen after midline pontine split. The results are summarized in Table I, which illustrates how the average percentages obtained during the first 2 weeks after bilateral pontine splitting are similar to those found in midline pontine cats except for desynchronized sleep, which is more reduced by the bilateral split than by the midline one. The histogram in Fig. 4 presents the time course of the average percentages of sleep and wakefulness in the two cats following bilateral splitting. Wakefulness always showed very high values up to 30 days after the operation. Synchronized sleep was drastically reduced and remained very low in each recording session. No asymmetry was ever seen during synchronization. Desynchronized sleep was absent for several days after surgery and, when it reappeared, had much lower values than those found in midline-split animals. An analysis of the sleep-wakefulness rhythms in a typical case on the sixth day after the bilateral split (Fig. 2, *C*) revealed that the EEG could be persistently desynchronized for long periods of time, interupted by short lasting phases of synchronization. No desynchronized sleep was normally found within 8–10 days after the splitting procedure. After this period desynchronized sleep was present in short episodes and sometimes directly followed a period of wakefulness.

The behavioural symptoms and loss of weight following the bilateral split, although more intense, were similar to those induced by the midline split.

Neurological symptoms also resembled those of midline-split cats except for abolition or marked reduction of corneal reflexes and more evident cerebellar symptoms.

c. *Unilateral pontine split*. Electrophysiological, behavioural and neurological changes, similar in all respects to those described in paragraph a were observed in one cat in which a complete unilateral longitudinal section of the pons was made at about 1.5–2 mm from the midline.

2. *Electrophysiological, behavioural and neurological changes induced by midline bulbar or mesencephalic split*

a. *Midline bulbar split*. After the cats had re-

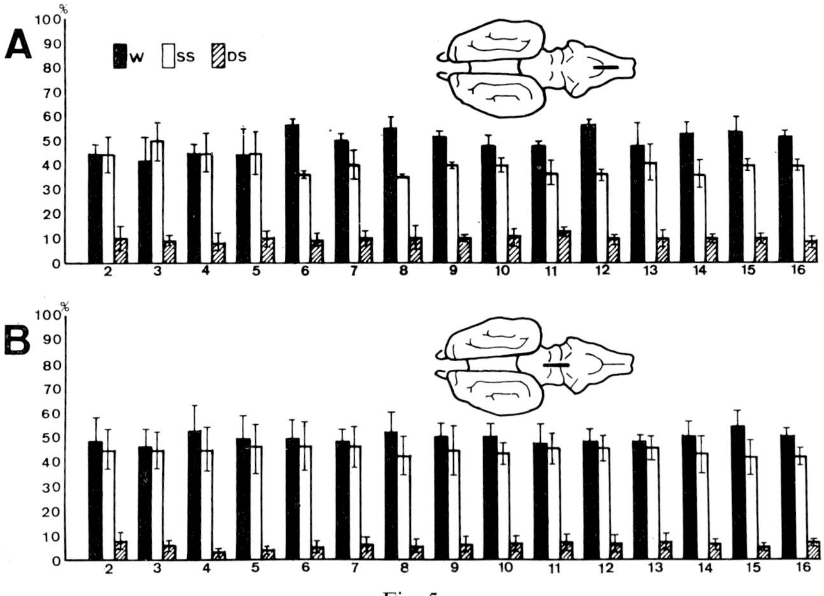

Fig. 5

Histogram showing average percentage values and standard deviations of wakefulness (W), synchronized sleep (SS) and desynchronized sleep (DS) for each day (22 h recording) in four midline-bulbar-split (*A*) and in five midline-mesencephalic-split (*B*) cats. Abscissa: days after operation. Drawings show position and extent of cuts (heavy lines). Note reduction of DS in B whilst all other percentages in *A* and *B* are close to normal.

covered from anaesthesia and started to breathe spontaneously, no changes in the sleep-wakefulness cycle could be found. The histograms of Fig. 5, *A* show that the percentages of wakefulness, synchronous sleep and desynchronized sleep during the 2 weeks after midline bulbar split is not consistently different from that of normal cats (Fig. 1, *A*). As determined by Student's *t* test the mean differences in bulbar-split cats were not statistically significant when compared with normal cats (Table I). A typical analysis of the sleep-wakefulness rhythm during 22 h recording after bulbar split is shown in Fig. 6, *A* where the amount of sleep (synchronized and desynchronized) and the length of its periods are very similar to normal (Fig. 2, *A*). Under these experimental conditions desynchronized sleep always followed a synchronized episode (Fig. 6, *A*). In some cats a rhythmic nystagmus appeared during wakefulness soon after the bulb had been cut (Fig. 7, *A*). The nystagmus disappeared during spontaneous EEG synchronization (Fig. 7, *B*), and was replaced by typical bursts of REMs during desynchronized sleep (Fig. 7, *C*); this phenomenon is comparable to that reported by Baldissera *et al.* (1967), after unilateral labyrinthectomy. In record *C* of Fig. 7 one can also see that nuchal EMG does not drop to zero, even when the cat is behaviourally asleep and shows twitching and eye movements typical of the desynchronized phase of sleep. This phenomenon was observed in some cats and alternated with other episodes in which the cervical tone was deeply depressed.

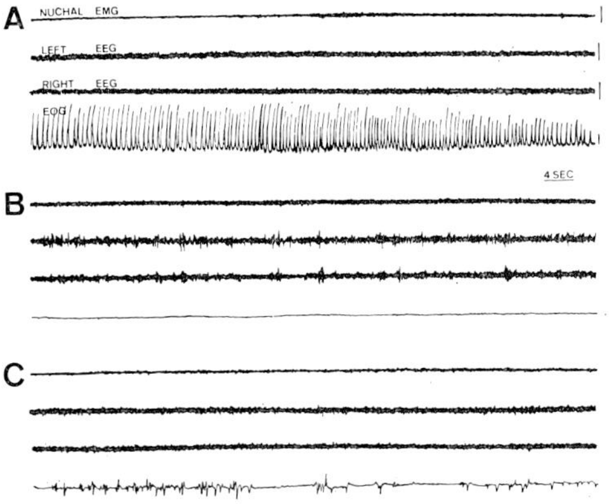

Fig. 7
EEG, EMG and eye movements (EOG) recorded in one cat 3 days after midline bulbar split. *A*: wakefulness; *B*: synchronous sleep; *C*: desynchronized sleep. Note intense nystagmus in *A* which disappears in *B* and is replaced in *C* by eye movements more typical of the desynchronized phase of sleep. Note also that muscular tone in *C* does not completely disappear. Calibration 200 μV.

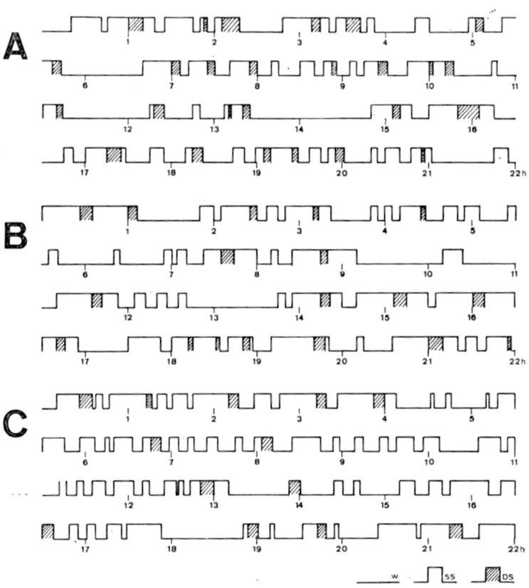

Fig. 6
Schematic representation of typical sleep-wakefulness rhythms of a midline-bulbar (*A*), midline-mesencephalic (*B*) and midline-bulbar-plus-mesencephalic-split (*C*) cat. Diagram represents periods of wakefulness (W), synchronous sleep (SS) and desynchronized sleep (DS) during 22 h recording of three animals on the third day after operation. Stages represented as indicated at the bottom of the figure. Time in hours. *A*, *B* and *C* appear normal (compare with Fig. 2,*A*). Note that desynchronized sleep always follows a synchronous episode.

Split-bulb cats did not present any particular behavioural change which could be comparable with those following a pontine split, nor did they lose weight after the operation.

As to the neurological signs, bulbar section induced hypertonus of all four limbs and a tendency to opisthotonus. The animal generally lay on its side; when helped to stand the postural hypertonus and opisthotonus became more evident. Cerebellar symptoms such as swaying of the body, incoordination of movements and dysmetria were present. After 6–10 days these motor symptoms were less evident and the animal could walk by itself. Muscular hypertonus was still evident 2 weeks after operation. The pupils were normal, isocoric and reactive to light. The eyes could move in all planes. Corneal reflexes were present. Facial movements were normal. Respiration became quite normal on the second day after the operation. The animals could swallow but were normally fed through a cannula.

b. *Midline mesencephalic split*. Because of the presence of the falx it was always very difficult to cut the midbrain tegmentum exactly along the midline. In most cases the spatula shifted 1 mm toward the left. Nonetheless, the damaging action of the cut usually reached the midline (Fig. 10, *right*) and it is therefore reasonable to refer to this preparation as a midline mesencephalic split.

The midbrain section did not consistently change the amount of wakefulness and synchronized sleep for the full period of observation (16 days) (Fig. 5, *B*). Desynchronized sleep was, however, significantly ($P < 0.05$, Table I) affected in all cats, being permanently reduced in comparison with the normal (Fig. 5, *B*).

Fig. 6, *B* represents diagrammatically a typical sleep-wakefulness rhythm over a period of 22 h 3 days after a midbrain splitting operation. It can be seen that the number of desynchronized sleep episodes is smaller than that of a normal cat (Fig. 2, *A*) or of a midline-bulbar-split animal (Fig. 6, *A*), but the episodes always follow a pattern of synchronization. In some cats, in the days immediately following the split, an EEG asymmetry could be observed during spontaneous synchronization. Spindles and slow waves prevailed on the right side, *i.e.*, on the side opposite to the one where the split was performed. An asynchrony in the appearance of spindles in the two hemispheres was also seen, similar to that reported by Berlucchi (1966) in cats with a brain section reaching the rostral part of the midbrain tegmentum. During desynchronized sleep the pattern of ocular movements changed as time passed. The large groups of REM which were present before the operation were replaced by infrequent, isolated, rapid movements soon after the split, but some REMs reappeared in bursts several days later.

From the neurological point of view the midbrain-split cats presented a slight muscular hypotonia, prevalent on the left side; they tended to move continuously in circles towards the left, and showed an abolition of the placing reaction of the left fore and hind limb. Vertical eye movements were permanently abolished whilst the lateral ones were unaffected. Pupils were sometimes anisocoric, with prevalent mydriasis on the left side, although they reacted bilaterally to light; corneal reflexes were present on both sides. A characteristic alteration of visual perception, resulting in apparent blindness, was observed after the midbrain split: when moving in circles the cats bumped into the objects they met. Nor did they respond to significant visual stimuli. No cat in this group lost weight. Some could eat spontaneously, and their diet did not differ from that given to normal animals or to other groups of operated animals.

c. *Midline bulbar plus mesencephalic split*. In the cat in which a bulbar plus a mesencephalic split were carried out the percentage values calculated from data recorded each day during the first 2 weeks after operation did not differ significantly from those recorded after mesencephalic split only. The alterations in pupil diameter and eye motility, as well as the change in visual perception, were also similar to those found in mesencephalic-split cats. The postural hypertonus and some lateral nystagmic movements resembled the signs present in cats after bulbar section.

3. *Control experiments*

In four cats electrodes alone were chronically implanted. Records were made for 15 days in the same conditions as for the split animals (data presented in Fig. 1, *A* and summarized in Table I). One cat in which the cerebellum was cut at the midline showed neither changes in wakefulness and sleep nor behavioural modifications.

4. *Histological controls and experiments*

An example of midline pontine section is presented in Fig. 8, *D–F* where the cut was exactly in the midline and did not produce haemorrhage. In Fig. 8, *A–C* serial sections of the brain-stem of a cat after bilateral pontine split are shown. Here one can see that the cut had produced bilateral damage to n.reticularis pontis caudalis and oralis.

The study of cellular changes induced by brain-stem splitting has been reserved essentially to the median and paramedian aspecific nuclei of the brain-stem, including n.reticularis gigantocellularis (GC), n.reticularis paragigantocellularis

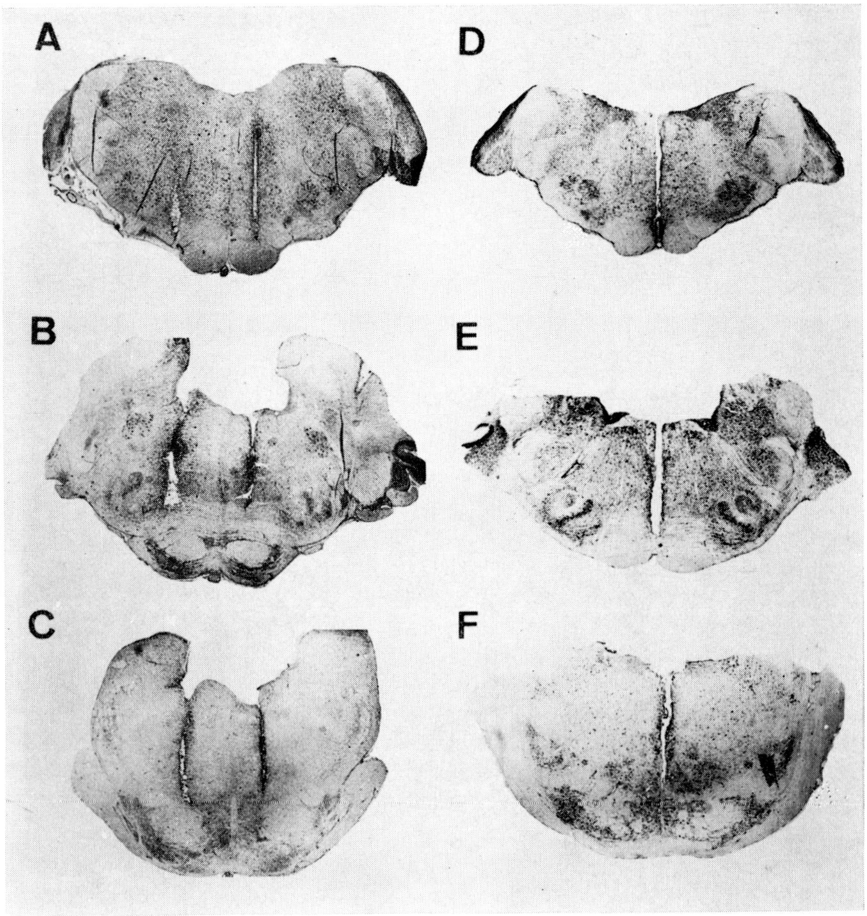

Fig. 8
Histological preparations of bilateral pontine split (*A–C*) and midline pontine split (*D–F*) in cats one month after operation.

dorsalis (Pgd) and lateralis (Pgl), n.parvocellularis (Pc), n.reticularis pontis oralis (PoO) n.reticularis pontis caudalis (PoC) and the raphe nuclei (RPA, RPO, RM) (see Brodal 1957; Brodal *et al.* 1960a, b; Taber 1961). Changes which could be observed in some specific brain-stem nuclei have been purposely neglected.

a. *Changes induced by pontine splitting.* The most consistent retrograde changes in the brain-stem have been found following a midline pontine split. As shown in Fig. 9 (*left*), important modifications following such a section were observed in n.reticularis gigantocellularis, paragigantocellularis dorsalis, pontis caudalis and pontis oralis, consisting in different degrees of chromatolysis up to severe atrophy with death of large, medium and small cells. Neurones close to the midline were most severely affected. Pontine raphe nuclei were evidently destroyed by the cut. A very few slightly degenerated elements could be found in the bulbar raphe nuclei while n.reticularis parvocellularis and parasagittalis lateralis, as well as midbrain raphe nuclei were unaffected. Comparable alterations occurred in brain-stem nuclei following bilateral pontine splitting, as can be seen in Fig. 9 (*right*). In these experimental conditions a large percentage of neurones belonging to n.reticularis parvocellularis as well as to n.reticularis pontis oralis and caudalis were directly destroyed by the cut and the remaining cells of this region underwent very severe chromatolysis with cellular death. Pontine and bulbar raphe nuclei were

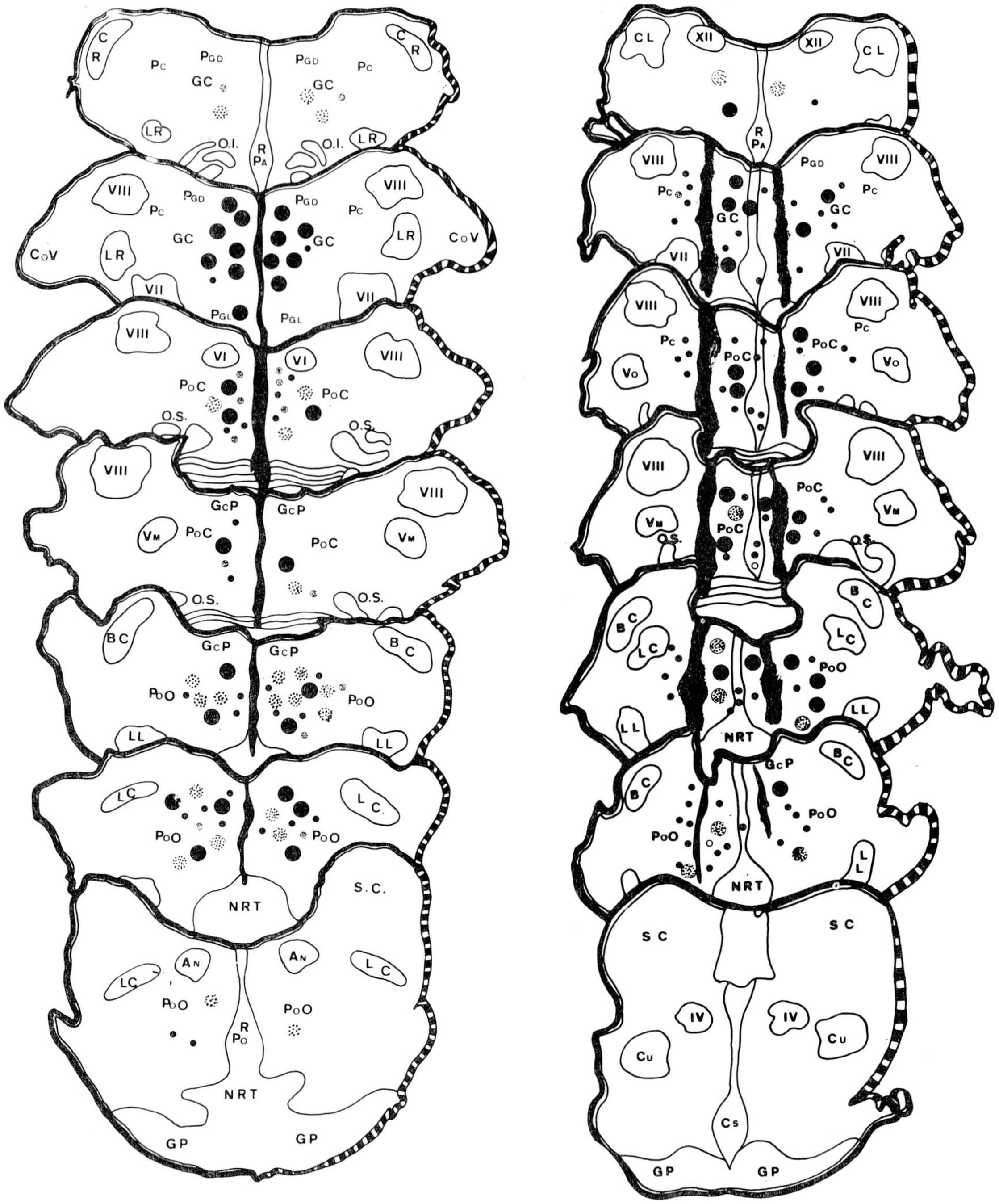

Fig. 9

Diagrammatic representation of retrograde changes occurring in brain-stem nuclei following longitudinal midline pontine (*left*) and bilateral pontine (*right*) sections. Severe degeneration is schematically represented by filled circles. Stippled circles indicate slight changes. Large circles: large cells. Small circles: small cells. Shaded area surrounding cut indicates extent of necrosis and glial reaction.

For this and Fig. 10 symbols are as follows: An = n.annularis; BC = brachium conjunctivum; CL = n.cuneatus lateralis; CoV = cochlearis ventralis; CR = corpus restiforme; Cs = n.centralis superior; Cu = n.cuneiformis; GC = n.gigantocellularis; GcP, Gcp = griseum centrale pontis; GP = griseum pontis; LC = locus coeruleus; LL = n.lemnisci lateralis; LR = n.lateralis reticularis; NRT = n.reticularis tegmenti pontis; O.I. = n. olivaris inferior; O.S. = n. olivaris superior; Pc = n.parvocellularis; Pgd = n. paragigantocellularis dorsalis; Pgl = n.paragigantocellularis lateralis; PoC = n.pontis centralis caudalis; PoO = n.pontis centralis oralis; Rm = n.raphe magnus; RPa = n.raphe pallidus; RPo = n.raphe pontis; SC = superior colliculus; IV = n.nervi trochlearis; Vm = n.nervi trigemini motorius; Vo = n.tractus spinalis trigemini oralis; VI = n.nervi abducentis; VII = n.nervi facialis; VIII = n.nervi vestibularis; XII = n.nervi hypoglossi.

largely unaffected by the bilateral cut, which induced only minor and inconstant alterations in a small number of their smallest cells.

b. *Changes induced by bulbar and mesencephalic splits*. The retrograde changes which were found in the brain-stem following a bulbar split are

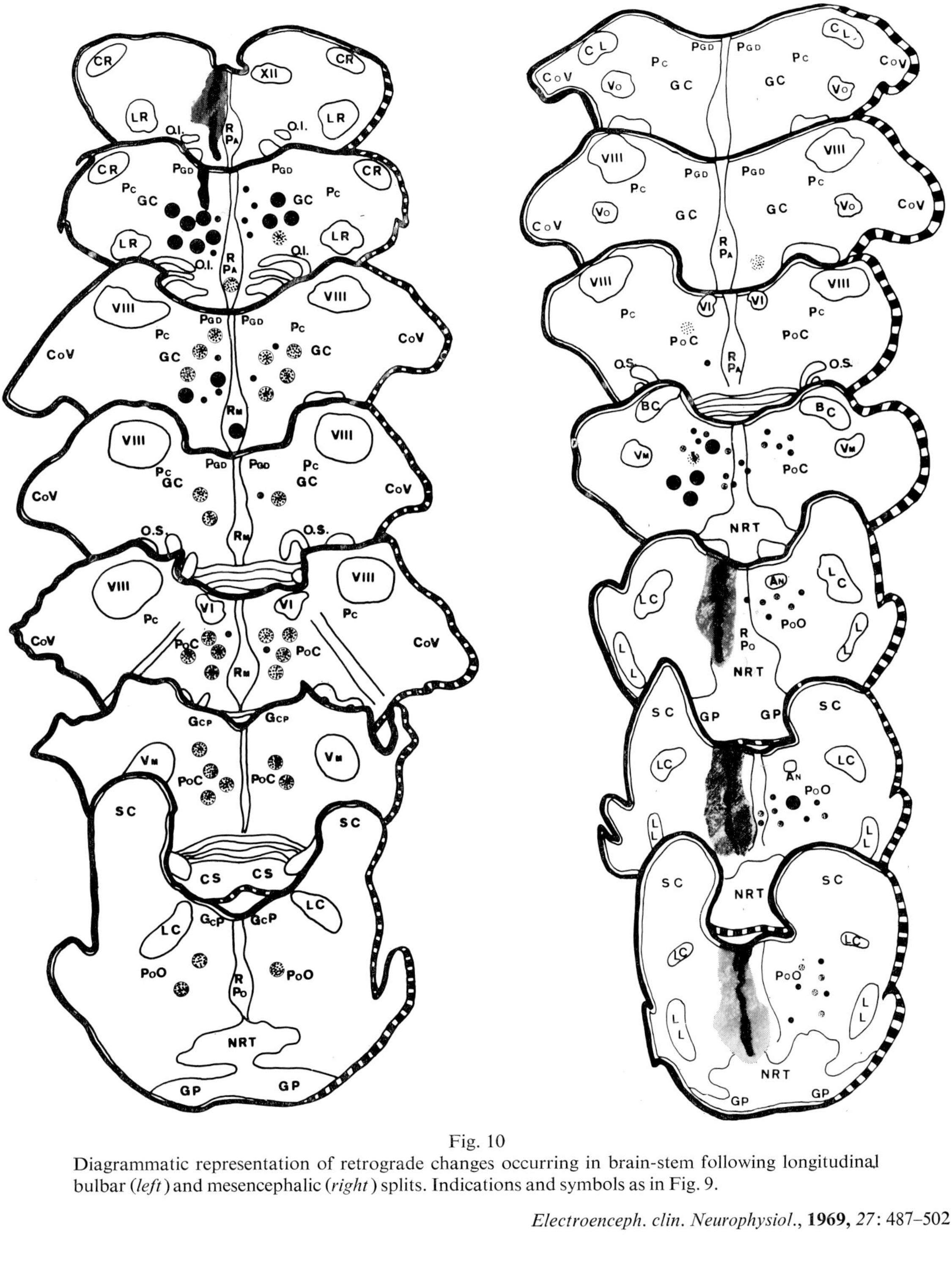

Fig. 10
Diagrammatic representation of retrograde changes occurring in brain-stem following longitudinal bulbar (*left*) and mesencephalic (*right*) splits. Indications and symbols as in Fig. 9.

presented in Fig. 10 (*left*). After this operation many large cells belonging to n.reticularis gigantocellularis were severely affected. Slight chromatolysis was found in some large neurones belonging to n.reticularis pontis oralis and caudalis. The raphe nuclei in the bulb were destroyed by the cut whereas only minor changes could be seen in the more rostrally situated raphe nuclei.

Fig. 10 (*right*) outlines the retrograde changes found in the brain-stem after the midbrain split. Here it may be observed that the section was not exactly in the midline although the midline structures were damaged. Retrograde chromatolysis was found in some large and small cells of the cranialmost part of n.reticularis pontis caudalis and of the entire n.reticularis pontis oralis. No cellular changes occurred in bulbar aspecific median and paramedian nuclei.

c. *Control experiments* performed on cats without any section, or on the cat with the cerebellar split alone, have shown that the brain-stem nuclei investigated were not affected by these procedures.

DISCUSSION

The results reported in this paper indicate that it is possible to induce a persistent EEG desynchronization and all signs of behavioural insomnia by a midline split of the pontine tegmentum. The profound changes in the sleep-wakefulness cycle which invariably followed such a procedure cannot be ascribed to a traumatic irritation of the nervous tissue separated by the cut since: (i) the EEG and behavioural insomnia could be observed for 4–5 weeks, and (ii) some reflex activities involving pontine structures were still present a few hours after the splitting operation. Therefore, the conclusion that a longitudinal midline section limited to the pons is responsible for the changes observed seems justified. Michel and Roffwarg (1967) found an increase in wakefulness and a reduction in sleep in cats following a complete brain-stem split from the bulb to the mesencephalon; Jouvet and Renault (1966) reported persistent insomnia with reduction of both synchronized and desynchronized sleep following electrocoagulation of midline raphe nuclei from bulb to mesencephalon. These authors, however, specified that "la lésion isolée des noyaux du raphé pontis n'a pas d'effet notable sur le sommeil lent", an observation which is in contrast with the results obtained in this research following midline pontine section. Jouvet *et al.* (1967) and Renault (1967) found a close relationship in their chronic cat preparations between, on the one hand, the extent of the lesion to the brain-stem raphe system and the reduction of cerebral serotonin, and, on the other, the percentage increase of wakefulness. Some histochemical investigations (Dahlström and Fuxe 1964), revealing the existence of monoamine-containing neurones in the various raphe nuclei of the brain-stem, might justify the conclusions of the above-mentioned authors (Jouvet and Renault 1966; Jouvet *et al.* 1967; Renault 1967) that the reduction or abolition of sleep after electrocoagulation of the entire raphe system was due to an alteration of the serotonine-producing mechanism in the brain. However, any electrocoagulation of the brain-stem along the midline, besides destroying the raphe system, will obviously cut all ascending crossing fibres coming from regions at the level of those which had been coagulated or from more caudal ones. It therefore seems reasonable to suspect that any changes in sleep and wakefulness following a midline brain-stem lesion may be partly or entirely due to section of ascending fibres crossing the midline. The persistent increase in wakefulness and reduction in both synchronized and desynchronized sleep, induced by pontine splitting, can be ascribed to suppression or reduction of a flow of physiological sleep impulses (synchronizing and desynchronizing the EEG) originating in regions at the level of, or caudal to, the pontine cut and ascending contralaterally to diencephalic and cortical regions. This conclusion is based on the following experimental facts: (i) the important and persistent changes in the sleep-wakefulness rhythms occurred following a midline longitudinal cut limited to the pons; (ii) similar results were also found when the pontine split was not strictly in the midline but a few millimeters to one side, so that the pontine raphe nuclei were largely spared; (iii) an increase in wakefulness, a marked reduction of synchronized sleep and abolition (at least for the first week) of desynchronized sleep were found when the pons was cut longitudinally on both sides about 3mm from the midline, so that the pontine raphe nuclei were untouched while the paramedian pontine nuclei (reticularis pontis oralis and caudalis) were largely destroyed by the cuts, together with most of the crossing ascending fibres; (iv) the increase in wakefulness and the reduction in sleep were less marked in the case in which the midline cut involved only the dorsal half of the pons; (v) no significant changes were seen after bulbar or mesencephalic splitting or in the cat with bulbar + mesencephalic split, in which the brain-stem raphe system was largely destroyed (60–70% at least in the latter case); (vi) the anatomical control and the histological investigations limited to the aspecific brain-stem structures (see Brodal 1957; Rossi and Zanchetti 1957; Taber 1961) revealed severe retrograde degeneration, particularly in large cells belonging to n.reticularis gigantocellularis, paragigantocellularis dorsalis, pontis oralis and pontis caudalis, following the midline pontine split. The bilateral pontine split, in spite of its highly significant persistent alterations of the sleep-wakefulness cycle, induced no consistent change in the raphe system, whilst neurones belonging to the above mentioned brain-stem nuclei were severely affected. These retrograde changes allow some anatomo-functional correlations: the aspecific brain-stem nuclei which underwent marked alterations after pontine splitting represent those structures located in the brain-stem (pons and rostral medulla) involved in the physiological processes of synchronized and desynchronized sleep. Although direct evidence is still lacking, several types of experiment (Batini *et al.* 1959; Cordeau and Mancia 1959; Jouvet 1962; Rossi and Zanchetti 1957; Rossi *et al.* 1963; Rosina and Mancia 1966) strongly support the hypothesis that neurones belonging to reticular structures of the rostral medulla and caudal pons, such as n.reticularis gigantocellularis, paragigantocellularis dorsalis and reticularis pontis caudalis are actively responsible through their long ascending fibres (Rossi and Brodal 1956; Brodal 1957; Nauta and Kuypers 1958; Scheibel and Scheibel 1958) for EEG synchronization.

Neurones belonging to the rostral part of n.reticularis pontis caudalis and the entire n.reticularis pontis oralis are considered to be actively responsible for desynchronized sleep (Jouvet 1962; Rossi *et al.* 1963; Carli and Zanchetti 1965; Rosina and Mancia 1966). Besides the results obtained in pontine-split cats, this hypothesis also finds support in our mesencephalic-split experiments in which the reduction of desynchronized sleep goes with retrograde changes in large cells in n.reticularis pontis caudalis (rostralmost part) and in n.reticularis pontis oralis.

It is worth emphasizing that, in the split pons experiments, several episodes of desynchronized sleep could occur directly following a state of intense alertness. This indicates the possibility that, under certain experimental conditions in which the animal undergoes severe sleep deprivation, the two mechanisms responsible for sleep (synchronized and desynchronized) may be dissociated, a situation which has never been reported in normal cats. Moreover, the appearance of an episode of desynchronized sleep, even when no signs of synchronization could be seen in the records, supports the idea of a "state of need" during sleep deprivation which is relatively more important for desynchronized than for synchronized sleep.

In bulbar-split cats it often occurred that during desynchronized sleep the nuchal EMG did not drop to zero as in normal animals. This phenomenon could be due to severance of crossing descending fibres coming from bulbar inhibitory structures (Magoun and Rhines 1946) which appeared to be severely damaged by the cut.

No explanations can at present be offered for the mixed electrographic pattern which was also seen in monkeys after sleep deprivation (Mancia *et al.* 1968). This pattern might represent a compensatory phenomenon brought about by lack of sleep.

The behavioural alterations which have been observed in pontine-split cats are quite comparable with those seen in monkeys (Mancia *et al.* 1968) except for the increase in appetite, which was not observed in cats. These behavioural changes are strictly related to the loss of sleep since they were never found in those split-brain-stem cats in which no alterations of sleep and wakefulness occurred.

The characteristic alteration of visual perception, resulting in apparently blind behaviour, which was seen in mesencephalic-split cats is similar to that reported by Voneida (1965) and Berlucchi (1966) following midline section of the midbrain tegmentum and by Michel and Roffwarg (1967) in their chronic split-brain-stem preparations. It is difficult to give a satisfactory explanation of this finding at present. Since the phenomenon occurred only after mesencephalic splitting, which may have damaged the superior colliculi or cut fibres coming from or going to the colliculi, the hypothesis might be advanced that the apparent blindness of the animals is due to a lesion of structures necessary for a more complex visual integration. Varied evidence indicates indeed that the superior colliculi are involved in visually guided behaviour (Sprague and Meikle 1965; Sprague 1966a, b) and collicular cells have been found to be driven by moving visual stimuli (Horn and Hill 1966; Marchiafava and Pepeu 1966; Straschill and Tagwavy 1967; Wickelgren and Sterling 1967; Humphrey 1968; McIlwain and Buser 1968; Sprague *et al.* 1968).

In conclusion, the pontine split induces insomnia parallel to EEG desynchronization. This phenomenon is probably due to abolition of incoming sleep impulses following the section of crossing ascending fibres coming from lower brain-stem nuclei.

SUMMARY

1. A midline pontine split induced a persistent alteration of sleep-wakefulness rhythms in cats; sleep (synchronized and desynchronized) was drastically reduced, reaching mean percentages of 16.7% (synchronized sleep) and 4.4% (desynchronized sleep). Wakefulness remained persistently very high (78.9%). These changes lasted 3–5 weeks after the splitting procedure. Similar changes in sleep and wakefulness were observed after bilateral pontine splits at 3 mm from the midline, in which the pontine raphe nuclei were spared, and after unilateral longitudinal pontine section at 1.5–2 mm from the midline.

2. A midline bulbar split did not cause any consistent change in the sleep-wakefulness cycle of the cat. A mesencephalic split significantly reduced the amount of desynchronized sleep whilst synchronized sleep was not modified. An apparent blindness was observed in this preparation.

3. Marked alterations in behaviour, such as restlessness and hyperirritability, together with a marked loss of body weight, were observed in cats with severe sleep deprivation induced by pontine splitting.

4. The retrograde changes in the aspecific brain-stem neurones brought about by midline and bilateral pontine splits suggest the hypothesis that the persistent increase in wakefulness and reduction of sleep (synchronized and desynchronized), induced by these cuts, may be ascribed to suppression or reduction of the flow of physiological sleep impulses (synchronizing and desynchronizing the EEG) originating in regions at the level of the pontine section or caudally to them, and ascending contralaterally to diencephalic and cortical regions.

RÉSUMÉ

MODIFICATIONS ÉLECTROPHYSIOLOGIQUES ET COMPORTEMENTALES APRÈS SECTION DU PONT CÉRÉBRAL CHEZ LE CHAT

1. Une section médiane du pont induit des altérations persistantes (pouvant durer jusqu'à 3–5 semaines) du rythme veille-sommeil chez le chat: une forte réduction des pourcentages de sommeil synchronisé (16.7%) et désynchronisé (4.4%) parallèle à une augmentation de la veille (78.9%). On observe des modifications pareilles après une section bilatérale pontique à 3 mm de la ligne moyenne qui ne lèse pas les noyaux du raphé et après section unilatérale longitudinale du pont à 1.5–2 mm de la ligne moyenne.

2. Une section médiane bulbaire n'est pas suivie par des modifications significatives du cycle veille-sommeil. La section mésencéphalique induit une réduction du sommeil désynchronisé tandis que le pourcentage de sommeil synchronisé reste inchangé. Dans cette préparation on observe une altération caractéristique de la perception visuelle.

3. Lorsque la section du pont est suivie par une privation significative de sommeil on assiste à de profondes modifications comportementales et à un amaigrissement progressif du chat.

4. Les modifications rétrogrades induites dans les noyaux du tronc cérébral par la section médiane et bilatérale pontique suggèrent l'hypothèse que l'augmentation persistente d'éveil et la réduction de sommeil (synchronisé et désynchronisé) peuvent être attribuées à une suppression ou une réduction des afférences responsables du

sommeil et provenant de portions plus caudales du tronc cérébral.

The author wishes to thank Dr. Aldo Rustioni for his contribution in preparing and studying the histological slides.

REFERENCES

BALDISSERA, F., BROGGI, G. and MANCIA, M. Nystagmus induced by unilateral labyrinthectomy affected by sleep-wakefulness cycle. *Nature (Lond.)*, **1967,** *215*: 62–63.

BATINI, C., MORUZZI, G., PALESTINI, M., ROSSI, G. and ZANCHETTI, A. Effects of complete pontine transections on the sleep-wakefulness rhythm: the midpontine pretrigeminal preparation. *Arch. ital. Biol.*, **1959,** *97*: 1–12.

BERLUCCHI, G. Electroencephalographic studies in "split brain" cats. *Electroenceph. clin. Neurophysiol.*, **1966,** *20*: 348–356.

BRODAL, A. *The reticular formation of the brain-stem. Anatomical aspects and functional correlations.* Oliver and Boyd, Edinburgh, **1957,** 87 p.

BRODAL, A., TABER, E. and WALBERG, F. The raphe nuclei of the brain stem in the cat. II. Efferent connections. *J. comp. Neurol.*, **1960**a, *114*: 239–259.

BRODAL, A., WALBERG, F. and TABER, E. The raphe nuclei of the brain stem in the cat. III. Afferent connections. *J. comp. Neurol.*, **1960**b, *114*: 261–281.

CARLI, G. and ZANCHETTI, A. A study of pontine lesions suppressing deep sleep in the cat. *Arch. ital. Biol.*, **1965,** *103*: 751–788.

CORDEAU, J. P. and MANCIA, M. Evidence for the existence of an electroencephalographic synchronization mechanism originating in the lower brain stem. *Electroenceph. clin. Neurophysiol.*, **1959,** *11*: 551–564.

DAHLSTRÖM, A. and FUXE, K. Evidence for the existence of monoamine-containing neurons in the central nervous system. *Acta physiol. scand.*, **1964,** *Suppl. 62*: 1–55.

HORN, G. and HILL, R. M. Responsiveness to sensory stimulation of units in the superior colliculus and subjacent tectotegmental regions of the rabbit. *Exp. Neurol.*, **1966,** *14*: 199–223.

HUMPHREY, N. K. Responses to visual stimuli of units in the superior colliculus of rats and monkeys. *Exp. Neurol.*, **1968,** *20*: 312–340.

JOUVET, M. Recherches sur les structures nerveuses et les mécanismes responsables des différentes phases du sommeil physiologique. *Arch. ital. Biol.*, **1962,** *100*: 125–206.

JOUVET, M., BOBILLIER, P., PUJOL, J. F. et RENAULT, J. Suppression du sommeil et diminution de la sérotonine cérébrale par lésion du système du raphé chez le chat. *C. R. Acad. Sci. (Paris)*, **1967,** *264*: 360–362.

JOUVET, M. et RENAULT, J. Insomnie persistante après lésions des noyaux du raphé chez le chat. *C. R. Soc. Biol. (Paris)*, **1966,** *160*: 1461.

MAGOUN, H. W. and RHINES, R. An inhibitory mechanism in the bulbar reticular formation. *J. Neurophysiol.*, **1946,** *9*: 165–171.

MANCIA, M. Changes in sleep and wakefulness following split of the brain stem in cats. *Psychophysiology*, **1968a,** *5*: 199.

MANCIA, M. Changes in sleep and wakefulness induced by brain-stem split. *Proc. XXIV Int. Congr. Physiol. Sci., Washington, D.C.*, **1968**b, *7*: 280.

MANCIA, M., CHHINA, G. S. e DESIRAJU, T. La preparazione "split brain-stem" nella scimmia: effetti sul ciclo sonno-veglia. *Boll. Soc. ital. Biol. sper.*, **1967,** *43*: 1626–1628.

MANCIA, M., DESIRAJU, T. and CHHINA, G. S. The monkey split brain-stem: effects on the sleep-wakefulness cycle. *Electroenceph. clin. Neurophysiol.*, **1968,** *24*: 409–416.

MANCIA, M. e RUSTIONI, A. Modificazioni del ciclo sonno-veglia indotte da split del tronco dell'encefalo in gatti: correlazioni anatomo-funzionali. *Boll. Soc. ital. Biol. sper.*, **1968,** *44*: 1750–1753.

MARCHIAFAVA, P. L. and PEPEU, G. The responses of units in the superior colliculus of the cat to a moving visual stimulus. *Experientia (Basel)*, **1966,** *22*: 51–55.

MCILWAIN, J. T. and BUSER, P. Receptive fields of single cells in the cat's superior colliculus. *Exp. Brain Res.*, **1968,** *5*: 314–325.

MICHEL, F. and ROFFWARG, H. P. Chronic split brain stem preparation: effect on the sleep-waking cycle. *Experientia (Basel)*, **1967,** *23*: 126–128.

NAUTA, W. H. and KUYPERS, H. G. J. M. Some ascending pathways in the brain stem reticular formation. In H. H. JASPER *et al.* (Eds.), *Reticular formation of the brain.* Little, Brown, Boston, Mass., **1958:** 3–30.

RENAULT, J. *Monoamine et sommeils. III. Rôle du système du raphé et de la sérotonine cérébrale dans l'endormissement.* Tixier, Lyon, **1967,** 143 p.

ROSINA, A. and MANCIA, M. Electrophysiological and behavioural changes following selective and reversible inactivation of lower brain-stem structures in chronic cats. *Electroenceph. clin. Neurophysiol.*, **1966,** *21*: 157–167.

ROSSI, G. F. and BRODAL, A. Corticofugal fibers to the brain-stem reticular formation. An experimental study in the cat. *J. Anat. (Lond.)*, **1956,** *90*: 42–62.

ROSSI, G. F., MINOBE, K. and CANDIA, O. An experimental study of the hypnogenic mechanisms of the brain-stem. *Arch. ital. Biol.*, **1963,** *101*: 470–492.

ROSSI, G. F. and ZANCHETTI, A. The brain-stem reticular formation. Anatomy and physiology. *Arch. ital. Biol.*, **1957,** *95*: 199–435.

SCHEIBEL, M. E. and SCHEIBEL, A. B. Structural substrates for integrative patterns in the brain stem reticular core. In H. H. JASPER *et al.* (Eds.), *Reticular formation of the brain.* Little, Brown, Boston, Mass., **1958**: 31–35.

SPRAGUE, J. M. Interaction of cortex and superior colliculus in mediation of visually guided behavior in the cat. *Science*, **1966**a, *153*: 1544–1547.

SPRAGUE, J. M. Visual acoustic and somesthetic deficits in the cat after cortical and midbrain lesions. In D. P. PURPURA and M. D. YAHR (Eds.), *The thalamus.* Columbia Univ. Press, New York, **1966**b: 391–417.

SPRAGUE, J. M., MARCHIAFAVA, P. L. and RIZZOLATTI, G.

Unit responses to visual stimuli in the superior colliculus of the unanaesthetized, mid pontine cat. *Arch. ital. Biol.*, **1968,** *106*: 169–193.

SPRAGUE, J. M. and MEIKLE, T. H. The role of the superior colliculus in visually guided behavior. *Exp. Neurol.*, **1965,** *11*: 115–146.

STRASCHILL, M. und TAGWAVY, A. Neuronale Reaktionen im Tectum opticum der Katze auf bewegte und stationare Lichtreize. *Exp. Brain Res.*, **1967,** *3*: 353–367.

TABER, E. The cytoarchitectony of the brain stem of the cat. *J. comp. Neurol.*, **1961,** *116*: 27–69.

VONEIDA, T. J. Visual loss following midline section through the mesencephalic tegmentum in cats. *Anat. Rec.*, **1965,** *151*: 429.

WICKELGREN, B. and STERLING, P. Receptive fields in cat superior colliculus. *Physiologist*, **1967,** *10*: 344.

Reference: MANCIA, M. Electrophysiological and behavioural changes owing to splitting of the brain-stem in cats. *Electroenceph. clin. Neurophysiol.*, **1969,** *27*: 487–502.

Electroencephalography and Clinical Neurophysiology
Elsevier Publishing Company, Amsterdam – Printed in The Netherlands

DISCRIMINATION OF BEHAVIORAL STATE IN THE CAT UTILIZING LONG-TERM EEG FREQUENCY ANALYSIS[1]

M. D. FAIRCHILD, D. J. JENDEN AND M. R. MICKEY

Veterans Administration Hospital, Long Beach, Calif. 90801 and Department of Pharmacology and Health Sciences Computing Center, Center for the Health Sciences, University of California, Los Angeles, Calif. (U.S.A.)

(Accepted for publication: March 24, 1969)

Since the introduction of automatic frequency analysis by Grass and Gibbs (1938) a variety of techniques have been employed to evaluate quantitatively alterations in spontaneous brain electrical activity (EEG). However, as pointed out by Burch (1959), "The most difficult and frustrating practical problem in working with frequency spectra is in the treatment of the analyzed data". While a number of useful univariate statistical techniques have been described for the processing of such data (Glesser 1954; Johnson and Ulett 1959; Lettich and Margerison 1961; Matoušek 1967) and a multivariate approach has recently been reported (Walter *et al.* 1967), none of these would appear adequate to handle the vast amount of data which would be generated should the research objective be a continuous frequency analysis spanning hours of time.

This report is concerned with a system for frequency analysis, automatic data collection, and multi-variate statistical processing which we believe makes feasible long-term EEG analysis. The particular problem to which this investigation is addressed is the identification of orthogonal patterns of frequency change which quantitatively describe spontaneous variations occurring in the EEG during the sleep-waking cycle of the cat.

METHODS

Electrode implantation

Six adult, female cats weighing between 2.9 and 3.4 kg were anesthetized with pentobarbital sodium and prepared with electrodes chronically implanted in the prepyriform cortex, olfactory bulb, dorsal and ventral hippocampus, lateral geniculate nucleus, midbrain reticular formation, and bilaterally in parietal bone.

Electrodes implanted in subcortical structures consisted of two 40-gauge, insulated, stainless steel wires affixed to a length of 26-gauge hypodermic tubing with epoxylite electrode insulator. One wire was sectioned 3.5 mm and the other 5.0 mm below the end of the central shaft. Insulation was scraped to expose an additional 0.5 mm of wire above each tip.

Electrodes recording cortical activity were $0 \times \frac{1}{4}$ inch nickel plated wood screws inserted into but not through the parietal bone. A similar electrode used for grounding was placed in the anterior aspect of the nasal bone.

Single lengths of stainless steel wire, insulated except at their looped ends, were employed for recording both eye movement and neck muscle electrical activity. The wires were led subcutaneously and the looped ends were sutured either to the fascia just above the supraorbital crest or into the body of the rectus capitis muscle. Placements were bilateral.

All electrode leads were soldered to a 20-pin miniature Winchester plug which was subsequently affixed permanently to the skull with acrylic plastic.

Electrodes were positioned in subcortical structures either by usual stereotaxic procedures or by observing characteristics of potentials evoked in the target site through electrical stimulation of afferent pathways.

Olfactory bulb stimulation induced potentials in the ipsilateral prepyriform cortex which were utilized to place the electrode tips directly across the pyramidal cell dipole generator in that struc-

[1] This research was supported in part by NIH Grant FR-3.

ture. The electrode was fixed in position when the potentials recorded monopolarly from the dorsal and ventral tips were approximately mirror images of each other. This technique has been described in detail by Freeman (1959).

An attempt was made to employ analogous techniques in placing electrodes in the dorsal and ventral hippocampus. The fornix was stimulated in the region of its commissure and mirror-image evoked potentials were sought across hippocampal pyramidal cell layers. Boudreau (1966) has utilized similar procedures in positioning hippocampal electrodes. Although mirror-image evoked potentials were obtained in the prepyriform cortex of all six animals, this was generally not realized in the hippocampus. Clear reversals were obtained in but two of six dorsal hippocampal placements and in only one ventral hippocampal site. The majority of electrodes were fixed in position when evoked potentials obtained maximum amplitudes on both the dorsal and ventral tips.

Lateral geniculate electrodes were positioned by maximizing potentials resulting from stimulation of the optic tract in the region of the chiasm. Stereotaxic procedures alone were used in placing reticular formation electrodes, since the diffuse structure of this area did not readily lend itself to localization based on evoked potentials.

At the termination of the experiments the disposition of all electrode tracts was determined from serial sections stained with thionin.

Experimental procedures

Electrical activity recorded from the left prepyriform cortex, right ventral hippocampus, left lateral geniculate and right midbrain reticular formation was selected for frequency analysis. Three experiments were performed with each of the six cats at 1 month intervals. Individual test sessions were conducted as follows: upon completion of its morning meal, a cat was placed in a sound-attenuated and electrically shielded chamber and attached to the recording and analyzing equipment (see Frequency Analysis, below). Continual observation was maintained through a one-way mirror, and each 1 min segment of the experiment was classified with regard to the sleep-waking cycle. Commonly employed behavioral and electrical criteria were utilized in defining states of slow sleep (S) and fast sleep (F). In the former, antigravity muscles appeared relaxed, neck muscle activity was reduced, large amplitude slow waves dominated the EEG, and few eye movements occurred. In the latter, low amplitude fast activity was recorded from cerebral electrodes in conjunction with theta rhythms in the hippocampus and spike-like potentials in the lateral geniculate; neck muscle leads were silent and numerous eye movements were observed. A given minute was classified as alert behavior (A) only when the cat was observed actively attending to various auditory and visual stimuli provided by the experimenter. All minutes of the experiment which did not fulfill the behavioral and electrical criteria for classification as S, F or A were placed in the undetermined (U) group. The latter category included minutes during which behavior fitted what is often termed "drowsy", as well as those periods involving obvious transitions between the three well-defined states. A fifth classification, "reject" (R), was applied to those infrequent periods when gross motor activity caused major artifacts to appear in the EEG recordings. These minutes were not used in the statistical calculations.

The first experiment with each animal was continued for a period of time sufficient to obtain at least 30 min in each of the three states, S, F and A. The 30 min classified as A were obtained in three separate 10 min segments which, so far as was possible, followed spontaneous alertings at the termination of sleep cycles. The second and third experiments with each cat were conducted at 1 month intervals. They were of a constant 240 min in duration, with observations and minute-to-minute behavioral state classification beginning at the start of a sleep cycle.

Frequency analysis

Recording electrodes in the brain of the cat were connected through a Lehigh Valley Co. 20-pin brush-block assembly to the pre-amplifiers of a Grass Model IV A electroencephalograph. Spontaneous electrical activity from the prepyriform cortex, ventral hippocampus, lateral geniculate and midbrain reticular formation was taken from the Grass amplifiers through appropriate coupling networks to FM recording circuits of an Ampex Model CP-100 tape recorder. Tape recorder output from one of the four brain areas was then led to a frequency analyzer. This instrument has been previously described (Fairchild *et al.* 1967) and consists essentially of eight tuned amplifiers covering the frequency range from 2.5 to 40 c/sec in half-octave steps and connected through rectifying circuits to integrators with essentially infinite time constants. At 1 min intervals a synchronous motor driving a cam triggers a series of cascading relays which sequentially connect the integrator outputs to an Infotronics Model CRS-30E digitizer and then reset the integrators. This device converts the analog voltage signal of the integrators to three-digit numbers representing the mean amplitude of the frequency components within the range of each of the eight tuned amplifiers. The digitizer is interfaced with both an IBM electric typewriter and Model 026 printing card punch.

Following on-line frequency analysis of the first brain area, similar data were obtained for the remaining three by a playback of their recorded electrical activity through the frequency analyzer. Temporal synchronization of initial and playback records was assured by tone generating and sensing circuits within the analyzer. During the on-line analysis, a 3000 c/sec tone of 1 sec duration was recorded on a separate tape channel simultaneously with initiation of output relay cascade; upon playback, the recorded tone was utilized to initiate the same relay cascade sequence.

The punched cards produced for each of the four brain areas for each minute of the experiment were compatible with the input devices of the large, high speed, digital computers employed in the statistical analysis of the data. These cards required no further processing prior to computer input since, in addition to digital information concerning frequency channel output, they also contained coded data relating to experiment identification, temporal sequence and behavioral state.

Data analysis

A goal of the analysis was to classify for each minute of the experiment the behavioral state of the animal using objective, numerical criteria in such a way as to correspond to the observed state. The data upon which the classification was to be based were the averages for each minute of the 32 amplitudes in the eight frequency bands in each of the four brain areas. The formal problem of constructing such classifications has been studied by statisticians, starting with R.A. Fisher (1936), and the general problem has been labeled "discriminant analysis". In general, one supplies "examples" of data for each classification category to be considered, and the calculation is to indicate the category to which any given case (minutes, in our problem) is "most similar". The recognition of categories in addition to those indicated is not considered part of the discriminant problem. Resolutions of the problem differ according to how the term "most similar" is to be defined.

The most common form of solution is the construction of numerical indices, scores or weighted sums of the values (more precisely, linear combinations), in our case, of the 32 amplitudes at any given minute. A separate score (discriminant function) is constructed for each classification group and the classification of the state of the cat at any given minute is based on which score has the largest value for that minute. For example, for each minute a score is computed corresponding to the state "sleep", one corresponding to "fast sleep", and one corresponding to "alert". If the largest of the three scores is that corresponding to "sleep" then the cat is classified, numerically, as having been in the state "sleep" for that minute.

Calculations of the appropriate weighting coefficients and scores would be exceedingly tedious by hand or with the aid of a desk calculator. With the aid of a large digital computer, the calculations and data manipulation become quite feasible. The discriminant analysis calculations were carried out using the computer program BMD 07M (Dixon 1967). The computer output provides a classification of each minute as well as a specification of the weighting coefficients with which the scores are constructed. An evaluation of the relative contribution of each variable (brain area—frequency band amplitude) is provided in the form of analysis of variance and covariance statistics for differences among classification groups. The program is multivariate in that it takes due account of the correlations among the variables as well as the differences among group means.

An additional feature of the program BMD 07M is that it creates a set of so-called canonical variables that are equivalent to the original set. These, like the discriminant functions, are weighted sums of the original set of variables. The characteristics of these canonical variables are: (1) all of the variables are uncorrelated or orthogonal in the sense that the "within groups" sample standard deviation is equal to 1 and the sample correlations are all zero, and (2) the first few canonical variables (one less than the number of categories) contain "all the information" for discrimination among groups; the other canonical variables have zero means. We have made use of this feature in analyzing the characteristics of the data for minutes not behaviorally classified into one of the three main states (for example, a minute during which there was a transition between "alert" and "sleep", so that the minute could not be classified as entirely sleep or entirely alert).

As a matter of detail, in order to allow for the possibility of drift in gain, the data were normalized by computing the logarithms of the amplitudes and then subtracting from each such value the average of the logarithms for that minute for the corresponding brain area. This was equivalent to forming the geometric mean for each area for each minute, dividing amplitudes by the corresponding geometric mean, and finally computing the logarithm of the ratio. In this way, any gain drift would be compensated for.

In addition to the method of discriminant analysis, use was made of linear regression analysis. Computations were done with computer program BMD 02R (Dixon 1967).

RESULTS

1. *Electrode placement*

Examination of the sectioned brains revealed that in all six cats the leading and trailing electrode tips in the prepyriform cortex straddled the pyramidal cell layer. This result had been expected since "mirror-image" evoked potentials were recorded from these electrodes at the time of implant. Spontaneous electrical activity was consistent with that described by Freeman (1959), and in the alert animal consisted of bursts of fast sinusoidal activity riding on lower frequency components.

Ventral hippocampal placements were less uniform. In the one animal exhibiting a clear mirror-image evoked potential at implant, the electrode tips were found to straddle the pyramidal cell layer in area CA_3. Other placements, however, were generally deeper, with leading tips either in the vicinity of the dentate gyrus or approaching the dorsal surface of pyramidal cell layer in areas CA_1 to CA_2. Large amplitude theta activity was recorded from four electrodes found to be in close proximity to pyramidal cell layers; theta rhythms were less pronounced in two electrodes located nearer the dentate gyrus.

Attempts to locate electrodes accurately within the lateral geniculate nucleus by evoked potential methods were largely unsuccessful. In only two of six placements were both electrode tips imbedded in nuclear tissue; the other four were off target in a ventro-lateral direction with their lead tips in fibers of the optic tract. Spike discharges in the lateral geniculate during the F state, as first described by Mikiten *et al.* (1961), reflected electrode position. High amplitude spiking was observed in the two animals with correctly placed electrodes; these potentials were either reduced or absent in the more ventrolateral positions. In the latter location, distinct theta rhythms were recorded from the underlying ventral hippocampus, and this fact was probably responsible for the similar frequency distribution observed in the lateral geniculate and ventral hippocampal electrodes during the F state (see Fig. 2).

TABLE I

Behavioral *vs.* statistical classification (see Data Analysis) of 2,252 one-minute epochs into slow sleep (S), fast sleep (F) and alert (A) states derived from 32 variables in each of 18 individual experiments in six cats

Behavioral classification	Statistical classification		
	S	F	A
S	1075	4	0
F	3	624	0
A	2	0	544

2. Classification of S, F and A minutes

Each experiment was individually subjected to a stepwise discriminant analysis (BMD program 07M) based on those 1 min epochs which had been behaviorally classified as S, F or A. Table I summarizes the statistical classification as compared to the behavioral classification for all 18 experiments. The agreement is obviously excellent. Of a total of 2,252 min, an identical classification was reached in 2,243 (99.6%).

Output from the statistical program includes the coefficients and values for each case of two canonical variables representing differences between the S, F and A groups. The EEG pattern in any given minute may be represented as a point projected onto the plane defined by the two canonical variables. Fig. 1 shows the data from a representative experiment depicted in this way. Minutes behaviorally classified as S, F or A appear as tightly clustered points with large intervals between the groups; U minutes are also represented in this figure and will be considered further below.

The remarkable stability of the frequency patterns and discriminant functions between different experiments on the same cat and even between different cats is indicated by the fact that even when the results of all 18 experiments were pooled (Table II) the discriminant analysis agreed with the behavioral classification in 98.0% of cases.

Both of the above analyses are retrospective in the sense that discriminant functions were used to classify the same data from which they were calculated. The excellent agreement implies that the results were consistent but does not adequately evaluate the predictive value of the discriminant analysis as applied to this type of data. This was accomplished by using the pooled results of the first two experiments on each cat to calculate discriminant functions which were then used to classify the minutes of the third experiment, conducted 1 month later. This classification agreed

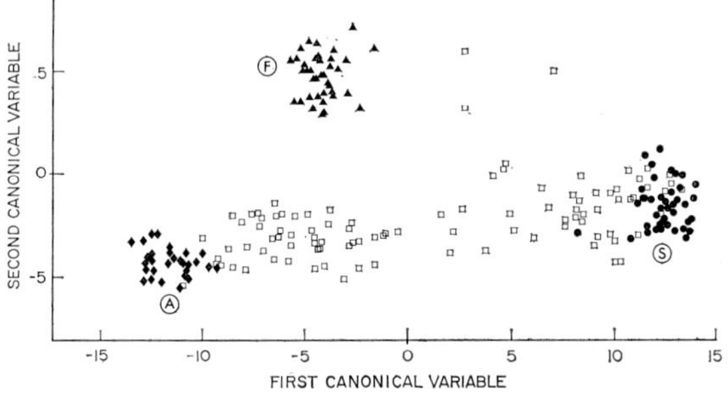

Fig. 1

Distribution of 1 min epochs from a representative experiment classified as either slow sleep (S, filled circles), fast sleep (F, filled triangles), alert (A, filled diamonds) or undetermined (open squares) behavior.

TABLE II

Behavioral *vs.* statistical classification (see Data Analysis) of 2,252 one-minute epochs derived from 32 variables in each of 18 experiments in six cats with the data pooled. Symbols are as in Table I

Behavioral classification	Statistical classification		
	S	F	A
S	1066	11	2
F	8	610	9
A	2	14	530

TABLE III

Behavioral *vs.* statistical classification (see Data Analysis) of 771 cases from six experiments on the basis of discriminant functions calculated from the pooled data of two prior experiments in each of the six cats. Symbols are as in Table I

Behavioral classification	Statistical classification		
	S	F	A
S	380	0	0
F	0	210	1
A	0	0	180

TABLE IV

Behavioral *vs.* statistical classification (see Data Analysis) of state utilizing discriminant functions derived from the data pooled in 15 experiments on five cats and applied to the data of three experiments on a sixth animal. The total of 2,252 cases represents the pooled results from all six analyses of this type. Symbols are as in Table I

Behavioral classification	Statistical classification		
	S	F	A
S	1052	16	11
F	12	553	62
A	3	20	523

with the entirely independent behavioral classification (Table III) in 770 of 771 cases (99.9%).

An even more severe test is to interpret the data from one animal using discriminant functions calculated from the pooled results of the other five cats. Agreement with the independent behavioral classification was obtained (Table IV) in 2128 of 2252 cases (94.5%). It may be concluded that the broad-band EEG frequency spectrum can be used to achieve an entirely objective classification of behavioral state which is stable over long periods of time (1–2 months) and is consistent from cat to cat.

3. *The individual S, F, A variables*

Fig. 2 represents the relative mean amplitude in each of eight frequency bands (see Table V) for S, F and A states in the four brain areas which were sampled. Calculations are from the pooled data of all 18 experiments comprising a total 2,252 one-min epochs. It can be seen from Fig. 2 that S patterns in the four brain areas were somewhat similar with lower frequencies having the greatest mean amplitude. Frequency distribution during F and A states had a number of common features within any given brain area, but tended to differ among the four sites tested. In the prepyriform cortex, higher frequencies were clearly predominant during both F and A, while in the ventral hippocampus and lateral geniculate, frequencies in the theta range were greater in amplitude (as discussed in 1. Electrode placement). The reticular formation, although exhibiting slightly more theta activity, had a relatively equal frequency distribution during those minutes classified as F or A.

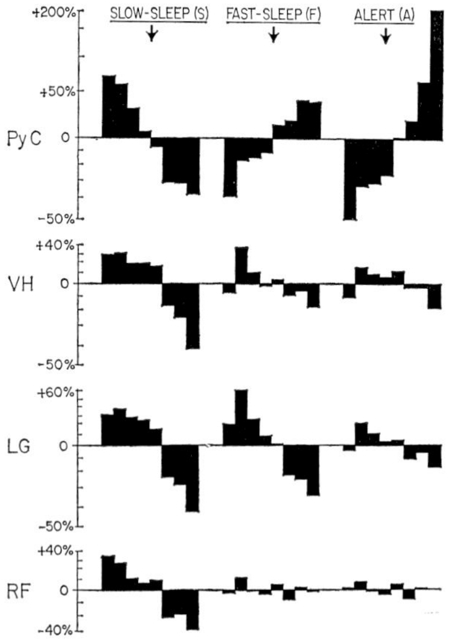

Fig. 2
Patterns representing the frequency distribution in the eight channels of the analyzer for the prepyriform cortex (PyC), ventral hippocampus (VH), lateral geniculate (LG) and midbrain reticular formation (RF) during S, F and A states. Low frequencies are to the left and high frequencies to the right (for band-passes see Table V). The ordinate represents the mean amplitude in each frequency band expressed as a percentage of the mean amplitude in all frequency bands in the corresponding brain area.

The first stage of the stepwise discriminant analysis provides variance ratios computed for each variable separately for between-state/within-state variation, and hence provides an assessment of the discriminative ability of each variable alone. Such variance ratios are presented in Table V for each of the eight frequency bands in the four brain areas. Although each of the variables considered independently provides highly significant variance ratios, it is evident that a clear hierarchy for discriminative ability exists, both among brain areas and among frequency bands within a given brain area. Thus the order prepyriform cortex > ventral hippocampus > lateral geniculate > reticular formation can readily be discerned from an inspection of Table V. In all four central structures frequencies at both the upper and lower ends of the spectrum yielded relatively high variance ratios in comparison to midrange frequencies. An exception was in the ventral hippocampus and lateral geniculate where 7–10 c/sec activity resulted in the highest values.

Linear combinations of 32 variables derived from the simultaneous measurement of frequency distribution in four brain areas have been employed in the multivariate statistical analysis. Although the automated system which has been developed makes the generation of this large data matrix comparatively simple and statistical processing is readily accomplished by high speed digital computers, the question arises as to whether fewer variables might suffice to provide comparable levels of discriminatory ability. While no systematic exploration of this question has yet been attempted, some preliminary calcu-

TABLE V

Between group/within group variance ratios (S, F and A states) calculated separately for each of the 32 variables used in the multivariate discriminant analysis

Channel number	Frequency (c/sec)	F ratio (D.F., 2-2249)			
		Prepyriform cortex	Ventral hippocampus	Lateral geniculate	Reticular formation
1.	2.5– 3.5	6581	729	264	489
2.	3.5– 5.0	5817	158	499	258
3.	5.0– 7.0	4729	175	314	268
4.	7.0–10.0	3449	1339	733	283
5.	10.0–14.1	1044	420	482	160
6.	14.1–20.0	5717	484	463	344
7.	20.0–28.3	6470	859	616	525
8.	28.3–40.0	5382	909	590	487

lations were made utilizing eight variables derived from the frequency distribution in each brain area separately. Results indicated that discriminatory ability of individual brain areas was high when data from a given animal were considered singly; values were found which ranged from 100% correct S, F, A classification for the prepyriform cortex to 96.7% for the reticular formation. When pooled data served as input, the level of discriminative ability was reduced; results from six cats pooled across the 18 experiments gave 95.8% correct classification for the prepyriform cortex, 79.9% for the ventral hippocampus, 78.9% for the lateral geniculate and 63.9% for the reticular formation. It is of interest to note that this order reflects the hierarchy of F ratios seen in Table V.

4. *Classification of the "undetermined" minutes*

The behavioral state in about half of the minutes in each experiment was classified as "U" or undetermined because no definitive assignment of behavioral state could be made or because this appeared to be transitional. This group undoubtedly includes minutes which should have been classified as S, F or A had it been possible to define the state observationally; it may also include minutes during which the animal was in a fourth discrete state for which insufficient criteria were available to specify it accurately. It is therefore of interest to determine whether the data provide evidence of a fourth discrete state or whether U minutes may be adequately represented on a continuum between S, F and A. The distribution of U minutes in Fig. 1 certainly suggests that most of these represent temporal or behavioral transitions between S and A, *i.e.*, different degrees of alertness.

To investigate this question, a second discriminant analysis was performed on each experiment between S, F and A minutes pooled as a single group, and U minutes, using as input residuals from the S-F-A discriminant analysis, *i.e.*, frequency patterns orthogonal to the plane defined by the first two canonical variables. In every experiment it was found that a highly significant discrimination could be made between S, F and A minutes and U minutes, suggesting that the latter in fact represented a discrete state definable in terms of a difference in the value of a third

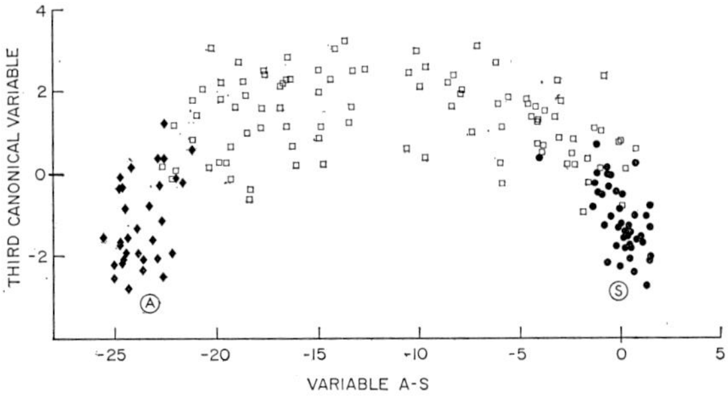

Fig. 3

Distribution of undetermined minutes (open squares) in the direction of canonical variable 3 between alert A and slow sleep S states. Variable A–S was obtained by an orthogonal rotation of canonical variables 1 and 2 in the direction defined by the group means for S and A.

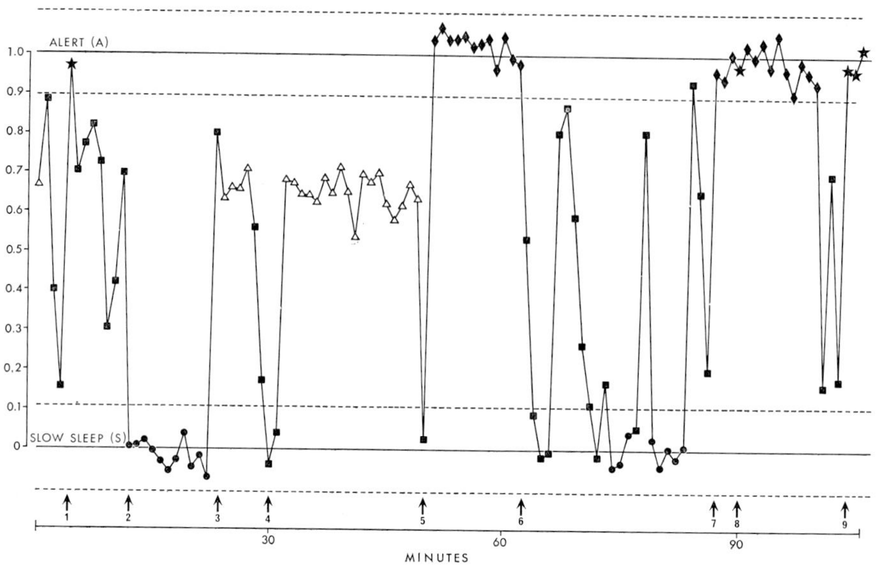

Fig. 4
Statistical estimates of alertness in a representative series of 1 min epochs plotted in temporal sequence. For details see text (Results, Section 5, The sleep-waking cycle).

canonical variable. Further analysis, however, showed this conclusion to be unjustified because a consistent and predictable relationship was found between the value of this third variable and the values of the first two. In every experiment this relationship could be expressed as a highly significant biquadratic regression. The meaning of this regression can perhaps best be understood by reference to Fig. 3, in which the value of the third canonical variable is plotted on the ordinate and the abscissa represents the projection of each point on to a line joining the S and A group means. Each point on Fig. 3 represents a minute of observation; the open squares were classified U, closed circles were S (right) and closed diamonds were A (left). It is apparent that all the points cluster about a smooth curve, which the regression analysis referred to above showed to be adequately represented as a parabola.

5. *The sleep-waking cycle*

The two-dimensional representation of behavioral state, Fig. 1, can be plotted so that one of the coordinate axes is related to alertness; the axis can be located and scaled so that the mean value of the coordinate is zero for the sleep state and unity for alert. A graphic representation of the sleep-waking cycle during an experiment (Fig. 4) can then be constructed by plotting the value of this variable against time and by indicating departure from the axis, in the direction of F in Fig. 1, by replacing solid by open symbols. The dotted lines on Fig. 4 represent 99% tolerance limits[1] for the S and A groups, and solid symbols within the bands indicate the statistically defined behavioral state. Points lying outside the bands plotted with solid symbols are interpreted as transitional states between S and A. All of the points in Fig. 4 plotted with open symbols correspond to states observationally classified as fast sleep (F). Of particular interest are the minutes for which the observer could not unequivocally assign either an S (circle), F (triangle) or A (diamond) designation on the basis of behavioral criteria; they are represented by the square

[1] A statistical tolerance interval is an interval that can be expected to contain the specified fraction of the population. The limits of Fig. 4 were calculated on the basis of the assumption that the canonical variables are normally distributed and independent with unit standard deviation and means equal to the means of the specified groups. On the scale of Fig. 1 the tolerance region considered for each group is a square oriented parallel to the line joining the S and A group means, centered at the group mean and of dimension $\pm$ z.0025 = $\pm$ 2.81. Since the distance between the S and A group means of Fig. 1 and 3 is 24.31, the limits for Fig. 4 are $\pm$ 2.81/24.31 = $\pm$ 0.115.

symbol and correspond to the "undetermined" or "U" classification. The "reject" category is depicted by star-shaped symbols and, as previously stated, designates minutes during which the animal was grooming or otherwise engaged in motor activity sufficient to cause gross artifacts to appear in the EEG recording.

The correspondence between the behavioral and statistical classification of minutes during the sleep-waking cycle can be visualized by reference to the sequentially numbered arrows appearing above the abscissa of Fig. 4. They can be interpreted as follows:

1. Following several minutes of U classification, the animal briefly groomed, causing major EEG record disruption. This minute was statistically classified with the A group.
2. The beginning of a 10 min period of S during which behavioral and statistical classifications were in agreement.
3. After 1 min of transition, S is replaced by F.
4. A 4 min interruption of F occurred with 2 min behaviorally classified as U falling within the confidence limits of the S group.
5. The F state was replaced during a 1 min period behaviorally classified as U but falling statistically within the S group. The animal was then alerted and maintained in the A state for a 12 min period.
6. The start of a 24 min period during 6 min behaviorally classified as U were statistically within the S or A group (5 in S and 1 in A).
7. The cat was again aroused and maintained in the A state for 14 min.
8. Motor activity produced gross EEG artifact resulting in a behavioral classification of R. The minute was within the confidence limits of the A group.
9. The beginning of grooming activity resulting in R behavioral classification which fell statistically within the A group (as in 1 and 8 above).

DISCUSSION

Frequency analysis of the EEG has been employed extensively in the last 30 years, and represents only one of many ways in which complex wave forms have been analyzed (Burch 1959; Dern and Walsh 1963; Matoušek 1967).

Most analogue methods of frequency analysis have employed narrow pass filters, and the Walter Analyzer (Walter 1943), as modified by Baldock (Baldock and Walter 1946) and subsequently by Ulett (Ulett and Loeffel 1953) has enjoyed wide popularity. Its disadvantages are the large amount of output because of the numerous filters which must be employed to cover the relevant frequency range, the inertia of the narrow pass filters, and persistent technical problems arising from instability of the filter circuits. Broad-band frequency analysis has recently received considerable attention (Kaiser *et al.* 1964; Selldén 1965; Matoušek *et al.* 1967; Volavka *et al.* 1967) and effectively divides the signal into components containing discrete frequencies. Similar results have been obtained by pooling data from narrow pass filters into groups (Glesser 1954; Fink 1961; Heusler *et al.* 1965; Itil 1965). While these systems lose some ability to detect small shifts in dominant frequency, the lower inertia of the broad-band filter and fewer variables for subsequent statistical treatment offer distinct advantages.

A great many studies employing EEG frequency analysis are subject to the criticism leveled by Knott (1953), "...an instrument designed to complement *visual* analysis should not lead just to further visual analysis". Additional treatment of the output is required in order to abstract from the data information relevant to the problem being studied in the form of a few specific parameters from which definitive statistical conclusions can be drawn. The methods which have been used are for the most part empirical (Glesser 1954; Kaiser *et al.* 1964; Selldén 1965) and there has been no widespread recognition of the essentially multivariate nature of the problem, despite the existence of powerful statistical techniques specifically developed to deal with such data. One promising study along these lines has recently been published (Walter *et al.* 1967) in which discriminant analysis was applied to EEG data which had first been subjected to spectral analysis by digital techniques. Digital techniques of spectral analysis are very powerful and make it possible to investigate phase relationships and coherence between signals from different brain areas (Walter 1963), but analogue to digital conversion of the raw EEG and subsequent spectral analysis are not feasible over long periods of observation with present equipment because of the immense amount of data involved.

The techniques described in this report represent a hybrid system designed for long-term analysis of the EEG. The initial broad-band frequency analysis is carried out by an analogue device, and subsequent interpretation employs a large computer to extract relevant information by multivariate statistical analysis. A digital voltmeter coupled to an IBM card punch machine provides the interface between the analogue and digital stages.

The work presently described represents the first stage of a project which has for its ultimate objective the quantitative analysis of drug effects on the EEG. Since most drugs have a time course of action of the order of hours or longer, this objective requires a system capable of prolonged and continuous analysis. Conversely, the intensity of drug effects is unlikely to show rapid alterations in time because plasma and tissue levels in general change slowly. Therefore little information is likely to be lost by averaging the frequency spectrum over sampling periods of 1 min.

The data presented show that this system is capable of reducing the observed EEG changes during spontaneous behavior to two relevant variables. The analysis and the results it yields are remarkably stable over long periods of time and from cat to cat. It therefore provides a satisfactory description of normal changes of EEG frequency distribution, so that drug effects may be quantitatively assessed, either as restrictions or extensions of the two-dimensional surface on which spontaneous changes may be represented or as time-dependent deviations from this surface in directions characteristic of each drug or group of drugs. Preliminary investigations of barbiturates and amphetamines have provided encouraging results along these lines.

SUMMARY

A hybrid system is described which makes feasible a continuous, long-term analysis of the EEG. A broad-band frequency analyzer is interfaced with a digital voltmeter which in turn drives a typewriter and card-punch machine. Data are thus generated in a form directly compatible with the input devices of a large, electronic computer used to extract relevant information by multivariate statistical analysis.

Spontaneous variations in the frequency spectrum of the EEG, as the result of changes in behavioral state, may be adequately represented as points on a two-dimensional surface. The location of a point corresponding to the spectrum during a given 1 min epoch allows an objective discrimination to be made between the states of slow sleep, fast sleep and alert. Minutes which are transitional between these three well-defined states can also be represented. This classification is in excellent agreement with independent behavioral assessment, is stable over long periods of time (1–2 months) and is consistent from cat to cat.

The reliability and stability of this technique should provide a means of quantitative assessment of drug effects on the EEG over long periods of time.

RÉSUMÉ

DISCRIMINATION DE L'ÉTAT COMPORTEMENTAL CHEZ LE CHAT À L'AIDE DE L'ANALYSE DE FRÉQUENCE EEG À LONG TERME

Les auteurs décrivent un système hybride qui rend possible une analyse continue, à long terme, de l'EEG. Un analyseur de fréquence à large bande est connecté avec un voltmètre digital qui, à son tour entraîne une machine à écrire et une machine à perforer des cartes. Les données sont ainsi produites sous une forme directement compatible avec le système d'entrée d'un grand calculateur électronique utilisé pour extraire les informations appropriées par analyse statistique de multivariables.

Les variations spontanées du spectre de fréquence de l'EEG, liées à des modifications de l'état comportemental peuvent être représentées de façon adéquate sous forme de points sur une surface à deux dimensions. La localisation d'un point correspondant au spectre pendant une époque donnée d'une minute, permet une discrimination objective entre les états de sommeil lent, de sommeil rapide et d'alerte. Les époques de transition entre ces trois états bien définis peuvent également être représentées. Cette classification est en accord complet avec l'appréciation indépendante du comportement; elle est stable sur de longues périodes de temps (1–2 mois) et est valable d'un chat à l'autre.

La validité et la stabilité de cette technique devrait fournir un moyen d'appréciation quantitative des effets des drogues sur l'EEG sur de longues périodes de temps.

The authors are indebted to Miss Cora Lee Yale for her significant contribution in conducting the calculations using the programs and equipment of the U.C.L.A. Health Sciences Computing Facility.

REFERENCES

BALDOCK, G. and WALTER, W. G. A new electronic analyzer. *Electron. Engin.*, **1946,** *18*: 339–344.

BOUDREAU, J. C. Computer measurements of hippocampal fast activity in cats with chronically implanted electrodes. *Electroenceph. clin. Neurophysiol.*, **1966,** *20*: 165–174.

BURCH, N. R. Automatic analysis of the electroencephalogram. A review and classification of systems. *Electroenceph. clin. Neurophysiol.*, **1959,** *11*: 827–834.

DERN, H. and WALSH, J. B. Analysis of complex waveforms. In W. L. NASTUK (Ed.), *Physical Techniques in biological research.* Academic Press, New York, **1963**: 99–216.

DIXON, W. J. (Ed.). *BMD biomedical computer programs.* University of California Press, Los Angeles, **1967.**

FAIRCHILD, M. D., ALLES, G. A., JENDEN, D. J. and MICKEY, M. R. The effects of mescaline, amphetamine and four ring-substituted amphetamine derivatives on spontaneous brain electrical activity in the cat. *Int. J. Neurophysiol.*, **1967,** *6*: 151–167.

FINK, M. Quantitative electroencephalography and human pharmacology. *Med. exp. (Basel)*, **1961,** *5*: 364–369.

FISHER, R. A. The use of multiple measurements in taxonomic problems. *Ann. Eugen. (Lond.)*, **1936,** *7*: 179–188.

FREEMAN, W. J. Distribution in time and space of prepyriform electrical activity. *J. Neurophysiol.*, **1959,** *22*: 644–665.

GLESSER, G. C. A method of statistical treatment for electronically analysed EEG data. *Electroenceph. clin. Neurophysiol.*, **1954,** *6*: 329–333.

GRASS, A. M. and GIBBS, F. A. A Fourier transform of the electroencephalogram. *J. Neurophysiol.*, **1938,** *1*: 521–526.

HEUSLER, A. F., WORD, T. J., ULETT, G. A. and BOWERS, C. A. Electronic analysis of drug induced EEG changes. *Int. J. Neuropsychiat.*, **1965,** *1*: 131–138.

ITIL, E. M. Quantitative EEG changes induced by anticholinergic drugs and their behavioral correlates in man. *Rec. Adv. Biol. Psychiat.*, **1965,** *8*: 151–174.

JOHNSON, L. C. and ULETT, G. A. Quantitative study of pattern and stability of resting electroencephalographic activity in a young adult group. *Electroenceph. clin. Neurophysiol.*, **1959,** *11*: 233–249.

KAISER, E., PETERSÉN, I., SELLDÉN, U. and KAGAWA, N. EEG data representation in broad-band frequency analysis. *Electroenceph. clin. Neurophysiol.*, **1964,** *17*: 76–80.

KNOTT, J. R. Automatic frequency analysis. *Electroenceph. clin. Neurophysiol.*, **1953,** *Suppl. 4*: 17–25.

LETTICH, E. and MARGERISON, J. H. Presentation of data from low frequency analysis to illustrate serial changes in the electroencephalogram. *Electroenceph. clin. Neurophysiol.*, **1961,** *13*: 606–611.

MATOUŠEK, M. *Automatic analysis in clinical electroencephalography.* Psychiat. Res. Inst., Research Reports, Rept. No. 9, Prague, **1967,** 240 p.

MATOUŠEK, M., VOLAVKA, J., ROUBIČEK, J. and ROTH, Z. EEG frequency analysis related to age in normal adults. *Electroenceph. clin. Neurophysiol.*, **1967,** *23*: 162–167.

MIKITEN, T. H., NIEBYL, P. H. and HENDLEY, C. D. EEG desynchronization during behavioral sleep associated with spike discharges from the thalamus of the cat. *Fed. Proc.*, **1961,** *20*: 327.

SELLDÉN, U. Electroencephalographic response to megimide as evaluated by routine EEG interpretation and by broad-band frequency analysis. *Acta neurol. scand.*, **1965,** *13*: 193–210.

ULETT, G. A. and LOEFFEL, R. G. A new resonator-integrator unit for the automatic brain wave analyser. *Electroenceph. clin. Neurophysiol.*, **1953,** *5*: 113–115.

VOLAVKA, J., GROF, P. and MRKLAS, L. EEG frequency analysis in periodic endogenous depressions. *Psychiat. Neurol. (Basel)*, **1967,** *153*: 384–390.

WALTER, D. O. Spectral analysis of electroencephalograms: Mathematical determination of neurophysiological relationships from records of limited duration. *Exp. Neurol.*, **1963,** *8*: 155–181.

WALTER, D. O., RHODES, J. M. and ADEY, W. R. Discriminating among states of consciousness by EEG measurements. A study of four subjects. *Electroenceph. clin. Neurophysiol.*, **1967,** *22*: 22–29.

WALTER, G. An automatic low frequency analyzer. *Electron. Engin.*, **1943,** *16*: 8–13.

Reference: FAIRCHILD, M. D., JENDEN, D. J. and MICKEY, M. R. Discrimination of behavioral state in the cat utilizing long-term EEG frequency analysis. *Electroenceph. clin. Neurophysiol.*, **1969,** *27*: 503–513.

Elsevier Publishing Company, Amsterdam – Printed in The Netherlands

RETICULAR MULTIPLE UNIT ACTIVITY DURING A PROGRESSION OF STATES INDUCED BY CNS EXCITANTS. III[1]

WALLACE D. WINTERS, KENJIRO MORI[2], MARSHALL B. WALLACH[3], ROBERT J. MARCUS AND CHARLES E. SPOONER[4]

Brain Research Institute and Department of Pharmacology, U.C.L.A. School of Medicine, Los Angeles, Calif. 90024 (U.S.A.)

(Accepted for publication: March 26, 1969)

Prior studies utilizing EEG, gross behavior and auditory evoked response techniques have demonstrated that some agents although reported to be "anesthetics" should be, in fact, classified as "epileptogenics" (Winters and Spooner 1965a, b; Winters *et al.* 1967a). In order to assess more critically the neuronal state induced by these agents, *e.g.*, phencyclidine and gamma-hydroxybutyrate, it is necessary to utilize methods which are more sensitive to changes in neuronal activity than those afforded by techniques such as the gross EEG and behavioral responsiveness (Winters and Spooner 1965a, b; Winters *et al.* 1967a), loss of the righting reflex (Marcus *et al.* 1967), and the size of the evoked response (Mori *et al.* 1968). Continuous monitoring of the activity of neuronal elements in the midbrain reticular formation which is very sensitive to changes in behavioral states (Moruzzi and Magoun 1949; French *et al.* 1953) has been useful in examining neuronal changes during wakefulness and sleep (Winters *et al.* 1967b) and during the various stages of anesthesia (Mori *et al.* 1968). The technique of monitoring the unit activity of a large population of neuronal elements described previously (Arduini and Pinneo 1962; Schlag and Balvin 1963; Buchwald *et al.* 1965; Winters *et al.* 1967b) seems particularly useful for the present study since drug-induced epileptoid states are phenomena which probably arise from changes in neuronal aggregates.

In the present study we will attempt to compare the action of six compounds which induce varying degrees of CNS excitation: amphetamine, lysergic acid diethylamide, mescaline, phencyclidine, pentylenetetrazol and gamma-hydroxybutyrate. The changes in reticular multiple unit activity (RUA) will be compared with the changes in gross behavior and EEG in an attempt to clarify some of the underlying processes involved in these induced states, and a continuum of excitatory states and two types of generalized seizures will be discussed.

METHODS

A total of 70 experiments was performed on ten adult cats of both sexes with chronically implanted cortical and subcortical electrodes. Prior studies described in detail the techniques utilized in the acquisition of the EEG, gross behavior (Winters 1964), and multiple unit activity (Winters *et al.* 1967b).

The behavioral criteria for each level of excitability were based on the assessment of the general activity, posture, and responsiveness of the animal to auditory or tactile stimulation. Salivation, defecation, pupil size, inappropriate behavior, abnormal posture, myoclonic jerking, and generalized clonic and/or tonic seizure ac-

[1] Supported in part by grants 5 TI-MH-6415, 1 RO1-MH-12121, 5 RO1 MH-10836 (U.S.P.H.S.), and NsG 237-62 (N.A.S.A.). Bibliographic assistance was received from the U.C.L.A. Brain Information Service which is part of the Neurological Information Network of N.I.N.D.B. and is supported under contract DHEW PH-43-66-59.

[2] Present address: Department of Anesthesiology, Tokyo Women's Medical College, Shinjuku, Tokyo, Japan.

[3] Present address: Department of Psychiatry, New York University Medical Center, 560 First Avenue, New York, N.Y. 10016.

[4] Present address: Department of Neurosciences, School of Medicine, University of California at San Diego, La Jolla, Calif. 92037.

tivity were noted. Inappropriate behavior was characterized by the animal moving its head as if visually tracking in space objects which were not visible to the observer.

EEG patterns induced by the drugs in the present study have been reported previously: *d*-amphetamine 2–8 mg/kg or methamphetamine 2 mg/kg (Bradley and Elkes 1957); lysergic acid diethylamide (LSD-25) 50–100 μg/kg (Heath and Mickle 1960; Adey *et al.* 1962); mescaline 20–30 mg/kg (Bradley and Elkes 1957); phencyclidine 2–8 mg/kg (Winters *et al.* 1967a); gamma-hydroxybutyrate 200–800 mg/kg (Winters and Spooner 1965a,b, 1966); and pentylenetetrazol 20–25 mg/kg (Ajmone Marsan and Ralston 1957; Okuma 1960).

Each agent induced similar results in a minimum of four different cats before a characteristic pattern of events was accepted; while each cat did not receive all of the drugs studied, all cats received gamma-hydroxybutyrate for comparison. No animal received drug more often than once every 10 days. Each agent was administered intraperitoneally in sufficient dosage to obtain the desired action rather than in pre-set doses. It was not the intent in this study to evaluate the potency or rate of action of each agent, but rather to examine the progression of induced states.

Saline, drug carrier, or ineffective doses of each drug were administered for control observation, and the slight activation of the EEG, RUA and behavior due to handling of the animal and/or peritoneal irritation disappeared within 5 min in all experiments. When the initial excitation exceeded 10 min, it was assumed that the excitation resulted from central activation rather than peritoneal irritation, since similar activation of the EEG accompanied by elevation of RUA was demonstrated in ten gallamine triethiodide (Flaxedil®) immobilized cats following either gamma-hydroxybutyrate (5 experiments) or pentylenetetrazol (5 experiments) given intravenously (unpublished). An animal with a jugular vein implant inserted chronically likewise demonstrated an initial period of excitation after gamma-hydroxybutyrate administration. In the acute studies (unpublished), the blood pressure rose minimally prior to the onset of generalized seizures; thus the initial excitation does not appear to be related to pressure changes.

Recordings of the multiple unit activities were obtained from the same gross electrode which was simultaneously recording the EEG in the midbrain reticular formation. The stereotaxic placement of the electrodes was either at A 3, L 3, H −1 or A 4, L 2, H −1 (Jasper and Ajmone Marsan 1953) and was verified histologically in six cats. The electrical activity obtained from each bipolar electrode (diameter 160 μ) was AC coupled into the first stage of the EEG machine (Grass Model 6). The high frequency components of the electrical signals were tapped off at the second amplifier stage (terminals J-3 and J-4) through a 100 pF capacitor; thus electrical activity above 500 c/sec was shunted through the capacitor. The electrical activity below 500 c/sec continued from the 1st stage amplifier to the final EEG amplifier stage with suitable filtering and amplification, and this standard EEG signal was expressed on the paper write-out of the EEG machine. Meanwhile the high frequency component, after passing through the 100 pF capacitor, was amplified and the component above 2500 c/sec shunted to ground by passing the signal through a Tektronix 122 preamplifier (set at 1 kc), resulting in a bandpass system centered at 1000 c/sec with −3 dB points at 500 c/sec and 2500 c/sec. This activity representing multiple unit activity was displayed on a Tektronix 502 oscilloscope. To obtain a continuous recording of the change in unit activity before and after drug administration, the filtered signals were passed through the cathode follower output of the oscilloscope, rectified, smoothed, and recorded continuously on a slow-moving strip chart recorder (Brush 280). Thus, the data were obtained as both a large population of raw units observed on the oscilloscope and the amplitude demodulated signal recorded on the strip chart recorder (Winters *et al.* 1967b). At the completion of each experiment the system noise was tested utilizing a dummy plug containing a 10 kΩ resistor across the input in place of the animal (see Winters *et al.* 1967b for a discussion of relationship of this signal to unit activity). The change in both the basal level of unit activity and the fluctuation of activity from this basal level was examined, since the basal level of the unit activity is directly related to the width of the envelope of raw units; when the envelope is wider the DC value of the basal level is higher and, conversely, when the envelope is smaller the basal level falls to a level closer to DC 0. As discussed previously (Winters *et al.* 1967b), the change in the envelope width suggests that the appearance of larger spikes indicates that a larger number of units are firing simultaneously, and the greater the number and frequency of units firing the greater the chance of summation of units due to coincident unit firing. The fluctuation in unit activity indicates that the firing pattern of the population of units alternates above the basal rate, and the height of these bursts of unit activity is a reflection of this pattern expressed as the fluctuation of unit activity.

Each experiment was preceded by control examination of the animal during rhombencephalic (paradoxical) sleep, wakefulness, and slow wave sleep. Following the establishment of control levels for these three states (Winters *et al.* 1967b), the drug was administered and the changes in the basal level and fluctuation of multiple unit activity were observed.

RESULTS

All of the agents studied induce a similar general pattern of EEG and behavioral change and differ mainly in the degree of progression (Fig. 1). The changes in the basal level and fluctuation of unit activity induced by each agent correlate with the changes in gross behavior and EEG. The progression of changes induced by each drug can be delineated according to the EEG patterns as follows.

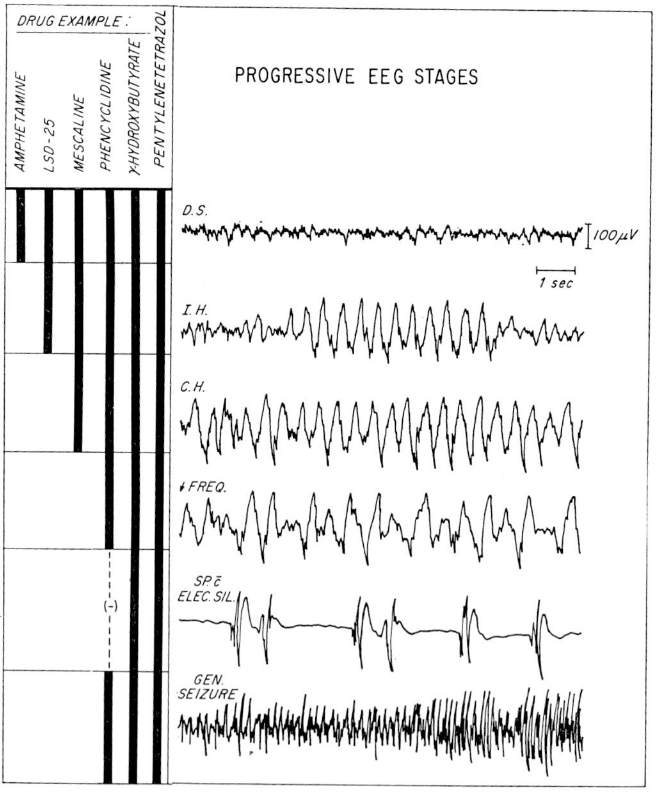

Fig. 1

A representation of the states and EEG stages induced by various drugs, as follows: desynchronization (D.S.); intermittent 2.5–3 c/sec hypersynchrony (I.H.); continuous 2.5–3 c/sec hypersynchrony (C.H.); reduced frequency (1.5 c/sec) hypersynchrony (↓ Freq.); spikes with electrical silence (Sp. c̄ Elec. Sil.); and generalized seizure (Gen. Seizure). The vertical bar under each drug represents the progressive state(s) which were induced by each agent in the present study. Spikes with electrical silence were rarely noted following phencyclidine. In general, the EEG patterns were similar and each agent differed mainly in the rate of progression and the total progression induced.

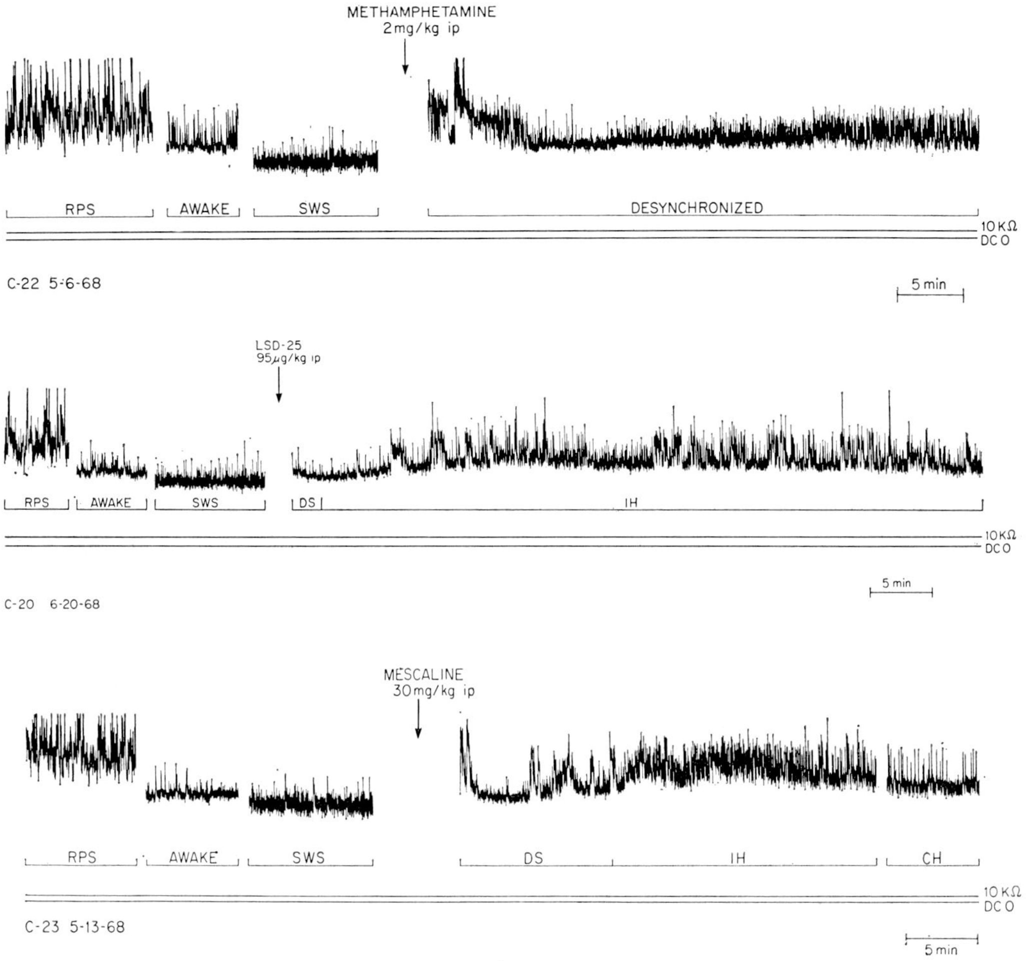

Fig. 2

Comparison of the amplitude demodulated signals of the midbrain reticular formation unit activity during the control states of RPS (rhombencephalic phase of sleep), Awake, and SWS (slow wave sleep) and following administration of methamphetamine, LSD-25 and mescaline. The lowest line (DC 0) represents the system balanced to zero; the 10 kΩ line represents the system noise level with a 10 kΩ resistor across the input. Changes in basal unit activity are measured as the distance from the base of the unit activity tracing to the 10 kΩ line. The fluctuation is the width of the excursion from the basal reticular unit activity level to the peaks. See legend to Fig. 1.

A. *Desynchronized*

Amphetamine, LSD-25, mescaline, phencyclidine, gamma-hydroxybutyrate, and pentylenetetrazol all induced EEG desynchronization, behavioral hyperactivity plus a slightly increased basal level of RUA above awake control levels and no significant change in fluctuation (Fig. 2 and 3).

B. *Intermittent hypersynchrony*

All of the agents examined except amphetamine induced EEG patterns of intermittent 2.5–3.5 c/sec hypersynchrony, inappropriate behavior, hyperactivity, pupillary dilation, salivation, occasional defecation and a slight increase in the level of RUA above the desynchronized state (Fig. 2 and 3). Pentylenetetrazol traverses this phase so rapidly that this phase is often not seen.

C. *Continuous hypersynchrony*

LSD-25 effects did not progress to this state.

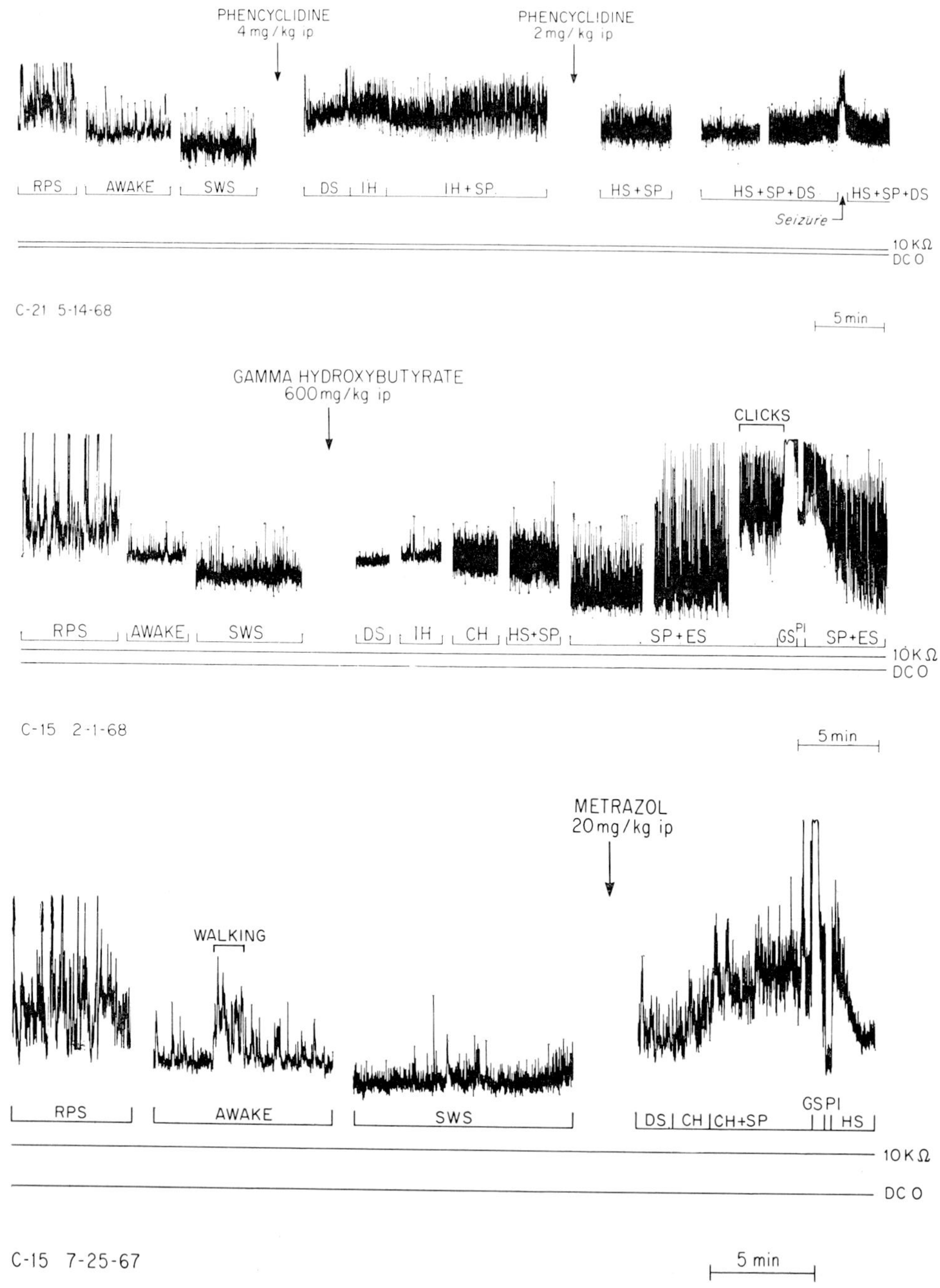

Fig. 3

Comparison of the amplitude demodulated signals of the midbrain reticular formation unit activity during control states and following phencyclidine, gamma-hydroxybutyrate and pentylenetetrazol (Metrazol). Intermittent hypersynchrony and spiking (IH + SP); hypersynchrony and spiking (HS + SP); hypersynchrony, spiking and desynchrony (HS + SP + DS); spiking and electrical silence (SP + ES); generalized seizure (GS); post-ictal depression (PI). See legends to Fig. 1 and 2.

Mescaline, phencyclidine, gamma-hydroxybutyrate and pentylenetetrazol all induced rigid postures with fixed gaze, pupillary dilation, reduced responsiveness to stimuli, inappropriate behavior and continuous 2.5–3 c/sec hypersynchronous EEG waves.

There were two types of RUA during this phase. Mescaline and pentylenetetrazol induced no change, or a slight elevation in basal unit level and no changes in the fluctuation compared to intermittent hypersynchrony; phencyclidine induced the same level as or slightly lower than intermittent hypersynchrony and reduced fluctuation, whereas gamma-hydroxybutyrate induced a decrease of the basal RUA level below the awake control level with an increased fluctuation (Fig. 2 and 3).

D. *Reduced frequency hypersynchrony with spikes*

This state was not achieved with mescaline. Gamma-hydroxybutyrate induced a state wherein the animal lay on its side with the head and limbs in abnormal positions and exhibited a fixed gaze, pupillary dilation, and unresponsiveness to stimuli; the EEG pattern was characterized by 1.5 c/sec slow waves and spikes and there was a

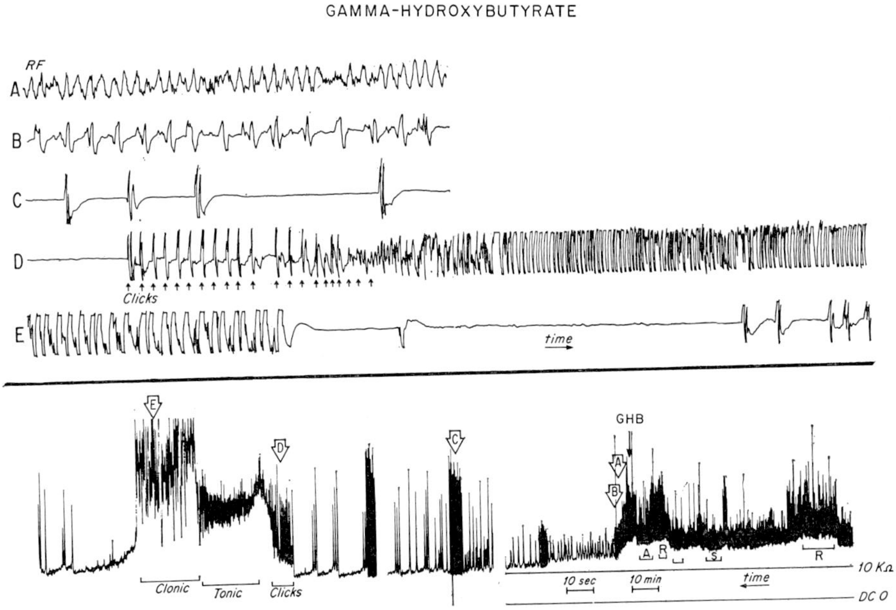

Fig. 4

Comparison of various stages (*A–E*) of gamma-hydroxybutyrate (GHB) induced EEG changes with the corresponding amplitude demodulated multiple unit activity recording (*A–E* in arrows) from the same electrode implanted in the midbrain reticular formation.

EEG (*upper portion*): 2.5 c/sec hypersynchrony (*A*), 1.5 c/sec hypersynchrony (*B*), spontaneous spikes bursts with varying periods of electrical silence (*C*), induction of generalized seizure bursts by presentation of clicks during *C* (*D*), termination of generalized seizure from *D* followed by post-ictal depression and a return to pattern noted in *C* (*E*).

Multiple unit activity (*lower portion*): Control unit activity during rhombencephalic sleep (R), slow wave sleep (S), and wakefulness (A) and following 800 mg/kg GHB. Arrows with letter inserts denote corresponding EEG patterns. Time runs from right to left. From start to *B* chart ran at slow speed: 7 mm = 10 min; then the chart speed was periodically increased to 7 mm = 10 sec to demonstrate the intermittent unit bursts. The 2 burst episodes prior to the onset of clicks and the entire seizure progression *D* and *E* were run at the faster chart speed. Note the large amplitude of summated spikes intermittently occurring on a markedly reduced basal firing level starting at *B* and most pronounced between *C* and *D*. The signal to noise ratio (computed by measuring the basal height above DC 0 *vs.* the height above DC 0 of a 10 kΩ dummy load at the input) in this animal was not as good as those noted in the cats shown in Fig. 2 and 3; however, the findings are representative.

fall in the basal RUA level below control slow wave sleep with an increased fluctuation (Fig. 3). Phencyclidine induced 1.5 c/sec slow waves with spiking and periods of desynchronization between slow wave bursts; the animal was rigid and immobile with a fixed gaze and abnormal postures; there was no change in the basal unit level and a reduction in the fluctuation (Fig. 3). Pentylenetetrazol induced behavioral immobility with fixed gaze and rigid abnormal posture, the EEG waves were 1.5 c/sec slow waves with spiking, and the basal RUA level increased above control rhombencephalic sleep level (Fig. 3).

E. *Spikes with electrical silence*

Gamma-hydroxybutyrate induced a period of polyphasic spike bursts separated by increasing intervals of electrical silence lasting up to 1–3 sec, associated with myoclonic jerks, fixed gaze, rigid abnormal posture and a marked fall in the basal RUA level with bursts of markedly increased fluctuations which occurred simultaneously with the appearance of EEG spike bursts (Fig. 3 and 4). Phencyclidine induced an increase in spiking and a slight increase in fluctuation but no change in basal level (Fig. 3). Pentylenetetrazol induced increased spiking, increased rigidity and a rise in the level of unit activity and fluctuation (Fig. 3).

F. *Generalized seizures*

Gamma-hydroxybutyrate, phencyclidine and pentylenetetrazol induced tonic-clonic generalized seizures with a high frequency, high amplitude EEG pattern. The seizure following either phencyclidine or pentylenetetrazol occurred without external stimulation. Following gamma-hydroxybutyrate, the seizure was induced by repetitive auditory, visual or tactile stimulation. The basal level of reticular unit activity was at or above the control rhombencephalic phase of sleep level following phencyclidine, gamma-hydroxybutyrate and pentylenetetrazol, and the fluctuation increased above the level noted during rhombencephalic sleep (Fig. 3 and 4).

G. *Post-ictal depression*

A brief post-ictal depression was noted with gamma-hydroxybutyrate or pentylenetetrazol, followed by a return to the activity noted just before the generalized seizure. During the post-ictal depression the basal level dropped markedly from the level noted during the seizure but did not fall below control levels (Fig. 3 and 4). The phencyclidine-induced seizure was not followed by a post-ictal period, but the pattern noted prior to the seizure reappeared (Fig. 3).

DISCUSSION

The progression of events induced by the agents in the present study implies that three basic states are induced; *i.e.*, an initial excitation, followed by a state characterized by abnormal posture and behavior, and finally, generalized seizures (Fig. 5). During the initial excitation the reticular unit activity changes in a manner similar to the initial excitatory stages (I and II) induced by general anesthetics (see Fig. 5 and Winters *et al.* 1967b; Mori *et al.* 1968).

While the initial state induced in the present study is clearly a behavioral and electrical excitatory state, the second induced state is less clearly understood. This state is characterized by inappropriate behavior coupled with abnormal postures indicative of "hallucinatory" behavior. Obviously one cannot be certain that this induced state in cats is the same hallucinatory phenome-

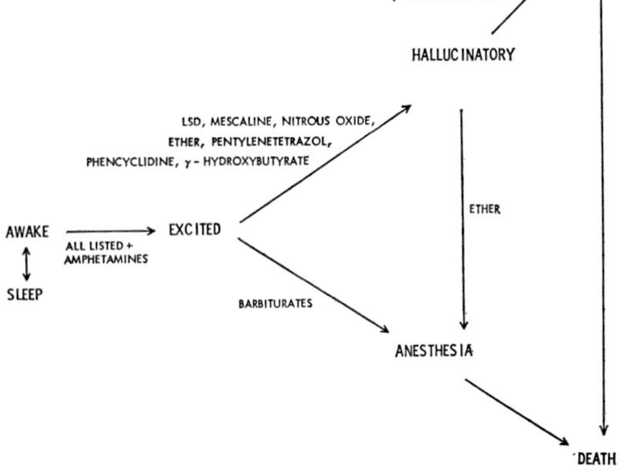

Fig. 5

A proposed schema of states induced by some CNS excitant and depressant agents. The data are compiled from data in the present study and a previous study (Mori *et al.* 1968). See discussion for details.

non that occurs in man; however, this behavior is pronounced in the cat following agents such as LSD-25, mescaline and psilocybin which induce profound hallucinatory actions in man. In addition to the induction of hallucinatory behavior in man, these agents induce 2.5–3 c/sec hypersynchronous EEG wave patterns during the hallucinatory state which appear to be similar to the hypersynchronous activity noted in cats with these agents (Heath and Mickle 1960). Further, Adey *et al.* (1962) demonstrated that LSD-25 induced an apparent intermittent loss of contact with the environment at the same time that the hypersynchronous 3 c/sec EEG waves appear in the EEG of the cats performing in a T maze. Thus there is strong presumptive evidence that the induced state of intermittent hypersynchrony, inappropriate behavior, and inappropriate postures are, in fact, evidence of a hallucinatory state. The hallucinoid activity preceding the generalized seizure activity induced by these convulsant agents may represent the aura noted clinically prior to a grand mal seizure.

With phencyclidine and pentylenetetrazol, the pre-seizure phase of CNS excitation is associated with a progressive rise in the level of reticular unit activity indicating a progressive rise in the frequency of reticular formation unit firing. However, during the pre-convulsant state induced by gamma-hydroxybutyrate, the basal level of reticular unit activity progressively falls while the intermittent fluctuation of unit activity is markedly increased; thus the units fire less frequently, but when they do fire, they do so synchronously both spontaneously and in response to stimuli (Fig. 4). In contrast, during Stage III anesthesia, the basal level of unit activity is likewise low but the fluctuation is markedly reduced, the units do not fire in bursts and are relatively unresponsive to stimuli (Mori *et al.* 1968). It appears that gamma-hydroxybutyrate induces episodes of refractoriness followed by periods of synchronous responsiveness to stimuli, whereas during general anesthesia the reticular units are continuously unresponsive, presumably due to a profound inhibition.

The amazing similarity of actions induced by the structurally different groups of agents listed in Fig. 5 may indicate that the system affected by these agents involved interference at one of a number of different levels of energy transfer. (See Marcus *et al.* 1967 for a discussion.)

As can be noted from the present and previous studies (Winters *et al.* 1967b; Mori *et al.* 1968) a combination of gross behavior, ongoing EEG, averaged evoked responses and multiple unit activity form a useful group of neuropharmacological techniques for the analysis of drug-induced states in cats with chronic brain electrode implants.

SUMMARY

The EEG, gross behavior and multiple unit activity were recorded during the continuous progression of states induced by amphetamine (*d*-, and meth-), lysergic acid diethylamide (LSD-25), mescaline, gamma-hydroxybutyrate, pentylenetetrazol or phencyclidine. The drugs appear to fall within a pattern of progressively increasing excitatory states. The least active agents induce only the initial phase, *i.e.*, excited: amphetamine; then hallucinoid: LSD-25 and mescaline. The more potent agents transcend these initial phases and induce generalized seizures: gamma-hydroxybutyrate, phencyclidine and pentylenetetrazol. The reticular multiple unit activity increased slightly during the initial two phases; then following gamma-hydroxybutyrate the basal level fell progressively while the fluctuation rose markedly, whereas following pentylenetetrazol the multiple unit activity progressively increased. During the generalized seizures the unit activity was markedly elevated in both of these groups; then the unit activity fell during the brief period of post-ictal depression followed by a return of each drug group to the unit activity levels noted during the pre-seizure state.

RÉSUMÉ

ACTIVITÉ UNITAIRE MULTIPLE DE LA FORMATION RÉTICULAIRE AU COURS D'UNE PROGRESSION D'ÉTATS INDUITS PAR DES EXCITANTS DU SYSTÈME NERVEUX CENTRAL

L'EEG, le comportement global et l'activité unitaire multiple ont été enregistrés pendant la progression continue d'états induits par: les amphétamines (*d* et meth), l'acide diéthylamide lysergique (LSD-25), la mescaline, le gamma-hydroxybutyrate, le pentylènetétrazol ou phencyclidine. Ces drogues provoquent des états d'excitation progressivement croissants. Les agents les moins actifs induisent seulement la phase initiale, c'est-à-dire l'excitation (amphétamines) puis des hallucinations (LSD-25 et mescaline). Les agents les plus puissants dépassent ces phases initiales et induisent des crises généralisées (gamma-hydroxybutyrate, phencyclidine et pentylènetétrazol). L'activité unitaire multiple réticulaire augmente légèrement pendant les deux phases initiales; puis, après gamma-hydroxybutyrate, le niveau de base tombe progressivement tandis que la fluctuation augmente de façon marquée; après pentylènetétrazol l'activité unitaire multiple augmente progressivement. Pendant les crises généralisées, l'activité unitaire s'élève de façon importante dans ces deux groupes, puis elle diminue pendant la brève période de dépression post-ictale, qui est suivie par un retour, pour chaque groupe de drogues, aux niveaux d'activité unitaire notés pendant l'état pré-critique.

The authors wish to thank Mrs. Susan Miller and Mrs. Merrilyn Kvam for their valuable technical assistance.

REFERENCES

ADEY, W. R., BELL, F. R. and DENNIS, B. J. Effects of LSD-25, psilocybin, and psilocin on temporal lobe EEG patterns and learned behavior in the cat. *Neurology (Minneap.)*, **1962,** *12*: 591–602.

AJMONE MARSAN, C. and RALSTON, B. L. *The epileptic seizure, its functional morphology and diagnostic significance; a clinical electrographic analysis of metrazol-induced attacks.* Thomas, Springfield, Ill., **1957,** 251 p.

ARDUINI, A. and PINNEO, L. R. A method for the quantification of tonic activity in the nervous system. *Arch. ital. Biol.*, **1962,** *100*: 415–424.

BRADLEY, P. B. and ELKES, J. The effects of some drugs on the electrical activity of the brain. *Brain*, **1957,** *80*: 77–177.

BUCHWALD, J. S., HALAS, E. S. and SCHRAMM, S. Comparison of multiple unit and electroencephalogram activity recorded from the same brain sites during behavioral conditioning. *Nature (Lond.)*, **1965,** *205*: 1012–1014.

FRENCH, J. D., VERZEANO, M. and MAGOUN, H. W. A neural basis of the anesthetic state. *Arch. Neurol. Psychiat. (Chic.)*, **1953,** *69*: 519–529.

HEATH, R. G. and MICKLE, A. W. Evaluation of seven years' experience with depth electrode studies in human patients. In E. R. RAMEY and D. S. O'DOHERTY (Eds.), *Electrical studies on the unanesthetized brain.* Hoeber, New York, N.Y., **1960**: 215–247.

JASPER, H. H. and AJMONE MARSAN, C. *A stereotaxic atlas of the diencephalon of the cat.* Nat. Res. Council of Canada, Toronto, **1953.**

MARCUS, R. J., WINTERS, W. D., MORI, K. and SPOONER, C. E. A comparison of gamma-hydroxybutyrate, gamma-butyrolactone and short chain fatty acids on the EEG and behavior of the rat. *Int. J. Neuropharmacol.*, **1967,** *6*: 175–185.

MORI, K., WINTERS, W. D. and SPOONER, C. E. Comparison of reticular and cochlear multiple unit activity with auditory evoked responses during various stages induced by anesthetic agents. II. *Electroenceph. clin. Neurophysiol.*, **1968,** *24*: 242–248.

MORUZZI, G. and MAGOUN, H. W. Brain stem reticular formation and activation of the EEG. *Electroenceph. clin. Neurophysiol.*, **1949,** *1*: 455–473.

OKUMA, T. Effect of metrazol on cortical and subcortical evoked potentials. *Electroenceph. clin. Neurophysiol.*, **1960,** *12*: 685–694.

SCHLAG, J. and BALVIN, R. Background activity in the cerebral cortex and reticular formation in relation with the electroencephalogram. *Exp. Neurol.*, **1963,** *8*: 203–219.

WINTERS, W. D. Comparison of the average cortical and subcortical evoked response to clicks during various stages of wakefulness, slow wave sleep and rhombencephalic sleep. *Electroenceph. clin. Neurophysiol.*, **1964,** *17*: 234–245.

WINTERS, W. D., MORI, K., SPOONER, C. E. and BAUER, R. O. The neurophysiology of anesthesia. *Anesthesiology*, **1967**a, *28*: 65–80.

WINTERS, W. D., MORI, K., SPOONER, C. E. and KADO, R. T. Correlation of reticular and cochlear multiple unit activity with evoked responses during wakefulness and sleep. I. *Electroenceph. clin. Neurophysiol.*, **1967**b, *23*: 539–545.

WINTERS, W. D. and SPOONER, C. E. A neurophysiological comparison of gamma-hydroxybutyrate with pentobarbital in cats. *Electroenceph. clin. Neurophysiol.*, **1965**a, *18*: 287–296.

WINTERS, W. D. and SPOONER, C. E. Various seizure activities following gamma-hydroxybutyrate. *Int. J. Neuropharmacol.*, **1965**b, *4*: 197–200.

WINTERS, W. D. and SPOONER, C. E. A neurophysiological comparison of alpha-chloralose with gamma-hydroxybutyrate in cats. *Electroenceph. clin. Neurophysiol.*, **1966,** *20*: 83–90.

Reference: WINTERS, W. D., MORI, K., WALLACH, M. B., MARCUS, R. J. and SPOONER, C. E. Reticular multiple unit activity during a progression of states induced by CNS excitants. III. *Electroenceph. clin. Neurophysiol.*, **1969,** *27*: 514–522.

EEG CHANGES IN WILSON'S DISEASE

P. HANSOTIA, RUTH HARRIS[1] AND JEAN KENNEDY

The National Hospital, Queen Square, London, W.C.1, and The Royal Free Hospital, Grays Inn Road, London, W.C.1 (Great Britain)

(Accepted for publication: March 29, 1969)

Recent advances in the knowledge of normal and abnormal copper metabolism (Osborn and Walshe 1964, 1965; Neumann and Silverberg 1966; Walshe 1967) and of the morbid anatomy and pathophysiology of hepatolenticular degeneration (Wilson's disease) (Bearn *et al.* 1957; Osborn and Walshe 1968; Shikata 1968; Shiraki 1968) reflect the considerable interest in this condition. This inborn error of metabolism is notable for insidious onset of hepatic, neural and renal involvement which may follow a fluctuating course in severity. The purpose of this study is to examine the relevance of the EEG in this illness.

There are few studies on the EEG in Wilson's disease, and these consist mainly in descriptive case reports in which the EEG findings are included. Heller and Kooi (1962) reviewed eighty case reports of Wilson's disease from the world literature, in addition to seven of patients of their own, in which the EEG interpretations were available. No specific EEG abnormality was associated with the disease and, in general, the degree of abnormality paralleled the severity of clinical involvement. EEG improvement with treatment was uncertain.

METHOD AND MATERIAL

Twenty-three patients and five asymptomatic siblings, all of whom showed the characteristic abnormalities of copper metabolism (Bearn 1960), were studied. The patients, fourteen male and nine female, ranged in age from 8 to 35 years. The average age of the group was 20 years. The asymptomatic siblings, one male and four female, ranged in age from 7 to 27 years and their average age was 15 years. Five families contributed seventeen cases; there was no family history in the remaining eleven. In thirteen patients the clinical features were mainly neurological and consisted of dysarthria, tremor, involuntary movements, ataxia and mental impairment. One patient had myoclonus and generalized convulsions in addition to other neurological abnormalities. Hepatic signs and symptoms, including haematemesis, melaena, hepato-splenomegaly and jaundice, were predominant in seven patients, in whom neurological disturbances were almost absent. Three patients showed both hepatic and neural clinical features. Kayser-Fleischer rings were present in all patients and absent from the asymptomatic siblings. The duration of the illness at the time of the first EEG studies varied from 2 months to 25 years.

Sixty-six EEG records were taken from these patients and examined for excess of slow activity (with regard for the patient's age) and focal or paroxysmal features. The clinical and biochemical states were noted at the time of these recordings in every patient. Serial EEGs, therefore, were accompanied by a corresponding follow-up of the patient's clinical and biochemical conditions.

The 10–20 system of electrode placement was used, with some modifications in a few cases. The usual gain was 10 μV/mm pen deflection; time constant 0.3 sec. The records were made on either an Elema Schonander 16-channel or an Offner type T 8-channel machine.

RESULTS

Ten patients had normal EEGs. Of the remaining thirteen patients with abnormal EEGs, eleven showed mild or moderate excess of bilat-

[1] Present address: Maudsley Hospital, Denmark Hill, London, S.E.5.

TABLE I

EEG results

	First EEG		Repeat EEGs (not obtained in all patients)			
				No change		
	Normal	Abnormal	Improved	Previously normal	Previously abnormal	Variable
Patients with hepatic symptoms	3	4	2	2		2
Patients with neurological disorders	7	6	1			
Patients with both neurological and hepatic symptoms	—	3			2	
Asymptomatic siblings	3	2	2			

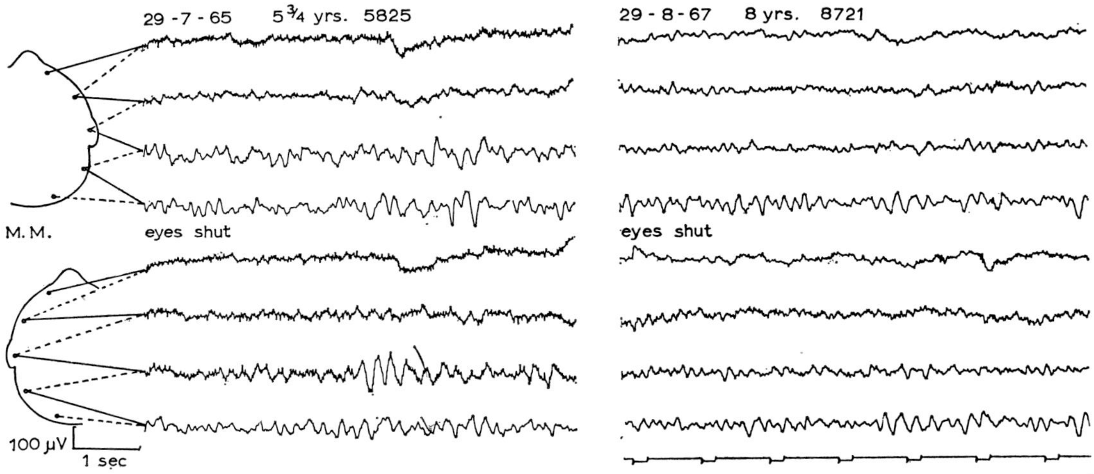

Fig. 1
M.M. Records from an asymptomatic sibling. *29.7.65*: An abnormal record. No definite alpha rhythm is recognizable and there is an excess of slow wave activity over the temporo-occipital regions. *29.8.67*: Two years later there is some evidence of maturation with an increase in the frequency of the rhythms over the posterior part of the head. Although there is a decrease in slow activity, the alpha rhythm is still poorly formed for a child of this age.

eral theta activity without any clear localizing or paroxysmal features (Table I). In this group some of the patients who had serial records showed improvement in the EEGs, with corresponding improvement in their clinical state, whereas the remainder showed little or no EEG change. Severe EEG abnormalities were found in cases with severe liver dysfunction and these recovered with improvement in liver function (Case report I, J.P.).

Seven patients with prominent neurological disturbances had normal EEGs. The remainder showed moderate EEG abnormalities, with the exception of one patient who had myoclonic and major motor seizures, a rare occurrence in this disease (Case report II, M.M.N.).

Two of the asymptomatic siblings had abnormal EEGs while the three others had normal records. Moderate or mild EEG abnormalities appeared to be shown more prominently by members of some families than by others. In one family with three siblings, only one of whom was clinically affected, the EEG abnormalities were similar in all the children. Over an interval of 2 years, during which they were treated with appropriate doses of penicillamine, the EEGs showed improvement in all three and this improvement has been maintained (Fig. 1).

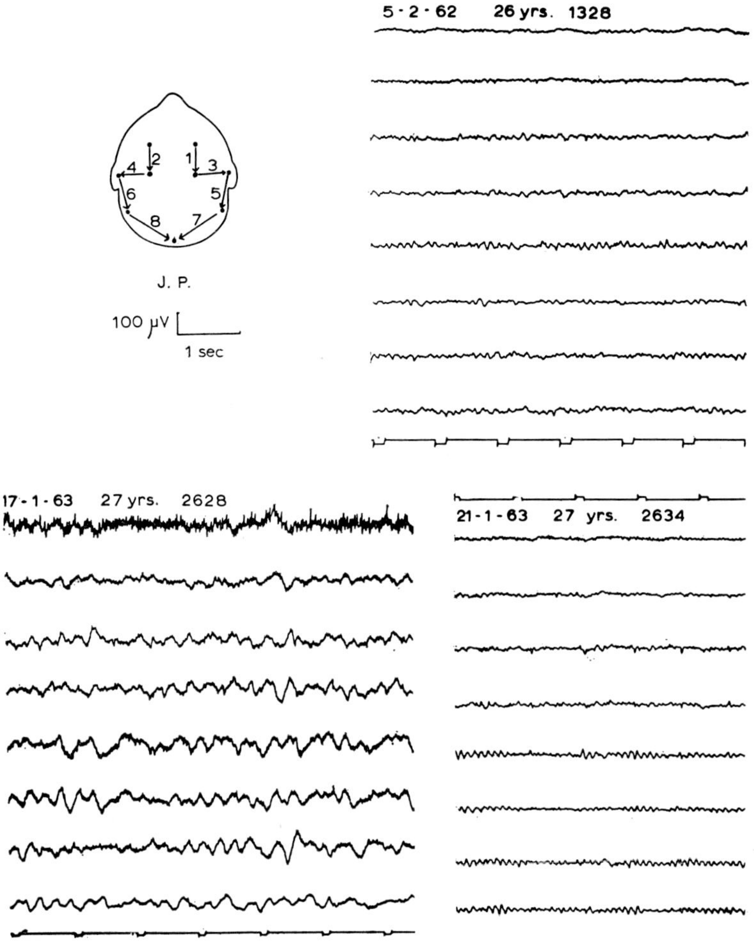

Fig. 2

J.P. Case No. 25. *5.2.62*: The record shows no special features. *17.1.63*: EEG during hepatic coma shows diffuse, high voltage slow activity. *21.1.63*: The record taken after recovery from coma shows striking improvement.

Case reports

Case No. I (J.P.). This man, 26 years of age, was seen at the Royal Free Hospital with melaena, jaundice, hepato-splenomegaly and Kayser-Fleischer rings, in October 1961. Investigations confirmed the diagnosis of Wilson's disease. His personality was said to be odd but he had no significant neurological abnormalities. Three months later, in January 1962, he was readmitted after a haematemesis. An EEG at the time showed no special features. About a year later he developed rapidly progressive hepatic insufficiency and became comatose. The EEG showed changes characteristic of hepatic coma. The patient recovered rapidly with the usual treatment for hepatic coma (Sherlock 1963). Within a few days he was conscious, alert and responsive. The EEG showed striking improvement (Fig. 2).

Case No. II (M.M.N.). This patient was 22 years old at the time of the EEG studies. There was a family history of the illness and he had had the clinical features of Wilson's disease from the age of 9. Generalized convulsions were first noted when the patient was 17, following a course of treatment with dimercaprol (BAL). His condition remained relatively stable until October 1967, when he was 21 years old. Thereafter he deteriorated progressively. He was admitted to the National Hospital in April 1968.

He was a mildly obese young adult, with a

vacant dull expression that broke into fatuous smiles on the slightest provocation. Mental impairment was marked. His speech had a scanning and slurred quality but there was no dysphasia. Broad grey-green Kayser-Fleischer rings were easily visible. Jerky dystonic movements were marked on the right but present on both sides. Myoclonic jerks of the trunk and limbs occurred very frequently and were more marked on the right than left side. All movement disturbances, including the myoclonus, were absent during sleep. The rest of the neurological examination was within normal limits.

There was marked gynaecomastia, with a normal distribution of hair, normal testicles and no evidence of hepato-splenomegaly or ascites. The rest of the general examination was normal.

Laboratory investigations showed: serum Cu=25 μg/100 ml (normal 90–120 μg/100 ml); caeruloplasmin=3.5 mg/100 ml (normal 20–40 mg/100 ml, Cummings 1968); urinary Cu and amino acid excretion patterns were also typical for Wilson's disease; liver function tests were within normal limits.

The patient was treated with 900 mg penicillamine daily for 2 weeks with little improvement. Two 5 day courses of BAL, 200 mg daily, were then given in conjunction with potassium sulphide 20 mg t.d.s. by mouth. No specific anticonvulsants were administered at any time.

After this course of treatment there was marked improvement in the patient's mental state and physical condition. His gait was steadier and he was able to perform activities, such as dressing himself, which had been difficult previously. The involuntary movements were considerably reduced and the myoclonic jerks were almost absent.

Serial EEGs were taken before and during this last course of treatment (Fig. 3). Initially the EEG showed a severe generalized abnormality with an excess of slow activity and frequent generalized and multi-focal spikes, usually related to the myoclonic jerks. The alpha rhythm was not recognizable. During treatment there was a progressive improvement, with a decrease in slow activity and disappearance of spike discharges, but the final EEG was still diffusely abnormal.

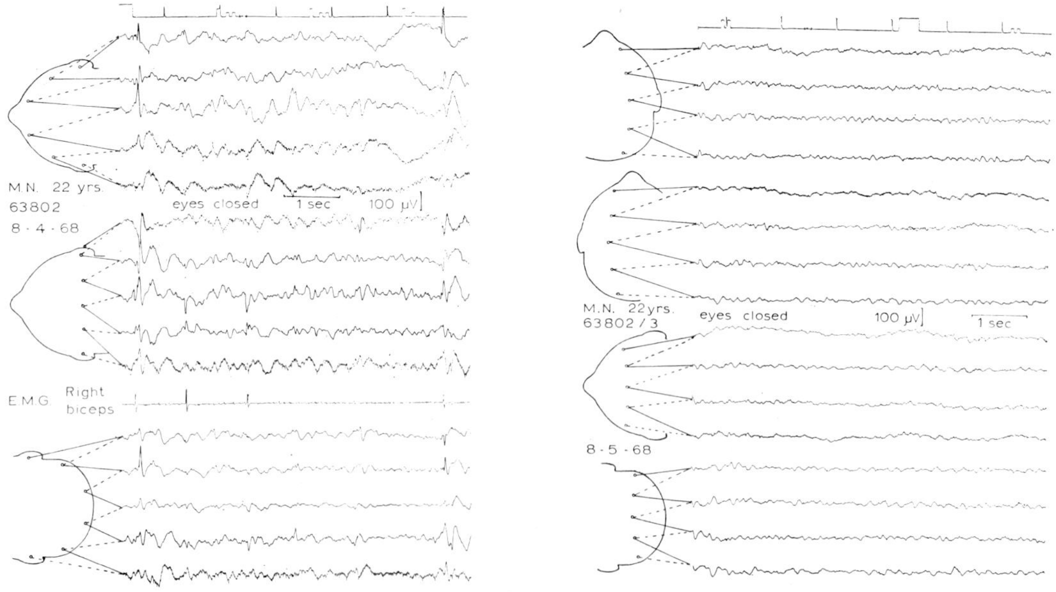

Fig. 3

M.M.N. *8.4.68*: The patient was alert but suffering from frequent myoclonic jerks. A surface EMG recorded over the right biceps muscle shows frequent large muscle action potentials occurring at the same time as the cerebral spike activity. Diffuse slow activity is present. *8.5.68*: The patient was much better, with virtually no myoclonus. No spike activity is seen and there is a marked reduction in slow wave activity.

DISCUSSION

The results of our study show that generalized non-specific EEG abnormalities may be seen in uncomplicated Wilson's disease. These abnormalities were seen in patients who had movement disorders or Kayser-Fleischer rings, with or without hepato-splenomegaly, in addition to the characteristic abnormality of copper metabolism. These patients did not have significant mental deterioration or seizures, or jaundice or other evidence of severe hepatic insufficiency. The EEG abnormalities did not appear to be related to a specific clinical state or to particular signs or symptoms; patients with predominantly hepatic or neural involvement showed identical EEG changes.

The two patients reported with complications of Wilson's disease (neural or hepatic) had associated severe abnormalities in the EEG which were appropriate for the complication. Both seizures and EEG spike discharges appear to be very rare in this disease. In our patient and in other cases reported (Streifler and Feldman 1953), in which the clinical seizure disorder and the EEG spike activity were associated with Wilson's disease, the clinical and EEG abnormalities responded to treatment of the disease rather than to specific anti-convulsant therapy. The EEG abnormalities associated with complications of the disease in the cases presented bear a close relationship with the clinical state and correspond with improvement in the clinical condition.

In our small number of asymptomatic siblings the EEGs appeared to follow a familial pattern. The asymptomatic siblings of patients with abnormal EEGs showed similar EEG disturbances, while siblings of patients with normal EEGs also had normal EEGs. Genetic studies have repeatedly shown similarity in the form of disease in the propositi and in their affected siblings (Arima and Sano 1968). In our experience this feature appears to hold true for the EEG as well.

The controversy over the prophylactic treatment of asymptomatic patients of Wilson's disease is well summarized in an editorial of the *Lancet* (1968)[1]. The author concludes: "All siblings of a proven case, all children who have a sibling with cirrhosis, and all young people with chronic liver disease should be screened. When evidence of a homozygous state is found, prophylactic treatment with Penicillamine should be instituted". All asymptomatic patients reported in the literature who have been on treatment, up to 6 years or more, remain symptom-free (Arima and Sano 1968; Sternlieb and Scheinberg 1968). The levels of copper in serum and in hepatic and renal tissues seem to fall with treatment of the disease (Walshe 1967). At present these biochemical studies remain as the only objective means of measuring change with treatment, particularly of the asymptomatic patients, of this disease. The EEG may offer another, albeit less exact, method for the same purpose. Of our asymptomatic siblings, all of whom were on prophylactic treatment with penicillamine, two had abnormal EEGs. The propositi showed improvement in their clinical states along with a reduction in serum Cu levels and improvement of the EEGs. The asymptomatic siblings showed a corresponding improvement in the EEG and Cu studies during the same period of time. This observation appears to strengthen the argument for the prophylactic treatment of asymptomatic cases of Wilson's disease.

SUMMARY

The EEGs of twenty-three patients and five asymptomatic siblings with Wilson's disease were correlated with their clinical states and biochemical studies related to liver function and copper metabolism. In uncomplicated cases of the disease the EEG may be normal or abnormal. When the EEG is abnormal there does not appear to be a clear correlation with a clinical or biochemical state.

Severely abnormal EEGs are seen with severe complications of the disease and are appropriate to the complication. These EEGs show improvement parallel with clinical improvement. Asymptomatic siblings with the characteristic biochemical defect of copper metabolism may also show normal or abnormal EEGs, a feature which seems to have a familial tendency. The abnormal EEGs of asymptomatic siblings show improvement with treatment, supporting the argument for prophylaxis in such cases.

[1] Effect of Penicillamine on failure of renal acidification in Wilson's disease. *Lancet*, 1968, *1*: 775.

RÉSUMÉ

MODIFICATIONS EEG DANS LA MALADIE DE WILSON

Les EEG de vingt-trois patients atteints de maladie de Wilson, et de cinq collatéraux asymptomatiques on été mis en relation avec les données cliniques et biochimiques relatives à la fonction hépatique et au métabolisme du cuivre. Dans les cas non compliqués de l'affection, l'EEG peut être normal ou anormal. Lorsque l'EEG est anormal, il n'apparaît pas de corrélation évidente avec un état clinique ou biochimique particulier.

Les EEG très anormaux sont rencontrés lors des complications graves de la maladie et correspondent à cette complication. Ces EEG montrent une amélioration parallèle à l'amélioration clinique. Les collatéraux asymptomatiques avec déficit biochimique caractéristique du métabolisme du cuivre peuvent également montrer des EEG normaux ou anormaux, donnée qui semble présenter une tendance familiale. Les EEG anormaux des malades asymptomatiques s'améliorent avec le traitement, ce qui constitue un argument en faveur d'une action prophylactique dans de tels cas.

We are most grateful to Professor Sheila Sherlock of the Royal Free Hospital, Dr. P. C. Gautier-Smith and other physicians of the National Hospitals for Nervous Diseases, for allowing us to study the patients under their care. We have had invaluable help from Dr. W. A. Cobb during the course of this study.

REFERENCES

ARIMA, M. and SANO, I. Genetic studies of Wilson's disease in Japan. *Birth Defects: original article series*, **1968**, *4*, *No. 2:* 54–59.

BEARN, A. G. Wilson's disease. In J. B. STANBURY *et al.* (Eds.), *The metabolic basis of inherited disease*. McGraw-Hill, Toronto, **1960**: 809–838.

BEARN, A. G., YU, T. F. and GUTMAN, A. B. Renal function in Wilson's disease. *J. clin. Invest.*, **1957**, *36*: 1107–1114.

CUMMINGS, J. N. Trace metals in the brain and in Wilson's disease. *J. clin. Path.*, **1968**, *21*: 1–7.

HELLER, G. L. and KOOI, K. A. The electroencephalogram in hepato-lenticular degeneration (Wilson's disease). *Electroenceph. clin. Neurophysiol.*, **1962**, *14*: 520–526.

NEUMANN, P. Z. and SILVERBERG, M. Active copper transport in mammalian tissues. A possible role in Wilson's disease. *Nature (Lond.)*, **1966**, *210*: 414–416.

OSBORN, S. B. and WALSHE, J. M. Studies with radiocopper (Cu^{64}) in Wilson's disease: the liver/thigh ratio. *Clin. Sci.*, **1964**, *27*: 319–328.

OSBORN, S. B. and WALSHE, J. M. Studies with radiocopper (Cu^{64}) in Wilson's disease: dynamics of copper transport. *Clin. Sci.*, **1965**, *29*: 575–581.

OSBORN, S. B. and WALSHE, J. M. Studies with radiocopper (Cu^{64} and Cu^{67}). A distinction between the hepatic and neurologic stages of Wilson's disease. *Birth Defects: original article series*, **1968**, *4*, *No. 2*: 41–44.

SHERLOCK, S. *Disease of the liver and biliary system.* Blackwell, Oxford, **1963**, 699 p.

SHIKATA, T. Morphogenesis of liver cirrhosis in Wilson's disease. *Birth Defects*: *original article series*, **1968**, *4*, *No. 2*: 88–91.

SHIRAKI, H. Comparative neuropathologic study of Wilson's disease and other types of hepatocerebral disease. *Birth Defects*: *original article series*, **1968**, *4*, *No. 2*: 64–73.

STERNLIEB, I. and SCHEINBERG, I. M. Prevention of Wilson's disease in asymptomatic patients. *New Eng. J. Med.*, **1968**, *278*: 352.

STREIFLER, M. and FELDMAN, S. Effect of dimercaprol (BAL) in hepatolenticular degeneration: Report of a case with clinical and EEG study. *Arch. Neurol. Psychiat. (Chic.)*, **1953**, *69*: 84–90.

WALSHE, J. M. The physiology of copper in man and its relation to Wilson's disease. *Brain*, **1967**, *90*: 149–176.

Reference: HANSOTIA, P., HARRIS, R. and KENNEDY, J. EEG changes in Wilson's disease. *Electroenceph. clin. Neurophysiol.*, **1969**, *27*: 523–528.

Electroencephalography and Clinical Neurophysiology
Elsevier Publishing Company, Amsterdam – Printed in The Netherlands

CLINICAL AND LABORATORY NOTES

EFFECTS OF *PARA*-CHLOROPHENYLALANINE ON SLEEP IN MAN

RICHARD J. WYATT, KARL ENGELMAN, DAVID J. KUPFER, JIMMY SCOTT, ALBERT SJOERDSMA AND FREDERICK SNYDER

Laboratory of Clinical Psychobiology, National Institute of Mental Health, and (K.E., A.S.) Experimental Therapeutics Branch, National Heart Institute, Bethesda, Md. 20014 (U.S.A.)

(Accepted for publication: March 3, 1969)

Considerable research effort has been expended in an attempt to elucidate the possible role of serotonin in the neuropharmacology of sleep (Koella 1967; Jouvet 1968). Non-specific reduction of brain serotonin (5-HT) levels with reserpine reduced both rapid eye movement (REM) and non-rapid eye movement (NREM) sleep (Jouvet 1968), while stereotaxic destruction of serotonin-containing neurons has produced insomnia in animals (Jouvet 1968). With the discovery of a specific inhibitor of 5-HT synthesis, *para*-chlorophenylalanine (PCP), it has been possible to deplete brain serotonin selectively in animals in the absence of neuro-anatomic lesions or changes in brain catecholamine content (Jequier *et al.* 1967; Koe and Weisman 1968). When PCP was administered to cats there was a marked reduction in NREM sleep, and while REM sleep was also reduced, the reduction was proportional to the change in NREM sleep (Delorme *et al.* 1966). Sleep studies of monkeys (Weitzman *et al.* 1968) given PCP revealed that while NREM sleep decreased there was no change in REM sleep, indicating that PCP produced varying effects in different species. Because of these species differences it was of particular interest to determine the effect of PCP administration on the sleep of man.

METHODS AND MATERIALS

To evaluate the possible effects of depleting brain 5-HT in man, it was necessary to study the sleep of patients with malignant carcinoid syndrome who received PCP for therapeutic purposes (Engelman *et al.* 1967), because administration of this drug to normal subjects has been restricted. Two male and two female patients (ages 42–54) were studied by continuous nightly recordings of their electroencephalogram (EEG), horizontal electro-oculogram (EOG), and submental electromyogram (EMG). The patients slept in their regular hospital rooms and were undisturbed until they were awakened after 8 h of possible sleep time. Except for patient M.R., who received 0.25 mg digoxin daily, all medications were discontinued 10 days prior to the study. A constant number of identical capsules containing either placebo or PCP were administered throughout the study on a daily schedule of 8 a.m., 12 a.m., 6 p.m. and 10 p.m., with a maximal drug dose range of 3.0–4.0 g/24 h[1]. The sleep records were evaluated according to modified Dement–Kleitman (1957) criteria by a scorer who was unaware of the patient's drug status. The first 2 nights of each sleep study were used to adapt the patient to the slightly unnatural sleeping conditions, and no data from these nights are included in the results. Each period of the study was comprised of at least 3 consecutive nights of sleep, with the majority being 5 nights or longer. Urinary excretion of 5-hydroxyindoleacetic acid (5-HIAA) was determined on 24 h urine specimens (Udenfriend *et al.* 1955). Bidirectional paper chromatography of urine aliquots (Jepson 1955) failed to reveal 5-HTP as a significant urinary excretion product of each of these tumors. The statistical significance of the sleep data was determined using a two-tailed Mann-Whitney Test (Siegel 1956).

D,L-5-Hydroxytryptophan monohydrate (600 mg/night, equivalent to 4 mg L-5-HTP/kg) was administered to one patient (W.F.) in equally divided oral doses at 9 p.m. and 11 p.m. for 7 consecutive nights, while he was also receiving PCP in a dose sufficient to reduce REM sleep by 40% (3.0 g/24 h).

RESULTS

The effect of PCP administration on NREM and REM sleep and the urinary excretion of 5-HIAA in patient W.G. is shown in Fig. 1. REM sleep and urinary 5-HIAA excretion declined gradually as PCP dosage was increased, but there was no change in NREM sleep. When the drug was discontinued REM sleep increased more slowly than urinary 5-HIAA, but did not return to normal levels during the 12 post-drug nights. Significant reduction of REM sleep occurred in all patients receiving PCP (Fig. 2),

[1] Supplied by Dr. Sheldon Gilgore, Chas. Pfizer and Co., Groton, Conn.

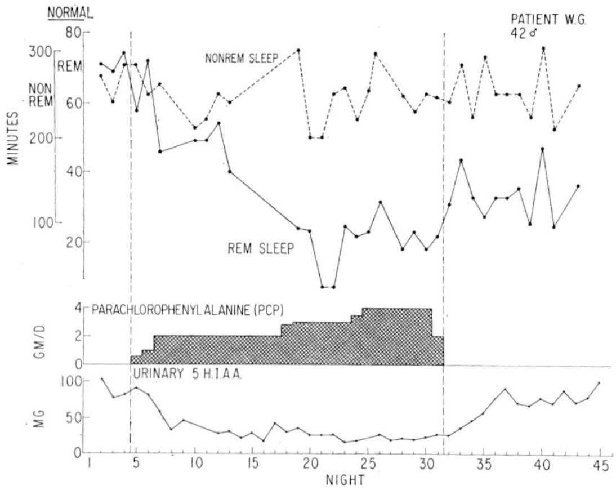

Fig. 1
Relative changes in rapid eye movement (REM) and non-rapid eye movement (NREM) sleep, and 24 h urinary 5-hydroxyindoleacetic acid (5-HIAA) excretion in a carcinoid patient receiving *para*-chlorophenylalanine.

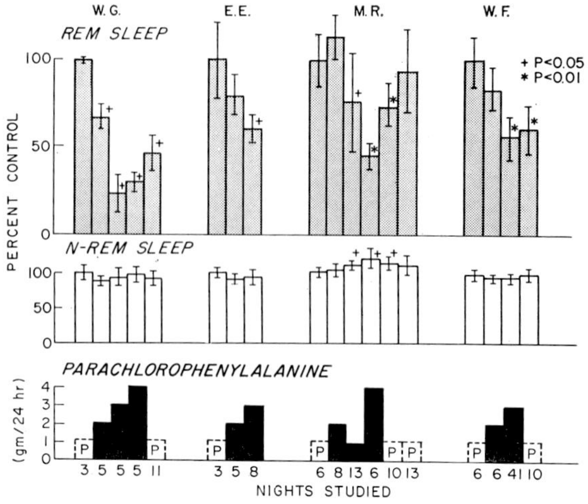

Fig. 2
para-Chlorophenylalanine (PCP) dose and sequence for the four patients studied. Upper two rows of vertical bars represent rapid eye movement (REM) and non-rapid eye movement (NREM) sleep as a percentage (mean ± S.D.) of control period. In the third row, P refers to placebo given during control period. PCP dosage is marked in black. Number of nights studied refers to total number of consecutive nights studied on dosage of PCP or P.

and REM sleep suppression was prolonged in the three patients who were studied following drug discontinuation[1]. In the patient (M.R.) studied for the longest post-drug period, the REM sleep did return to control values several weeks after PCP was discontinued, but she did not compensate for REM sleep deprivation by a subsequent increase above baseline, as is seen under other conditions of REM sleep suppression (Dement 1965).

In contrast to the effects observed in REM sleep, there was no significant change in NREM in three of the patients. In the fourth subject (M.R.) there was a slight but statistically significant increase in NREM ($P < 0.05$), while REM was markedly reduced ($P < 0.01$) from control values (Fig. 2).

As had been previously observed in similar patients (Engelman *et al.* 1967), the urinary excretion of 5-HIAA was reduced by as much as 80% when these patients received PCP. Despite the fact that mean urinary 5-HIAA excretion increased from 87 to 197 mg/24 h when the patient received 5-HTP and PCP, there was only a slight, but not statistically significant, increase in the mean duration of both REM (from 44 to 52 min) and NREM (from 316 to 343 min) sleep. Despite these findings, when a measure of the amount of eye movement was examined, there was a statistically significant increase ($P < 0.05$) when patient W.F. received 5-HTP.

[1] Subsequently patient W.G. was maintained on a 2 g/24 h dosage of PCP for 380 days. At the end of this period a 5-night sample of his sleep showed that REM sleep (21 min/night) was one-third of his baseline levels and NREM sleep remained unchanged from pre-drug levels. This prolonged REM suppression appeared to have caused no gross psychological problems.

DISCUSSION

The decrease in REM sleep of patients taking PCP was accompanied by a decrease of urinary 5-HIAA levels. Although the excretion of 5-HIAA in these patients mainly resulted from tumor production, we consider it reasonable to assume a parallel decrease in the 5-HT production of other tissues, including brain. This is reflected in the reduced 5-HIAA excretion previously documented in normal subjects receiving PCP (Cremata and Koe 1966). Brain levels of 5-HT were not thought to be affected by the secretory products of the tumors since 5-HT does not cross the blood-brain barrier (Axelrod and Inscoe 1963), and, as is usually the case in patients with carcinoid tumor (Oates and Sjoerdsma 1962), the four tumors in question were shown not to produce significant quantities of 5-HTP.

PCP inhibits only the first step in 5-HT biosynthesis, the enzymatic conversion of tryptophan to 5-HTP. 5-HTP has been shown to reverse the depletion of brain 5-HT in animals receiving PCP (Koe and Weisman 1968). Oral 5-HTP administration did not reverse the decrease in REM sleep when given at the same time as the PCP. This is in contrast to the observation in cats that parenteral 5-HTP (20 mg/kg) reversed the sleep changes induced with PCP (Jouvet 1968). Failure of 5-HTP to affect sleep in our patient could be attributed to the difference in route of administration or the small dose (4 mg/kg *vs.* 20 mg/kg; larger doses of 5-HTP in man are limited by symptoms of nausea and diarrhea), and a possible utilization of the 5-HTP by the tumor in this patient cannot be excluded[1].

The correlation between inhibition of 5-HT synthesis (as reflected by changes in urinary 5-HIAA excretion) and the changes observed in the sleep EEG is not fully explained by our data. While 5-HIAA excretion returned to control values within the first week following PCP withdrawal, the return of REM sleep to baseline conditions was more delayed (Fig. 1). It is possible that this reflects a difference in the inhibition of tryptophan hydroxylase produced by PCP in carcinoid tumor and the human brain. Precedent for this possibility exists from the finding that administration of PCP to rats produces irreversible inhibition of brain tryptophan hydroxylase while competitive inhibition of shorter duration occurs in rabbit brain-stem (Robinson and Lovenberg, personal communication). Since the urinary 5-HIAA excretion in these patients reflects mainly tumor metabolism, it is possible that more prolonged inhibition of tryptophan hydroxylase in normal tissue is masked.

In contrast to the high incidence of neuropsychiatric responses observed previously in patients receiving PCP (Engelman *et al.* 1967), only one of these patients (M.R.) showed similar effects during this study. While receiving 4 g/24 h she became very frightened, agitated and on several occasions was incontinent of urine during sleep; there was no evidence of hallucination or delusion as we had noted in the prior study. Although she claimed that she slept poorly during the time of these abnormal responses, the NREM sleep for her 2 most disturbed nights was not decreased, even though her REM sleep was reduced by 60% (from 68 to 24 min) during this period (Fig. 2).

The effects of PCP on sleep in man appear to differ from those observed in other species. In cats (Delorme *et al.* 1966) PCP administration (300 mg/kg) abolished both NREM and REM sleep. However, when dosages of 50 mg/kg (our maximum dosage) were administered to cats, only a slight reduction in both REM and NREM sleep was observed (Koella *et al.* 1968). Weitzman *et al.* (1968) reported that PCP (330–1000 mg/kg) selectively decreased NREM while not affecting REM sleep in monkeys. Thus, even the results in this primate were exactly opposite to those we observed in man.

It is evident that considerable species variation has been observed in the response of sleep mechanisms to brain 5-HT depletion. Therefore, establishment of any general significance of serotonin in the neuropharmacology of sleep will require detailed investigation of the species in question.

SUMMARY

The effect of depleting brain serotonin with *para*-chlorophenylalanine (PCP), a selective inhibitor of serotonin synthesis, was studied on the sleep of man. PCP markedly decreased rapid eye movement (REM) sleep. Non-rapid eye movement (NREM) sleep remained either unchanged or was slightly increased. This is in contrast to the reported effect of PCP in other mammals, which is to decrease NREM sleep. In one subject, at a time when PCP had maximally reduced REM sleep, psychological disturbances were produced similar to those previously described in patients taking PCP. These data and the results of other reported investigations suggest that the establishment of any general significance of serotonin in the neuropharmacology of sleep will require detailed investigation of the species in question.

RÉSUMÉ

EFFET DE LA *PARA*-CHLOROPHÉNYLALANINE SUR LE SOMMEIL DE L'HOMME

L'effet de la diminution de la sérotonine cérébrale par la *para*-chlorophénylalanine (PCP), inhibiteur électif de la synthèse de la sérotonine, a été étudié sur le sommeil de l'homme. La PCP diminue de façon marquée les stades de sommeil avec mouvements oculaires rapides (REM). Le sommeil sans mouvements oculaires rapides (NREM) reste inchangé ou est légèrement augmenté. Ceci est en contradiction avec les effets rapportés de la PCP chez d'autres mammifères, qui serait de diminuer le sommeil sans mouvements oculaires rapides. Chez un sujet, au moment où la PCP a réduit au maximum le sommeil avec mouvements oculaires rapides, on observe des perturbations psychologiques semblables à celles qui ont été décrites antérieurement chez des malades prenant de la PCP. Ces données et les résultats d'autres investigations rapportées suggèrent que l'attribution d'une signification générale quelconque à la sérotonine dans la neuropharmacologie du sommeil requiert une investigation détaillée des espèces en question.

REFERENCES

AXELROD, J. and INSCOE, J. K. The uptake and binding for circulating serotonin and the effects of drugs. *J. Pharmacol. exp. Ther.*, **1963**, *141*: 161–165.

CREMATA, V. Y. and KOE, B. K. Clinical-pharmacological evaluation of *p*-chlorophenylalanine: a new serotonin depleting agent. *Clin. Pharmacol. Ther.*, **1966**, *7*: 768–776.

DELORME, F., FROMENT, J. L. et JOUVET, M. Suppression du sommeil par la p. chlorométhamphétamine et la p. chlorophénylalanine. *C. R. Soc. Biol. (Paris)*, **1966**, *160*: 2347–2351.

DEMENT, W. Recent studies on the biological role of rapid eye movement sleep. *Amer. J. Psychiat.*, **1965**, *122*: 404–408.

DEMENT, W. and KLEITMAN, N. Cyclic variations in EEG during sleep and their relation to eye movements, body motility and dreaming. *Electroenceph. clin. Neurophysiol.*, **1957**, *9*: 673–690.

ENGELMAN, K., LOVENBERG, W. and SJOERDSMA, A. Inhibition of serotonin synthesis by para-chlorophenylalanine in patients with the carcinoid syndrome. *New Engl. J. Med.*, **1967**, *277*: 1103–1108.

[1] Similar studies in two subsequent patients receiving PCP revealed that 600 mg 5-HTP/evening resulted in a return of REM sleep to control values while NREM sleep was unchanged.

JEPSON, J. B. Paper chromatography of urinary indoles. *Lancet*, **1955,** *269*: 1009–1011.

JEQUIER, E., LOVENBERG, W. and SJOERDSMA, A. Tryptophan hydroxylase inhibition: the mechanism by which *p*-chlorophenylalanine depletes rat brain serotonin. *Molec. Pharmacol.*, **1967,** *3*: 274–278.

JOUVET, M. Mechanisms of the states of sleep: a neuropharmacological approach. In S. S. KETY *et al.* (Eds.), *Sleep and altered states of consciousness.* Williams and Wilkins, Baltimore, **1967**: 86–126.

JOUVET, M. Insomnia and decrease of cerebral 5-hydroxytryptamine after destruction of the raphe system in the cat. In S. GARATTINI and P. A. SHORE (Eds.), *Advances in pharmacology.* Academic Press, New York, **1968**: 265–279.

KOE, B. K. and WEISMAN, A. *p*-Chlorophenylalanine: a specific depletor of brain serotonin. *J. Pharmacol. exp. Ther.*, **1968,** *154*: 499–516.

KOELLA, W. P. *Sleep.* Thomas, Springfield, Ill., **1967,** 199 p.

KOELLA, W. P., FELDSTEIN, A. and CZICMAN, J. S. The effect of *para*-chlorophenylalanine on the sleep of cats. *Electroenceph. clin. Neurophysiol.*, **1968,** *25*: 481–490.

OATES, J. A. and SJOERDSMA, A. A unique syndrome associated with secretion of 5-hydroxytryptophan by metastatic gastric carcinoids. *Amer. J. Med.*, **1962,** *32*: 333–342.

SIEGEL, S. *Nonparametric statistics for the behavioral sciences.* McGraw-Hill, New York, **1956,** 312 p.

UDENFRIEND, S., TITUS, F. and WEISSBACH, H. The identification of 5-hydroxy-3-indoleacetic acid in normal urine and a method for its assay. *J. biol. Chem.*, **1955,** *216*: 499–505.

WEITZMAN, E. D., RAPPORT, M. S., MCGREGOR, P. and JACOBY, J. Sleep patterns of the monkey and brain serotonin concentration: effect of *p*-chlorophenylalanine. *Science*, **1968,** *160*: 1361–1363.

Reference: WYATT, R. J., ENGELMAN, K., KUPFER, D. J., SCOTT, J., SJOERDSMA, A. and SNYDER, F. Effects of *para*-chlorophenylalanine on sleep in man. *Electroenceph. clin. Neurophysiol.*, **1969,** *27*: 529–532.

Electroencephalography and Clinical Neurophysiology
Elsevier Publishing Company, Amsterdam – Printed in The Netherlands

TECHNICAL CONTRIBUTIONS

ON-LINE ANALYSIS OF EEG WITH A SMALL COMPUTER (PERIOD–AMPLITUDE ANALYSIS)[1]

H. LEGEWIE AND W. PROBST

Abteilung für Neurophysiologie, Max-Planck-Institut für Psychiatrie, Munich (West Germany)

(Accepted for publication: March 11, 1969)

The chief methods of power spectral density and frequency correlation coefficient determination which have been used up to the present time for automatic EEG analysis possess the following disadvantages: (1) the extent to which the basic assumptions of these methods are met is controversial; (2) the analysis requires considerable storage space and calculating time; (3) the results are not clearly interpretable within the conceptual framework of traditional electroencephalography. Since small and inexpensive program-controlled computers are available, simpler methods of analysing the major EEG components should be sought.

In our laboratory a modification of the well-known period analysis based on the zero-crossing method (Burch 1959) has been shown to be highly satisfactory. (Results were reported by Creutzfeldt *et al.* 1969; Legewie *et al.* 1969; Scheich 1969.) Period analysis can be carried out with the help of electronic elements (Burch 1959; Schwarzer and Reetz 1966) or an appropriately programmed medium-sized computer (Burch 1964; Bente and Ferner 1969). In comparison with previous methods, the method suggested here possesses a high degree of flexibility at relatively low cost.

[1] Supported by the Deutsche Forschungsgemeinschaft (Grant Cr30).

METHOD

The basic measurement procedures are shown in Fig. 1, *a*. After a suitable base line has been set, a single EEG wave is defined as the segment of the curve between two successive zero-crossings which are positive in direction. The periods of the EEG waves are then given by

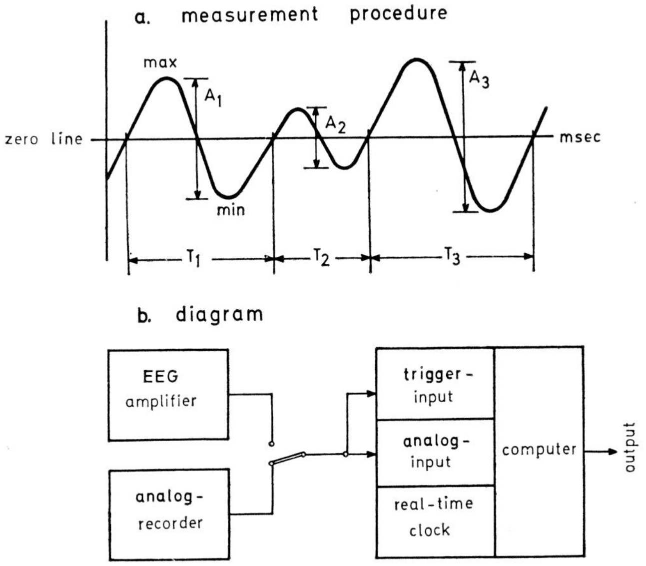

Fig. 1
Period–amplitude analysis with the digital computer. *a*: shows the measurement procedure and the definition of periods (T) and amplitudes (A); *b*: shows a block diagram of the apparatus.

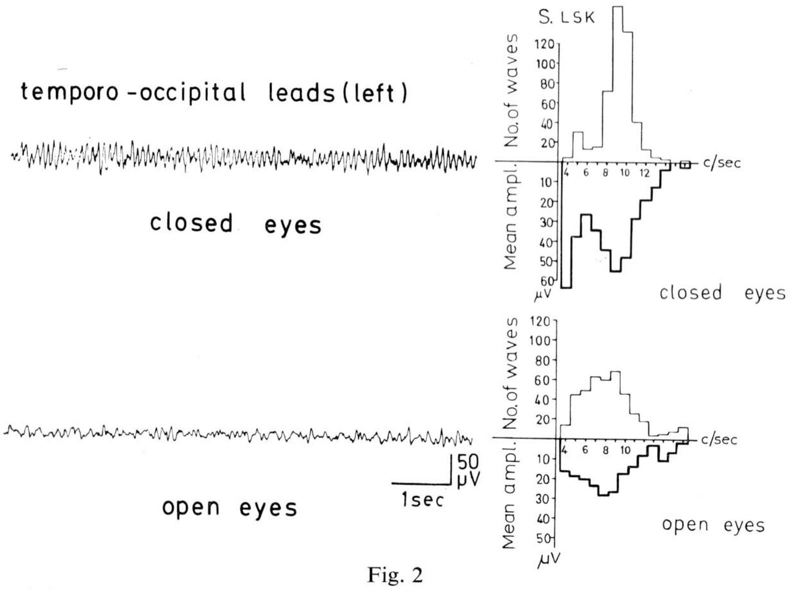

Fig. 2

Example of the analysis. Two samples of 8 sec EEG at the left, the corresponding histograms of 1 min EEG activity at the right. In the histograms, periods are converted into the usual frequency classes. Above the abscissa the ordinates of each histogram show the number of waves per frequency; below the abscissa the mean amplitudes per frequency are shown.

the time intervals between two zero-crossings (T1, T2, ...) and the amplitudes by the differences in maximal and minimal potential (max — min) occurring between successive zero-crossings (A1, A2, ...).

As shown in Fig. 1, *b* the output to be analysed, from the EEG amplifier or the analogue tape recorder, is fed into the computer by both a Schmitt trigger and an analogue–digital converter simultaneously (the computer must be provided with an interface possessing suitable input channels and a millisecond clock; see Färber and Probst 1968). To avoid slow base line shifts it is recommended to pass the record through an appropriate broad-band filter. In the example below we used a Schwarzer filter (4–16 c/sec, 12 dB/oct.) to analyse the frequencies in the alpha range.

After passing through the trigger input (the threshold is adjustable by hand) the zero-crossings are identified by the program[1] and the intervals between them are stored. Amplitudes are computed simultaneously by the analogue input. When a chosen period of measurement is completed, an interval histogram and a histogram of average amplitudes become available for oscilloscopic display or for printed output. Also, whatever statistical parameters based on the histogram are desired can be computed separately.

As an example, Fig. 2 presents two original records and frequency and amplitude histograms (durations of intervals were converted into frequency classes).

DISCUSSION

The procedural simplicity and low costs of this method make it suitable for routine analysis in the clinical EEG laboratory as well as for experimental questions. In addition, the on-line processing allows considerable concentration of data prior to their statistical evaluation by a large computer. One particular application is that of monitoring over extended periods of time (during sleep, narcosis and intensive therapy); here any criteria chosen can be applied to the on-line parameters available (intervals and amplitudes), appropriate warning signals being provided by the computer.

Certain disadvantages must be taken into account, however, when this method is employed in its simple version: (1) the arbitrary choice of the zero-line can influence the results; (2) the EEG must be recorded with a short time constant or be passed through a suitable filter prior to analysis, in order to avoid slow fluctuations of the zero-line. The latter disadvantage makes the method unsuitable for analysing slow EEG components. One solution to this problem is the repeated analysis of a given record with different settings of broad-band filters; this technique, based on the principle of the Schwarzer analyser (Schwarzer and Reetz 1966), allows superimposed waves, such as sleep spindles on delta waves, to be separated.

[1] With little increase in program complexity, the zero-crossings can be calculated by the program; this obviates the need of the trigger input, although it increases computation time.

Thus, if the simple form of the method reported here is chosen, the disadvantages mentioned must be tolerated; with use of additional programming and apparatus these can be avoided.

SUPPLEMENT

Our suggestions for a program are based on the capacity of the cheapest commercially available small computers (*e.g.*, PDP 8L) for which the manufacturers are ready to construct whatever interface is required. The total costs of the equipment (including the display screen) should be approximately $15,000. The program suggested here can be altered or enlarged as required.

1. Start of program!
   Read analysis time!
   Storage zero!
   (H(T) for frequencies of individual periods, A(T) for amplitudes, T = 1, ... 50)
2. Wait for start of analysis!
3. Wait for first zero-crossing!
4. Time 1 = 0!
   (Real time)
5. Time 2 = time 1!
   (Time of last zero-crossing)
6. Analysis time exceeded?
   No: Continue 7.
   Yes: Continue 10.
7. Determine MAX and MIN of analogue potential!
8. Zero-crossing?
   No: Continue 6.
   Yes: Continue 9.
9. Store results:
   T = (Time 1 − Time 2)/10!
   (T is interval class, class range 10 msec)
   Limit T to maximal 50!
   H(T) = H(T) + 1!
   (Frequency is increased in period class T)
   A(T) = A(T) + MAX − MIN
   (Addition of peak-to-peak amplitude in class)
   Return 5!
10. Output:
    H(T) = histogram of period frequencies
    A(T)/H(T) = histogram of mean amplitudes in each frequency class
11. End.

SUMMARY

A simple method for automatic analysis of the EEG is described, suitable for use with the smallest digital computers presently available (period–amplitude analysis by the zero-crossing method). The computer program suggested supplies complete period and amplitude histograms for any analysis time chosen. Applications of this flexible and economical method for clinical and scientific purposes are discussed; an illustrative example is given.

ZUSAMMENFASSUNG

ON-LINE-ANALYSE DES EEG AUF KLEINCOMPUTERN (INTERVALL–AMPLITUDEN-ANALYSE)

Es wird eine einfache automatische Analysemethode des EEG für den Einsatz der kleinsten z. Zt. verfügbaren Digitalrechner beschrieben (aperiodische Intervall–Amplituden-Analyse nach dem Nulldurchgangs-Verfahren). Das vorgeschlagene Rechnerprogramm liefert vom laufenden EEG (on-line) in frei wählbaren Analyseabschnitten ein vollständiges Intervall- und Amplituden-Histogramm. Die Anwendungsmöglichkeiten dieses flexiblen und gleichzeitig ökonomischen Verfahrens für wissenschaftliche und klinische Fragestellungen werden diskutiert und an einem Beispiel belegt.

We gratefully acknowledge the help of Dr. Goldsmith in preparing the English manuscript.

REFERENCES

BENTE, D. und FERNER, U. Digital amplitude–interval analysis. A new method of quantitative analysis of the EEG. *Electroenceph. clin. Neurophysiol.*, **1969,** *27*: 628P.

BURCH, N. D. Automatic analysis of the electroencephalogram: a review and classification of systems. *Electroenceph. clin. Neurophysiol.*, **1959,** *11*: 827–834.

BURCH, N. R. Period analysis of the electroencephalogram on a general-purpose digital computer. *Ann. N. Y. Acad. Sci.*, **1964,** *115*: 827–843.

CREUTZFELDT, O. D., GRÜNEWALD, G., SIMONOVA, O. and SCHMITZ, H. Changes of the basic rhythms of the EEG during performance of mental and visuomotor tasks. In C. R. EVANS and T. B. MULHOLLAND (Eds.), *Proceedings of the conference on attention in neurophysiology*, Butterworth, London, **1969** (in press).

FÄRBER, G. und PROBST, W. Automatische Versuchssteuerung und Versuchsauswertung mit dem IBM System 1130, dargestellt an einem Beispiel aus der Medizin. *IBM Nachrichten*, **1968,** *18*: 126–131.

LEGEWIE, H., SIMONOVA, O. and CREUTZFELDT, O. D. EEG changes during performance of various tasks under open- and closed-eyed conditions. *Electroenceph. clin. Neurophysiol.*, **1969,** *27*: 470–479.

SCHEICH, H. The behaviour of the alpha rhythm under defined motor and pharmacological conditions. *Electroenceph. clin. Neurophysiol.*, **1969,** *27*: 626P.

SCHWARZER, F. and REETZ, H. Machines for EEG analysis. *Electroenceph. clin. Neurophysiol.*, **1966,** *20*: 278P.

Reference: LEGEWIE, H. and PROBST, W. On-line analysis of EEG with a small computer (period–amplitude analysis). *Electroenceph. clin. Neurophysiol.*, **1969,** *27*: 533–535.

Electroencephalography and Clinical Neurophysiology
Elsevier Publishing Company, Amsterdam – Printed in The Netherlands

OSCILLOSCOPIC RECORDING OF MUSCLE FIBER ACTION POTENTIALS. THE WINDOW TRIGGER AND THE DELAY UNIT

JAN CZEKAJEWSKI, JAN EKSTEDT AND ERIK STÅLBERG

Department of Pharmacology, Department of Clinical Neurophysiology and Wallenberg Laboratory, University of Uppsala, Uppsala (Sweden)

(Accepted for publication: March 12, 1969)

In recording single muscle fiber action potentials in voluntarily activated human muscle (Ekstedt 1964; Stålberg 1966) it is essential, for various reasons, to trigger the oscilloscope sweep from the action potentials themselves. One reason is that the shape of the action potential must be studied with a time base of 20–100 μsec/cm during the experiment, and this cannot be done with a free running sweep. Another is that comparison of consecutive action potentials with each other can only be accomplished by superimposing them on the oscilloscope screen. This is also necessary when measuring the jitter, *i.e.*, the variability in the time intervals between action potentials from two different fibers from the same motor unit (Ekstedt 1964) and the propagation velocity of single muscle fibers (Stålberg 1966).

The use of the delay unit was described by Stålberg (1966). A similar device has recently been published by Nissen-Petersen *et al.* (1969).

This paper deals with some technical aspects of oscilloscope triggering, especially with regard to the problem of selecting action potentials from only one muscle fiber.

The parameters of single muscle fiber action potentials

The single muscle fiber action potential, recorded with a needle multi-electrode with 25 μ circular platinum leading-off surfaces in the side of the needle, appears as a smooth positive–negative action potential. Ekstedt (1964) gave the following values for the action potentials from about 300 fibers: *voltage*: median value 5.6 mV, range 0.7–25.2 mV; *duration of fast positive–negative deflection*: median value 112 μsec, range 67–200 μsec; *total duration*: median value 470 μsec, range 265–800 μsec. However, a bias in the sampling in favor of large action potentials might have arisen because, when large and small action potentials are present simultaneously, only the large ones can be made to trigger the oscilloscope with ordinary triggering methods. This will be discussed below.

Ordinary oscilloscope triggering

Triggering of the oscilloscope from an action potential does not in itself present any problems because most modern oscilloscopes have a built-in trigger circuit by means of which the sweep can be started from any desired point on the recorded signal. Often the trigger level control knob can only be rotated three-quarters of a turn, making adjustments rather difficult. It is therefore advantageous to increase the resolution of the trigger level control by, for example, replacing the one-turn with a ten-turn potentiometer.

To select the action potential of largest amplitude from several different ones, the trigger level is set sufficiently high so that only the initial positive phase of the largest action potential passes the trigger level. If one decreases the trigger level, another muscle fiber action potential might also reach the trigger level and start the sweep. Thus, it is not possible to obtain a clean oscilloscopic recording of any other potential than the largest of those present.

The delay unit

To study that part of the action potential preceding the triggering point, the delay unit was constructed. The oscilloscope sweep is triggered by the original action potential which, before being displayed on the screen, is delayed for a pre-set period of up to 500 μsec. The delay unit has two independent channels in each of which the delay is adjustable in steps of 10 μsec within the interval 0–100 μsec and in steps of 100 μsec in the interval 100–500 μsec. The two channels may be coupled in series and a total delay of 1 msec thus obtained.

The delay unit is based on two identical electromagnetic delay lines (5T200G Ad Yu Electronics Lab Inc., Passaic, N.J.) consisting of a number (in this case 100) of LC networks in series. A signal at one end of this series will be propagated with a certain velocity along the delay line and may be picked up anywhere along it and the original wave form regained. However, along the delay line there is a continuous attenuation of the signal, especially of the high frequency components. When feeding a square wave into the input, the plateau value decreases by 15% at the output, where the rise-time (10–90%) is 15 μsec. The frequency response curve is flat between 0 and 25 kc/sec and 3 dB down at 35 kc/sec at 500 μsec delay. The phase shift is linear up to about 70%

of the cut-off frequency. A slight overshoot, with a damped oscillation with a fundamental frequency of about 50 kc/sec is observed when a square pulse is fed into the delay line (Fig. 2). There is no measurable variability of the wave form of consecutive pulses.

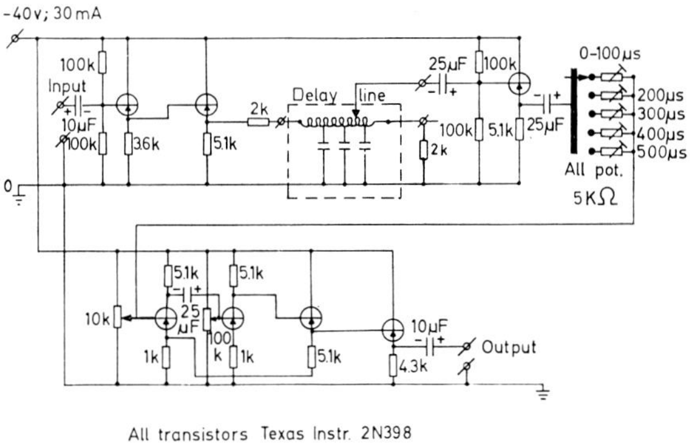

Fig. 1

The electronic design of the delay unit. The electronic delay line (Ad Yu 5T200G) is represented by the broken lines. The five 5 kΩ variable resistors are used for compensation of the signal loss along the delay line and are coupled in with the same selector that selects the different delay positions on the delay line. The 10 kΩ potentiometer is used to adjust the over-all gain to unity.

The electronic design of the delay unit is shown in Fig. 1. The input amplifier feeds the delay line from a source of 2000 Ω output impedance and the delay line is terminated with a 2000 Ω resistor which prevents reflections and oscillatory responses in the delay line. The tappings of the delay line are sampled by a multipolar switch, by which also resistors are switched in to compensate for the continuous loss of signal amplitude along the delay line. Although it is technically feasible, no attempt to compensate for the high frequency loss has yet been made. In the final stages the signal is amplified so that the whole device has unity gain. The input is designed for signals of amplitude ±10 V. For an action potential with a fast positive–negative deflection of 100 μsec, the delay unit increases this by 1 μsec but on comparing the delayed and undelayed signals no other distortion can be detected (Fig. 2).

By means of the delay unit it is also possible to trigger the signal from a point on the steep positive–negative deflection of the action potential, the slope of which is 3–4 times steeper than that of the initial phase, and the stability of the recording is much improved. The best point for triggering is the baseline intersection, because here small variations in wave form due to variations in the electrode–fiber relationship will be at a minimum (Stålberg 1966). However, the baseline intersection cannot generally be used for triggering, because all other action potentials and all noise signals also pass the zero line and can cause triggering. The two most urgent problems

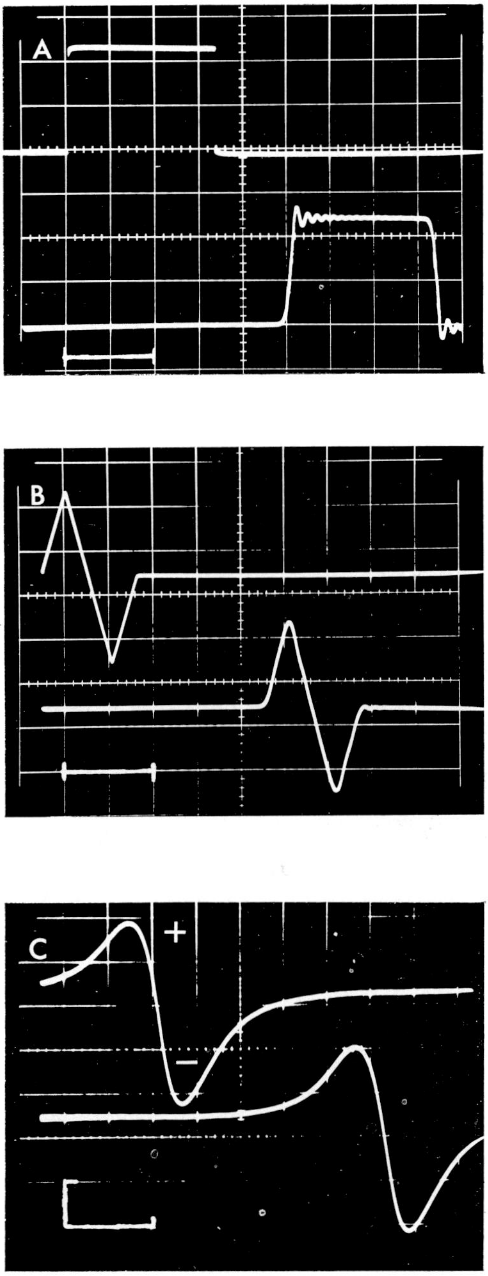

Fig. 2

Distortion of signals caused by the delay unit. Signals at the input of the delay unit (upper beam on each photograph) and at the output after 500 μsec delay (lower). The rise time of the square pulse (*A*) has increased by 15 μsec. There is a slight overshoot and a damped oscillation with fundamental frequency 50 kc/sec. The alteration of the shape of a synthetic action potential (*B*) and of a single muscle fiber action potential (*C*) is hardly noticeable. The rise time has been lengthened by about 1 μsec. Calibration: 3 mV and 200 μsec.

still remaining therefore are: (a) how to record only the *small* action potentials when large action potentials are present simultaneously; (b) how to trigger exactly at the zero intersection point of the rising phase of an action potential. These problems are both solved with the window trigger.

The "window trigger"

The principles are illustrated in Fig. 3. The oscilloscope trigger level is set exactly at zero voltage. When an action potential reaches a certain value, determined by the potentiometer P1, during its positive phase, it will cause a one-shot multi-vibrator (MV1) to release a pulse

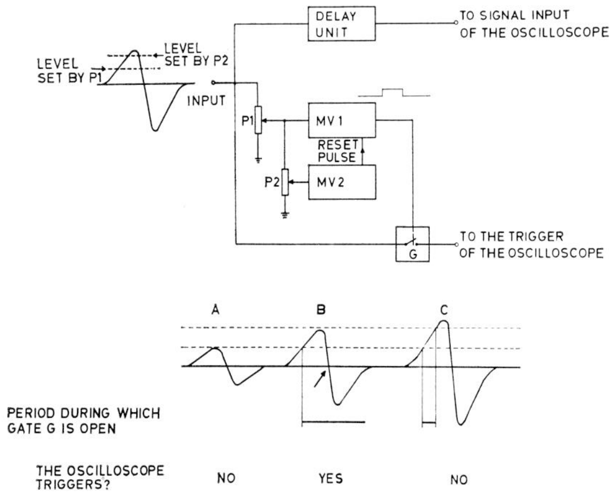

Fig. 3

The principles for the window trigger. An action potential is fed to the input. At the voltage level determined by P1, the one-shot multi-vibrator MV1 gives a pulse that opens the gate G for the action potential to the oscilloscope trigger circuit. However, if the action potential voltage exceeds the level set by potentiometer P2, the one-shot multi-vibrator MV2 gives a pulse that immediately resets MV1 and thus the gate G closes again. The action potential is fed to the vertical input of the oscilloscope via the delay unit.

of 800 μsec. This in turn will open the gate (G) to the oscilloscope trigger circuit for 800 μsec. Thus, the gate is open when the action potential positive–negative deflection crosses the baseline, where the oscilloscope sweep will be triggered. The oscilloscope will remain untriggered for all signals that do not have a positive phase large enough to activate MV1. To prevent larger action potentials from triggering the oscilloscope another one-shot multi-vibrator (MV2), giving a pulse at a voltage level determined by the potentiometer P2, is added. This pulse will immediately block the gate-opening pulse from MV1, thus shutting the gate G again.

In order to trigger the oscilloscope the initial positive peak of the action potential must thus fit into a given *window*. The size of the window may be estimated directly on the oscilloscope by incorporating an extra amplifier which serves to brighten the oscilloscope beam when the gate to the oscilloscope trigger circuit is open. The window size will be indicated by a vertical bright line on the oscilloscope screen each time the action potential exceeds the desired value.

The detailed circuit diagram is given in Fig. 4.

The counter gate

Stålberg (1966) has described methods for measuring the time intervals between the baseline intersections of two action potentials, using a time interval counter (Hewlett Packard Electronic Counter 5245L with time interval unit 5262A). The readings of the time interval counter are automatically recorded on a digital magnetic tape recorder (Dymec 2564A) that can record up to 250 characters per second. The tape is fed into the computer. The measurements can be made between any two points on the action potentials, but zero intersections are usually used because the measurements are then least influenced by changes in the needle position. The disadvantage of using zero intersections for measurement and for triggering the oscilloscope is, however, that action potentials from other motor units and all noise signals will also pass the zero level and be measured by the time interval counter. To overcome these problems, the counter is blocked for all signals except those coincident with the special "unblanking pulse" from the oscilloscope, *i.e.*, the pulse used within the oscilloscope to brighten the beam during a sweep. The unblanking pulse is of the same duration as the sweep and therefore the counter only functions for signals that are displayed on the oscilloscope. Thus, all selection facilities offered by the delay unit and the window trigger are extended to the time interval measurements which, in this way, can be made with an accuracy better than ± 0.3 μsec.

SUMMARY

This paper deals with some technical problems in connection with the oscilloscopic recording of single muscle fiber action potentials. The action potentials trigger the sweep of the oscilloscope to permit a fast time base and comparison of the shapes of consecutive action potentials. By means of the *delay unit* it is possible to record on the oscilloscope the part of the action potential appearing up to 500 μsec before the triggering point. With this unit it is also possible to trigger the oscilloscope sweep on the fast positive–negative deflection of the action potential, thereby obtaining a much steadier display than when triggering on the initial positive phase.

By means of the *window trigger* it is possible to record action potentials of any given size. Only action potentials having a positive peak lying within two fixed limits (which can be selected) will trigger the oscilloscope.

The *counter gate*, which allows automatic time interval measurements only of those action potentials that are displayed on the oscilloscope, is finally described.

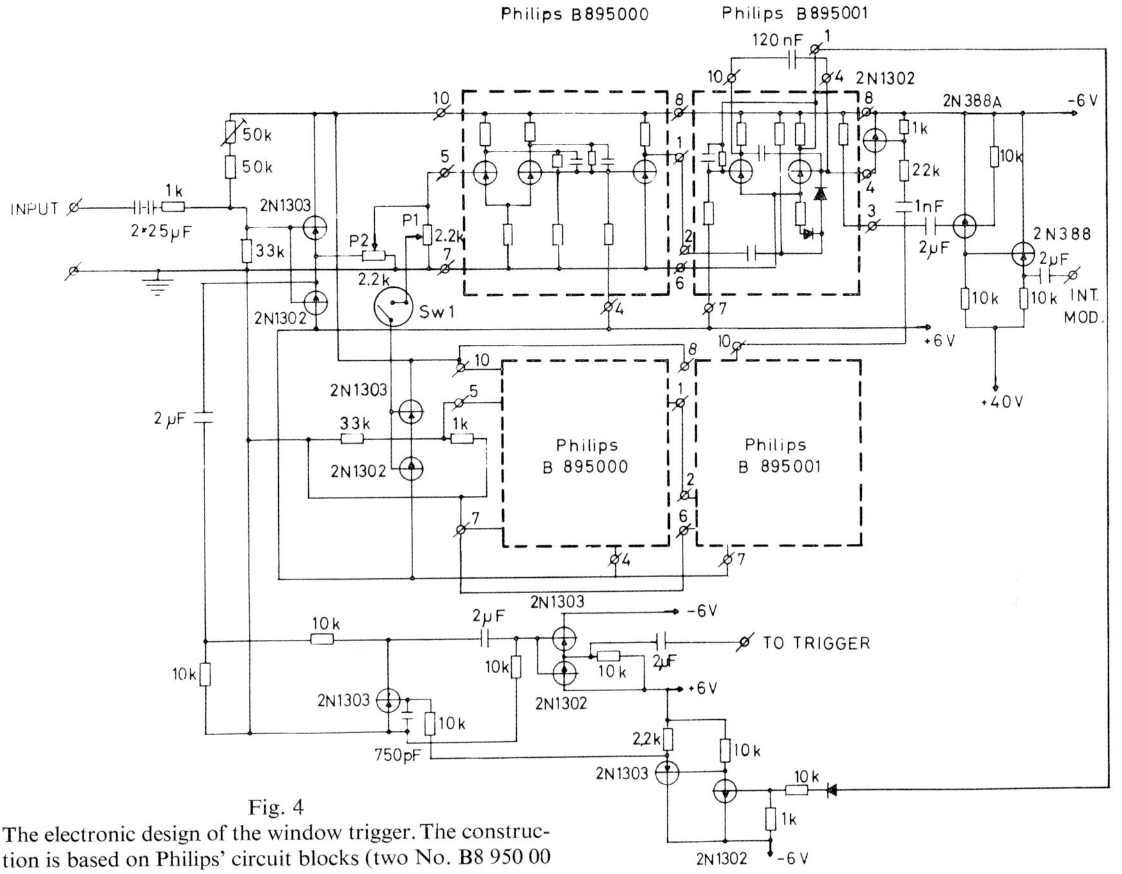

Fig. 4
The electronic design of the window trigger. The construction is based on Philips' circuit blocks (two No. B8 950 00 and two No. B8 950 01).

RÉSUMÉ

ENREGISTREMENT OSCILLOSCOPIQUE DES POTENTIELS D'ACTION DE LA FIBRE MUSCULAIRE. DÉCLENCHEMENT PAR UNE FENÊTRE ET CIRCUIT DE DÉLAI

Ce travail concerne quelques problèmes techniques en connection avec l'enregistrement oscilloscopique des potentiels d'action de la fibre musculaire unique. Les potentiels d'action déclenchent le balayage de l'oscilloscope de façon à permettre une base de temps rapide et une comparaison des potentiels d'action consécutifs. Au moyen du *circuit de délai*, il est possible d'enregistrer sur l'oscilloscope la partie du potentiel d'action qui apparaît jusqu'à 500 μsec avant le point de déclenchement. Avec ce circuit il est également possible de déclencher le balayage de l'oscilloscope sur la déflexion positive–négative rapide du potentiel d'action, obtenant ainsi une présentation plus stable que lorsque le déclenchement est fait sur la phase positive initiale.

Au moyen de *déclenchement par une fenêtre* il est possible d'enregistrer les potentiels d'action de n'importe quelle dimension. Seuls les potentiels d'action ayant un pic positif situé entre deux limites fixées (qui peuvent être sélectionnées) déclenchent l'oscilloscope.

La *porte de comptage* qui permet des mesures automatiques des intervalles de temps des seuls potentiels d'action qui sont présentés sur l'oscilloscope est décrite.

This work was supported by the Swedish Medical Research Council (Grant No. 14x-135), the Magnus Bergwalls Foundation and the Swedish Association against Poliomyelitis.

REFERENCES

EKSTEDT, J. Human single muscle fiber action potentials. *Acta physiol. scand.*, **1964,** *61*, *Suppl. 226*: 1–96.

NISSEN-PETERSEN, H., GULD, C. and BUCHTHAL, F. A delay line to record random action potentials. *Electroenceph. clin. Neurophysiol*, **1969,** *26*: 100–106.

STÅLBERG, E. Propagation velocity in human muscle fiber *in situ*. *Acta physiol. scand.*, **1966,** *70*, *Suppl. 287*: 1–112.

Reference: CZEKAJEWSKI, J., EKSTEDT, J. and STÅLBERG, E. Oscilloscopic recording of muscle fiber action potentials. The window trigger and the delay unit. *Electroenceph. clin. Neurophysiol.*, **1969,** *27*: 536–539.

Electroencephalography and Clinical Neurophysiology
Elsevier Publishing Company, Amsterdam – Printed in The Netherlands

THE CONSTRUCTION OF NEEDLE MULTI-ELECTRODES FOR SINGLE FIBER ELECTROMYOGRAPHY

JAN EKSTEDT, PER HÄGGQVIST AND ERIK STÅLBERG

Department of Pharmacology, Department of Clinical Neurophysiology and Wallenberg Laboratory, University of Uppsala, Uppsala (Sweden)

(Accepted for publication: March 12, 1969)

This paper deals with the construction of the needle multi-electrodes used by Ekstedt (1964) and Stålberg (1966) for the recording of single muscle fiber action potentials and for measurements of propagation velocity in muscle fibers. Buchthal *et al.* (1957) used a multi-electrode for the analysis of the spike of the motor unit potential and this gave the idea for this work. The needle used by Buchthal *et al.* had a diameter of 1.0 mm and each of the twelve leading-off surfaces in the side of the needle had a diameter of 50 or 100 μ. In the multi-electrodes developed by us the outer diameter of the needle is 0.5–0.6 mm and fourteen platinum leading-off surfaces of 25–30 μ diameter are mounted in the side of the needle (Fig. 1 and 2).

General considerations in the construction of needle multi-electrodes

In order to decrease muscle fiber damage and minimize pain during insertion of the needle it is necessary that its outer diameter should be as small as possible. However, with a diameter of less than 0.5 mm the needle becomes too flexible and brittle. For that reason no attempt was made to employ diameters less than 0.5 mm. A needle length of 60 mm has been found to be sufficient in most cases.

The array of leading-off surfaces was mounted in the side of the needle so that the desired arrangement could be obtained and an accurate positioning of the needle in relation to the muscle fiber was possible. Neither of these conditions could be fulfilled with the leading-off surfaces in the bevel of the needle. The array was inlaid in the side of the needle opposite to the bevel mainly on the assumption that the fibers from which the recording should be made would be less liable to damage if they did not have to slide over the bevel. In the multi-electrode used by Buchthal *et al.* (1957) and those manufactured by Disa (Herslev, Denmark) the array is on the same side as the bevel.

In order to minimize disturbance of the electrical field around the muscle fiber, the diameter of the leading-off surfaces ought to be small. The diameter was, in our case, determined by the smallest diameter of insulated platinum wire that was commercially available at the time of construction (30 μ for the first electrode, there-

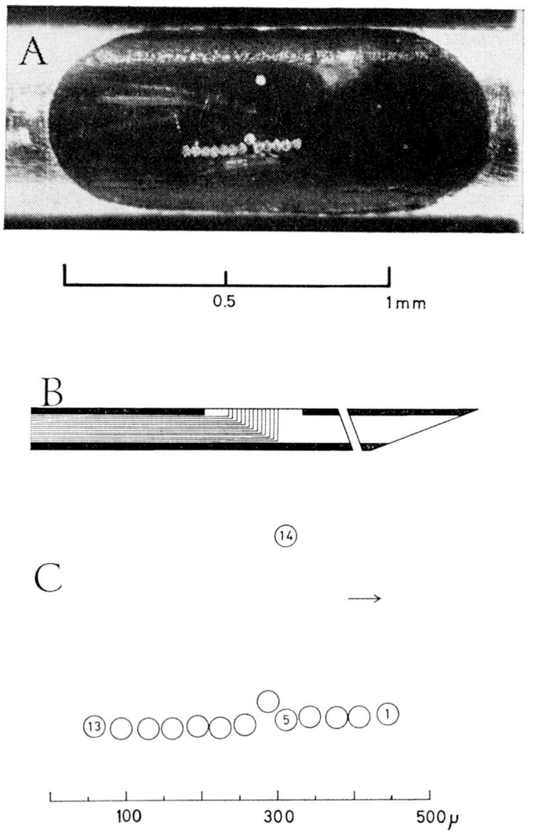

Fig. 1
A needle multi-electrode. The needle used by Stålberg (1966) for the measurement of the propagation velocity of single muscle fiber action potentials. There is a row of 13 round platinum leading-off surfaces of diameter 25 μ, with one electrode displaced by about 250 μ from the center of the row. The diameter of the needle is 0.5 mm. *A*: microphotograph of the array of leading-off surfaces with surrounding epoxy resin; *B*: schematic drawing of the needle, and *C*: electrode array redrawn after a microphotograph.

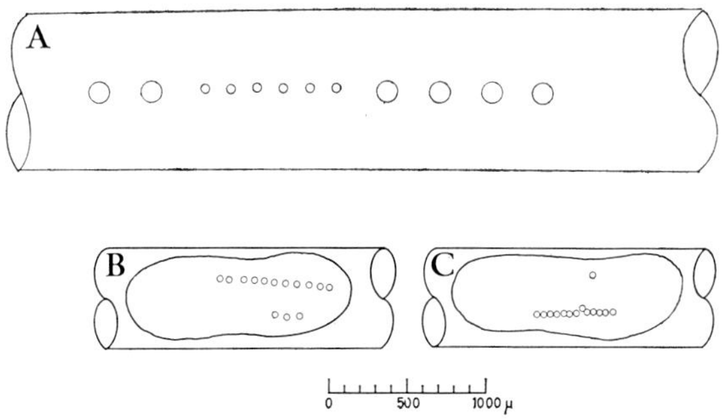

Fig. 2
Drawings of the multi-electrodes used by Buchthal *et al.* (1957) (*A*), Ekstedt (1964) (*B*) and Stålberg (1966) (*C*).

after 25 μ). Platinum wire, coated with Diamel, was obtained from Johnson Mathey, London.

Construction procedures

The array of leading-off surfaces. 25 μ platinum wire is difficult to handle. Watchmaker's forceps leave impressions on the wire and damage the insulation and therefore must not be used on any part of the wire that will be within the multi-electrode. Ordinary Scotch tape or double-faced Scotch tape has proved to be an excellent tool for handling the wire in situations where it is not possible with the unaided fingers.

The array is arranged outside the needle on a stand made from metal rods tied together with laboratory clamps according to Fig. 3. To the middle rod a piece of Teflon (10 × 10 mm) with a flat upper surface is fastened. To the two outer rods double-faced tape is attached.

Platinum wires of appropriate length (about 15 cm) are placed side by side on the Teflon plate and fastened to the double-faced tape on the outer rods, with just sufficient tension to keep them in the correct position. All the wires that will constitute the electrode row are mounted in this way. A piece of ordinary tape is placed over the wires on the double-faced tape on the outer

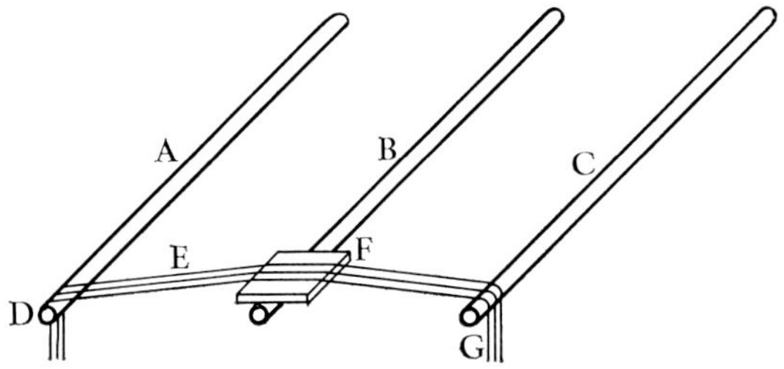

Fig. 3
The mounting stand for arranging the wires in the electrode array. A schematic drawing. A, B and C are metal rods on which the wire array (E) is fastened with double faced Scotch tape at D and G. The wire array passes over a Teflon plate (F) fastened to rod B.

rods. By continuously turning one of the outer rods in its clamp, it is possible to obtain the same tension in all the wires, because the resistance from the adhesive mass of the tape is approximately the same for all of them.

The array is now arranged under a binocular dissection microscope at a magnification of 6–20 times. The arrangement is made partly with the bare fingers and partly by means of a sharp sewing needle, taking care that no part of the wire that is to be incorporated in the multi-electrode is touched with the needle. When the desired arrangement has been obtained the wires are degreased with carbon tetrachloride and ethanol.

For fixation of the wires an epoxy resin is used. We use Araldite (Ciba, Basel), resin F with hardener 972, in the proportions 100 parts by weight of resin and 27 parts by weight of hardener. The mixture is thoroughly stirred and placed in an oven at a temperature of 60° C for 5–10 min to decrease the viscosity and allow all the air bubbles to disappear. At this temperature the viscosity of the mixture is about the same as that of water. A drop of the mixture is taken on a glass rod and allowed to cool until the viscosity is such that when it is applied in the middle of the Teflon plate the mixture is not drawn by capillary forces between the wires outside the plate. A great deal of experience is necessary to choose the right moment for placing the drop; if the viscosity of the resin is too high, the wires may be inadequately covered. The resin layer should be less than 0.5 mm thick.

The resin is allowed to harden at room temperature for 5–6 h. After this time, heat can usually be applied by means of an infra-red lamp, but the temperature must initially be low, 40–50° C. The process must be supervised under the microscope to prevent too much heat being applied too soon, because this results in decreased viscosity of the resin, which may then be drawn up between the platinum wires. When the initial hardening stage is complete the temperature is increased to about 150–180° C by bringing the lamp closer, and this temperature is maintained for at least half an hour. The temperature is more easily controlled if the whole assembly is put in an oven at 180° C for half an hour.

The next step, trimming the Araldite plate, is performed by means of a scalpel under the microscope. The thickness is reduced by scraping to about 0.2 mm; should it happen to be less than 0.2 mm more resin must be applied and the procedure repeated.

More wires may now be arranged on the trimmed Araldite plate to form the second electrode row. New double-faced Scotch tape is applied to the two outer rods and a new arrangement of the wires is made, exactly as described above. The Araldite is translucent and therefore this operation can easily be performed with a high degree of precision. A new drop of Araldite is applied and the hardening repeated.

After this, the plate is trimmed as small as possible with the scalpel and the array is bisected perpendicular to the wires, thus giving material for two multi-electrodes. Finally, the two halves are carefully dissected free from the Teflon plate by means of the scalpel.

The wires must now be bent individually through 90° at the point where they leave the Araldite plate. This must be done very carefully with the fingers, under microscope control.

Preparation of the needle

Ordinary injection needles of stainless steel of good quality are used. Needles with an outer diameter of 0.5 mm usually have too small a bore; therefore, 0.65 mm needles are used and later reduced in diameter by grinding. A small hole is made in the side of the needle either with a conventional drill or with a dentist's drill. The aperture is made even and smooth by means of dentist's drills of different shapes, manipulated by hand. The syringe mount of the needle is cut off and the opening at this end of the needle carefully ground to remove any edges and avoid subsequent damage to the wires. A copper wire of 0.7 mm diameter, a few centimeters long, is soldered to this end of the needle and to one of the contacts in a multiway plug, as shown in Fig. 4 and 5. A Cannon or McMurdo plug (Dee-Range) with 15 pins is usually used. To each of the mounting tags of the plug

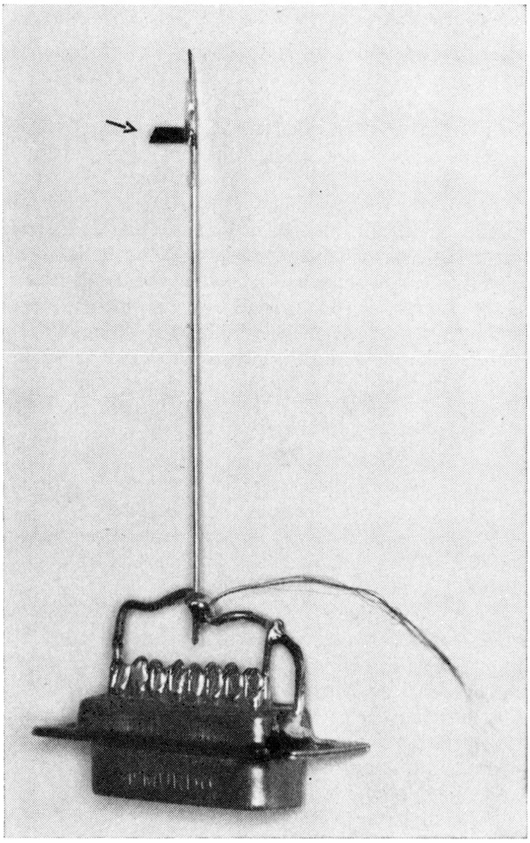

Fig. 4

The needle multi-electrode at a stage when the platinum wires have been introduced in the needle. The Araldite plate (arrow) with the electrode array is inserted in the hole in the side of the needle but not yet fixed.

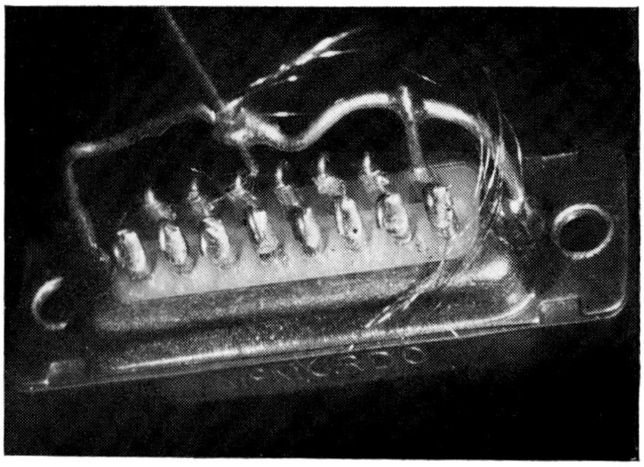

Fig. 5

The multi-way plug. Small hooks of copper have been soldered to the mounting tags of the plug and the platinum wires are to be connected to their appropriate tags.

is soldered a copper wire (diameter 0.2 mm), shaped as a small hook, for attaching the platinum wires.

Mounting of the electrode array in the needle

The free ends of the platinum wires are hooked over a loop of 25 μ tungsten wire and drawn by means of this through the hole in the needle. Ethanol is used as lubricant. The Araldite plate is then placed in its correct position in the hole in the needle with the electrode row exactly parallel to the long axis of the needle. Scotch tape is used to prevent the position of the wires altering during the subsequent procedures.

A small amount of Araldite at a temperature of 70° C is placed in the openings and allowed to be drawn up by capillary forces within the needle. This procedure is repeated until the needle, including the point, is filled. An infra-red lamp is focused on the needle so that a temperature not higher than 70° C is obtained, otherwise the Scotch tape may be damaged and the position of the array altered. During the following few hours additional drops of resin are applied as required. When the hardening procedure has reached the stage at which the Araldite is no longer mobile, the needle is transferred to an oven and kept for 2 h at a temperature of 160° C.

The resin and the platinum wires that extend outside the hole in the side of the needle are now ground flush with the needle surface with emery paper. The grinding procedure may be continued until the outer diameter over the whole needle is reduced to about 0.5 mm. The final grinding is performed with a fine emery polishing paper (No. 3/0, Behr-Manning Co., Troy, N.Y.) which gives an extremely smooth surface.

Identification of the leading-off surfaces and mounting of the plug

The plug and needle are adjusted to their final positions and the platinum wires are cut to appropriate lengths. The outer few millimeters of the wires are de-insulated by rapidly dipping them into concentrated sulfuric acid, after which they are thoroughly rinsed in water so that no acid is left which could later damage the insulation and the wires.

The needle is inserted through the wall of a small rubber cap (the plug of an injection bottle) until the array of leading-off surfaces occupies the center of the cap, which is then filled with 0.9% NaCl. A platinum needle is also inserted into the cap. The positive pole of a 4.5 V battery is connected to the platinum needle (the shaft of the needle electrode must not be used for this purpose as this will cause corrosion of the stainless steel). The negative pole of the battery is connected via a 100 kΩ resistor to a watchmaker's forceps. The electrode array is studied in the microscope and, one by one, the platinum wires are held at their uninsulated ends with the forceps. The respective leading-off surfaces can easily be recognized by the small gas bubbles that form on its surface. The wire can then be applied to the correct pin in the multi-way plug. The wires are twisted tightly around the small hooks in the plug, previously described.

The wires are difficult to solder to the hooks because the surface forces prevent them from tinning. Hence, the electrical connection is made by applying a drop of silver color to each connection. The silver color (Leitsilber 200, Deutsche Gold- und Silber-Scheideanstalt, Frankfurt am Main or E-KOTE 40, Epoxy Products, Irvington, N.J., U.S.A.) consists of silver particles, of a size less than 1 μ, suspended in an organic solvent.

A mold is then formed with Scotch tape around the multi-way plug and Araldite is added to the mold. As the needle is subject to most strain at the point where it emerges from the Araldite, this part is strengthened with a stainless steel tube, of outer diameter 1 mm and length 1 cm, which slides over the needle and extends down into the Araldite mold.

After thermal hardening, the plug is trimmed with a knife. A layer of silver color is applied in order to ground the plug. A thin layer of Araldite is applied over the silver color after it has been allowed to dry for 24 h.

Care of the needle

For recording from single muscle fibers it is necessary that the point of the needle is kept as sharp as possible. Any slight upward deflection of the point will damage the muscle fibers immediately in contact with the needle. Therefore, the needle is usually reground before each experiment and this is carried out either with polishing paper or by means of an Arkansas stone. This procedure takes about 15 min.

Buchthal *et al.* (1957) suggested that the electrical noise from the leading-off surfaces could be considerably reduced by electrolytic treatment. The technique described above for identifying the electrodes is used and 10 μA passed through each leading-off surface (which will be the negative pole) for 10 sec before each experiment.

SUMMARY

This paper describes the construction of a needle multi-electrode in which fourteen 25 μ platinum leading-off surfaces are mounted in epoxy resin in an opening in the side of an injection needle, 0.5–0.6 mm in diameter.

RÉSUMÉ

CONSTRUCTION D'AIGUILLES MULTI-ÉLECTRODES POUR L'ÉLECTROMYOGRAPHIE DE LA FIBRE UNIQUE

Ce travail décrit la construction d'une aiguille multi-électrodes dans laquelle quatorze surfaces de contact en platine de 25 μ sont montées sur résine époxique dans une ouverture latérale d'une aiguille à injection de 0,5–0,6 mm de diamètre.

This work was supported by the Swedish Medical Research Council (Grant No. 14x-135), the Magnus Bergwalls Foundation and the Swedish Association against Poliomyelitis.

REFERENCES

BUCHTHAL, F., GULD, C. and ROSENFALCK, P. Volume conduction of the spike of the motor unit potential investigated with a new type of multielectrode. *Acta physiol. scand.*, **1957,** *38*: 331–354.

EKSTEDT, J. Human single muscle fiber action potentials. *Acta physiol. scand.*, **1964,** *61*, *Suppl. 226*: 1–96.

STÅLBERG, E. Propagation velocity in human muscle fibers *in situ*. *Acta physiol. scand.*, **1966,** *70*, *Suppl. 287*: 1–112.

Reference: EKSTEDT, J., HÄGGQVIST, P. and STÅLBERG, E. The construction of needle multi-electrodes for single fiber electromyography. *Electroenceph. clin. Neurophysiol.*, **1969,** *27*: 540–543.

Electroencephalography and Clinical Neurophysiology
Elsevier Publishing Company, Amsterdam – Printed in The Netherlands

SOCIETY PROCEEDINGS

EASTERN ASSOCIATION OF ELECTROENCEPHALOGRAPHERS

New York, December 4, 1968

Secretary: M. TARLAU

80-02 Kew Gardens Road, New York, N.Y. 11415 (U.S.A.)

1. EEG abnormality in first grade children with "soft" neurological signs. — M. A. Kennard (Manchester, N.H.).

For about 30 years the findings reported by Jasper and Bradley concerning EEG abnormalities in young children with disorders of behavior have been discussed in relation to organic brain disorders. Short span of attention, easy distractibility, and some delays in learning occur in many of these children. This has been closely related in older children to behavior disorders, many of them primary and without any suggestion of organic brain disorder in the history.

In the present study a group of 80 normal first grade children has been compared with children of similar age brought to a psychiatrist for school difficulties. Both groups have been rated for "soft" neurological signs; *e.g.*, speech defects, left–right confusion, mixed dominance, difficulty in hopping, and in fine manipulation of fingers.

There is a significant difference in EEG between the two groups: those (ages 5 or 6 and in first grade) who were developmentally younger in motor coordination and those who, although not chronologically different, show a more mature motor system. Abnormal EEGs are significantly greater among the children with "soft" neurological signs.

In an older group of patients, ages 7 through 9 inclusive, "soft" neurological signs diminished. This was much more marked among girls than among boys. Since there are relatively 3–4 unsuccessful boy children in first grade, as compared to girls, this may be significant.

The abnormal EEG recognized for many years becomes thus an immature EEG and the explanation of more EEG abnormalities with boys in this group is now explicable.

2. Prolonged recording of EEG by radiotelemetry: an aid to localization and treatment of epilepsy. — J. R. Stevens, V. M. Milstein and S. Dodds (Portland, Ore.).

Not infrequently, particularly in patients with psychomotor epilepsy, scalp, sphenoidal, and even chronic subdural or intracerebral electrodes give ambiguous information with respect to the localization of the primary seizure focus. Activation procedures, including i.v. or intracarotid analeptics or barbiturates may only add to the confusion by producing inconsistent results, both with one another and upon successive occasions. If localizing radiological changes are also equivocal or absent, surgical intervention is generally inadvisable. Electrical monitoring of EEG by radiotelemetry has been undertaken from chronic scalp, intracranial or sphenoidal sites from patients hospitalized and maintained on reduced anticonvulsant medication. The technique requires little supervision and results have been unexpectedly rewarding: spontaneous attacks with clearly lateralized onset have been recorded in all cases studied to date. 24–48 h recordings from freely moving patients also greatly assist in the rapid evaluation of drug regimens, particularly in young or retarded patients with frequent minor seizures largely unrecognized by medical supervisory personnel. Details of technique, data analysis, and results are presented.

3. EEG changes after intravenous diazepam (Valium). A preliminary report. — E. Niedermeyer (Baltimore, Md.).

The most impressive effect of diazepam on the EEG was noted with recurrent generalized synchronous seizure discharges. Hyperventilation-induced bursts of 3/sec spike-wave complexes were completely suppressed when overbreathing was repeated immediately after the injection of 5 mg diazepam (when the patient was still sufficiently alert to perform satisfactory hyperventilation). Flicker-induced paroxysmal bursts were also completely suppressed when this activation was repeated immediately after administration of 5 mg.

Patients with bilateral synchronous seizure discharges in the routine sleep EEG showed a burst-free period lasting from 5 to 20 min when sleep was induced with 10 mg diazepam. During this period there was a depression of vertex waves and K complexes while spindles were present. The induced fast activity was detectable for a variable length of time.

Patients with inter-ictal generalized synchronous seizure activity failed to show any response to i.v. diazepam.

Focal spikes were either slightly reduced or unchanged after the i.v. administration of diazepam. In one patient with depth electrodes, sharp activity in the right peri-amygdaloid region was enhanced after the injection.

Diazepam was also used for muscular relaxation in tense patients and for reduction of local muscle spasm in patients with sphenoidal electrodes; the technical quality of the record was greatly improved during the following period of 10–20 min.

There is reason to assume that diazepam will provide us with further insight into the mechanisms involved in generalized epilepsies. The long-term therapeutic value of diazepam cannot be assessed on the basis of our data.

4. Observations on DC potentials in the human EEG. — R. Cohn (Bethesda, Md.).

Negative DC shifts are by far the most usual finding with DC recordings during paroxysmal activity. Positive DC shifts, however, do occur. Positive DC shifts have been observed in the frontal regions in two cases of Dawson's inclusion body encephalitis, usually as part of the "periodic" bursts. Positive DC shifts are also recognized in some individuals in both the frontal and occipital regions during paroxysmal activity. The positive discharges from the occipital regions of the head during the electric discharge appear to be an expression of a "dipole" action in that a concomitant high voltage negative shift is seen in the frontal regions. Negative DC shifts are observed in the great majority of individuals who generate frontal slow activity during hyperventilation. Positive and negative DC shifts, generally of small amplitude, are observed during certain phases of intermediate depth sleep. DC shifts, of either polarity, appear to be the consequence of high voltage synchronized cortical activity.

5. Studies on the pathophysiology of "centrencephalic" epilepsy. — E. Rodin, T. Onuma, S. Wasson and J. Porzak (Detroit, Mich.).

The pathophysiologic mechanisms underlying grand-mal seizures that appear to be generalized from the start are still inadequately understood. A common concept is that these seizures are due to excessive firing of the brain-stem reticular formation or its thalamic counterpart.

A series of cats with chronic electrode implantations in various deep cerebral structures, as well as in cortical regions, were subjected to intraperitoneal injection of Megimide. The electrical seizure activity started in nearly all instances in the cortex and not in thalamus or brainstem. Among cortical structures, the cingulate gyrus showed usually largest amplitude seizure activity. The spikes accompanying myoclonic jerks which preceded the seizure were also usually of largest amplitude in the cortex rather than in the depth. Photic stimulation during seizure induction showed that the spikes which preceded generalized seizures were related to normal photic evoked response characteristics and consisted of a marked exaggeration of the secondary response components. The hypothesis is therefore advanced that the electrical expression of "centrencephalic" epilepsy is a cortical phenomenon related to those neuronal populations that deal with the elaboration of the secondary evoked response characteristics. Instead of postulating excessive activity in deeper structures of the brain, it is proposed that normal impulses coming from the depth find the cortex in a hypersensitive state leading to seizure production.

6. Some observations on the electrophysiology of timing in the nervous system. — J. S. Barlow (Boston, Mass.).

In previous work evidence was found suggesting that occasionally omitted flashes in a periodically presented series of click–flash pairs were accompanied by EEG "responses" time-locked to the absent or "limped" stimuli and the same phenomenon occurred when flashes alone were presented periodically, occasional flashes being deleted.

The present experiments were carried out to explore the latter phenomenon. Vertex, midparietal and occipital EEGs referred to linked ears, as well as vertical EOGs (electro-oculograms) were recorded in 6 subjects with eyes closed under different experimental conditions. Stimuli were 500 flashes at a 1 f/sec among which 100 flashes were deleted in a semi-random manner. The EEGs and EOGs were averaged so as to display, on a single 2.5 sec time base, events time-locked to the flashes immediately preceding and immediately following as well as to the deleted flashes themselves.

Most subjects showed a positive deflection at the vertex, beginning approximately 100–150 msec and peaking some 300 msec following the instant at which the deleted flash would have occurred. The positivity, much less evident at the occiput, was most prominent during attention to the flashes (*e.g.*, counting the actual or the "limped" flashes), being little or not evident at rest. Simultaneous averaging of the EOGs clearly eliminated eye movements as an explanation.

These findings, which indicate a form of temporal conditioning of the EEG, are discussed in relation to the general problem of the neurophysiological basis of timing in the nervous system in its two aspects; *i.e.*, basic rhythmic mechanisms and accumulating or totaling mechanisms.

7. Intracellular studies of amygdaloid neurons: synaptic events initiated by caudate and thalamic stimulation. — M. Santini and D. P. Purpura (New York, N.Y.).

Intracellular recordings (K^+-citrate filled micro-pipettes) were obtained from neurons in the amygdaloid complex during low frequency stimulation of the caudate nucleus and different medial and intralaminar thalamic nuclei. Amygdaloid neurons characteristically exhibit prominent depolarizing after-potentials whereas post-spike hyperpolarizations are rarely observed. Approximately 30–40% of amygdaloid neurons exhibit 4–10 msec latency EPSPs of 15–30 msec duration. EPSPs are invariably succeeded by IPSPs of 60–100 msec duration. Frequently the first caudate stimulus is ineffective in eliciting an IPSP but subsequent stimuli of a repetitive train produce IPSP augmentation. Some cells exhibiting this PSP sequence are also responsive to thalamic stimulation, but latencies and temporal characteristics of thalamic evoked PSPs differ considerably. IPSP alternation patterns observed in previous studies of thalamic neurons are also noted in amygdaloid neurons during thalamic stimulation. Spontaneously occurring IPSPs of long duration are common in amygdaloid neurons during their spontaneous activity. Inactivation responses are frequently observed in amygdaloid neurons. These may be interrupted by caudate stimulation which induces an EPSP–IPSP sequence. Double and triple spikes of progressively increasing amplitude and duration are also encountered in amygdaloid neurons. These and other features of amygdaloid neuron spike potentials and synaptic events differ from characteristics of caudate, lenticular, neocortical and thalamic neurons. Events reminiscent of the activities of hippocampal pyramidal neurons and "climbing fiber responses" of Purkinje cells are detectable in amygdaloid neurons. Evidently these events are not referable to unique features of the geometry of amygdaloid neurons or their excitatory synaptic input.

8. Comparison of synaptic effects of internal capsule and caudate stimulation on thalamic neurons. — T. L. Frigyesi and J. Machek (Bronx, N.Y.).

Intracellular studies were performed in neurons of the dorsal thalamus during low frequency (8/sec) stimulation of the head of the caudate nucleus (Cd) and of adjacent internal capsule (IC). Stimulation of Cd commonly generated polysynaptic EPSPs and succeeding IPSPs in these neurons. IPSPs elicited by stimulation of Cd generally exhibited shorter latencies (20–40 msec) in neurons in the medial and dorso-lateral thalamus than in neurons in the VA–VL region (40–60 msec). Latencies of Cd evoked IPSPs as short as 8 msec were observed in the intralaminar nuclei. On the other hand, stimulation of IC elicited antidromic potentials and/or oligosynaptic EPSPs in the VA–VL region and generally complex, polysynaptic EPSPs in medial and dorso-lateral thalamus. IPSPs elicited by capsular stimulation exhibited shortest latencies of 4–8 msec in these thalamic nuclei. PSPs evoked by IC and Cd stimulation differed not only in terms of latencies but also in mode of development. PSPs generated through caudatofugal and through cortico-thalamic synaptic pathways could be distinguished in each neuron by temporal properties of build-up. The data indicate synaptic pathways arising in the head of the caudate produce excitatory and inhibitory PSPs in medial, dorsolateral, and ventro-lateral thalamus. Caudatofugal synaptic pathways involved in the production of both EPSPs and IPSPs in the dorsal thalamus are distinct from those capsular elements which also generate PSPs in neurons in the same thalamic regions.

9. Applications of interpolation and area display in EEG. — F. E. McGee Jr., R. G. Lee, J. A. Harris, G. Melby and R. G. Bickford (Rochester, Minn.).

During the last 2 years Harris and Melby have developed CDC 3200 computer programs and associated hardware in this laboratory which allow: (1) viewing the potential field data contained in the EEG as a four-dimensional "hill-valley" display in space and time; (2) mathematical interpolation of the data from 16 (4×4) sampling points of the scalp array to develop 400 "statistical electrodes" (with an acceptable error) covering the area. Computer techniques can then be used to sample the conventional EEG between any of these 400 data points within the array and by any desired montage. Looking at EEG fields in a space domain is novel to the electroencephalographer and has required the re-investigation of potential fields occurring in saline models, in evoked potentials of normal subjects, in spike discharges from the strychninized cortex of animals and in those from patients with epileptic lesions.

Advantages of the system are: (1) transferring the 16 voltage time graphs of the conventional EEG to a potential field plot on the scalp is performed automatically and the result is evident without special EEG training; (2) it provides a generalized approach to problems of electrode placement and montage. Thus, the investigator can test the EEG appearance with individual laboratory placements, with the International System, and by any required montage; (3) spatial and time components of evoked potentials can be effectively separated and many apparent problems in standardization of evoked potentials disappear; (4) conduction of spike foci can be followed spatially, providing important insights into their origin not apparent from the conventional EEG.

10. Distribution of eye movement and eyeblink potentials over the scalp. — D. A. Overton and C. Shagass (Philadelphia, Pa.).

Detailed knowledge of the scalp distribution of orbital potentials resulting from eye movements and eyeblinks is helpful in interpreting surface evoked response recordings. Voltages induced by voluntary blinks following an auditory click and eye movements associated with following a moving light source were recorded in 8 subjects at 25 electrode locations. Amplifier time constant was 10 sec and a CAT averager was used. Inter-subject differences were noted in the size of the potentials recorded but not in the pattern of distribution over the head. Right and left movements produced equal but opposite potentials at all electrodes; a similar trend was noted for up and down movements. The potentials accompanying a 45° diagonal eye movement could be accurately predicted by summing the potentials resulting from movements in the horizontal and vertical planes. Vertical eye movements and eyeblinks produced different patterns of potential distribution over the head. Upward rotation of the cornea induced a positive potential on the forehead and an almost equal negative potential on the face below the eyes. Eyeblinks produced a larger positive forehead potential but only a small negative potential on the lower face. This difference between eye movement and eyeblink potentials recorded near their source was reflected in an altered distribution of these potentials over the entire head. If voltages resulting from eye movements or eyeblinks are measured at vertical and horizontal electrodes placed near the eyes, the data allow a prediction of the propagated potentials recorded between electrodes at other locations on the head.

11. Slow potential shifts in dorsal hippocampus during "epileptogenic" perfusion of the inferior horn with high K^+ CSF. — E. C. Zuckermann and G. H. Glaser (New Haven, Conn.).

Slow potential shifts and responses to ipsi- and contralateral hippocampus stimulation were recorded from basal and apical dendritic layers of dorsal hippocampus in 15 awake cats, using chronically implanted pipettes (50 μ tip) filled with NaCl agar. Perfusion of the inferior horn with CSF in which K^+ concentration was raised from normal 3 mequiv/l to 9–18 mequiv/l induced, after 20–50 sec, an early DC shift (1–3 mV) only in the basal dendritic layer, reaching a plateau after 2–3 min. During this time no changes in the pattern of hippocampal evoked responses were observed. In the following period, while the DC level was constant, large potentials, negative in basal dendrites and positive in apical dendrites, gradually developed in response to single shock stimulation, reaching a peak in 6–15 min when a seizure was triggered. During the last minute preceding the paroxysmal discharge, the main transient of each response was followed by a long lasting negative wave from basal dendrites and a synchronous positive wave from apical dendrites. At this moment a DC shift occurred by the overlapping of the long late waves. Paroxysmal discharges then were superimposed on this DC shift.

It is assumed that the initial DC shift, recorded only from the periventricular electrodes, was connected with changes in ependymovascular membranes, and that the K^+ increased epileptogenic excitability by another mechanism than a global gradual depolarization of neurons. The slow potential shift accompanying the seizure was generated apparently by the development of "paroxysmal depolarization and hyperpolarization shifts" at the level of basal and apical dendrites.

12. Anatomical substrates of descending hippocampal influences. — F. K. Redding (Detroit, Mich.).

The effects of repetitive stimulation of the hippocampus upon visual cortical evoked potentials have been studied in the *encéphale isolé* cat. Previous studies produced evidence for mixed facilitatory and inhibitory effects on upper and lower parts of the brain-stem arousal system, respectively. Routes of transmission of these influences were investigated by comparing the effect of hippocampal stimulation before and after bilateral lesions in the fornix or upper part of the septum. Previously this type of evaluation in the *cerveau isolé* preparation, in which the facilitatory effect alone is manifest, has shown that the effect is transmitted bilaterally in the fornix to some rostral elements of the brain-stem arousal system.

In some experiments the amplitudes of all waves of the visual evoked potential decreased during and after hippocampal stimulation, while in other experiments amplitudes increased. In a minority there was no significant change. In almost every instance, the change in amplitude produced by stimulation was abolished or markedly attenuated after bilateral fornix or septum lesions. Hippocampal stimulation produced no significant changes in blood pressure, pulse, temperature, and only slight and inconsistent changes in neocortical electrical activity. This was true both before and after fornix and septum lesions.

These results are interpreted as further confirmation of a dual counter-balancing effect transmitted from the hippocampus: facilitatory on upper brain-stem or thalamic centers, and inhibitory on lower brain-stem structures. In the *encéphale isolé* preparation sometimes one and sometimes the other predominates. Both facilitatory and inhibitory influences are transmitted from the hippocampus bilaterally via septum and fornix.

13. Effects of brain-stem stimulation, rapid eye movements and alerting of LGB transmission in monkeys. — B. Cohen, M. Feldman and S. Diamond (New York, N.Y.).

Lateral geniculate body (LGB) potentials induced by optic tract shocks were not significantly affected by reticular formation, saccades, or quick phases of nystagmus in alert animals in darkness. The initial portion of calcarine cortex potentials induced by optic tract stimuli were similarly unaffected. On the other hand retrograde optic tract potentials evoked by LGB stimulation were enhanced in alert monkeys after stimulation of the brain-stem reticular formation. This appeared to be due to a process associated with alerting since, after administration of amphetamine, retrograde optic tract potentials were continuously close to maximum amplitude and enhancement associated with brain-stem stimulation was reduced. In any state of alertness, retrograde optic tract potentials induced by LGB stimuli were not affected by rapid eye movements (REMs). In the drowsy monkey, orthograde LGB, calcarine, and retrograde optic tract potentials were concurrently enhanced by reticular formation stimulation or by sensory stimulation which produced alerting.

From these data it would appear that stimulation of the brain-stem reticular formation activates at least two processes in LGB. One produces the LGB negativity associated with REMs. The second is responsible for the enhancement of retrograde optic tract potentials induced by LGB shocks. It has been postulated that depolarization of retinal ganglion cell axon terminals in LGB causes the enhancement of retrograde optic tract potentials after brain-stem stimulation. This implies that pathways originating in the brain-stem mediate pre-synaptic inhibition onto retinal ganglion cell axons in LGB. If this were true, then some inhibition of orthograde LGB and calcarine potentials should be demonstrable when there was enhancement of retrograde optic tract potentials. Since this did not occur in the alert monkey, this explanation of the phenomena may be incorrect.

14. Analysis of acoustically evoked scalp potentials by cross correlation of EEG with prescribed template. — A. J. Derbyshire, S. B. Osenar, L. R. Hamilton and M. E. Joseph (Chicago, Ill.).

Psychological events are a sequence of individual, continually varying phenomena. To study the relation of EEG to such central processes as perception, it is essential to have a method which reliably detects an EEG response to a single stimulus. Cross correlation acts as a highly specific filter for patterns of complex form and could therefore describe an EEG response which occurs to any single verbal stimulus. Since interest here is centered on that part of the event which is common to all men, it is expedient to use several subjects at each experiment. This procedure algebraically sums the EEGs of the several subjects into one tracing (a "group noodle") and creates an experimental procedure which is identical and simultaneous for all subjects. The correlograms that result from the cross correlations between a template, the ideal response filter, and a "group noodle" EEG permit a promising degree of detection of signal. Ratio of probability of detecting signal when present to detecting signal when not present is 0.7(d^1). Detection of signal is a function of (1) the sound structure of the word within its first 100 msec; (2) the composition of the subject group and its variation in age, sex, etc.; and (3) the shape of the template.

15. Occipital alpha activity during accommodative vergence, pursuit tracking and saccadic eye movements. — T. Mulholland (Bedford, Mass.).

Occipital alpha rhythm was evaluated during various eye movements recorded using the EOG technique. A subjective estimate of target clearness was also recorded. Alpha activity occurred more often and with larger amplitude under all conditions where there was no pursuit tracking of the moving target. More alpha activity occurred during continuous saccadic movement compared to continuous pursuit tracking movements.

The duration of successive alpha and no alpha events were evaluated for each condition. These yield the familiar habituation functions:

$$\Delta t_{\text{alpha}} = aN + b;\ \Delta t_{\text{no alpha}} = \frac{c}{N} + d$$

N is the serial number of successive events (Mulholland and Runnals, *Electroenceph. clin. Neurophysiol.*, 1964, *17*: 371). The values of the parameters of the habituation functions were different for the various viewing conditions: b for pursuit tracking was smaller than for conditions of relaxed accommodation and no tracking; for the same conditions, c and d were larger. No definite change occurred for a. Thus alpha rhythm was observed to occur in a regular way, though less frequently, for the condition of focussing and pursuit tracking a moving target. Conversely, there was increased alpha activity and a greatly reduced initial "activation" or alpha blocking for the condition of relaxed accommodation and no pursuit tracking.

16. A biopotential analog. — G. Schuler (Ottawa, Ont., Canada).

A biopotential analog presently under construction is a device which will acquire and process numerous body surface signals to effect a more sensitive and discrete means for their study.

In a prospective EEG study, 100 electrodes would be applied to acquire the variety of signals found on all areas of the scalp. 100 ultra low-noise amplifiers with interconnected input stage emitters, simulating a common average-signal reference, amplify and condition the signals so that with matched gains and matched upper and lower frequency attenuation curves, the 100 output signals represent the signal voltages existing between each scalp electrode and the average of all electrodes. These 100 signals are then applied to the periphery of a resistive homolog of the head so that the scalp potential pattern is duplicated in a greatly amplified form upon the periphery of the resistive homolog. The homolog, a weakly saline aqueous solution enclosed within a plastic replica of the head, has its volume available for signal exploration by probes placed through the neck of the homolog. In theory, the sites of particular electrical signals might be localized, or the signals of particular sites might be examined.

With special low-noise amplifiers having about one-tenth the noise of present day EEG amplifiers, and with the benefits of parallel averaging inherent in a 100-channel biopotential analog, an equivalent noise level in the low nanovolt region should reveal many useful signals heretofore undetectable.

The employment of this technique should greatly facilitate the detection and localization of epileptic sites, the origin and propagation path of evoked potentials, and perhaps aid in non-mechanical communication with the brain.

17. Background activity in evoked potentials. — J. Woods and R. J. Broughton (Montreal, P.Q., Canada).

Summation of an evoked response allows the signal to be identified while the non-stimulus-lock background activity is increasingly cancelled. The interaction between this background activity, or biological "noise", and the evoked potential is difficult to assess but cannot be ignored.

The techniques currently used to estimate the noise at the time of the response are not reliable because they fail to consider the effect of the stimulus on the background activity. This difficulty is especially obvious in excitability cycles when the inter-stimulus interval is shorter than the duration of the response to single stimuli. The overlapping portions of the two responses are greatly altered by superimposition and biological interaction. Subtracting summated responses to single stimuli from the combined responses to the paired stimuli only increases distortion of the response.

Different types of background activity produce different effects on the evoked responses. Failure to recognize this seriously weakens any attempt to ascribe physiological or pathological significance to alterations in the form of responses evoked under different conditions (*e.g.*, during wakefulness, sleep, or during epileptic seizures). Efforts must be directed toward understanding the effects of stimuli on background cerebral activity before such interpretations can be made.

18. EEG and cerebral death. The neurologist's view.— D. Silverman and R. Masland (Philadelphia, Pa.), M. G. Saunders (Winnipeg, Man., Canada) and R. S. Schwab (Boston, Mass.).

Analysis of a questionnaire sent to neurologists on EEG criteria of cerebral death (irreversible coma) revealed that of 344 neurologists, 31 had no experience with this problem. 54 maintained the only criterion of death was cessation of cardiac function but an equal number accepted the state of coma *dépassé* with an isoelectric record of 1 h duration sufficient, while 63 would wait 12 h; 90, 24 h; and 43, 48 h. The majority (173) would not accept the EEG alone as a criterion but 94 would. Almost all who answered believed that a new definition of brain death was important in case of donor for transplants (285) and in the case of an irreversible coma patient on a respirator (270). Most (201) did not feel these concepts were premature. Potential dangers or errors were seen in the following categories: medico-legal complications (48), unsuspected CNS depressants (41), overlooked extreme hypothermia (4), misjudging of the irreversibility of the coma (33), removal of organs from live persons (15), lack of unequivocal clinical findings (31), and inaccurate EEG apparatus, technique or interpretation (35). Interesting individual comments from the respondents were discussed.

Electroenceph. clin. Neurophysiol., **1969,** *27*: 544–549

SOUTHERN ELECTROENCEPHALOGRAPHIC SOCIETY

Birmingham, Ala., October 25–27, 1968

Secretary: R. L. GREEN, JR., M.D.

Veterans Administration Hospital, Durham, N.C. 27705 (U.S.A.)

1. Electroencephalography's increasing debt to technology. — M. A. B. Brazier (Los Angeles, Calif.).

The increasing capabilities for EEG analysis that computers have made available in the last two decades were described. Emphasis was given especially to clinical applications with examples of 9 categories of computer analysis that have been applied in disease states.

The 9 categories are: time series; frequency spectra; cross-correlation and cross-spectra; evoked potentials; variability; unit analysis; pattern recognition; spatio-temporal distribution; and tremendously accelerated ability to test hypotheses.

What emerges for the clinical worker is the need for, and a trend towards analysis in both time and space. The early methods treated the EEG as a single voltage-time curve; the next step was to a study of the interrelation between pairs of electrode locations, but now the most important advance for clinical EEG is the ability to analyze, quantify and display potentials from many electrode positions simultaneously in both time and space. Four different methods for achieving this end were illustrated (the methods of Rémond, of Harris, of Estrin and of the author).

One characteristic of all the categories illustrated is that they present averaged data and the result derived is in terms of probability. This parallels the recognition of a great change that has taken place in scientists' thinking; *i.e.*, the change from the old deterministic view of the nervous system to a probabilistic one. The concept of statistical probability, rather than one-to-one cause and effect, is now recognized as closer to the mechanisms of the nervous system — and this information is what our computers can easily give us.

2. EEG findings in Devic's disease. — E. L. Reilly and W. P. Wilson (Durham, N.C.).

Devic's disease, or neuromyelitis optica, is a rare syndrome which clinically presents with the association of sudden vision loss and associated involvement of the spinal cord. In this country, the combination of symptoms has been felt by many to represent a variety of multiple sclerosis.

A total of 15 EEGs were done on 9 patients with this syndrome. Six of the 9 patients had one or more abnormal tracings. Five of the patients were males with an age range of 9–37 years. The median age of the males was 10. Four females with an average age of 6 were examined. Four EEGs were obtained a week or less after the onset of vision loss. Three were normal and one demonstrated diffuse slowing with temporal region attenuation. Seven records were done more than a week, but less than 2 months, after the onset of visual symptoms. One of these records was borderline normal and the other 6 were abnormal records with excessive slowing. Most commonly, this slowing consisted of mixed theta and delta waves; on several occasions, the delta activity was paroxysmal. From these observations it would appear that diffuse abnormal slowing is considerably more frequent in Devic's disease than is generally seen in multiple sclerosis. This difference may relate to the age range of the patients involved or to the observation of others that Devic's disease is associated with more gray matter involvement than multiple sclerosis.

3. Long-term prognosis of petit mal epilepsy. — D. A. Barnhart, T. D. Newsom, J. W. Crawley and T. E. Zion (Houston, Texas).

Before the advent of EEG, almost any type of minor seizure

short of a fully developed tonic-clonic convulsion was labeled "petit mal". In 1935, Gibbs and Gibbs described the 3/sec spike and wave EEG pattern which is now considered to be essential to the clinical diagnosis of petit mal epilepsy. Because "petit mal" was once a collective term for many types of seizure disorders, the long-term prognosis of petit mal epilepsy is obscure. Previous studies attempting to define the natural history of petit mal epilepsy have been inadequate because the samples have been small, the duration of follow-up has been short, and many of the patients have been prepubescent.

The present study is of a group of 50 patients in whom the diagnosis of petit mal was made using the following criteria: (1) the onset in childhood of clinical petit mal "absence" seizures; (2) demonstration of the 3/sec spike and wave pattern in the EEG; and (3) the absence of any neurological abnormality on examination. All of the patients included in this study were 16 years of age or older.

Our data demonstrate that the probability of the persistence of petit mal epilepsy into adult life is greatly increased in a child who has had grand mal as well as petit mal seizures. Specifically, 83% of those patients whose petit mal seizures persisted into adult life had associated grand mal convulsions. Of the patients who had petit mal seizures alone, only 13% continued to have seizures at the time of re-evaluation.

In addition, the following observations were made: the age of onset of petit mal epilepsy is rarely, if ever, before 3 years of age, or later than puberty. If cessation of seizures does occur, it will occur before 20 years of age. The hormonal and physiological changes associated with puberty do not appear to be the cause of cessation of attacks. The preponderance of petit mal seizures in females gives reason to question the contention that petit mal is an autosomal dominant trait. Petit mal patients are generally of average intelligence.

4. The EEG in subacute sclerosing panencephalitis (SSPE). — H. Lemmi (Memphis, Tenn.).

Eight patients from the Memphis area, all males ranging in age from 2 years and 8 months to 12 years, were studied by serial EEGs for a period of 2 years. In addition to the clinical picture, the diagnosis was established by elevated gamma globulin in the CSF and elevated titers for measles on both hemagglutination inhibition and complement-fixation tests in the CSF and serum. Brain biopsy in 3 cases demonstrated changes compatible with encephalitis, and the presence of virus-like inclusion bodies was verified by electron microscope.

Forty-two tracings were analyzed and the following were noted: (1) irregularity and slowing of the background activity was in every case present early in the disease: in all cases which were followed through the full course of the disease the background abnormality improved in the later phases of the evolution; (2) SSPE complexes appeared within the first month of the disease and persisted throughout the follow-up period, becoming less prominent in the later phases; (3) in general, a greater frequency of recurrence of the SSPE complexes was associated with the progression of the disease; (4) sharp and spike waves, independent of the SSPE complexes, were seen in *all* patients and were unrelated to the evolution of the disease; (5) slow foci, not related to sites of biopsies were seen in 4 patients; in one the focus disappeared in a follow-up study; (6) suppression bursts were seen in 3 patients.

These observations of the EEG evolution of SSPE have revealed changes in cortical electrical activity paralleling the clinical condition in more consistent fashion than previously reported.

5. Temporal lobe seizures and exhibitionism. — H. Hooshmand (Richmond, Va.).

Two cases suffering from temporal lobe seizures, and having automatisms simulating "exhibitionism", are reported. Both cases were involved in legal suits for "exhibitionism". In the first case, with a sole manifestation of indecent public exposure strongly simulating exhibitionism, the scalp EEG showed a left temporal spike focus. Medical treatment has controlled the patient's symptoms for the past year. In the second case, the patient had a right temporal glioblastoma. Scalp EEGs were not significant. Electrocorticography revealed slow arrhythmic waves, and spike activity at the edge of the tumor. After partial removal of the tumor and radiotherapy, the patient has been rendered free from the attacks of "exhibitionism".

The second patient is the sixth reported case with brain tumor and evidence of focal ventricular dilatation on air studies.

Major points of differentiation between true exhibitionism and ictal indecent exposure are discussed. EEG may be very helpful in achieving a more accurate diagnosis.

6. Photically evoked responses in the subcortex of man. — W. P. Wilson and B. S. Nashold (Durham, N.C.).

A study of direct visual inputs to the mesencephalon and diencephalon of man was performed using multiple contact stainless steel electrodes which were implanted in a variety of subcortical nuclei including the lateral geniculate nuclei. Single and multiple flashes were presented on several occasions and a plot of the response areas was made. It was observed that responses could be recorded from the medial tegmentum, tectum, and ventral medial diencephalon. These responses were of short latency. Stimulation of these same nuclei resulted in eye movement, emotional, autonomic and sensory responses. On one occasion, stimulation of the colliculus resulted in a sensation that was described as resembling scintillating scotomata.

It was concluded that these findings confirm similar observations in animals. As stimulation responses were varied, it seems likely that sensory motor integration occurs in these structures.

7. Statistical analysis of EEG–single neuron relationships. — J. D. Frost Jr. (Houston, Texas).

A statistical method for analyzing relationships existing between EEG activity and neuronal spike discharges is described. A three-dimensional selective amplitude histogram shows the frequency of occurrence of EEG amplitudes as a function of single unit discharge time. This graph and related statistical derivations permit detection and quantification of non-random EEG–single unit correlations.

Analysis of data obtained from the cat cerebral cortex under a variety of experimental conditions (neuronally isolated cortex, midpontine-pretrigeminal preparation, barbiturate anesthesia, ether anesthesia) has shown that consistent and statistically significant correlations often exist between the discharge time of a single neuron and the surface EEG amplitude. These relationships are commonly not evident to the human observer of photographic records.

This method appears to offer a means for classifying a particular neuron in terms of its behavior as a member of a larger population, and thus neighboring neurons, recorded at different times, may be compared with each other in terms of their mutual participation in the process producing EEG activity.

8. Diencephalic lesion effects on EEG sleep patterns. — M. F. Jurko and O. J. Andy (Jackson, Miss.).

The objective of the present study was to correlate various scalp EEG sleep patterns with their respective site of thalamic origin.

Sleep EEG patterns were studied in 20 Parkinson patients following thalamotomy. A major objective was to determine whether or not frontal sleep spindles were primarily associated with medial dorsal, and parietal spindles with lateral thalamic lesions.

Results: The lesions placed in the medial anterior thalamus which implicated the intralaminar structures and medial dorsal nucleus were primarily accompanied by ipsilateral changes in the EEG sleep pattern. Those lesions in the lateral thalamus were accompanied by bilateral changes in the sleep pattern. The parietal spindles were more attenuated than the frontal spindles following placement of lesions in both the medial and lateral thalamic areas. Parietal humps and K complexes were also attenuated but not differentially affected with respect to their scalp distribution. In a third group of patients the lesions were placed in the area of the centrum medianum nucleus. It is of special interest to note that lesions implicating the latter nucleus were not accompanied by changes in spontaneous EEG sleep patterns.

9. Clinical electroencephalography and the law. Moot trials. — *Presiding Judge, 10th Judicial Circuit of Alabama*, **Honorable T. E. Huey Jr.**; *Lawyers*: **T. E. Embry, H. W. Peterson, R. Beddow Jr. and R. T. McDonald (Birmingham, Ala.)**; *Clinical electroencephalographers*: **W. P. Wilson (Durham, N.C.), C. E. Henry (Cleveland, Ohio), R. M. Paddison (New Orleans, La.) and J. Knott (Iowa City, Iowa)**; *EEG technician*: **Mrs. S. Sharp (Birmingham, Ala.)**; *Discussants of proceedings*: **Honorable S. H. Lynne (Birmingham, Ala.), D. D. Daly (Dallas, Texas) and S. C. Little (Birmingham, Ala.).**

A. Civil case. This is a tort action wherein the plaintiff is seeking damages for personal injuries sustained in an automobile accident from the defendant in the amount of $50,000. Patient experienced transient period of unconsciousness when his head struck the windshield. Brief hospitalization revealed no noticeable injuries. Three months post-accident, plaintiff developed headaches and dizziness, within 6 months marked personality changes were noted. Decrease in intellectual functioning making it impossible for plaintiff to satisfactorily perform his job as an executive was also noted. Local medical doctor of 20 years duration reports plaintiff to be in good health until the head injury except for mild hypertension, mild diabetes mellitus and possibly general arteriosclerosis. Due to impairment of intellectual functioning and personality changes, the local medical doctor requested an EEG as a diagnostic aid. Moot trial carried out with utilization of electroencephalographers as expert witnesses for both the plaintiff and defense. Judgement rendered by jury.

B. Criminal case. Defendant accused of first degree murder of 3 persons following a minor automobile accident in which the defendant was involved with the 3 victims. Following the accident the defendant suddenly began to use profane language, became very aggressive and waved his arms in a threatening manner. He attacked the victim with a tire iron and battered him to death. Three of the victim's family remaining in the car observed the assault and began to scream, whereupon the defendant turned his attention to them and proceeded to beat them savagely with the tire iron. Two additional persons died of the assault but one recovered to testify to the details of the other three deaths. History revealed numerous episodes of behavior in the past characterized by sullenness, aggressiveness, argumentiveness, ideas and statements suggesting paranoid distortion. In preparation of the defense, psychiatric evaluation was obtained and EEG studies were done. The EEG suggested psychomotor epilepsy. Both prosecution and defense offered testimony from electroencephalographers. Jury verdict, EEG findings and implications were discussed in detail.

Electroenceph. clin. Neurophysiol., **1969**, *27*: 549–551

Electroencephalography and Clinical Neurophysiology
Elsevier Publishing Company, Amsterdam – Printed in The Netherlands

UDRUŽENJE ZA ELEKTROENCEFALOGRAFIJU I KLINIČKU NEUROFIZIOLOGIJU JUGOSLAVIJE

Split, October 19, 1968

Secretary: Dr. V. Dürrigl

Mental Hospital Vrapce, Zagreb (Yugoslavia)

1. Present-day trends in examination of sleep mechanisms. — F. Hajnšek (Zagreb).

Anatomical studies have changed considerably our concept of so called "sleep and wakefulness centres". Presently, several regions in the midline responsible for sleep mechanisms can be differentiated. The main characteristics of rhombencephalic and telencephalic sleep are reported together with various external and internal factors which influence them. These factors may interfere with cyclic periodicity and the shifting of rapid eye movement phases. Sleep studies have become an important parameter in evaluation of, *e.g.*, drug action on the CNS, assessing sleep disturbances in both insomnias and hypersomnias. Recently several promising reports on epilepsy and sleep mechanisms have appeared. Lastly, the results of more recent research in this field are presented.

2. Glycogenic response of CNS to paradoxical sleep deprivation in cats and rats. — V. Karadžić and B. Mršulja (Belgrade).

Selective paradoxical sleep deprivation and its neurochemical effects are not identified clearly. By the finding that telencephalic acetylcholine changes in response to paradoxical sleep, while the norepinephrine and serotonine levels remain unchanged (Bowers *et al.*, *Science*, 1966, *153*: 1416), it was confirmed that paradoxical sleep deprivation leads to certain changes in CNS chemistry.

Our study defines the effects of paradoxical sleep deprivation on glycogen levels in various structures of the brain in cats and rats (especially in those structures which were noted to participate neurophysiologically in paradoxical sleep) because there are "*de norma*" differences in glycogen content. Glycogen fractions were determined, as various fractions can have various functional meanings.

The total of 42 cats and 36 rats was divided into the following groups: (1) normal controls; (2) stress controls; (3) PS-deprived animals; this group was further divided into subgroups, according to the duration of paradoxical sleep deprivation and duration of the post-deprivational period.

The experiments led to the following conclusions: (1) Brain glycogen in cats which were deprived of paradoxical sleep for 96–192 h fell in all the structures examined; this glycogen fall occurred because of the decrease in bound glycogen. (2) 24, 48 and 72 h of PS deprivation in cats did not lead to significant changes of glycogen content in the brain. (3) 72 h of PS deprivation in rats led to a significant fall in total glycogen content on account of the bound glycogen. (4) The control stress group did not show any deviations of glycogen content. (5) In the post-deprivational period glycogen continued to fall during the first 3 h of recuperative sleep and during the next 6 h it reached the pre-deprivational level. (6) As the sleep physiology of rats is similar to that of cats (and man) it seems that rats operate on a shorter time base, because the short PS deprivation in rats is equivalent to a long PS deprivation in cats, at least from the point of view of glycogen changes. (7) Changes in glycogen content represent a biochemical event, not uniformly in the whole brain, but in certain of its structures.

As the glycogen content in the control stress situation remained unchanged, it is very probable that PS deprivation is a specific stress.

3. Clinical and diagnostic significance of the EEG in the course of sleep. — V. Dürrigl (Zagreb).

In the introductory part of this review the diagnostic value of the EEG in the course of sleep was described. Various disturbances of sleep and the outstanding value of the EEG in the differential diagnosis were reviewed. Various classifications, both from the clinical and the pathophysiological points of view, were listed. For a better understanding of the mechanisms of the disturbances of sleep, the following division was accepted: (1) general disturbances of sleep; (2) hypersomnia; (3) hyposomnia. In each group we attempted to present the pathophysiological basis and the corresponding therapy. Enuresis, somnambulism and narcolepsy were presented in more detail, owing to their clinical significance. Hyposomnia of various types allows detailed classification within the group of depressions, as well as the differential diagnosis in a schizophrenic group which, from the therapeutic point of view, is of outstanding importance. In conclusion: (1) the EEG in sleep is often a more valuable method than in the waking state; (2) the EEG in sleep allows a more subtle diagnosis, both scientific and practical neurophysiological. (3) It is thus possible to establish a more precise differential diagnosis within each group of diseases; and (4) the application of an adequate therapy.

4. An electrophysiological study of spinal reflex activity in normal man during sleep. — M. Dimitrijević, J. Faganel and M. Janko (Ljubljana).

Spinal reflex excitability was tested by the Achilles jerk or H reflex and by a polysynaptic reflex, *i.e.*, the flexor response to a noxious cutaneous stimulus, during the various stages of sleep and wakefulness. The stages of sleep were determined by continuous monitoring of EEG, EMG of mental muscles and oculogram. Electromyographically detected H and tendon reflexes, elicited at a rate of 1/5 sec, were recorded on tape and subsequently analysed on a Computer of Average Transients, so that sequential histograms of mean EMG response output were obtained. Latency histograms of polysynaptic reflexes were also computed.

Three investigations out of 18 performed on 14 healthy adults covered all stages of sleep. During the REM stage the H reflexes were completely depressed, while other stages were associated with wide variation in H reflexes. In the case of tendon reflexes, variation was even wider. Polysynaptic flexor reflexes could not be evoked in stages III and IV. The response, which was ample in wakefulness, appeared only when the subjects were brought into light sleep or wakened, which happened after two or three stimuli.

5. Diurnal and nocturnal EEG in patients with insomnia caused by affective psychosis. — K. Barjaktarević-Nikolić and J. Veljković (Belgrade).

In 20 patients with clinical manifestations of endogenous depression and in 10 patients with maniacal psychosis EEGs were recorded. Patients of both groups suffered from insomnia. They were examined during their first hospitalization, and were not treated with drugs. In the analysis of their EEGs, special attention was given to the waking nocturnal EEG trace, recorded all night and analysed every hour. These findings are graphically presented in the paper.

These nocturnal types of EEG trace were the following: (a) low voltage, continuous alpha rhythm in posterior regions with persistence of beta activity anteriorly; (b) generalized alpha activity with short desynchronization periods lasting about 4 sec (maximum 10 sec); (c) generalized desynchronization lasting about 10 min, with short-term hypersynchronous alpha activity for 2–5 sec; (d) uniform generalized slow alpha activity with periodical appearance of low voltage and high frequency spindles; (e) hypersynchronous, generalized alpha activity with generalized theta activity lasting 4–5 min; (f) hypersynchronous alpha activity with short-term phases of delta activity, lasting up to 4 min.

Some differences in the EEG sequences and frequencies found by the authors in the examined clinical categories were: patients with maniacal psychosis showed, in the second half of the night, (e) and (f) types of EEG and, on the contrary, the depressive patients had in the same period (b) and (c) types of EEG traces.

6. Disturbances of wakefulness in narcolepsy. — P. Fildiševski (Skopje).

The author reviews the main clinical characteristics of narcolepsy, stating that, besides attacks of sleep, within the boundaries of the disease can also be found cataplexy, sleep paralysis and nightmares. Contrary to some authors, who recognize "symptomatic" and "genuine" narcolepsy, the author acknowledges full authenticity only of the latter. The work is based on the study of genuine narcolepsy, which is rarely met, so that the author had the opportunity to observe only 14 cases in the past 10 years.

The work deals only with disturbances in the rhythm of wakefulness and sleep which represent the basic characteristics of narcolepsy, offering firstly a description of narcoleptic attacks from the clinical point of view and then presenting the EEG findings. The author regularly found normal alpha rhythm ("hypernormal", according to Gastaut) in the intervals between narcoleptic attacks. The attacks of neuroleptic sleep were manifested by changes seen in stages A and B (according to Loomis, Harvey and Hobart) of the normal sleep of healthy persons. The most characteristic features of narcoleptic sleep are the non-physiological conditions under which a narcoleptic falls asleep.

The work presents some pathophysiological assumptions concerning narcoleptic disturbances of the rhythm of wakefulness. In this sense, the author's opinion is that these are caused by a permanent blockade of the reticular system as the basic pathophysiological disturbance of narcolepsy.

7. Electrogenesis of sleep. — P. Žeškov (Zagreb).

Electro-clinical studies of two types of sleep (slow sleep and paradoxical fast sleep) show a certain parallelism between them from early childhood until death. From this aspect a mechanism of physiological sleep is analysed.

8. Epileptic crises during sleep. — P. Žeškov (Zagreb).

Different epileptic seizures show a certain regularity in appearing during sleep. The author presents two basic types of epileptic discharges, one in slow sleep and the other in paradoxical sleep. Bilaterally synchronous discharges, like spike and wave complexes, seem to appear more as the first type, whereas the focal psychomotor epileptic attacks occur as the second type.

9. Some characteristics of all-night sleep recordings in schizophrenic patients. — V. Rogina, V. Dürrigl and N. Madjarević (Zagreb).

The techniques of all-night sleep polygraphic recording and the methods of analysis and processing of the observed data were described. Twenty-four 8-hour all-night recordings were made on 6 subjects (3 normal healthy persons and 3 acute schizophrenic patients). Prior to therapy the schizophrenics showed reduced total sleep time and REM percentage, but increased total REM time and REM latency, as compared with healthy controls.

After 3 weeks of drug treatment, total sleeping time and REM percentage were within the range of the normal controls, with total REM time, and particularly REM latency, still significantly reduced in comparison with the normal group.

10. Spectral analysis of the sleep-wakefulness mechanism in a case of apallic syndrome. — F. Hajnšek (Zagreb).

A 32-year-old patient in a state of coma for more than 5 years following a cardiac arrest during abdominal surgery is presented. She belongs broadly to the apallic syndrome. Routine day EEG recording revealed only a flat baseline with rare slow waves in the theta range.

Round the clock examinations, including all-night recording, showed some new aspects which may be summarized as follows: (a) there were some differences between "day and night" recording, although a clear tendency to the so-called "prolonged night type" prevailed; (b) sleep cycles were found to be similar to those of normal persons, but less regular and less stable; (c) rapid eye movement (REM) periods were found, of shorter duration and with a lower stimulus threshold; (d) 48–66% of the total night recording period showed intensive tooth grinding, which simulated REM phenomena according to spectral analysis, ECG and EEG changes; (e) there was a general feeling that the remaining parts of functionally still active telencephalon were taking part in discharges of spike-and-wave-like graphoelements. Some neurophysiological bases for such phenomena were discussed.

11. Behaviour of free amino acid pool in various brain structures of cats deprived of paradoxical sleep. — D. Mičić, V. Karadžić and L. Rakić (Belgrade).

The role of free amino acids (FAA) in brain functions has been already stressed. The pool of FAA in the brain is the source for the formation of amines and proteins; amino acids liberated by the breakdown of proteins are returned to it. The FAA pool is characterized by stability under particular physiological conditions, and in particular brain structures, and instability when functional requirements are changed.

Experiments were carried out on adult cats, completely deprived of paradoxical sleep for 72 h by the water tank technique. The animals were decapitated and their heads were quickly put into liquid air. Various brain regions were taken from the frozen tissue in the cool chamber (Mičić *et al.*, *Nature*, 1967, *215*, No. 5097: 169).

Amino acids were determined by two-dimensional paper chromatography. The following regions were investigated: cerebral cortices (frontal-Fr Cx and occipital-Occ Cx), caudate nucleus (Cd), thalamus (Th), hippocampus (Hippo) and brain-stem reticular formation (RF).

The results showed that the changes in amino acids in cats deprived of paradoxical sleep have a high regional specificity and do not include all amino acids. Statistically highly significant changes were: GABA (increase in Fr Cx, Th, Hippo and RF and decrease in Cd); aspartic acid (increase in Fr Cx, Th, Hippo and RF); glycine (increase in Cd, Hippo and RF); histidine (increase in Fr Cx and RF and decrease in Th); cysteine (increase in Th and RF); lysine (increase in Fr Cx and decrease in Cd); threonine (increase in Fr Cx, Hippo and RF) and glutamic acid (increase only in Th). Other FAA did not show significant changes in the brain structures examined. The results are discussed in connection with the participation of FAA metabolism in different brain regions and sleep genesis.

12. The effect of JB-329 (Ditran) on sleep in the cat. — V. Karadžić and R. Veskov (Belgrade).

The effect of JB-329 (Ditran; ethotrimeprazine) on sleep was investigated in adult male cats, prepared for chronic sleep recording.

The following results were obtained: JB-329 at 10 mg/kg body weight was found to have a very potent suppressor effect on REM sleep; the time spent in wakefulness was increased; the EEG was dominated by synchronization; there was a dissociation between behaviour (hyperactivity) and EEG manifestations (synchronization); the cat's behaviour in the course of drug administration appeared to be "hallucinatory"; complete suppression of REM sleep was not followed by REM rebound during the 10 day recovery period. Results were discussed in the light of a possible connection between lack of REM rebound and the psychotomimetic properties of the drug.

Electroenceph. clin. Neurophysiol., **1969,** *27*: 552–554

Electroencephalography and Clinical Neurophysiology
Elsevier Publishing Company, Amsterdam – Printed in The Netherlands

BOOK REVIEWS

Edited by H. Petsche *and* John R. Hughes

Atlas des Mittel- und Zwischenhirns des Kaninchens. Atlas of the mes- and diencephalon of the rabbit. — L. Gerhard. (Springer, Berlin–Heidelberg–New York, 1968, 64 Fig., 184 p., U.S. $44.50).

Up to the present time, Winkler and Potter's atlas, published in 1911, had to be consulted in problems concerning the topography of the rabbit's brain. It is, therefore, no commonplace to say that this book fills a true gap in the literature. There are, it is true, several short guides through the highly intricate structures of the rabbit's di- and mesencephalon, but all these booklets were primarily meant to assist the stereotaxic approach in experiments. They were usually of little value to support the investigator in analysing, after the experiment, the exact structures of the brain which the recording or stimulating electrodes were in touch with. The main aim of Gerhard's atlas is, therefore, not to give coordinates still more exactly than before, but rather to spread out a detailed picture of the very landscape of the brain. After a thorough study of this work, one may conceive why this author, *a priori* and intentionally, dispensed with trying to "maintain exactly reproducible levels of section since this would only be attainable imperfectly". Accordingly, in combination with one of the few available stereotaxic guides, this book represents the best thinkable instrument to know one's way about the depths of the rabbit's brain.

A short description may show its over-all organization. The book is introduced by sketches and X-ray diagrams of the rabbit's skull from different sides with the brain drawn in. Sketches and photos of the brain from different sides and with partially removed cortex and hippocampus follow. Next comes the main bulk of sections: 12 frontal levels, 6 horizontal and 3 parasagittal levels are pictured. Generally, cellular and fibre stainings (cresyl violet and Heidenhain, respectively) are arranged on each of two contiguous pages of the volume. All the anatomical names occurring in the region depicted are enlisted on the same side, as well as a short description of this zone, in English and in German. The quality of the preparations and of the printing is superior, the size of the pictures sufficiently large.

This part of the book is followed by a detailed description and illustration of certain diencephalic and mesencephalic nuclei with their cellular patterns (magnification up to 100 ×). This part of the atlas will probably be of highest practical importance for exact location of electrodes.

After some remarks about macroscopic anatomy and Rose's cytoarchitectonic fields, material and methods are treated. It is remarkable that the material collected in this volume was chosen from 20 rabbits (2100–3195 g, 8 months – 3 years). Fourteen complete serial sections at 18–20 μ intervals were performed.

What follows is an attempt to go beyond the strictly topographic goal of the book and to treat the different nuclei and pathways from a functional point of view. The author wanted, in this chapter, nothing less than to present a broad neuroanatomico-functional aspect. Such an attempt would perhaps have been promising if it could have been pursued in collaboration with several neurophysiologists. Otherwise, it was bound to fail. Thus the neurophysiologist who is most interested in getting an answer to questions of pressing importance will be more or less disappointed when reading this chapter: no word about the function of intralaminar nuclei, about today's views on pathways directly connecting them and the cortex etc. On the other hand, the long-abandoned suppressor zones are discussed anew. Moreover, several physiological statements are claimed without reference (whereas every anatomical proposition is well backed up by literature). This part of the book is written only in German.

This relatively minor drawback, however, is not at all bound to reduce the high value of this work, elaborated as extensively and thoroughly as it is. It is beyond any doubt that this atlas will remain, for a long time, the standard reference book on this topic.

H. Petsche
Neurological Institute,
University of Vienna (Austria)

Electroenceph. clin. Neurophysiol., **1969,** *27*: 555

Chemische, physikalische und radiologische Probleme in der Neurochirurgie (Beiträge zur Neurochirurgie, Heft 13). G. Merrem (Editor). (J. Ambr. Barth, Leipzig, 1966, 225 p., 174 Fig. Price unknown).

This very well edited Congress Report contains 36 papers on modern trends in Neurosurgery. The book consists of three parts: chemical, physical and radiological problems. Several free topics are also discussed. Most of the papers have short summaries. The radiological chapter is followed by a tight report of a symposium. One chapter is dedicated to the equipment necessary for neurosurgical policlinics.

In the first chapter experimental and clinical observations on metabolic disturbances and dietetics of patients in neurosurgical clinics are thoroughly discussed. Different ways of using radioactive substances in diagnosis are reported, as well as special methods of treatment, *e.g.* selective brain perfusions with antitumoural agents in cases of glioblastomas and the method of intravenous oxygenation. In this, particular techniques of brain perfusion are critically discussed, comparing them with intra-arterial applications.

The part entitled "Physical problems in neurosurgery" contains diagnostic methods such as echoencephalography, the usefulness of fluorescence phenomena for the diagnosis of brain tumours, questions concerning post-operative care of brain-operated patients by using special techniques, such as implanted electrodes, measuring the oxygen content of the CSF as an index of the oxygen supply to the brain, and the "tele-EEG". Reports are given on therapeutic methods such as selective cooling of the brain, measuring oxygen pressure in the CSF and the filling up of CSF after surgical interventions in the posterior fossa, to avoid post-operative oscillations of intracranial pressure. One paper deals with the possibilities of recording tremor.

In the chapters on radiological problems, questions of X-ray therapeutics in cases of brain tumours, combined with surgical interventions and anti-tumoural agents, are extensively discussed. Several papers deal with vertebral angiography. One of them discusses the indications for ventriculography with positive contrast media.

This report, as a whole, gives a good survey of modern trends in neurosurgery and may be recommended to neurosurgeons and neurologists.

A. Ross
Neurological Clinic of the University,
Munich (W. Germany)

Electroenceph. clin. Neurophysiol., **1969**, *27*: 555–556

Membranes, ions, and impulses.—K. S. Cole. (University of California Press, Berkeley and Los Angeles, Calif., 1968, 569 p., $15.00).

What Dr. Cole has done in this extraordinary and interesting book is to look at the beginning, the development and the full flowering of that aspect of biophysics concerning the behavior of excitable membranes. Cole calls his book a "chapter in classical biophysics". Indeed it is that, but it is also far more.

"Membranes, Ions, Impulses" is an inventory of and source-book to a wealth of theoretical and technical information about excitable membranes that is available nowhere else. There are also many original and new contributions to the field within this book. These are of very high quality, and each is almost a paper in itself. The book is a personal close-up description of one man's scientific progress. The reader is figuratively taken along with Cole as he moves from physics, to physiology, to biophysics, as he proceeds in time from red cells and marine eggs with their passive properties to algal cells and squid giant axons with their dynamic electrical characteristics. Throughout the book the presence of the prime movers of a given time is felt. We go back into the past as Cole visits in a colleague's laboratory. The work and the researcher are observed, the exchanged information is digested, stored, and perhaps commented on in terms contemporary with the visit. Then, in a giant step into the present, all is re-evaluated in the context of today's knowledge and insight. At this point, it is necessary to state that the book is not a history, nor is it a memoir in any sense of the word. To understand what Cole has done, the over-all format should be considered.

The format of the book follows three interlocking main lines. The first trend concerns itself with the elements making up excitable membranes. These are more often discussed and analyzed as analogous components from electrical circuit theory (resistance, capacitance, inductance and solid state elements) than as molecular building blocks. In this area the book contains many contributions to membrane biophysics that are completely unique and specifically reflect Cole's approach to the over-all problem. In this respect, the book follows Cole's personal scientific style. Impedance measurements obviously lead to the classical electric analog circuits, just as voltage clamp measurements lead to a mosaic of specific ionic conductances. The background for these discoveries is electrochemistry. Our guides to the field are Helmholtz, Kelvin, Nernst, Boltzman, Planck and DeBye.

The second main line concerns the historical development of the field. In this respect Cole pays close attention to the role that both theory and experimental technique play in the advancement of understanding. With great skill, Cole blends these two trends in such a way that the field remains alive and interesting while the over-all approach is kept within the bounds demanded by scientific rigor.

The third approach which appears in the form of a set of subdivisions is based on a number of the major preparations now being used in the excitable membrane field. Squid giant axons predominate, but medullated axons, cell bodies as well as various skins, bladders and plaques are also included.

Tying all these lines of approach together is the overwhelming consideration that the book should function primarily as a lesson in science. It is obvious that Cole believes that the best instructional approach is enthusiasm for and love of the subject being taught.

I recommend this book to all who work in biophysics, neurophysiology, membrane physiology and related fields. It is a very beautiful book and has been written with loving care. The book reflects the triumph and anguish of the intellectual process; it burns with honesty and personal integrity. I am sure it will provide many hours of joyful reading to all who are involved in any way with science.

William J. Adelman, Jr.
Department of Physiology,
School of Medicine,
University of Maryland,
Baltimore, Md. 21201 (U.S.A.)

Electroenceph. clin. Neurophysiol., **1969**, *27*: 556

THE EFFECT OF NON-PARALYTIC DOSES OF D-TUBOCURARINE ON INDIVIDUAL MOTOR END-PLATES IN MAN, STUDIED WITH A NEW ELECTROPHYSIOLOGICAL METHOD

JAN EKSTEDT AND ERIK STÅLBERG

Department of Pharmacology, Department of Clinical Neurophysiology and Wallenberg Laboratory, University of Uppsala, Uppsala (Sweden)

(Accepted for publication: March 12, 1969)

The conventional methods for the study of neuromuscular transmission in man are mainly based upon electrical stimulation of a motor nerve and the measurement of either the mechanical response of the muscle or the amplitude of the compound action potential generated by a great number of muscle fibers. In this way it is possible to estimate the development of total block in a certain percentage of the motor endplates during the course of stimulation (Harvey and Masland 1941).

Ekstedt (1964) has described methods for recording single muscle fiber action potentials in voluntarily activated human muscle by means of a needle multi-electrode. If action potentials from two muscle fibers belonging to the same motor unit were picked up simultaneously, the time intervals between the potentials were slightly different for consecutive discharges. This variability, the jitter, was normally 10–30 μsec (expressed as standard deviation about the mean interval). Experimental evidence was presented in favor of the assumption that the main part of the normal jitter was due to variability in the synaptic delays of the two motor end-plates involved.

The authors have found that the jitter increases in myasthenia gravis (Ekstedt and Stålberg 1965, 1967) and under the influence of ischemia (Stålberg *et al.* 1966). The present paper is an attempt to apply the method to the study of motor end-plate pharmacology.

METHODS

The methods are essentially those described by Ekstedt (1964) with the modifications described by Stålberg (1966), who has also described the methods for propagation velocity measurements. The single fiber action potentials were recorded with a needle multi-electrode (outer diameter 0.6 mm) in which were mounted fourteen 25–30 μ platinum leading-off surfaces (Ekstedt *et al.* 1969). A subcutaneous concentric needle electrode was used as reference.

The action potentials were recorded on oscilloscopes and they themselves triggered the sweeps of the oscilloscopes. The single fiber action potentials were identified by the criterion that, under recording conditions in which it was possible to detect time differences of at least 10 μsec, consecutive discharges resulted in potentials of identical shape (Ekstedt 1964). The methods used in the present paper permitted the detection of a variability in time of less than 1 μsec.

The time intervals between the action potentials from two different fibers belonging to the same motor unit were measured between the zero intersections of the fast positive–negative deflections of the potentials by means of an electronic time interval counter (Hewlett-Packard Electronic Counter 5245L with Time Interval Unit 5262A). A special gating device prevented other signals than those displayed on the oscilloscopes from being measured by the counter. The maximal error of measurements did not exceed 0.5 μsec. The readings of the time interval counter were automatically recorded on a digital tape recorder (Dymec 2546A). The tape was fed into a computer on which all calculations were made. Further details are given in Czekajewski *et al.* (1969). The jitter was calculated as the standard deviation of the mean time interval between the two fiber action potentials for 50 consecutive discharges. The recording conditions are described in Fig. 1.

Twelve experiments were performed on five males, aged between 28 and 34 years, without signs or symptoms of disease. The needle multi-electrode was inserted between the end-plate zone and the tendon in the distal part of the short head of the right brachial biceps muscle in seven experiments and in the right extensor digitorum of the third finger in five experiments. The motor unit was voluntarily activated and the discharge rate was kept as even and constant as possible during the whole experiment. During partial neuromuscular block the discharge rate, of course, decreased and became irregular. When action potentials from two fibers from the same motor unit were found ("a potential pair"), the jitter between the two fiber potentials was recorded for about 10 min (about 2000–3000 data were collected for the calculation of the jitter, divided in series of 50 consecutive items). Next, 15 μg/kg body weight D-tubocurarine (Abbott) was rapidly injected in a cubital vein in the left arm. During the following 10 min the jitter was recorded as above. After this 30 μg/kg D-tubocurarine was injected and jitter recordings were made during the next 10–20 min. In two cases repeated injections were given until one or the other of the fiber potentials in the action potential pair was frequently lacking (as a sign of occasional neuromuscular block).

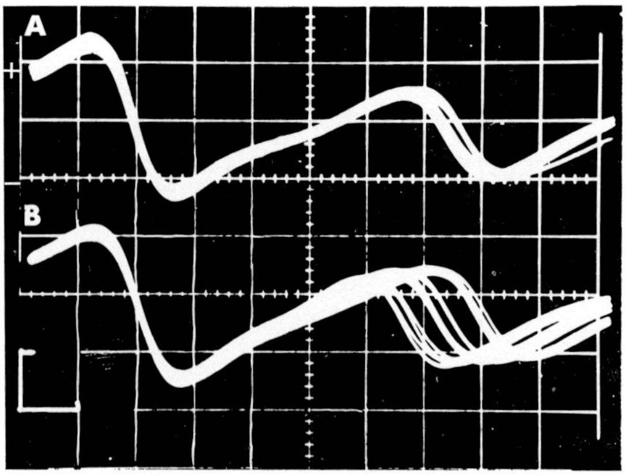

Fig. 2
Oscilloscope pictures of the jitter in a potential pair. *A*: Superimposition of 9 discharges before injection. *B*: The same potential pair 5 min after the injection of 30 μg/kg body weight of D-tubocurarine. Superimposition of 12 discharges. Calibration: 1 mV and 100 μsec.

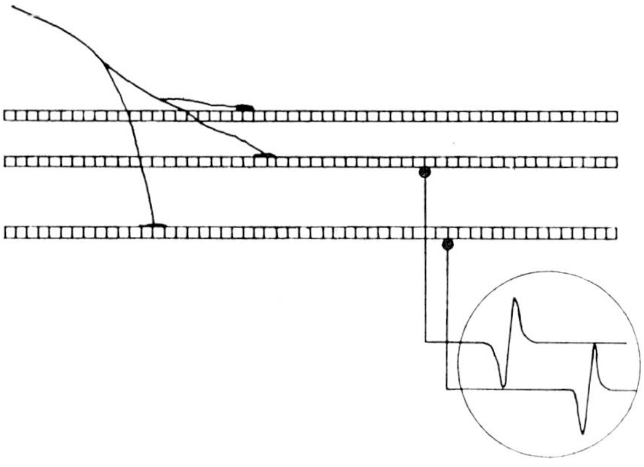

Fig. 1
The recording conditions. The action potentials from two fibers are picked up with the multi-electrode. The two fibers are innervated by branches of the same nerve fiber and thus the two action potentials must always be linked to each other in consecutive discharges. Two such fiber action potentials are called a potential pair. The variability in the arrival time of the two action potentials at the electrodes results in variability in the time interval between the action potentials, *the jitter*.

RESULTS

In all experiments the jitter increased by about 5–15 μsec after the injection of 15 μg/kg D-tubocurarine. The peak value was obtained 3–5 min after injection and then the value declined slowly during the following 10–15 min. There was no blocking of any of the potentials in the potential pair at this dose level. The subjects sometimes complained of disturbed eye coordination and heavy eyelids, but there were no signs of muscular weakness in any other muscles.

When injecting 30 μg/kg of D-tubocurarine the jitter had usually not recovered to the basal value and the increase was more pronounced. The values reached a peak (40–80 μsec) 2–5 min after the injection and then gradually decreased. Occasional blocking of one or other of the potentials in a potential pair was noticed. This seemed to occur only when the jitter exceeded

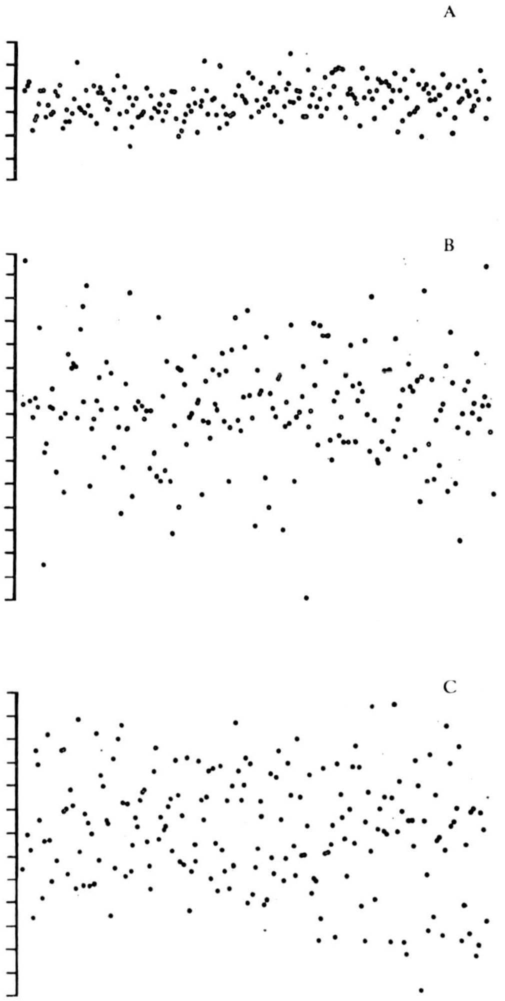

Fig. 3
Sequential histograms of the time intervals between first and second fiber action potentials of a potential pair. Abscissae: discharge number. 200 consecutive discharges are plotted in each histogram. Ordinates: time intervals of a potential pair. Each division corresponds to 5 μsec. *A*: Jitter before the injection of D-tubocurarine. The jitter, expressed as the standard deviation of the potential intervals, = 14.6 μsec. *B*: 8 min after the injection of 15 μg/kg body weight D-tubocurarine. Jitter = 25.3 μsec. *C*: 5 min after the additional injection of 30 μg/kg D-tubocurarine. Jitter = 65.6 μsec. Histograms taken from the experiment shown in Fig. 4.

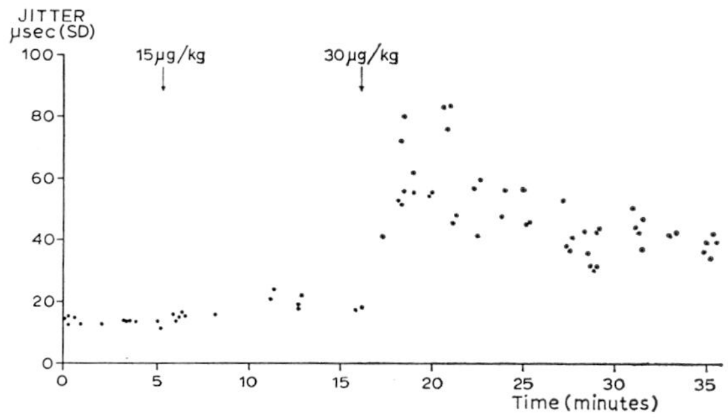

Fig. 4
The size of the jitter during one experiment. Abscissa: time in minutes from the beginning of the experiment. Ordinate: the size of the jitter. Each plotted value is the standard deviation of the time intervals for 50 consecutive potential pairs of discharges.

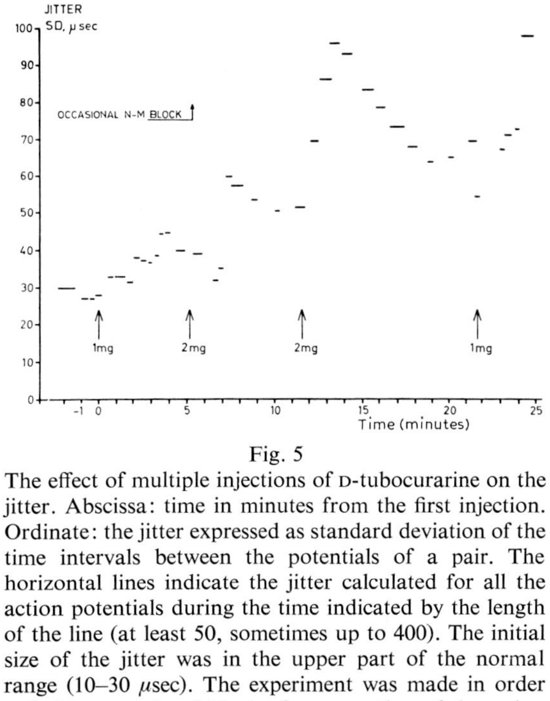

Fig. 5
The effect of multiple injections of D-tubocurarine on the jitter. Abscissa: time in minutes from the first injection. Ordinate: the jitter expressed as standard deviation of the time intervals between the potentials of a pair. The horizontal lines indicate the jitter calculated for all the action potentials during the time indicated by the length of the line (at least 50, sometimes up to 400). The initial size of the jitter was in the upper part of the normal range (10–30 μsec). The experiment was made in order to induce occasional block of one or other of the action potentials in a pair. This occurred frequently when the jitter exceeded 70–80 μsec. The diagram is based upon about 10,000 time interval measurements.

70–80 μsec. At the highest dose level diplopia and slight ptosis were sometimes evident, but there were no other signs of muscle weakness. The results of two experiments are shown in Fig. 2–4.

In two experiments frequent potential blocking was observed after repeated injections of 30 μg D-tubocurarine. Here it was also found that occasional blocking of potentials did not occur until the jitter exceeded 70–80 μsec.

Usually, one of the potentials in a pair blocked more frequently than the other. An example is shown in Fig. 5. An action potential in a potential pair was either present or absent. No fractionation or splitting of the action potentials was seen in thousands of those observed in the curarized subjects.

In two of the cases the propagation velocity in the muscle fibers was also studied, according to the methods described by Stålberg (1966). Curarization did not seem to alter the propagation velocity, nor did it change the interval-dependent variability of the propagation velocity.

DISCUSSION

Fig. 1 illustrates schematically the authors' view of the recording conditions in the muscle. Ekstedt (1964) considered the main cause of the jitter between the two muscle fiber action potentials to be variability in the synaptic delay in the motor end-plate. This conclusion was mainly based on the finding that there seemed to be no difference in the size of the jitter when recorded close to the end-plate zone or near the tendon, where delay changes, arising from variability in muscle fiber propagation velocity, ought to be more pronounced. However, Stålberg (1966) showed that there *was* variability in the propagation velocity of the muscle fibers, dependent on the time interval between the action potential discharges. At the ordinary voluntary innervation frequency an action potential always fell within a time interval which was less than that required for the muscle fiber membrane properties to be fully restored after the preceding impulse. A short interval gave a higher propagation velocity than a longer. The delay changes due to variations in propagation velocity for the two fibers in a jitter recording ought to be approximately the same for the two muscle fibers, provided that the distance between the end-plate and recording site is the same for the two fibers. If the innervation frequency is regular, as during the present recordings, the variability of the muscle fiber propagation velocity is also minimized. When the distance between the end-plate and the recording electrode increases unequally for the two fibers, the influence of propagation velocity variability on the jitter increases; Stålberg (1966) recorded jitter with two needle electrodes placed some centimeters from each other (the propagation length for the two fibers involved thus being different) and found a jitter exceeding that obtained with the method of Ekstedt (1964) (which is the method used in this paper). Graham (1934) showed that the propagation velocity in the nerve is time interval dependent. For the terminal nerve twigs this parameter probably contributes to the total jitter only slightly within the range of inter-spike intervals (50–500 msec) obtained during voluntary contraction, because the conduction velocity in nerve has nearly completely recovered after 100 msec.

The fact that the propagation time variability is time interval dependent, whereas the neuromuscular jitter seems to be mainly random (see below) affords a possible means of distinguishing the two factors.

Variability in the synaptic delay has been shown for the frog motor end-plate by Katz and Miledi (1965).

Fractionation of the *motor unit potential* during curarization has been reported by Locke and Henneman (1960) and this seems to be the equivalent of the blocking of action potentials found in the present investigation. The action of D-tubocurarine is generally considered to be localized to the motor end-plate without any action being exerted on the excitable membranes in muscle and nerve. Stålberg (1966) was unable to detect any change in propagation velocity or its variability in human or in rabbit muscle during curarization and this was also confirmed in the present investigation. Even if a part of the normal jitter is due to variability of the propagation velocity in the muscle fibers the increase in jitter during curarization must be ascribed to increased variability in the synaptic delay in the motor end-plates, because the propagation velocity variability did not increase during the experiment. It must be stressed that *two* end-plates are involved in the recording of the jitter and therefore it is not possible to detect any systematic changes in the synaptic delay, for example an equal increase in the delay for both of them. Only *differences* in the synaptic delay contribute to the neuromuscular jitter.

The normal neuromuscular jitter probably

depends on several factors. The propagation of the impulse in the terminal nerve twig might vary. The amount of acetylcholine might vary and thus also the gradient in the rising phase of the end-plate potential. The time for transmitter release might vary; the sensitivity of the post-synaptic receptors might vary; the rate of restitution of normal conditions in the synaptic cleft after an impulse might vary and the trigger level of the muscle fiber membrane might be subject to fluctuations. Which of these factors is the most important for the normal jitter cannot at present be evaluated.

D-Tubocurarine probably acts by competitively blocking the receptors for acetylcholine without causing depolarization; the rate of increase of the end-plate potential at the trigger level decreases and the end-plate potential decreases in amplitude. If the decrease in amplitude is great enough, the trigger level is not reached and transmission is blocked. The increase of jitter during curarization indicates that there is an increase of the variability of the synaptic delay. The exact mechanism cannot at present be settled. The quantitative aspects of the action of D-tubocurarine on the jitter will not be treated here, but is the subject of an extended investigation.

The present methods can be used only when there is such a slight alteration in neuromuscular transmission that most of the impulses pass. With other methods (Harvey and Masland 1941) used in man or animal it is not possible to detect any changes in neuromuscular transmission under these conditions. Furthermore, with the present method only two end-plates are studied and a reliable and reproducible quantitative measure of the uncertainty of transmission is obtained. The method seems thus to be a complement to the conventional method involving stimulation of the whole nerve and electrical recording from a large area of the muscle, which gives conclusive results only if *total* block develops in a certain percentage of the muscle fibers during stimulation.

It should be noted that it is possible to detect occasional blocking of action potentials even when recording from only one muscle fiber. The doubling of some time intervals may be easily heard in the loudspeaker and is confirmed by subsequent analysis of the inter-spike intervals. This has also frequently been observed in myasthenia gravis (Ekstedt and Stålberg 1965, 1967).

SUMMARY

The authors have used a new method for the study of synaptic transmission in individual motor end-plates in man. Single muscle fiber action potentials are recorded and the method is based upon the following principle: when *two* muscle fibers, belonging to the same motor unit, are recorded at the same time, there is always a variability in the time interval between the two action potentials for consecutive discharges. This variability, of 10–30 μsec, is called the *jitter* phenomenon and has been used in this investigation to study D-tubocurarine.

It has been found that the jitter increases with doses of D-tubocurarine far below those required to give any neuromuscular block. With a dose of 15 μg/kg D-tubocurarine the jitter increased by 5–15 μsec from the normal. A dose of 30 μg/kg increased the jitter to more than 70 μsec, when occasional blocking occurred. This seems to be the first *in situ* method for obtaining quantitative information concerning synaptic transmission in individual motor end-plates in man.

RÉSUMÉ

EFFET DE DOSES NON-PARALYTIQUES DE D-TUBOCURARINE SUR LES PLAQUES MOTRICES INDIVIDUELLES CHEZ L'HOMME ÉTUDIÉ AVEC UNE NOUVELLE MÉTHODE ÉLECTROPHYSIOLOGIQUE

Les auteurs ont utilisé une méthode nouvelle pour l'étude de la transmission synaptique dans les plaques motrices individuelles chez l'homme. Les potentiels d'action de la fibre musculaire sont enregistrés et la méthode est basée sur le principe suivant: lorsque *deux* fibres musculaires, appartenant à la même unité motrice, sont enregistrées en même temps, il y a toujours une variabilité dans l'intervalle de temps entre les deux potentiels d'action pour des décharges consécutives. Cette variabilité de 10–30 μsec est appelée phénomène de "jitter" et a été utilisée dans cette investigation pour étudier la D-tubocurarine.

Les auteurs ont observé que le "jitter" augmente avec des doses de D-tubocurarine bien nettement inférieures à celles qui sont nécessaires pour obtenir un blocage neuromusculaire. Avec une dose de 15 μg de D-tubocurarine par kilo le "jitter" augmente de 5–15 μsec par rapport au normal. Une dose de 30 μg/kg augmente le "jitter" à plus de 70 μsec lorsqu'un blocage occasionnel survient. Ceci paraît être la première méthode *in situ* d'obtention d'informations quantitatives sur la transmission synaptique dans la plaque motrice individuelle de l'homme.

The investigation was supported by The Swedish Medical Research Council (Grant No. 14x-135), the Magnus Bergvalls Foundation and the Swedish Association against Poliomyelitis.

REFERENCES

CZEKAJEWSKI, J., EKSTEDT, J. and STÅLBERG, E. Oscilloscopic recording of muscle fiber action potentials. The window trigger and the delay unit. *Electroenceph. clin. Neurophysiol.*, **1969,** *27*: 536–539.

EKSTEDT, J. Single muscle fiber action potentials. *Acta physiol. scand.*, **1964,** *61*, *Suppl. 226*: 1–96.

EKSTEDT, J., HÄGGQVIST, P. and STÅLBERG, E. The construction of needle multi-electrodes for single fiber electromyography. *Electroenceph. clin. Neurophysiol.*, **1969,** *27*: 540–543.

EKSTEDT, J. and STÅLBERG, E. The diagnostic use of single muscle fiber recording and the neuromuscular jitter in myasthenia gravis. *Proc. 6th int. Congr. EEG clin. Neurophysiol.*, **1965**: 669–672.

EKSTEDT, J. and STÅLBERG, E. Myasthenia gravis. Diagnostic aspects by a new electrophysiological method. *Opusc. med. (Stockh.)*, **1967,** *12*: 73–76.

GRAHAM, H. T. Supernormality, a modification of the recovery process in nerve. *Amer. J. Physiol.*, **1934,** *110*: 225–242.

HARVEY, A. M. and MASLAND, R. L. A method for the study of neuromuscular transmission in human subjects. *Bull. Johns Hopk. Hosp.*, **1941,** *68*: 81–93.

KATZ, B. and MILEDI, R. Propagation of electric activity in motor nerve terminals. *Proc. roy. Soc. B*, **1965,** *161*: 453–482.

LOCKE, S. and HENNEMAN, E. Fractionation of motor units by curare. *Exp. Neurol.*, **1960,** *2*: 638–651.

STÅLBERG, E. Propagation velocity in human muscle fibers *in situ*. *Acta physiol. scand.*, **1966,** *70*, *Suppl. 287*: 1–112.

STÅLBERG, E., EKSTEDT, J. och DAHLBÄCK, L.-O. Ischemiska effekter på den neuromuskulära transmissionen och på propagationshastigheten i muskelfibrer. *Nord. Med.*, **1966,** *75*: 764–765.

Reference: EKSTEDT, J. and STÅLBERG, E. The effect of non-paralytic doses of D-tubocurarine on individual motor end-plates in man, studied with a new electrophysiological method. *Electroenceph. clin. Neurophysiol.*, **1969,** *27*: 557–562.

A CORRELATION OF EEG, RETICULAR MULTIPLE UNIT ACTIVITY AND GROSS BEHAVIOR FOLLOWING VARIOUS ANTIDEPRESSANT AGENTS IN THE CAT. IV[1]

MARSHALL B. WALLACH[2], WALLACE D. WINTERS, ARNOLD J. MANDELL[3] AND CHARLES E. SPOONER[4]

Brain Research Institute and Departments of Pharmacology and Psychiatry, U.C.L.A. School of Medicine, Los Angeles, Calif. 90024 (U.S.A.)

(Accepted for publication: April 7, 1969)

The most effective drugs for the treatment of mental depression are the tricyclic agents. The available neurophysiological data on these agents are limited but indicate that they induce some EEG slow wave activity and an elevated EEG arousal threshold (Bradley and Key 1959; Monnier and Krupp 1959; Sigg 1959; Van Meter *et al.* 1959; Kaneko *et al.* 1960; Rubio-Chevannier *et al.* 1961; Vernier 1961). Studies utilizing gross behavior, EEG and electromyograph (EMG) monitoring techniques were instituted in our laboratory to investigate the actions of these agents. In addition, studies demonstrated that monitoring the activity of a large population of neurons in the midbrain reticular formation (reticular unit activity) (Winters *et al.* 1967b, 1969; Mori *et al.* 1968) was a further useful method for assessing states of CNS excitation and/or depression. The actions of three tricyclic antidepressant agents, *i.e.*, imipramine, amitriptyline, and desmethylimipramine, were assessed and compared with the actions of several other groups of clinically useful antidepressant agents, *i.e.*, a monoamine oxidase inhibitor, pargyline; a psychomotor stimulant, methamphetamine; and two substituted phenothiazines, perphenazine and chlorpromazine (Kline 1964; Klerman and Cole 1965; Náhunek 1966; Hollister *et al.* 1967; Kielholz and Poeldinger 1968).

[1] Supported by U.S. Public Health Service Grants 5 TI-MH 6415-11, MH 12121-02 and MH 10836-03.

[2] Present address: Department of Psychiatry, New York University, Medical Center, 560 First Avenue, New York City, N.Y. 10016.

[3] Present address: School of Medicine, University of California at San Diego, La Jolla, Calif. 92037.

[4] Present address: Department of Neurosciences, School of Medicine, University of California at San Diego, La Jolla, Calif. 92037.

METHODS

Fifty-one experiments were performed on twenty-two adult cats of either sex chronically implanted with monopolar cortical and bipolar subcortical electrodes. Gross behavior, electroencephalogram, midbrain reticular formation multiple unit activity (RUA; A3, L3, Hc−1), and cervical neck muscle tone (EMG) were recorded as previously reported (Winters *et al.* 1967b). Recordings of the RUA were obtained from the same gross electrode which was simultaneously recording the EEG in the reticular formation. The data are recorded as the amplitude demodulated signal recorded on a slowly moving strip chart recorder (Brush Recorder Mark 280). The basal RUA was arbitrarily set at 100% during the rhombencephalic phase of sleep (RPS — paradoxical sleep) and all values obtained during control and drug-induced states were adjusted accordingly. During these studies, RUA and EMG were recorded continuously while EEG recordings were sampled intermittently. At least 24 hours of control recordings were obtained prior to drug administration, and the recordings were continued for 3–8 days after drug administration. At least 14 days elapsed between periods when the animal received a drug. Amitriptyline (Elavil ®), 5–50 mg/kg (13 experiments; 10 cats); imipramine (Tofranil ®), 5–50 mg/kg (11 experiments; 10 cats); desmethylimipramine (Pertofrane ®), 5–50 mg/kg (9 experiments; 8 cats);

pargyline (Eutonyl®), 10–100 mg/kg (5 experiments; 5 cats); methamphetamine (Methedrine®), 2–4 mg/kg (4 experiments; 4 cats); perphenazine (Trilafon®), 4 mg/kg (2 experiments; 2 cats); or chlorpromazine (Thorazine®), 3–15 mg/kg (10 experiments; 6 cats) were administered by the intraperitoneal route. Four to eight cats were utilized for each drug except for the perphenazine studies which were performed on two cats.

RESULTS

Amitriptyline, desmethylimipramine and imipramine

Convulsant action. Administration of 25–50 mg/kg of amitriptyline, desmethylimipramine or imipramine induced an initial slight elevation in the RUA level, the animals were alert, the EMG increased, and the EEG desynchronized for about 15 min. This activity was replaced by a drop in the RUA level down to or slightly below the control slow wave sleep level while the animals were lying quietly with head up and EEG slow wave activity. Within 20–30 min all three agents induced a subconvulsant phase characterized by an elevated RUA level, an increased EEG slow wave pattern with spiking, and an increase in EMG activity; the animals were excited, hyperventilating, rigid and exhibited myoclonic jerks during the EEG spiking (Fig. 1). The RUA reached its highest levels during the ensuing generalized seizures. Following lower doses (25 mg/kg) the seizures began with violent facial and neck twitching; then recurrent clonic-tonic seizures occurred. Following higher doses (50

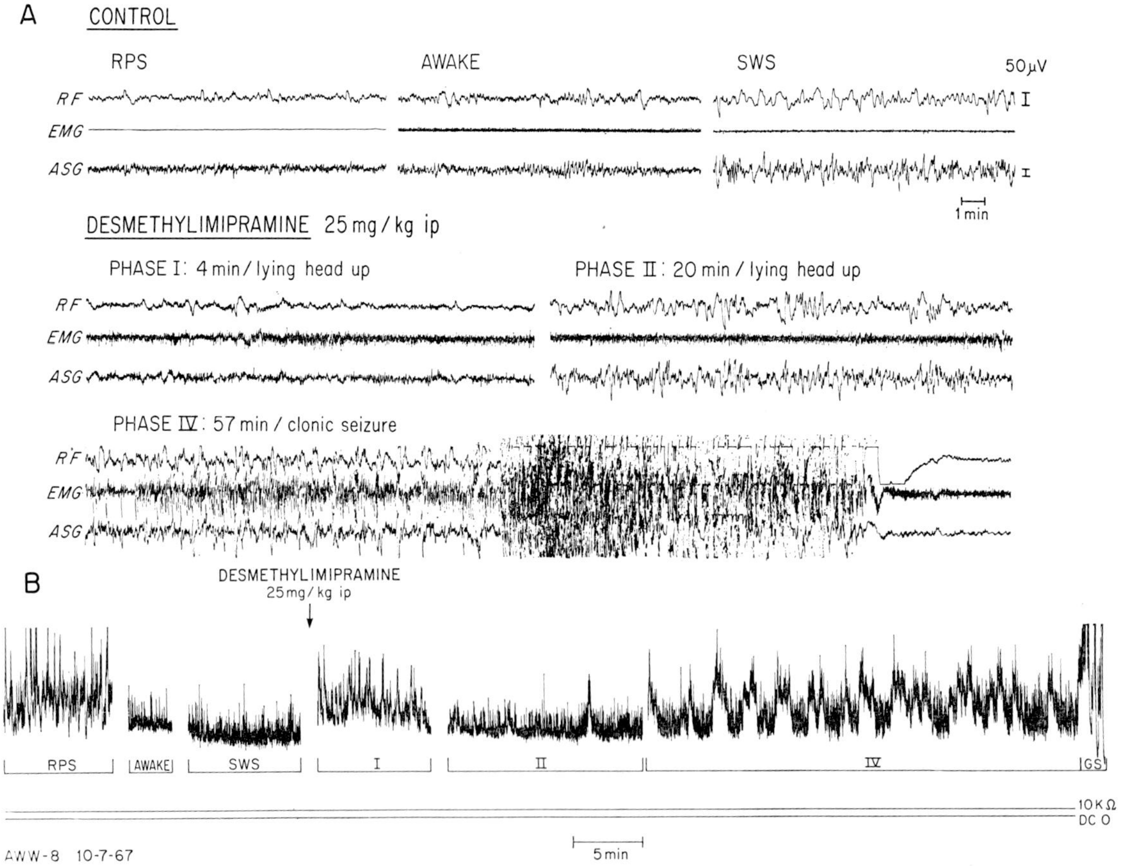

Fig. 1

Comparison of EEG (*A*) and reticular multiple unit activity (*B*) during the control states of wakefulness and sleep and following a single administration of desmethylimipramine, 25 mg/kg. Anterior suprasylvian gyrus (ASG), generalized seizure (GS) interspersed with periods of post-ictal depression characterized by the fall in unit activity towards DC 0. See also legend for Fig. 2.

mg/kg) only the recurrent clonic-tonic seizures were noted. Post-ictal depression followed each seizure and was characterized by EEG electrical silence and a reduced RUA level.

Subconvulsant actions. Following lower doses of these agents (5–15 mg/kg) two phases of drug action could be differentiated for amitriptyline, desmethylimipramine and imipramine; however,

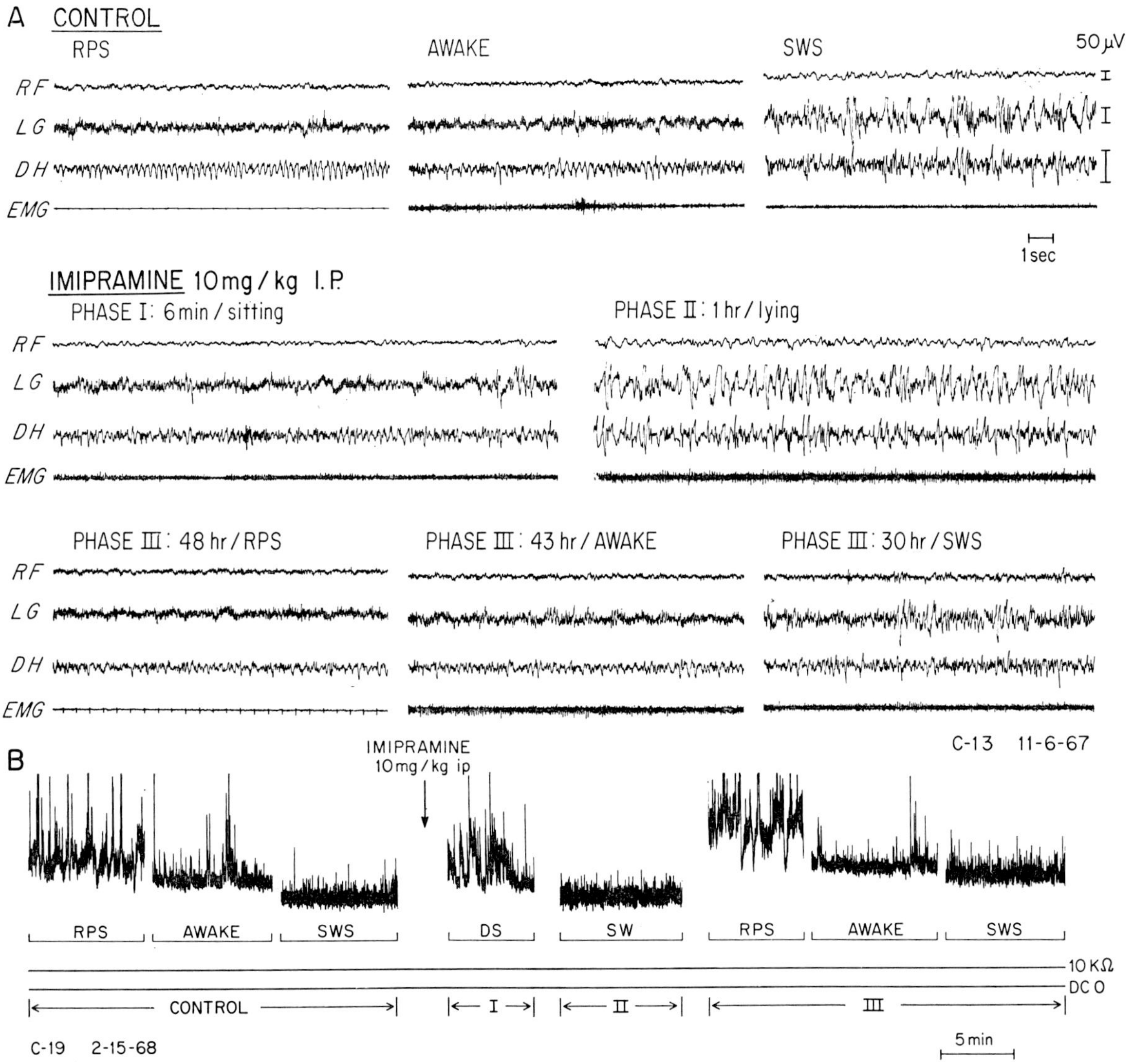

Fig. 2

Comparison of EEG (*A*) and reticular multiple unit activity (*B*) during control states of rhombencephalic sleep (RPS), awake, and slow wave sleep (SWS) and during Phase I (I), Phase II (II), and Phase III (III) following a single administration of imipramine, 10 mg/kg i.p.

A: EEG recordings from the midbrain reticular formation (RF), lateral geniculate nucleus (LG), dorsal hippocampus (DH), and cervical neck muscle (EMG).

B: Recordings of the amplitude demodulated signals of the midbrain reticular formation unit activity. The lowest line (DC 0) represents the system balanced to zero; the 10 kΩ line represents the system noise level with a 10 kΩ resistor across the input. Changes in basal unit activity are measured as the distance from the base of the RUA tracing, to the 10 kΩ line. Desynchronized EEG (DS), slow wave EEG (SW), slow wave sleep (SWS).

imipramine induced a third phase at a time when amitriptyline and desmethylimipramine were returning to the control state.

Phase I: Within 2–5 min following amitriptyline, desmethylimipramine or imipramine administration, 5–15 mg/kg i.p., Phase I began and was characterized by a minimal rise in the RUA above the control awake level (Fig. 2; Table I). The EEG was desynchronized, and the animal was alert, exhibiting excessive use of the litter pan, licking of the face, and occasional retching.

Phase II: The second phase appeared within 30 min after drug administration and was characterized by a fall in RUA to a level equal to or slightly below the level observed during slow wave sleep (Fig. 2; Table I). The EEG was characterized by slow wave activity similar to control slow wave sleep; however, the EMG activity was higher than would be expected during slow wave sleep (Fig. 2), and behaviorally the animal did not appear to be asleep, *i.e.*, the eyes were open, the animal was lying prone, and the head was either elevated or resting on the forelegs. Following amitriptyline or desmethylimipramine, Phase II peaked during the first day and then the RUA level, EEG, EMG, and be-

TABLE I

Comparison of basal midbrain reticular formation unit activity (RUA) level during control states and following drug administration. Figures represent mean percentage of RPS (100%) ±S.D.

Drug	Control		Post-drug		Approximate duration
	State	RUA level (% RPS)	Drug phase	RUA level (% RPS)	
Imipramine, 10 mg/kg $N = 4$	Awake	85.0±3.0	I	82.3±2.8	< 30 min
	SWS	60.8±4.6	II	56.0±6.6	18–24 h
	RPS	100	III	R 124.8±6.0	5–6 days
				A 99.0±6.0	
				S 83.0±10.8	
Amitriptyline, 10 mg/kg $N = 4$	Awake	85.3±4.6	I	86.8±4.6	< 30 min
	SWS	63.0±3.2	II	61.8±2.6	1–2 days
	RPS	100			
Desmethylimipramine, 10 mg/kg $N = 3$	Awake	84.0±2.6	I	89.0±3.4	< 30 min
	SWS	66.7±0.5	II	67.3±4.9	1–2 days
	RPS	100			
Chlorpromazine, 15 mg/kg $N = 2$	Awake	83.5±4.9	I	95.0±2.2	15 min
	SWS	66.0±1.4	II	60.0±3.5	2 days
	RPS	100			
Perphenazine, 4 mg/kg $N = 2$	Awake	88.5±4.9	I	89.5±2.1	< 30 min
	SWS	67.0±3.5	II	67.0±2.8	12 h
	RPS	100			
Methamphetamine, 2 mg/kg $N = 2$	Awake	83.5±4.9	I	86.2±11.5	2–10 h
	SWS	66.0±5.6			
	RPS	100			
Methamphetamine, 4 mg/kg $N = 2$	Awake	86.5±2.1	I	101.0±2.5	20–36 h
	SWS	68.0±4.2			
	RPS	100			
Pargyline, 50 mg/kg $N = 3$	Awake	82.0±3.1	I	84.3±3.2	1 h
	SWS	62.0±4.9			
	RPS	100			
Pargyline, 100 mg/kg $N = 2$	Awake	83.0±1.0	I	91.3±1.3	4–6 h
	SWS	63.0±2.8			
	RPS	100			

Slow wave sleep (SWS) (S), rhombencephalic phase of sleep (RPS) (R) and awake (A).

havior returned to more normal patterns within the next 2 days. However, after imipramine, Phase II lasted 18–24 hours; then a third phase appeared.

Phase III: The third phase would not have been easily noted without assessing the RUA and EMG, since the behavior and EEG following imipramine appear to be similar to the control states of wakefulness and sleep. The RUA was markedly elevated compared to the control levels (Fig. 2; Table I) during what appears grossly to be the comparable states of "RPS", "slow wave sleep", and "awake". In Phase III the RUA levels during these three states differed from each other qualitatively to about the same degree as was noted in control states (Table I). It appears that the level of RUA was elevated for all three states without affecting the relationship between states. Notable differences do appear between the control states and Phase III, such as: the hippocampal theta activity is less apparent during the "RPS" state than is normally noted during control RPS; the "slow wave activity" is less pronounced and the EMG activity is higher than

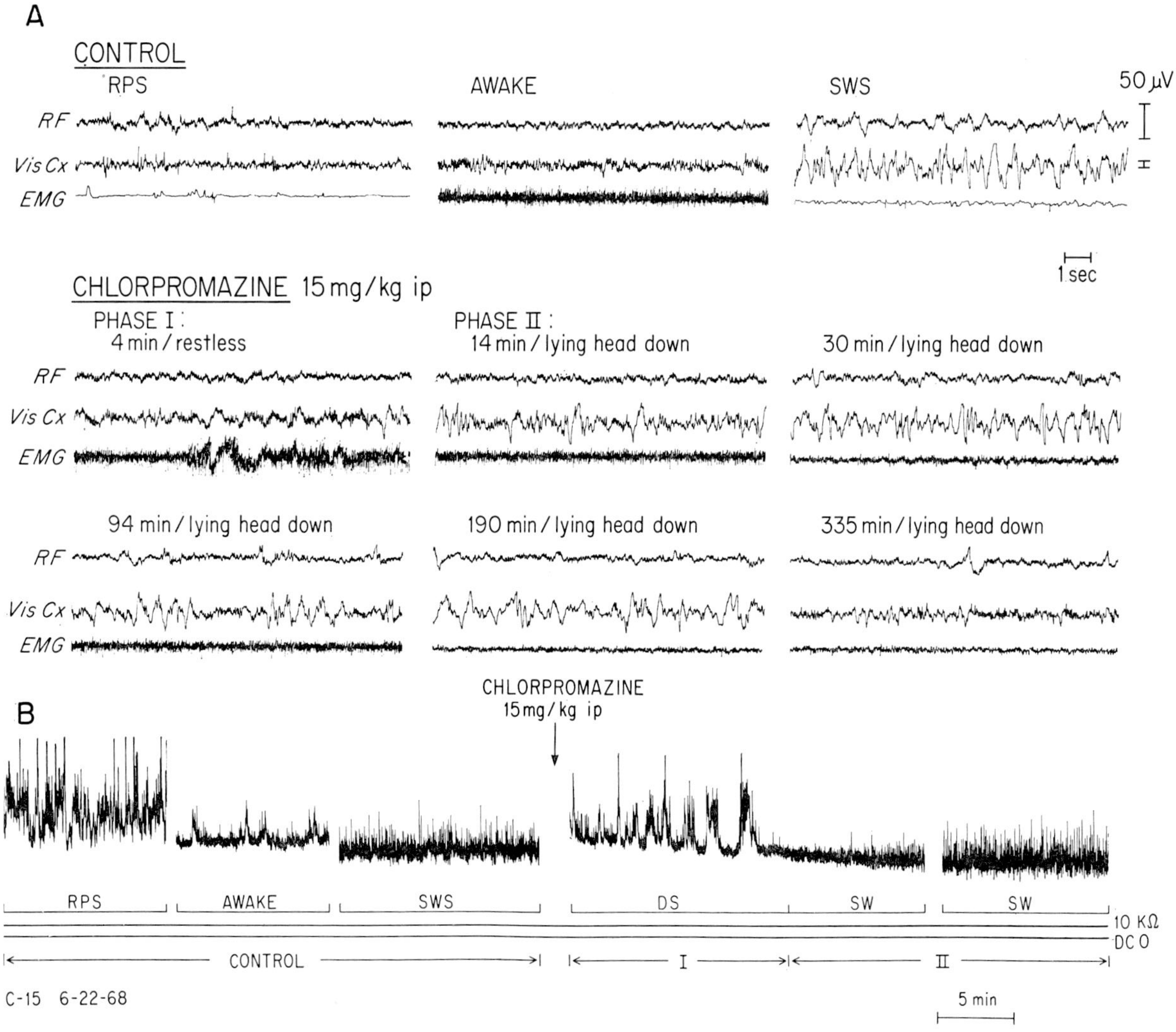

Fig. 3

Comparison of EEG (*A*) and reticular multiple unit activity (*B*) during the control states of wakefulness and sleep and following a single administration of chlorpromazine, 15 mg/kg. Visual cortex (Vis Cx). See also legend for Fig. 2.

that noted during the control slow wave sleep. The RUA, EEG, and EMG returned to levels identical with pre-drug control states approximately 6 days after imipramine administration.

Chlorpromazine

Phase I: Following the administration of 3–15 mg/kg of chlorpromazine (the dose range comparable to that used for the above tricyclic agents) the cats were initially restless and continuously moved about. The EEG during Phase I was desynchronized (Fig. 3) and the RUA rose slightly higher than the awake level (Table I).

Phase II: This phase began about 10–15 min after the administration of the drug. The EEG was dominated by slow waves, higher EMG activity than control slow wave sleep, and the RUA dropped slightly below the control slow wave sleep level. The animal assumed a prone posture similar to the posture noted following the tricyclic agents. The EEG desynchronized and the RUA level increased if the cat was disturbed by noise, or spontaneously arose to change position or to eat. Phase II was most profound on the

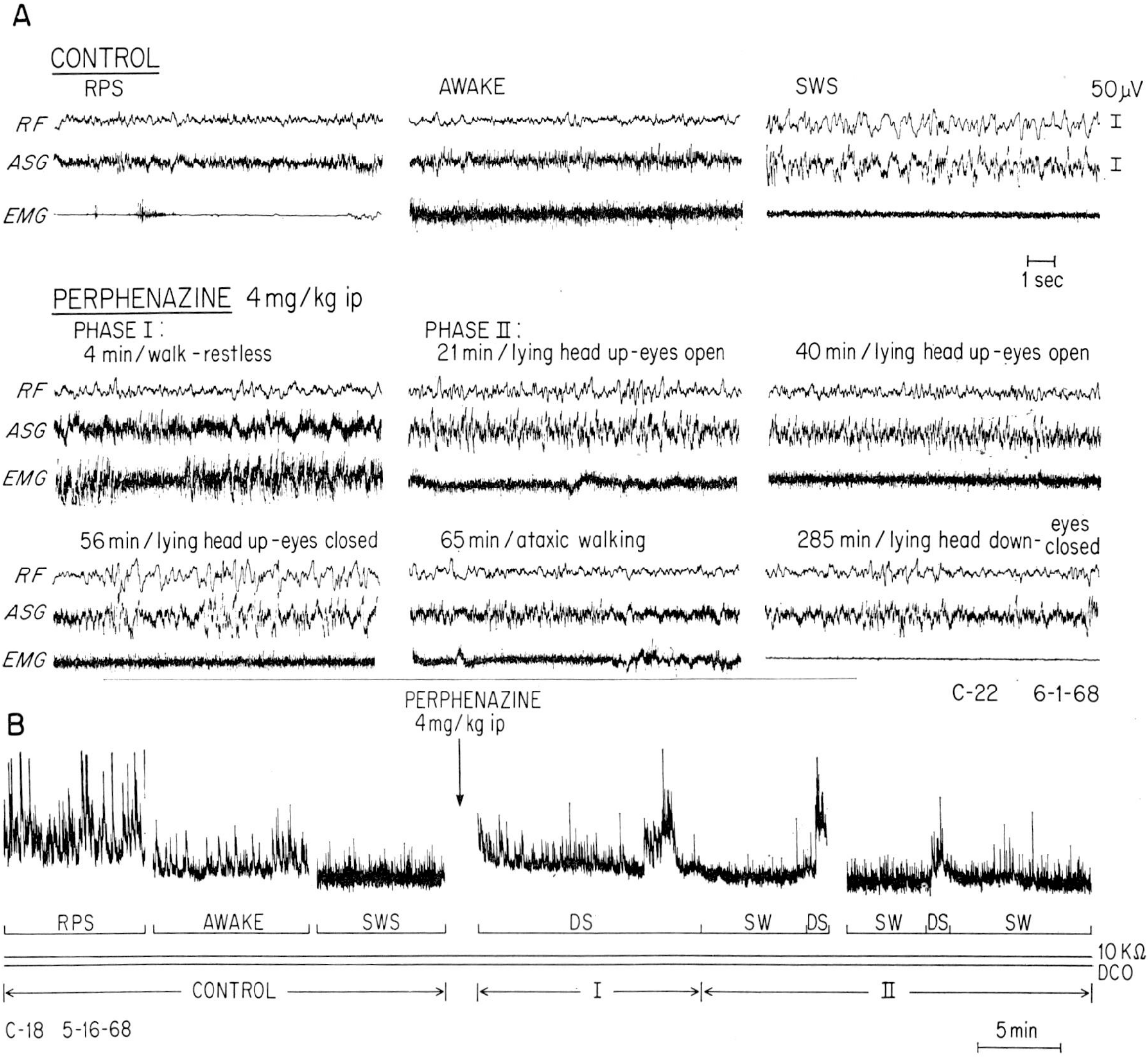

Fig. 4

Comparison of EEG (*A*) and reticular multiple unit activity (*B*) during the control states of wakefulness and sleep and following a single administration of perphenazine, 4 mg/kg.

first day; then the RUA level, EEG and behavior gradually returned to normal within the next 2 days.

Perphenazine

Phase I: Perphenazine, 4 mg/kg, induced similar but milder effects as compared with chlorpromazine. The EEG desynchronization markedly increased and EMG and behavioral restlessness lasted up to about 30 min (Fig. 4; Table I).

Phase II: During this phase, lasting 12 hours, the EEG was characterized by slow wave activity and higher EMG activity than control slow wave sleep. The RUA level was similar to the control slow wave sleep level. The animals elicited marked ataxia; consequently higher doses were not used.

Methamphetamine

Following methamphetamine 2–4 mg/kg, the cat was highly alert and moved about for the initial 10 min after drug administration. This was followed by a period of 2–10 hours during which the animal assumed a fixed immobile body position with frequent head movements. After this period of immobility, the animals receiving 2 mg/kg began to move about normally; however, the cats receiving 4 mg/kg remained highly excited, and exhibited circling movements, panting and salivating for more than 12 hours, and returned to control levels in 20–36 hours. During the excited states the EEG was desynchronized, EMG activity was increased, the basal RUA level was higher than the control awake level, and the RUA fluctuation was markedly increased (Fig. 5; Table I) (see Winters *et al.* 1967b; Mori *et al.* 1968 for discussion of unit fluctuation).

Pargyline

Phase I: Within 5 min after the administration of 50–100 mg/kg pargyline, the animal was markedly excited, *i.e.*, running about, exploring

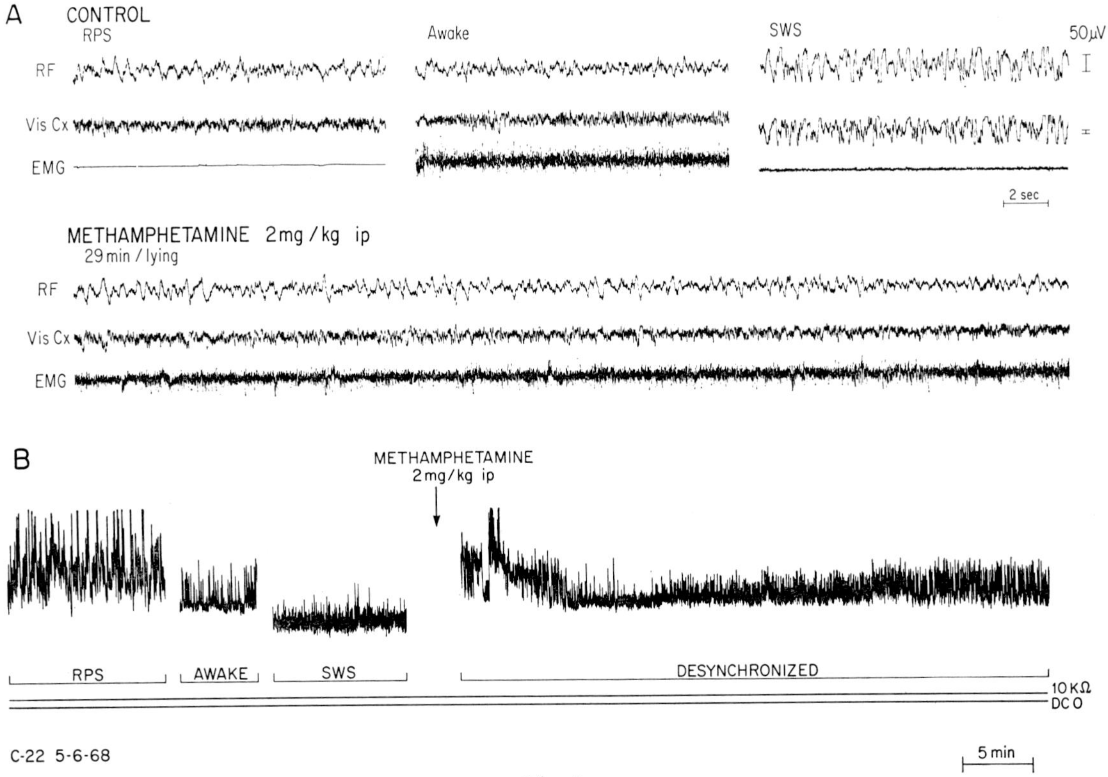

Fig. 5

Comparison of EEG (*A*) and reticular multiple unit activity (*B*) during the control states of wakefulness and sleep and following a single administration of methamphetamine, 2 mg/kg.

and attempting to bite objects in the cage. The initial period of excitement following pargyline differed from the Phase I induced by the tricyclic agents in that pargyline-induced excitement appeared to be more intense and was dominated by excessive exploratory behavior similar to the initial excitatory behavior noted following methamphetamine. The EEG was desynchronized, the EMG activity was increased, and the RUA level was similar to or higher than the active awake level (Fig. 6; Table I).

After about 1 hour following 50 mg/kg and 4–6 hours following 100 mg/kg the active phase ceased; the animal appeared drowsy and the EEG, EMG, and RUA levels were alternating between desynchronization and slow wave activity with comparable cycling of the RUA (Fig. 6; Table I). Control EMG and RUA levels of slow wave sleep appeared approximately 4–6 hours following 50 mg/kg pargyline, and 24 hours following 100 mg/kg. This curious cycling of states at a rate of about 0.5–1.0 c/min was not

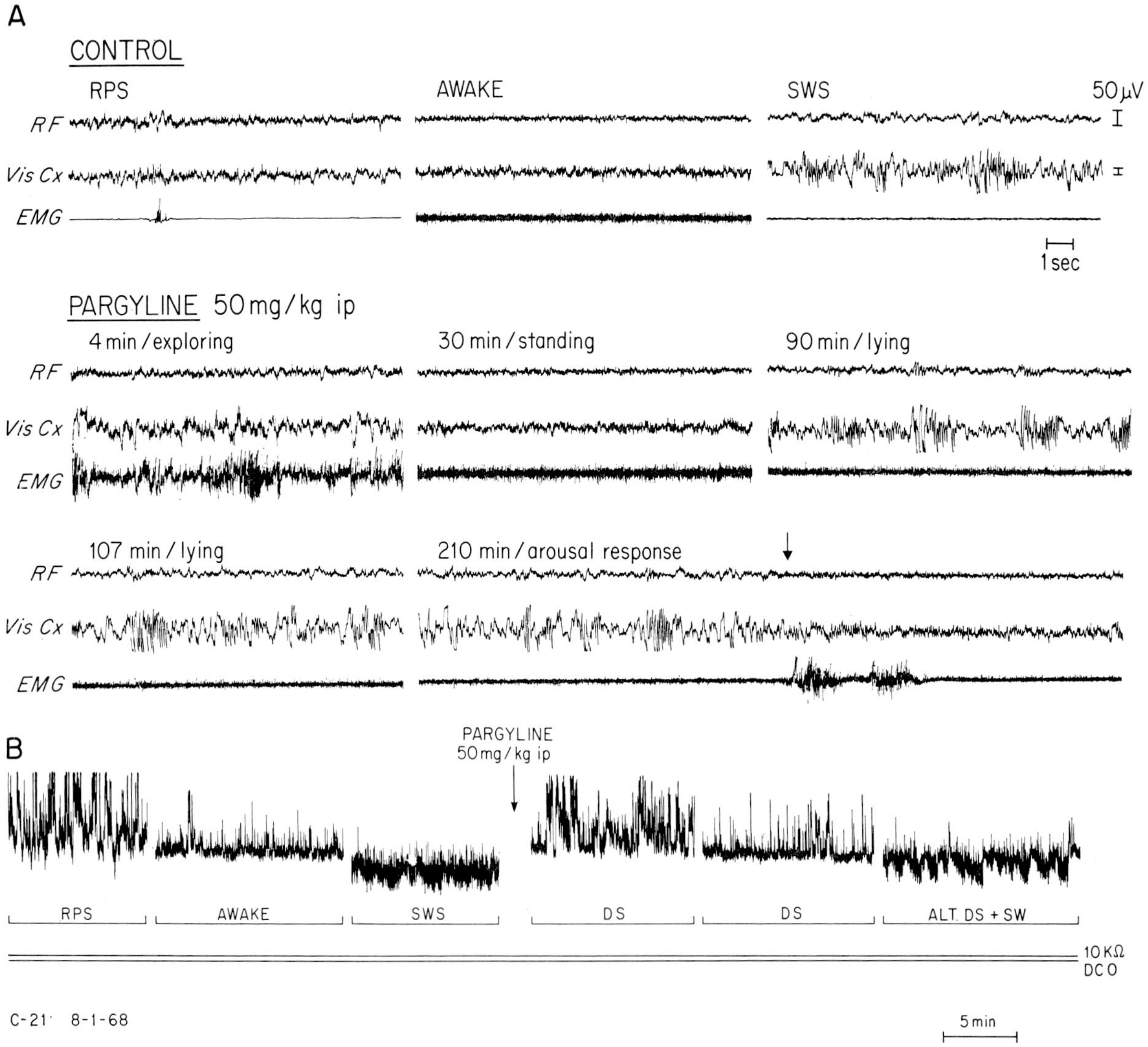

Fig. 6

Comparison of EEG (*A*) and reticular multiple unit activity (*B*) during the control states of wakefulness and sleep and following a single administration of pargyline, 50 mg/kg. ALT. DS + SW, alternating desynchronization and slow waves; ↓, indicates touching door of observation box.

noted during control states or following other drugs.

DISCUSSION

With the exception of the prolonged excitation induced by methamphetamine or pargyline, the induced states are manifested by quite subtle behavior and neurophysiological changes. Whereas Phase I is probably a manifestation of mild CNS excitation, Phase II appears to be a prolonged "sleep-like" state with EEG slow wave patterns and RUA levels both comparable to slow wave sleep. However, Phase II is obviously not the same as slow wave sleep since the animals do not have the normal sleep posture, the EMG activity is elevated, and there is a marked suppression of RPS (Hishikawa *et al.* 1965; Okuma and Akimoto 1966; Okuma *et al.* 1967; Wallach *et al.* 1969) rather than a rise in the percent RPS as would be expected if an increase in duration of spontaneous slow wave sleep had occurred.

The rise in the RUA level following imipramine (Phase III) is of interest since an apparently normal physiological state co-exists with the increased RUA during Phase III. The rise in the RUA level during this phase differs from the increased unit activity induced by methamphetamine and other CNS excitant agents which induce a psychomotor excitation associated with a suppression of the normal states of wakefulness, RPS, and slow wave sleep (Wallach *et al.* 1969). It is not presently clear what Phase III represents physiologically. The rise in RUA during Phase III associated with states similar to control RPS, awake, and slow wave sleep is curious and was not observed previously following CNS depressant or excitant agents (Mori *et al.* 1968; Winters *et al.* 1969).

The chlorpromazine-induced Phase II appeared to be similar to the tricyclics, whereas the perphenazine-induced state was not as profound as the tricyclic agents.

Pargyline, like methamphetamine, induced only Phase I; however, the subsequent state of vacillating quiet awake and drowsy behavior which persisted for several hours is curious. It is enticing to propose biogenic amine actions to explain the cyclic activity noted after Phase I; however, it does not appear that there are sufficient data on brain amine levels during various time intervals following pargyline in the cat to make such assumptions.

The difference in neuropharmacological action of desmethylimipramine *vs.* imipramine is curious in view of the studies (Gillette *et al.* 1961; Sulser *et al.* 1961) demonstrating that in the rat the major metabolite following imipramine is desmethylimipramine. Some investigators postulate that the pharmacological action of imipramine is by virtue of a conversion of imipramine to the active metabolite desmethylimipramine (Brodie *et al.* 1961; Gillette *et al.* 1961; Sulser *et al.* 1961). Since desmethylimipramine does not induce Phase III but imipramine does, it would appear that imipramine action is, in part at least, independent of any desmethylimipramine action in the cat. Perhaps these findings represent a species difference in demethylating enzyme activity between the cat and rat.

All three tricyclic agents induce seizure activity; however, the general EEG progression leading to seizures is not similar to Phase III nor to those patterns noted following pentylenetetrazol, gamma-hydroxybutyrate, or phencyclidine (Winters and Spooner 1965; Winters 1967; Winters *et al.* 1967a, 1969). It is curious that while these tricyclic agents all induce seizure activity, imipramine has been shown to block pentylenetetrazol seizures at lower doses (Piette *et al.* 1963).

The prolonged duration of action of the three tricyclic agents following a single dose is of interest. This clearly illustrates that varying actions can be induced by a single drug administration, and assessment of drug action depends on the time of observation. Certainly in attempts to relate the observed drug action to clinical efficacy this prolonged and varying action should be kept in mind. An example of the danger of not assessing the time course of drug action resulting in completely different interpretations of data can be noted in the biochemical studies of Schildkraut *et al.* (1968), Mandell and Spooner (1968) and Mandell *et al.* (1968). Each investigator reported opposite results and interpretations of their data; however, the former apparently performed the biochemical analysis shortly after drug administration, presumably during Phase II imipramine action, whereas the latter investigators performed their studies during what appears to be the equivalent of Phase III.

Studies describing the influence of these antidepressant agents on the diurnal cycle of cats will be described in detail in the following report (Wallach *et al.* 1969).

SUMMARY

Reticular formation multiple unit activity (RUA), EEG, EMG, and gross behavior were recorded from cats chronically implanted with cortical and subcortical electrodes. Following the administration of various antidepressant agents three phases of drug-induced action were described, as follows:

Phase I — a short period of excitement accompanied by increased EMG, a desynchronized EEG, and increased RUA.

Phase II — characterized by a prolonged lowering of the RUA to the slow wave sleep level, EEG slow wave activity and behavioral quiescence without the behavioral concomitants of sleep, lasting for 1–3 days.

Phase III — characterized by EEG and gross behavior comparable to control wakefulness, RPS and slow wave sleep; however, the RUA levels for each state were elevated above control levels.

Amitriptyline, desmethylimipramine, imipramine, chlorpromazine and perphenazine all induced Phases I and II. Imipramine was the only compound studied to elicit Phase III. Convulsions were observed following high doses of amitriptyline, desmethylimipramine and imipramine.

Methamphetamine and pargyline induced changes characteristic of Phase I. Methamphetamine induced a prolonged period of alertness with an increased RUA level and desynchronized EEG. Pargyline elicited a period of alertness followed by a prolonged period of vacillating wakefulness and drowsy behavior.

RÉSUMÉ

CORRÉLATION ENTRE EEG, ACTIVITÉ UNITAIRE MULTIPLE RÉTICULAIRE ET COMPORTEMENT GLOBAL APRÈS DIFFÉRENTS AGENTS ANTIDÉPRESSEURS CHEZ LE CHAT

L'activité unitaire multiple de la formation réticulaire, l'EEG, l'EMG et le comportement global sont enregistrés chez des chats ayant des électrodes corticales et souscorticales implantées chroniquement. Après administration de divers agents antidépresseurs, 3 phases d'action induite par les drogues sont décrites:

Phase I: courte période d'excitation accompagnée d'une augmentation de l'EMG, d'un EEG désynchronisé et d'une augmentation de l'activité unitaire multiple réticulaire.

Phase II: abaissement prolongé de l'activité unitaire multiple réticulaire jusqu'à un niveau qui correspond au sommeil lent, ondes lentes EEG et tranquillité comportementale sans les concomitants comportementaux du sommeil, durant 1–3 jours.

Phase III: EEG et comportement global comparables à ceux de l'état de veille de contrôle, PMO, et sommeil avec ondes lentes; cependant, le niveau d'activité unitaire multiple réticulaire pour chaque état est supérieur aux niveaux de contrôle.

L'amitriptyline, la desméthylimipramine, l'imipramine, la chlorpromazine, et la perphénazine, induisent toutes les phases I et II. L'imipramine est la seule drogue étudiée qui permette de faire apparaître la phase III. Des convulsions ont été observées après doses élevées d'amitriptyline, de desméthylimipramine et d'imipramine.

La méthamphétamine et la pargyline induisent les modifications caractéristiques de la phase I. La méthamphétamine entraîne une période prolongée d'alerte avec augmentation du niveau d'activité unitaire multiple réticulaire et EEG désynchronisé. La pargyline fait apparaître une période d'alerte suivie d'une période durable d'oscillations entre état de veille et somnolence.

The authors wish to thank Mrs. Susan Miller and Mrs. Merrilyn Kvam for their valuable technical assistance, Dr. G. Everett of Abbott Laboratories for generous supplies of pargyline (Eutonyl ®), and Geigy Pharmaceuticals for supplies of imipramine (Tofranil ®) and desmethylimipramine (Pertofrane ®).

REFERENCES

BRADLEY, P. B. and KEY, B. J. A. A comparative study of the effects of drugs on the arousal system of the brain. *Brit. J. Pharmacol.*, **1959**, *14*: 340–349.

BRODIE, B., PICK, P., KIELHOLZ, P., POELDINGER, W. and THEOBALD, V. Preliminary pharmacological and clinical results with desmethylimipramine (DMI) G35020, a metabolite of imipramine. *Psychopharmacologia (Berl.)*, **1961**, *2*: 467–474.

GILLETTE, J. R., DINGELL, J. V., SULSER, F., KUNTZMAN, R. and BRODIE, B. B. Isolation from rat brain of a metabolic product, desmethylimipramine, that mediates the antidepressant activity of imipramine (Tofranil). *Experientia (Basel)*, **1961**, *17*: 417–418.

HISHIKAWA, Y., NAKAI, K., IDA, H. and KANEKO, Z. The effect of imipramine, desmethylimipramine and chlorpromazine on the sleep-wakefulness cycle of the cat. *Electroenceph. clin. Neurophysiol.*, **1965**, *19*: 518–521.

HOLLISTER, L. E., OVERALL, J. E., SHELTON, J., PENNINGTON, V., KIMBELL, I. and JOHNSON, M. Drug therapy of depression: amitriptyline, perphenazine, and their combination in different syndromes. *Arch. gen. Psychiat.*, **1967**, *17*: 486–493.

KANEKO, Z., HISHIKAWA, Y., SHIMIZU, A., FUKUI, S. and HIDAKA, Y. [Effects of imipramine on the electrical activity of the brain of the cat.] (in Japanese). *No to shinkei (Tokyo)*, **1960**, *12*: 698–705.

KIELHOLZ, P. AND POELDINGER, W. Pharmacotherapy of endogenous depression. *Comprehens. Psychiat.*, **1968**, *9*: 179–186.

KLERMAN, G. L. and COLE, J. O. Clinical pharmacology of imipramine and related antidepressant compounds. *Pharmacol. Rev.*, **1965**, *17*: 101–141.

KLINE, N. S. The practical management of depression. *J. Amer. med. Ass.*, **1964**, *190*: 732–740.

MANDELL, A. J. and SPOONER, C. E. Psychochemical research studies in man. *Science*, **1968**, *162*: 1442–1453.

MANDELL, A. J., SPOONER, C. E., WINTERS, W. D., CRUIKSHANK, M. and SABBOT, I. M. Imipramine antagonism of the CNS effects of norepinephrine: behavioral and biochemical correlates. *Life Sci.*, **1968**, *7*: 1317–1324.

MONNIER, M. and KRUPP, P. Elektrophysiologische Analyse der Wirkungen verschiedener Neuroleptica (Chlorpromazin, Reserpin, Tofranil, Meprobamat). *Schweiz. med. Wschr.*, **1959**, *89*: 430–433.

MORI, K., WINTERS, W. D. and SPOONER, C. E. Comparison of reticular and cochlear multiple unit activity with auditory evoked response during various stages induced by anesthetic agents. II. *Electroenceph. clin. Neurophysiol.*, **1968**, *24*: 242–248.

NÁHUNEK, K. The antidepressive action of phenothiazines and imipramine substances. *Activ. nerv. sup. (Praha)*, **1966**, *8*: 353–354.

OKUMA, T. and AKIMOTO, H. Fundamental and clinical studies on the neural mechanism of sleep. *Progr. Brain Res.*, **1966**, *21B*: 208–229.

OKUMA, T., FUJIMORI, M., HAYASHI, A. and NAKAMURA, K. The effect of some psychotropic drugs on the electrical acivity of the brain and sleep cycle pattern of the cat. *Folia psychiat. neurol. jap.*, **1967**, *21*: 1–17.

PIETTE, Y., DELAUNOIS, A. L., DE SCHAEPDRYVER, A. F. and HEYMANS, C. Imipramine and electroshock threshold. *Arch. int. Pharmacodyn.*, **1963**, *144*: 293–297.

RUBIO-CHEVANNIER, H., BACH-Y-RITA, G., PEÑALOZA-ROJAS, J. and HERNÁNDEZ-PEÓN, R. Potentiating action of imipramine upon "reticular arousal". *Exp. Neurol.*, **1961**, *4*: 214–220.

SCHILDKRAUT, J. J., KOPIN, I. J., SCHANBERG, S. M. and DURELL, J. Norepinephrine metabolism and psychoactive drugs in the endogenous depressions. *Pharmakopsychiat. Neuro-psycho-pharmak.*, **1968**, *1*: 69–92.

SIGG, E. G. Pharmacological studies with Tofranil. *Canad. psychiat. Ass. J.*, **1959**, *4*: S75–85.

SULSER, F., BICKEL, M. H. and BRODIE, B. B. On mechanism of the antidepressant action of imipramine. In W. D. M. PATON (Ed.), *Pharmacological analysis of central nervous action.* Macmillan, New York, **1961:** 123–129.

VAN METER, W. G., OWENS, H. F. and HIMWICH, H. E. Effects of tofranil, an antidepressant drug on electrical potentials of rabbit brain. *Canad. psychiat. Ass. J.*, **1959**, *4*: S113–119.

VERNIER, V. G. The pharmacology of antidepressant agents. *Dis. nerv. Syst.*, **1961**, *22*: 7–13.

WALLACH, M. B., WINTERS, W. D., MANDELL, A. J. and SPOONER, C. E. Effects of antidepressant drugs on wakefulness and sleep in the cat. *Electroenceph. clin. Neurophysiol.*, **1969**, *27*: 574–580.

WINTERS, W. D. Neuropharmacological studies and postulates on excitation and depression in the central nervous system. In J. WORTIS (Ed.), *Recent advances in biological psychiatry.* Plenum, New York, **1967:** 313–345.

WINTERS, W. D., MORI, K., SPOONER, C. E. and BAUER, R. O. The neurophysiology of anesthesia. *Anesthesiology*, **1967**a, *28*: 65–80.

WINTERS, W. D., MORI, K., SPOONER, C. E. and KADO, R. T. Correlation of reticular and cochlear multiple unit activity with auditory evoked responses during wakefulness and sleep. I. *Electroenceph. clin. Neurophysiol.*, **1967**b, *23*: 539–545.

WINTERS, W. D., MORI, K., WALLACH, M. B., MARCUS, R. J. and SPOONER, C. E. Reticular multiple unit activity during a progression of states induced by CNS excitants. III. *Electroenceph. clin. Neurophysiol.*, **1969**, *27*: 514–522.

WINTERS, W. D. and SPOONER, C. E. Various seizure activities following gamma-hydroxybutyrate. *Int. J. Neuropharmacol.*, **1965**, *4*: 197–200.

Reference: WALLACH, M. B., WINTERS, W. D., MANDELL, A. J. and SPOONER, C. E. A correlation of EEG, reticular multiple unit activity and gross behavior following various antidepressant agents in the cat. IV. *Electroenceph. clin. Neurophysiol.*, **1969**, *27*: 563–573.

Electroencephalography and Clinical Neurophysiology
Elsevier Publishing Company, Amsterdam – Printed in The Netherlands

EFFECTS OF ANTIDEPRESSANT DRUGS ON WAKEFULNESS AND SLEEP IN THE CAT[1]

MARSHALL B. WALLACH[2], WALLACE D. WINTERS, ARNOLD J. MANDELL[3] AND CHARLES E. SPOONER[4]

Brain Research Institute and Departments of Pharmacology and Psychiatry, U.C.L.A. School of Medicine, Los Angeles, Calif. 90024 (U.S.A.)

(Accepted for publication: April 7, 1969)

Most drug-sleep studies on freely moving cats report control data for several hours prior to and less than 24 hours after drug administration. These studies do not account for normal circadian changes during the control and/or drug-induced periods and, furthermore, do not adequately follow the total duration of drug action (for example, see Hishikawa *et al.* 1965).

Observation of the daily wakefulness and sleep pattern of the laboratory cat indicates that episodes of slow wave sleep and rhombencephalic phase of sleep (RPS — paradoxical sleep) occur many times in 24 hours. Although the rate of cycling is not constant during each 24 hour period, it is reasonably constant from day to day. Approximately 50% of the daily quota of RPS occurs in the 8 hours between 9:00 a.m. and 5:00 p.m. and 50% of the daily spindle burst sleep occurs in a 9 hour period between 9:00 a.m. and 6:00 p.m. (Sterman *et al.* 1965).

The difficulties in both obtaining continuous recordings of the EEG for several days and scoring the records are formidable. The recently developed technique for recording reticular formation multiple unit activity (RUA) (Winters *et al.* 1967) is a useful method for recording and analyzing the continuous sleep-wakefulness cycle in laboratory animals for long periods of time.

Our previous paper described the prolonged action of various antidepressant agents (Wallach *et al.* 1969). Since these drug studies were followed 24 hours per day, for 3–8 days after drug administration, it was possible to examine the percent change in daily wakefulness, RPS and slow wave sleep throughout the study; the present report represents this analysis. These data are of interest in view of the reported relationship (Hartmann 1968a–c) between these states and the severity of mental depression. The purpose of this report is to examine the effects of antidepressant agents on the sleep-wakefulness cycle of cats as well as the relationship of these changes to the various phases of drug action reported previously (Wallach *et al.* 1969).

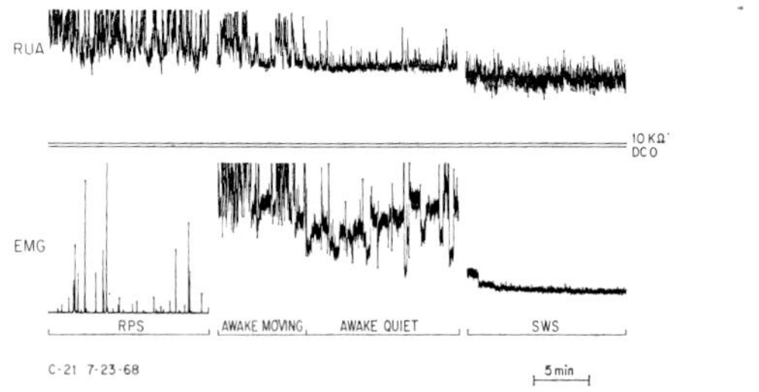

Fig. 1

Recordings of the amplitude-demodulated signals of the midbrain reticular formation unit activity (RUA) and cervical neck muscle tone (EMG). The lowest line (DC 0) represents the system balanced to zero; the 10 kΩ line represents the system noise level with a 10 kΩ resistor across the input. Changes in basal unit activity are measured as the distance from the base of the RUA tracing to the 10 kΩ line. The fluctuation is the width of the excursion from the basal RUA level to the peaks. The RUA and EMG are recorded during the control states of rhombencephalic phase of sleep (RPS), wakefulness and slow wave sleep (SWS). (See also Winters *et al.* 1967.)

[1] Supported by Grants 5 TI-MH 6415-11, 1 RO 1-MH-12121, and 5 TI-MH-10836 from the U. S. Public Health Service.

[2] Present address: Department of Psychiatry, New York University Medical Center, 560 First Avenue, New York, N. Y. 10016.

[3] Present address: School of Medicine, University of California at San Diego, La Jolla, Calif. 92037.

[4] Present address: Department of Neurosciences, School of Medicine, University of California at San Diego, La Jolla, Calif. 92037.

METHODS

Thirty-one experiments were performed on nine adult cats of either sex, chronically implanted with bipolar subcortical and monopolar cortical electrodes and cervical neck muscle leads (EMG). Midbrain reticular formation (A3; L3; Hc −1) unit activity and EMG activity were continuously recorded on a Brush Recorder (Mark 280) as previously reported (Winters *et al.* 1967), and the EEG and gross behavior were monitored intermittently. The RUA and EMG recordings were used to determine the time the animal was awake, in slow wave sleep, or in RPS (Fig. 1). Differences in the level of RUA characteristic of each phase of wakefulness and sleep have been reported previously (Winters *et al.* 1967). Recording the EMG in the same manner as the RUA results in an integration of the EMG envelope expressed as a DC level. By observing the changes in the level of EMG activity simultaneously with the RUA, an added degree of accuracy was obtained for assessing behavioral states (Fig. 1). The duration of each phase of wakefulness and sleep was determined by measuring the duration of each episode to the nearest millimeter on the Brush recorder run at 6 mm/min. These millimeter measurements were expressed as a percentage of the total millimeters in 24 hours. A 24 hour record could be scored in less than 1 hour by this technique.

Measurement of the change in the RPS time was more accurate than the determination of wakefulness and slow wave sleep since the determination of the beginning and end of the transitional states, *i.e.*, drowsy and light sleep, are more gradual than the abrupt start and end of RPS. Slow wave and desynchronized EEG activity post-drug was assumed to represent states similar to the comparable control states of slow wave sleep, wakefulness and RPS; however, there were significant differences indicating that the post-drug states are similar but not identical to the control states (Wallach *et al.* 1969) prior to recovery.

At least 24 hours of control recordings were obtained prior to drug administration, and at least 14 days elapsed between each drug administration. Amitriptyline (Elavil ®), 5–15 mg/kg (5 experiments; 5 cats); desmethylimipramine

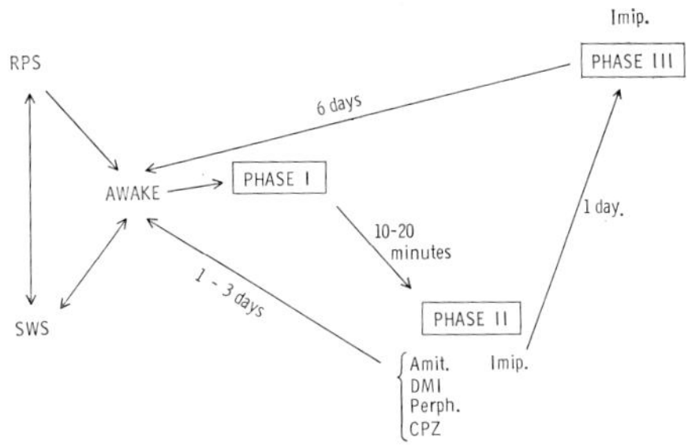

Fig. 2

Schema representing control states of awake, rhombencephalic phase of sleep (RPS) and slow wave sleep (SWS) and the induced phases following amitriptyline (Amit.), desmethylimipramine (DMI), perphenazine (Perph.), chlorpromazine (CPZ), and imipramine (Imip). The durations following each phase represent the time the drug-induced phase lasts prior to passing to the next phase.

(Pertofrane ®), 5–25 mg/kg (6 experiments; 6 cats); imipramine (Tofranil ®), 10–15 mg/kg (6 experiments; 6 cats); chlorpromazine (Thorazine ®), 15 mg/kg (2 experiments; 2 cats); perphenazine (Trilafon ®), 4 mg/kg (2 experiments; 2 cats); methamphetamine (Methedrine ®), 2–4 mg/kg (4 experiments; 4 cats); or pargyline (Eutonyl ®), 50–100 mg/kg (6 experiments; 5 cats) were administered by the intraperitoneal route. See prior report (Wallach *et al.* 1969) for induced EEG, EMG, behavior and RUA following these agents (Fig. 2).

RESULTS

Control: Correlation of all control 24 hour data demonstrates that the cats spend approximately 47.0 ± 7.8% (± S.D.) of the day in slow wave sleep ($N=31$ days), 40.6 ± 7.8% either awake or drowsy ($N=31$ days), 12.5 ± 3.1% in RPS ($N=60$ days) and 33.5±9.4% RPS episodes occur during each control 24 hour period.

Tricyclic antidepressant agents

Amitriptyline, desmethylimipramine, and imipramine: During the initial 24 hours following the administration of amitriptyline, desmethylimipramine, or imipramine, 5–15 mg/kg, RPS was completely suppressed and progressively returned to control values by the fourth day. The number of RPS episodes was likewise reduced during the first post-drug day and progressively increased until control levels were reached on day 4 (Fig. 3,

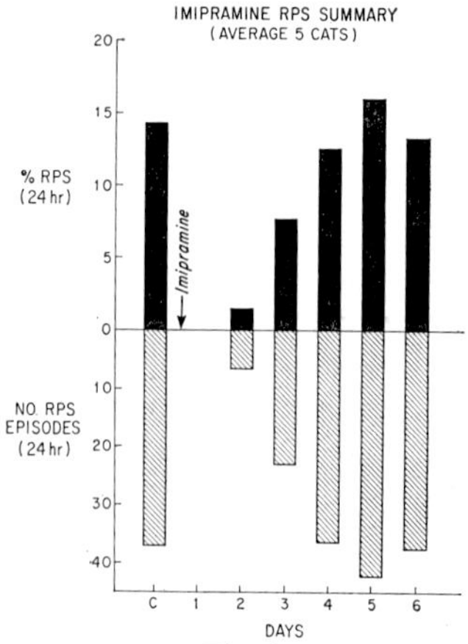

Fig. 3
Graphic representation of the percentage of RPS and the number of RPS episodes recorded for each 24 hour period during control and following imipramine. C = control.

Table I). The awake drowsy period was markedly reduced on the first day and likewise returned to control levels on the fourth day (Fig. 4; Table II). During the initial 3 days there was an increase in EEG slow wave activity (Fig. 4; Table III) which was similar to slow wave sleep; however, the EMG activity was higher than expected during slow wave sleep, and the animal did not assume the normal sleep posture (Wallach *et al.* 1969). Following imipramine the daily pattern of RPS suppression was similar to amitriptyline and desmethylimipramine; however, the awake desynchronized activity returned to control levels on day 2 (Fig. 4; Tables I–III). No evidence of significant RPS rebound was observed following these agents.

Amitriptyline, desmethylimipramine, and imipramine, 5 mg/kg, failed to completely suppress RPS during the initial 24 hours, while cats receiving a convulsant dose of 25 mg/kg desmethylimipramine exhibited complete RPS suppression for over 48 hours without evidence of RPS rebound by day 6 post-drug.

TABLE I

Rhombencephalic phase of sleep

Drug	Control	Day 1	Day 2	Day 3	Day 4	Day 5	Day 6
Amitriptyline, 10–15 mg/kg $N = 2$	11.6±1.5*	0	2.3±2.1	4.2±2.0	10.9±2.1	14.5±4.1	
Desmethylimipramine, 10 mg/kg $N = 3$	12.4±3.3	0	1.4±1.5	5.6±3.6	12.2±4.2		
Imipramine, 10–15 mg/kg $N = 4$	14.9±1.0	0	1.1±1.2	6.5±3.4	12.7±4.0	16.6±3.8	13.0±2.0
Chlorpromazine, 15 mg/kg $N = 2$	13.5±2.4	1.3±0.9	7.5±1.7	12.1±1.7	14.0±3.7	10.6±0.4	
Perphenazine, 4 mg/kg $N = 2$	10.6±4.9	8.6±1.6	10.9±5.1	11.7±2.7			
Methamphetamine, 2 mg/kg $N = 2$	11.2±6.1	1.9±2.7	14.7±0.9				
Methamphetamine, 4 mg/kg $N = 2$	11.5±0.4	0.4±0.6	12.0±5.9	14.3±5.6			
Pargyline, 50 mg/kg $N = 2$	15.0±2.3	2.4±2.5	12.6±1.0	13.7±2.1			

* % of the day ± S.D.

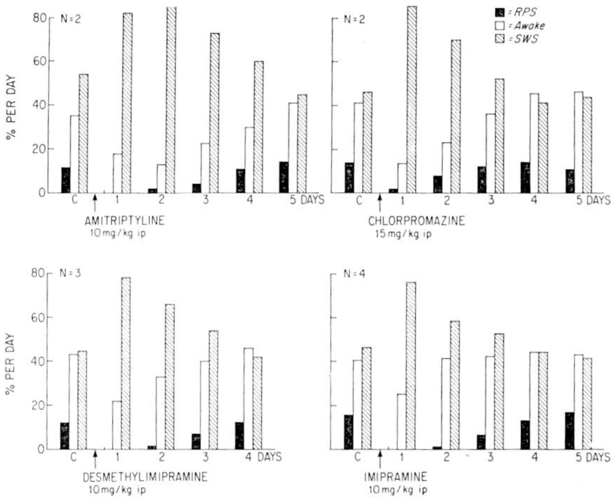

Fig. 4
Graphic representation of daily percentage of rhombencephalic phase of sleep (RPS), wakefulness, and slow wave sleep (SWS) during control (C) and each day following a single administration of amitriptyline, chlorpromazine, desmethylimipramine or imipramine. Day = 24 hours. See Methods for discussion of SWS following drug administration.

Chlorpromazine and perphenazine

Following chlorpromazine, 15 mg/kg, RPS was almost completely suppressed on day 1 (Fig. 4; Table I) and returned to control levels by day 3 with no apparent RPS rebound. The slow wave activity was increased on day 1 and day 2 while awake desynchronized activity was reduced during these days. Both states returned to normal levels on day 3.

Following perphenazine, 4 mg/kg, RPS was minimally suppressed during the first 24 hours and returned to control levels by day 2. On day 1 slow wave activity was markedly increased and returned to control levels on day 2 (Tables I–III).

Methamphetamine

Following methamphetamine, 2–4 mg/kg, both slow wave activity and RPS were sharply reduced and awake desynchronized EEG and behavior were markedly increased (Fig. 5; Tables I–III). The RPS which was observed occurred in

TABLE II

Awake

Drug	Control	Day 1	Day 2	Day 3	Day 4	Day 5	Day 6
Amitriptyline, 10–15 mg/kg $N = 2$	34.5±12.0*	18.0±1.4	12.5±2.1	22.5±6.4	30.0±2.8	41.0±14.1	
Desmethylimipramine, 10 mg/kg $N = 3$	43.3±8.1	22.3±5.5	32.7±9.2	40.0±18.4	45.7±6.8		
Imipramine, 10–15 mg/kg $N = 4$	40.0±8.4	24.5±7.6	41.3±6.6	42.0±7.2	43.5±6.8	43.3±1.2	50.8±6.4
Chlorpromazine, 15 mg/kg $N = 2$	41.0±7.1	13.5±3.5	23.0±1.4	36.0±2.8	45.0±4.2	46.0±5.5	
Perphenazine 4 mg/kg $N = 2$	42.0±4.2	29.0±5.6	57.0±14.0	44.5±13.4			
Methamphetamine, 2 mg/kg $N = 2$	51.0±1.4	90.0±14.1	42.5±6.4				
Methamphetamine, 4 mg/kg $N = 2$	36.5±9.2	88.5±16.2	29.5±30.3	27.5±16.2			
Pargyline, 50 mg/kg $N = 2$	41.5±4.9	53.0±14.1	44.5±12.0	47.0±8.5			

* % of the day ± S.D.

TABLE III

Slow wave sleep

Drug	Control	Day 1	Day 2	Day 3	Day 4	Day 5	Day 6
Amitriptyline, 10–15 mg/kg $N=2$	54.0±14.1*	82.0±1.4	85.0±1.4	73.5±7.8	59.5±0.7	44.5±17.6	
Desmethylimipramine, 10 mg/kg $N=3$	44.3±6.7	77.7±5.5	66.0±10.4	54.0±19.1	42.0±10.8		
Imipramine, 10–15 mg/kg $N=4$	45.8±7.0	75.5±6.4	57.8±6.0	57.5±7.6	43.8±9.8	41.3±2.8	36.3±6.0
Chlorpromazine, 15 mg/kg $N=2$	45.5±4.9	85.0±2.8	69.5±0.7	52.0±4.2	41.0±8.5	43.5±9.2	
Perphenazine, 4 mg/kg $N=2$	47.5±0.7	63.0±4.2	32.0±14.1	43.0±10.7			
Methamphetamine, 2 mg/kg $N=2$	38.5±4.9	8.5 ±12.0	43.0±7.0				
Methamphetamine, 4 mg/kg $N=2$	52.0±9.0	11.0±15.4	58.0±23.8	58.5±21.7			
Pargyline, 50 mg/kg $N=2$	43.5±7.8	44.5±12.0	42.5±12.0	39.5±10.7			

* % of the day ± S.D.

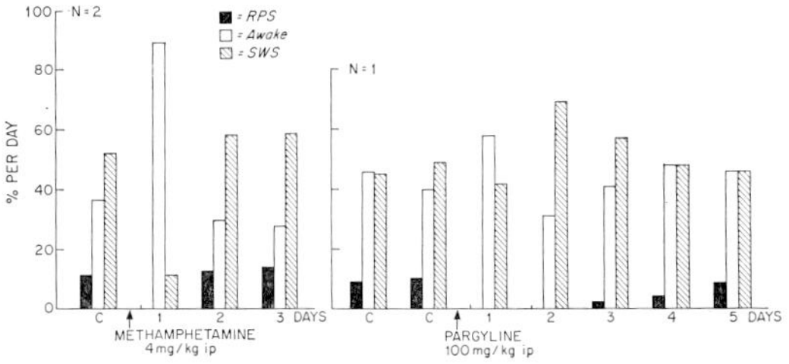

Fig. 5

Graphic representation of daily percent of rhombencephalic phase of sleep (RPS), wakefulness, and slow wave sleep (SWS) during control (C) and each day following a single administration of methamphetamine or pargyline. Day = 24 hours.

the last part of the initial 24 hour period. Control values of RPS, slow wave sleep and wakefulness were noted on days 2 and 3 post-drug.

Pargyline

RPS was completely suppressed for approximately 1 day following 50 mg/kg of pargyline (Table I), and 2 days following 100 mg/kg. There was no evidence of rebound following recovery of RPS. Following the 50 mg/kg injection of pargyline there was considerable variability in desynchronization *vs.* slow wave activity (Tables II, III); however, following 100 mg/kg there was an increase in desynchronization on day 1, an increase in slow wave activity on day 2 and a return to control levels on day 5 (Fig. 5).

DISCUSSION

Each of the agents examined in the present study induced an initial RPS suppression as well as changes in the ratio of wakefulness, RPS and slow wave sleep. The agents differed in the duration of the RPS suppression, the rate of recovery of RPS, and the amount of slow wave *vs.* awake activity during the post-drug period. Correlation of the wakefulness and sleep data with the induced phases of drug action described earlier (Wallach *et al.* 1969) clearly demonstrates that the altered sleep patterns are apparently unrelated to the appearance of the various induced phases. For example, following amitriptyline and desmethylimipramine Phase II continued for several days beyond the period of peak RPS suppression, whereas following imipramine the RPS suppression continued during an entirely different state, Phase III (Fig. 2). In spite of the differences in action between amitriptyline or desmethylimipramine and imipramine, the daily pattern of RPS suppression was the same for all three agents at comparable dose levels (Fig. 4). These findings indicate that the mechanisms involved in the generation of the three observed phases are unrelated to the mechanism involved in the generation of RPS suppression.

The phenothiazine agents induced changes in wakefulness, RPS, and slow wave sleep which were similar to those of the tricyclic agents; however, the phenothiazine-induced action was of shorter duration than that of the tricyclics. Since chlorpromazine induced an equivalent lowering of RPS during Phase II compared with the tricyclics, but a lesser degree of RPS suppression, it is again clear that there is apparently little direct correlation between the induced phases or RUA levels and the ensuing RPS suppression.

Pargyline and methamphetamine generally induced a prolonged period of wakefulness with elevated RUA levels along with the period of suppression of RPS and slow wave sleep.

It is apparent that, unlike the relationship of midbrain reticular formation activity with wakefulness, sleep and induced states of CNS excitation and depression, there is little correlation between RPS suppression and RUA activity.

RPS suppression in cats following desmethylimipramine, imipramine, and chlorpromazine has been reported by Hishikawa *et al.* (1965); however, the cats were observed only for a maximum of 10 hours and therefore the duration of the suppression could not be ascertained. Okuma *et al.* (1967) administered the tricyclic and phenothiazine agents to cats in divided doses, one-third of the daily dose in the morning and two-thirds in the late afternoon. They recorded for two 7 hour periods immediately after administration of the drugs; therefore the drug action was examined only for 14 hours of each day. Obviously these techniques will not adequately evaluate the total drug action.

It is interesting to note that whereas all of the drugs examined in the present study induce RPS suppression, methamphetamine induces an increase in total wakefulness during the suppression whereas the other agents studied induce an increase in slow wave activity during RPS suppression. It is possible that methamphetamine induces RPS suppression by suppressing slow wave sleep; thus no RPS occurs, since RPS occurs only after a period of slow wave sleep but does not appear immediately after wakefulness (Hubel 1960). The increased slow wave activity during RPS suppression induced by the other drugs studied does not appear to be identical to slow wave sleep; thus this group may likewise block RPS via a reduction in slow wave sleep or via a specific block on the system necessary for the induction of RPS.

All of the antidepressant agents studied induce a suppression of RPS with no evidence of RPS rebound. It is difficult to agree with the premise of Hartmann (1968c) that mental depression is characterized by an increased need for RPS and these agents act via a reduction of the need for RPS. He has, in fact, demonstrated that manic-depressives have relatively normal sleep patterns during depression. As stated in the present study, RPS was suppressed during either increased wakefulness or increased Phase II and/or III; thus there may not be any direct relationship between wake–sleep cycles and the therapeutic efficacy of drugs in treating mental depression. Lacking in all of these studies is an examination of the action of chronic antidepressant drug administration. This approach would be most valuable since it is well known clinically that antidepressant therapy is ineffective during the initial 5–7 days of daily administration.

SUMMARY

Wakefulness–sleep cycles were determined for each 24 hour period during control days and each day following the administration of various antidepressant agents; *i.e.*, amitriptyline, desmethylimipramine and imipramine; chlorpromazine and perphenazine; pargyline; or methamphetamine. All of the agents induced an initial suppression of RPS. Methamphetamine induced an increase in total wakefulness during the suppression, whereas the other agents studied induced an increase in slow wave activity during the suppression. None of the agents induced a clear RPS rebound. The normal wake–sleep cycle reappeared in 3–4 days following the tricyclics and phenothiazines, in 4–5 days following pargyline, and in 2 days following methamphetamine.

RÉSUMÉ

EFFETS DES DROGUES ANTIDÉPRESSIVES SUR L'ÉTAT DE VEILLE ET DE SOMMEIL CHEZ LE CHAT

Les cycles veille–sommeil sont étudiés tout au long de périodes de 24 heures pendant plusieurs jours de contrôle et pendant chaque jour suivant l'administration de divers agents antidépresseurs, *i.e.*, amitriptyline, desméthylimipramine et imipramine; chlorpromazine et perphénazine; pargyline, ou méthamphétamine. Tous ces agents induisent une suppression initiale des phases de mouvements oculaires du sommeil (PMO). Pendant cette suppression la méthamphétamine induit une augmentation du temps total de veille, tandis que les autres agents étudiés induisent une augmentation de l'activité lente. Aucun des agents ne provoque de rebound net de PMO. Le cycle normal veille–sommeil réapparaît en 3–4 jours après les tricycliques et les phénothiazines, en 4–5 jours après la pargyline et en 2 jours après méthamphétamine.

The authors wish to thank Mrs. S. Miller and Mrs. M. Kvam for their valuable technical assistance, Dr. G. Everett of Abbott Laboratories for generous supplies of pargyline (Eutonyl ®) and Geigy Pharmaceuticals for supplies of imipramine (Tofranil ®) and desmethylimipramine (Pertofrane ®).

This work has been assisted by the U.C.L.A. Brain Information Service which is a part of the National Information Network of the National Institute for Neurological Diseases and Blindness and supported under Contract PH-43-66-59.

REFERENCES

HARTMANN, E. Antidepressants and the need for D. *Psychophysiology*, **1968**a, *4*: 390–391.

HARTMANN, E. The effect of four drugs on sleep patterns in man. *Psychopharmacologia (Berl.)*, **1968**b, *12*: 346–353.

HARTMANN, E. Longitudinal studies of sleep and dream patterns in manic-depressive patients. *Arch. gen. Psychiat.*, **1968**c, *19*: 312–329.

HISHIKAWA, Y., NAKAI, K., IDA, H. and KANEKO, Z. The effect of imipramine, desmethylimipramine and chlorpromazine on the sleep-wakefulness cycle of the cat. *Electroenceph. clin. Neurophysiol.*, **1965**, *19*: 518–521.

HUBEL, D. H. Electrocorticograms in cats during natural sleep. *Arch. ital. Biol.*, **1960**, *98*: 171–181.

OKUMA, T., FUJIMORI, M., HAYASHI, A. and NAKAMURA, K. The effect of some psychotropic drugs on the electric activity of the brain and sleep cycle pattern of the cat. *Folia psychiat. neurol. jap.*, **1967**, *21*: 1–17.

STERMAN, M. B., KNAUSS, T., LEHMANN, D. and CLEMENTE, C. D. Circadian sleep and waking patterns in the laboratory cat. *Electroenceph. clin. Neurophysiol.*, **1965**, *19*: 509–517.

WALLACH, M. B., WINTERS, W. D., MANDELL, A. J. and SPOONER, C. E. A correlation of EEG, reticular multiple unit activity and gross behavior following various antidepressant agents in the cat. IV. *Electroenceph. clin. Neurophysiol.*, **1969**, *27*: 563–573.

WINTERS, W. D., MORI, K., SPOONER, C. E. and KADO, R. T. Correlation of reticular and cochlear multiple unit activity with evoked responses during wakefulness and sleep. I. *Electroenceph. clin. Neurophysiol.*, **1967**, *23*: 539–545.

Reference: WALLACH, M. B., WINTERS, W. D., MANDELL, A. J. and SPOONER, C. E. Effects of antidepressant drugs on wakefulness and sleep in the cat. *Electroenceph. clin. Neurophysiol.*, **1969**, *27*: 574–580.

EFFECTS OF LOWERED BODY TEMPERATURE ON HYPEROXIC SEIZURES

M. L. GIRETTI[1], F. S. RUCCI AND M. LA ROCCA

Istituto di Fisiologia Umana, Istituto di Clinica Chirurgica, Università di Sassari, Sassari, Sardinia (Italy)

(Accepted for publication: April 4, 1969)

Several investigators have pointed out a protective action of hypothermia against oxygen poisoning. Campbell (1937a, b) first showed that lowering the body temperature increases the survival time of rats exposed to hyperbaric oxygen. Such a finding was confirmed and extended by other researchers, not only on mammals (Bean 1945; Grossman and Penrod 1949; Popovic *et al.* 1964), but also on invertebrates (Rosenbaum and Wittner 1960) and protozoa (Cleveland and Burke 1956; Wittner 1957). However, no one has considered up to now the effects of body cooling on the EEG alterations induced by high O_2 pressure, which are notoriously the first symptom of oxygen poisoning. The present investigations were undertaken to analyse the influence of cold on the convulsive activity elicited by hyperbaric oxygen in unrestrained, unanaesthetized rats.

In previous investigations carried out in this laboratory the influence of hyperbaric oxygen on the electrical activity of the cerebral cortex and of some subcortical structures was studied (Rucci *et al.* 1967). In another paper the role of the cerebellum in the mechanism of starting and developing hyperoxic seizures was analysed (Rucci *et al.* 1968). Thus it seemed advisable to continue such series of papers dealing with electrophysiological aspects of the hyperbaric seizures.

MATERIAL AND METHODS

Ninety male rats of the Sprague-Dawley strain, weighing 200–300 g, were employed in the present research. Under metoxyflurane anaesthesia two extradural electrodes, consisting in iron screws, were located on the cerebral cortex (usually on the frontal lobes) and two deep tungsten needles were placed in the subcortical structures (thalamus and mesencephalon) according to the technique used in our previous papers (Rucci *et al.* 1967, 1968).

The animals were cooled in a refrigerating unit a few days after insertion of the cerebral electrodes. The rectal temperature could be lowered to 35–15° C within 3–8 hours. A Grass polygraph model 7 recorded continuously and simultaneously the electrical activity of the cerebral cortex (bipolar) and of the brain-stem (Rucci *et al.* 1967, 1968), the EKG and, in many instances, the rectal temperature by means of a copper-constantan thermocouple. In other cases the rectal temperature was measured by means of a mercury thermometer. No measurements of cerebral temperature were carried out. The technique of hyperbaric oxygenation was the same as that used in our previous papers (Rucci *et al.* 1967, 1968); the O_2 pressure was 5 atm. abs. In the hyperbaric chamber the temperature was brought, by means of crushed ice, to the same level as that of the rectal temperature obtained in the cooling unit.

However, it was difficult to keep steady the rectal temperature of the rats inside the hyperbaric chamber throughout hyperoxia. In regard to this, the rats which underwent cooling in the hyperbaric chamber exhibited a relatively steady temperature, with only modest variations (mean 0.7°C $\pm$ 0.36 SE/h), during hyperbaric oxygenation. All other rats which showed larger variations in temperature were neglected.

At the end of the experiments the positions of the deep electrodes were marked by electrolysis. The animals were killed by means of a dose of Nembutal. The brain was fixed in alcohol, cleared

[1] Fellowship of C.N.R.

TABLE I

Rats classified by temperature

Groups	N	Rectal temperature (° C)
A	18	Euthermic
B	11	35–30
C	12	30–27
D	18	27–21
E	12	21–15

in xylene, embedded in paraffin, serially cut and stained according to the Nissl method to show the sites of recording. The effects of the low body temperature on the development of hyperoxic seizures were studied in 5 groups of rats (Table I) and the following parameters were analysed in each group: (1) incidence of seizures; (2) latency of the first attack. The statistical analysis was carried out by calculating the chi square for parameter 1 and Student's t test for parameter 2.

RESULTS

Effects of hyperbaric oxygen on euthermic rats

Eighteen normal rats (rectal temperature 37°C) subjected to hyperbaric oxygen were taken as a control. Hyperoxic seizures appeared in fifteen out of eighteen animals (83 %) with a mean latency of 54.26 min ± 9.16 SE.

Effects of hypothermia on the electrical activity of some cortical and subcortical structures of rats at normal air pressure

Nineteen normal animals underwent hypothermia (35°–15° C) while breathing air at normal pressure. A progressive decrease in voltage and in frequency of the cerebral electrical activity was observed during cooling.

Pre-epileptic activity, consisting of sharp waves and isolated spikes synchronous in all leads or only in cortical leads, was present when the rectal temperature attained 24° C. Eight rats out of thirteen (61%) whose rectal temperature was between 21° and 15° C (mean 17.4° C ± 1.01 SE) exhibited epileptic seizures (Fig. 1).

The attacks induced by cooling showed a lower discharge frequency and a longer duration than those elicited by hyperoxia and were not followed by post-ictal electrical silence. On the other hand hyperbaric oxygenation was capable of blocking hypothermic attacks: in fact in three animals the seizures induced by cooling disappeared at the beginning of hyperbaric oxygenation (Fig. 1, *C*).

Effects of hyperbaric oxygen on hypothermic rats (Fig. 2 and 3)

Fifty-three rats were exposed to hyperbaric oxygen at different rectal temperatures. The results in this group of animals were compared with those in the animals under hyperbaric oxygen alone (Table II). A significant decrease in the incidence of seizures was obtained when the rectal temperature was 35–27° C (groups B and

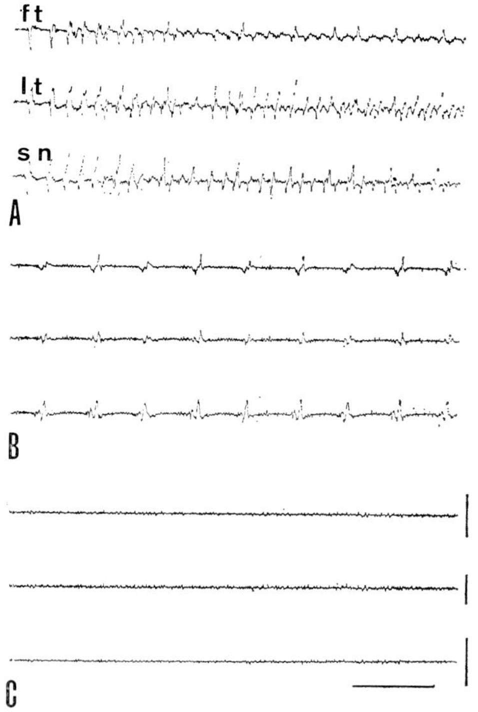

Fig. 1

Effect of hyperbaric oxygen on hypothermic attacks. Rat No. A95. Rectal temperature: in *A* and *B* 17°C , in *C* 15° C. *A*: onset of hypothermic seizure. *B*: 2 min after *A*, just before the beginning of hyperbaric oxygenation. *C*: immediately after the beginning of hyperbaric oxygenation. Note the disappearance of spikes. Calibrations: 2 sec and 200 μV.

Abbreviations in this and in the following figures: cc: crus cerebri; ekg: electrocardiogram; ft: frontal transverse; lt: n.lateralis thalami; mrf: mesencephalic reticular formation; sga: substantia grisea periaqueductalis; sn: substantia nigra; vt: n.ventralis thalami.

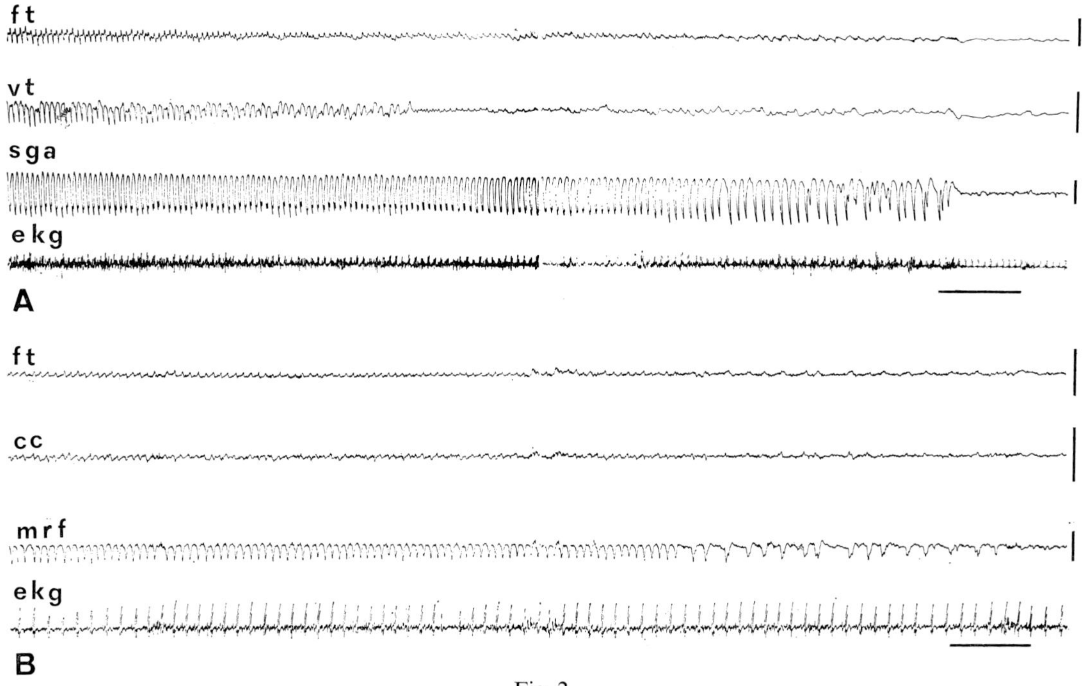

Fig. 2

Low body temperature and hyperoxia. *A*: rat No. A60. Rectal temperature 22°C. Record taken 57 min after the beginning of hyperoxia. *B*: rat No. A61. Rectal temperature 25.5° C. Record taken 40 min after the beginning of hyperoxia. Both *A* and *B* show the end of the first attack. The two seizures were predominantly subcortical. Calibrations: 2 sec and 400 μV.

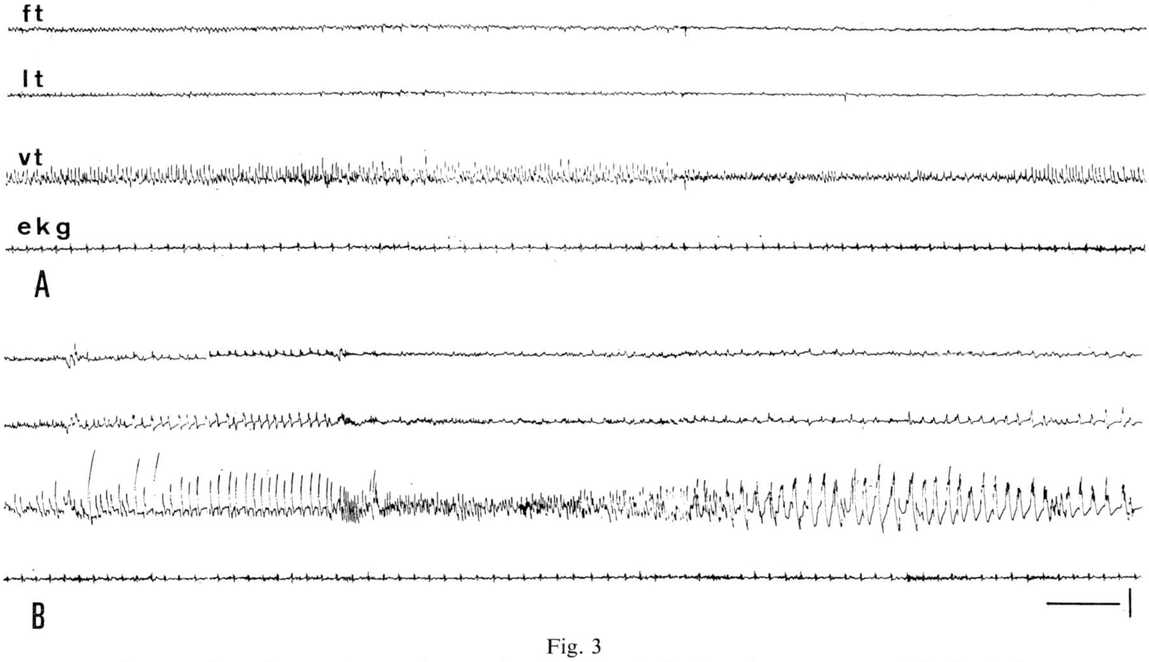

Fig. 3

Influence of cooling on hyperoxic attacks. Rat No. A49. Rectal temperature: 22° C. *A*: first attack 64 min after the beginning of hyperoxia; *B*: second hyperoxic attack 1 min after *A*. The appearance of the two attacks was evident in the subcortical formations. Calibrations: 2 sec and 400 μV.

TABLE II

Incidence of hyperoxic seizures in hypothermic rats

	A	B	C	D	E	Totals	Comparison	*df*	χ^2	*P*
Attack	15	5	5	12	3	40	A *vs.* D	1	1.32	N.S.
No attack	3	6	7	6	9	31	B *vs.* C	1	0.03	N.S.
Totals	18	11	12	18	12	71	B + C *vs.* E	1	1.13	N.S.
% Attack	83	45	42	67	25		A + D *vs.*B+C+E	1	10.32	< 0.005
							Total	4	12.46	< 0.015

C) and 21–15° C (group E). The rectal temperature of 27–21° C (group D) was particularly critical: at such a level the percentage of animals (67%) which exhibited attacks was similar to that of the euthermic control animals (group A).

Table II summarizes the incidence of hyperoxic seizures in the various groups of hypothermic and euthermic animals.

The statistical analysis (χ^2) showed that the cooled animals did not represent a homogeneous population and the most significant differences were found between the control rats (group A) and those (group D) whose rectal temperature was 27–21° C *versus* the other groups ($P < 0.005$).

The latency of the first attack (Table III) was related to the incidence of the seizures. Lowering rectal temperature (groups B and C) induced a progressive and significant increase in latency of the first attack (maximal value: 137 min ± 7.76 SE, group C). Between 27 and 21° C (group D) the increase in incidence was accompanied by a highly significant decrease in latency ($P < 0.001$) *versus* group C. The number of rats which exhibited a hyperoxic attack below 21° C (group E) was too small for statistical analysis.

TABLE III

Effects of hypothermia on the latency of hyperoxic seizures

Groups	A	B	C	D	E
N	15	5	5	12	3
Mean	54.26	80.40	137.20	76.16	109.66
S.E.	9.16	16.86	7.76	5.50	11.26

Student's *t* test

Groups	B	C	D	E
A	0.88	4.96**	1.92	3.33
C	3.06*		6.20**	2.09

*$P < 0.02$.
**$P < 0.001$.

The cooled rats exhibited some peculiarities in the ECoG aspects, more evident in those with rectal temperature below 27° C: (1) in some instances the first epileptic attack appeared first in the subcortical structures and then in the cortex; (2) the cortex showed a lower voltage than the subcortical formations; (3) sometimes the attacks faded away first from the cortex and then from the subcortical leads (Fig. 2); (4) in some instances the seizures were exclusively subcortical (Fig. 3).

DISCUSSION

It is well known that hypothermia is capable of decreasing the electrical activity of the normal cerebral cortex. However, there is no agreement on a possible role of hypothermia in provoking epileptic activity.

Hypothermic spikes were seen in dogs at 22° C (Ferrari and Amantea 1955), in kittens at 17° C (Jouvet *et al.* 1956) and in cats at 22–21° C (Lipp 1964). Spontaneous spikes were recorded by Lourie *et al.* (1960) in cooled dogs, while a pre-convulsive state was recorded by Noell and Briller (1953) in hypothermic rabbits. Conversely, other investigators have observed an increase in convulsive threshold in hypothermic monkeys (Baldwin *et al.* 1956) and progressive disappearance of the seizures following local cooling of the human cerebral cortex (Ommaya and Baldwin 1963). No seizures were observed by Battista (1967) in hypothermic cats. We are in agreement with those who claimed hypothermic attacks: at rectal temperatures of 25–21° C isolated spikes were seen; however, seizures occurred only at rectal temperatures of 21–15° C. Thus, under such experimental conditions, a clear-cut pre-seizure activity was present in all the animals, whereas epileptic seizures appeared only in 61% of the animals when the rectal temperature was lowered below 21° C.

That no seizures were observed under cooling by some researchers could be explained by their animals not being subjected to a sufficiently deep hypothermia: in fact also Belsey *et al.* (1968) recently described seizures in man only when the rectal temperature was 15° C in the course of deep hypothermia for cardiac surgery.

It should be noted that the seizures induced by cooling could be related to the concomitant hypoxia caused by lowering of breathing rate and of blood pressure. In fact the spikes induced by hypothermia faded away when the animals were exposed to hyperbaric oxygen. Thus Belsey *et al.* (1968) did not observe seizures in man during hypothermia when the pCO_2 was maintained at a steady level of 40 mm of Hg.

By combining hypothermia with hyperoxia in the present research a decrease in the appearance of hyperoxic seizures occurred; also the latency of the seizures was longer. However, at rectal temperatures of 27–31° C the incidence and latency of the seizures were similar to those observed in normal animals. Thus the hypothermia seemed to have an inhibitory role on the development of hyperoxic seizures except when the body temperature was 27–21° C. It is difficult to explain such an effect. However, a probable explanation could be that lowering the body temperature decreased metabolic activity of the whole organism and of the nervous system (Grossman and Penrod 1949; Popovic *et al.* 1964). It is more difficult to explain why, at rectal temperatures of 27–21° C, the behaviour of the animals submitted to hyperbaric oxygen was about the same as that of euthermic rats. Further investigations are necessary in regard to this. Particularly the variations in the pH, pO_2 and pCO_2 of the cerebral structures should be analysed. On the other hand one could suppose that at this rectal temperature the inhibition of seizures by some cerebral structures could be removed. Previous investigations showed that the cerebellum has an inhibitory role in experimental epilepsy induced by hyperbaric oxygen (Rucci *et al.* 1968). Other investigators (Chatfield *et al.* 1951) pointed out a hierarchy in the inhibition of the various brain structures by hypothermia.

SUMMARY

The influence of hypothermia on the mechanism of hyperoxic seizures in unrestrained, unanaesthetized rats was investigated. In a first group of animals the effect of simple hypothermia on the cerebral electrical activity was analysed: a pre-epileptic activity, consisting of isolated spikes and sharp waves, occurred at a rectal temperature of 24° C, and spontaneous convulsive activity was recorded in 61% of animals when the body temperature was below 21° C (mean 17.4° C ± 1.01 SE). Hyperbaric oxygen stopped the hypothermic seizures. The starting and development of hyperbaric seizures were investigated in a second group of hypothermic rats (rectal temperatures of 35–15° C) in comparison with euthermic animals submitted to simple hyperoxia. Hypothermia provoked a decrease in the incidence of seizures and an increase in their latency. A probable explanation for this could be that, by lowering the body temperature, a decrease in the metabolic activity of the whole organism and of the nervous system was induced. The rectal temperature of 27–21° C was particularly critical; at such a level the percentage of animals which exhibited attacks, and the latency of the first attack, were similar to those shown by euthermic control animals.

Seizures in cooled rats submitted to hyperoxia were more evident in subcortical than in cortical structures.

RÉSUMÉ

EFFETS DE L'ABAISSEMENT DE LA TEMPÉRATURE CORPORELLE SUR LES CRISES HYPEROXIQUES

L'influence de l'hypothermie sur le mécanisme des crises hyperoxiques a été étudiée chez des rats libres et non anesthésiés. Dans un premier groupe d'animaux, l'effet de l'hypothermie simple sur l'activité électrique cérébrale a été analysé: une activité pré-épileptique, consistant en pointes ou ondes pointues isolées survient à une température rectale de 24° C et une activité convulsive spontanée est enregistrée chez 61% des animaux quand la température corporelle est inférieure à 21° C (moyenne 17.4° C ± 1.01 SE). L'oxygène hyperbare arrête les crises hypothermiques. Le début et le développement des crises hyperbares sont étudiés dans un second groupe de rats en hypothermie (température rectale de 35–15° C) par comparaison avec des animaux à température normale soumis à l'hyperoxie simple. L'hypothermie provoque une diminution dans la survenue des crises et une augmentation de leur latence. Une explication probable de ces données pourrait être que, en abaissant la température corporelle, on induit une diminution de l'activité métabolique de l'organisme global et du système nerveux. La température rectale de 27–21° est particulièrement critique; à ce stade, le pourcentage d'animaux qui présentent des crises et la latence de la première crise sont semblables à ceux que l'on observe chez les animaux de contrôle à température normale.

Chez les rats en hypothermie soumis à l'hyperoxie, les crises sont plus évidentes dans les structures sous-corticales que dans les structures corticales.

REFERENCES

BALDWIN, M., FROST, L. L., WOOD, C. D. and LEWIS, S. A. Effect of hypothermia on epileptiform activity in the primate temporal lobe. *Science*, **1956,** *124*: 931–932.

BATTISTA, A. F. Effect of cold on cortical potentials in the cat. *Exp. Neurol.*, **1967,** *19*: 140–155.

BEAN, J. W. Effects of oxygen at increased pressure. *Physiol. Rev.*, **1945,** *25*: 1–143.

BELSEY, R. H. R., DOWLATSHAHI, K., KEEN, G. and SKINNER, D. B. Profound hypothermia in cardiac surgery. *J. thorac. cardiovasc. Surg.*, **1968,** *56*: 497–509.

CAMPBELL, J. A. Oxygen poisoning and tumour growth. *Brit. J. exp. Path.*, **1937**a, *18*: 191–197.

CAMPBELL, J. A. Body temperature and oxygen poisoning. *J. Physiol. (Lond.)*, **1937**b, *89*: 17P.

CHATFIELD, P. O., LYMAN C. P. and PURPURA, D. P. The effects of temperature on the spontaneous and induced electrical activity in the cerebral cortex of the golden hamster. *Electroenceph. clin. Neurophysiol.*, **1951,** *3*: 225–230.

CLEVELAND, L. R. and BURKE JR., A. W. Effects of temperature and tension on oxygen toxicity for the protozoa of Cryptocercus. *J. Protozool.*, **1956,** *3*: 74–77.

FERRARI, E. and AMANTEA, L. Convulsive electrocortical discharges in hypothermic dogs. *Electroenceph. clin. Neurophysiol.*, **1955,** *7*: 441P.

GROSSMAN, M. S. and PENROD, K. E. Relationship of hypothermia to high oxygen poisoning. *Amer. J. Physiol.*, **1949,** *156*: 177–181.

JOUVET, M., BENOIT, O., COURJON, J. and TANCHE, M. The EEG during hypothermia in paralyzed cats. *Electroenceph. clin. Neurophysiol.*, **1956,** *8*: 708P.

LIPP, J. A. Effect of deep hypothermia on the electrical activity of the brain. *Electroenceph. clin. Neurophysiol.*, **1964,** *17*: 46–51.

LOURIE, H., HOLMES, T. G., WEINSTEIN, W., SCHWARTZ, H. G. and O'LEARY, J. L. Observations on selective brain cooling in dogs. *Arch. Neurol. (Chic.)*, **1960,** *3*: 163–176.

NOELL, W. K. and BRILLER, S. A. *The effects of hypothermia on brain activity.* Project No. 21/1202-0003, Rep. No 1,1–33, Air Univ., U.S.A. School of Aviation Medicine, Randolph Field, Texas, **1953.**

OMMAYA, A. K. and BALDWIN, M. Extravascular local cooling of the brain in man. *J. Neurosurg.*, **1963,** *20*: 8–20.

POPOVIC, V., GERSCHMAN, R. and GILBERT, D. L. Effects of high oxygen pressure on ground squirrels in hypothermia and hibernation. *Amer. J. Physiol.*, **1964,** *206*: 49–50.

ROSENBAUM, R. M. and WITTNER, M. The effects of hyperatmospheric oxygen concentration on early cleavage in the sand dollar, *Echinarachnius parma*. *Exp. Cell Res.*, **1960,** *20*: 416–427.

RUCCI, F. S., GIRETTI, M. L. and LA ROCCA, M. Changes in electrical activity of the cerebral cortex and of some subcortical centers in hyperbaric oxygen. *Electroenceph. clin. Neurophysiol.*, **1967,** *22*: 231–238.

RUCCI, F. S., GIRETTI, M. L. and LA ROCCA, M. Cerebellum and hyperbaric oxygen. *Electroenceph. clin. Neurophysiol.*, **1968,** *25*: 359–371.

WITTNER, M. Effects of temperature and pressure on oxygen poisoning of Paramecium. *J. Protozool.*, **1957,** *4*: 20–23.

Reference: GIRETTI, M. L., RUCCI, F. S. and LA ROCCA, M. Effects of lowered body temperature on hyperoxic seizures. *Electroenceph. clin. Neurophysiol.*, **1969,** *27*: 581–586.

PRIMARY AUDITORY EVOKED POTENTIALS AFTER SECTION OF BRACHIUM OF THE INFERIOR COLLICULUS[1]

JERZY MAJKOWSKI[2] AND PILAR P. MORGADES[3]

Brain Research Laboratories, Department of Psychiatry, New York Medical College, New York, N.Y. 10029 (U.S.A.)

(Accepted for publication: April 14, 1969)

There is rather general agreement that the first positive component of the cortical positive-negative primary sensory evoked potentials depends on the lemniscal system; the negative component depends on the multi-synaptic unspecific system.

In our previous studies, the disappearance of primary auditory evoked potentials (PAEPs) in the auditory cortex was considered as an indicator of completeness of the section of the brachia of the inferior colliculus (BIC) (Majkowski and Jasper, unpublished; Majkowski 1964). Galambos *et al.* (1961) confirmed this finding in experiments in which Nembutal (pentobarbital) anesthesia was used. However, with chloralose or in the absence of anesthetics, the auditory evoked potentials in auditory cortex persisted unchanged after section of BIC. Recently, Adrian *et al.* (1966) using chloralose came to the conclusion that the section confined to the lateral quadrant of the midbrain may abolish the evoked potentials from auditory areas, but they stated also that the short latency, positive-negative potentials may be recorded from auditory cortex after complete section of BIC. The same conclusion was reached by Goldberg and Neff (1961).

On the other hand, there is agreement that the secondary evoked potentials with long latency, duration and lability, which can be recorded outside of primary auditory areas, *e.g.*, in middle suprasylvian, anterior lateral gyri and in somatomotor cortex (Lombroso and Merlis 1957; Buser and Borenstein 1959; Buser *et al.* 1959; Thompson and Sindberg 1960), are not influenced, in recordable way, by section of BIC.

The question of the mediation of auditory impulses by the specific or unspecific systems is very important from the point of view of neurophysiological mechanisms of auditory discriminative learning in cats with section of BIC (Kryter and Ades 1943; Raab and Ades 1946; Goldberg and Neff 1961; Majkowski 1964). It seems that the phylogenetically newer lemniscal pathways, with their fast conduction fibers, play an important role in carrying meaningful information. It was found that after section of BIC the learning to clicks took 2–3 times longer than in intact cats (Majkowski 1964). However, when the section was not complete, even on one side, and some fibers (about 10%) were not cut, the learning was not changed. Thus, the extent of the lesion seems to be very critical for behavioral and electrophysiological results.

The purpose of these experiments was to study the PAEPs in acute and chronic preparation, before and after section of BIC, with Nembutal and chloralose anesthesia, without anesthesia, and after electrical stimulation of inferior colliculi (IC).

MATERIAL AND TECHNIQUE

The experiments were performed on twenty adult, healthy male and female cats, which seemed to have normal hearing. The weights of the cats were between 2.5 and 3.5 kg. Nembutal (40 mg/kg, i.p.) or chloralose anesthesia (65–70 mg/kg, i.p.) was used. In some cats the PAEPs were studied chronically without any anesthetics,

[1] This work was supported by U.S. Public Health Service Grant MH 08579.

[2] Present address: Clinical and Experimental EEG Laboratory, Department of Neurology, Medical Academy, Warsaw, Poland.

[3] Present address: Department of Neurology, Columbia University, 630 W. 168th Street, New York, N.Y. 10032.

in the period up to 5 months after section of BIC. In addition to auditory stimulation, electrical stimulation of the IC was performed before and after section of BIC. The PAEPs were studied on both sides in auditory cortex (A1), medial geniculate body (MGB), and in IC. Small 0.5 mm holes were drilled in the skull over the projection area of A1. When PAEPs with the shortest latency and the largest amplitude were found, the wire electrodes were fixed by cement epidurally or cortically. Bipolar depth electrodes were placed in MGB (coordinates: A5, L8, H1) and in IC (P1, 5, L5, H3). Pictures of single and superimposed evoked potentials were taken using a Grass kymograph camera C4J or a polaroid camera from the Tektronix dual-beam oscilloscope (Type 502) or storage oscilloscope (Type 564) with Tektronix pre-amplifier (Type 122). In some chronic experiments, the PAEPs were recorded on magnetic tape and then studied on a CAT computer.

Different types of wire electrodes were used for depth recording but mostly consisted of two stainless steel wire electrodes (0.25 mm diameter) with a 1 mm spacing between contacts. The epoxylite insulation was removed about 0.5 mm from the tip of the electrodes. The cortical electrodes were made from the same wire. The dis-

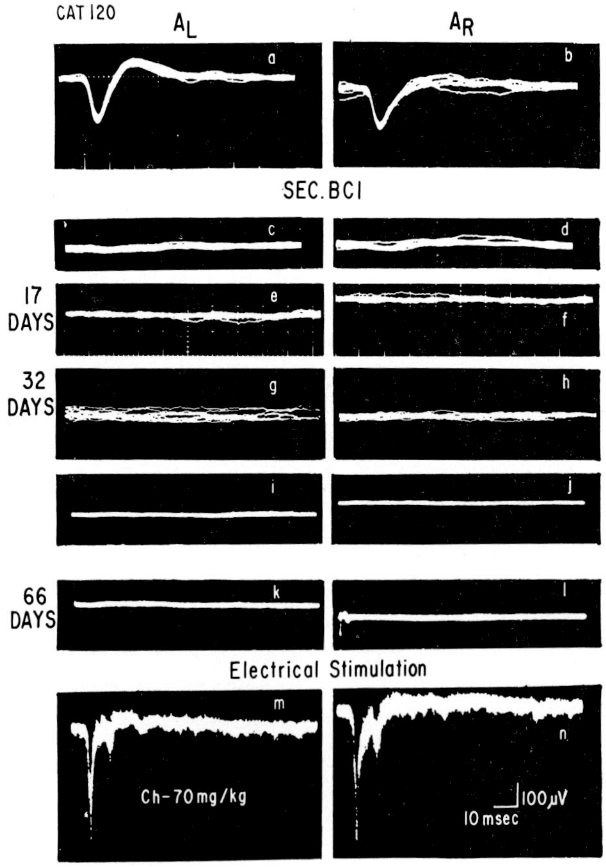

Fig. 1

Cat C-120. The PAEPs from A1 (left and right) are seen at *a* and *b*. At *c* and *d*, after section of BIC, the PAEPs disappeared (some delayed response disappeared in a few minutes). Control records taken 17 days later under chloralose (*e* and *f*); 32 days later under Nembutal (*g* and *h*) and 66 days later under chloralose anesthesia (*i* and *j*). All records show no PAEPs in auditory cortex. At the time electrical stimulation of IC was performed with the same result (*k* and *l*). The PAEPs from IC were not changed (*m* and *n*). All records with exception of *i*, *j*, *k* and *l* represent 10 superimposed evoked responses.

tance between them was 2–3 mm. All records shown were taken with bipolar electrodes.

The section of BIC was performed either after complete removal of the skull bone or after making a round opening on each side of the skull of about 2 cm in diameter, anterior to the tentorium. In the first procedure, dura was removed completely and the brain was immersed in paraffin oil of appropriate temperature. In the second procedure, dura was cut along the occipital lobe. In both cases, the occipital lobe was slightly retracted forward and upward in order to approach the BIC. The space between the tentorium and the retracted hemisphere was about 3 mm. After visualization of the BIC, the section was performed on one side and auditory responses were studied. Next, the section was performed on the other side and auditory responses were studied on both sides. Cortical and sometimes MGB electrodes were not changed after section, but the electrodes in IC had to be implanted again after every BIC section.

A loudspeaker emitting clicks at a frequency of 1 c/sec, 0.5 msec duration, and about 70 dB intensity, was placed in front of the cat's head at a distance of 40 cm. Clicks were delivered through hollow earpieces inserted into the external auditory canals. For electrical stimulation of IC, a Grass stimulator S4 was used, delivering single, unidirectional, rectangular impulses of 0.3–1 msec, 6–12 V at 1/sec. The same electrodes were employed for stimulation and recording. In chronic experiments, the cats were tested for auditory responses with anesthesia and without, during a period of up to 5 months. At the end of each experiment, perfusion of the brain with 10% formalin solution was performed and the lesion was examined by histological methods (Luxol fast blue–PAS–hematoxylin).

RESULTS

From this experimental material, five chronic cats with complete section of the BIC and with observations over several months after operation were chosen for presentation.

C-120

Section of the BIC was performed under alpha-chloralose anesthesia (70 mg/kg, i.p.). Fig. 1 shows the PAEPs before (*a*, *b*) and after (*c*, *d*) section of the BIC. Recordings were taken 17 days later (*e*, *f*) under alpha-chloralose anesthesia (70 mg/kg), and 32 days after section (*g*, *h*) under Nembutal anesthesia (40 mg/kg). They showed no PAEPs.

Electrical stimulation was performed 66 days later (*k*, *l*) and auditory stimulation (*i*, *j*) showed no PAEPs under alpha-chloralose anesthesia. The PAEPs in IC were not changed (*m*, *n*).

Histological studies show section of both BIC and the lesion extending to central gray on the right side (see Fig. 2).

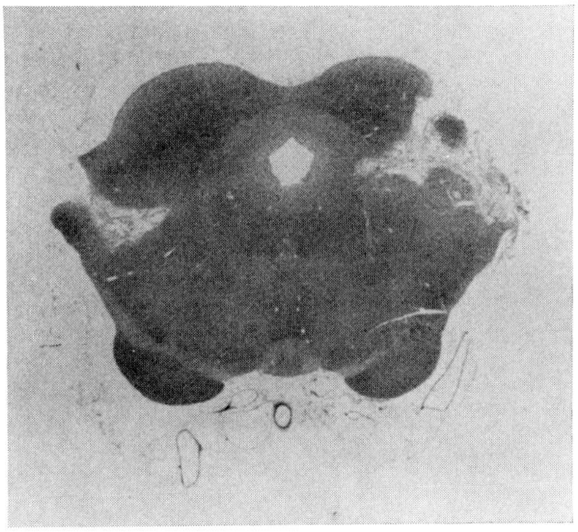

Fig. 2
Cat C-120. Histological preparation showing bilateral lesions in BIC. On the right side, the lesion extends to central gray.

C-51

Section of the left BIC under alpha-chloralose anesthesia (70 mg/kg, i.p.) resulted in disappearance of cortical PAEPs on the side of the section (Fig. 3, *a*, *b*). However, there was some delayed response on the left side which disappeared after subsequent section of the right BIC. Section on both sides resulted in disappearance of the PAEPs on both sides (*c*).

The PAEP in IC (Fig. 3, *d*–*f*) before and after section of the BIC has a different shape, amplitude and duration. This is due to reimplantation of electrodes after section of the BIC. However, the latency of these responses (about 4 msec) was unchanged. The PAEP in this cat was tested several times under Nembutal and alpha-chloral-

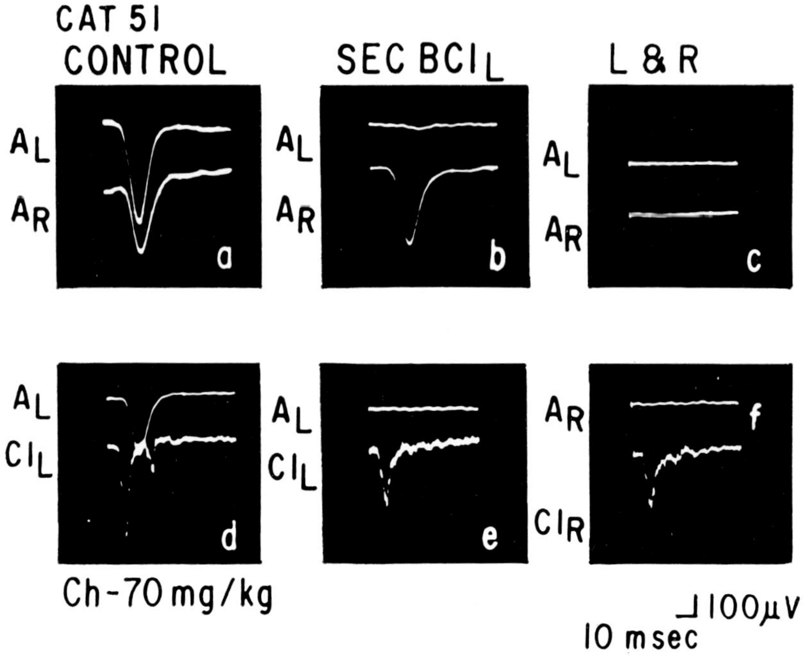

Fig. 3
Cat C-51. Control PAEP before BIC (*a* and *d*). After section of left BIC, there is a trace of response with longer latency in left auditory cortex (AL). On the right side, there is slight increase of amplitude of the PAEP (*b*). The additional section of the right BIC resulted in disappearance of both PAEPs (*c*, *e*, *f*). The change of PAEP in CI is due to reimplantation of electrodes in CI (compare *d* with *e* and *f*).
Abbreviations: AL and AR, cortical auditory areas A1 on left and right side. CIL and CIR, colliculus inferior left and right, respectively. Ch, chloralose. L & R, section of left and right BIC.

ose anesthesia and also without anesthetics, always with the same results. Fig. 4 shows absence of the PAEPs in the cortex and in the MGB 4 months after section of the BIC, with recordings from the unanesthetized, awake animal. Histological studies of this cat showed complete section of the BIC on both sides.

C-119

Section of the BIC performed under alpha-chloralose (70 mg/kg, i.p.) resulted in bilateral disappearance of the PAEP. The PAEP from the IC was not changed. Ninety days after section of the BIC, there were no PAEPs in the cortex

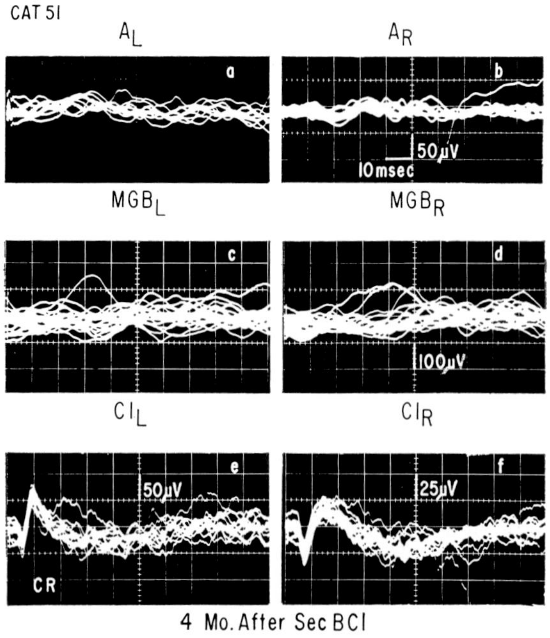

Fig. 4
Cat C-51. Control records of the same cat as in Fig. 1, 4 months after section of BIC, taken without any anesthetics. There are no PAEPs in auditory cortex (A1) and in MGB on both sides (*a–d*) and there are PAEPs in IC (*e*, *f*). All records represent the mean of 25 superimposed responses. (Amplification in *a* as in *b*; in *c* as in *d*.)

and MGB (recording without anesthetics). However, good responses were recorded from the IC. Histology shows complete demyelinization of both BIC.

C-138

PAEPs were studied in both auditory cortex, in response to auditory stimulation. After section of the BIC, there were no PAEPs to auditory or electrical stimulations of the IC, performed under Nembutal anesthesia. However, a weak response, suggestive of a residual PAEP, persisted on the right side.

Histological studies indicated that some fibers ventral to the BIC were not completely demyelinized on the right side, whereas the left side lesion was more extensive and the section was complete. Electrical stimulation of the left or right IC after section of the left BIC revealed no PAEP in the left auditory cortex. However, stimulation of the left IC and recording from the right auditory cortex revealed normal response, indicating commissural transmission between the IC.

C-141

Section of the BIC was performed under alpha-chloralose anesthesia (65 mg/kg). The PAEP disappeared after the operation. Three and 5 weeks later, the PAEPs were tested again under chloralose anesthesia and there were no PAEPs. Histological examination shows complete section of both BIC.

DISCUSSION

The PAEP seems to be sensory specific since the bilateral section of auditory pathways at the level of BIC resulted in its disappearance. The effect was permanent for several months and could be observed under Nembutal or alpha-chloralose anesthesia as well as without any anesthetics. Moreover, the electrical stimulation of IC failed to evoke the responses in MGB and in auditory cortex A1. The same conclusion was reached by Nieder and Strominger (1965) with pentobarbital anesthesia and without it by Adrian and Goldberg (1962) and to some extent by Adrian *et al.* (1966) with alpha-chloralose anesthesia. Thus, these results are not in agreement with those of Galambos *et al.* (1961).

On the other hand, it is known that cats with section of BIC can learn to respond to tones (Goldberg and Neff 1961) and to clicks (Majkowski 1964). In such cats the clicks used as conditioned stimuli evoke a conditioned rhythmical activity in mesencephalic reticular formation and in motor cortex. This activity is similar to that obtained in cats with intact auditory pathways (Majkowski and John, unpublished), indicating that auditory impulses are mediated by neurons below the section, propagating to motor and other cortical areas through the so-called unspecific system with the long latency and other characteristic features of the non-primary types of evoked potentials. There are known collaterals from auditory pathways (below section of BIC) which enter the reticular formation of the brain-stem (Jungert 1958), mesencephalic reticular formation (Moore and Goldberg 1961) and central gray matter (Moore and Goldberg 1963).

It seems to us that unchanged PAEPs after section of BIC reported by Galambos *et al.* (1961) might have been due to incomplete section of BIC. Alternatively, the postulated extra-lemniscal route parallel to this lemniscal system might be so close to BIC that it would be included anatomically in the same bundle of fibers. The same possibility might be considered to account for the results described by Adrian *et al.* (1966), who recorded "short latency" positive-negative potentials after complete section of BIC, suggesting that impulses can reach auditory cortex by other than BIC pathways. It is possible that in our studies the section was more extensive than in those of Galambos *et al.* (1961). However, no difference was observed between influence of Nembutal and alpha-chloralose and between anesthetized and non-anesthetized animals on the PAEP before and after section. Thus, it seems that the very attractive hypothesis about fast conducting "poly-synaptic pathways" in reticular formation is rather questionable.

Majkowski (1962, 1964) had suggested the possible formation in reticular formation (after section of BIC) of new, relatively specific pathways, which were called "para-specific". This formation or rather transformation of potentially existing pathways to functionally transmitting, relatively specific routes, would result from the learning process; that is, repetition of conditioning auditory stimuli. The learning in cats after section of BIC took 2–3 times longer than in intact cats. Indication of the possible existence of such systems in the mesencephalic reticular formation was shown recently by Kadjaya and Narikashvili (1966). However, the long latency of such responses indicates slow-conducting multisynaptic pathways.

SUMMARY

The primary auditory evoked potentials (PAEPs) were studied in acute and chronic experiments before and after section of the brachia of the inferior colliculus (BIC) under Nembutal and alpha-chloralose anesthesia, without anesthesia and during electrical stimulation of inferior colliculi (IC). Out of twenty cats, five were chosen for detailed presentation.

The section of BIC resulted in disappearance of PAEPs recorded from auditory cortex A1, regardless of the type of anesthesia and in cats without anesthetics, during auditory and electrical stimulation of IC. This effect lasted for several months.

The results are discussed from the point of view of relative specificity of the pathways in reticular formation which would transmit the auditory impulses to levels above section of BIC.

RÉSUMÉ

POTENTIELS ÉVOQUÉS AUDITIFS PRIMAIRES APRÈS SECTION DU BRAS DU TUBERCULE QUADRIJUMEAU INFÉRIEUR

Les potentiels évoqués auditifs primaires (PAEPs) ont été étudiés dans des expériences aiguës et chroniques avant et après section du bras du tubercule quadrijumeau inférieur sous anesthésie au Nembutal et à l'alpha-chloralose, sans anesthésie et pendant la stimulation électrique du tubercule quadrijumeau inférieur. Dans une série de vingt chats, cinq ont été sélectionnés pour une présentation détaillée.

La section du bras du tubercule quadrijumeau inférieur aboutit à la disparition des PAEPs enregistrés au niveau du cortex auditif A1, quel que soit le type d'anesthésie ou en l'absence d'anesthésie, au cours de la stimulation auditive et de la stimulation électrique du tubercule quadrijumeau inférieur. Cet effet dure plusieurs mois.

Ces résultats sont discutés du point de vue de la spécificité relative des voies situées dans la formation réticulaire qui transmettraient les influx auditifs à des niveaux situés au-dessus de la section du bras du tubercule quadrijumeau inférieur.

We wish to express our gratitude to Dr. E. R. John who provided us with the facilities to perform these studies.

REFERENCES

ADRIAN, H. O. and GOLDBERG, J. M. Cortical potentials evoked by auditory stimuli after section of the brachium of the inferior colliculus in the cat. *Anat. Rec.*, **1962,** *142*: 207.

ADRIAN, H. O., GOLDBERG, J. M. and BRUGGE, J. F. Auditory evoked cortical potentials after lesions of brachium of inferior colliculus. *J. Neurophysiol.*, **1966,** *29*: 456–466.

BUSER, P. et BORENSTEIN, P. Réponses somesthésiques, visuelles et auditives, recueillies au niveau du cortex "associatif" suprasylvien chez le chat curarisé non anesthésié. *Electroenceph. clin. Neurophysiol.*, **1959,** *11*: 285–304.

BUSER, P., BORENSTEIN, P. et BRUNER, J. Étude des systèmes "associatifs" visuels et auditifs chez le chat anesthésié au chloralose. *Electroenceph. clin. Neurophysiol.*, **1959,** *11*: 305–324.

GALAMBOS, R., MYERS, R. E. and SHEATZ, G. C. Extralemniscal activation of auditory cortex in cats. *Amer. J. Physiol.*, **1961,** *200*: 23–28.

GOLDBERG, J. M. and NEFF, W. D. Frequency discrimination after bilateral section of the brachium of the inferior colliculus. *J. comp. Neurol.*, **1961,** *116*: 256–290.

JUNGERT, S. Auditory pathways in the brain stem. *Acta oto-laryng. (Stockh.)*, **1958,** *Suppl. 138*: 183–185.

KADJAYA, D. V. and NARIKASHVILI, S. P. Topography of electrical responses to different peripheral stimuli in the mesencephalic reticular formation of the cat. *Physiol. and Behav.*, **1966,** *1*: 209–213.

KRYTER, K. and ADES, H. Studies on the function of the higher acoustic nervous centers in the cat. *Amer. J. Psychol.*, **1943,** *56*: 501–536.

LOMBROSO, C. T. and MERLIS, J. K. Suprasylvian auditory responses in the cat. *Electroenceph. clin. Neurophysiol.*, **1957,** *9*: 301–308.

MAJKOWSKI, J. Aspura rolului sistemului specific şi al celui asanumit nespecific, in conditionare. *Stud. Cercet. Neurol.*, **1962,** *7*: 157–171.

MAJKOWSKI, J. Wplyw niszczenia dróg sluchowych kota na proces uczenia się odpowiedzi na bodźce dźwiękowe. *Rozpr. Wydz. Nauk. med. pol. Akad. Nauk*, **1964,** *9*: 59–108.

MOORE, R. Y. and GOLDBERG, J. M. Midbrain auditory connections in the cat. *Anat. Rec.*, **1961,** *139*: 256.

MOORE, R. Y. and GOLDBERG, J. M. Ascending projections of the inferior colliculus in the cat. *J. comp. Neurol.*, **1963,** *121*: 109–136.

NIEDER, P. C. and STROMINGER, N. Evoked potentials in auditory cortex after bilateral transection of the brachium of the inferior colliculus in the cat. *J. Neurophysiol.*, **1965,** *28*: 1185–1194.

RAAB, D. and ADES, H. Cortical and midbrain mediation of a conditioned discrimination of acoustic intensities. *Amer. J. Psychol.*, **1946,** *59*: 59–83.

THOMPSON, R. and SINDBERG, R. Auditory response fields in association and motor cortex of cat. *J. Neurophysiol.*, **1960,** *23*: 88–105.

Reference: MAJKOWSKI, J. and MORGADES, P. P. Primary auditory evoked potentials after section of brachium of the inferior colliculus. *Electroenceph. clin. Neurophysiol.*, **1969,** *27*: 587–593.

Electroencephalography and Clinical Neurophysiology
Elsevier Publishing Company, Amsterdam – Printed in The Netherlands

A TEST OF AN "EFFERENT MODEL" OF THE FUNCTION OF INFEROTEMPORAL CORTEX IN VISUAL DISCRIMINATION[1]

PHILIP A. SCHWARTZKROIN[2], ALAN COWEY[3] AND CHARLES G. GROSS

Department of Psychology, Harvard University, Cambridge, Mass. 02138 (U.S.A.)

(Accepted for publication: April 4, 1969)

A series of investigations over 30 years has revealed that ablation of specific regions of "association" cortex of the rhesus monkey produces specific impairments in discrimination learning (see references in Pribram 1954; Mishkin 1966). Specifically, inferotemporal cortex appears necessary for normal visual discrimination, superior temporal cortex for auditory discrimination, posterior parietal cortex for somesthetic discrimination, anterior temporal cortex for olfactory discrimination, and the insula for gustatory discrimination.

The impairment of visual discrimination following inferotemporal lesions has been the most intensively studied of these dysfunctions. Recently two models of the inferotemporal deficit have been suggested. The first may be called a "serial processing model". It is based primarily on the facts that: (a) inferotemporal cortex receives input from prestriate cortex (Kuypers *et al.* 1965); (b) this input is necessary for normal visual discrimination (Mishkin 1966); and (c) single units in inferotemporal cortex are specifically responsive to visual stimuli (Gross *et al.* 1967). The model suggests that inferotemporal cortex is a further stage in the hierarchy of processing mechanisms for visual information that Hubel and Wiesel (1962, 1965) have demonstrated in the retina, lateral geniculate body, striate cortex and prestriate cortex. Unlike these processing stations, inferotemporal cortex is hypothesized also to receive previously stored information about the visual world; *e.g.*, past associations of visual stimuli, responses to them, and the consequences of such responses.

The second model of inferotemporal function is an "efferent" one (Spinelli and Pribram 1966, 1967; Pribram 1967). It is based primarily on the facts that: (a) inferotemporal cortex sends projections to several subcortical sites (Whitlock and Nauta 1956); (b) undercutting of inferotemporal cortex impairs visual discrimination (Pribram *et al.* 1966); and (c) chronic stimulation of inferotemporal cortex alters the recovery cycle of striate cortex evoked responses to paired flashes so that the striate evoked response to a second of two light flashes is depressed (Spinelli and Pribram 1966). Pribram and collaborators suggest that inferotemporal cortex exerts an inhibitory influence on the visual system; chronic stimulation is hypothesized to enhance this efferent inhibition and hence depress the recovery cycle. According to the model, inferotemporal lesions remove this inhibitory influence, and thereby impair visual discrimination performance. Spinelli and Pribram (1966) and Pribram (1967) specifically predict that after inferotemporal lesions this disinhibition will be reflected in an enhanced striate evoked response to the second of two light flashes.

The present experiment is a direct test of this prediction from the efferent model of inferotemporal cortex: recovery functions of evoked responses recorded from striate cortex to paired flashes were measured before and after bilateral removal of inferotemporal cortex. The monkeys

[1] Supported by United Cerebral Palsy Research and Educational Foundation Grant R-213-67, National Institute of Mental Health Grant MH-14471, National Science Foundation Grant GB-6999 and, for A. Cowey's travel expenses, the H. E. Durham Fund of King's College, Cambridge (England).

[2] Now at Stanford University, Stanford, Calif. 94305, U.S.A.

[3] Now at Institute of Experimental Psychology, Oxford University, Oxford, England

were also trained on a visual discrimination task before and after the inferotemporal ablation in order to determine whether they showed the classical inferotemporal syndrome of impaired visual discrimination.

METHOD

Subjects and electrodes

Three rhesus monkeys were implanted with transcortical bipolar electrodes in the foveal projection area of lateral striate cortex. The electrodes were constructed of 300 μ diameter Formvar coated stainless steel wire. The tips were sharpened to a 45° taper, and the distance between tips of each electrode pair was approximately 2 mm. The upper electrode was placed on the pial surface and the lower electrode penetrated cortex. The electrodes were soldered to a miniature plug cemented to the skull. Recordings were made at the upper tip with respect to the lower tip.

Recording methods

Recording did not begin until at least 3 weeks after implantation or ablation. The monkeys sat in a restraining chair during recording sessions. Single or paired light flashes were produced by a Grass PS-2 photostimulator at a rate of 1/sec unless specifically mentioned otherwise. Three testing conditions were used: (1) *Alert in globe.* The restraining chair was placed in a dark cabinet, and a white translucent globe (diameter 13 in.) was placed over the animal's head. The photostimulator bulb was placed behind the globe where it fairly uniformly illuminated the entire globe. The animal was kept awake by allowing him to grasp a rod inserted into the cabinet and constantly moved by the experimenter. (2) *Drowsy in globe.* The stimulus conditions were the same as in condition 1, but no attempt was made to keep the monkey awake, and observation of the monkey through a peephole and examination of its EEG indicated that the monkey was at least drowsy and often asleep. (3) *Alert and outside globe.* No globe was placed over the animal's head and the animal was able to observe the experimenters and apparatus through a 9 in. × 12 in. aperture in the front of the testing cabinet. The ambient level of light in the room was about 1 foot-lambert. The photostimulator was placed 36 in. in front of the animal at eye level. Condition 3 is similar to that used by Spinelli and Pribram (1966), whereas the other two conditions were similar to those used in a previous study of the effect of lesions on visual evoked responses (Vaughan and Gross 1969).

The cortical potentials were amplified by a Schwarzer polygraph with high and low frequency cut-off at 2,000 and 5.0 c/sec, displayed on an oscilloscope and averaged on a Mnemotron Computer of Average Transients. The average was written out on a Hewlett-Packard X–Y recorder.

With short inter-flash intervals, the response to the second flash was superimposed on the response to the first, and its amplitude was difficult to measure. To reduce this difficulty, we obtained records in which the response to the first flash was eliminated by subtracting from the record the response to a single flash. This was usually done by subtracting the averaged response to a block of 50 single flashes from the averaged response to a block of 50 pairs of flashes. In addition, in monkey No. 3, 50 double and 50 single flashes were alternated trial by trial, and the responses to the latter were subtracted from the responses to the former. This second method usually yielded more consistent records and a more complete subtraction of the response to the first flash, although it took much longer to perform. In this case, the inter-trial interval was 10 sec rather than 1 sec.[1]

The different inter-flash intervals were randomized in each daily session, which lasted from 3–6 h. From 2–5 averages at each inter-flash interval were collected each day, but on any particular day all intervals were presented equally often.

In all animals, recovery cycles were computed from the peak-to-peak amplitude of the first negative-positive deflection of the averaged

[1] Both these subtraction methods involve the assumption that the responses to the two flashes add in a linear fashion (*cf.* Donchin *et al.* 1963). However, in this study, the effects of the lesions were the same whether a subtraction method was used or not, except that measurements were difficult or impossible at the shortest intervals without using a subtraction procedure.

response. In addition, recovery cycles were also computed from the amplitude of the first negative deflection, as measured from the base-line. Measurements on the response to the first flash were always made on the original averaged response to the paired flashes. Measurements on the response to the second flash were made both before and after the first response was subtracted. Recovery cycles were obtained by plotting the amplitude of the second response relative to the amplitude of the first response as a function of inter-flash interval. For each animal all pre- and post-operative data were obtained from the same pair of electrodes.

Behavioral methods

Only two of three subjects (RC2 and RC3) were used for the behavioral part of the study. They had received no previous discrimination training. Their performance was compared to that of six normal animals, also experimentally naive. The third subject (RC1) could not be used for this part of the study because it had received extensive previous experience and no data on monkeys with identical experience were available.

The behavioral apparatus was a sound-insulated box. Two translucent keys, $1\frac{1}{8}$ in. in diameter and 12 in. apart, were mounted in one wall. A reward of 0.25 ml of orange juice was provided by a liquid dispenser mounted below and between the keys. *S*s were first trained on a preliminary discrimination to a criterion of 5 errors in 50 trials. The positive stimulus was a white square measuring 0.5 in. × 0.5 in. and the negative stimulus was a blank key. They were then trained to discriminate two $\frac{1}{8}$ in. wide horizontal white stripes (positive) from the same stripes vertically oriented (negative) for 100 trials per day to a criterion of 10 errors or less on 2 successive days. Two weeks after receiving inferotemporal lesions, the subjects were retrained on the horizontal *vs.* vertical discrimination for 100 trials per day until they reached the same criterion.

Surgical and histological methods

The intention was to remove all inferotemporal cortex extending dorso-ventrally from the bottom of the inferior bank of the superior temporal sulcus to the occipito-temporal sulcus, with the anterior limit close to the temporal pole and the posterior limit 5 mm in front of the inferior occipital sulcus.

Following completion of the experiment, the monkey was anesthetized, the electrode site marked with lesions, and the monkey perfused with saline and then with formol saline. The

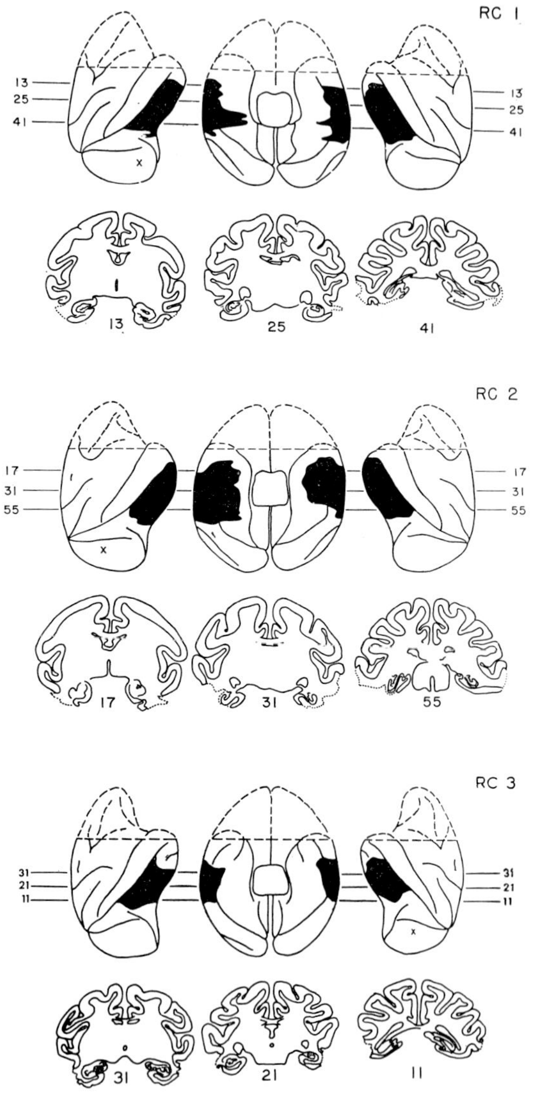

Fig. 1
Reconstructions of the brains of the experimental animals together with representative cross-sections. On the reconstructions, the electrode sites are marked with an X, the lesions in black, and the dashed outline represents areas not sectioned but drawn from photographs of the brain. On the cross-sections, the borders of the lesions are indicated with dotted lines.

brain was blocked in stereotaxic coordinates, embedded in albumin, cut in 25 μ or 50 μ frozen sections and stained either with cresyl violet or according to the method of Klüver and Barrera.

Reconstructions and cross-sections of the lesions are shown in Fig. 1. They were essentially identical to the usual inferotemporal cortex ablation used in behavioral studies (*cf.* Pribram 1954; Mishkin 1966).

RESULTS

Behavioral results

Prior to operation, monkeys RC2 and RC3 reached criterion on the discrimination of vertical and horizontal lines after making 210 and 148 errors, well within the normal range of the many experimentally naive monkeys previously trained on this discrimination. After their inferotemporal lesions they were severely impaired on retention of this task, as measured both by the number of errors they made in reaching their pre-operative level of performance and in their savings scores (*i.e.*, post-operative errors minus pre-operative errors divided by post-operative errors plus pre-operative errors). Animals RC1 and RC2 made 219 and 84 post-operative errors, giving them savings scores of 0.00 and 0.06, whereas for a group of matched unoperated monkeys the corresponding mean and range for post-operative errors were 17 and 0 to 51, and for savings 0.78 and 0.24 to 1.00.

Electrophysiological results

There were no discernible effects of the inferotemporal lesions on either the EEG or visual evoked responses recorded from striate cortex.

The visual evoked response at striate cortex remained fairly constant for any given testing or subject condition. The response to a single flash always consisted of an initial surface negative deflection followed by a surface positive wave. Always in RC3, and sometimes in RC1 and RC2, this was followed by a second prominent surface negative wave (see Fig. 2).

At inter-flash intervals of 63 msec or less, the response to the second flash was usually not simply a reduced version of the response to a single flash, but had an altered wave form. Indeed, at the shortest intervals it may be more meaningful to sepak of a single response to a pair of closely spaced flashes rather than the sum of two independent responses (see Fig. 2).

In all subjects, and under all stimulus conditions and measuring methods, there was a fairly smooth decline in recovery down to the 50 msec intervals with a flattening or even a rise in the curve at lower intervals. A similar rise at

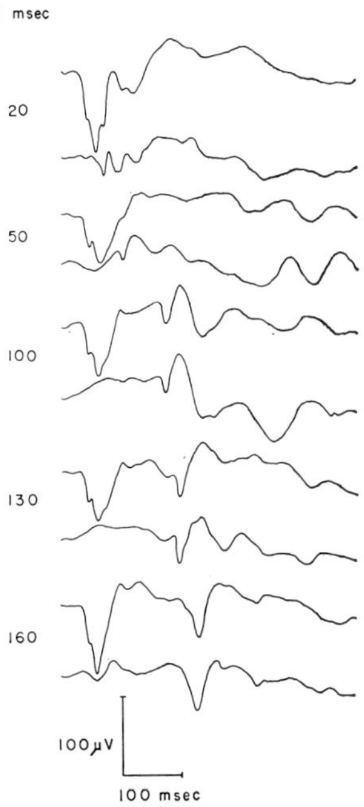

Fig. 2
Average evoked responses to paired light flashes in subject RC3 after bilateral inferotemporal lesion. At each interval the upper trace is the response to 50 paired flashes. The lower trace was obtained by subtracting the response to 50 single flashes from the upper trace.

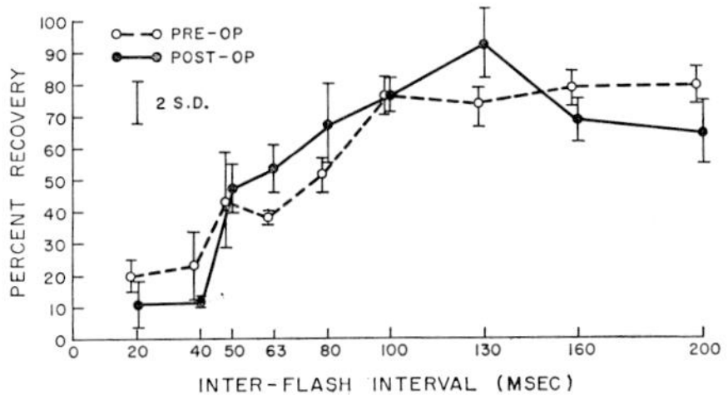

Fig. 3
Recovery functions in Monkey RC1 before and after bilateral inferotemporal lesions. Subject was alert and in the globe. Each point is a mean of seven recovery ratios taken over 7 days. Each ratio was based on an average of 50 trials. Measurements were peak-to-peak (see text).

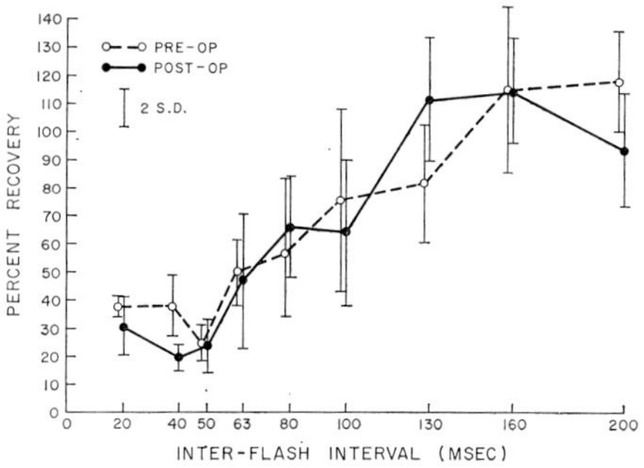

Fig. 4
Recovery functions in Monkey RC2 before and after bilateral inferotemporal lesions. Subject was alert and facing the photostimulator. Each point is a mean of six recovery ratios taken over 3 days. Each ratio was based on an average of 50 trials. Measurements were peak-to-peak (see text).

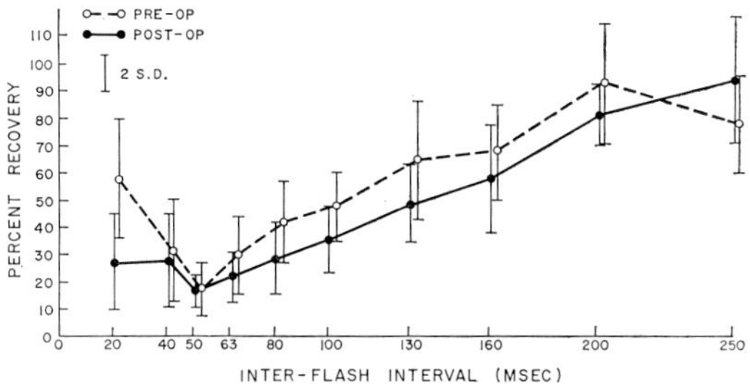

Fig. 5
Recovery functions in Monkey RC3 before and after bilateral inferotemporal lesions. Subject was alert and in the globe. Each point is a mean of 18 recovery ratios taken over 7 days. Each ratio was based on an average of 50 responses. Measurements were on the first deflections (see text).

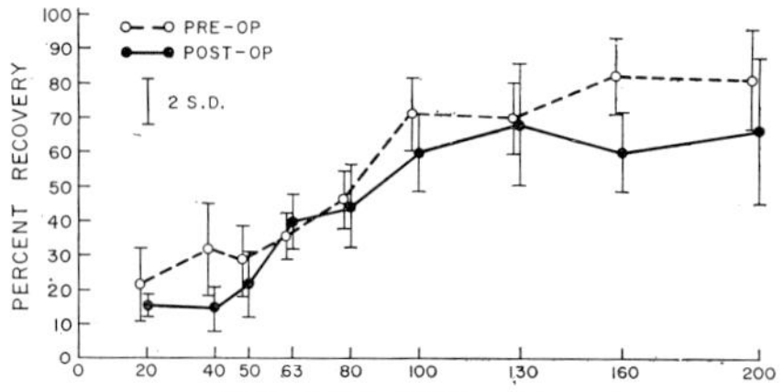

Fig. 6
Recovery functions in Monkey RC2 before and after inferotemporal lesions. Subject was in the globe and not alert, but drowsy or asleep. Each point is a mean of eight recovery ratios taken over 4 days. Each ratio was based on an average of 50 responses. Measurement was peak-to-peak (see text).

short inter-stimulus intervals has been reported by Supin (1966).

Finally, and most important, the inferotemporal lesions had no effect whatsoever on the recovery cycle of any animal. This was true under all three testing conditions and with all measuring procedures (Fig. 3–6).

DISCUSSION

The impairment in retention of the visual discrimination after the inferotemporal lesions was similar to that previously found and indicates that the animals in this study showed the typical "inferotemporal syndrome".

The absence of any effect of the bilateral inferotemporal lesions on visual evoked responses recorded from striate cortex extends the previous finding that unilateral inferotemporal lesions do not affect striate evoked responses (Vaughan and Gross 1969). This finding in itself fails to support an efferent influence of inferotemporal cortex on the retino-geniculo-calcarine system.

If one accepts that recovery cycles of evoked responses from striate cortex provide a measure of efferent inhibitory influences impinging on the visual system, then the absence of any effect of the inferotemporal lesions on the recovery cycle of striate cortex argues strongly against the suggestion that inferotemporal cortex exerts an inhibitory influence on the visual system (Pribram 1967). More specifically, with our stimulating and recording conditions we were unable to confirm the prediction of Spinelli and Pribram (1966) that inferotemporal lesions would facilitate recovery of striate evoked responses. Their prediction was based on two findings. The first was Spinelli and Pribram's (1966) observation that chronic electrical stimulation of inferotemporal cortex decreased the amplitude of the response of striate cortex to the second of a pair of flashes. They suggested that removal of inferotemporal cortex would have the opposite effect, namely facilitation of recovery. However, there is no reason to expect ablation of cortex to have the opposite effect to its stimulation. Indeed, the behavioral effects of stimulation and ablation of association cortex are often identical (Chow 1961; Stamm 1961; Weiskrantz *et al.* 1962). Furthermore, if Spinelli and Pribram's mode of stimulation did have effects opposite to ablation, their animals should have been superior to controls in visual discrimination performance, whereas they were not. Pribram's second justification for his prediction was the finding of Dewson *et al.* (1966) that removal of insular-temporal cortex in the cat shortened recovery time of evoked responses to paired clicks recorded from the cochlear nucleus. However, it is not clear that insular-temporal cortex in the cat is in any way homologous or analogous in function to inferotemporal cortex in the monkey.

In conclusion, the present results fail to confirm the prediction of the efferent model of inferotemporal cortex and, furthermore, they call into serious question the relevance to that model of Spinelli and Pribram's finding of an effect of inferotemporal stimulation on the excitability of striate cortex. Our results, of course, do not disprove the more general idea that inferotemporal cortex may have an efferent function.

NOTE ADDED IN PROOF

Relevant to the question of the function of inferotemporal cortex is the recent finding that neurons in inferotemporal cortex of the monkey had visual receptive fields which were very large (greater than $10° \times 10°$) and almost always included the fovea. Some extended well into both halves of the visual field while others were confined to the ipsilateral or contralateral side. These neurons were differentially sensitive to several of the following dimensions of the stimulus: size and shape, color, orientation, direction of movement (C. G. Gross, D. B. Bender and C. E. Rocha-Miranda, 1969, submitted for publication).

SUMMARY

Paired flashes of light were presented to monkeys under a variety of testing conditions. The amplitude of the evoked response at striate cortex to the second flash was expressed as a percentage of the response to the first flash and plotted against inter-flash interval to yield a recovery function. Bilateral removal of inferotemporal cortex failed to change the recovery function. This result fails to confirm the hypothesis that inferotemporal cortex exerts an inhibitory influence on the visual system.

RÉSUMÉ

TEST D'UN "MODÈLE EFFÉRENT" DE LA FONCTION DU CORTEX TEMPORAL INFÉRIEUR DANS LA DISCRIMINATION VISUELLE

Des éclairs lumineux couplés sont présentés à des singes dans toute une série de conditions expérimentales. L'amplitude de la réponse évoquée au second éclair au niveau du cortex strié est exprimée en pourcentage de la réponse au premier éclair, et dessinée en fonction de l'intervalle interéclair pour mettre en évidence la fonction de récupération. L'ablation bilatérale du cortex temporal inférieur ne modifie pas cette fonction de récupération. Ce résultat ne confirme pas l'hypothèse que le cortex temporal inférieur exerce une influence inhibitrice sur le système visuel.

We would like to thank D. Bender for helpful discussions and continued assistance, and K. Domoto for assistance in gathering the data.

REFERENCES

Chow, K. L. Anatomical and electrographical analysis of temporal neocortex in relation to visual discrimination learning in monkey. In J. R. Delafresnaye (Ed.), *Brain mechanisms and learning*. Blackwell, Oxford, **1961**: 507–525.

Dewson, J. H. M., Nobel, K. W. and Pribram, K. H. Corticofugal influence at cochlear nucleus of the cat: some effects of ablation of insular-temporal cortex. *Brain Res.*, **1966**, *2*: 151–159.

Donchin, E., Wicke, J. D. and Lindsley, D. B. Cortical evoked potentials and perception of paired flashes. *Science*, **1963**, *141*: 1285–1286.

Gross, C. G., Schiller, P. H., Wells, C. and Gerstein, G. L. Single-unit activity in temporal association cortex of the monkey. *J. Neurophysiol.*, **1967**, *30*: 833–843.

Hubel, D. H. and Wiesel, T. N. Receptive fields, binocular interaction, and functional architecture in the cat's visual cortex. *J. Physiol. (Lond.)*, **1962**, *160*: 106–164.

Hubel, D. H. and Wiesel, T. N. Receptive fields and functional architecture in two nonstriate visual areas (18 and 19) of the cat. *J. Neurophysiol.*, **1965**, *28*: 229–289.

Kuypers, H. G. J. M., Szwarcbart, M. K., Mishkin, M. and Rosvold, H. E. Occipito-temporal cortico-cortical connections in the rhesus monkey. *Exp. Neurol.*, **1965**, *11*: 245–262.

MISHKIN, M. Visual mechanisms beyond the striate cortex. In R. RUSSELL (Ed.), *Frontiers of physiological psychology*. Academic Press, New York, **1966**: 93–119.

PRIBRAM, K. H. Toward a science of neuropsychology: (method and data). In R. A. PATTON (Ed.), *Current trends in psychology and the behavioral sciences*. University of Pittsburgh Press, Pittsburgh, **1954**: 115–142.

PRIBRAM, K. H. The limbic systems, efferent control of neural inhibition and behavior. In W. R. ADEY and T. TOKIZANE (Eds.), *Progress in Brain Research, Vol. 27, Structure and function of the limbic system*. Elsevier, Amsterdam, **1967**: 318–336.

PRIBRAM, K. H., BLEHERT, S. R. and SPINELLI, D. N. Effects on visual discrimination of crosshatching and undercutting the inferotemporal cortex of monkeys. *J. comp. physiol. Psychol.*, **1966,** *62*: 358–364.

SPINELLI, D. N. and PRIBRAM, K. H. Changes in visual recovery functions produced by temporal lobe stimulation in monkeys. *Electroenceph. clin. Neurophysiol.*, **1966,** *20*: 44–49.

SPINELLI, D. N. and PRIBRAM, K. H. Changes in visual recovery functions and unit activity produced by frontal and temporal cortex stimulation. *Electroenceph. clin. Neurophysiol.*, **1967,** *22*: 143–149.

STAMM, J. S. Electrical stimulation of frontal cortex in monkeys during learning of an alternation task. *J. Neurophysiol.*, **1961,** *24*: 414–426.

SUPIN, A. Y. [Cortical and thalamic contributions to recovery cycle of evoked potentials in visual cortex.] *Fiziol. Zh. (Leningr.)*, **1966,** *52*: 1297–1304. [Translated from Russian in *Neurosci. Transl.*, **1967–68,** *No. 4*: 411–417].

VAUGHAN, H. G. and GROSS, C. G. Cortical response to light in unanesthetized monkeys and their alteration by visual system lesions. *Exp. Brain Res.*, **1969,** *8*: 19–36.

WEISKRANTZ, L., MIHAILOVIĆ, L. J. and GROSS, C. G. Effects of stimulation of frontal cortex and hippocampus on behavior in the monkey. *Brain*, **1962,** *85*: 487–504.

WHITLOCK, D. G. and NAUTA, W. J. H. Subcortical projections from the temporal neocortex in *Macaca mulatta*. *J. comp. Neurol.*, **1956,** *106*: 183–212.

Reference: SCHWARTZKROIN, P. A., COWEY, A. and GROSS, C. G. A test of an "efferent model" of the function of inferotemporal cortex in visual discrimination. *Electroenceph. clin. Neurophysiol.*, **1969,** *27*: 594–600.

Electroencephalography and Clinical Neurophysiology
Elsevier Publishing Company, Amsterdam – Printed in The Netherlands

CLINICAL AND LABORATORY NOTES

THE KLEINE-LEVIN SYNDROME WITH INTERMITTENT ABNORMALITY IN THE EEG

MARTA ELIAN AND BERNARD BORNSTEIN

Department of Neurology, Beilinson Medical Center, Tel-Aviv University Medical School, Petah Tikva (Israel)

(Accepted for publication: April 4, 1969)

Disturbances of a periodic nature have always been of special interest to most physicians. Periodic hypersomnia, best known as the Kleine-Levin syndrome, is a benign syndrome usually occurring in young males in the second decade of life. It is characterized by a sudden onset of sleeping attacks which last for several days and which are often, but not necessarily, associated with increased food and fluid intake. In the intervals between attacks, which always subside without treatment, these patients act completely normally.

The very nature of the disease makes its investigation, both aetiologically and therapeutically, most difficult. Though some authors emphasize the importance of psychiatric factors (Pai 1950; Critchley 1962; Jaffe 1967), the organic nature of the disease is not questioned. From mainly clinical observations the disease is considered to be a dysfunction of the diencephalon. Some patients may have normal results in all laboratory investigations, whereas others may show slight deviation from the normal in the glucose tolerance curve, protein-bound iodine, steroid excretion, cholesterol level or electrolyte balance (Critchley 1962; Gallinek 1962; Gilbert 1964; Garland *et al.* 1965).

Most reports of cases of the Kleine-Levin syndrome note that the EEG was normal. Critchley (1962), in his extensive review, noted slight, diffuse, non-specific changes in the EEG in some patients and Takahashi (1965) found a clear abnormality in three of his patients' tracings. In the case presented here we had the opportunity to study daily tracings during several attacks as well as in the intervals between attacks. The pathological findings in the EEG of our patient, and particularly their dynamic nature, prompted the publication of this case report, since they may throw some light on the aetiology of the disease. The report is based on a 5 year observation period which began in 1963 and extends to the present (1968).

Case report (Michael P.)

In February 1963 a 13-year-old boy was referred by the Mental Health Clinic to our department for examination. He had always been healthy but about 4 months prior to admission he had begun to suffer from regular attacks of headaches and hypersomnia which occurred every 3–4 weeks and which lasted about 10 days. At the end of the attack there was a sudden return to his usual, normal, healthy state. None of the psychological or psychiatric tests which were carried out in the "normal" period between attacks showed any deviation from the normal.

The attacks began with the sudden appearance of a headache, and his behaviour would immediately change. If he happened to be in school, this usually well-mannered boy would leave the classroom without saying a word to his teacher, find his way home and immediately go to sleep with no explanation. During the attack he hardly ever left his bed. He became apathetic and could not bear the company of people. He slept most of the time, taking no interest whatsoever in what was taking place around him. The family also reported an increase in his appetite.

We saw him several times during attacks. He was very pale, with a puffy face, and he sometimes perspired profusely. He slept all the time if he was not disturbed but was easily awakened. He rose by himself to take care of his needs, but otherwise made no purposeful actions. He ate well, but we did not see the greatly increased appetite described by his mother, and he never ate ravenously. On the other hand, several times he was offered a second meal shortly after he had eaten, which he also finished. It is possible that he had already forgotten the first. He did not talk spontaneously, but when questioned gave laconic answers. He had no orientation in time or space. Particularly noticeable was his disorientation and uncertainty as to personal details, for example where he had been on the last school excursion, what presents he had received for his birthday, the date of his birthday, etc. He remembered nothing of the events taking place during the attacks, such as who had visited him or how he had reached the hospital, whether or not a blood sample had been taken, etc. On the other hand, he gave relatively quick answers to simple arithmetic problems and to such questions as "Who is the president of this country?" or about the dates of historical events. To the question "What is wrong with you?" he stereotypically answered "Headache and nausea." His speech was slow. He was noticeably apathetic and at times torpid. When we stopped putting questions to him, he immediately fell asleep again.

This condition continued for 10 days, at the end of which there was a startling change in his manner. We would suddenly find him one morning fully awake, reading a book with great interest, or walking in the ward talking to other patients. The colour of his face became normal and there was no way whatsoever in which he could be differentiated from any ordinary boy. He remembered nothing of what had taken place during this period, the length of which he was unable to estimate and which he described as having been erased from his life.

At the beginning these states appeared every 1–2 months, the intervals between attacks gradually lengthening to a year and a half. His last attack was in June 1965. He was last in hospital in November 1966 as an emergency case because he had developed torsion movements of the neck and spasms of the face and oral muscles, including the

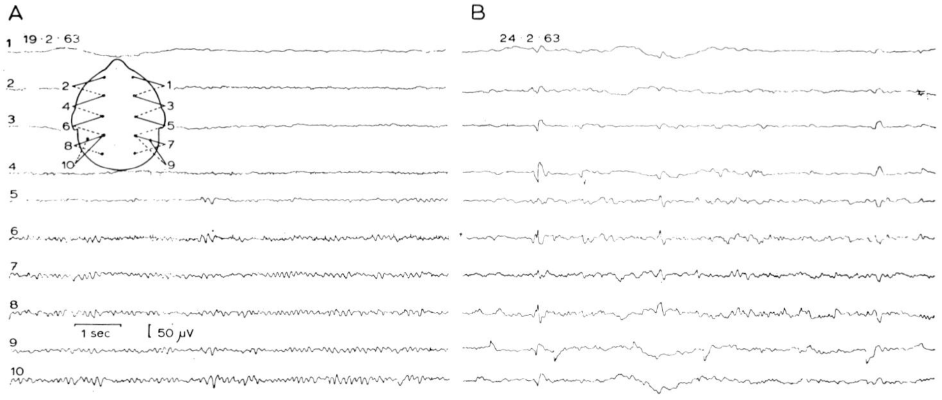

Fig. 1

A: Feb. 19th: Normal waking record between attacks. *B*: Feb. 24th: Sleep record between attacks, revealing single diphasic spike discharges, more prominent on the left.

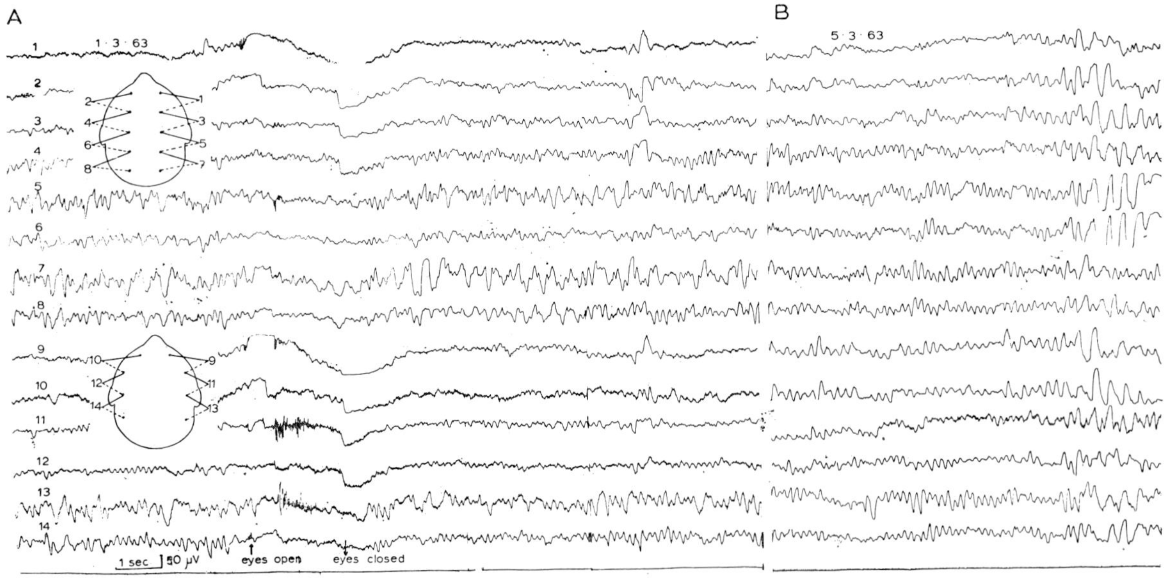

Fig. 2

A: March 1st: Record on the first day of an attack. A somewhat irregular background activity is seen, with 3–5 c/sec irregular high voltage slow waves. These are somewhat more prominent in the posterior leads and on the left, disappearing with opening of the eyes. In the second part of this sample a short burst of high voltage irregular slow waves is seen. *B*: March 5th: Record on the fifth day of the same attack. Alpha activity is seen, though it is somewhat irregular and of higher voltage than in the patient's normal record. One of the very frequent bursts of irregular high voltage slow waves is shown.

tongue, symptoms which typically appear in persons sensitive to phenothiazine, which he was taking. He was afterwards seen during the summer of 1968 when he had just finished high school.

All the laboratory tests, including CSF, electrolytes, liver function, protein-bound iodine and ketosteroids were repeatedly within normal limits, except for a flat sugar load curve during and after an attack.

Large numbers of EEG records were obtained; daily records were made during several attacks while he was in hospital, and several others were made in the intervals between attacks. Only a few of these tracings, most apt to throw light on the evolution of the attack, have been chosen to be presented here.

Feb. 19th: (Fig. 1) Between 2 attacks, a normal waking record was obtained, with symmetrical alpha activity, but with an interspersion of scattered low voltage slow waves. Hyperventilation was also normal.

Feb. 24th: (Fig. 1) One week later, during a sleep record, several single spike discharges were seen, more prominent to the left.

March 1st: (Fig. 2) The record obtained on the first day of an attack. The background activity is somewhat irregular. High voltage 3–5 c/sec slow waves appear almost continuously, mostly in the posterior leads, somewhat more prominent on the right. These disappear when the eyes are opened. 1–2 sec high voltage slow wave bursts appear later in the record. During hyperventilation an abnormal reaction is seen with several bursts of high voltage slow waves.

March 5th: (Fig. 2) Background activity is more organized and alpha activity, though somewhat irregular, appears. The high voltage slow waves in the posterior region disappeared. High voltage irregular slow waves appear in very frequent bursts.

March 9th: (Fig. 3) Background activity exhibits a lower voltage and is more organized. Several high voltage slow wave bursts appear, but they are shorter and much less frequent than in previous records. Normal response to hyperventilation.

March 11th: (Fig. 3) The attack stopped the previous day. Background activity somewhat irregular and 6–7 c/sec. bursts are seen all through the record.

March 12th: Within normal limits — as seen on Feb. 19th.

It is of note that a record obtained on the 5th day of another attack showed a tracing similar to that described on March 5th.

COMMENT

The most obvious clinical signs, *i.e.*, the episodes of somnolence lasting for several days, with a history of increased food intake during some of the attacks, occurring in an otherwise normal, healthy adolescent male, and with a spontaneous recovery, is in accordance with the diagnosis of Kleine-Levin syndrome. All the classical criteria are fulfilled in this patient. The disturbance in the mechanism of sleep, the bulimia and the disturbed glucose tolerance curve, are all in accordance with the concept of diencephalic dysfunction.

The point of interest in this case is the EEG findings.

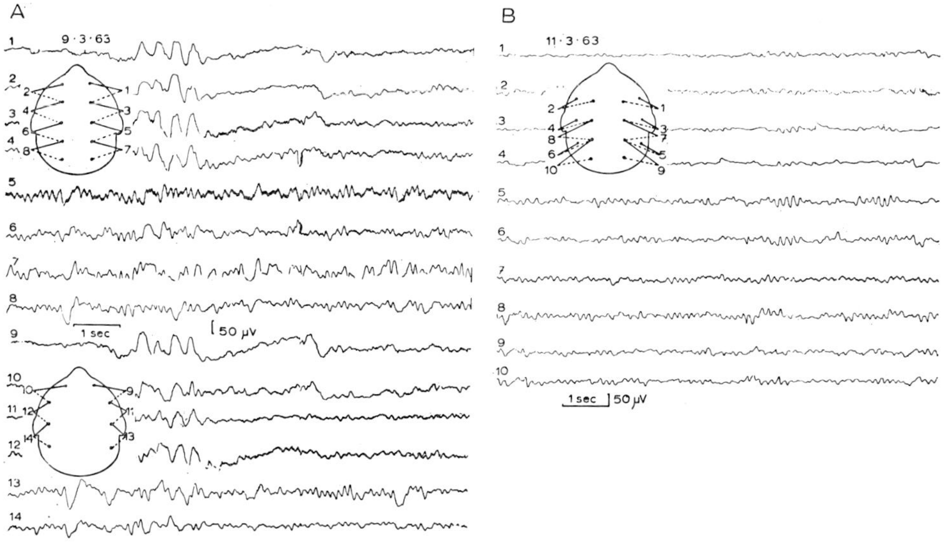

Fig. 3

A: March 9th: Record on the ninth day of an attack. It is basically similar to Fig. 2, *B*, which was obtained 4 days previously. Irregular alpha rhythm with a burst of irregular high voltage slow waves (the difference is mainly quantitative; see text). *B*: March 11th: Record on the first day after the attack had stopped. The tracing is within normal limits. Compared with Fig. 1, *A*, it is somewhat slower and more irregular.

Morphologically, the abnormality is of a paroxysmal nature: bursts of high voltage slow activity lasting several seconds, the background activity between bursts being normal or somewhat slow. Chronologically, the abnormality also appeared to be paroxysmal, that is, during periods of clinical health the waking records were entirely normal, whereas those made during the attacks were pathological. Moreover, there was a relationship between the amount of abnormality seen in the EEG and the duration of somnolence, which were proportional to each other: at the beginning of the attack the records invariably contained more abnormal bursts than they did near the end of the somnolent period. It should be noted that during the tracings the patient was kept awake, opening and closing his eyes and answering simple questions. In our opinion, this fact excludes the possibility that the tracings simply represent drowsy records. Rosenkötter and Wende (1955) described a case in which the clinical and EEG findings were similar to those in our case. They were of the opinion that the EEG records represent different stages of a sleep pattern. This would seem to be mostly a difference in interpretation. In our view, the paroxysmal quality of the many tracings is further supported by the one sleep record obtained during a normal wakeful period, *i.e.*, several weeks after, and several months before, an attack. This record contained spike discharges.

As noted in the introduction, the aetiology of the Kleine-Levin syndrome is still unknown. The paroxysmal nature of the attacks, with an abrupt onset and sudden termination, raises the question of its relationship to convulsive disorders. Support for such a relationship may be found in our case, with its paroxysmal clinical picture and the paroxysmal EEG findings. Additional support for this view is contained in the report made by Takahashi (1965), who found a lowered threshold for evoking paroxysmal discharges by Metrazol in ten of his patients. Three of his cases showed an epileptic abnormality in the EEG. Furthermore, some of Critchley's cases (1962) showed varying degrees of abnormality, and that of Jaffe (1967) had a brother suffering from epilepsy.

SUMMARY

A case is presented of Kleine-Levin syndrome observed over 5 years in which a large number of EEG records were made both during and between attacks. In contrast with most reported cases the serial records made during an attack revealed an abnormality. This consisted in bursts of slow waves, more prominent in the posterior region, with a quantitative decrease of the abnormality towards the end of the attack. Waking records between attacks were entirely normal. A sleep record made between attacks revealed distinct spike discharges, more prominent on the left.

The possibility that there is a relationship between the Kleine-Levin syndrome and the convulsive disorders is considered and discussed.

RÉSUMÉ

LE SYNDROME DE KLEINE-LEVIN — ANOMALIE EEG INTERMITTENTE

Les auteurs présentent un cas de syndrôme de Kleine-Levin observé sur une période de 5 ans au cours de laquelle un grand nombre d'enregistrements EEG ont été effectués pendant les attaques et entre les attaques. Contrairement à ce qui est rapporté dans la littérature, les tracés en série effectués au cours d'une attaque ont mis en évidence des anomalies consistant en bouffées d'ondes lentes, prédominant au niveau des régions postérieures, et qui diminuent quantitativement vers la fin de l'attaque. Les tracés de veille entre les attaques étaient entièrement normaux. Un enregistrement de sommeil effectué entre les attaques a montré de nettes décharges de pointes prédominant du côté gauche.

La possibilité d'une relation entre syndrôme de Kleine-Levin et maladies convulsives est prise en considération et discutée.

REFERENCES

CRITCHLEY, M. Periodic hypersomnia and megaphagia in adolescent males. *Brain*, **1962,** *85*: 627–656.

GALLINEK, A. The Kleine-Levin syndrome: hypersomnia, bulimia and abnormal mental states. *Wld Neurol.*, **1962,** *3*: 235–243.

GARLAND, H., SUMMER, D. and FOURMAN, P. The Kleine-Levin syndrome: some fuller observations. *Neurology (Minneap.)*, **1965,** *15*: 1161–1167.

GILBERT, G. J. Periodic hypersomnia: the Kleine-Levin syndrome. *Neurology (Minneap.)*, **1964,** *14*: 844–850.

JAFFE, R. Periodic hypersomnia and bulimia. *Israel Ann. Psychiat.*, **1967,** *5*: 43–52.

PAI, M. N. Hypersomnia syndromes. *Brit. med. J.*, **1950,** *1*: 522.

ROSENKÖTTER, L. und WENDE, S. EEG Befunde beim Kleine-Levin Syndrom. *Mschr. Psychiat. Neurol.*, **1955,** *130*: 107–121.

TAKAHASHI, Y. Clinical studies in periodic somnolence. *Psychiat. Neurol. jap.* **1965,** *67*: 853–889, cited by *Excerpta med. (Amst.), Sect. VIII*, **1966,** *19*: 969.

Reference: ELIAN, M. and BORNSTEIN, B. The Kleine-Levin syndrome with intermittent abnormality in the EEG. *Electroenceph. clin. Neurophysiol.*, **1969,** *27*: 601–604.

Electroencephalography and Clinical Neurophysiology
Elsevier Publishing Company, Amsterdam – Printed in The Netherlands

THE EEG IN A CASE OF PERIODIC HYPERSOMNIA

V. R. THACORE, MOHAMMAD AHMED AND IAN OSWALD

Department of Medicine, King George's Medical College, University of Lucknow, Lucknow (India) and Department of Psychiatry, University of Edinburgh, Edinburgh (Great Britain)

(Accepted for publication: April 8, 1969)

A number of cases of apparent abnormal sleepiness with overeating were described by Kleine (1925) and Levin (1929), after which other reports appeared describing patients with clinical features of greater or less similarity, mainly male adolescents. In a critical review, Critchley (1962) considered fifteen of the cases to conform to his criteria of a *syndrome*, and detailed nine new cases. He rejected many reports, including all female cases, though Duffy and Davison (1968) have described a female case of the "Kleine-Levin syndrome" which otherwise conformed to Critchley's criteria. Not all Critchley's own cases showed overeating. Their only remaining common feature was "sleep", described as excessive during self-limiting periods. The present case is reported because of its similarity to many of the cases in the literature, because of the early onset age and because the EEG was recorded in an attack and was not characteristic of sleep.

CASE

A boy, aged 13, had had bouts of excessive "sleep" for 5 years. The first episode lasted 7 days, as did a second 3 months later, and after each he recovered spontaneously. Two years later they began again, lasting 10–15 days and recurring about monthly, always with subsequent amnesia. He was alert and sociable in the intervals. The episode during which the patient was brought to the hospital was the second in one month.

The family history revealed little of relevance apart from an uncle who had attempted suicide after asocial acts. There was no history of significant physical disorder in the patient who was, however, described as stubborn and short-tempered.

He was of average build, afebrile, pulse 80/min, blood pressure 120/70 mm Hg and drowsy when first seen. Haemoglobin 12 g%, blood picture normal, with leucocytes 12,000/mm^3, neutrophils 66%, lymphocytes 32%. Fasting blood sugar 48 mg%. Liver function tests, serum cholesterol and protein, normal. Corrected ESR (Wintrobe) 6 mm for first hour, packed cell volume 38%. Cerebro-spinal fluid clear, normal tension, proteins 30 mg%, chloride 650 mg%, sugar 70 mg%. cells 5/mm^3. Wassermann reaction and Venereal Disease Reference Laboratory serological test negative. X-ray chest and skull, normal.

He was difficult to rouse and would follow instructions for only a few seconds before lapsing back into his inattentive state. He lay curled up, was irritable if disturbed, but would waken or be roused for toilet and meals (during each he would often fall asleep). He did not overeat but continually chewed his lips. There was no incontinence. He was disorientated and indifferent to his surroundings, his memory appeared defective and he just stared when asked questions. He said he felt different but denied hallucinations or delusions. He repeatedly dozed off during interviews and appeared to sleep a total of 20 hours per day.

The EEG (Fig. 1) recorded during the "sleep" state was dominated by generalized and symmetrical theta and delta activity, including bursts of delta waves of up to 220 μV at 2.5–3 c/sec, lasting about 10 sec. Brief periods of alpha rhythm were interspersed with theta activity. Slow wave activity continued when the eyes were open. No sleep spindles were present.

Six months later his father reported that he had remained well and resumed school. Contact was then lost.

DISCUSSION

Prolonged sleep-like states may be found in association with lesions of the brain-stem, in metabolic disorders and psychiatric conditions such as hysteria and depressive or catatonic stupor.

In the present patient the low single fasting blood sugar suggests the possibility of a hypoglycaemic state but, with no clinical signs of hypoglycaemia and intake of food being without effect, hypoglycaemia as a primary aetiological factor appears out of the question.

The youth looked as if he were asleep but, in contrast to true sleep, he could not be fully roused and his EEG was not that of sleep. Only two of Critchley's (1962) cases had EEGs performed during an attack and in neither case was the EEG that of sleep or, apparently, even that of drowsiness. His Case 7 had alpha rhythm, a hallmark of wakefulness, *mixed* with "post-central moderate voltage, slow waves", some of the last still being present after the attack. Case 3 "while he was in a state of somnosis" had alpha rhythm and W.A. Cobb was quoted as being "surprised at the slightness of the change during an attack compared with those of a comparable state of natural drowsiness". Critchley nevertheless wrote "the sleep does not differ in any obvious fashion from the normal". Criticism of Critchley's criteria of sleep has been made elsewhere (Oswald 1969).

Bonkalo (1968) described what he considered a case of the "Kleine-Levin syndrome" showing "*true* sleep". However, the description of "episodic or continuous high

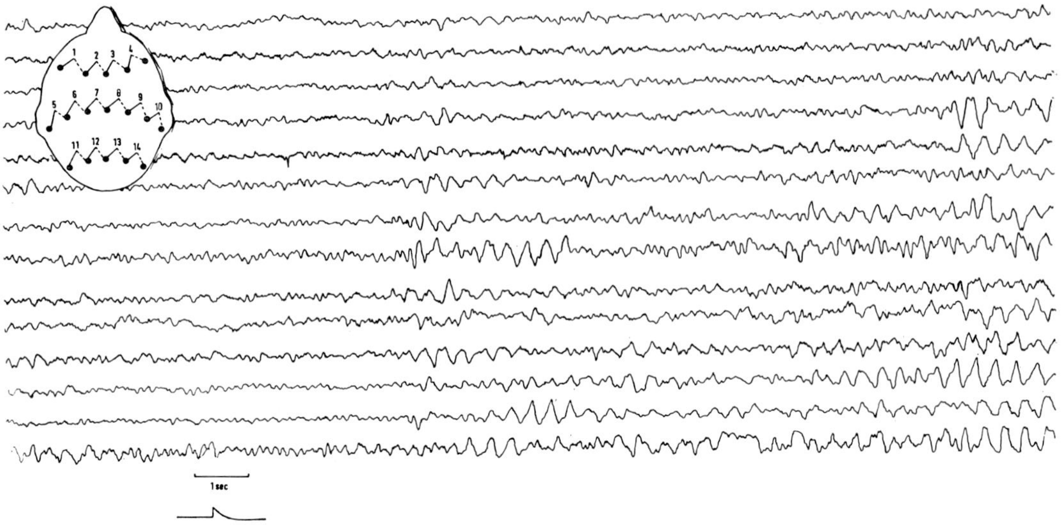

Fig. 1
A representative excerpt of the EEG of the patient during the "sleep" state. Bursts of diffuse delta waves of high voltage are interspersed in a record consisting predominantly of theta rhythm. No sleep spindles are present. Calibrations: 50 μV and 1 sec.

amplitude 5–6 cycles per second slow waves occurring in both frontal and temporal leads of the EEG" is not that of sleep. The only instance of a sleep EEG, with typical spindles illustrated, is to be found in a case of the Kleine-Levin syndrome, unmentioned by Critchley (1962), and described by Rosenkötter and Wende (1955).

The literature contains reports of patients of both sexes, not all of whom were adolescents, who suffered recurrent periods of altered consciousness, with inertia and unresponsiveness, appearing and disappearing spontaneously. Only some exhibited overeating and among those who looked as if they were asleep, a number would seem to have been awake. It would appear that any attempt to delineate a nosological entity must, in large measure, be dictated by idiosyncratic preference.

SUMMARY

A case of periodic hypersomnia, conforming to descriptions of the Kleine-Levin syndrome, is reported in a male of 13, the age of onset being 8 years. Overeating did not occur. The attacks, which lasted 1–2 weeks and ended spontaneously, were accompanied by a state which resembled sleep, but from which arousal to normal alertness was not possible. In an attack the EEG showed diffuse delta and theta abnormalities which did not resemble the EEG of sleep. Attention is drawn to the heterogeneity of other published cases.

RÉSUMÉ

L'EEG DANS UN CAS D'HYPERSOMNIE PÉRIODIQUE

Les auteurs rapportent un cas correspondant aux descriptions de syndrome de Kleine-Levin chez un sujet mâle de 13 ans, syndrome ayant débuté à l'âge de 8 ans. L'hyperphagie n'a pas été notée. Les crises qui ont persisté pendant 1–2 semaines et se sont terminées spontanément, s'accompagnaient d'un état ressemblant au sommeil; mais l'éveil à un niveau vigile normal n'était pas possible, et au cours de l'un de ces états, l'EEG montrait des anomalies theta et delta diffuses qui ne ressemblaient pas à l'EEG du sommeil. L'hetérogénéité des autres cas publiés est soulignée.

We thank Dr. B. C. Chatterjee for his co-operation.

REFERENCES

BONKALO, A. Hypersomnia. *Brit. J. Psychiat.*, **1968,** *114*: 69–75.

CRITCHLEY, M. Periodic hypersomnia and megaphagia in adolescent males. *Brain*, **1962,** *85*: 627–656.

DUFFY, J. P. and DAVISON, K. A female case of the Kleine-Levin syndrome. *Brit. J. Psychiat.*, **1968,** *114*: 77–84.

KLEINE, W. Periodische Schlafsucht. *Mschr. Psychiat. Neurol.*, **1925,** *57*: 285–320.

LEVIN, M. Narcolepsy and other varieties of morbid somnolence. *Arch. Neurol. Psychiat. (Chic.)*, **1929,** *22*: 1172–1200.

OSWALD, I. Sleep and its disorders. In P. J. VINKEN and G. W. BRUYN (Eds.), *Handbook of clinical neurology, Vol. 3.* North-Holland Publ. Co., Amsterdam, **1969**: 80–111.

ROSENKÖTTER, L. und WENDE, S. EEG-Befunde beim Kleine-Levin-Syndrom. *Mschr. Psychiat. Neurol.*, **1955,** *130*: 107–122.

Reference: THACORE, V. R., AHMED, M. and OSWALD, I. The EEG in a case of periodic hypersomnia. *Electroenceph. clin. Neurophysiol.*, **1969,** *27*: 605–606.

Electroencephalography and Clinical Neurophysiology
Elsevier Publishing Company, Amsterdam – Printed in The Netherlands

ABNORMAL CONNECTIONS BETWEEN SKELETAL MUSCLE FIBERS

JAN EKSTEDT AND ERIK STÅLBERG

Department of Pharmacology, Department of Clinical Neurophysiology and Wallenberg Laboratory, University of Uppsala, Uppsala (Sweden)

(Accepted for publication: March 12, 1969)

Reports indicating that two muscle fibers may have a direct electrical connection have not so far been published. However, in the present paper two recordings will be described which show that such a connection may exceptionally exist. The findings were made incidentally during two experiments on the jitter phenomenon (Ekstedt 1964), which is the variability for consecutive discharges in the time intervals between action potentials from two muscle fibers belonging to the same motor unit. The jitter, normally 10–30 μsec, increases under the influence of small doses of D-tubocurarine (Ekstedt and Stålberg 1969) as a result of increased variability in the synaptic delay of neuromuscular transmission.

METHODS

The methods are described in Ekstedt and Stålberg (1969) in this issue.

RESULTS

Case 1. A 33-year-old healthy man. He had served as an experimental subject several times previously and hundreds of needle insertions had been made in his right brachial biceps muscle, which was also investigated this time. Several hundred normal jitter recordings had been made previously. One of the potential pairs obtained consisted of two single muscle action potentials with amplitudes of 6 mV and 9 mV, respectively, when recording from two electrodes 60 μ apart. The mean time interval between the action potentials was 350 μsec. Even when observing the oscilloscope signal visually, it was evident that the jitter between the action potentials was strikingly small, and after the calculation of standard deviations for 3000 action potentials, divided in groups of 200–300 consecutive items, it was found to be 2–3 μsec, *i.e.*, far less than the normal 10–30 μsec (Ekstedt 1964). The jitter and the mean time interval between the action potentials in the potential pair were unaffected by change of the innervation frequency.

15 μg D-tubocurarine/kg body weight was injected into a cubital vein in the other arm. The jitter was not affected in the 20 calculations of 200–300 consecutive items that were made during the subsequent 10 min. 30 μg D-tubocurarine/kg body weight was then injected. Not even this dose affected the jitter during the subsequent 10 min, as revealed by 20 calculations made as above.

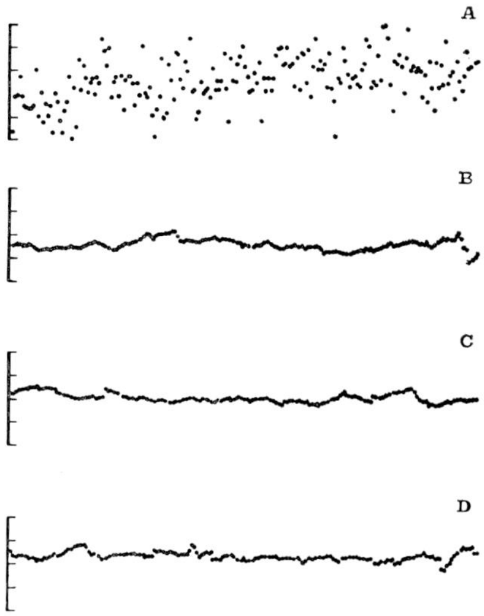

Fig. 1
Sequential histograms of jitter recordings from Case 1. *A*: A normal jitter recording. Jitter = 20.3 μsec. *B*: The abnormal jitter recording before the injection of D-tubocurarine. Jitter = 3.2 μsec. *C*: 3 min after the injection of 15 μg/kg body weight of D-tubocurarine. Jitter = 2.9 μsec. *D*: 5 min after the injection of 30 μg/kg body weight. There were occasional blockings of both action potentials of the potential pair simultaneously, not shown in the figure. Jitter = 3.0 μsec. Each division on the ordinate corresponds to 5 μsec.

About 5–7 min after the injection, however, the previously regular innervation frequency became irregular; there were occasional inter-discharge intervals that were double the usual, as if one discharge now and then was missing. Such failures affected the two fiber action potentials simultaneously and thus differed from the occasional blocking, ordinarily seen after the injection of D-tubocurarine (Ekstedt and Stålberg 1969) or in myasthenia gravis (Ekstedt and Stålberg 1965, 1967), in which only one of the two potentials periodically fails. This experiment is illustrated in Fig. 1.

Case 2. A 25-year-old man. He had also served as a subject before and hundreds of needle insertions had been made in his right brachial biceps muscle. Several hundreds of normal jitter recordings had been made previously. The same muscle was used in this experiment. In this case, a two-fiber recording was obtained from electrodes at a distance of 30–60 μ from each other. The mean time interval between the potentials was 600 μsec. The jitter was about 3 μsec and it was unaffected by injection of 15 and 30 μg D-tubocurarine/kg body weight respectively and, at the higher dose level, occasional failures of both fiber action potentials were observed, exactly as in Case 1. Neither the mean time interval between the potentials nor the jitter altered with different innervation frequencies.

DISCUSSION

Ekstedt and Stålberg (1969) have shown that the injection of 15 μg/kg D-tubocurarine i.v. under the same experimental conditions as in the present investigation increases the jitter from the normal 10–30 μsec to 20–40 μsec and the 30 μg/kg dose increases it to 40–80 μsec.

The present findings of a very small jitter, unaffected by curare, and of periodic blocking of both fiber action potentials simultaneously during curarization have not been previously encountered. It is unlikely that two fibers with separate motor end-plates, belonging to the same motor unit, would behave in this manner. The jitter should then be increased by curarization and the two fibers should not always block simultaneously. The findings are best explained by the assumption that the two muscle fibers were connected with each other electrically and the activity was thus always propagated along both fibers from one motor end-plate. The very small jitter seems to indicate that the impulses are transmitted between the two fibers directly and not by any ephaptic mechanism of the type that may occur between nerve fibers under some extreme experimental conditions (Arvanitaki 1942). An ephaptic transmission between muscle fibers *in situ* has not been reported in the literature. It seems then more reasonable that there was anatomical continuity between the respective muscle fibers.

The experimental results may be interpreted in two ways (Fig. 2). In the first, it is assumed that two, initially separate, fibers have grown together at one point, and in the second, that one fiber during its course has divided into two. One might feel tempted to try to explain either of these hypothetical conditions as an effect of muscle fiber damage caused by previous insertions of the needle multi-electrode. Adjacent damaged fibers might grow together transversely. Alternatively, when there had been a total break of continuity of the muscle fiber, the subsequent development of several buds could give rise to branching. Each original fiber could obviously have a functioning motor end-plate, the innervation of which would be either from the same or from different anterior horn cells. This has been shown in histological investigations (Henriksson 1960; Pearson 1963). According to this mechanism, one part of a severed muscle fiber grows into the sarcolemma of the other part. Splitting of muscle fibers into two longitudinal parts has also been described as a degenerative phenomenon in myopathy (Adams *et al.* 1962).

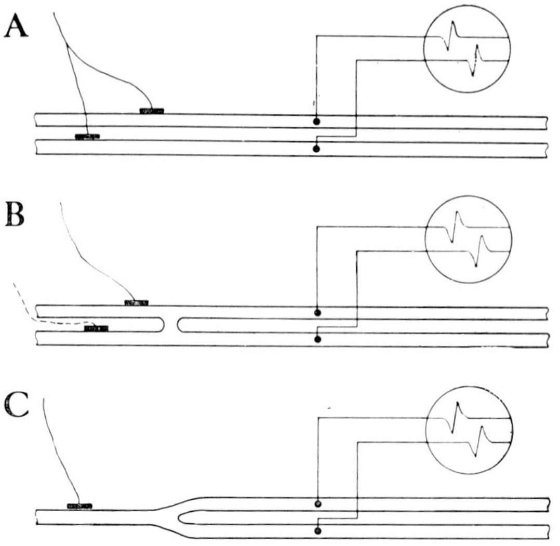

Fig. 2

Possible explanations for the records obtained. *A*: A normal jitter record: two muscle fibers from the same motor unit are recorded. There is variability in the arrival time at the electrodes of the two action potentials because of variable transmission times in the two end-plates involved. The jitter is then normally 10–30 μsec. *B*: illustrates a connection between the two fibers so that an impulse from one end-plate will always be transmitted directly to both fibers. *C*: illustrates branching of one original fiber with one motor end-plate. In both *B* and *C* the jitter ought to be small because there is only one end-plate involved and this may give no jitter. An increase of jitter should not be possible during curarization and with blocking of the motor end-plate both fibers must be affected.

A systematic search will now be made for this phenomenon in order to identify and study its causes.

SUMMARY

In two apparently healthy subjects EMG findings have been made of a type not previously encountered. The jitter between the muscle fiber action potentials from two different muscle fibers belonging to the same motor unit was only 2–3 μsec (S.D.), which is far less than that normally obtained (10–30 μsec). The jitter was unaffected by i.v. injection of 15 and 30 μg D-tubocurarine/kg body weight. Normally, a considerable increase of the jitter is seen at these doses. At the dose level 30 μg D-tubocurarine/kg, blocking of occasional discharges was seen, affecting both the fiber potentials simultaneously. Normally either one or the other of the two fiber potentials blocks in any one discharge.

A hypothesis is presented whereby an abnormal connection existed between two or more fibers, so that activation of one fiber via its motor end-plate also activated the other fiber.

Electroenceph. clin. Neurophysiol., **1969**, *27*: 607–609

RÉSUMÉ

CONNECTIONS ANORMALES ENTRE LES FIBRES MUSCULAIRES STRIÉES

Chez deux sujets apparemment bien portants, des données électromyographiques d'un type jamais rencontré auparavant ont été faites. Le "jitter" entre les potentiels d'action de deux fibres musculaires différentes appartenant à la même unité motrice n'était que de 2–3 μsec (S.D.), ce qui est nettement moindre que ce qui est obtenu normalement (10–30 μsec). Le phénomène de "jitter" n'était pas affecté par l'injection intraveineuse de 15 et de 30 μg de D-tubocurarine/kg de poids. Normalement, une augmentation considérable du phénomène de "jitter" est observée à ces doses. À la dose de 30 μg de D-tubocurarine par kg, on observe occasionnellement le blocage des décharges, affectant simultanément les potentiels des deux fibres. Normalement, les potentiels d'une seule des fibres se bloquent au cours d'une décharge.

Les auteurs font l'hypothèse qu'une connection anormale peut exister entre deux ou plusieurs fibres de telle sorte que l'activitation d'une fibre par l'intermédiaire de sa plaque motrice activerait également l'autre fibre.

The investigation was supported by the Swedish Medical Research Council (Grant No. 14x-135), the Magnus Bergvalls Foundation and the Swedish Association against Poliomyelitis.

REFERENCES

ADAMS, R. D., DENNY-BROWN, D. and PEARSON, C. M. *Diseases of muscle*, 2nd ed., Harper and Row, New York, **1962**: 350, 363 and 365.

ARVANITAKI, A. Effects evoked in an axon by the activity of a contiguous one. *J. Neurophysiol.*, **1942,** *5*: 81–108.

EKSTEDT, J. Human single muscle fiber action potentials. *Acta physiol. scand.*, **1964,** *61*, *Suppl. 226*: 1–96.

EKSTEDT, J. and STÅLBERG, E. The diagnostic use of single muscle fiber recording and the neuromuscular jitter in myasthenia gravis. *Proc. 6th int. Congr. EEG clin. Neurophysiol.*, **1965**: 669–672.

EKSTEDT, J. and STÅLBERG, E. Myasthenia gravis. Diagnostic aspects by a new electrophysiological method. *Opusc. med. (Stockh.)*, **1967,** *12*: 73–76.

EKSTEDT, J. and STÅLBERG, E. The effect of non-paralytic doses of D-tubocurarine on individual motor end-plates in man, studied with a new electrophysiological method. *Electroenceph. clin. Neurophysiol.*, **1969,** *27*: 557–562.

HENRIKSSON, K.-G. Muskelnervförändringar vid progressiv muskeldystrofi. *Nord. Med.*, **1960,** *63*: 289–292.

PEARSON, C. Pathology of human dystrophy in man and animals. In G. H. BOURNE and N. GOLARZ (Eds.), *Muscular dystrophy in man and animals*, Karger, Basel, **1963**, p. 4, 14 and 15.

Reference: EKSTEDT, J. and STÅLBERG, E. Abnormal connections between skeletal muscle fibers. *Electroenceph. clin. Neurophysiol.*, **1969,** *27*: 607–609.

Electroencephalography and Clinical Neurophysiology
Elsevier Publishing Company, Amsterdam – Printed in The Netherlands

TECHNICAL CONTRIBUTIONS

MICRO-ELECTRODE TIP POSITION MARKING IN NERVOUS TISSUE: A NEW DYE METHOD

B. B. Lee[1], G. Mandl[2] and J. P. B. Stean

National Institute for Medical Research, Mill Hill, London, N.W.7 (Great Britain)

(Accepted for publication: May 2, 1969)

Currently available methods for the marking of micro-electrode tip position can be divided into two groups, firstly techniques depending on the local destruction of tissue by passage of current and secondly techniques using iontophoretic deposition of dyes or metals from the electrode tip. Included in the second group are methods involving intracellular deposition of dyes.

Tissue destruction

Methods based on this technique have considerable shortcomings. The lesions produced have to be inconveniently large to be easily identified, the destruction of the tissue at the site from which electrical records were obtained is undesirable and the large currents necessary to produce such lesions may block a micro-pipette. One variation of the tissue coagulation method consists in passing relatively small currents (less than 1 μA) from the electrode tip. This results in negligible tissue coagulation and few cases of electrode damage, but the local injury inflicted causes the migration of polymorph cells to the affected site. With suitable histological staining procedures a small cluster of these cells can usually be detected near the site where the electrode tip had been lodged (Schwartz 1965). Since these cells become visible only after sectioning and staining, many sections have to be examined in order to find this mark. A further disadvantage of this method arises from the accumulations of polymorph cells that often line the borders of the entire electrode track.

Iontophoretic deposition of dyes or metals

Recently some authors have reported the use of various ionizing histological dyes for producing discrete coloured spots in the tissue close to the tip of the recording micro-pipette or within the recorded cell (Thomas and Wilson 1965, 1966; Kaneko and Hashimoto 1967). Of the metal deposition methods, the simplest and most reliable are those based on the release of ferrous or ferric ions into tissue (Rayport 1957; Talbot *et al.* 1967). With subsequent suitable chemical treatment of the tissue, either Prussian blue (ferric ferrocyanide) or Turnbull's blue (ferrous ferrocyanide) is formed at the sites of ion deposition, resulting in brilliant blue spots. This method can be used with steel electrodes as well as with micro-pipettes filled with the appropriate salt solutions. Table I contains a comparison of some of the marking methods quoted in the literature. The main advantage of all these iontophoretic methods lies in the ease with which spots can be detected on the block of tissue during sectioning on the microtome. Nevertheless some shortcomings should be listed: (a) The currents necessary to produce adequately coloured spots with extracellular micro-pipettes are in the range 5–12 μA, resulting in tissue coagulation. The coagulated, stained tissue may attach itself to the electrode tip and be subsequently torn out when the electrode is withdrawn. Some authors (Holubar *et al.* 1967), using methyl blue for intracellular staining, attribute their low success rate (25%) to this cause. (b) Some dyes produce spots which gradually disappear from the sites of deposition in the live tissue. For this reason it is necessary to kill the experimental animal within a few hours after the coloured spot has been produced (Holubar *et al.* 1967). (c) Some coloured spots do not withstand treatment with histological reagents. For example Prussian blue and Turnbull's blue do not survive Golgi-Cox impregnation. The shortcomings of the methods summarized in Table I led us to search for a new more satisfactory dye marking method for extracellular use. A list of requirements for such a method might read as follows: (1) the method should produce a discrete intensely coloured spot, the size of which should be roughly controllable between, say, 30 and 80 μ; (2) the current intensity necessary to produce such spots should not exceed 0.5 μA; (3) the duration of current flow should not exceed 1 min; (4) the spot produced should not diffuse from the site of deposition in the living tissue for at least 48 hours; (5) the spot should still be identifiable after any subsequent histological treatment of the tissue; (6) the dye–salt solution should not have a pH value so unphysiological as to affect tissue close to the electrode tip.

---

[1] Medical Research Council Scholar.

[2] Carnegie Fellow; present address: Aviation Medical Research Unit, McIntyre Science Center, Montreal, P.Q., Canada.

TABLE I

A comparison of some micro-electrode tip marking methods

Method	Dye concentration	Electrolyte in pipette	pH	Typical marking parameters		Type of recording	Comments	Reference
				μA	min			
Iontophoretic								
Alcian blue	8% or 3%	0.5 *M* Sodium acetate	5.8	(+) 0.5–1.0	0.5–1.0	Extra-cellular		
Fast green, FCF	Saturated	2 *M* Sodium chloride	5.1	(−) 10–12	5–10	Extra-cellular	Marks pale; disappear within a few hours of deposition	Thomas and Wilson 1965
Methyl blue	Saturated	0.5 *M* Potassium acetate	8.7	(−) 1–3	1–3	Intra-cellular		Thomas and Wilson 1966
	Saturated	1 *M* Potassium acetate	8.6	(−) 1–3	1–3	Intra-cellular	Marks often disappear due to diffusion or attachment of tissue to electrode	Holubar *et al.* 1967
	4%	1 *M* Sodium citrate	8.3	(−) 10	2	Extra-cellular	Marks often disappear after tissue sectioning	
Pontamine blue	2%	0.5 *M* Sodium acetate	8.3	(−) 5	5	Extra-cellular	Satisfactory	Kaneko and Hashimoto 1967
Prussian blue	—	0.7 *M* Potassium ferricyanide and 2 *M* potassium chloride	8.3	(−) 5–10	10–15	Extra-cellular	Tissue requires perfusion with developing solution	Talbot *et al.* 1967
Turnbull's blue	—	3 *N* Ferric ammonium sulphate	3	(+) 0.05	60	Extra-cellular	Tissue requires perfusion with developing solution	Rayport 1967
Tissue coagulation								
Lesions				(+) 2–15	5–10	Extra-cellular	For good visibility lesions must be large (100–400 μ)	
"Polymorph" marks				(+) 1	5–10	Extra-cellular	Mark invisible before histological staining; not specific for electrode tip	Schwartz 1965

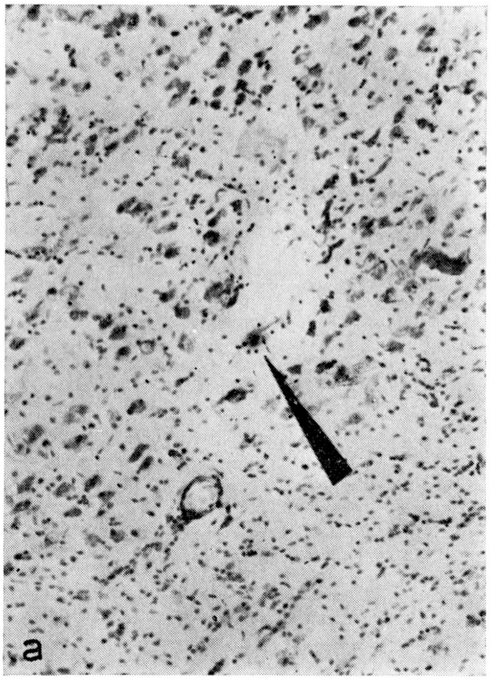

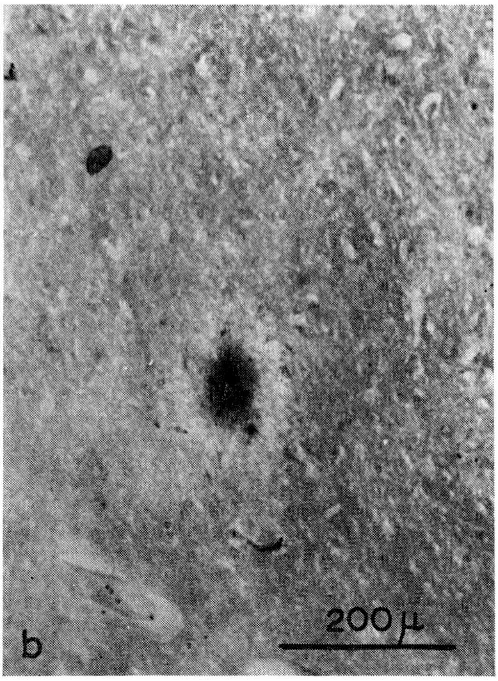

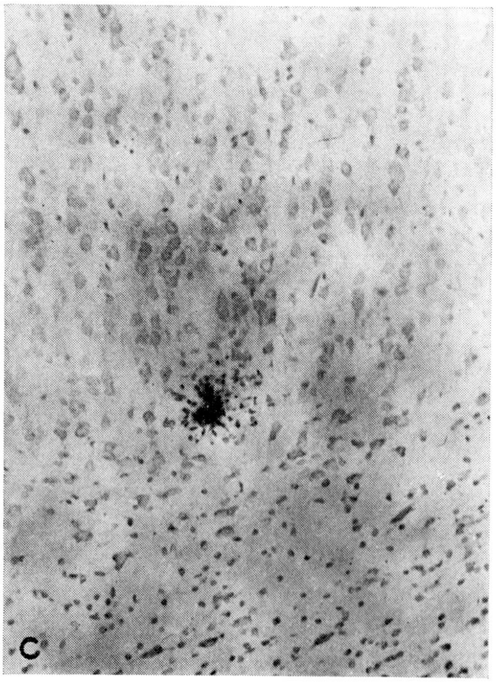

Fig. 1
Three methods of extracellular micro-electrode tip position marking. *a*: Fast green FCF. 10 μA, 10 min, tip negative. Rat thalamus, counterstain cresyl fast violet. *b*: Pontamine blue. 10 μA, 2 min, tip negative. Rabbit hypothalamus, counterstain phloxine. *c*: Alcian blue. 0.5 μA, 2 min, tip positive. Cat cortex, counterstain cresyl fast violet.

METHOD

Alcian blue 8GX has properties which have enabled us to meet most of these requirements. It is an amphoteric water-soluble derivative of copper phthallocyanin, having a tetraalkylisothiouronium group attached to each of the four peripheral benzene rings of the phthallocyanin chromophore (Scott *et al.* 1964). The isothiouronium group is unstable in alkaline solution. We found that the commercial product contains approximately 60% dyestuff by weight. The remaining constituents are apparently diluents and wetting agents (Alcian blue 8GX, obtained from G. Gurr, Colour Index No. 74240). Fifty-four attempts were made to mark the positions of the tips of extracellular recording glass micro-pipettes. Of these, 44 were in the cerebral cortex of cats, 4 in the cortex of rabbits and 6 in the hippocampus of rabbits. Tip diameters of the pipettes ranged between 1 and 4 μ. Dye solutions used consisted of either 3% or 8% Alcian blue in 0.5 *M* sodium acetate. All solutions were filtered through a 0.45 μ Millipore filter. Micro-pipettes were filled through the butt end, by pressure from a syringe, the solution being filtered again, using a Millipore syringe-fitting filter assembly (pore size 0.45 μ) (Millipore Cat. No. SX 0001300). With this procedure the resistance of the micro-pipette did not exceed 10 MΩ. The discharge patterns of cortical neurones, recorded with these dye-filled micro-pipettes, were indistinguishable from those obtained with pipettes filled with saturated sodium chloride solution. In order to determine the optimum marking parameters currents between 0.5 and 10 μA were passed for 0.5–10 min. The tip of each pipette acted as the anode. Of the 54 attempts, 45 were successful.

Three factors affected the size of the spots produced: (1) dye concentration; (2) current duration; (3) current intensity. Twenty-four spots were produced with 8% dye and 1 μA current, the duration of current flow varying between 30 sec and 10 min. Spot diameters varied between 30 and 120 μ and there was a correlation between current duration and spot diameter. With the same current (1 μA) and a similar range of current durations (2–10 min), but using a 3% dye solution, spot diameters ranged between 10 and 40 μ (5 spots). Thus, as would be expected, the size of a spot can be controlled either by duration of current flow or by dye concentration. We found that changing the current intensity was the less reliable method. This was partly due to the increase in electrode resistance that often accompanied high current intensities. Also, high current intensities had the disadvantage of causing tissue damage. Of the nine failures, most were associated with a rapid rise in electrode resistance on beginning to pass current.

More recently we have used a 5% solution of the dyestuff fraction extracted from the commercial product (Scott *et al.* 1964) in 0.5 *M* sodium acetate. Blockage of the micro-pipette has been minimized by using this modified dye solution. Using an 8% dye solution, we found that the optimum parameters were a 0.5–1 μA current passed for 1 min, producing a spot of about 40 μ diameter. All spots, irrespective of current intensity, current duration or dye concentration, were opaque, very sharply defined and readily visible during histological sectioning of the tissue. After passage of the "marking" current, time periods varying between 2 and 30 hours were allowed to elapse before the experimental animals were killed. No variation in the quality of the spots was observed. For 44 of the spots produced the tissue was perfused with formol–saline, soaked in a 30% sucrose solution, frozen and sectioned, and the sections were mounted using the gelatine method of Olt (1906). Sections were then stained by a variety of standard techniques. One spot preparation was subjected to Golgi-Cox impregnation. None of the histological reagents used caused any deterioration of the density or colour of the spots.

We believe that the discrete nature of an Alcian blue spot may be due either to the formation of electrostatic complexes with polyanions in the nervous tissue or to the decomposition of the isothiouronium groups at the pH of nervous tissue.

Fig. 1 shows photomicrographs of the three most satisfactory dye marking methods.

SUMMARY

Some methods of micro-electrode tip position marking are briefly discussed. Alcian blue, extruded iontophoretically with low current intensities (0.5 μA) and short time intervals (1–2 min) produces well-defined, non-fading spots in nervous tissue. We have succeeded in producing 45 spots in 54 attempts.

RÉSUMÉ

MARQUAGE DE LA POSITION DE L'EXTRÉMITÉ DE MICRO-ÉLECTRODES DANS LE TISSU NERVEUX; UNE NOUVELLE TECHNIQUE PAR COLORANT

Les auteurs décrivent brièvement plusieurs méthodes de marquage de la position de l'extrémité d'une électrode. Le bleu Alcien extrait par ionophorèse avec des intensités de courant faibles (0.5 μA) et des intervalles de temps courts (1–2 min) produit dans le tissue nerveux des taches bien définies et ne s'effaçant pas. Nous avons réussi à produire 45 taches en 54 essais.

We would like to thank Phil M. Waite and R. F. Hellon for two of the slides reproduced in Fig. 1.

REFERENCES

HOLUBAR, J., HANKE, B. and MALIK, V. Intracellular recording from cortical pyramids and small interneurons as identified by subsequent staining with the recording microelectrode. *Exp. Neurol.*, **1967,** *19*: 257–265.

KANEKO, A. and HASHIMOTO, H. Recording site of the single cone response determined by an electrode marking technique. *Vision Res.*, **1967,** *7*: 847–851.

OLT. Das Aufkleben mikroskopischer Schnitte. *Z. wiss. Mikr.*, **1906,** *23*: 323.

RAYPORT, M. Anatomical identification of somatic sensory cortical neurons responding with short latencies to specific afferent volleys. *Fed. Proc.*, **1957,** *16*: 104.

SCHWARTZ, S. T. *An analysis of resting activity in the cuneate nucleus.* Ph.D. Thesis, Albert Einstein College of Medicine, Yeshiva University, New York, **1965.**

SCOTT, J. E., QUINTARELLI, G. and DELLOVO, M. C. The chemical and histochemical properties of Alcian Blue. 1. The mechanism of Alcian Blue staining. *Histochemie*, **1964,** *4*: 73–85.

TALBOT, R. E., TOWE, A. L. and KENNEDY, T. T. Physiological and histological classification of cerebellar neurons in chloralose-anaesthetised cats. *Exp. Neurol.*, **1967,** *19*: 46–65.

THOMAS, R. C. and WILSON, V. J. Precise localisation of Renshaw cells with a new marking technique. *Nature (Lond.)*, **1965,** *206*: 211–213.

THOMAS, R. C. and WILSON, V. J. Marking single neurons by staining with intracellular recording microelectrodes. *Science*, **1966,** *151*: 1538–1539.

Reference: LEE, B. B., MANDL, G. and STEAN, J. P. B. Micro-electrode tip position marking in nervous tissue: a new dye method. *Electroenceph. clin. Neurophysiol.*, **1969,** *27*: 610–613.

Electroencephalography and Clinical Neurophysiology
Elsevier Publishing Company, Amsterdam – Printed in The Netherlands

A STEREOTAXIC FRAME ASSEMBLY FOR INVESTIGATING THE CAT AUDITORY SYSTEM[1]

C. W. Dunlop

Brain Research Unit, Department of Physiology, University of Sydney, N.S.W. 2006 (Australia)

(Accepted for publication: March 24, 1969)

A survey of stereotaxis for the cat has been made by Blum and Feldman (1964). Fixation of the head to the instrument is generally achieved by inserting bars into the external auditory meati and clamping bars over each inferior orbital ridge and behind the incisor teeth upward against the upper jaw. Jasper and Ajmone Marsan (1960) described a commonly used stereotaxic instrument and the principles of the method. However, this type of instrument is not satisfactory for the study of various regions of the auditory system.

The use of ear bars causes variable damage to the tympanic membrane and associated structures and prevents ready access to the bullae and other peripheral auditory structures. The ear bars are hollow for the transmission of sound and the nearest the acoustic transducers can be placed is approximately 8 cm from the tympanic membrane (the length of the ear bars), thus creating resonance problems when delivering the acoustic stimulus. The nearness of the calibrated side bars of the conventional frame assembly (approximately 15 cm) on which the electrode holders ride restricts the movement of the electrodes for penetration of laterally situated brain structures such as the auditory and associated cortices; therefore a tangential penetration of the cortex is often prevented.

A stereotaxic frame assembly is described here which permits fixation of the cat's head without ear bars, and more flexibility of electrode movement is achieved than in the conventional apparatus by further spacing of the side bar assembly to a distance of 25 cm (Fig. 1).

Construction and operation of the apparatus

Fixation of the cat's head in the apparatus requires more time than in the conventional apparatus; however, the procedure is a simple one. The head holder (Fig. 2) can be considered to consist of three parts:

1. A lower platform (LP) consisting of a cross-bar on which the upper jaw immediately behind the incisors rests.

2. A vertical rod (R) capable of being moved up and down and fixed in position by a screw clamp (C).

3. An upper platform (UP) which is attached to this vertical rod. This platform has a cross-member (CM) which can be moved in an antero-posterior direction and tilted to any angle by the manipulation of two screws (S1, 2). This cross-member is attached to the cat's skull by another two screws (S3, 4) which are screwed into two 2 cm threaded brass tubes (T) situated on the cat's skull and embedded in dental acrylic (see below).

The side bars of the frame assembly were constructed to carry the base block of a Trent Wells probe drive electrode carrier (Trent Wells, Mechanical Development, Southgate, California).

Fixation of cross-member to the cat's skull

The skin overlying the cat's cranium is incised in the midline from the supra-orbital ridge to the external occipital protuberance. The skin flaps are retracted, underlying fascia removed, and the temporal muscles reflected as far laterally as possible. The exposed skull is cleaned of blood and muscle. Two stainless steel screws (S5), size 6/32, length 3/16 in. are firmly screwed into and through the bone (Fig. 2, *b*), 1 cm each of the sagittal suture, in the region rostral to the coronal suture. The two internally threaded brass tubes are now firmly attached to the cross-member (CM) by way of the two brass screws (S3, 4). The area around the two screws in the skull is now thoroughly dried, the cross-member assembly is held in position (approximately 1.5 cm

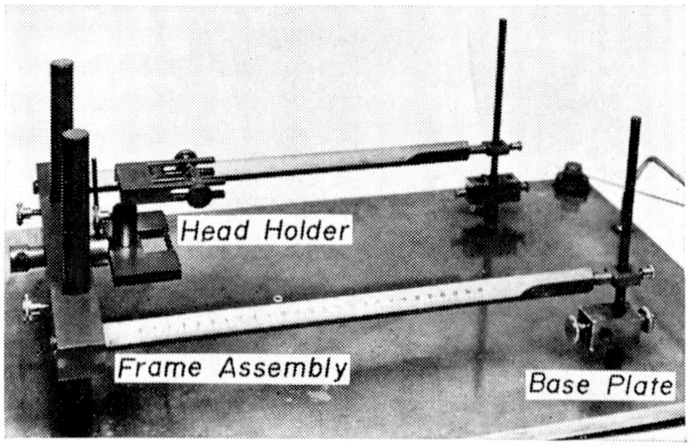

Fig. 1
A side-view photograph of the stereotaxic frame assembly consisting of a base plate, frame assembly and head holder.

[1] Supported by grants from the National Health and Medical Research Council of Australia and the University of Sydney.

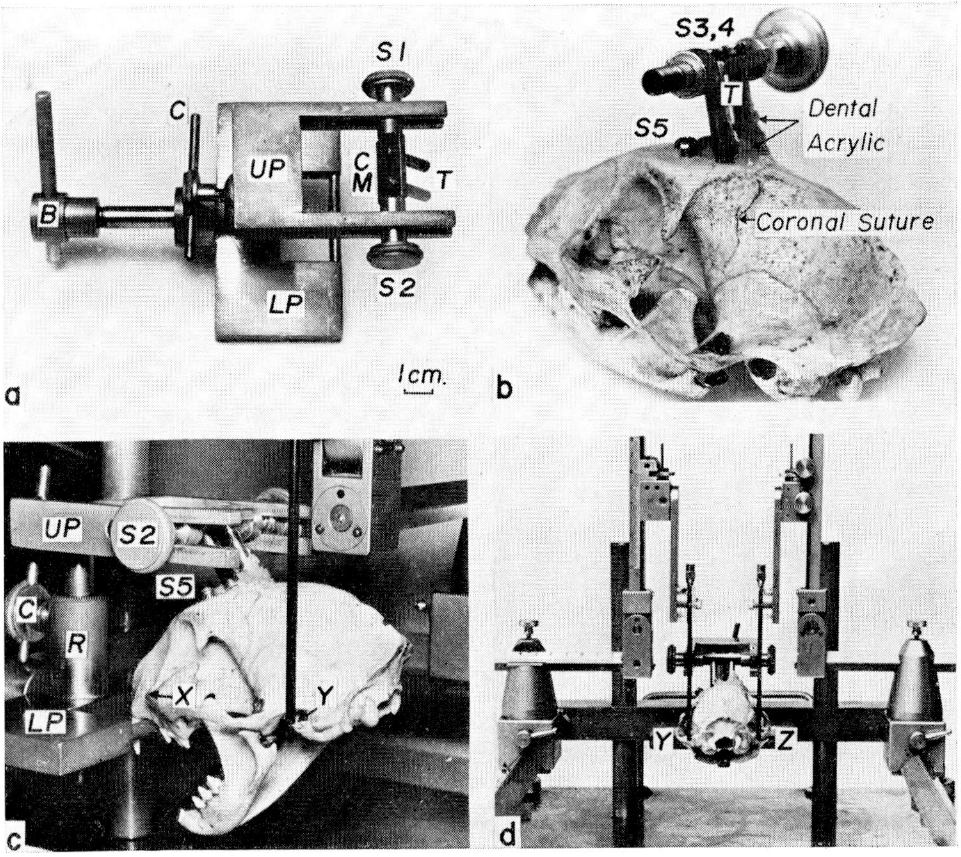

Fig. 2
a: Head holder removed from stereotaxic frame assembly. *b*: Arrangement of cross-member (CM), threaded brass tubes (T), screw (S5) and dental acrylic on surface of skull anterior to bregma. *c*: Skull positioned in head holder in the basal horizontal plane by manipulation of clamp (C) and screws (S1, 2) so that electrode at Y was at same height at X. *d*: Establishment of inter-aural line parallel to side bars of frame assembly by having electrodes at Y and Z at same height.

anterior to the bregma and at an angle of approximately 50° to the horizontal), and a dental acrylic preparation (Texton) is poured around the screws and brass tubes. During hardening of the dental acrylic care must be exercised in preventing movement of the preparation so that a rigid and strong cross-member fixation is obtained.

Orientation of cat's head for stereotaxic electrode placement

In all experiments the pinna are removed. For stereotaxic electrode placement, the inter-aural basal plane (XY, Fig. 2, *c*) is obtained by rotating the head holder by loosening clamp (C) so that the inter-aural line (YZ, the line connecting the center of each external auditory meatus, Fig. 2, *d*) is in a plane horizontal to the side bars of the stereotaxic frame. Having established this plane, the basal horizontal plane of the instrument (a plane through the inter-aural line and the centers of the inferior orbital ridges) is obtained by manipulation of the cross-member and the vertical rod of the head assembly, thus altering the degree of tilt of the head in an antero-caudal direction.

The zero frontal plane and the zero horizontal plane (1 cm above the inter-aural basal plane) are measured at the inter-aural line. These measurements are then referred to the bregma so that future electrode coordinates can be easily assessed. The midline of the brain serves as the zero plane for designating locations left and right in the brain.

Different planes of electrode penetrations of a given auditory region can be achieved by the combination of trigonometry and the use of the stereotaxic coordinates. Here the electrode holder may be tilted to an angle or kept in a vertical position with the horizontal plane of the cat's head set to a certain angle by loosening the clamp (C) attached to the head holder and rotating the assembly to that angle.

This apparatus has been successful in electrode penetrations of the auditory cortex, medial geniculate body, and inferior colliculus of the cat.

SUMMARY

A stereotaxic frame assembly for investigating the cat auditory system is described. Ear bars are not used. This allows the acoustic transducers to be placed adjacent to the tympanic membrane, and avoids damage to this membrane by conventional ear bars. The apparatus also allows for a much greater flexibility of electrode movement, especially in regard to different angular penetrations of laterally located central nervous regions.

RÉSUMÉ

CADRE STÉRÉOTAXIQUE POUR L'INVESTIGATION DU SYSTÈME AUDITIF DU CHAT

L'auteur décrit un cadre stéréotaxique destiné à l'investigation du système auditif du chat et dans lequel les barres d'oreille ne sont pas nécessaires. Ceci permet de placer les capteurs contre la membrane du tympan et évite les lésions de cette membrane par les barres d'oreille conventionnelles. L'appareil permet également une beaucoup plus grande liberté de mouvement des électrodes, spécialement en raison des différentes pénétrations angulaires des régions nerveuses centrales situées latéralement.

Acknowledgement is made to Mr. R. Munns for technical assistance.

REFERENCES

BLUM, B. and FELDMAN, B. A mountable stereotaxic apparatus for the cat. *Electroenceph. clin. Neurophysiol.*, **1964,** *16*: 403–408.

JASPER, H. H. and AJMONE MARSAN, C. *A stereotaxic atlas of the diencephalon of the cat.* Nat. Res. Council of Canada, Ottawa, **1960**.

Reference: DUNLOP, C. W. A stereotaxic frame assembly for investigating the cat auditory system. *Electroenceph. clin. Neurophysiol.*, **1969,** *27*: 614–616.

Electroencephalography and Clinical Neurophysiology
Elsevier Publishing Company, Amsterdam – Printed in The Netherlands

SOCIETY PROCEEDINGS

DEUTSCHE EEG-GESELLSCHAFT

Münster, June 13–16, 1968

Secretary: ST. KUBICKI

Abteilung für klinische Elektroencephalographie, Freie Universität, 1 Berlin 19 (W. Germany)

1. Mechanisms of origin of the EEG. — R. F. Schmidt (Heidelberg).

The following elementary processes of neuronal activity can be detected by electrophysiological methods: (a) *Generator potentials* of the receptors. These are non-transmitted depolarizations of the receptor membrane, by virtue of which extent and duration of depolarization depend on the characteristics of the receptors and the stimulus. (b) The *action potentials* of the neurones, which are set up either peripherally at the receptor or by means of synaptic activity and, obeying the all-or-none principle, are transmitted along the axon. A short spike potential is followed by more or less recordable after-potentials. (c) *Excitatory post-synaptic potentials, EPSP*. At the axo-somatic and axo-dendritic excitatory synapses a pre-synaptic action potential leads to the liberation of a transmitter substance which causes depolarization of the post-synaptic cell through a change of conductivity of the subsynaptic membrane. Depolarization to threshold liberates a transmitted action potential. (d) *Inhibitory post-synaptic potentials, IPSP*. By analogy with the events at the excitatory synapses, there is a hyperpolarization and increase of conductivity of the post-synaptic membrane at the inhibitory axo-somatic and axo-dendritic synapses by means of the liberated transmitter substance. The membrane potential becomes farther from the threshold because of the hyperpolarization, while at the same time, owing to the conductivity change, the effectiveness of the excitatory subsynaptic currents is diminished. Through activation of axo-axonic synapses, *pre-synaptic inhibition* of the posterior root fibres gives a depolarizing potential. For the duration of the depolarization a decreased amount of transmitter substance is liberated by a pre-synaptic action potential. (e) *Standing potentials*. These are relatively constant DC potentials which can be recorded between different points in the central nervous system.

In conventional EEG recordings, because of the biological and technical actualities, neither the generator potentials, nor the standing potentials, nor the spike potentials of the action potentials are detected. Apart perhaps from the after-potentials of the action potentials, it is chiefly the excitatory and inhibitory post-synaptic potentials which set the EEG pens in motion.

2. Mixing excitatory and inhibitory components in polysynaptic post-synaptic potentials. — M. R. Klee, A. Wagner and W. Papajewski (Frankfort/M.).

Because of the possible separation of its mono-, bi-, and polysynaptic entries, the already known definition of its post-synaptic potentials and the markedly feeble interference from "spontaneous" excitation, the motoneurone of the cat is better suited than the cortical cell to investigation of the possible mixing of PSPs. In relation to the motoneurone as a model, it should be explained, on account of findings relating to the interaction of different EPSPs on the cortical cells (to be explained by different localization of the excited synapses on the somata or dendrites of the cells) or on account of much more not already included in these complex PSPs, for example the "augmenting" and "recruiting" EPSPs, that polysynaptic EPSPs and IPSPs are possibly mixed.

Intracellular recordings were made with conventional techniques from motoneurones in the region L_2–S_1, chosen from the nuclear region of the biceps–semitendineus muscle. The anterior roots and the corresponding motor nerves were stimulated and, in some experiments, also the posterior roots. For puncturing, single or theta capillaries filled with K citrate or KCl were used. The recorded post-synaptic potentials were averaged directly on a CAT 400B.

The use of different methods of testing (homonymous and heteronymous interaction on mono- and polysynaptic EPSPs, interactions between EPSPs and antidromic action potentials, interactions between EPSPs and IPSPs, injections of Cl ions and application of current) showed that 70% of the polysynaptic EPSPs were mixed with IPSPs at the motoneurones, whose presence could be demonstrated, with the methods used, 4–8 msec after the commencement of the EPSPs, and whose latency was frequently shorter than the peak latency of the EPSPs. In heteronymous interaction it was shown in relation to the enhancement or reduction of test EPSPs that these findings corresponded with the interactions of "recruiting" and "augmenting" EPSPs of cortical cells. Also, the polysynaptic EPSPs to be observed in strychnine convulsions show clear conformity with the corresponding PSPs at cortical cells.

Such mixed polysynaptic EPSPs/IPSPs could also

explain why, after injection of strychnine, some postsynaptic potentials imposed as IPSPs are converted into EPSPs at the cortical cells following stimulation of a polysynaptic pathway. By blocking of the inhibitory components in the connected interneurones by strychnine, the polysynaptic potential recorded at the motoneurone as the sum of excitations arriving from the interneurones is changed to an exclusively or at least preponderantly excitatory potential. However, IPSPs could also be demonstrated in the discharge of these polysynaptic "EPSPs" after strychnine injection. Accordingly, in the action of strychnine there is likewise a blocking of strychnine-sensitive short-duration IPSPs and not a reversal of the action of the inhibitory transmitter substance.

3. The action of raised CO_2 pressure on the excitability of spinal motoneurones. — W. Papajewski, M. R. Klee and A. Wagner (Frankfort/M.).

Although the significance of CO_2 tension in the tissues for the excitability of neuronal structures is known, the action of CO_2 on the membrane potential has, with the exception of a short experiment of Krnjević and co-workers on the cat, only been investigated so far in the nerve cells and nerve and muscle fibres of cold-blooded animals. The results are not uniform: raising the CO_2 tension, for example, produces in the spinal ganglion cells a decrease of the membrane potential and in cortical cells an increase. In frog muscle fibres both effects can be observed to be dependent on the membrane potential, while the motoneurone of the cat does not react to changes of CO_2 tension.

Recordings from spinal motoneurones of cats were carried out with conventional techniques. The anterior and posterior roots were stimulated, or the corresponding muscle nerves. The animals were narcotized with Nembutal and kept still with Flaxedil; they were artificially ventilated and the following gaseous mixtures were administered under constant ventilatory frequency and volume: (1) 5% CO_2, 50% O_2, 45% N_2; (2) 10% CO_2, 50% O_2, 40% N_2; (3) 100% O_2. In some experiments ventilation was interrupted for 2–5 min. Measurement of arterial gas tension with glass electrodes showed, for mixture (1), an increase in pCO_2 of some 10 mm Hg with a corresponding pH reduction and an increase in pO_2 to about 1.5 times the initial value.

45 motoneurones could be recorded for 15–60 min without mechanical artefacts, despite tissue movement from the attendant changes in blood pressure. Nearly all cells showed a decreased excitability 1–3 min after starting to give increased CO_2 mixtures. On the other hand there were 3 types of change in the membrane potential: (a) In about half of the cells investigated a reduction of the membrane potential and of the action potential by 6–10 mV was observed, together with a reduction of the steepness of ascent and descent of the spikes and an increase in amplitude of the hyperpolarizing after-potentials. (b) On the contrary, in 30% of the cells we found a hyperpolarization of 7–12 mV. (c) 20% of cells showed a delayed hyperpolarization. The average membrane potentials of the cells described (a–c) were 71, 62 and 60 mV. Simultaneous measurements of electrotonic potentials (electrode resistances by the bridge method) demonstrated that movement artefacts, and thus damage to cells, were not the cause of the depolarization. It was also revealed by this measurement that the resistance of the cell membrane increased independently of the wave form of the membrane potential; on the contrary—equally for de- and hyperpolarization—the amplitude of the PSPs markedly decreased. Antidromic excitation was often blocked completely, not only at the generator of the B-spikes, and it could be shown in some cases that the stimulus strength must be raised or a depolarizing current be simultaneously applied. We obtained similar results with orthodromic excitation.

The increase of anion permeability and the proportion of free calcium ions, as well as the reduction of calcium concentration in the interior of cells, which are produced by increased CO_2, determined by the simultaneous change in H^+ concentration, partly clarify these findings.

4. Experimental single-cell investigations of a summatory excitatory picture (with reference to genesis of the EEG). — H. K. Oehlschlägel and B. von Westernhagen (Göttingen).

In the acoustic system large numbers of receptors can be studied relatively easily, both in a varied manner and in order of size, by means of variation of the stimulus parameters of adequate stimulation. This opens up the possibility of analysis in association with recording of single-cell activity. We thus have an experimental summatory excitation picture over primary and secondary convergence regions as well as beyond these.

Single-cell findings in the cochlear nucleus of the waking cat (type 1 cells of von Westernhagel *et al.* 1968) after stimulation of the intact hearing system with noise bands of variable bandwidth are reported and interpreted. In the excitatory pattern of the recorded cells the individual convergence regions of different neural processing stages are clearly traced, while efferent back-flow of the excitation obviously influences the whole acoustic system in a very wide-band manner.

By changing the stimulation conditions these effects shift relative to one another in such a way that some initial insight is possible into the mechanism of these special systems in regard to the wide-band, and practically the whole, system of the detecting summatory excitation picture. A synoptic estimation of this relationship under assumed diffuse stimulation must, in certain hypotheses, lead to rhythmic discharges which can take place in the same phase within the entire system. The question is discussed whether this is also applicable to the genesis of the EEG.

5. Findings in regard to spread of excitation in spinal motoneurones and motor cortex cells. — H. D. Lux (Munich).

The following observations were made by means of simultaneous recording of field potentials and membrane potentials of antidromically and directly stimulated motoneurones. On near-threshold stimulation of anterior root bundles there often appeared, during the usual negative field potential, exclusively with the occurrence of a soma-dendritic (SD) spike, a clear supplementary positive field potential which was followed by a short negative fluctuation. This potential might outlast the intracellularly recorded SD spike for about 1 msec. On direct stimulation of the same motoneurone through a second intracellular electrode action potentials continually appeared with similar extracellular potentials. These findings indicate that important differences may exist between the field potential of an individual neurone and that of a synchronously activated nucleus of nerve cells with overlapping dendrites. Intracellular separate double micro-electrodes show, indeed, that at least main dendrites of motoneurones may be excitable, yet it is concluded on the basis of field potential determinations, in agreement with other investigations, that the active spread of excitation is confined to an interval of about 2 msec. An excitation spread in peripheral dendrites appears unlikely.

For pyramidal cells of the motor cortex a comparison of electrophysiological and morphological findings suggests that active and passive spread of excitation in dendrites can take only a little more time. In the formation of the primary surface-negative deflection of the cortical evoked potential after orthodromic and antidromic stimuli, for example on the basis of latency relationships, there are far less active or passive excitatory transmissions in dendrites than excitatory and inhibitory activity of other neurones. In long-lasting synaptic events soma-dendritic potential spread appears less important in the determination of field and surface potentials.

6. Cortical recruiting and desynchronization by stimulation of the putamen and pallidum of cats. — G. Dieckmann (Frankfort/M.).

Near-threshold bipolar stimulation of the putamen and pallidum in 47 cats under Nembutal or Flaxedil influenced the cortical electrical activity in the form of a non-specific activation. This gave the comparative experiment of 71 stimulus points in the putamen, pallidum and nucleus entopeduncularis, with a further 96 subcortical stimulus points localized mainly in the internal capsule. There was direct EEG pen recording.

Unilateral putamen and pallidum stimulation with lower frequencies (6–10/sec; 0.6–1.0 V) gave, in the drowsy state, recruiting or recruiting-like responses, release of spindle activity, single bursts (stimulus frequency 0.5–1/sec) and generalized synchronization. The recruiting responses were found over the anterior and posterior sigmoid gyri of both hemispheres, and the remaining non-specific responses also over the suprasylvian gyrus, chiefly ipsilaterally. 30–100/sec stimuli could desynchronize synchronous cortical activity.

Low frequency stimulation in the internal capsule above the pallidum and nucleus entopeduncularis gave augmenting responses or augmenting-like discharges over the anterior and posterior sigmoid gyrus as well as over the coronal gyrus. Stimulation at higher frequencies was likewise followed by desynchronization. The ipsilateral cortical activity was affected by capsular stimulation.

Under the synchronized discharges, the recruiting responses for the putamen and pallidum seem to be locally specific, whereas augmenting responses seem so for the stimulated part of the internal capsule. The possibility is discussed of differentiating between responses to basal ganglia and capsule stimulation by means of cortical unit recordings in regard to antidromic spikes of 0.5–2.0 msec latency. The stimulus-induced desynchronization proceeds on the other hand from the capsule and investigated basal ganglia in similar ways.

7. On inter-hemispheric transfer in "corpus callosum cats". — K. A. Hossmann (Cologne).

The "corpus callosum cat" is an acute *cerveau isolé* preparation in which the midline of the brain below the corpus callosum is divided. The sole remaining anatomical connections between the two hemispheres are the corpus callosum and the psalterium. In the resting state a sleep EEG was recorded from both hemispheres; stimulation of the mesencephalic reticular formation (similarly divided at the midline) produced a unilateral arousal effect, which spread to the frontal region of the opposite hemisphere in only a few cases.

The surface positive transcallosal potentials (TcP) after electrical stimulation of the cortex or a specific thalamic nucleus were modified neither by an ipsilateral nor by a contralateral arousal. The TcP frequently followed a spindle, during which some of the cortical cells were activated and others inhibited. During the TcP itself only a very small percentage of the neurones was activated. The relationships between the TcP and the primary evoked potential recorded from the same area were described in detail.

8. Optokinetic and vestibular ear nystagmus in rabbits. — D. Schott, G. Koppen and K. P. Schaefer (Göttingen).

The optokinetic and the per- and post-rotatory reactions of the eye and ear were tested on an electronically controlled rotating chair (Tönnies, Freiburg) in 12 waking rabbits fixed at the head and extremities. The following were recorded oscillographically: the nystagmogram of the eyes, the myogram of the ear muscles and, through a transducer, the ear movements. Nystagmus occurred regularly in response to per-rotatory acceleration stimuli. Nystagmic ear movements could, however, only be observed sporadically. More frequently a tonic ear reaction occurred, which corresponded to the direction of the slow phase of the ocular nystagmus. Post-rotatory acceleration stimuli, on the other hand, resulted in a longer-lasting aural nystagmus, which occurred synchronously in each phase with the simultaneously recorded ocular nystagmus. Even with irregular expression of the ocular nystagmus the synchronization of the two events remained. The aural nystagmus merely died away somewhat earlier than the ocular nystagmus. In narcosis

(30–40 mg/kg Evipan i.v.) the post-rotatory aural nystagmus disappeared somewhat faster than the ocular nystagmus. Also, under these conditions the synchronization of the two events remained. This finding demonstrates that both events have a common substrate in the lower brain-stem. Vestibular afferents for directional hearing, *i.e.*, the acoustic spatial constant and also a co-ordination of the acoustic sense organs with spatial orientation, can be considered as proved.

9. Stimulation experiments on the tectum opticum of freely moving decorticate cats. — G. Hopf, H. Heller and K. P. Schaefer (Göttingen).

In 15 decorticate cats the superior colliculus was stimulated unilaterally with micro-electrodes, 121 times in all, using a triangular–rectangular stimulator (Tönnies, Freiburg); in a further 7 experiments both colliculi were stimulated simultaneously. The motor reactions of the animals were recorded in protocols and partly photographically and cinematographically, or else myographically. All movements of ears, eyes, head and body were thus recorded. All reactions showed, in addition to dependence on the strength of the stimulating current, a regular dependence on the locus of stimulation, related to the surface of the colliculus, *i.e.*, the projection area of the quadrants of the visual field. In 110 cases unilateral stimulation was followed by contralateral head turning which was stronger the nearer the stimulus point lay to the posterior pole of the colliculus. For 31 of these points there was an additional raising component, which increased as the stimulus point was shifted laterally. The experimental animal turned eleven times ipsilaterally, namely, on stimulation in the medial part of the colliculus. These movements occurred with a clear latent period. Conjugate eye movements were seen simultaneously, which corresponded to the direction of the head turning, and, as already described by Hess and co-workers, preceded the head movement. With increase of stimulus intensity the reactions described became movements of flight or other defensive reactions. On simultaneous punctate stimulation of both colliculi with two microelectrodes the single elicited movements were added together vectorially if they were similarly directed (for all raisings and lowerings) and were subtracted if they were in opposite directions (contralateral turning). For 68 of these points movements of one or both ears were observed to be regularly dependent on the site of stimulation, before eye and head movements occurred (threshold stimulus was 0.5–2 V, width of single pulse 10–20 msec and frequency 20–30 c/sec). On stimulation in the anterior pole there was a movement of both ears forward and on stimulation in the posterior pole there was a movement of the contralateral ear backwards.

These investigations correspond largely to the normal behaviour of the animal on visual environmental stimulation. The significance of the tectum opticum as a multisensorial integration centre is demonstrated afresh. Motor reactions of the ear allow us to recognize that monaural directional audition and binaural audition possess a biological significance, even in organisms with frontally directed eyes.

10. On extension of the diagnostic power of the EEG by micromotor tone recording. — H. D. Weigeldt (Bremen).

The unsatisfactory conclusions or ambiguity, especially in the late phase of evaluation of the EEG by an expert, and also the insufficient correlation between psychopathological findings and the shape of the curve, are generally known. To make good this lack micromotor tone recording, reported by F. Steinwachs in April 1961 in Kiel, seems to us appropriate. Since April 1962, in patients with organic cerebral and neurotic disturbances, investigations performed at first with an improved mechanical, and later with an electrical, writing pressure transducer confirmed the diagnostic possibility of separating psychic and organic disturbances. In the majority of our clinical comparative experiments we found the functional relationship suggested by Steinwachs between characteristic criteria of the curves of micromotor activity on the one hand and the psychopathological findings and changes in performance on the other. Furthermore, micromotor recording resulted in localization of temporofrontal, occipito-parietal or diffuse organic cerebral disturbances. Also, we carried out longitudinal studies in characteristic cases, partly without medication, in which the rate of progress of constitutional disturbances or alcoholic delirium were demonstrated strikingly in the form of curves.

Micromotor tone recording seemed to us especially informative in the evaluation and adjustment of medication in ictal disorders, because, on the background of constitutional specific reactivity, the expression of overdosage and its side-effects is recognizable in the micromotor curves.

For a few months we have studied by means of synchronous EEG and tone recording the influence of paroxysmal spike and wave outbursts. From this we have observed that spike and wave discharges of different forms, even of very short duration, exert effects on the regulation of peripheral tone. The change in the micromotor curve occasionally occurs before the onset of the spike and wave discharges in the EEG and seems to display a fixed dependence on the type, localization and organization of the spike and wave (bilaterally synchronized 3–4 c/sec spikes and waves, poly-spikes and waves or more focal spike and wave complexes).

The method of micromotor tone recording, as further developed by Steinwachs in respect of apparatus and evaluation, using 43 criteria of measurement, with numerous statistical safeguards in the clinical domain, is considered by us, from the point of view of apparatus and low time consumption, as a suitable supplement to the synchronous recording of the diagnostic EEG.

11. Results of micromotor tone research in the clinical neurological field. — F. Steinwachs (Aachen).

After statistically valid measurement criteria of micromotor function (pen pressure tracings) in healthy persons had been set up, and at the same time the effects of constitution, illness, age and development had been symptomatically clarified, distal tonus diagnosis, in association with other clinical methods in the clinico-pathological sphere in organic cerebral, endocrine and vegetative changes, was demonstrated in many systematic experiments to be informationally rich for the establishment of a differential diagnosis. In statistically representative comparative investigations of healthy and known brain-damaged persons (Itani) as well as of schizophrenics (Herzmann) there were significant syndromes, which also showed relationships to the degree of severity of the disease.

Within 9 sec of the start of oxygen deprivation in a reduced pressure chamber, adynamic curve symptoms occurred, followed by increasingly marked pathological symptomatic changes, while immediately after addition of oxygen the original normal curve appeared again. Further, it could be shown in 245 applicant pilots that there were significant functional relationships between micromotor curve symptoms and the physiological results of reduced respiration of CO_2 (Seiffert).

Adynamic reactions after cerebral trauma, which, as decreased efficiency in daily and weekly work, were regarded as questionably psychogenic, were measurable by motor recording, using 120 test word curves with continual retardation of tempo and special adynamic curve-course symptomatology, as organically determined changes in motive structure and as motivatory, not compensatable, changes.

Cerebro-organically determined changes of distal tone regulation could also be demonstrated, as in representative serial investigations on criminals (Philippen) and in clinically static treated organic neuroses (Merx). By synchronous electronic multiple curve scanning (Scheffler and Hohlweck) in association with statistical symptom evaluation of digitalized values with a computer (Korten, Burmeister) a new phase of research into distal micromotor tone is introduced, which is equally significant for precise basic research, clinical diagnosis and neurophysiological complementary diagnosis, together with EEG and EMG (Weigeldt).

12. Electronic analysis of EEG and other curves.— H. Hohlweck (Aachen).

Nearly all branches of science, research and technical work is concerned with curves and diagrams whose analysis by hand and eye is very time-consuming and prone to subjective errors. The desire for speedy, automatic analysis led to the development of the fully automatic electronic curve and diagram analyser (VAK 68). With this apparatus the request of science is satisfied, namely, a maximal objectivization of information from existing graphical material. In one second, 200 or more measurements can be digitalized and produced, according to the capacity of the connected printer or puncher. The frequently very thin and not always homogeneous EEG, EKG etc. curves present no difficulty to the analyser. The underlying graph paper may have any desired colours. Also, set markings for desired outputs or stimulus conditions may be had. For simultaneously plotted biological data, for example EEG, EKG, EMG, respiration and skin resistance, correlations between the results are obtainable because the analyser also makes possible the synchronous analysis of several curves.

13. EEG and cerebral circulation. — E. Betz (Tübingen).

Activation of the EEG is often associated with circulatory increase of the entire brain. Adequate analyses of the relationship between EEG and circulation make necessary local recordings of both measures, from which it is shown that in normal waking persons good correlations are obtained between frequency spectra of the EEG and circulatory values from the same region. In local hypoxia, in sleep or in different CO_2 concentrations in the blood, however, circulatory level and EEG are not correlated. Measures of the energy-rich phosphate in the cortex, the cortical circulation, the cortical pO_2 and pCO_2, as well as the EEG showed that there is no causal connection between local circulation and EEG, if one considers the circulation as a regulating factor of the adjustment for an optimal energy state of the brain. There were no indications that a direct causal relationship exists between the mean EEG frequency and local cerebral vascular resistance.

By the breathing of a CO_2-containing gas mixture (50–70% CO_2) the EEG is caused to disappear completely for some time, with the circulation remaining normal or even raised and the energy-rich phosphate of the cerebral cortex high. The smooth muscle of the blood vessels and the cells which are responsible for the cessation of the EEG have their individual autonomies which are normally harmonized with each other. This agreement is, however, not found in all experimental situations.

14. Correlation between regional cerebral blood flow (rCBF) and EEG frequency spectrum. — I. A. Sulg and D. H. Ingvar (Lund, Sweden).

There exist in animals and man significant correlations between cerebral circulation and the spectral frequency distribution of the EEG. A reduction of the blood flow is in general associated with a slowing of the EEG and *vice versa*. This relationship can be clarified in the case of metabolic disturbance of the cerebral circulation. In a group of 116 patients with various neurological diseases the frequency spectra, obtained by frequency analysis, and the mean EEG frequency (frequency index) were correlated with the hemispheral circulation. An extensive correlation was shown. The association was closer for rCBF of grey than of white matter. The above-mentioned physiological association between the EEG and blood flow can be obliterated by cerebral anoxia. In the anoxically damaged brain cerebral hyperaemia develops as a result of the disturbed metabolism, together with slowing of the EEG. In this post-anoxic state the normal autoregulation of the cerebral vascular resistance is also reduced or abolished. Apparently there exists after the post-anoxic hyperaemia and oedema a tissue acidosis. This acidosis should be the prime cause of the so-called "luxury circulation".

After acute apoplexy it ought to be possible to find, in different cerebral regions and in consecutive post-ischaemic stages, the normal "auto-regulative" EEG/rCBF relationship, as well as a decoupling of these parameters. A group of 6 cases with thrombosis of the middle cerebral artery was specially studied in this respect. It was shown that beyond the lesion and in the subacute and chronic state the above EEG/blood flow correlation exists. In the acute stage, decoupling of the EEG/blood flow correlation is found in the neighbourhood of the lesion. In one case these relationships occurred in 5 consecutive investigations.

There is in general a close correlation between EEG and cerebral circulation. This physiological coupling can be abolished by cerebral anoxia. Therefore the possibilities of drawing reliable inferences from the EEG about the cerebral circulation are limited. A very slow EEG in brain injury means, although it can coexist with relatively higher blood flow, that a severe tissue disturbance is present, and thus the slow EEG signifies a reduction of the cerebral tissue metabolism.

15. On hyperventilation changes in the EEG and their relationships to blood gases, hydrogen-ion concentration and electrolytes. — M. Kohler, R. Ferlinz and H. Sieprath (Bonn).

Bioelectric brain activity and respiration are bound together in many ways. Characteristic EEG changes can be elicited by hyperventilation. The aim of our experiments was to study the influence of the EEG, in 26 subjects, of an acute respiratory alkalosis induced by maximal, voluntary, alveolar hyperventilation. Simultaneously the levels of pO_2, pCO_2, pH, standard bicarbonate, magnesium, phosphorus, potassium, sodium, haematocrit, dry weight of the erythrocytes and total protein were measured in the arterialized capillary blood of the hyperaemic ear lobe. The analysis of the EEG allows formulation of two groups; in one group of cases the characteristic frontal high voltage 3 c/sec delta waves were found, while the other group did not show this feature. The EEG changes were related to the haematochemical findings of respiratory alkalosis.

16. On the development of the EEG in the course of treatment of diffuse cerebral vascular and atrophic processes. — E. W. Funfgeld (Homburg/Saar).

The possibilities of treating patients with diffuse organic cerebral atrophic syndromes, which may manifest themselves in a picture of dynamic reduction, personality change and dementia of manifold and different expressions and symptomatology, have for some years been extended through methods which can influence cerebral metabolism other than by the psychotropic drugs used until now. We have directed our aim according to the clinical observation of systematic serial EEG studies. These extended to 240 patients, of whom 114 were treated with Pyrithioxin, 90 with Actihaemyl and 36 with the two combined. The following were the initial EEG findings: (1) moderate to severe generalized changes in 110 cases; (2) borderline findings in 87 cases and (3) tracings in the normal range in 43 cases.

In 63% of cases the initially altered EEG tracings showed, after 2 weeks to several months, faster frequencies compared with the first EEG. In the majority of *all* cases, and also in those that were initially within the normal range, signs of an improved synchronization (amplitude-activation) were found. In many cases there were regularities and localizing peculiarities, *e.g.* remarkable frontal, and sometimes also temporal, activation. These regularities (synchronization-steps in regard to frequency *and* amplitude) were especially clear under Pyrithioxin treatment. The influence of Pyrithioxin on the EEG was dose-dependent, and in some cases this was also true with respect to Actihaemyl.

17. Serial studies of cerebral vascular processes by means of interval analysis. — G. Prull (Giessen).

Diagnosis and therapy concerning the increasing importance of prolonged intensive care place new demands on clinical electroencephalography. From lengthy recordings and frequent EEG studies conclusions are expected which are possibly of value for therapy and prognosis. In this connection a technical aid to evaluation is introduced which leads, by the application of statistical methods, to values which are comparable inter- and intra-individually and can supplement in functional diagnosis the more localizing visual evaluation. A centro-occipital recording from each hemisphere is stored on tape over 10 min and analysed by interval analyser (Schwarzer) in 12 frequency bands. The resulting values are summated and, for each frequency band, placed in a transformed ordinate scale (probability network) and compared with a collection of healthy probands. This method is demonstrated with the changes (measured as standard deviations) of the frequency distribution of the individual frequency bands in the form of interval histograms; these are obtained in the serial study of cerebro-vascular processes in neurological intensive care. The method employed serves not for simplification but for quantification of the measures.

18. EEG changes in cerebral vascular occlusions. Differential diagnostic considerations.— M. Mortillaro (Homburg/Saar).

The most frequent EEG changes are described in more than 40 cases of angiographically verified carotid and middle cerebral occlusions. Grouped, intermittently occurring slow waves were particularly noted, whose morphology and distribution showed certain characteristics. From this, differential diagnostic considerations were set up, especially in contrast with acute space occupying processes. In this connection, besides these slow waves, the changes of background activity were also of great significance. By contrast to diffuse vascular processes, vascular occlusions showed, as expected, more localized changes, which were dependent on the collateral supply.

19. Influence of hyperbaric oxygenation on the recovery of the rabbit brain after cerebral ischaemia. — W. Bushart, P. Forner and P. Rittmeyer (Hamburg).

Inspection of 40 case histories of patients with cerebro-electrical silence after successful restoration of the circulation following temporary cardiac arrest showed that of these 40 patients 7 (17.5%) recovered completely. In 6 patients (15%) the electrical silence persisted and clinically no signs of cerebral activity returned. 27 resuscitated patients (67.5%), on the other hand, showed after a shorter or longer latent period returning cortical activity and parallel to it clinical recovery of the brain, followed by a renewed deterioration, this time to the final end. It was ascertained that in some cases peripheral disturbances (pulmonary oedema, heart failure) were the cause, in others cerebral oedema was found post mortem. In some cases the cause was never clarified. An important fact appeared to be that in all 27 investigated cases the brain obviously began to recover from electrical silence after, at the longest, 48 h.

It is worth clarifying the basis which makes this development possible and, if necessary independently of it, assisting the tendency to recovery of the brain. For this the use of hyperbaric oxygen is available. We produced cerebral ischaemia for a duration of 15–20 min in experiments on rabbits by means of the Opitz technique. After restoration of the cerebral circulation those animals recovered quickly and completely which, after release of the compressing cervical collar, breathed pure oxygen for 2–3 h in the pressure chamber at 3 atmospheres pressure. The control animals survived no longer than 14 h, while the animals from the experimental group recovered completely.

20. EEG flattening and spinal reflex excitability. — H. E. Reichenmiller and E. A. Zysno (Tübingen).

Electrically released monosynaptic reflexes (Hoffman) were studied in the stage of complete electrical silence and total areflexia in 2 patients with anoxic damage who later died. In one case, after one hour of electrical silence in the EEG, there were still well defined H reflexes in the triceps surae, with depression by multiple stimuli and with post-tetanic potentiation, while after 20 h only small potentials with F wave characteristics (Magladery) were elicitable. In other cases with over 24 h of isoelectric EEG, only F waves were demonstrated. Two further patients (intoxication by a hypnotic and cardiac infarction with transient respiratory and circulatory arrest) displayed, during a flattened EEG with intermittent discharges, small inconstant late potentials on supramaximal stimulation, which showed an increase in amplitude on repetitive stimulation.

The questions are discussed of the extent to which a true reflex spinal excitability exists and of whether it is a matter of antidromically released discharges from motoneurones.

21. The role of electroencephalography in resuscitation. — St. Kubicki (Berlin).

Between 1959 and 1968 1214 patients in the intensive care division had EEGs (3636 recordings). Excluded from the following were 787 cases of poisoning. In the other cases (mostly brain damage, anoxia and hypoxia due to a variety of causes) the EEGs obtained were classified according to their prognostic significance, as "moribund", "doubtful", "dangerous", "acceptable" and "favourable".

Moribund: isoelectric EEG and absence of cortical potentials with painful stimulation (100% mortality).

Doubtful (practically moribund but where cortical discharges were still found): (a) isoelectric sections of over 5 sec duration and short bursts; (b) unilateral isoelectric picture, nearly always with silent areas and contralateral bursts; (c) extremely flat EEG; (d) subdelta, less than 0.3 c/sec; (e) more or less steep and periodic discharges bilaterally, with at times isoelectric pauses of 0.3–0.5 sec; (f) sudden potential collapse with slower recovery.

Dangerous (still high mortality): (a) flat intervals of less than 5 sec duration; (b) unilateral periodic discharges; (c) delta and steep waves; (d) delta below 1.5 c/sec.

Acceptable: (a) delta sections acoustically provokable; (b) theta activity with delta groups; (c) accentuated fronto-temporal 6–15 c/sec.

Favourable: (a) basic alpha rhythm with scattered theta waves; (b) flat alpha; (c) slow alpha; (d) normal EEG.

As criteria for establishing cerebral death we require a totally isoelectric appearance as well as areflexia with advanced impairment of vegetative functions (breathing, circulation, temperature regulation, etc.). The recording must continue for at least 30 min and must be repeated after 3 and 6 h. Periodically amplifications up to 20 mm/50 μV should be chosen. The resistance between two electrodes should not exceed 10 kΩ and electrode separation should not be more than 8 cm. Artifacts should be eliminated by removing sources of electrical disturbance, control of EKG and by transient curarization. As additional tests we recommend electromyography and cortical evoked potentials. The effects of hypothermia and hypnotics must be carefully considered. The presence of death should only be declared after consultation. The author also holds the view that, with an isoelectric state for 12 h (after ruling out extreme hypothermia and hypnotics), all efforts will be futile, even with incomplete impairment of brain-stem signs, as irreversible cortical death has superseded.

22. Experimental investigations on newborn and young kittens, especially on animals with chronic epileptogenic foci in different locations. — K. Schmalbach (Hamburg).

Based on 160 kittens from 40 litters of own breeding, multilateral investigations were carried out with EEG, electrostimulation, strychnine stimulation, alumina foci and micro-recordings. A comparison of adults and juveniles shows a stimulation response which is more differentiated and extended in the young. Isolated afterdischarges may be seen at an early age; EEG seizures, however, occur later. Clinical convulsions follow only after some time. Various stimuli produce comparable results. The pattern of appearance of convulsions following alumina cream application in the young differs from the normal course in adult cats. There are two culmination points, one in the course of the fourth decade after the application and, with some individual cases of intermediate seizure outbreaks, another in the tenth decade. All these differences reflect the process of cerebral maturation in the kittens.

Combined micro- and macro-EEGs show the possibilities as well as the difficulties of coordinating these methods, which have two completely different dimensions.

23. Neurophysiological and biochemical investigations on cats with epileptic seizures. — K. Schmalbach and A. H. Kottler (Hamburg).

Cats received alumina foci by a standardized method and following this developed epileptic seizures. Their brain tissue was freshly taken out, divided and examined chemically. Subsequent tests were carried out on the aluminium content of focal and other regions of the brains. Special attention was given to the electrophysiologically established regions of mirror foci. In addition, the tissues were examined for possible changes in the sodium and potassium content. The following findings were made: (1) the aluminium was only partly preserved in the focal areas. No traces of the metal were found contralaterally; (2) there was a clear rise of the sodium content in the focal region. The potassium content was lowered strongly in the same area. Possible consequences of these findings are discussed briefly.

24. A twilight state or focal sensory attack? — H. Helmchen, I. Hoffmann and S. Kanowski (Berlin).

We describe a 25-year-old woman who, after infantile brain damage with persisting slight right-sided signs and severe retardation of development, has had since the second year of life ballisto-tonic unilateral attacks on the right side and, since the tenth year of life, major attacks beginning focally and becoming generalized. The patient came to be admitted on account of previously unrecognized transient states of very striking behaviour. In these she was absorbed in herself, fully given up to the experience of visual illusory perceptions which she followed with her eyes and enumerated. She was not distracted by them. This picture seemed closest to a twilight state, especially if it occurred directly in connection with a severe convulsive attack. Precise observation, however, showed that the hallucinatory experience lasted at times for only seconds or minutes. In the intervals between these very frequent and rapidly recurring states, which started and ended abruptly, the patient recognized objectively and critically the illusory character of her paroxysmal experiences.

Five EEG recordings during the 8-week hospital admission showed a constant delta and theta focus with a maximum in the right occipital and right posterior temporal areas. Only once, during the above described state, did there occur up to 35 sec of a persistent episode of regular, large spikes in the same focal region. Synchronously with this series of focal spikes the patient experienced visual illusory perceptions during the EEG recording. The view is expressed, in relation to the literature, that we are dealing with a state of focal sensory attacks, diagnostically separated from a post-paroxysmal twilight state.

25. The significance of extremely fast beta waves (> 30 c/sec) in conventional surface EEG in man. — K. A. Flugel (Erlangen).

Extremely high frequency beta waves of 30 c/sec and more were found in 1.15% of cases in a collection of 10,000 EEG tracings (predominantly neuropsychiatric investigations). 90% of the repeatedly investigated persons showed this pattern in several recordings. Constancy of the waves was observed over a maximal period of 10 years. Relationships between this feature of the EEG and clinical data were not established; there was, however, a relatively high proportion of psycho-vegetative disturbances in comparison with a control group without beta waves. These findings were compared with the various attempts at classification of beta activity and with the investigations of other authors on extremely fast beta waves.

26. Syndromes of hypochondriasis and the EEG. — G. Paal (Münster).

Using the EEG of 89 hypochondriac patients we posed the question whether any light could be thrown on the underlying disease in these syndromes. Clinically 3 groups were distinguished: 45 patients without organic pathology; 19 patients with cerebral atrophy; 21 with evidence of cerebro-vascular insufficiency. In 59 cases the EEG was considered pathological. The most evident changes were found in the first group (39 out of 49). The observed deviations were always non-specific. In the forefront was an irregular low voltage background rhythm, a frequency lability or increased intermediate waves. Differences between the two sides or focal changes were never seen. Definite differences between the individual groups were not found.

In 25 cases the EEG could be compared with pneumoencephalographic and CSF findings. Such cases were mainly concerned with demonstrable cerebral atrophic processes. These EEGs showed no higher incidence of pathological changes as compared with the other patients. Widespread EEG changes were more consistently associated with CSF changes. As, according to Habeck, a pathological CSF generally antedates lesions shown by pneumoencephalography, the high incidence of pathological EEG findings in patients without (yet) demonstrable cerebro-organic findings could be of greater significance than the pneumoencephalogram in early cerebral atrophic processes or vascular insufficiency. Such EEG changes should at least be an indication for regular control of such patients.

27. Supplementary investigations on the question of the influence of hypothyroidism on the central nervous system. — K. Schmalbach, O. Encinoza and Y. Alajmo (Hamburg).

Following a series of investigations on motor behaviour and the action potentials of peripheral nerves in the hypothyroid rat certain peculiar findings led us to re-examine our experimental data. As a regular assessment of body temperature of the experimental animals had been carried out by measuring both rectal and muscular temperatures, and as there was a clear lowering of these temperatures by 7°C on average, a new series was prepared for (a) the control of these findings and (b) for the examination of the influence of low temperatures on the recruiting potentials recorded after electrical stimulation of n. medio-dorsalis thalami. In hypothyroid rats temperatures of 29 and 27°C could frequently be recorded under Nembutal narcosis, whereas in normals it only led to a lowering to 35°C. Temperatures of 29 and 27°C led to similar findings for recruiting potentials as for action potentials. For this reason we consider the phenomena described by Bradley and others for recruiting potentials, and by us for the action potentials of the hypothyroid rat, as parts of one process, *i.e.* the influence of hypothyroidism, not directly on the cortex but merely indirectly, possibly via the intermediary of hypothalamic regulation.

28. The "tracé alternant" of the sleeping EEG in full-term, premature and hypotrophic neonates. — R. Nolte, F. J. Schulte, U. Weisse and R. Gruson (Göttingen).

The "tracé alternant" or episodic sleep activity, is a characteristic electroencephalographic activity during restful sleep in neonates. Its presence can be shown at 32–34 weeks and at 37–38 weeks it is fully developed; it disappears gradually and almost simultaneously with the appearance of the first "sleep spindles" at the age of 44–46 weeks. This phenomenon was examined quantitatively by measuring the intervals of sleep groups. Several polygraphic sleep records of 24 neonates formed the basis of this analysis. The evaluation comprised descriptive and statistical comparison of frequency distribution and occurrence of intervals in 3 groups of children: (1) full-term neonates of normal weight (38–42 weeks); (2) prematures of 34–37 weeks; (3) full-term, underweight neonates in the same age group as (1) and the same weight group as (2). The findings are discussed with reference to normal and abnormal cortical maturation.

29. Polygraphic recording in children with phenylketonuria. — H. P. Gross and F. J. Schulte (Göttingen).

Polygraphic recordings of 1.5–2.5 h duration, showing EEG, respiration, eye movements and muscle activity during sleep, were made in children with phenylketonuria. In comparison with normal children of equal age groups an increase of spindle activity during restful sleep (non-REM), and to some extent even during active sleep (REM), was found. In some cases there was nearly continuous beta activity at the frequency of spindles, so that a clear separation was not always possible.

30. Electroencephalographic manifestations of cerebral attacks and intellectual development in phenylketonuria. — A. Lutcke and H. Bickel (Marburg/Lahn).

From 1955 to 1968 we had the opportunity to examine neurologically, psychiatrically and with EEG 81 children suffering from phenylketonuria. Single examinations were made on 11 children. Regular examinations continued for 1 year in 17 children, for 2 years in 15 children, for 3 years in 11, for 4 years in 10, for 6 years in 11 and for 11 years in 2 children. In all these examinations more than 460 EEGs and more than 400 psychometric tests were undertaken. This material was analysed with reference to the age at examination at the commencement of treatment of the children and to the contents of their diet. Clear correlations were shown between intellectual development, certain EEG appearances and the clinical manifestations of attacks on the one hand, and the age at which a consistent alanine-free diet was started on the other.

31. Investigations on the genetics of photosensitivity. — H. Doose, H. Gerken, E. Volzke and Ch. Volz (Kiel).

144 siblings of patients with generalized irregular spikes and waves during photic stimulation and 268 children with clinically normal brains were examined electroencephalographically under standardized conditions. The tracings examined blind gave the following results: (1) photosensitivity with the appearance of spikes and waves during intermittent photic stimulation showed a definite age relationship, being found mainly in children between the ages of 5 and 15 years; (2) the normal siblings showed photosensitivity considerably more frequently than the control group (average 28% compared with 7%); (3) photosensitivity is considered as a symptom of a genetic susceptibility to centrencephalic epilepsy; the mode of inheritance is still uncertain; (4) the clinical picture of epilepsy in children with photosensitivity is varied. The attacks and clinical behaviour distinguish well recognized forms; so-called photogenic epilepsy merely represents a special and rare variety.

32. Hypsarrhythmia, spike and wave variants and petit mal status in childhood. — R. Kruse (Heidelberg).

Typical hypsarrhythmia—generalized, multifocal and asynchronous diffuse epileptic potentials—occurring mainly in infancy, shows with aging a tendency towards increased synchronization, a paroxysmal behaviour and predominance of tracings described as "slow spikes and waves" and "sharp and slow wave complexes", constituting the EEG entity "spike and wave variant" (syn: petit mal variant). A practically continuous spike and wave variant associated with clouding of consciousness is called petit mal status. Such a petit mal status may have a benign course ("benign petit mal status"; "spike and wave stupor") or be associated with epileptic symptoms such as absences, myoclonic and drop attacks ("myoclonic-astatic petit mal status"). This form of petit mal status, with the EEG pattern of spike and wave variant, is mainly found in childhood, much more commonly than the classical petit mal absence status, with 3 c/sec spikes and waves in the EEG, or the pure myoclonic petit mal status with a poly-spike and wave pattern. As the spike and wave variant pattern during a petit mal status more often shows a transition to hypsarrhythmia, we venture the hypothesis that hypsarrhythmia may also be a cause of (benign) clouding of consciousness in infancy and thus a petit mal status. This question requires careful clinical research.

33. Electrocerebral findings in closed head injuries in childhood. — H. W. Steinmann (Cologne).

166 children, aged 8 to 14 years, were examined electrocerebrally in the acute, and in some cases later, post-traumatic periods. Primary loss of consciousness was present in 136 patients. In the subacute phase 25 children had epileptic attacks. Skull fractures were found in 73 cases. Typical sequences were analysed in sample tracings. In particular, the local and unilateral depressions of the subacute phase are discussed in relation to their differential diagnostic significance.

34. The regulation of the heart rate during sleep. — W. Baust, B. Bohnert and O. Riemann (Düsseldorf).

Experiments were carried out on cats with chronically implanted electrodes. For the differentiation of individual sleep and waking periods simultaneous recording of EEG, EMG and eye movements was used. The heart rate was measured by an electrical counter coupled to the EKG. In contrast to intact cats, cats with bilateral vagotomy showed an increase in heart rate in all sleep and waking stages, though the range of frequency was more restricted. The fall in heart rate in the REM stage remained unchanged. The rise in heart rate seen in intact cats during the waking reaction disappeared in cats with bilateral vagotomy. The phasic heart rate changes coinciding with the bursts of rapid eye movements were quantitatively decreased after vagotomy and this was particularly the case for the initial rise in heart rate. In cats with denervation of the heart by bilateral vagotomy and stellate extirpation, practically no change in heart rate related to sleep-waking periods remained. From the findings the deductions are made that the tonic changes associated with the different sleep and waking stages are predominantly sympathetic, while the phasic changes are in the first case under parasympathetic control.

35. Differential diagnostic applicability of the EEG in comatose patients. — E. A. Zysno and H. E. Reichenmiller (Tübingen).

In the sphere of intensive care and resuscitation the EEG plays a considerable role regarding essential diagnostic and therapeutic measures. This is indicated during prolonged EEG examinations of comatose patients with diverse aetiology. The pathology is divided into three large groups: coma after head injury; coma due to intoxication (particularly after attempted suicide), and coma due to metabolic causes, *e.g.*, hepatic, uraemic, diabetic, thyrotoxic and major electrolyte disturbance. The differential diagnostic evaluation of the EEG in these diseases, in conjunction with clinical data, can clarify certain coma types and depth of coma, with facilitation of prognostic judgement.

36. The periodicity of erection during sleep in healthy men. — U. J. Jovanovic (Würzburg).

This contribution is concerned with the problem of erections in men under known and unknown situations during the whole of natural sleep. The erections were recorded by phallograph (PLG), examined statistically and correlated with the usual signs of paradoxical sleep. The findings showed that in healthy men (aged 20–42 years; 20 healthy subjects) erections occurred 3–6 times during a 7–8 h sleep (average 5.1 times) and lasted from 8–40 min (average 15–30). More than 70% of the erection duration was correlated with the phase of paradoxical sleep. In a few cases erections were registered without signs of the dream phase. The erections of 20 patients with a variety of symptomatologies were examined and the results compared with those of healthy subjects. Slight to marked deviations from the normal were found and these are discussed. Amongst others, the relation of erections to mental, motor and vegetative processes during sleep is examined.

37. The behaviour of the alpha rhythm under defined motor and pharmacological conditions. — H. Scheich (Munich).

The basis of the present work is the analysis of EEG samples by automatic, so-called aperiodic, interval analysis, with subsequent digitalization of the intervals. During rest the alpha rhythm was analysed according to average frequency, standard deviation of the frequency and number of waves per time unit; the correlation of these parameters was used in an attempt to establish situation characteristics. An increase or decrease of alpha waves with motor activity or administration of drugs resulted in changed parameter characteristics which will be explained by the use of the example of a technical channel.

38. Considerations on the relationship between alpha rhythm and so-called expectancy waves. — U. Heinemann and H. Scheich (Munich).

The experiments were concerned with the recording of basic rhythm and expectancy waves before a conditioned and an unconditioned hand movement. Subsequent treatment was by methods of frequency analysis, averaging and correlative pattern recognition. The subjects pressed against a lever with a controlled resistance. By means of the recorded myogram or the lever pressure the subject set up either a continuous optical or auditory signal which varied in pitch, intensity, timbre or duration, or according to the experimental situation. As a control the analysis included lever pressure without subsequent stimulation. Further tests were carried out as described by Grey Walter.

The trigger pulses caused by the myogram and the EEG were recorded on a tape recorder and analysed further, after analogue–digital conversion, on an IBM 1130 computer. At least 50 one-second sections before and after the trigger were analysed by means of a program developed by us, from the following points of view: (1)

mean and distribution of 50 trigger sections were calculated; (2) with cross- and partial auto-correlation the phase constancy and basic frequencies between both hemispheres were tested; (3) correlation with a sine wave in the region of the alpha rhythm made it possible to determine the phase relationship of the alpha rhythm to the trigger, before and after the myogram trigger; (4) correlation with a specimen of the averaged expectancy wave before each trigger allowed clarification of the distribution of the time relationship between the expectancy waves and movements. The findings are discussed.

39. EEG changes under different conditions. — O. Simonova and H. Legewie (Munich).

In the previous projects EEG changes under different conditions, but with open eyes, were examined. In contrast, the present examination compares the effects of comparable tasks on the alpha rhythm with the eyes open and closed. Eight healthy subjects had EEG tracings recorded by telemetry under conditions of rest and 5 different states of activity. Automatic analysis of the left temporo-occipital EEG activity showed the following findings: (1) with the eyes open, in contrast to closed eyes, signs of increased desynchronization were found, without exception; (2) the changes during mental activity showed a greater than chance tendency to reach a mid level between extreme synchronization and extreme desynchronization. With the eyes closed this mid level was arrived at by an increase in desynchronization; with open eyes by synchronization; (3) the increase in synchronization with open eyes would appear to be mainly independent of whether visual components were immediately involved.

40. EEG frequency analysis in the examination of groups. A study of the EEG of old people. — K. Suwelack and F. Abbink (Münster).

Problems which arise in EEG frequency analysis have been discussed for many years. Starting from the standpoint that methods of frequency analysis have something to say about the genesis of the EEG and can help pragmatically in a fuller interpretation of the clinical EEG, it will appear that it may be useful in clinical practice and in several statistical correlation questions. Critics mainly attack the inaccuracy of much frequency analysis as it either ignores amplitude or is unable to identify interference potentials. Such objections can be countered by the argument that such mistakes are constant under standard conditions and for purposes of comparison are of no consequence. The advantage of our method of frequency analysis, adapted from that developed by Dr. van Gogh, is that the histograph appears well defined and that EEG background activity thus analysed can easily be compared.

This is even more the case when the background activity is very irregular and covers broad spectra of varying frequency, widely dispersed. The histographic picture of the background activity thus obtained is useful, *e.g.*, to show discrete contralateral differences often not evident to the trained eye. Also, a tendency to frequency increase or decrease during prolonged recordings, which may have prognostic significance, may be found. EEG similarities in the examination of groups are also readily demonstrated with this useful procedure. In the context of a larger geriatric research project this was applied to a group of very old people. Noteworthy agreement was found between the frequency analysis curve, the usual EEG conclusion and other clinical data, particularly cardio-vascular. Using histographic curves groups were established which showed similarities reflected in the usual EEG findings as well as in the cardio-vascular symptoms.

41. Frequency analysis of the flat EEG. — A. E. Adams (Freiburg/Br.).

The expression "flat EEG" is used to describe tracings with irregular, low voltage mixed frequencies (7–35 c/sec, under 20 μV). The usual visual assessment of such EEG tracings is inadequate. Therefore such tracings obtained during rest, mental activity, sleep and narcosis and in cerebral diseases were subjected to automatic frequency analysis. The flat EEG appears with physical maturation and then remains as an unchanging EEG feature, characteristic for that individual, in about 10% of healthy waking adults. Flat EEGs are rare in healthy children or adolescents. This EEG type is, however, not so uncharacteristic as suggested by the absent background frequency. With automatic analysis the minimum frequency is shown to be in the region 6–9 c/sec and, after visual stimulation, shows a transient, limited reactivity with response frequency from 3.5 to 6 c/sec, persisting about 4–5 sec following the stimulus. It would appear as if the flat EEG represents the outward sign of a stable electrocortical reactivity—and irritability—barrier.

The originally flat EEG can be changed to a tracing with normal potentials during sleep from stage C, anaesthesia and generalized disease processes. It will then be virtually indistinguishable from an alpha EEG originally of normal amplitude, changed by the same processes. This leads to doubts about hypotheses of a consistent relationship between EEG macro-potentials and cerebro-physiological component mechanisms. Focal changes in the flat EEG are increasingly considered ("amplitude too small, thus focus not clearly demonstrable") as a good localizing activation, with slowing of the frequency and larger amplitude. These can be provoked by sleep or brief anaesthesia. The flat EEG is not merely a negative variation resulting in difficult EEG diagnosis because of the small amplitude. It is more a special form of the normal EEG which behaves somewhat differently from the usual alpha EEG under physiological and disease processes.

42. Comparison of the Fourier and aperiodic interval analysis of EEG tracings. — O. Creutzfeldt, W. Probst and H. Schmitz (Munich).

The EEG was recorded in healthy persons under a variety of psychological and motor conditions. With the aid of aperiodic interval analysis (Schwarzer system) the EEG was analysed automatically with subsequent digital data-processing and independently with the use of Fourier analysis. The findings of the two methods were then compared. In the main the two methods gave similar results but the aperiodic analysis allowed a better estimate of the number of waves of a certain frequency. The advantage of Fourier analysis lies in the better over-all representation of the curve, while the aperiodic analysis is partly dependent on amplitude. The disadvantage of the Fourier analysis is the time required. The possibility of digital interval analysis is discussed.

43. Automatic recognition of pattern groups in the EEG. — W. H. Probst (Munich).

The programable digital computers available in medical science today, with the possibility of recording analogue data on several channels simultaneously, make it possible to analyse the EEG not only as regards frequency (Fourier analysis, power spectrum) and intervals (interval histograms) but also for special patterns (*e.g.* spindles, spike and wave, etc.). The technique described here, similar to the estimation of the cross-correlation function, handles selected patterns and shifts stepwise along the EEG curve to be examined. For each shift step we measure the two quantities

$$r(\tau) = \frac{\frac{1}{n}\sum_{i=1}^{n}(x_i - \bar{x})(y_{i+\tau} - y_\tau)}{Sx \cdot Sy\tau}$$

and

$$r(\tau) \cdot Sy\tau$$

We then have measures of the similarity with the comparison pattern and of the amplitude of the desired patterns. Some illustrative samples are shown and the data possibly of interest for research in automatic EEG diagnosis are discussed.

44. Visual evoked potentials in epilepsy. — C. H. Lucking (Munich).

Visual evoked potentials were obtained in various brain regions in a large sample of patients with cerebral epilepsy of a variety of forms and aetiologies. Besides regular and irregular slow flashes more rapid flash frequencies were used, corresponding to the range more liable to involve the driving phenomenon and patterns of discharges. The properties of the visual evoked potentials, including their dependence on the site of recording and the rate of stimulation, were compared in the different types of epilepsy as well as with a group of healthy individuals. No deviation from the norm was found in epileptics though in healthy as well as epileptic subjects a dependence was found in relation to the background activity. The findings are discussed in connection with the present contradictory evidence found in the literature.

45. Digital amplitude interval analysis. A new method of quantitative analysis of the EEG. — D. Bente and U. Ferner (Erlangen).

In contrast to the customary methods of interval analysis this digital method results in the determination of amplitudes and intervals on a reference level which is drawn through the mean value of the time function representing the electrical activity and therefore results from its total characteristic. The following steps are undertaken: analogue to digital conversion (IBM System 1800) and storage of the EEG, determination of the instantaneous values and calculation of their mean values, determination of the signal zero crossings ("intervals") and extremes ("amplitudes"), and reproduction of the distribution of the instantaneous values, intervals and amplitudes in the form of histograms. By a further step one may calculate continuously the arithmetic and quadratic means over equidistant sections of the investigated random sample function and thus obtain data which allow inferential statistical explanations of the structure of the underlying stochastic processes, and make it possible to check the hypotheses which are decisive for the statement capacity of the auto-covariance analytical methods (auto-correlogram, power spectrum). Examples of the application are demonstrated and the inferences arising from these are discussed.

46. EEG analysis using the signal comparator procedure. — O. Vatter, R. Rischmaui and J. Muller (Göttingen).

With the signal comparator we can determine: (1) intervals between points of intersection of the EEG with any voltage level; (2) EEG voltage changes during any chosen time lapse (*e.g.* 5–500 msec). In the first procedure the time base must be long enough to cope with the measurements of slow EEG waves; in the guinea pig this should be at least 0.5–1 sec. A line of intersection varying in voltage from sweep to sweep has, in contrast to a fixed intersection line, the advantage of picking up the smaller from the overlying background activity consisting of waves of higher frequency. We measure the distance between the first and third points of intersection and thus the entire wave length. Advantageous is automatic addition by the use of an electronic counter and the summation of hundred sweeps. The second procedure is particularly useful for showing the participation of stated frequencies in the EEG; to determine the participation of very slow waves interval histography can be used. With special electro-mechanical counting of time intervals as well as voltage changes occurring in freely chosen low, middle and high zones, further information is obtained. As the peak latencies of evoked potentials during only moderate changes of stimulation intensity vary only slightly, the second procedure can also be applied to measure amplitude. In contrast to the averaging procedure this has the advantage that with small responses the relation of the response amplitude to the stimulus-independent spontaneous EEG voltage can easily be determined. In addition, the average size of the deflections lying in the direction of the expected response peaks (a) is determined and from this the average size of deflections in the opposite direction (b) are deducted. The response amplitude then consists of (a — b)/(a + b) c/sec of the average EEG voltage.

47. The possibilities of telemetry of physiological data. — A. Kofes (Berlin).

For the telemetry of physiological data two methods are generally considered, cable-telemetry and radio-telemetry. In both cases practically the same apparatus is used. The two methods only differ as regards the conduction medium. In the one the signal passes along a cable (telephone) and in the other by radio. In both cases the possibility exists of carrying several channels simultaneously (2, 4 or 8). The separate channels are mixed in transmission, through a cable or from a v.h.f. transmitter, to a receiver, there to be separated again and recorded on appropriate apparatus. The problems such as frequency bands, interference, range, etc. which arise with this method are further discussed.

48. EEG and reanimation. — H. Hirsch (Cologne).

According to animal experiments, reanimation time of the entire organism after complete asphyxia at normal temperature is 3.5–5 min. The cause of this short reanimation time is asphyxial damage to the heart. The aim of all reanimation measures must be to limit this cardiac damage and if possible to attain rapidly the hypercritical increase in blood pressure necessary for recovery. The reanimation time of the entire function of the brain is 8–10 min after complete ischaemia at normal temperature. The tolerance time of the heart is 15–20 min; the metabolism of the heart is maximally decreased by cardiac arrest for the duration of the O_2 deficiency. The time for complete revival of the electrocorticogram after complete cerebral ischaemia is 8–10 min at normal temperature. An incomplete, *i.e.* temporally limited, recovery of the electrocorticogram is attained at up to about 15 min after complete cerebral ischaemia. The time for recovery of respiration after complete cerebral ischaemia is at normal temperature more than 20 min. Reanimation of the organism will then be only incomplete or limited in time. In complete cerebral ischaemia the electrocorticogram can be transiently inactive for up to 3–4 h. In incomplete cerebral ischaemia there have until now been no quantitative data on the recovery time and the maximal duration of a temporarily isopotential electrocorticogram. No conclusion about possible recovery of the entire function of the brain can be drawn from cortical steady potentials. Recovery time is shortened by hyperthermia and lengthened by hypothermia.

Electroenceph. clin. Neurophysiol., **1969**, *27*: 617–629

RUMANIAN GROUP OF ELECTROENCEPHALOGRAPHY AND CLINICAL NEUROPHYSIOLOGY

9th Annual Meeting

Bucharest, December 6–7, 1968

Secretary: DR. V. NEȘTIANU

Str. Progresului 8, Bucharest (Rumania)

1. EEG investigations in aircraft crews. — V. Filcescu and C. Cristescu (Bucharest).

The present report discusses the results obtained following more than 3500 polygraphic recordings (EEG, ECG, EDG, REG) in aircraft crews during the last 5 years. Study by polygraphic recording of a chiefly healthy population raised interest in questions concerning the classical criteria of appraisal of normal EEG tracings.

The significance of the EEG temporal tracing, fairly frequent among the authors' cases (4%), was discussed in terms of its organic origin. A neurotic state has an activating effect the same as overbreathing, lack of sleep, hypoxia, etc., reflecting a latent, sequelar disturbance.

Apart from the standard recordings systematic studies were carried out under conditions of specific aeronautic stress: hypoxia, hypocapnia, respiration of pure oxygen under high pressure and lack of sleep. The polygraphic method facilitated differentiation of the paroxysmal manifestations of syncopal and epileptic types. Longitudinal polygraphic recordings confirmed once again the incompatibility of subjects with a spasmophilic background and the stress of flying in supersonic aircraft, and showed the utility of this method in the dynamic follow-up of craniocerebral injuries.

2. EEG contributions to problems in industrial medicine. — I. M. Lupu, C. Ittu and E. Ittu (Sibiu).

The present paper reports on electro-clinical correlations in 50 cases of disease, in various fields of activity, which required individual and collective medico-social measures of protection. Epilepsy was found in a high proportion of the cases (76%). Close agreement was noted between the clinical and EEG examinations in 84% of the cases. However, the priority of the former is accepted since a diagnosis cannot be exclusively based on the EEG. For the sake of safety, it is considered that even those who simulate a disease should be removed from dangerous places or highly responsible situations, if for no other reason than that of the psychological alteration of their personalities.

Electroenceph. clin. Neurophysiol., **1969**, *27*: 629–639

3. Critical view on the possibility of using the rheoencephalogram in medico-aeronautical expertise. — I. Pintilie, C. Cristescu and V. Filcescu (Bucharest).

In spite of difficulties of a technical order, the rheoencephalogram can be used as an auxiliary method of investigation in medico-aeronautical expertise, especially for a good appraisal of the functional state of the brain in stress tests (hypoxia tests in a low pressure chamber or breathing oxygen under pressure). The rheoencephalogram makes it possible to assess the compensatory mechanisms and reflects the effects of different cardiovascular diseases upon the cerebral circulation. It was also used as a means of controlling the correct adjustment of the high altitude compensation equipment. Among the criteria of interpretation of the rheoencephalogram, the relative pulse-volume/1000, the celerity index and calculation of the rheoencephalographic wave surface appear to be more significant than pulse velocity or rise time.

4. Certain electroencephalographic aspects in accidental poisoning with Ecatox in children. — G. Puskás, C. Rusnac and C. Rusnac (Tîrgu-Mureş).

The present work refers to a total of 19 children (15 boys and 4 girls) aged 6 months to 15 years, admitted during 1963–1968 to the Clinic of Pediatrics, Tîrgu-Mureş, with a diagnosis of accidental poisoning with Ecatox, involving a number of severe clinical aspects, such as coma, convulsions, pulmonary oedema, etc. In the interpretation of the EEG account was taken of the clinical picture of the disease and the age of the children. The main EEG findings were the following: normal records in 5 children; modified background rhythm in 14 children, either slow arrhythmia (in 7) or severe diffuse disorganization (in 7); focal abnormalities in 9 children (in 6 of a lesional type and in 3 of an irritative type); diffuse alterations in 5 children (lesional in 3 and irritative in 2) and slight inter-hemispheric asymmetry in 3 children. The EEG alterations appeared to be polymorphic, almost constant and quite uncharacteristic of poisoning with Ecatox. They failed to show any significant correlation with the clinical phenomena, their gravity or the children's ages. The EEG revealed the existence of cerebral disease (as a consequence of hypoxic encephalopathy) even in children without evident clinical nervous symptoms. The evolving EEG aspects differed: in 9 children there was a certain improvement, in 5 children the alterations persisted, leading to electrical sequelae in spite of the apparent clinical recovery of all the children. The possibility of EEG sequelae and their detection prior to their clinical manifestation underlines the prognostic value of EEG and the severity of accidental intoxications in children and points to the necessity of treatment continued in out-patient units in order to prevent possible clinical sequelae.

5. Electroencephalographic investigations of workers in a chemical coke plant. — F. Schneider and C. Ursoniu (Timişoara).

EEG investigations carried out in a coke plant by means of a 4-channel portable "Galileo" electroencephalograph, included 71 workers aged on average 30 $\pm$ 1 years and having a length of service of 4.6 $\pm$ 0.4 years at the same working site.

The gross appearance of the records, processed statistically, revealed a predominant alpha rhythm, with a prevailing frequency of 10.4 $\pm$ 0.1 c/sec, a mean amplitude of 29.4 $\pm$ 1.4 μV in posterior and of 11.2 $\pm$ 0.2 μV in anterior derivations, with an alpha index of 83 $\pm$ 3% and an incidence of theta waves of 6.4 $\pm$ 1.3%. The reactivity to overbreathing was low, the increase of theta waves alone being noteworthy (10.7 $\pm$ 2.2%). Analysis of the individual tracings permitted grouping of the cases into six lots: (1) without pathological elements in 13 cases (18.3%); (2) dysrhythmic tracing in 5 cases (7%); (3) irritative tracing in 4 cases (5.6%); (4) dysrhythmic and irritative in 36 cases (50.8%); (5) tracing indicating diffuse cerebral disturbance in 11 cases (15.5%); (6) tracing with waves reflecting injuries in 2 cases (2.8%).

Investigation of the environment revealed the presence of benzene, toluene and sometimes of carbon sulphide in the air, their concentrations varying over a fairly wide range, which may be accounted for by the character of the working conditions at different stages of the working process, periodically attaining a value as high as 1.5, up to 10 times the maximum concentration permitted for benzene. This might be one of the reasons for the disturbances mentioned and justifies the necessity of periodical EEG examination of men employed in an environment containing benzene and its homologues.

6. The electroencephalogram in medico-legal assessment. — M. Terbancea, G. Călcăianu, I. Quai and V. Dragomirescu (Bucharest).

The value of EEG examination in medico-legal assessments is discussed with reference to 223 cases, of which 112 were adult and 111 juvenile delinquents. In adults, the patients were grouped according to the diagnosis and the clinical manifestations: psychopaths (33.92%), craniocerebral injuries with neuropsychical manifestations, as well as recent cranial injuries with medico-legal implications (25.89%), epilepsy with paroxysmal and interparoxysmal psychical disorders (12.15%) and malingerers (28.04%).

In juvenile delinquents the EEG examinations were performed in order to define the morbid influences determining the behavioural disturbances and the tendency toward delinquency. Normal tracings were noted in only 18% of the total number of cases, whereas in the others electrographic alterations with a pathological significance were found, such as EEG aspects below the chronological age, denoting neuropsychical retardation, functional rhythms characterizing the state of neuronal hyperexcitability and discharges of epileptic type with clinical manifestations, not diagnosed previously. The great majority of the delinquents were in the 14–15 year age group and their numbers decreased toward the age of 18.

Serial EEG examinations and the use of drug activation permitted delimitation of the pathological events which may, within the clinical context, account for the tendency to infraction.

7. Clinico-electroencephalographic correlations in psychiatric expertise of juvenile delinquents — E. Stanciu and K. Szücs (Tîrgu-Mureş).

In psychiatric forensic expertise it often appears very difficult to integrate from a medical standpoint the infractions committed by youngsters, particularly when the conclusions are drawn solely from the data contained in the files, or from a simple medical and psychiatric examination. In this connection reference is made to 48 delinquents between the ages of 8 and 18 years, most of them in the pubertal or pre-pubertal age and adolescence. The psychopathology of these cases was characterized by polymorphism, which could however be classified along general lines within the vast field of disorders affecting the individual's character and behaviour. From the standpoint of nosological integration particular attention is paid to the contribution of the EEG. In terms of the role played by the latter in establishing the diagnosis, the cases were divided into three groups. The first included the cases in which elucidation of the correct diagnosis was primarily due to the medico-psychiatric examination, the EEG examination playing only a complementary role. This group included a total of 15 youths of whom 9 proved to be psychopathic or cases with an unharmoniously developed character and 6 cases of mental debility. The second group comprised the cases in which the EEG examination played an essential role in establishing the diagnosis. It included 2 cases of schizophrenia in the initial phases, 4 cases of temporal epilepsy, and 2 cases of epileptoid episodic psychosis of poriomanic type, a group in which the EEGs were considered as characteristic and very significant. The third group included a certain number of behavioural disorders that had developed against a pubertal background, psychopathic with a limited intellect and hypomanic condition, in which the EEG recordings appeared to be normal or insignificant. The conclusions point to the necessity of close cooperation between the specialists carrying out the forensic-psychiatric examinations and EEG specialists. The results of these examinations may also shed new light and reveal interesting aspects in the various psychical diseases.

8. Penicillin epilepsy in man. — C. Arseni and I. Tudor (Bucharest).

Three clinical cases of convulsive manifestations induced by penicillin are reported. The first consists in the appearance of generalized status epilepticus with Jacksonian onset after mild surgery on the neurocranium, with application of penicillin to the wound. After the remission of status epilepticus, the patient still had rare Jacksonian seizures. The second case was that of a generalized status epilepticus in a patient with uraemia, on massive penicillin treatment. In this case, interruption of the penicillin suppressed the status epilepticus. The last case was a patient with generalized convulsions resulting in death after the intraspinal injection of penicillin. Penicillin epilepsy in man is discussed in the light of the authors' experience and the data in the literature.

9. A 7-year-old boy with akinetic mutism after cerebral contusion. — F. Bogdan and I. Bozsodi (Oradea).

Cerebral contusion caused by a traffic accident was manifested in a 7-year-old boy by a syndrome of akinetic mutism. During the first 10 days he sat in his bed with wide open eyes, but without spontaneous movements or attention. He did not answer any question. After 10 days he progressively improved; 30 days after the accident his behaviour became normal in all respects.

The EEG was recorded 6 times. During the first 10 days the basic activity was represented by delta (3 c/sec) and theta waves (4–6 c/sec), 50–100 μV, without any difference between the hemispheres but frequently interrupted by paroxysmal activity (predominantly bilateral or generalized sharp waves). Basic activity was without paroxysms in only 15% of the recording time. Paroxysmal activity gradually disappeared.

The great vulnerability of the hippocampus to traumatic cerebral lesions and the very low threshold which permits stimulation of the hippocampus up to paroxysmal electrical discharge are well known. Pampiglione and Falconer stimulated the hippocampus in man and produced, for a few seconds up to 1 min, a state of unresponsiveness to sensory and verbal stimuli with amnesia for this period. In this case, and probably in others, it may be assumed that functional inhibition of the hippocampus had a role in the appearance of akinetic mutism.

10. The significance of EEG anomalies refractory to treatment in epileptic children. — E. Broşteanu (Bucharest).

A discrepancy sometimes exists between the favourable clinical evolution and the persistence of EEG anomalies during anticonvulsive treatment. Abnormal tracings were found in a group of 73 epileptic children under treatment, followed up for 8 years. Apart from the paroxysmal anomalies evoked in 8 cases only by overbreathing, the following anomalies persisted with age: (a) increased amplitude of the tracing; (b) dominant occipital rhythm at the lower limit; (c) increased proportion of low voltage, diffuse or localized slow waves.

Two electro-clinical cases are reported, with an excellent response to treatment and disappearance of the paroxysmal anomalies, but persistence of the high voltage tracing. In the first, a typical petit mal developed at the age of 6.5, with synchronous bilateral spike and wave discharges; in the second case, a little girl, the seizures had a focal onset with secondary generalization and the EEG showed a focus of isolated, high voltage spikes and waves at the right mid-temporal derivation. EEG examination of the members of the families revealed minor dysrhythmias in the mother and the mother's brother in the first case, and in both parents in the second case. In both cases, puberty led to progressive improvement of the tracings with a decrease in amplitude. Gradual diminution and then suppressing of the treatment did not result in the reappearance of EEG anomalies or in clinical seizures, after 2 years.

In these cases the increased amplitude raised the question of the existence of certain metabolic alterations against a genetic background of increased convulsive reactivity, improved at puberty.

11. The value of electrophysiological investigations in the rehabilitation of former tuberculous patients. — R. Broşteanu (Bucharest).

The main conditions of rehabilitation in tuberculosis are: stability of the pathological process, maintenance of a respiratory capacity compatible with the necessary physical effort and the neuropsychic possibility of adaptation to the process of production. A survey which included various pneumological, cardiological, neuropsychic, biochemical and electrophysiological aspects showed that useful information was obtained by electrophysiological investigations.

Apart from the severely altered EEG tracings, whose proportion does not change, and those within normal limits, there were 61% of tracings with discrete and moderate alterations before the resumption of work. During the first weeks of work the proportion of these tracings increased by 18% (79%) showing the existence of a period of difficult adaptation. After one year's activity only 62% of modified tracings were found. In the well adapted subjects hyperventilation after rest altered the tracings in 8.8% (70.8%) and hyperventilation after effort brought them back to 62%. Thirteen per cent of the reactivated tuberculosis cases belonged to the group with marked EEG alterations and 9% to the group with discrete alterations: no normal tracing was recorded.

12. Gammaencephalographic investigations in cerebral tumour diagnosis. — E. Câmpeanu and E. Dumitru (Cluj).

The authors examined clinically a group of 30 patients suffering from surgically verified brain tumours; gammaencephalography had been also performed in view of the diagnosis. Radio iodine serum albumin (^{131}I) was used, the impulses being recorded with the help of a scintillation counter. Analysis of the results showed, in 26 of the 30 examined patients, gammaencephalographic alterations, *i.e.* foci of hyperactivity (22) and hypoactivity (4). The best results were obtained in cases of superficial tumours, whereas with the deeply located tumours or those at the base the results were not always conclusive. From the histological viewpoint glioblastomata and cerebral metastases gave more accurate data.

13. Motor, electrographic and vegetative reactivity to slight vestibular stimulation. — E. Crighel and I. Poilici (Bucharest).

The motor (nystagmus), electrographic (EEG and flash-evoked potentials: EP) and vegetative (rheoencephalography: REG; digital plethysmography: PL; ECG; electrodermogram: EDG, and pneumogram: PN) reactivity to a slight vestibular caloric stimulus was investigated in controls and in patients with cerebrovascular diseases: diffuse cerebral atherosclerosis, carotid and vertebro-basilar insufficiencies and neocortical and capsular vascular lesions.

The most constant responses were the EP and PL. In the controls and in diffuse atherosclerosis and cerebral circulatory insufficiency the EPs were enhanced, whereas in patients with neocortico-diencephalic lesions the EPs were depressed by ipsilateral vestibular stimuli. Neither quantitative nor qualitative differences in PL were found between the controls and the patients with cerebrovascular diseases. The REG showed the same reaction frequency to slight vestibular stimulation as the PL but the reaction in the majority of the cases was reversed: vasodilatation in the former and vasoconstriction in the latter. Nystagmus was less constant. In vertebro-basilar insufficiencies the latency was long and the nystagmus small and periodically interrupted.

The ECG and PN were more modified by the vestibular caloric stimulus in the initial period (orienting reaction) than 50 sec after the beginning of stimulation. No qualitative changes were found between the controls and the patients with different types of cerebrovascular diseases. The EDG and EEG showed a very inconstant response to the vestibular stimulus.

The results of the investigation suggest that the differentiated motor, electrographic and vegetative reactivity to slight caloric vestibular stimuli is determined by the different levels of connection of vestibular afferent impulses with the motor and vegetative outflow and the level of interaction between vestibular and photic efferent impulses. The modulating influence of the reticular formation on vestibular inputs and on the above mentioned reactivities is discussed.

14. EEG aspects in craniostenosis. — C. Cristian, C. Arseni, A. Terzi and I. Roman (Bucharest).

A study was carried out on 44 cases of craniostenosis admitted to the Clinic of Neurosurgery during 1964–1968. The EEG was recorded pre- and post-operatively in order to mark the effect of the operation. Correlations were established between the EEG and the age group, sex, raised intracranial pressure syndrome, neurological signs, the presence of epileptic seizures, psychical disturbances, radiological signs, the presence of exophthalmos and the circumference of the head. No correlation could be established between the raised intracranial pressure syndrome and the EEG.

Three parameters were taken into consideration (amplitude, frequency and morphology) in analysing the electrical activity. A high voltage tracing was recorded in 28 cases, and medium voltage in 16 cases. Spontaneous electrical activity showed dominant delta and theta rhythms in 39 cases and, apart from the dominant theta rhythm, groups of alpha and beta waves in 5 cases. The morphology of the tracings showed pathological aspects with bisynchronous discharges in 19 cases, inter-hemispheric asymmetry of lesional type in 5 cases and spike and wave complexes in 2 cases of paroxysmal abnormalities. In the cases with exophthalmos the electrical abnormalities in the background tracing were accentuated and accompanied by electrical signs pointing to involvement of the deep formations (hypersynchronous slow wave discharges).

15. Electro-clinical considerations on some cases of van Bogaert's subacute leukoencephalitis. — I. M. Lupu (Sibiu).

A clinical and EEG study was carried out on 3 cases of van Bogaert's subacute sclerosing leukoencephalitis, emphasizing the importance of the EEG examination for an early diagnosis, especially in cases with a prolonged psychiatric symptomatology. The high specificity of Radermecker's complexes is discussed, since some authors subsequently found these formations in other leukoencephalitides (Schilder's diffuse sclerosis, Dawson, etc.), which would be an argument lending support to the unity of these encephalitides. The specificity of these complexes is, however, less certain for the group of sclerosing encephalitides, since they were also found in other dementing states (general juvenile paralysis, for instance) and in a case of Ramsay-Hunt cerebellar myoclonic dyssynergism. Hence, electro-clinical comparison appears very useful for elucidation of the diagnosis, even in the cases where it is impossible to carry out a histo-pathological examination.

16. A case of epilepsia partialis continua. — A. Naghiu and F. Bogdan (Oradea).

A 24-year-old male presented, from the age of one year, continous localized myoclonic seizures of the first two fingers of the right hand. At the age of one year he had suffered from encephalitis. The myoclonic movements were permanent and of greater amplitude during emotion or effort, but only once became generalized into a grand mal seizure. The EEG permanently presented frontal and central spikes at 150–200 μV on the left side and, occasionally, in the temporo-parietal region. On the right side the basic activity was represented by alpha waves at 12 c/sec and 50 μV. It is likely that a cortical focus developed, with a permanent activity due to a reverberating circuit with the ventro-lateral nucleus of the thalamus. It is surprising that after more than 20 years of constant activity in the motor area the discharges did not generalize to the opposite side and permitted the appearance of a normal alpha rhythm.

17. The role of the central monoamine oxidase systems in the determination of EEG alterations in Graves disease. — A. Nicolescu-Catargi (Bucharest).

To high voltage alpha rhythms (100–150 μV) and high frequencies (12–13 c/sec), an increased variability coefficient of the alpha spindle (sudden oscillations in amplitude with a sharp alpha appearance) and a tendency to synchronization over the whole scalp are characteristically added. This aspect was encountered in 70% of over 300 cases of Graves disease. Paroxysmal discharges sometimes (20% of the cases) appeared in the tracings (high voltage discharges of variable frequency, from 6 to 10 c/sec).

To determine whether relative blocking of cerebral monoamine oxidases interferes in the production of these EEG anomalies, small Niamide (nialamide) doses (100 mg/day, for 7 days) were administered. The EEG showed a definite increase in the spontaneous anomalies described, even in the slightly modified basic EEG tracings. Triiodothyronine, administered in the Werner test during 10 days, produced effects that were similar but less evident than those induced by Niamide.

In contrast with euthyroid patients with normal EEGs, monoamine oxidase inhibitors produced rapid alteration of the tracings in Graves disease, lending support to the existence of an instability of the cerebral regulation of electrogenesis in this disease. Since the appearance described is also encountered in patients with a high LATS (long-acting thyroid-stimulator) titre, who respond by intense thyroid secretion, the deficit of the cerebral monoamine oxidase system is considered to be an intermediate link in the alterations produced in the hypothalamo-reticulo-mesencephalic integration pathways, reflected in the cortex.

The genetic factor (pathology of the central and thyroid monoamine oxidase systems) and the interference of thyroid and hypothalamo-hypophyseal polypeptide hormones (thyroid-releasing factor, thyroid-stimulating hormone) in these enzymatic systems appear to be the basis of the EEG alterations, in the proportion found.

18. Polygraphic investigations of sleep in nocturnal ambulatory automatisms. — L. Popoviciu and L. Szabó (Tîrgu-Mureș).

Various polygraphic examinations were carried out during sleep (EEG, EMG and ocular movements) by means of continuous nocturnal recordings (4–8 h) in 20 patients suffering from nocturnal ambulatory automatisms, divided into four groups, according to the incidence of these automatisms, either singly or combined with other nocturnal manifestations (night terror, enuresis, somniloquy, masticatory automatisms) or temporal diurnal manifestations. In 8 cases the standard EEG recordings by day revealed the presence of certain diffuse anomalies, not specific of epilepsy, in 4 cases temporal epileptic anomalies, in 4 patients moderate inter-hemispheric asymmetries and in the other 4 cases normal EEGs.

In the majority of the cases important modifications were noted in the development of sleep, *i.e.*, agitated sleep, with the predominance of light slow wave sleep, an evident decrease in the proportion of REM sleep in 13 cases (5.5%–12.5%) or an increase in the proportion of REM in 4 patients (between 27.8% and 31.3%). During sleep recordings there were discharges of poly-spikes and of poly-spikes and waves in all the cases, either with temporal foci or in all derivations, predominantly or exclusively during slow wave sleep, particularly deep sleep (15 cases), or on the contrary, predominantly or exclusively during REM (5 cases). The abnormalities noted during sleep, substantiated by the clinical and historical data, led to the conclusion that these non-convulsive nocturnal manifestations are of epileptic origin.

19. EEG investigatons on the action of Chlordelazine, Oxypertin and Fluanxol in chronic schizophrenia. — V. Predescu and I. Roman (Bucharest).

Investigations were carried out on 48 cases of schizophrenia exhibiting the following clinical aspects: isolation, autism, inactivity, inaffectivity, restricted verbal communications summed up in the apatho-abulic syndrome, stability without remissions. The age of the patients ranged between 20 and 56 years, average 34 years, the disease dating back 5–18 years, average 10 years. The patients, divided into three equal groups, received no medication for 14–20 days and were then given psycholeptics for the following 30 days, *i.e.* Fluanxol, 10–15 mg daily (average length of illness 10 years), Oxypertin 80–120 mg doses (average duration 10 years) and Chlordelazine 200–300 mg doses (average duration 11 years).

The results were appraised according to Larr's multidimensional scale and a series of psychological tests. After one month's treatment favourable results were obtained with Fluanxol in 75% of the cases, with Oxypertin in 37.5% and with Chlordelazine in 31.2%. EEG recording was done before, during and after the treatment. Significant EEG changes were obtained with Fluanxol: decrease in alpha frequency below 8 c/sec, disorganization of the tracing following increase in the theta and delta indices in all the leads, mainly occipital and frontal, and on overbreathing bursts of delta waves and slow synchronous spikes in all leads. These EEG changes corresponded to evident clinical improvement (in 4 cases the tracing was not modified). The EEG was only slightly and insignificantly altered following treatment with Oxypertin, affecting the amplitude and decrease in alpha frequency and improving the tracing in 6 cases (10 cases not modified). Chlordelazine produced evident initial changes in the alpha rhythm, increasing its amplitude and area, then becoming slow, monomorphous, with transition to 7 c/sec. Slow theta waves and paroxysms of monomorphous delta waves were induced by overbreathing towards the end of the treatment in 3 cases. The discrete EEG changes following Oxypertin and the over-all alpha rhythm changes after Chlordelazine corresponded clinically with promising improvement in only one-third of the cases.

20. Contributions to the EEG study of W.Y. 3498. — V. Predescu and I. Roman (Bucharest).

34 patients, admitted to the Psychiatric Clinic and suffering from anxiety states within the framework of various types of neurotic diseases, were treated with W.Y. 3498. The results were appraised by clinical observation, psychometric criteria (Hamilton's scale for evaluating anxiety states) and serial EEG recording. After the administration of daily doses of 45 mg for several weeks, the clinical and psychometric tests showed diminution or disappearance of anxiety; the EEG was similarly modified. The control EEG before treatment showed an activity of low voltage and poor alpha rhythm (15 cases), flat tracings dominated by diffuse fast activity (9 cases), rapid alpha rhythm with a relatively predominant theta rhythm in the temporal leads (6 cases) and low voltage, diffuse theta waves (4 cases).

After the administration of W.Y. 3498 the following changes were noted: (a) synchronization of the flat, desynchronized tracings; (b) increase in the incidence of alpha rhythm, which became synchronous with the fast rhythms in the Rolandic region; (c) the alpha rhythm extended its distribution to the anterior regions; (d) the EEG with an average alpha rhythm (within normal limits) underwent a process of supernormalization by increase in the alpha index, the regional differences disappearing in almost 95% of the cases; (e) the immature tracings changed their morphology towards slow, monomorphous alpha rhythm, the temporal predominance disappearing. Following treatment with W.Y. 3498 EEG criteria of anxiety, *i.e.*, poor rapid, low voltage alpha rhythm, diffuse beta rhythm and immature tracings disappeared, the EEG becoming normal and corresponding clinically with the disappearance of anxiety.

21. The significance of minor EEG abnormalities focal in the left temporal region. — I. Roman (Bucharest).

From 10,000 patients with psychiatric diseases admitted to the Psychiatric Clinic, Bucharest, and followed up for 7 years, repeated EEG recordings revealed left temporal abnormalities, *i.e.*, bursts of sinusoidal or sharp theta waves, sharp large alpha waves, groups of low voltage delta waves, slow fast spikes of medium amplitude, at rest and after overbreathing, in 250 cases (2.5%). The clinical material was selected by excluding all cases of epilepsy, encephalopathy, psychiatric disturbances with cerebral tumours and abiotrophic processes. The patients were divided into 3 groups: (a) psychiatric patients with combined, mild organic and functional signs: affective syndromes in cerebral atherosclerosis (CAS), post-traumatic syndrome, chronic psychotic alcoholism, involution melancholia, etc.; (b) patients with depressive states: neurosis, endogenous depression, pre-involution depression etc.; (c) patients with personality disturbances, children with temper tantrums and children with affective fits and stammering.

Left temporal EEG abnormalities, exacerbated by overbreathing and by activation with Ahyponon (3-ethyl-3-methylglutarimide) and persistent in the course of many years, in some cases without aggravation or not influenced by the treatment, were considered lesional and encountered in neurotic disturbances in CAS, in the post-traumatic syndrome and in 5% of psychopathic alcoholics (activated with alcohol per os).

The temporal abnormalities that changed their morphology in the course of the disease, variable in terms of the treatment and disappearing in the remission periods, were considered to be functional alterations (theta rhythm projected from the rhinecephalon and hypothalamus to the temporal leads), *i.e.*, neurotic, pre-involutional and endogenous depressions, affective disturbances in CAS, neurotic disturbances in ethylism (disappearing with abstinence from alcohol) and in schizophrenia.

In the third group EEG abnormalities underwent changes with age and in terms of cerebral maturation, having a functional character and being closely linked to the maturation of electrogenesis.

The functional aspects of the EEG must be viewed critically. The clinical evolution and dynamic EEG aspects should be followed up during treatment and drug activation for several years. Use of the term "left functional temporal focus" after only one or two EEG examinations has no practical value and leads to confusion, to the detriment of the patient.

22. EEG data in intracranial metastases. — I. Roman, C. Cristian and A. Terzi (Bucharest).

EEG investigations were carried out in 100 patients with intracranial metastases, admitted to the Service of Neurosurgery during 1964–1968, checked intra-operatively and at the post mortem examination in 85% of the cases. These investigations were carried out in view of the increased incidence of cerebral metastases (over 10%), of the clinical polymorphism with intricate focal neurological signs, raised cranial pressure, signs of irritation and important psychiatric manifestations, and in order to find objective electrical signs for the diagnosis of multiple intracranial metastases, to establish an indication of non-intervention. Most cerebral metastases were located supratentorially and involved 1–2 lobes in 55 cases; multiple metastases were found in 25 cases, deep and midline in 8 cases and in the posterior fossa in 12 cases.

Focal EEG abnormalities were found in 74 cases, *i.e.*, polymorphous delta waves, 2–3 c/sec, with an amplitude of 70–150 μV against a background of generalized disturbance, with degradation of the alpha rhythm and increase in the slow theta and delta wave indices. With deep tumours, diffuse alterations of various degrees were found, depending upon the incidence of the polymorphous delta rhythm and the bilateral appearance of monomorphous theta and delta discharges. Metastases in the posterior fossa gave general alterations in 8 cases with accentuation in the occipital and temporal leads in 2 cases. With multiple metastases polymorphous delta abnormalities were noted, extending to a whole hemisphere (corresponding to metastases found in that hemisphere). As a rule the abnormalities were generalized and seldom perifocal. Electro-clinical correlations were established with the following parameters: epileptic seizures, psychic disturbances, raised intracranial pressure, the size and nature of the metastatic process, acute or subacute evolution of the tumour. Significant correlations were found between confusional states, raised intracranial pressure and multiple tumours giving general alterations. Normal tracings were only observed in a few cases: 2 metastases of the posterior fossa and 4 deep metastases of small size.

23. The place and the importance of EEG and rheoencephalography in the pathology of the operated stomach. — T. Spîrchez and E. Broşteanu (Bucharest).

A study was carried out on 634 patients operated on for ulcer; 143 presented an early post-prandial syndrome. In 75 cases the early post-prandial syndrome was produced by the administration, through a jejunal tube, of hypertonic glucose solution. The EEG, ECG, rheoencephalogram, digital plethysmogram and blood pressure were recorded concomitantly (Boucke-Brecht method). In a control group cerebral circulation was determined with radioactive chrome during the early post-prandial syndrome. The background EEG showed deviations from the normal average type: (a) increase in the proportion of flat tracings, of the LVF type; (b) increase in the proportion of fast rhythms and of rhythms in the Rolandic area; (c) the apparently spontaneous appearance of spikes of the vertex.

During the early post-prandial syndrome a vegetative "storm" is produced, with collapse of the cerebral circulation (clearly seen in the rheoencephalogram in average cases) paradoxical peripheral vasodilatation, tachycardia and EEG alterations, with progressive increase of the slow components linked to disturbances in the distribution of blood leading to cerebral anoxia.

It is concluded that, apart from the background EEG aspects of the ulcerous disease, the administration of hypertonic glucose solution by jejunal tube, with concomitant recording of the EEG and rheoencephalogram, in cases proposed for surgery, permits detection of neurovegetative disorders whose presence make it necessary to prolong conservative treatment.

24. ERG and EEG changes in Steinert myotonic dystrophy. — B. Stănescu and E. Wawernia (Bucharest).

ERG and EEG examinations were performed in 6 patients with myotonic dystrophy. The recordings revealed subnormal electroretinograms and morphological changes in the b wave. All the patients presented diffuse alterations of the EEG, some with slow dysrhythmia and others with a flat tracing. These changes are similar to those found in retinitis pigmentosa. The implications of these facts are discussed.

25. EEG study of hypophyseal dwarfism. — D. Stoian, S. Poenaru, V. Stănescu and L. Stefănică-Moţoc (Bucharest).

EEG recordings were taken in 70 cases of hypophyseal dwarfism, aged 5–19, with tumoural lesions in 8 cases, non-tumoural lesions in 18 cases and idiopathic form in 44 cases. The results were referred to age and correlated with the aetiopathogenesis, statural hypotrophy indices, psychical development and endocrine factors associated with the hypophyseal deficit (hypothyroidism, hypoglycaemia, diabetes insipidus).

Normal EEGs were only found in 4 cases, with marked incidence of deficient modulation of the basic rhythm (85.70% of cases), high voltage tracings in 58.55%, increase in the sensitivity to overbreathing in 58.55% and the presence of spikes in 48.57% of the cases. Spontaneous predominance of slow (theta) dysrhythmia was noted in 27.14% of the cases, epileptiform changes in 13.43% and inter-hemispheric asymmetry in 5.75% of the patients. The incidence of EEG alterations was proportional to the statural hypotrophy indices, with the presence of signs of hypothyroidism, hypoglycaemia and diabetes insipidus, also showing certain correlations with the psychical deficit. The results are of importance for the elucidation of certain aspects of the aetiopathogenesis of the syndrome (idiopathic forms) and for assessing the value of the EEG in following up the patients' evolution under treatment.

26. Clinical EEG and polygraphic investigations of sleep in children with simple enuresis or associated with other non-convulsive nocturnal episodic manifestations. — L. Szabó and L. Popoviciu (Tîrgu-Mureş).

The authors analyse the data obtained in a polygraphic study of sleep (EEG, EMG and ocular movements) by continuous nocturnal recordings (4–8 h) in 20 enuretic children, of whom 8 had simple enuresis, 5 enuresis, somniloquy and nocturnal automatisms, and 7 had enuresis, somnambulism, nocturnal terror, masticatory automatisms, etc. Important disorders were noted in the development of sleep. In most of the cases studied (17) sleep was extremely agitated, uneasy, with considerable alternation in the waking and sleep phases. There was a predominance of slow wave light sleep over slow wave deep sleep, which was seldom recorded. Moreover, there was a considerable decrease in the proportion of REM sleep (between 6.9 and 16%), with only 2 cases showing a normal proportion between the two types of sleep (slow and REM).

In all the cases in which enuresis was combined with other non-convulsive nocturnal episodic manifestations, as well as in some non-associated cases, the EEG showed diffuse (3 cases) or focal (10 cases) epileptic abnormalities, particularly in the course of slow wave sleep, with a marked predominance in the C phase which, in correlation with the history and clinical data of this group, pleads in favour of their epileptic origin. The 3 c/sec spike and wave complexes noted in one case in the course of slow wave light sleep (B phase) proves the existence of certain clinical forms of "petit-mal enuresis". On the other hand, the psychoreactive origin of enuresis may be suspected in those non-associated in which the EEG recording of sleep failed to show any epileptic changes, while clinically the patients presented psychical syndromes with reactive psycho-affective elements.

In 5 children enuretic episodes were noted during the D phase, preceded in all cases by a series of discharges of poly-spikes or poly-spikes and waves and followed by alternative sleep and transitory B phase.

27. Electroencephalograms in meningitis. — A. Vâţă, E. Brauner, I. Petrovanu, V. Mihul, A. Baltiev, S. Dimitriu, T. Turcu and I. Cercel (Iassy).

EEGs were repeatedly recorded in 23 patients with viral meningitis, in 8 patients with tuberculous meningitis and in one case with leptospiral meningitis. Most cases were young adults. In 25 cases the tracings were pathological, with abnormal basic rhythms, hypersynchronous sinusoidal discharges, irritative abnormalities and changes in amplitude. The alpha rhythm was generally absent or with reduced incidence. The appearance of theta or delta waves was the most common feature, reflecting the diffuse character of the cerebral disturbance. Involvement of centro-diencephalic structures, manifested by hypersynchronous sinusoidal discharges, was found in 2 cases.

Persistence of irritative elements in the late control tracings was significant for the appearance of sequelae. The incidence of abnormalities was greater in the acute period, their intensity running parallel to the gravity of the clinical condition. The recorded changes had no aetiological specificity. The EEG investigation, useful for appraising cerebral impairment in the acute period, is a necessary criterion for prognosis.

28. Cerebral electrical investigations in raised blood pressure in children and youths. — L. Zarea (Bucharest).

Cerebral electrical activity was studied in 67 patients with raised blood pressure, aged 3–40 years. The patients formed 3 groups: essential hypertension, 22 cases; secondary hypertension due to congenital coarctation of the aorta, 24 cases; secondary hypertension due to other causes, 21 cases. Pathological alterations were recorded in 46% of the cases, in an approximately equal proportion in the first and second groups (41% and 42%) and in a somewhat higher proportion in secondary hypertension due to other acquired causes (57%). The EEG alterations were discrete and represented in general by the appearance of slow waves. Borderline tracings were recorded in 34% of the cases and normal tracings in 20%. An agreement was found in 57–77% of the cases between cerebral electrical changes and the results of examination of the fundi. The pathogenetic mechanisms that might explain EEG alterations in young patients with raised blood pressure are discussed.

29. The applications of electromyography in stomatology. — E. Costa and V. Bodnar (Bucharest).

The authors show that EMG tracings are indispensable for an accurate diagnosis and for the control and follow-up of treatment in a great number of dental disorders, especially in prosthetic treatment and in investigations. A description is given of the most important prosthetic EMG applications.

30. Electromyography in the determination of certain aetiopathogenic aspects of scoliosis. — A. Denischi and G. Panait (Bucharest).

EMG examinations of 37 patients with scoliosis supplied objective evidence of a functional imbalance in the paravertebral musculature, in the dynamics of its evolution in terms of the clinical degree of scoliosis and the mode in which it was influenced by the orthopaedic and surgical treatment. The EMG data lend support to the existence of inapparent forms of poliomyelitis as aetiological factors in idiopathic scoliosis.

31. The EMG picture of diuretic therapy in hypothyroidism. — V. Mareş, M. Morariu and L. Gozariu (Cluj).

Ionic and EMG alterations, occurring in hypothyroidism during diuretic treatment with Clopamide (1-(4-chloro-sulfamoylbenzamido)-2,6-dimethylpiperidine), administered in doses of 40 mg/day for 3 days, were followed up. In addition to its major diuretic effect, Clopamide alters the EMG, pointing to repeated activity, and the ionogram, the most constant effect observed being a tendency to hypopotassaemia. The authors emphasize the importance of EMG control during diuretic therapy in hypothyroidism, as it might prevent the onset of a spasmophilic condition and, in addition, some major accidents.

32. Study of the latency of the response in chronic tetany. — S. Poenaru, D. Stoian and L. Stefănică-Moţoc (Bucharest).

The present paper refers to 11 cases of chronic tetany, 6 children and 5 adults, in which the EMG, performed according to the Alajouanine technique, evidenced activity characteristic of tetany. Supramaximal electrical stimulation of the cubital nerve in the epitrochlear groove was done with surface electrodes, and recordings with bipolar, double wire electrodes at the level of the first dorsal interosseous muscle before the two facilitating tests for tetany (reference determinations) and immediately after the onset of electrical activity specific to tetany.

In the reference determinations the latency of the response ranged between 3 and 12.3 msec, the parameters of the motor response being: in 8 cases an amplitude of 300 μV and in 3 cases of 300–580 μV; duration 4–12.5 msec; shape, normal in 3 cases and polyphasic in 8 cases. Stimulation-detection in the ischaemic period (2 cases), post-ischaemic period (7 cases) and during hyperpnoea (3 cases) revealed an increase in latency in 7 cases and diminution in 2 cases; changes were likewise found in the parameters of the motor response. Stress is laid on the importance of continuing studies on the latency of the response in chronic tetany, according to aetiologic criteria, for the elucidation of certain aspects of the pathological physiology of tetany.

33. Study of conduction velocity in motor fibres of peripheral nerves in toxic polyneuritis produced by carbon disulphide. — C. Vasilescu (Bucharest).

The conduction velocity was determined in the motor fibres of the median, ulnar and peroneal nerves, in 60 patients with toxic polyneuritis produced by carbon disulphide. The respective cases were divided into two groups according to the clinical gravity of the disease: group I, with objective clinical signs of the disease; group II with subjective phenomena only. The average age, 24.5 years, was the same for each group and all nerves. In group I the mean conduction velocity in the median and ulnar nerves was 44.1 m/sec (78% of control mean) and in the peroneal nerve 36.5 m/sec (70% of control). In group II the corresponding figures were 49.5 m/sec (89%) and 42.3 m/sec (82.4%).

In group II the diagnosis was exclusively based on determination of the conduction velocity and the EMG. Dynamic study showed that in the cases in which the diagnosis was made in the early subclinical stage of the disease, rapid recovery without sequelae was obtained when the patients were removed from the toxic environment and an adequate medication was prescribed.

34. Effects of noise on EEG latency changes in an auditory vigilance task. — E. Gulian (Bucharest).

Latency of alpha blocking to correct detections (CD), false alarms (FA) and missed signals (MS) was investigated under different types (continuous and intermittent) and intensities (70 dB and 90 dB) of noise, the first experiment being performed in conditions of quiet. The subjects (15) had the task of detecting a signal among 4 other acoustic stimuli which appeared randomly, at irregular intervals. EEG was recorded continuously from the T–O and T–T leads, during the whole session (1 h 30 min). It was found that: (1) the latency of CD is shorter than that of FA and MS under all experimental conditions; (2) the mean latency of CD and FA varies (decreases) mainly as a function of the type of noise and only secondarily of its intensity (in continuous noise the latency is greater than in intermittent noise); (3) the longest EEG latencies for all performance indicators were recorded in the course of weak continuous noise. It is suggested that differences in background noise elicit variations in mean latency scores for each category of indicators, but that the general level of latencies (longer or shorter) is determined by the response type. Thus, background noise exerts an unspecific influence which mainly induces changes in the cerebral tone, whereas a task, which implies continuous attention, has a predominantly specific arousing effect.

35. The effects of suppressing the paradoxical phase of sleep on the metabolism of cerebral ammonia. — I. Hăulică, L. Ababei, C. Teodorescu, C. Costan, V. Roşca, M. Moisiu and C. Haler (Iaşi).

Using the technique of the swimming pool devised by Jouvet *et al.* (1964), adapted for rats by Cohen and Dement (1965), it was found that removal of the paradoxical phase of sleep during 10 days brings about a 56% increase in cerebral ammonia (Conway micro-method). Intensification of glutaminesynthetase activity ran parallel to the increase in ammonia, rising from an average value of 13.85 to 16.15 μg/mg/h, which corresponds to 96.11 and 112.15 μmole glutamine synthesized per g/h, respectively. After only 6 days of suppressing paradoxical sleep, glutaminesynthetase activity increased by 16%, without significant changes in cerebral ammonia, probably due to its neutralization by the mechanism of glutamine formation.

In contrast to ammonia and glutaminesynthetase, the brain nucleic acids (RNA and DNA) presented a significant decrease both after 10 and after 6 days of depriving the animals of paradoxical sleep. Increase in cerebral ammonia is caused by intensification of the proteolytic and deamination processes. The decrease in nucleic acids and the increase in AMP-deaminase in the brain lend support to this point of view.

36. Induced depressant influences from the centrum medianum (Luys) upon the evoked activity of the amygdalo-hippocampal complex. — A. Kreindler, D. Florescu, D. Volanschi and G. Popescu-Tismana (Bucharest).

In acute experiments on non-anaesthetized cats immobilized with Flaxedil (gallamine) and artificially respired, the influence of high frequency (150 c/sec) electrical stimulation of the centrum medianum (CM) on the following responses was investigated: (1) the ventral hippocampal (Hcv) and entorhinal evoked responses elicited by single, slightly supraliminal, stimulation of the ipsilateral parvocellular basal amygdaloid nucleus (Abp) and (2) the Hcv local response to single supraliminal stimulation. CM high frequency stimulation induced marked diminution, tonic in character, of the Hcv responses to Abp shocks. The amygdalo-entorhinal responses were not influenced. The late components and the tendency to after-discharge of the local Hcv response were also depressed by CM stimulation.

The depressant influence induced by CM high frequency stimulation was similar to those exercised by high frequency stimulation of the mesencephalic and pontine reticular formations and of the posterior hypothalamus, previously described. The mechanisms by which high frequency stimulation of the CM depresses the amygdalo-hippocampal and local hippocampal responses are discussed.

37. Transistorized neuro- and myostimulator with impulse memory. — J. Nagy and R. A. Silveanu (Timişoara).

A transistorized apparatus was developed by the authors for experimental and clinical investigation of the nervous and muscular tissues. The apparatus generates constant rectangular pulses with adjustable parameters. It also permits the measurement of tissue excitability and contains a memory of the generated impulses.

38. EEG alterations in athletes in the barochamber at 5000 m altitude. — V. Neştianu, A. Demeter, C. Cristescu, I. Pintilie and V. Filcescu (Bucharest).

The EEG, EKG, EDG, respiration and flicker fusion threshold to intermittent photic stimulation (IPS) were recorded in 30 athletes, in the plains and at 5000 m altitude (30 min) simulated in the barochamber. In the plains, at rest, the alpha rhythm (9–12 c/sec frequency, 25–80 μV amplitude) with an incidence in the occipital tracing of 40–70%, exhibited an evident arrest reaction and often a rebound on closing the eyes. The fusion threshold, with broad individual variations, was 24–48 c/sec.

At 5000 m the amplitude of the alpha rhythm decreased with the time spent in the barochamber, *i.e.*, up to 50%, and sometimes even more after isometric work, the frequency increased by 0.5–1 c/sec, the arrest reaction and the rebound visibly decreased, the incidence gradually diminished, especially after isometric contraction, and the fusion threshold fell by 30% on average. The alpha rhythm was no longer organized in bursts. In cases of modified respiration, with periodic apnoea, in the individuals with a low resistance to high altitudes, the arrest reaction appeared in the EEG simultaneously with apnoea. In some cases isolated synchronous or asynchronous (localized) spikes, extrasystoles in the EKG and even theta rhythm in bursts developed (sign of deep disturbance and low resistance to hypoxia); they appeared in a European sports champion who, at the Olympic Games in Mexico City, had to give up in the first few minutes, as foreseen by the doctors.

In conclusion, well trained athletes are far more resistant to hypoxia at an altitude of 5000 m, in comparison with most of the population, owing to repeated exposure to hypoxia during training. In general, signs of inhibition do not appear (except for a fall in the flicker fusion threshold). Stress is laid on the particular value of EEG testing in the barochamber for the selection of athletes in view of resistance to hypoxia and hence, to prolonged aerobic exercise.

39. Interaction between the substantia nigra and nucleus caudatus in evoking recruiting-like cortical responses. — A. Nicolescu-Catargi, M. Coculescu, S. Petrescu and M. Petrescu (Bucharest).

Acute experiments were carried out on 15 non-anaesthetized cats under Flaxedil (gallamine), recording the ECoG with bipolar electrodes introduced stereotaxically in the substantia nigra (SNg) and nucleus caudatus (NCd). Stimulation of NCd with electrical impulses of 7 c/sec, 10–40 V, induced recruiting-like cortical responses with spindles of 8–10 cycles and variations in amplitude of approximately 50%. Stimulation of the NCd by a single pulse induced a spindle of slow cortical waves. Stimulation of the SNg with 7 c/sec, 10–30 V, 0.10–0.5 msec, synchronized the ECoG, predominantly sigmoid. In 50% of the cases the cortical evoked potential presented a recruiting-like waxing and waning, with spindles of 5–6 cycles and variations in amplitude of about 40%. The phenomenon was maintained in the *encéphale isolé* preparation. In 2 animals a cortical rhythm of 3–4 c/sec built up, although the SNg was stimultated at 7 c/sec.

Simultaneous stimulation of the SNg and NCd with 7 c/sec, 10–20 V, induced recruiting-like cortical responses, with waxing and waning in 10–15 cycle periods and variations in amplitude of the initial and maximum waves by about 70% (50%–80%), more persistent and regular than following separate stimulation of NCd. These responses appeared even to simultaneous stimulation of insufficient intensity to induce cortical recruitment in the case of isolated NCd stimulation.

Simultaneous stimulation of the NCd and SNg with single pulses of 0.1 c/sec, 30–40 V, brought about disappearance of the spindle of slow cortical waves induced by stimulation of NCd alone with the same parameters. Therefore, the electrically stimulated SNg dissociated the activity of the NCd, potentiating the recruitment-like cortical response, but suppressing the spindle of slow cortical waves induced in the NCd. These phenomena are considered to express the existence of different systems of neurones (dopaminergic, cholinergic, etc.) in the NCd and SNg.

40. Polygraphic method of investigation of the complex reactivity to slight caloric vestibular stimulation. — I. Poilici and E. Crighel (Bucharest).

Some authors (Kreindler 1932; Carmichael 1958; Karbowsky 1966; Barac 1967; Fischer 1967 etc.) reported on the influence of caloric vestibular stimulation on the electrical activity of the brain and on vegetative disturbances during the test, accounted for by the rich vestibular connexions with many integrating structures in the CNS.

Simultaneous polygraphic recording of the motor (electronystagmogram), electrical cerebral (EEG and flash-evoked potential) and vegetative (REG, ECG, digital plethysmogram, electrodermogram and pneumogram) activity during and after caloric vestibular stimulation by the Hallpike-Fitzgerald method (1942) showed reactivity differences between normals and patients with cerebrovascular diseases. Complex reactivity is analysed in detail for each of the mentioned functions during three different periods:

1. At the beginning of caloric stimulation. The vegetative and electric alterations at this moment represent the reactivity to an exteroceptive stimulus and can be compared with the orientation reaction to a sudden visual or auditory stimulus. The inconstant and slight EEG and EDG modifications suggest that the stimulus is liminal and does not inconvenience the subject.

2. After 40–60 sec, just at the appearance of the motor reaction (nystagmus), electrographic (especially EP) and vegetative alterations were observed. This moment represents the actual vestibular influence.

3. After 150–200 sec the motor activity (nystagmus) ceased and the vegetative and electrical spontaneous and evoked activities usually returned to normal. A neurohumoral influence acts at this moment, restoring the homeostatic balance of the functions examined.

The normal limits of reactivity during the three periods of the slight caloric vestibular stimulation test are discussed.

41. EEG in rabbits following glucose infusion. Simple quantitative analysis. — R. Racotta (Bucharest).

Pairs of electrodes were chronically implanted in various regions of the rabbit brain: cortex (Cx), hypothalamic and mesencephalic areas and dorsal medulla (BD). EEG recordings were made before, during and at various moments after glucose infusion (GI) in the ear vein (1 g/kg). A new quantitative technique was used in order to determine alterations in amplitude and period of EEG waves. The following results were obtained: (1) no consistent and comparable period changes in any region except in BD at 12–20 min after GI; (2) no significant amplitude changes in the lateral hypothalamic area; (3) significant amplitude increase in Cx and mesencephalic central grisea in most of the animals and in the ventromedial hypothalamic area (VHM) in all the animals; (4) amplitude changes began 20–50 min after GI and had dissimilar evolutions in different animals; (5) two recordings from the same rabbit produced similar results as regard the initial moment of amplitude changes.

The lack of concordance in time between changes in central nervous activity and glycaemic level seem to be relevant to Russek's theory of peripheral intracellular afferentation. Such peripheral receptors could signal in this case "cellular satiety". That would account for: (a) the lack of strict specificity of glucose loading on VMH recordings, and more especially (b) the belated effect of glucose infusion, starting at various time intervals in different rabbits.

42. EEG investigations with micro-electrodes in the primary acoustic areas. — O. Sager, I. Cincă and A. Serbănescu (Bucharest).

Recording with micro-electrodes (0.5 μ glass tip) in the cat, from the median ectosylvius gyrus (MEG), supplied evidence of cells whose spontaneous activity is activated, or inhibited or not influenced by click acoustic stimulation. The latency of single discharges to clicks in MEG is about 25 msec, whereas in EA, EP and the anterior pseudosylvian gyrus it is about 100–160 msec.

Tonotopic investigations revealed a caudo-oral location in AI–AII, from low (200 c/sec) to high frequencies (3600 c/sec); in EP the responses to low frequencies were predominant. The application of tones of the same frequency (800 c/sec) and intensity (40 dB), lasting 2.5 sec, repeated at 5 sec intervals, induced in the middle of AI and AII, unitary activity that gradually diminished at the moment of application up to complete disappearance at the 12th–14th repetition, but persisted when the tone was suppressed (in the graphic representation suppression of the tone follows a slope, it is not sudden). The application of short duration tones of 40 msec, with an intensity of 40 dB and frequency of 800 c/sec, repeated every second, produced a unitary activation which, however, gradually disappeared towards the 15th repetition. Whether these findings may be attributed to a process of adaptation at the unitary level is discussed.

43. The transmission pathways of acoustic stimulation to the anterior sigmoid gyrus. — O. Sager, V. Florea-Ciocoiu and V. Neştianu (Bucharest).

Single acoustic stimuli (clicks) evoked electrical potentials in the anterior sigmoid gyrus (aSG) (with slight individual latency variations) in 9 animals with bilateral topectomy of the primary auditory areas (BTAA), with (4) or without (5) chloralose injection. Histological examination showed bilateral retrograde degeneration of the median geniculate ganglion (mGG). Hence, acoustic stimulation could only be transmitted to the aSG by extrageniculate pathways.

In 18 *normal animals* clicks evoked potentials in the aSG, whether chloralose was injected (5) or not (13), but with a wide range of latencies. Single electrical stimuli to the mGG evoked a potential in the aSG (with slight individual latency variations). Stimulation by single shocks to the midbrain reticular formation evoked a potential in the aSG with a similar latency in both normal and BTAA animals.

From the data obtained it results that in *normal animals* electrical stimulation applied to mGG is transmitted to the median ectosylvian gyrus and from there to the aSG by two pathways: a cortico-subcortico-cortical pathway with a long conduction time and a cortico-cortical pathway with a shorter conduction time between mEG and aSG; stimulation induced by click may also be transmitted to the aSG by a third extra-geniculate pathway with a starting point in the MRF, as in BTAA animals, apart from the two forementioned pathways.

44. Electrocortical and autonomic balance induced by vegetative afferents. — E. Wawernia and A. Faibiş (Bucharest).

The influence of pulmonary cardiovascular reflexes on electrocortical activity was investigated under certain experimental conditions. In dogs anaesthetized with chloralose electrocortical activity, EKG, blood pressure and the respiratory rate were recorded after rapid 10% bleeding. In some cases, concomitant to an increase in the respiratory rate and tachycardia, haemorrhage gave rise to intermittent hypersynchrony and finally to desynchronized activity (arousal reaction). Intermittent hypersynchrony was characterized by desynchronized activity in the expiratory phase and spindles in the inspiratory phase (electrocortical activity balance).

Electroencephalography and Clinical Neurophysiology
Elsevier Publishing Company, Amsterdam – Printed in The Netherlands

BOOK REVIEWS

Edited by H. PETSCHE *and* JOHN R. HUGHES

The dizzy patient.—J. C. Elia. (C. C. Thomas, Springfield, Ill., 1968, 95 p., $7.50).

Over the years the house of Charles C. Thomas has published a number of outstanding classics, such as D. Cogan's *Diseases of the ocular muscles*, and F. Ford's *Diseases of the nervous system in infancy, childhood and adolescence*. In addition, they have served the medical profession by publishing scholarly monographs on topics of interest to a limited audience of physicians or medical scientists. Unfortunately, *The dizzy patient*, by J. C. Elia is not in the same tradition of excellence and represents a trivial approach to this difficult problem.

The author begins by briefly discussing the anatomy and physiology of the vestibular system in a fashion that reveals his lack of attention to the details of nervous system structure and function. His clinical approach to the classification and diagnosis of dizziness is similarly superficial. Even beginning medical students must surely be put off by such statements as, "No measure is more important in meeting the diagnostic challenge of dizziness than a good chronological history and a thorough otological and neurological examination".

The book is principally concerned with labyrinthine vertigo, rather than with all aspects of dizziness, despite a few references to other causes of this complex of symptoms. Among others, epilepsy, as a cause of dizziness is alluded to, either as an aura, or as isolated "vertiginous epilepsy". In discussing the role of electroencephalography in this entity, the author writes, "Positive electroencephalographic findings will usually confirm the diagnosis". An example of the speculative material included is the author's discussion of the importance of "dental factors" in producing dizziness. He states, "Dizziness is not infrequently a complaint in cases of dental occlusal and temporomandibular joint abnormalities... The dizziness... is likely to be continuous, of progressing severity, and associated with increased cranial pressure and paralysis of muscles supplied by the facial cranial nerve." The inappropriateness, not to mention hazard, of evaluating dental factors in the face of "increased cranial pressure and paralysis of muscles supplied by the facial cranial nerve" scarcely requires emphasis.

There is a rather simple description of such techniques as caloric testing. Unfortunately the table distinguishing the characteristics of *canal paresis* from those of *directional preponderance* in 15 diseases has the headings reversed, and will surely serve as a source of confusion to anyone who relies upon it. A list of rules for the interpretation of electronystagmograms is given, including such vague notations as, "Hypoactive responses associated with bilaterial (sic) gaze paralysis suggest positive pathology". The discussion includes numerous photographs of "black box" instruments containing impressive arrays of dials and knobs, with the manufacturers' trademarks prominently displayed; one, for example, is a picture of an oscilloscope, with the legend reading, "Oscilloscope".

The major thrust of the book is a discussion of the role of the microcirculation in the causation of Menière's disease, and the possible usefulness of beta-histidine (Serc®) in its treatment. There is an emotional appreciation of the importance of microcirculation: "The discoveries made to date in this comparatively new branch of medicine, microcirculation, may constitute the most important development in medicine in the century ... The belief is gaining ground that the microcirculatory approach is the most promising path to the diagnosis, prevention, or treatment of a wide range of illness that continue to mystify medical science and defy definite therapies."

Inserted in the middle of the book are five pages of half-tone reproductions of an original article written by Prosper Menière in the *Gazette Médicale de Paris* in 1861. Unfortunately, the print is almost unreadable in certain areas. However, there is a useful English translation of Menière's article, and this is undoubtedly the high point of the book.

The format of the book is pleasant, and many of the illustrations are sharply printed. The book contains more than its share of grammatical and typographical errors. In all there is too little scientific or medical information, too many serious omissions, and too many speculations and errors of fact to recommend it to any group of readers.

DAVID A. DRACHMAN
Northwestern University Medical Center, Chicago, Ill. 60611 (U.S.A.)

Electroenceph. clin. Neurophysiol., **1969**, *27*: 640

VIIth International Congress of Electroencephalography and Clinical Neurophysiology

SAN DIEGO, CALIFORNIA, SEPTEMBER 13–19, 1969

Pre-publication Committee:

DAVID D. DALY (Chairman), COSIMO AJMONE MARSAN
MICHAEL SAUNDERS, RICHARD D. WALTER

Editorial Assistant:

SUZANNE MARTIN

CONTENTS

Common Sessions 643
Free Communications in Electroencephalography 655
Free Communications in Electromyography 713
Demonstrations and Exhibits 729
Author Index 737

INVITED PAPERS
COMMON SESSIONS

1. Electroencephalography in neurosurgery.—**A. E. Walker (Baltimore, Md., U.S.A.).**
Electroencephalography is of significant help to the neurosurgeon in the management of both acute and chronic conditions. The diagnosis of the comatose patient who is admitted to the neurosurgical service without adequate history may be suggested by an electroencephalogram which indicates the presence of a focal lesion, a toxic condition, or some other specific abnormality. Even if the electroencephalogram only has lateralizing findings, it is of considerable value to the neurosurgeon who may then be able to instigate other diagnostic procedures to give a more precise localization.

In the routine neurological workup, electroencephalography is of considerable value, not only in localization of lesions but also in providing information relative to their nature. The fairly typical findings in epilepsy, in certain toxic states, and at times in neoplastic conditions, makes the electroencephalogram particularly useful. This is true even though isotopic studies may be needed to establish a localizing diagnosis.

In patients suspected of having a convulsive diathesis, the electroencephalogram with activating techniques becomes of great importance. The number of activating techniques has so increased it is possible in most cases to establish electroencephalographic evidence of epilepsy in any patient so suspected. With sphenoidal leads the medial temporal structures may be explored. If these recordings are not satisfactory, depth electrodes inserted into the temporal regions, either by an anterior or posterior approach, will enable the electroencephalographer to record over a period of time and to stimulate various subcortical structures which may reveal a hyperactive focus. During such stimulations, observations may be made of attention, mentation, memory, etc.

In addition, polarographic determinations of oxygen tension, changes in cerebral blood flow, pH, etc., may be made, to demonstrate abnormally functioning areas of the cerebral cortex.

During craniotomies, especially for epilepsy, the neurosurgeon has the opportunity of recording directly from the cerebral cortex under a number of conditions. Although the findings may be of limited surgical value, they may provide an insight into the physiology of the cortex.

There is no doubt that the surgeon who attempts to expand the borders of electroencephalography is able to obtain much more information than one who uses the technique only sporadically.

2. Clinical medicine and the neurosciences discuss the value of clinical neurophysiology.—**H. Gastaut (Marseilles, France).**
The topic director of this session has access to information on the activity of all the Clinical Neurophysiology services in the city of Marseilles available to the specialties represented here. In order to simplify the task of the neurologist, psychiatrist, neurosurgeon, pediatrician, general physician and psychologist who have to give their opinions on the value of Clinical Neurophysiology to their specialties, the director has supplied them, in an introductory report, with data concerning:

—the annual number of requests for EEGs in Marseilles from 1947 to 1967.
—the distribution of these EEGs amongst the specialties requesting them.
—the ratio of requests between public health service doctors (hospital staff) and doctors in private practice.
—the approximate value of the information supplied by the EEG for each of the requesting specialties.
—the number of Clinical Neurophysiology examinations, other than EEG, requested annually in Marseilles.

As these facts result from assessing *all* recordings carried out during 20 years in all the Clinical Neurophysiology labs in a city of a million inhabitants, they have the advantage of great homogeneity. Their analysis leads to the following conclusions:

I EEG is by far the most often used Clinical Neurophysiology method.
 a) In the public service the EEG is used especially
  1—by neurologists and neurosurgeons who have used it faithfully for 20 years and always expect the same information from it: principally the diagnosis and therapeutic management of attacks, mainly epileptic; secondly, the diagnosis of all cerebral disturbances particularly tumoral, vascular and infectious.
  2—in internal medicine where the EEG is used more and more to assess the cerebral effects of visceral or metabolic disturbances.
  3—by pediatricians who increasingly call on the EEG both for neuropediatric problems and for cerebral effects of visceral or metabolic disorders.

4–psychiatrists, however, rarely use the EEG.

b) In private practice, the EEG is used particularly by general practitioners for neurological problems in adults and children with which they feel able to deal without specialist help. These problems comprise mainly the diagnosis of attacks which are cerebral or thought to be so, and the assessment of consequences of benign cranial trauma (in an attempt to make objective the post traumatic subjective syndromes).

II After EEG, gamma-encephalography is the most often used Clinical Neurophysiology method. This is carried out only in the public service, although requests come from private specialists as well as from the hospitals, for investigation of cerebral tumors.

III Echoencephalography is used less than gamma-encephalography, which indicates a very small interest in this easily applied method.

IV Polygraphy is used a great deal by the neurologists mainly for studying the pathology of sleep and the myoclonic syndromes.

V Radio-isotope clearance, which has only been in current use for less than six months in the public service, has had some success with neurologists and neurosurgeons studying cerebrovascular disorders.

VI Stereoencephalography is restricted to some very specific neurosurgical procedures. Recording of average evoked potentials with summation methods is scorned by clinicians who see no practical value in it.

3. Electroencephalography in the study of sensory thresholds.—E. N. Sokolov (Moscow, U.S.S.R.).

Electroencephalography as a science and specific method can be used in psychology for the study of learning, attention, sleep and wakefulness, individual differences and, finally, for the investigation of detection and recognition of signals.

The response consisting in a blockade of the alpha-rhythm is very helpful in the study of thresholds—a classical problem in psychology.

In the study conducted by N. N. Korzh and myself the parallel recording of human EEG (occipital lobe) and EMG (flexors of the fingers) was used in the situation of detection of visual and acoustic signals of low intensity. Subjects were given an instruction to respond continuously throughout the perception of the signals. Because of the spontaneously emerging intersignal EEG and EMG responses, the complete record was used for an evaluation of probabilities of hits and false alarms according to the criteria characterizing the EEG and EMG responses. Due to the weakening of visual stimuli, the probabilities of hits of the EEG and EMG responses decreased. The latencies of these responses increased in such a way that the beginning of the EMG activity became more and more postponed as related to the beginning of the blockade of the alpha rhythm. The duration of an aftereffect measured from the moment when the signal was switched off up to the end of the reaction increased with a weakening of the stimuli, too. The latencies of the EMG responses and the durations of the aftereffects were linearly correlated.

An instruction to respond by making a fist only to the signals which equalled or exceeded the intensity of the standard stimulus presented beforehand, did not modify the psychometric function based on the EEG responses. At the same time the psychometric function based on the EMG responses was shifted toward more intensive signals in respect to the given standard one. Thus, the decision-making threshold was increased up to the level of standard stimulus, without a modification of the threshold of an analyser. The latencies of the EEG responses were not modified. Those of the EMG responses increased for the signals close to the standard stimulus. This increase was so large that they assumed the corresponding values for previously threshold signals. The duration of the EMG aftereffects for the same signals remained unchanged, however.

Analogous phenomena complicated by a habituation of the EEG responses were observed in the case of the measurement of auditory thresholds. During the extinction of the EEG responses to all intensities an increase of the EEG responses to the signals with the values close to that of the standard one was evident.

A model for the sequential analysis of the signals perceived by a subject is suggested as an explanation of the obtained data.

Having the threshold of an analyser (indicated by the EEG responses) already reached, the signals reach as well a decision-making threshold (indicated by the EMG), kept in memory as a trace of standard stimulus. The latencies depend upon the time required for the sequential analysis used in detection and decision-making processes when the background excitation (noise) is transformed into excitation evoked by the stimulus (signal + noise). The duration of an aftereffect is determined by the sequential analysis employed by the subject in detection and decision-making processes in a situation when the excitation is replaced by the background activity. When the threshold of the decision-making is close to the threshold of an analyser, the latencies of the EMG responses and durations of the EMG aftereffects are equal. If the decision-making threshold is artificially elevated, the latencies of the EMG responses increase since the subject now compares the "signal + noise" with the memory trace evoked by the standard stimulus. The durations of the aftereffects did not increase because of the very pronounced differences between "signal + noise" and "noise" in the subject's decision-making system.

The evaluation of the data showed that the EEG responses are influenced by three main types of excitations arising in the CNS during the handling of information: energy effect, which depends upon the stimulus intensity; novelty effect, depending upon the expectancy of stimulus; and discrimination effect, which is proportional to the difficulty for the decision-making in the verbally controlled responses.

The study of single unit responses in rabbit showed that the mechanism of threshold responses could be represented by neural networks comprising the intensity and novelty detectors.

4. The future of clinical neurophysiology.—W. G. Walter (Bristol, G.B.).

The future of Clinical Neurophysiology is as intricate as its clumsy name, since it is bound up with the other disciplines engaged in brain research, and also with the structure and evolution of human society. The possibilities of this latter relationship are particularly bewildering since the more significant and effective our efforts the more we may hope to influence the social mechanisms within which we operate. We may explode into a new world force or collapse into a vestigial technology.

We also share with other young sciences the embarrassment of having outgrown our strength. In spite of the inspired and dedicated efforts of our organisers, our corporate structure could be described as gangling—a term which is only phonetically related to the ganglia in our heads. At whatever cost we must find better ways of exchanging discoveries and opinions; our contributions should, as it were, be rectified and integrated on-line so as to achieve some sort of mutual amplification. Between us we have spent several million dollars to meet together here and this is the scale on which we must think, both in our technical operations and in our efforts to transcend the barriers of language, pride and indolence.

Clinicians, Computers and Charity are essentials for brain research. Clinicians, because the pressure of human misery is needed to fire our imagination, Computers because we have always used them, in our simplest amplifiers or in the most elaborate calculating engines, Charity because we depend on taxes or private generosity to promote innovation.

As Clinicians become more adventurous and more confident, so our functions in the clinic develop fresh responsibilities and demand intense technical and ethical exploration. The gruesome task of assisting in the definition of death is complemented by the even more delicate duty of deciding what sort of lives are worth living. The pride of doctors, surgeons and scientists in their new-found ability to manipulate the human organism evokes a corresponding prejudice against interference with "natural" processes. We must share with our colleagues both the pleasure of achievement and the discomfort of popular suspicion. When molecular biologists learn how to control human heredity, the relation between genetic and neural coding may well become the most explosive issue we have ever had to face.

As technical advances make computing machinery more accessible and elaborate, we shall have to solve the same problems of redundancy and re-deployment that are disturbing industry and commerce. The intimacy of contact between men and machines can be exciting or embarrassing; as they absorb more of our talents, it becomes more difficult for us to look through our artefacts rather than at them. Delegation of human faculties to machinery tends to turn experiments into tests by extracting assumptions from hypotheses. We can already see the danger that our exploratory urge may turn in on itself to become parochial, conceited and sterile.

The forerunners of the instruments we must learn to control were designed for the destruction, not the enlightenment, of our fellow-men. "War is the father of everything", of our money as well as our machines, whatever the nominal structure of our society. Our future depends on the continuation and intensification of conflict, but our duty is so to enhance respect for the electric jelly in our heads that no human can be alien to us. We have won our spurs in skirmish with human ailments; now we can claim our rightful place in the decisive battles with the obscure and sinister contradictions in human nature.

5. Properties and activities of dendrites.—D. P. Purpura (New York, N.Y., U.S.A.).

The morphological characteristics of dendrites of mammalian neurons are determined in part by the nature and origin of presynaptic pathways and intrinsic genetically controlled events. The latter operations are demonstrable in the case of basilar dendritic growth of neurons in isolated immature neocortex. Presynaptic influences are illustrated in the bizarre alterations in cerebellar Purkinje cell dendritic morphogenesis following extensive destruction of the granule cell-parallel fiber system of the molecular layer. Disturbances in synaptogenesis have important consequences for dendritic function as evidenced by the development of excitability characteristics which are not ordinarily encountered in immature Purkinje cells.

Important clues to special activities of dendrites may be derived from knowledge of the predominant distribution of major afferent projections to dendrites. In a number of neuronal organizations in which intracellular studies have been correlated with light and electron microscopic investigations, evidence has been obtained that powerful axodendritic excitatory synaptic inputs may initiate partial or all–or–none spikes in dendrites. These recent findings are considered in respect to the generally accepted views of dendrites as passive receptor surfaces for linear and non-linear summation of postsynaptic potentials (PSPs). The latter hypothesis has been amply confirmed and extended as a result of a large number of intracellular studies in adult animals. From these investigations it is evident that axodendritic PSPs exert their major effects on neuronal excitability by electrotonic extension to low threshold impulse generation sites in the initial axonal segment–axon hillock region. Spikes initiated in these regions exhibit variable invasion of proximal dendritic membrane as inferred from characteristics of post-spike delayed depolarizations and conditioning effects of soma–dendritic EPSPs. The "single impulse trigger site" hypothesis is central to the Rall dendritic compartment model whose application to problems of spinal motoneuron, olfactory bulb and neocortical pyramidal cell PSP interactions has greatly advanced analysis of the location and functional consequences of different axodendritic synaptic inputs.

Intracellular studies of immature neocortical neurons suggest that passive membrane properties of dendrites are acquired during postnatal ontogenesis. In these elements in which axodendritic synapses constitute the major mode of excitatory afferent engagement suppression of primary impulse trigger sites by prolonged IPSPs or induced membrane hyperpolarization may result in a shift of impulse initiation to dendrites. Under these conditions orthodromic spikes may be generated which lack characteristic depolarizing prepotentials. Axodendritic EPSPs which trigger dendritic spikes are frequently not detectable even under conditions of strong membrane hyperpolarization sufficient to block somatopetal spikes of dendritic origin. Particularly clear examples of this are found in fish oculomotor neurons in which vestibular nerve stimulation elicits axodendritic EPSPs and spikes which lack depolarizing prepotentials. Such spikes are not blocked by hyper polarizing currents threshold for suppressing spikes generated by other afferent inputs.

Partial and all–or–more spikes in dendrites are demonstrable in hippocampal pyramidal neurons after brief tetanization of axodendritic synaptic pathways. However, abnormal states of excitability are not prerequisite for dendritic spiking in hippocampal neurons or other elements such as thalamic and mesencephalic reticular neurons. In the case of specific thalamic neurons dendritic spike initiation occurs in response to powerful axodendritic synapses effected by lemniscal or brachium conjunctivum projections which terminate largely in relation to dendrites of VB or VL thalamic neurons, respectively. Partial dendritic spikes may also be observed in VL neurons during and following prolonged low–frequency stimulation of lenticular outflow pathways. Such alterations in dendritic excitability provide a mechanism for facilitating transmission in pathways with predominant axodendritic synaptic inputs. Additional examples of local dendritic spike initiation are to be seen in reticular neurons and cerebellar Purkinje cells of some lower vertebrates. The capacity for spike initiation and propagation in dendrites greatly expands the repertoire of neuronal behavior and introduces complexities in neuron modeling that have not as yet been sufficiently appreciated or explored.

6. Somatic sensation: transfer and processing of information iii spinal cord.—M. Hugon (Marseille-Saint-Jerome, France).

The grey dorsal spinal and (medullary) substance forms a neuronal relay in which the somatic sensory message is deeply changed before its transfer in the ascending pathways. This transfer mainly depends on the spinal organization and supraspinal centers. A few points should be emphasized:

1. *Dorsal horn regions are characterized by specific structures.* The *gelatinosa substantia Rolandi* (GSR) is an association of radial sheets. Differently, cells of the transitional lamina IV have a three-dimensional dendritic tree. Cells of the lamina V and VI belong to transverse elementary chips. Detailed analyses suggest anatomical opportunities for pre- and post-synaptic phenomena. Cervical nuclei and medullary grey also have a particular organization.

2. *Specific neuronal structures exhibit specific neural activities.* GSR generates the depolarization of primary cutaneous and some other axons (PAD) and the correlated pre-synaptic inhibition. The lamina IV is a relay between specialized cutaneous afferents and the spino-cervical tract, and/or the lamina VI. The lamina V cells exhibit a particular sensitivity to the thin myelinated axons

from skin, muscle or viscera. The lamina VI receive in-put from articular and probably muscular afferents too. Ascending pathways in the anterolateral quadrant apparently arise from these lamina V and VI.

3. *Spinal activities are under control from supraspinal centers.* PAD can be elicited by descending fibers from vestibular, ponto-medullary or post-central cortical areas. From post-central area also proceeds depressive post-synaptic spinal control, through pyramidal pathways.

Rather from pre-central areas proceed excitative effects on the lamina V and VI. These controls seem to act through reflex loops.

4. Two general ascending somesthetic pathways arise from spinal relays. The "lemniscal" ascending pathways should especially be topic and has modality specificity. The "extra-lemniscal" system should be diffuse, nonspecific and deeply involved in nocioceptive sensitivity, affect and alertness.

Processing sensory information in spinal cord relies on increasingly clear anatomical arrangement and synaptic properties. Description of related patterns of neuronal activities, by both physiology and mathematical tools, is another way to elucidate the principles of sensory information. Understanding supposed general principles in sensory processing and special understanding in somesthetic discrimination are two close targets in these studies.

7. Interest of electrophysiology in reanimation and resuscitation.—F. H. Bostem and M. L. Lamy (Liège, Belgium).

Reanimation and resuscitation have been, in the last ten years, a subject of exceptional interest and expense. This resulted in the conception and realization of the modern "intensive care units".

As a result, the caricatural frontier who still in the early 50's shared life and death, progressively became less clear, creating a gap of undefinition.

This needed more or less arbitrary definition.

A report of R. Naquet in this congress will deal with the criteria of death. Consequently in turn, life must receive a satisfactory definition for our field.

Legally and medically we now agree that cerebral irreversible functional exclusion is a sufficient and necessary criterion of death. We thus must conclude that life is characterized by an efficient cerebral function; it is:

—sensory data acquisition.

—sensory pattern recognition and processing.

—reaction.

It appears thus that every effort devoted to the maintenance of the principal phsyiological systems has no goal in itself, but the preservation of the brain functions, every physiological main system having to be considered as an ancillary of the master cerebral function. In such a situation, the numerous involved methodologies in the field of reanimation must be given an order of priority.

I *Physiologic survey:*

Every main physiologic system (cardiovascular, pulmonary, metabolic, etc.) is submitted to a survey to maintain its function within definite limits, by:

a) Direct survey of the parameters:

This presents no other difficulty than a good choice of transducer and adaptation.

We must however point out that in such a survey, human vigilance may fail particularly when extensive periods of duration are required. It may even become dangerous, and the development of some automatic alarm system was soon necessary. This unfortunately results in numerous false triggering by erroneous data acquisitions (*e.g.*, transducers mismatching). Some improvements were necessary:

1) Progress is now achieved by performing an autocoherence and cross-coherence index between the main parameters (pulse rate, temperature, arterial blood pressure, photoelectric sphigmogram). This avoids alarm triggering by a transistory shift of a single parameter, and improves the reliability of the system, but involves simple real-time data processing.

2) Starting from the alarm point, the information available to the physician, should be dramatically evident. It is a necessity for him to know not only the present situation but also to appreciate the characteristics of evolution in the past few moments. As a result, temporary or permanent memorization of the main parameters appears as a necessity just like their possible display at any time. Thus, special techniques of recording must be conceived.

3. In some applications, particularly when conclusions have to be extracted from the complete evolution of some patients, continuous recording is done. However, in such cases, only few epochs of limited duration were significant. Human analysis of such recordings is possible but often results in the same unsatisfactory and unreliable results as by direct survey.

Extraction of significant patterns of data may require automatic data processing.

b) *Survey of indirect data:*

In some cases, a first data processing yield original and significant data. For example, cardiac output measurement until now was practically impossible in a permanent clinical use. Recent research has demonstrated that a close value could be obtained by complex processing of the averaged plethysmogram (electrically measured) combined with the isomorph ballistocardiogram.

II. *Cerebral function survey:*

The brain is generally considered as the most precious organ we have. We must also consider it as the most sensitive transducer we possess, the functional analysis of which gives priceless information about integrated physiological functioning.

a) The spectral density of electrical brain activity discloses sensitive variation with almost every change of the main parameters.

The spectral density may be visually appreciated by a well-trained electroencephalographer, but his availability for each patient is uncertain. Real time analysis by small computers performing the "Fast Fourrier Transform" offers a better solution.

b) The brain reactions to sensory stimulations (evoked potentials) are sensitive to most pathological situations, *e.g.* anoxia. Averaging allows the detection of those activities, but only experienced neurophysiologists can extract the significance of the observed changes in the pattern, thus limiting its clinical application.

A more sophisticated approach would consist of data reduction with display of patterns of limited complexity, easily recognizable by less specialized physicians, *e.g.*, integrated chronograms or topograms.

8. Evolution of clinical neurophysiology since Hans Berger, the past 40 years of EEG.—W. A. Cobb (London, G.B.).

The term "clinical neurophysiology" can be made to include human experimental EEG studies but precludes more than passing mention of the vast fertile investigation of the animal brain. Though we are rightly honoring Berger's achievement of 40 years ago, for most of us the EEG began in 1934 with the paper by Adrian and Matthews and we should not forget that it was in that same year that Bremer was working on his paper on the *cerveau* and *encéphale isòles* of the cat, which was the starting point for so much of modern cerebral physiology.

In fact we could go back a few years further to recall that Bartley and Bishop in America, Fischer, Kornmuller and Tönnies in Germany, Adrian and Buytendijk in England and others elsewhere had recorded the spontaneous and evoked activity of mammalian brains during the early 1930s.

1934 brought not only the Adrian-Matthews paper but the beginning of EEG work in a number of countries, including that of Jasper at Brown, of Forbes and his colleagues at Harvard, of Fessard in Paris and, of course, of Fischer and Kornmuller in Berlin. Within a remarkably short space of time the first clinical fruits began to come in and by the coming of war in 1939 most of the major topics had already been attempted. In retrospect, the observations of that time, thirty years ago, have for the most part survived remarkably well the more sophisticated appraisal of later years. Looking now at the records of those days one can only wonder that the authors extracted so much valid information from their often crude and usually limited records.

Here in America it seems that the War only slowed developments, whereas in some of the countries of Europe they came to a standstill. Its ending brought a tide of young men looking for an interesting carreer, surplus apparatus to be used by the ingenious and great advances in technology. By 1947 old laboratories were rejuvenated and new ones were multiplying.

This year was momentous. Through the initiative of Grey Walter and others the First International Congress was held in London. Small, amateur and impoverished by today's standards it brought together for the first time many of those who were to play leading roles in the next 20 years and during it were discussed the publication of a journal of clinical electroencephalography and the formation of an international society. By the second congress in Paris in 1949 Jasper was able to hand over to the International Federation of Societies, which was there set up, the ownership of the Journal which he and a devoted band of colleagues had already brought into being.

The growth and perfecting of clinical EEG has been steady, if unspectacular, since that time, still unfortunately deriving little from the new knowledge of how the brain works and still almost wholly empirical—therein lies the hope for the future. An exception perhaps might be made of the study of human and animal sleep, where interaction has been close and fruitful.

On the other hand, experimental EEG has taken on a new look in the past 20 years, stemming mainly from the proposal of Dawson in 1951 for the extraction of small signals from a larger random background. While variations of this technique are everywhere in use the older methods of analysis and quantification of the EEG are giving place to new, which the computer has made possible. Where, if anywhere, this will lead it is still too early to say.

9. The work of Hans Berger.—P. Gloor (Montreal, Canada).

As a scientist, Hans Berger was heir to the thinking of the 19th century German psychophysical school made famous by Fechner, Wundt and others. His search for the electroencephalogram of man was motivated by his desire to find a physiological method that might be applied successfully to the study of the age-old problem of the relationship between the mind and the brain. Berger's entire scientific career was oriented towards the elucidation of the psychophysical relationship in terms of principles that would stand the acid test of natural sciences and would not have to rely upon vague philosophical or mystical principles which will forever remain beyond the grasp of scientific understanding. During his early career, Berger attempted to study psychophysical relationships by plethysmographic measurements of changes in the brain circulation of patients with skull defects. Later he investigated temperature changes occurring in the human brain during mental activity and the action of psychoactive drugs. However he became disappointed by the dearth of psychophysical understanding generated by these investigations.

He therefore turned to the study of the electrical activity of the brain and, in the 1920s, set out to search for the human electroencephalogram. He believed that the electroencephalogram at last provided him with a physiological method capable of providing insight into mental functions and their disturbances.

He first set out to prove that the electrical oscillations he succeeded in recording extradurally from skull defects or from the intact skull indeed represented electrical signals generated by the brain, rather than by muscles, blood vessels or some other extracerebral source. Undaunted by the numerous critics who were unwilling to accept the carefully assembled evidence in favor of the cerebral origin of the oscillations he had discovered, he then addressed himself to what had always been foremost in his mind, namely, the investigation of psychophysical relationships by means of the electroencephalogram. He demonstrated the electroencephalographic correlates of attention, as represented by the arrest of the alpha rhythm and the modification of the electroencephalogram by general anesthetics, hypoxia and hypoglycemia. He investigated the electroencephalographic changes induced by pathological conditions affecting mental functions such as epileptic seizures and structural brain lesions. In the course of these studies he was the first to propose a physiological model of attention and conscious perception based on verifiable physiological observations. In the course of his studies on this subject he developed what is probably the first physiological model of such modern concepts known today by the terms of "surround inhibition" and "signal–to–noise ratio". He was also the first to prove the correctness of the Jacksonian hypothesis that clinically observable epileptic manifestations result from excessive discharge of brain tissue in an area related to the function involved in the clinical seizure.

Berger conceived of the electroencephalogram as a rhythmic sequence of activity cycles of large groups of cortical neurons. He believed that this activity was controlled by a regulatory center in the upper brainstem region, presumably in the thalamus. He attributed the manifestations of sleep, generalized epileptic seizures, anoxia, barbiturate anesthesia and hypoglycemia to an interference with the function of this hypothetical thalamic regulatory center.

Although many of the specific concepts which Berger elaborated in his papers are now dated, his thoughts on the physiological interpretation of the human electroencephalogram and on its relationship to the integrated function of the brain as a whole are still fascinating today. We have to admit that many of the questions he asked himself with the greatest insistence still remain unanswered and represent a challenge for future investigators in this field.

10. Clinical neurophysiology and neurological practice.—R. P. Schmidt (Gainesville, Florida, U.S.A.).

Neurological diagnosis may be compared roughly to the "black-box" experiments of electronics. Through the neurological history, mental and physical examinations, the neurologist makes inferences with respect to function and structural integrity of the organ within the cranial box. The greater the number of actual measurements, the more highly refined the diagnostic process. Aside from the physical and psychological examinations performed by the clinician, there are few tests which directly reflect the dynamic function of the brain. The electroencephalogram provides such a measure, and the information derived from its proper study continues to be improved through application of computer techniques of analysis, and by continued research in clinical correlation, and by advances in activation techniques. In clinical neurological practice, the electroencephalogram has achieved such status so that in many of the types of disease states it is indispensable and the examination of a patient cannot be complete without it.

Several of the major areas of usefulness of electroencephalography to the neurologist are:

1) The diagnosis of epilepsy and the differentiation and definition of the anatomical and physiological substrates of the various seizure types and syndromes.

2) The detection or confirmation of organic pathological processes or structural lesions involving the brain.

3) As a monitor of brain function in a variety of conditions which alter cerebral function. These include such examples as infections and drug administration.

In clinical neurology the electroencephalogram is used as a dynamic tool. It provides a record of the course of disease and information of prognostic and therapeutic value may be derived from an interpretation of changes which take place with respect to time and in correlation with the patient's evolving symptoms and signs.

In this paper, the value of the electroencephalogram to the neurologist will be emphasized through demonstration of the types of information which can be obtained through its proper application. Emphasis will be placed upon electroencephalographic examination in the epilepsies and in organic pathological processes either localized or diffuse. In addition, the types of information which may be developed by the clinical neurophysiologist for increased value to neurology will be discussed. The clinical neurophysiologist must continue in the development of new ways of examining old information and new ways of clinical neurophysiological testing. These will include the application of computer techniques of quantification and comparison, the study of averaged sensory evoked responses, polytest correlations and more accurate behavioral monitoring. In the United States, most of the electroencephalography is performed by physicians who devote only part of their time to it. These individuals can and do perform adequately but will in the future be called upon increasingly to become more than electroencephalographers. They must become clinical neurophysiologists in the true sense of the term.

11. Somatic sensation: transfer and processing of information. 1. Peripheral receptors.—E. R. Perl (Salt Lake City, Utah, U.S.A.).

A premise concerning specificity of sense organ response is fundamental to any theory correlating receptor activity to modality of somatic sensation. For cutaneous sense, early arguments favoring the concept that excitation of a given receptor leads to a particular sensation came from psychophysical observations indicating the presence of separate punctate regions for touch, warmth, cold or pain. The advent of electrophysiological techniques made it possible to obtain a direct indication of the way in which sense organs transmitted information about the stimulus. Following the pioneer efforts of Adrian, analyses based upon discharges recorded from single primary afferent fibers have shown that the somatic receptors exhibit systematic differences in their responsiveness to various stimulus types and parameters. Considering the common use of electrical stimuli as a means of exciting primary afferent fibers, it must be pointed out that their conduction velocity and therefore, electrical threshold do not reliably indicate the functional characterisitcs of somatic afferent units.

A major attack on the link between cutaneous receptor mechanisms and sensory experience has come from recent experiments comparing the effects of equivalent stimuli (vibration or tactile pressure) upon receptors in monkey and perception in man. The correlation between stimulus intensity and subjective experience on the one hand and stimulus intensity and the discharge of certain receptors on the other has been found to be similar, implying that a given set of receptive characteristics are closely tied to sensory modality.

Periodically, it is emphasized that the role of receptor activity is least clear in mechanisms associated with pain. The fact that electrical excitation of slowly-conducting myelinated or unmyelinated fibers of peripheral nerves causes pain or pain-like responses in both man and animals is well established; however, most studies of receptors with slowly-conducting fibers have reported many low-threshold (responsive to weak stimuli) units and few, if any, types demanding strong stimulation (high-threshold). The absence of convincing data on specific nociceptive elements led to hypotheses assuming that intense stimulation causes unusual patterns of activity in low-threshold sensory units and so initiates "pain reactions". During the past several years, new data has clarified this picture, beginning with the demonstration that a significant proportion of cutaneous receptors with slowly-conducting myelinated fibers in the cat and monkey stemmed from mechanoreceptors requiring intense to frankly damaging stimuli for liminal excitation. In these species, such high-threshold mechanoreceptors are the only sensory elements with myelinated afferent fibers capable of signalling the difference between innocuous and noxious mechanical stimulation. When the receptors of unmyelinated (C) fibers from hairy skin were similarly surveyed for responsiveness to noxious stimuli, a large fraction were noted to have elevated thresholds for thermal and/or mechanical stimuli. The most common high-threshold unmyelinated units respond well to more than one kind of noxious stimulation, including elevated temperature, marked mechanical distortion and chemical irritation. Moreover, these polymodal nociceptors exhibit a persistent enhancement of sensitivity following activation by heat, reminiscent of certain hyperalgesias. In contrast, a number of other C fiber receptors are easily excited by weak mechanical stimuli, and do not convey activity which distinguishes gentle from damaging stimuli. In the face of such evidence, concepts of pain mechanisms must presume activation of "nociceptors" as an essential step.

These two examples indicate that in the somatic senses, as in others, the particular kinds of receptor activated by an environmental change represent a crucial part of the code indicating the nature of the stimulus.

12. Clinical medicine and neurosciences discuss the value of clinical neurophysiology.—S. Thieffry (Paris, France).

Our purpose is to identify and specify the contribution of clinical electroencephalography to pediatric practice, with respect to diagnosis, prognosis and treatment. This work summarizes the experience acquired for the past 20 years in General Pediatrics, Neuropediatrics and Child Reanimation.

Our study deals only with infantile "convulsions" and epilepsy without extending to other organic brain diseases which may lead to epilepsy (infections, tumors, malformations, degenerative diseases).

We shall examine the most positive aspects: 1) Outline of the precise limits of epileptic seizures in child. 2) Clinical and electroencephalographical semiology of the seizures especially in young children before the end of cerebral maturation. 3) Isolation of some specific syndromes. 4) Reconsideration of the problem of infantile convulsions and epilepsy. 5) Possibility of brain damage arising after delayed seizures and importance of the *status epilepticus* in Neuropediatrics.

1) Convulsive seizures must be formally distinguished from other acute seizures: cerebral fits caused by anoxia, ischemia, asphyxia, psychic fits. The clinical diagnosis has to deal with: accidental falls, syncopal falls, sleep fits, disorders of consciousness and vigilance, disorders of behavior, vertigo fits, spasms of sobbing in the infant.

In such instances, the EEG appears frequently as indispensable. Let us recall that a false interpretation of nonspecific anomalies of the EEG record, especially during sleep, can lead to a prognosis or treatment prejudicial to the patient.

2) In the outline of the pediatric practice, the EEG has permitted establishment of an elementary semiologic list of epileptical phenomena and in numerous instances a valuable electroclinical correlation.

Even if partial nonclonic seizures are less characteristic than in adult patients, especially in younger children, they nevertheless exist (inhibitory, adversive, sensory, vegetative fits).

On the other hand, seizures with generalized EEG expression are frequent and particular.

Grand mal tonic-clonic seizures are observed only from a certain age. In early childhood, there are pure clonic or pure tonic seizures or hypotonic seizures.

In the case of generalized or partial myocloniae, the polyspikes and the clinical event do not always synchronize.

The real *absence* (or *absence petit mal*) presents such a characteristic tracing that the EEG acquires a particular value in distinguishing the real *absence* from the atypical one (spike, slow wave).

Particular attention must be directed to the frequency of unilateral seizures in children: directly hemigeneralized, partial or unilateral secondary generalized seizures, whatever their type may be: *grand mal,* tonic or clonic.

In newborns, seizures (to be distinguished from tremors) present very frequently an erratic clinical and electroencephalographical character.

3) A correlation exists undoubtedly between the type of the convulsive manifestations and the age of the patient. Furthermore, some cerebral diseases appear at a characteristic age with specific epileptic manifestations orienting to a clearly defined syndrome.

In newborns, the clonic generalized and particularly hemigeneralized fits prevail.

Around the age of six months, West's syndrome appears. Clinically, it includes flexor spasms and generalized psychomotor regression. The typical interictal hypsarhythmic EEG tracing is always present. Another particular aspect of this type of epilepsy is the marked effect of corticoids on the spasms and on the EEG pattern and a less complete effect of these drugs on the psychic development.

Around the age of three years, an epilepsy of particular type can be distinguished as the Lennox's syndrome: short tonic spasms and different types of *absences* with or without motor manifestations become more and more frequent (akinetic fits) while the child progresses no more and presents behavior disorders. The interictal tracing is rather characteristic: spikes and slow or very slow waves (described by Gibbs as *petit mal variant*).

This syndrome must be formally distinguished from *absence petit mal.* These *absences* rarely appear before the age of three years.

4) The pediatric tradition outlines the frequency of the "convulsions" in the infants and insists on their benignity. On the other hand, an interrelation between infantile convulsions and subsequent epilepsy undoubtedly exists. Finally, the very early beginning of epilepsy can be recognized thanks to the EEG.

The infant tends to react by an occasional convulsion to an exceptional or transitory situation: dehydratation, hypo- or hyperelectrolytemia, hypocalciemia, hypomagnesiemia, hypoglycemia, pyridoxine deficiency. In general, the prognosis remains good, unless correction occurs too late.

On the other hand, the prognosis of the recurrent febrile convulsions, whatever their origin may be, is far from clear. Even restricting consideration to the pure forms, the rate of subsequent cases of chronic seizures, though small, is nevertheless greater than the average rate.

For treatment and control of these patients, periodic EEG examinations are indispensable during the first years.

5) The pediatric practice discloses the particular frequency of the *status epilepticus* and its seriousness, especially in the three first years of life.

This is a possible complication of common infantile convulsions and especially of plain febrile convulsions. In fact, *status epilepticus* by its local cerebral effects (edema, damage due to anoxia) can cause death or can leave neuropsychic sequellae.

A most significant example is the hemiplegia consecutive to hemiconvulsive *status epilepticus* (Gastaut's HHE syndrome).

The treatment of the *status epilepticus* in spite of all the possibilities of respiratory, circulatory, metabolic reanimation, remains difficult. Continuous EEG monitoring remains the best criterion for treatment.

13. Somatic sensation: transfer and processing of information. iii. Spinal cord.—M. Hugon (Saint Jerome, France).

With the exception of the dorsal column system, ascending sensory information from the body undergoes at least one synaptic relay in the grey matter of the spinal dorsal horn or its medullary equivalent. The sensory messages from the primary afferent neurons are modified to a greater or lesser extent at these synaptic transfers depending upon the functional organization there and descending effects from supraspinal centers. Several concepts, derived from recent work, deserve emphasis:

I. *The spinal horn is characterized by specific structural arrangements.* Anatomically, the dorsal horn is formed by distinctive layers. The most superficial layer, lamina I, consists of sparsely distributed large cells with dendritic processes in the deeper cellular layers and an axon extending into the lateral column white matter. Laminae II and III, the *substantia gelatinosa* complex, cap the deeper layers with a sheet(s) of small cells while lamina IV is a transitional zone consisting of cells with dendritic tree extending up into the *substantia gelatinosa* as well as medially and laterally. Laminae V and VI contain neurons which seem to be part of a transversally oriented organization in contrast to the longitudinally arranged superficial layers. The structural features of the dorsal horn cells and the manner in which primary afferent and other synaptic connections are made to them suggest that opportunities exist for both presynaptic and postsynaptic interactions. Nuclei at the cervical level of the spinal cord and in its medullary extension also show a high degree of morphological specialization.

2. *Specific neuronal structures have specific functions.* Certain lamina I cells are excited only by nociceptive primary afferent fibers and may be part of modality-specific pain mechanisms. It has been argued that *substantia gelatinosa* cells (laminae II and III) are part of the process generating depolarization of primary afferent fibers (PAD), and thereby causing presynaptic inhibition. Lamina IV neurons have ascending processes in the dorsolateral funiculus (forming the spinocervical tract) and/or projections to deeper layers. Lamina V neurons are particularly responsive to activity in thin myelinated fibers from skin, muscle or viscera. Lamina VI receives input from certain articular (and probably muscle) receptors. Ascending fibers of the anterolateral quadrant apparently arise from cells of laminae I,V and VI.

3. *Spinal activity is under the control of supraspinal centers.* Depolarization of primary afferent fibers can be elicited by excitation of descending fibers of vestibular, ponto-medullary or postcentral cerebral cortical regions. To whatever extent PAD and presynaptic inhibition are related, such PAD indicates supraspinal influences on ascending sensory information as well as local spinal mechanisms. Postsynaptic depressive effects upon spinal cells also originate from cortical somatosensory regions and are mediated by axons traveling in the pyramidal tracts. In contrast precentral (motor) areas give rise to excitatory effects upon laminae V and VI neurons.

4. At least two general types of ascending activity for somesthetic processes are transmitted from spinal sources. One carries information coded for stimulus type and location and matches the characteristics input provided by the medial lemniscus to the ventral thalamus ("lemniscal"). The spinal trajectory of lemniscal systems may be

either in the dorsal or lateral column. A second kind of sensory information is provided by pathways without detailed differentiation for stimulus type or location. Such "extralemniscal" projections are presumed to be important for reactions and sensations associated with affect, alertness and avoidance.

Thus, it has become increasingly clear that sensory information processed by spinal systems is dependent both upon specific anatomically defined connections and upon synaptic interactions. So far, only a beginning has been made in deciphering how fluctuating activity in populations of neurons provide the basis of somesthetic mechanisms and further understanding undoubtedly will depend upon mathematical as well as physiological and morphological tools.

14. Advances in the design and implementation of automated techniques for hemodynamic measurements on patients.—M. H. Weil, R. Martin, J. H. Carrington, H. Shubin, E. Peterson and N. Palley (Los Angeles, Calif., U.S.A.).

In the past decade, experience gained from the investigation of hemodynamic defects during acute life-threatening illnesses have proven directly useful for clinical management of patients. The incentive for the availability of practical techniques of hemodynamic monitoring to support routine care of patients has been great. Yet it has proven to be a technically formidable undertaking because of the complexity of available instrumentation and the operational difficulties that are encountered in its routine use.

The physical restraint imposed by sensors and transducers, particularly by the cables with which they are connected to the remainder of the system, compromise access to the patient. The routine operation of commercially available amplifiers usually imposes a requirement for repetitive adjustment of five or more controls. The accuracies of the measurements themselves are limited by inconsistencies in technical operation, the variability of calibration standards, and the formidable procedures involved in error checking. These problems are magnified in the critical care environment in which the technical demands for operation of monitoring equipment is construed as competitive with the professional needs for superior patient care.

With the resources provided by an interdisciplinary team of physician-physiologists, engineers, and biomathematicians, major improvements in the operational design of a system for measuring intravascular pressures, electrocardiographic signals, and body temperatures was achieved. Sensors and tranducers were connected by short cables to an instrument island which was so constructed that access to the patient and mobility of the bed were retained. The transducers themselves were housed in movable receptacles so that their position in relationship to the body of the patient and the maintenance of their connection to the remainder of the system were optimized. Sizable electronic components were maintained in a remote position adjacent to, but without impingement on, the bedside area. All amplifiers were designed to have very low output impedances to minimize incompatibilities that would result from multiple inputs into a common data acquisition system. Full-scale values were standardized in all amplifiers and provisions were made to safeguard against short circuits and imperfect grounding.

With special reference to the blood pressure amplifiers, calibration adjustment is accomplished by two internal servo motors and servo loops. These serve to control valves which open the system to reference pressures which are applied to the transducers. Motor drive control relays are activated and these sense the completion of the calibration procedure. By these techniques, a zero reference pressure is translated into a zero voltage output and a reference pressure of 200 mm Hg is translated, by servo adjustment, to a 4V output. Since the pressure source had an inconsistency of only 0.1%, this simplified calibration procedure also provides notable improvement in accuracy of the pressure reference. The entire automated procedure is accomplished by the sequential depression of two switches, one for the zero reference signal and the other for the 200 mm Hg calibration signal. The amplifier is also provided with a test circuit which activates a light indicator in the event that the calibration procedure is not accomplished. The amplifiers are physically small and of modular configuration to allow clinical staff to conveniently exchange units in case of failure during the period of clinical use.

The electrocardiographic amplifier is completely isolated from ground and the patient circuit operates at a maximum of 6 volts. Again, only two controls are provided, a calibration switch and a lead selector. Comparable concepts are inherent in the design of amplifiers for measurement of temperature and for measurement of urine flow. Maximal ease of calibration, error checking methods and compatibility to data acquisition equipment are assured.

In its present configuration, these components were designed to operate as part of a larger and digital computer controlled patient monitoring system. However, the components of the system and particularly the amplifier designs which have been developed quite apart from their relationship to the computer serve as examples of designs by which operational simplification and error checking is achieved. Such simplification and insurance of reliability is an important goal if hemodynamic measurements are to be rountinely available at the bedside of the critically ill.

15. Somatic sensation: transfer and processing of information. Peripheral nerve.—A. Rosenfalck (Copenhagen, Denmark).

That peripheral nerves contain fibers with different diameters, thresholds and velocities of conduction has been known since the pioneer work of Gasser and Erlanger. Their finding has been confirmed in man in excised human nerves most recently by Lambert and Dyck.

Only in man can the different groups of fibers be related to perception. Heinbecker found that a stimulus strong enough to evoke pain was sufficient to activate the fibers as small as those conducting at 25 m/sec but not the smallest fibers conducting at 1.5 m/sec. Collins stimulated and recorded from the exposed sural nerve in man. The largest threshold (A α and β) subserved touch and strong tapping, and the small fibers (A Υ and C) subserved pain.

We have addressed ourselves to the problem: how many fibers are activated by an electrical stimulus at threshold strength, and what is their size, or conduction velocity? To this purpose we have delivered electrical stimuli to the fingers, the method first used by Dawson, and have recorded the potential from the median nerve with needle electrodes placed close to it at the wrist, elbow and the upper arm. The number and the diameter of the fibers in the median nerve were measured histologically, and the potentials evoked by threshold and by supramaximal stimuli were constructed. As a result we could deduce that the potentials evoked by supramaximal stimuli (average 20-40 μV) originated from fibers conducting at 30-60 m/sec (5-12 μ) with components (0.1-0.4 μV) from fibers conducting at 10-30 m/sec (2-5 μ).

The number of activated fibers fell out gradually as the stimulus current was diminished with no abrupt change at threshold. When all random stimuli could just be felt, the potentials had amplitudes of 0.1-0.15 μV and originated from 3-6 fibers conducting at 30-35 m/sec (5-12 μ). None of the stimuli were perceived when the current was 10% below threshold, and at half threshold strength the potentials were from one or two fibers.

Hensel and Boman recorded from single fibers in the exposed nerve of man and delivered mechanical stimuli, and they concluded that the mechanical stimulus required for a threshold sensation is of the same order as that which evokes a single potential in a single fiber. Hence, the fibers we found could be activated by current below sensory threshold may be proprioceptive. That few fibers suffice to convey the threshold is consistent with the experience in patients that touch may appear unimpaired even when 99% of the fibers are lost. Denny-Brown reported a case of sensory neuropathy with anesthesia in whom some cells remained in the dorsal roots. We have recorded the action potential in a similar case and found 1% intact fibers despite the anesthesia, the remaining fibers may have been proprioceptive.

That few fibers suffice to mediate touch at threshold was confirmed during recovery from local anesthesia. We blocked the median nerve, and measured the sensation of touch, two-point discrimination and of electrical stimulation and the action potentials evoked by supramaximal stimuli. The first fibers which recovered gave potentials similar to the response in normal nerve at threshold. The log amplitude of the potential was plotted against the log sensory threshold during recovery. The slope of the curve for electrical stimuli was 4, close to the slope of Steven's plot of perception of electrical stimuli against stimulus strength. The slopes of the curves for touch were much lower, 0.3 in our and 1.1 in Steven's subjects.

Sears and McLeod recorded potentials evoked from the nerve by tapping the nail. Knutsson and Widen recorded the potentials elicited from single fibers by striking the skin or moving the joint. Both methods open a possiblity of recording the response of peripheral nerve to the adequate stimulus and relating it to perception.

FREE COMMUNICATIONS IN EEG

1. Cerebral vasomotor responses to stimulation of the posterior hypothalamus and mesencephalic reticular formation.—**C. Sterman-Marinchescu (Bucharest, Rumania).**

Simultaneous recording of central retinal artery (CRA) and femoral artery pressures have been made in spinal and intact cats during electrical stimulation of vaso-pressor areas in the posterior hypothalamus and mesencephalic reticular formation. Changes in CRA pressure independent of femoral artery pressure changes have been observed. During stimulation in intact animals, even with very weak stimuli, CRA pressures rose with the appearance of EEG desynchronization but femoral artery pressures only increased by 16%. Stimulation in spinal animals produced similar central responses but peripheral pressor effects were suppressed.

From these results the possibility of a direct influence of the areas stimulated on cerebral circulation will be discussed. The existence of vasomotor neurones in the posterior hypothalamus and mesencephalic reticular formation suggests that these structures may act as part of a cerebral vaso-motor reflex system. It is also possible that effects on the cerebral vessels are mediated through vaso-motor fibers in the cranial nerves.

2. Interseizure activity in the EEG of patients with grand-mal epilepsy.—**A. Kreindler and G. D. Popescu-Tismana (Bucharest, Rumania).**

The purpose of the work to be presented has been to examine the EEG changes in patients with clinically confirmed *grand-mal* epilepsy. From 100 randomly selected patients changes in normal background patterns, effects of overbreathing and photic stimulation, appearance of paroxysmal patterns, possible focal origins of epileptogenic discharges and reactivity of the patterns were studied.

In 31 patients the EEG was within normal limits and in 22 typical *grand-mal* patterns were seen. Of the latter, only 68% showed paroxysmal anomalies as well. In 78% of patients alpha activity was present, in 59% theta activity and in 18% spike-wave discharges. The appearance of spike-wave discharges superimposed on background activity or between paroxysmal anomalies was frequent in patients whose epilepsy had appeared in the first two decades of life (15 out of 18 patients).

The most frequent paroxysmal anomalies were grouped spiked discharges (50%), theta waves (24%) or high voltage isolated spikes (22%). Anomalies in the delta band were very infrequent.

Cortical focal origin of paroxysmal discharges was demonstrable in 41% of cases, although clinically the attacks commenced as generalized convulsions. In 29 of these cases the focal origin was in the rolandic area with grouped spike discharges the most characteristic anomaly in 27. In 12 other patients the focal origin was temporal and in 4 patients parieto-occipital.

It is noteworthy that there appear to be no definite relations between age, duration of disease, seizure frequency, total number of seizures or the EEG findings.

3. Contribution of "vertical" montages to the interpretation of routine EEG recordings.—**L. Sorel (Uccle-Bruxelles, Belgium).**

The results to be discussed are based on simultaneous bipolar longitudinal and transverse recordings with a "vertical" recording using the neck as a reference. By this technique one can establish if the reference electrode is active or inactive. A standard EEG machine can be used provided the pens write on recti-linear coordinates and are exactly aligned. All recordings in this work were made on a 24 channel Schwarzer EEG.

The spike-wave discharge never affects the neck electrode and one may consider the "vertical" montage as truly monopolar for (typical or atypical) spike and wave complexes. It is possible to establish the potential gradients with great precision and measure time differences as short as 5 msec when using paper speeds of 200 mm/sec.

With spike activity, bipolar montages may hide patterns demonstrable with the "vertical" montage. With the latter it is possible to differentiate between spike fields which remain negative and those which are simultaneously positive in some areas and negative in other areas. The former are related to organic focal lesions whereas the latter are presumably of a functional nature.

The use of the "vertical" montage as a referential technique will avoid errors of interpretation of the distribution of the background rhythm that occur with conventional bipolar montages. The background (or dominant) rhythm originates normally in the parieto-central areas. It may extend towards the frontal poles or the occipital poles and then influence the neck electrode. The forward and backward displacements are related to certain organic or functional conditions.

4. The influence of partial bilateral fornicotomy on auditory evoked potentials.—**J. Ungher, R. Rogozea and S. Sirian (Bucharest, Rumania).**

In an earlier paper, we reported that bilateral

hippocampal lesions in cats induced important alterations in the orientating reaction to auditory stimuli. At the first presentation of a prolonged tone the EEG showed a generalized desynchronization with absence of theta activity in the hippocampus. Habituation was also more delayed than in controls. Similar changes have been noted after bilateral fornicotomy.

To estimate the effects quantitatively following fornicotomy, cats with partial chronic bilateral lesions in the *corpora* and *columnae fornicis* were tested with paired clicks at 300, 500, and 1000 msec intervals. The EEG responses were recorded from the right and left median ecto-sylvanian gyrus and the dorsal hippocampus with silver or stainless steel insulated electrodes. The electrodes were placed under oscilloscopic control and electrolytic or mechanical lesions were made in the fornix from the stereotaxic coordinates of the Atlas of Jasper and Ajmone Marsan.

After recovery from the operative procedures, the evoked potentials to the paired stimuli were of larger amplitude and shorter duration in the control cats than in those with the fornicotomy (150-200 vs. 50-60 μV and 200-300 vs. 300-500 msec).

Morphological differences were also found with the control animals showing overt spikes and the damaged animals rounded waves often lacking the negative or positive phase. Also in the damaged animals, the second click failed to produce an evoked potential especially when the interval between the pairs was less than 500 msec. The changes between control and damaged animals are statistically significant.

The functional implications of hippocampal-neocortical relationships through the fornix will be discussed.

5. Polygraphic investigations of sleep in patients with ischemic cerebro-vascular disease.—I. Popoviciu, I. Pascu, B. Asgian, and C. Sipos (Tirgu-Mures, Rumania).

During sleep periods lasting eight hours continuous recordings were made of eye movements, the EMG and the EEG on 20 patients with cerebro-vascular insufficiency. Seventeen patients had basilar artery and 3 had carotid artery insufficiency.

Of the 17 cases of basilar artery insufficiency 4 had intermittent changes, 6 had bulbar or bulbar-pontine syndromes, 2 had penduncular syndromes, 2 had subthalamic syndromes, and 1 each had a thalamic syndrome, akinetic mutism and bilateral posterior cerebral artery thrombosis. Disorganization of the various phases of sleep appeared as well marked increases or decreases in the REM stages. A variety of anomalies of EEG activity also appeared sometimes only in certain stages of sleep.

The changes in sleep behavior and EEG activity from continuous polygraphic recordings will be discussed and related to the anatomico-clinical aspects of lesions of the brain stem and thalamus.

In the 3 cases of carotid artery insufficiency changes in organization of sleep behavior and EEG activity also appeared particularly when the temporal lobe was involved. These changes will also be discussed.

6. The transmission pathways of acoustic stimuli to the anterior sigmoid gyrus.—O. Sager, V. Florea-Ciocoiu and V. Nestianu (Bucharest, Rumania).

Single acoustic stimuli (clicks) evoked electrical potentials in the anterior sigmoid gyrus in 9 animals with bilateral topectomy of the primary auditory areas. Slight individual variations in latency of the responses appeared in the animals, of which 4 were with and 5 without chloralose anesthesia. Histological examination showed bilateral retrograde degeneration of the medial geniculate body indicating that acoustic stimuli in these animals could only be transmitted to the anterior sigmoid gyrus by extrageniculate pathways.

In 18 normal animals clicks evoked potentials in the anterior sigmoid gyrus whether chloralose was injected (5) or not (13) but a wide variability of latencies appeared. Single electrical stimuli to the medial geniculate body evoked potentials in the anterior sigmoid gyrus but with only slight latency variations. Stimulation of the midbrain reticular formation evoked potentials in the anterior sigmoid gyrus both in normal animals and those with bilateral topectomy of the primary auditory areas. These experiments suggest that in normal animals stimulation of the medial geniculate body is transmitted to the median ectosylvian gyrus and from there to the anterior sigmoid gyrus by two pathways: a cortico-subcortico-cortical pathway with a long conduction time and a cortico-cortical pathway with a shorter conduction time between the medial geniculate body and the anterior sigmoid gyrus. On the other hand, acoustic stimuli may also be transmitted to the anterior sigmoid gyrus by a third extrageniculate pathway starting in the midbrain reticular formation.

7. Lithium and the EEG: an analysis of behavioral, biochemical and electrographic changes.—G. Johnson (New York, N.Y., U.S.A.).

This study was designed to investigate the effect of the lithium ion on the electrical activity of the brain using the scalp EEG, following acute and chronic administration, and the association, if any, between EEG and behavioral change. Changes in electrolyte metabolism occurring with lithium, and the relationship of these to EEG changes were also analyzed.

Ten patients were selected who were either receiving lithium as part of a double blind controlled evaluation of lithium and chlorpromazine in manic states, or who were undergoing investigation of electrolyte metabolism during lithium administration.

A 16-channel Grass EEG was used and the EEGs were analyzed visually by two electroencephalographers, one of whom was blind to the medication the patient was receiving.

Acute administration of 750 mg of lithium carbonate did not produce any significant changes in the EEG or in behavior 1½ h following ingestion. Chronic administration of lithium carbonate at doses from 1 to 2.5 g per day produced EEG changes in 70% of the patient group.

These were characterized by decrease in the dominant frequency and an increase in amplitude. On two occasions, a decrease in responsiveness of the alpha rhythm was discernible. No focal or paroxysmal activity was induced. All cases showing EEG changes manifested toxic effects predominantly of central nervous system type. Serum levels of lithium ranged from 0.846 to 2.8 milliequivalents per litre in this group. EEG changes were not associated with behavioral changes. Patients without toxic symptoms did not show changes in the EEG although blood levels ranged from 1.12 to 1.73 milliequivalents per litre.

No consistent alterations in serum sodium, potassium or magnesium sufficient to account for the changes in the EEG or toxic symptoms were observed, although individual fluctuations in electrolyte balance occurred.

These findings will be discussed in relation to the mode of action of the lithium ion in manic depressive illness.

8. The electroretinogram, visual evoked potentials and spike discharges in the visual cortex of the albino rat.—M. Ebe, I. Hamma and Y. Ishiyama (Tokyo, Japan).

Experiments were performed on albino rats lightly anesthetized with intraperitoneal urethane. Their weights ranged from 50 g in young animals to 200 g in the adults. The electroretinograms (ERG) were recorded from a silver ring electrode attached around the edge of the cornea and when of small amplitude the signal was summed 30 times by an averaging computer. The visual evoked potentials (VEP) recorded with the animal in the dark were led from area 17 by a micro-electrode inserted successively from the surface to the deep layers of the cortex. The VEP was summed 30 times by the averaging computer and for both the ERG and VEP a Xenon strobe light was used to stimulate the responses. In certain cortical layers spike discharges on the VEP were recorded photographically from an oscilloscope and on magnetic tape. This permitted interval histograms of the spike discharges to be made. The EEG was recorded to check that the VEPs were taken during the waking state.

The amplitude of the "a" plus "b" wave of the ERG was under 100 μV even in the young rats and became smaller with increase in age. In the adult the "a" wave was particularly difficult to discern even with increased stimulus intensity.

The VEP from the surface of the cortex generally consisted of a positive followed by a negative deflection as a later component, with or without an initial small negative deflection as the early component. Peak latency and amplitude varied from animal to animal. When the microelectrode was inserted into the cortex the early component became more conspicuous and at 1 mm spike discharges superimposed on it. Peak latency of the early component shortened as the stimulus intensity was increased but the frequency of the spike discharge was not always increased although the unit discharges in the lateral geniculate body are the cause of the spikes.

9. Modification of sensation evoked by skin stimulation during CNS stimulation.—J. Gybels, F. Peluso and P. Cosyns (Leuven, Belgium).

In the lemniscal system, descending inhibitory influences have been demonstrated with stimulation of the reticular formation, the ventral anterior vermis, the precentral motor area, the post central and secondary sensory areas and the anterior cingulate area. In the extralemniscal system caudate nucleus stimulation inhibits ascending nonspecific sensory activity. In the experiments to be described an attempt was made to find out if in conscious man, stimulation of these structures would modify touch or pain sensation.

In 7 patients with Parkinsonism the finger was stimulated through 1 mm diameter bipolar electrodes with 300 msec trains of rectangular pulses (80 p/sec, 3 msec duration). The stimulus strength for touch was 0.11 mA (S.D.=0.04) and for the threshold of pricking pain 0.53 mA (S.D.=0.13). A method was developed permitting computer calculation of the electrode position in the brain and determining the trajectory to reach two target areas with one insertion. The CNS structures were stimulated monopolarly with 10 sec trains of rectangular pulses (5 or 50 p/sec, 1 msec duration). The maximal stimulus strength was 2.0 mA. The subjects were asked to compare identical skin stimuli before and after CNS stimulation.

The results of the experiments showed that: 1) no difference in touch or pain sensation was reported after stimulation of the precentral or postcentral cortex, the corpus of the caudate nucleus, the n.L.P. or n.V.L. thalami, 2) stimulation of the cortex posterior to the sensory areas, while not eliciting paresthesiae, caused diminution of sensation of the skin stimulation and 3) after stimulating the n.V.P. thalami the subject reported paresthesiae and there was a diminution of the sensation of skin stimulation for up to 500 msec.

10. The differential effects of minor and major tranquilizers on digital computer sleep prints and REM.–T. Itil (St. Louis, Mo., U.S.A.).
To answer the question of whether the effect of minor and major tranquilizers can be better discriminated with digital computer analyzed resting EEG, sleep EEG, or REM activity, various studies have been carried out in chronic schizophrenic patients with single as well as chronic oral administration of compounds. Both the resting and sleep EEGs have been analyzed using digital computer period analysis and the sleep EEGs have been classified according to the "sleep print". The length of the REM periods as well as the number of samples with single and burst REM activity have been evaluated by visual means.

Our studies indicate that the evaluation of REM periods or REM activity is not discriminative in determining the drug effect. The length of sleep stages, evaluated through computer classification, gives more reliable information about the type of drugs. While minor tranquilizers increase deep sleep stages, the major tranquilizers, particularly those effective in chronic schizophrenics such as haloperidol and fluphenazine, decrease the deep sleep stages. The problems involved in sleep studies of chronic schizophrenics and the clinical means of evaluating the physiological findings will be discussed.

11. Alterations in quantitative EEG and behavior during smoking deprivation.–G. A. Ulett (St. Louis, Mo., U.S.A.).
Because of our interest in the relationship between EEG and behavior and because of recent publications concerning cigarette smoking, this study has been carried out to evaluate the effects of smoking withdrawal upon the brain function as reflected in both the quantitative EEG and behavior.

Thirty male volunteers who have been classified as heavy smokers were included in this study. Six different EEG recordings were taken for each subject: an initial adaptation recording, two baseline recordings in weekly intervals and the third baseline recording one week later, immediately prior to smoking deprivation; and another recording after 24 h of smoking deprivation, and a final recording after three cigarettes were smoked within a period of 10 min. During each recording, right occipital to right ear combination was analyzed for a total period of 10 min using both analog frequency analysis and digital computer period analysis. Various statistical procedures were applied to determine the EEG alterations during smoking as compared to the smoking deprivation period.

As seen in a previous pilot study which was carried out in a small group of young male volunteers, in this study also there were quantitative as well as qualitative EEG changes during the smoking deprivation period. In the group an increase of slow waves, decrease of fast activity, and increase of amplitude was seen during the smoking deprivation period. To resume smoking reversed these trends. The changes were more marked in subjects who exhibited various kinds of behavior symptoms due to withdrawal.

12. A moving topological display of the EEG.–T. Estrin and R. Uzgalis (Los Angeles, Calif., U.S.A.).
We have developed a new technique to automatically display topological EEG information as a motion picture.

An electrode helmet records 30 channels of EEG data. These signals are amplified, digitized at a suitable sampling rate, and stored on magnetic tape. The digital tape is processed by an IBM 360/91 computer to produce a series of contour maps. Each map is essentially a snapshot of the potential distribution over the area of head covered by the recording electrodes, at a known instant of time. The map is displayed on the cathode ray tube of an IBM 2250 graphics station. It is photographed by a modified movie camera under computer control to yield one frame of a motion picture.

Successive maps represent the voltage distribution at instants of time differing by a multiple of the sampling rate at which the EEG was originally digitized. Hence, a 2-sec alpha burst digitized at 100 samples /sec would produce 200 movie frames. If the film is projected back at the conventional rate of 24 frames /sec, a slow motion picture of the alpha burst is provided.

Representing the surface of the head on the plane of a tube distorts the head and information associated with it. This distortion is minimized by employing projection equations developed by cartographers to map the earth.

Our technique is being used to compare spatio-temporal characteristics of the alpha burst with the rhythmic after-discharge evoked by light flash in order to better discriminate the cortical areas involved. A short movie illustrative of this will be shown.

13. Regional activities within the human hippocampus.—M. A. B. Brazier (Los Angeles, Calif., U.S.A.).

The electrical activity and functional connectivities of the hippocampus have received considerable study in lower mammals but have until lately been less accessible in man. Yet the clinical need for some direct information about the relationship of the subcortical structures within the temporal lobe to the activity at the temporal convexity is paramount in some cases of epilepsy and especially in those being considered for therapeutic surgery.

The electrical signs of temporal lobe epilepsy require an understanding, not only of the anatomical pathways established by post-mortem studies and the impairment produced by lesions, but also the electrophysiological connections demonstrable *in vivo*. In man, the studies have been scattered and the information derivable from them unclear. From current studies carried out in collaboration with Dr. P. H. Crandall and Dr. R. D. Walter of the Divisions of Neurosurgery and Neurology, it seems likely that some of the disparities may be due to profound regional differences within the morphological structure known as the hippocampus or Ammon's horn, consisting of the dentate gyrus and the hippocampal pyramids.

Several methods for studying regional activities of the human hippocampus will be reported. These include:

(a) response to sensory stimulation.
(b) response to electrical stimulation of the amygdala.
(c) coherence of on-going EEG activity in the hippocampus with that in the amygdala.
(d) coherence of on-going EEG activity between zones within the hippocampus.
(e) coherence of on-going EEG activity between the hippocampal gyrus and various zones within the hippocampus.

14. EEG changes in patients with metastatic carcinoma.—J. Dorazco-Valdes (Mexico City, Mexico).

From personal experience and reports in the literature it is known that both primary cerebral tumors and cerebral metastases cause EEG changes. It is also observed that EEG abnormalities can be found in the absence of cerebral dissemination of the tumor. We have collected a series of 21 patients of the latter type on whom one or more EEGs were taken under the suspicion that they had cerebral metastases. Although the group is small, some observations of interest were made.

All 21 patients had abnormal EEGs. Eleven showed diffuse abnormality, 8 showed asymmetric abnormality, 2 showed paroxysmal abnormality and one showed both paroxysmal and diffuse abnormality. Those patients showing diffuse abnormality presented qualitative and quantitative clinical changes of consciousness. Those with asymmetric abnormalities showed changes in motor function and those with paroxysmal abnormalities unconsciousness and convulsions. The average time interval between the appearance of clinical signs and the first EEG and then to death was 4 days for the former and 6 months for the latter. It was shortest in the group with paroxysmal abnormality who showed the most profound clinical changes but showed no abnormalities with other procedures and no evidence of cerebral changes at autopsy.

One patient with the paroxysmal abnormalities had transient improvement under treatment and one showed EEG abnormalities similar to those seen in the leucoencephalopathies.

The findings suggest that the metastatic process, special properties of metastatic cells or even the primary itself induces some metabolic or chemical changes related to the EEG abnormalities.

15. Sleep studies in depression.—J. Mendels (Philadelphia, Penn., U.S.A.).

We have studied the sleep patterns of 21 depressed patients on a cross-sectional basis and of six depressed patients on a longitudinal basis. The data obtained from the latter will constitute the basis for this report. The patients were studied for a total of 154 nights during hospitalization. This allowed us to plot changes in sleep patterns with changes in course of the illness and the administration of various therapies (drugs and electroconvulsive therapy).

Our initial findings of a very variable and diffuse disturbance of sleep in depressed patients were confirmed. In addition, the following significant observations emerged:

1. The disturbance in slow wave sleep was very severe (levels approximately 10% of normal values were frequently seen).
2. The disturbances of slow wave sleep tended to persist beyond improvement in other stages of sleep and beyond clinical remission in some cases.
3. The evidence from the sleep studies (together with other studies of neurophysiological function and depression) lead to the hypothesis that depressed patients have a state of central nervous system hyperexcitability in spite of the behavioral psychomotor

retardation frequently seen.

4. Sleep study on a hypomanic patient showed disturbances very similar to those seen in the depressed patients. In particular, there was a gross disturbance of slow wave sleep. This, together with other evidence, leads to the postulate that neurophysiologically and biochemically, depression and mania are variants of the same condition and not polar opposites.

16. EEG in arterial hypertension.—H. Mitschke (Berlin, W. Germany).

The paper is based on 4000 EEG records of 850 hypertensives, each record consisting of a routine mono- and bipolar registration followed by 3 min of hyperventilation.

In a statistical evaluation the following results were obtained: There are no specific changes of the EEG in arterial hypertension. However, patients up to 30 years with no other diseases than unstable essential hypertension, lasting for only one year and still untreated, differed significantly from a control group of healthy people of the same age, the patients showing less frequently a predominant regular alpha rhythm and more frequently an increased response to hyperventilation; different forms of general pathological findings also were observed more frequently in the hypertensive group than in the controls. A comparison between four groups of hypertensives classified with regard to clinical aspects and findings (complaints, level of blood pressure, cardiac, renal, retinal and neurological state) indicating various degrees of severity of the disease showed a significantly augmenting number of general and focal disturbances mostly in form of slow wave activity and evidently in relation to increasing cardiovascular and particularly cerebrovascular insufficiency. Besides these relations to the clinical aspects no significant correlation was found between EEG findings, level of blood pressure and duration of the hypertensive disease. The age of patients when hypertension was first detected, however, seems to have some influence on the development of the EEG disturbances. In most cases there was no significant difference in the EEGs before and after hospital treatment, in spite of definite clinical improvement, and in general no prognostic prediction could be made from pretreatment records with respect to improvement or impairment of the EEG under therapy.

17. Visual evoked potentials in prematures, newborns, infants and children by stimulation with colored light.—H. Fichsel (Bonn, W. Germany).

The evoked potentials by stimulation with red, green and blue light were studied in 256 prematures, newborns, infants and children. They were compared with the evoked potential to white light. A CAT 400 C was used as averager.

The evoked potentials by stimulation with light of different wave-lengths in prematures are identical in shape for each component. The shape of the evoked potentials by colored light corresponds with those of white light. In newborns, infants and children there are also no remarkable differences in shape and chronological sequence of each component of the evoked potentials by stimulation with colored light from those evoked by white light. The most striking and important change is the prolongation of latency compared with the evoked potentials by white light. The stimulation with red light shows a slight, with green light a moderate, and with blue light a considerable prolongation of latency. The prolongation of the latency is seen in all discernable deflections of the evoked potentials. The amplitudes of all deflections show a small reduction on stimulation with colored light in each age. From fetal to school age the decrease of latency for the evoked potentials to red, green or blue light runs parallel to that of white light.

The minor number of retinal cones in newborns and their following increase in the first 4-5 months of life does not result in a dissociated shortening of the latency by stimulation with colored light; *i.e.*, during the change from scotopic to photopic vision. The parallelism with the changes of latency by white light stimulation is preserved. It can be said that the increase of cones is not the decisive factor in the sudden shortening of latency during the first 2-3 months of life. Other factors such as the progresssive myelinisation, thickening of fibers, shortening of the transmission time of synapses, increasing number of dendrites and their connections in visual cortex must be responsible.

18. Cerebral commissurotomy in man: EEG findings.—L. B. Mann, J. E. Bogen, P. J. Vogel and R. Saul (Los Angeles, Calif., U.S.A.).

Patients with seizure disorders refractory to medication had section of the entire corpus callosum and anterior commissure at a single operation, in the hope of deterring the spread of seizure activity. EEGs before operation showed in most cases multiple foci, and in some there had been demonstrated over the years a progression from focal to generalized disturbances. Following operation new abnormalities appeared; these gradually regressed, the two hemispheres tending to follow separate courses of subsidence. In several cases the EEGs have become essentially normal, the patients continuing on medication.

19. Electrophysiological studies of the olfactory bulb in man—a model for EEG investigation. —J. R. Hughes, D. E. Hendrix and N. Wetzel (Chicago, Ill., U.S.A.).

The electrical activity from electrodes chronically implanted in the human olfactory bulb has been recorded to study coding mechanisms within this system and to provide a model for analysis of rhythms from the CNS.

Twelve patients were studied with four 120 μ diameter electrodes implanted in the bulbs. Activity was recorded on a Grass model 6 EEG machine and a Mnemotron FM magnetic tape system.

Many different odorants were introduced to the patients through a 2 channel olfactometer with appropriate controls and compensators. The electrical responses to the odorants consisted mainly of rhythmical, sinusoidal activity. This was analysed from tape loops continuously playing into a Heterodyne Wave Analyzer and the responses were plotted on an X-Y recorder. This method of analysis indicates that each odorant is associated with a distinctive set of frequency components.

The results have led to the Frequency Component Hypothesis, suggesting that the coding for odour quality is represented by specific frequency components. However, some components are common to different stimuli and this varies with the similarity of stimuli from the stereochemical and vibrational frequency mode aspects of the stimulus. The coding for detection of odour intensity appeared to be related to the amplitude of the different frequency responses.

The olfactory bulb is an example *par excellence* of reverberating feedback loops, especially onto the mitral cells and their projections. Granule cells possibly represent structures, functioning as a mechanism for recurrent inhibition and evidence exists for both a specific and non-specific projection system onto different portions of cortical and subcortical regions. The glomeruli of the olfactory bulb may represent structures analogous to the thalamus in its projection to the cortex and its control over cerebral rhythms.

20. Documenting the human fetal EEG during birth.—M. G. Rosen and J. Scibetta (Rochester, N.Y., U.S.A.).

The human fetal EEG has been a source of interest for many years. Studies have been infrequent and generally unsuccessful due to technical difficulties in attaching electrodes to the fetal head prior to birth. A successful system is presented for the study of the human fetal EEG continuously during labor with the use of bipolar scalp electrodes, isolated from the maternal environment, and screening out electrical artifacts present during this time.

The documentation of human fetal EEG demonstrates patterns and voltages analogous to those found after birth. The wave frequencies vary between ½-25 c/sec with a preponderance of slower frequencies in the theta and delta range. Alpha frequencies are occasionally seen. Voltages vary from 5 to 50 μV. The use of an auditory sound stimulus is used to average the fetal EEG and provide a fetal auditory evoked response. Brain wave tracings and evoked response studies are duplicated in the newborn for comparison.

The application of this technique as a method to study gross metabolic changes produced by drugs or by asphyxia is presented in a still preliminary way. As an example of this application the fetal EEG changes produced following maternal intravenous meperidine injection will be demonstrated. Further use of this technique may find more widespread application in the study of fetal brain stress incurred prior to and during birth and its relation to the later appearance of brain damage in infancy.

21. Intravenous diazepam (valium) as a deactivation test in epileptics.—E. Niedermeyer (Baltimore, Md., U.S.A.).

Diazepam (valium) was administered i.v. during EEG recording in 80 epileptics with good evidence of either focal or generalized spikes. Small amounts (2 to 5 mg in children, 5 to 10 mg in adults) were injected at a rate of 5 mg/min. Seven patients had implanted depth electrodes (frontal lobes, limbic structures). The reduction of seizure activity was graded: excellent, good, fair, marginal and no response.

Out of 20 patients with clinical evidence of Common Generalized Epilepsy (also called "centrencephalic" or "idiopathic"), six had an excellent, eleven a good, two a fair and one had no response. There were 13 patients with a severe type of childhood epilepsy characterized by slow spike-wave complexes (Lennox-Gastaut syndrome); one had an excellent, four a good, three a fair and five had no response. Most of the tracings with poor responses were characterized by prolonged slow spike-wave bursts. Forty-three patients had focal seizure discharges; one had an excellent, eleven a good, seven a fair, six a marginal and 18 had no response. Most of the patients with focal spikes and good responses were children (7 to 10 years). Six of the seven patients with depth electrodes feil into the focal category and showed no response. The remaining four patients formed a heterogeneous group.

There is good evidence that i.v. diazepam is most effective in the suppression of generalized-synchronous seizure discharges; it also acts strongly against focal spikes in children. These focal (predominantly central) spikes are generally regarded as unstable and likely to disappear in adolescence. Stable focal spikes, however, respond poorly to such small amounts and might require larger dosages.

It is felt that this de-activation test might provide us with new insights into basic epileptic mechanisms.

22. Statistical procedures for relating one or more dichotomous responses to maturation and electrophysiological measurements.—D. R. Jensen and R. Engel (Blacksburg, Va., and Portland, Oregon, U.S.A.).

Statistical procedures are developed for assessing the projective value of latencies of evoked neonatal photic responses with regard to such abilities as locomotion and phonation. Because of the dichotomous nature of the latter, individuals first are grouped according to photic latencies, whereupon standard statistical procedures are used for making compilations of the proportions among groups. Some discussion is given to the problem of grouping. In practice, however, the analysis usually is complicated further by the fact that the dichotomous responses are observed at different conceptional ages which necessarily influence the responses observed. A statistical procedure is described for preparing proportions among photic latency groups while accounting for differences in conceptional ages at time of observation. An iterative numerical process is required which adapts readily to electronic computations. The entire statistical procedure is discussed in terms of the analysis of co-variance, which it resembles in some respects.

Further statistical problems arise when two or more dichotomous responses are recorded for each individual, and then the corresponding proportions for all responses are compared among photic latency groups. Suitable statistical procedures are described, including the case when conceptional ages differ at time of observation. These procedures are constructed in such a way as to preserve separate conclusions regarding each type of response.

The statistical procedures are illustrated numerically by examples involving latencies and the dichotomous responses, locomotion and phonation. However, these procedures apply equally well to other electrophysiological measurements used for projective purposes in the case of dichotomous responses.

23. Effects of attention modification by television viewing on somatosensory recovery functions.—C. Shagass, D. A. Overton, G. Bartolucci and J. J. Straumanis (Philadelphia, Penn., U.S.A.).

Our previous studies of somatosensory recovery function have demonstrated consistent differences between psychiatric patients and non-patient controls. Amplitude recovery of early components appears generally reduced in patients. However, since many evoked response characteristics may relate to attentiveness, this factor could produce differences between patients and controls. The work to be described examined the effects of variations of attentiveness on the somatosensory recovery functions and also the relation between the EEG amplitude changes with attentiveness and the evoked response amplitude.

Somatosensory functions were recorded in 18 subjects employing five interstimulus intervals: 10, 15, 20, 50 and 100 msec. The measurements were made alternately while resting in a reclining chair with eyes closed and while watching television. EEG amplitude was measured with a Drohocki-type integrator. Evoked responses to median nerve shocks were recorded from three pairs of leads placed over the contralateral hemisphere.

Television viewing markedly reduced EEG amplitude in all subjects except those with low voltage fast records and the degree of reduction was highly correlated with the base line measurement at rest. No consistent changes in amplitude or latency of the evoked responses were observed from the primary area to early (to 40 msec) and late (to 80 msec) responses while television viewing. The data were also analysed to determine whether the degree of EEG change was correlated with changes in evoked response amplitude and recovery functions. No significant relations were demonstrated.

The demonstration that somatosensory evoked responses and their recovery functions are not significantly altered by changes in attentiveness suggests that patient-nonpatient differences in recovery are not attributable to differences in attention. Also, it appears that the relationship between the EEG and evoked response amplitude which holds for a group of subjects does not extend to the individual subjects in the waking state.

24. Influence of spontaneous generalized and focal temporal epileptic EEG discharges on the contingent negative variation.—R. Zappoli, M. Papini and P. Cabras (Florence, Italy).

Polygraphic research was undertaken to establish whether the so-called sub-clinical spontaneous generalized and focal temporal epileptic EEG discharges can negatively influence the particular condition of conscious attentiveness manifested in the EEG by the "expectancy wave" (CNV) which precedes determined operant responses. Twenty-three carefully selected epileptic patients were examined: 12 with generalized "centrencephalic" seizures, 11 with well localized temporal epileptogenic lesions. Eight of the 12 cases with "centrencephalic" epilepsy, on 18 different occasions, presented generalized paroxysmal discharges coinciding with conditional stimuli (clicks), or during conditional (CS) and imperative stimuli (US) intervals. It was especially difficult to establish whether these discharges can really provoke transitory suppression or clear disorganization of CNVs. Difficulties are due to these discharges masking almost completely CNVs preceding operant responses. As, however, on 10 occasions the discharges proved able to disorganize operant responses, it is presumable they also disturb somehow the "expectancy waves".

On the other hand, when focal epileptic discharges of temporal lobe origin casually coinciding with acoustic CS or CS-US intervals tended to be prolonged (3.5 sec) and assuming a pseudorhythmic course, but apparently sub-clinical and strictly localized, they sometimes provoked transitory suppression or considerable disorganization of CNVs and operant responses. This phenomenon was observed only in 3 of 11 subjects with temporal lobe epilepsy on 5 occasions. Interestingly, the inhibitory effect on the CNVs was particularly evident only in the hemisphere not involved by the epileptic discharges.

These results show that epileptic EEG discharges of certain duration, especially when focal in the temporal area, can sometimes negatively influence the "expectancy waves" and operant responses. Hence they should not be considered truly sub-clinical even though they do not produce an appreciable disturbance of consciousness or behavior. This particular effect appeared, however, less evident and constant than that produced by similar discharges, both generalized and focal temporal, on first-order conditioned responses as observed in previous research.

25. Binocular addition of the visual evoked response with different stimulus intensities in man.—L. Ciganek (Bratislava, Czechoslovakia).

High intensity and very dim flashes elicit visual evoked responses of different forms interpreted as foveal-cone and peripheral-rod responses. The increase in size from monocular to binocular responses to bright flashes was found to be only 42% on the average while the increase for dim flashes was 100% or more. The reduction of evoked response amplitude in binocular addition for foveal-cone responses to bright flashes is explained by the occlusion effect of cone signals projecting bilaterally to both hemispheres and converging on the same cortical neurons. Since the occlusion effect is absent with unilateral transmission of peripheral-rod signals, binocular addition of this case results in at least an increase of 100%. However, binocular addition of responses to dim stimuli results sometimes in an amplitude larger than the sum of the two monocular responses and this suggests the presence of some facilitatory mechanism.

26. Effects of experimental control of the hippocampal theta rhythm on learning and extinction in the free-moving rat.—J. A. Gray and G. G. Ball (New York, N.Y., U.S.A.).

Rats were chronically implanted with bipolar electrodes in the dorsal hippocampus and in the medial septal area. Records of hippocampal activity were obtained during acquisition and extinction of a running response for water reward, under continuous and partial reinforcement schedules. Changes in both frequency and amplitude of the theta rhythm were observed during performance of this response. It was possible to drive the hippocampal theta rhythm by low-frequency stimulation in the septal area and to block it by high-frequency septal stimulation. Driving of the theta rhythm during extinction enhanced exploratory behavior and increased the speed of extinction. Effects of driving the theta rhythm during acquisition of the runway response and of blocking the theta rhythm during both acquisition and extinction are also described.

In other experiments rats were subjected to electrolytic lesions of the medial septal area, permanently disrupting the theta rhythm. These lesions also disturbed the normal rhythmic movements of the vibrissae seen in the exploring rat and sometimes caused a pronounced septal irritability syndrome. The behavior of the lesioned animals during acquisition and extinction of the running response will be reported.

The reinforcing effects of theta-driving and theta-blocking, and the effects of sodium amobarbital on driving and blocking thresholds, have also been investigated.

27. Recruiting responses in the cerebral cortex produced by putamen and pallidum stimulation.—G. Dieckmann and K. Sasaki (Frankfurt am Main, W. Germany).

Repetitive stimulation of the putamen and pallidum at a frequency of 6-10/sec elicited incrementing responses in the anterior sigmoid gyrus. These responses were studied mainly by laminar field potential analysis. Characteristic features of the field potentials set up by the putamen and pallidum stimulation were similar to those evoked by stimulation of nonspecific thalamic nuclei and typical as recruiting responses. The possiblity of stimulating current spread to the internal capsule and some adjacent structures was checked by moving stimulating electrodes to those structures. When the electrode was shifted by 2 mm and situated in the internal capsule, stimulation with the same electrical parameters evoked augmenting responses in the cerebral cortex as identified by laminar field potential analysis.

The recruiting response induced by the putamen and pallidum stimulation was not so widely distributed as that by nonspecific thalamic nucleus stimulation, but concentrated mainly in area 6a of the ipsilateral hemisphere. Area 7, for instance, yielded recruiting responses on stimulation of the centrum medianum but not with that of putamen and pallidum. Latency of recruiting responses produced by putamen stimulation was about 30 msec and always several milliseconds longer than that on the pallidum stimulation; the latter latency was comparable to that of the response from stimulation of the centrum medianum. Intracellular recording from cortical cells in area 6a revealed EPSPs followed by IPSPs which were similar to those reported by many authors with stimulation of nonspecific thalamic nuclei. The electrophysiological results seem to indicate that the putamen and pallidum are intimately related with the nonspecific thalamic system as previously suggested on anatomical grounds.

28. The CNV phenomenon and selective attention.—R. R. Ellis (Omaha, Neb., U.S.A.).

The purpose of this study was to demonstrate a relationship between the CNV phenomenon and attention. Attention is conceptualized as an active process by which the organism facilitates or attenuates afferent input to higher CNS levels. In this experiment the presence or absence of the CNV was the independent variable. The CNV was manipulated by having the subject press or not press a thumb switch at the offset of 500 c/sec 36 db tone of 1000 msec duration (the "cue stimulus"). Amplitudes of the late components of the vertex response evoked by a "test stimulus" was the dependent variable, considered to be a measure of attention, which is consistent with considerable evidence in the literature.

Eighteen male university students were randomly assigned to 3 groups of 6 each, based upon 3 different test stimuli to which they were to be exposed. The test stimuli, differed from the "cue stimulus" on one of the following dimensions: (1) intensity, (2) quality (frequency), or (3) modality (visual flash).

The CNV was first developed or extinguished to the "cue stimulus". Each subject served as his own control and order of CNV presence or absence was counter-balanced. in 1/3 of the subsequent trials one of the 3 "test stimuli" was superimposed upon the "cue stimulus" 500 msec after the onset of the "cue stimulus."

A significant ($P<0.05$) increase in amplitude of a surface positive vertex wave approximately 180 msec following the "test stimulus" occurred during the presence of the CNV as compared with its absence for the group in which the test stimulus was a 500 c/sec tone of increased intensity. No significant changes in vertex responses were found in the other 2 groups.

The fact that the ER change is specific only to the "test stimulus" of identical quality to the "cue stimulus" is consistent with a selective attention process and inconsistent with predictions derived from general arousal or response mobilization hypotheses.

29. The effects on learning and memory of alumina-induced spike foci in the parietal region of the monkey.—A. M. Moffett, M. Driver, P. St. John-Loe and G. Ettlinger (London, G.B.).

It has been shown that aluminium hydroxide gel placed on posterior parietal cortex produces, in the monkey, a spike focus and an impairment of learning on tactile tasks given in the dark after surgery. However, there was no impairment of memory on comparable tasks first learnt before surgery. The present study investigated further the relationship between such spike foci and tactile learning and memory. In addition, the effects of continuous spike activity were compared with those following ablations of comparable areas of cortex.

Twenty-three rhesus monkeys were taught two tactile tasks following which 6 had aluminium hydroxide gel placed unilaterally on posterior parietal cortex. Four others were given unilateral posterior parietal ablations and 13 were left as controls. All surgical procedures were performed on the hemisphere opposite to the hand preferred during discrimination training. Scalp EEGs were recorded both pre- and post-operatively from all animals. Those with alumina gel applications developed spike foci at 3-8 weeks post-operatively. Both the animals with discharging lesions and those with ablations were impaired on learning and memory tasks when compared with control animals. However, impairment was more severe in animals with ablations than in those with spike foci. Histological examination showed variable cortical destruction in the posterior parietal regions of the animals with alumina applications. Thus the behavioral deficit in the group showing focal spikes might be attributed to cortical damage rather than to electrical abnormalities.

30. Protracted cerebral evoked potentials driven by rhythmic auditory stimuli presented at a slow rate.—W. T. Liberson (Hines, Ill., U.S.A.).

We reported in the past that in about 50% of normal individuals, presentation at a constant rate of brief auditory stimuli or mono-syllabic words every 5 to 30 sec is followed by a slow, positive deviation over the vertex region (ear reference electrodes). In some cases the expected stimulus is preceded by a negative deviation. In the present paper further data concerning this finding of a driven, protracted cerebral potential, elicited by rhythmic auditory clicks, with the stimuli occurring at a very slow rate (1/5 sec), will be discussed. We found this phenomenon present in nearly all subjects when this rate of stimulation was used. The interference of the artefacts from the skin galvanic activity and eye movements will be considered in detail in relation to the geometry of driven slow potentials. The relationship of this phenomenon to the expectancy waves of Grey Walter will also be discussed. The importance of this finding for time perception and time conditioning will be stressed.

31. Cerebral events related to real and imaginary stimuli.—H. Weinberg, W. G. Watler, and H. J. Crow (Bristol, G. B.).

The subjects used were primarily patients at the Burden Neurological Institute who were under treatment for obsessive and anxiety disorders. Intracerebral electrodes chronically implanted in orbital, cingulate and parietal cortex were used for recording.

We instructed subjects to guess whether or not they would hear a click (or in some cases see a flash or feel an electric stimulus). If they expected the stimulus they depressed a small lever to the right. If they did not expect a stimulus, they depressed the same lever to the left. Whenever a stimulus did occur it always occurred upon switch closure. Thus, there were four possibilities: expected and occurrence of the stimulus, expected non-occurrence, not expected occurrence, not expected non-occurrence. Switch closure was used to trigger a LINC 8 computer which separately averaged the EEG corresponding to the above conditions. Since the stimulus always occurred upon switch closure, subjects had a precise index of when the stimulus should occur, if it was going to occur, and could determine if their guess was correct. For each 3 successively correct guesses they received sixpence.

The results suggest the presence of a clear cerebral event when an external stimulus is expected but does not occur. Of particular interest is the similarity of these events to responses evoked by stimuli for it suggests that these potentials may reflect a memory process corresponding to the stimulus. A second observation is a large and long latency positive component (200-250 msec) which has been reported by others who have used related paradigms and scalp electrodes. It has also been seen in CNV experiments when the imperative signal carries discriminative meaning. We think this deflection might be related to the resolution of uncertainty. Finally, several observations suggest a shortening of latency when the subject makes a guess before the stimulus, as if the general level of cortical excitability is increased. This is further supported by the evidence of an expectancy wave preceding the response.

32. The averaged photopalpebral reflex in man. —K. Inanaga and E. Yamaguchi (Kurume City, Japan).

The orbicularis oculi muscle contracts reflexly to a sudden change in light intensity in the visual field. This response to a photic stimulus has been termed the photopalpebral reflex. The authors have investigated variations in the reflex using digital computer techniques on normal subjects and on patients with neurological and psychiatric disorders.

All subjects lay recumbent in a dark quiet room. The digital computer was connected to a photic stimulator in such a way that the program caused stimuli to produce a flash once every second. The bulb of the photic stimulator was placed 10 cm away from the eyes. Contraction of the palpebra was recorded from a transducer loosely placed on the center of the upper eyelid to demonstrate acceleration changes and from electrodes placed between the upper eyelid and the inside corner of the lower eyelid. The signals picked-up were amplified and then averaged by the computer. As a rule 100 samples were averaged and sampling time for each was 250 msec.

The photopalpebral response was found to have a close correlation with the level of arousal. As examples, mental activity, administration of stimulants and emotional excitation facilitated the reflex. On the other hand the reflex was inhibited by drowsiness and the administration of hypnotics. In various organic brain diseases, changes in the reflex were observed.

33. An EEG analysis using simple arithmetic.—G. H. Byford (Fornborough, G.B.).

The detail in EEG recordings may be examined by any of a variety of established techniques. Such techniques involve assumptions which for the EEG are sometimes easier to refute than to accept, and their use to analyse the gross characteristics of records may lead to complications which the results do not always justify.

The method described here establishes a numerical classification for the observable characteristics of EEG recordings, illustrates the time course of EEG changes and provides a series of statistical decisions whose significance will draw attention to "abnormalities". There is no attempt to provide a "diagnosis"; concise evidence is presented, but its medical or physiological significance remains a matter for experienced clinical or research opinion.

There are two basic premises:

1) It is easier to point to the normal EEG than to characterize quantitatively the abnormal recording.

2) Since the nature of the EEG is essentially statistical, only "significant"/"non-significant" results are necessary; additional numerical information does not alter that decision once the level of significance has been established.

The first allows one to discard "normal" results and to draw attention only to the significant or "abnormal". The second permits the storage of results in a yes/no form ideally suited to digital computers.

Results appear in two forms:

a) Continuous curves representing the amount of activity in the frequency bands of recorded channels.

and

b) A framework of computer words, representing statistical decisions based on histograms derived from measurements along each channel individually and between the same time span on different channels.

The process may proceed on-line or by high speed replay from magnetic tape; the immediate provision is for 8 channels. A parallel-serial hybrid computer is used; it has an analogue bandwidth of 20 kc/sec and a digital transfer rate of 250,000 samples/sec. The technique will be illustrated by the results of studies concerning the effects of brief profound hypoxia on the time course and spatial distribution of the EEG.

34. Evoked cerebral sensory responses in relation to ongoing EEG activity.–E. W. Poole (Oxford, G.B.).

The usual averaging method for extracting evoked cerebral responses to sensory stimulation tends to eliminate differences in the response which might be associated with moment-to-moment spontaneous EEG activity. It seems of interest to consider such possible interaction between evoked responses and spontaneous wave forms as a means of determining the significance of such wave forms in nervous system economy.

Methods have been devised to assess the average cerebral responses from peripheral nerve or photic stimulation in relation to various types of EEG activity (*e.g.*, arousal/encephalitic complexes) or to other electrophysiological events. Stimuli to a digital nerve or photic stimuli are applied continuously (1-4/sec) and later from magnetic tape recordings average responses are extracted for those stimuli falling before, during, or after selected recurring EEG wave forms. Averages are obtained for comparison for each successive stimulus member of trains (*e.g.*, of 16 stimuli) related to EEG events which have been selected subsequently. This process of "partitioning" from sustained stimulation can be applied to many types of event in the one record (*e.g.*, K complexes, sleep spindles, EKG), these events being identified visually and marked from usual ink records, unless sufficiently distinctive to be instrumentally self-recognizing (*e.g.*, the EKG).

In a case of subacute encephalitis in the waking state and sleep, somatosensory responses were found to be greatly modified during the complexes, being reduced and then enhanced, and photic responses were also changed. With arousal complexes in sleeping normal subjects, somatosensory responses were increased during such complexes; but the situation is less clear for photic responses. Further studies on sleep spindles and slow activity also favor some modulation of sensory responses in association with ongoing EEG events, but it is not yet certain whether all components are affected equally. Further studies should show if this is a general effect, or related to the particular type of stimulus and brain areas involved in the response and EEG activity respectively.

35. Cerebral evoked responses in epilepsy.–J. B. Green (Indianapolis, Ind., U.S.A.).

Previous studies of visually evoked responses (VER) in photosensitive epilepsy have been extended to include auditory and somatosensory evoked potentials. This paper will present the results of repeated examinations in several closely followed cases.

A 12-year-old girl with a family history of Huntington's chorea was admitted because of frequent myoclonic seizures. She was markedly photosensitive with a VER of 225 μV at the left occiput compared to values in normals which rarely exceed 20 μV. A remission occurred with a disappearance of spontaneous seizure activity; after lagging several days behind the clinical improvement, the VER dropped to 100 μV. With recurrence of symptoms one week later the VER had increased to 275 μV.

A 14-year-old boy has been followed for four years because of *petit mal* attacks. Complexes of spikes and slow waves were readily produced on the EEG by changing the room illumination, by speaking to or touching the patient. The VER was a complex wave form and was 210 μV. The auditory response (AER) to pure tone (2000 c/sec) measured 100 μV and resembled the VER remarkably in wave form.

The VER in many photosensitive epileptics is characterized by a large positive spike at 60-80 msec, best recorded at the occiput. A later negative component is often recorded over the temporal regions. This pattern is not invariable and in some patients there are prominent frontal waves.

In the second case described above the similar wave form and distribution of the response to both visual and auditory stimuli suggests a diffuse increase in excitability.

Photosensitivity may in some cases represent an abnormality more or less confined to the visual system, while in others may be part of a more generalized over-reactivity to all sensory modalities.

36. The relation of pre- and perinatal pathology to the adult EEG.—J. Volavka and M. Matousek (Prague, Czechoslovakia).

Mild non-specific abnormalities found in subjects who do not show any neurological signs or symptoms are difficult to interpret. This problem poses a particular challenge to electroencephalographers working with psychiatric patients. The purpose of this study was to assess what portion of the abnormalities in the adult EEG could be explained to be a result of minimal pre- or perinatal brain damage.

Eighty-five adults were studied (mean age, 27 years). Seventy-five percent of these subjects were psychiatric patients; 25% were symptom-free volunteers. Psychiatric, neurological and EEG examinations (using broad-band frequency analysis) were carried out on all subjects. Mothers of all subjects were interviewed. A questionnaire describing the pre- and perinatal pathology was used.

Visual evaluation of the tracings showed that EEG abnormalities occurred with significantly greater frequency in subjects whose mothers reported a complicated gestation and/or delivery. There was a significant positive correlation between the occurrence of low voltage recordings and reported birth weights. Automatic frequency analysis supported these findings. Moreover, this analysis revealed an increase of beta activity in subjects with reported pregnancy and/or birth complications. Prematurely delivered subjects had significantly slower alpha activity than other persons.

37. Findings of a study devoted to the analysis of averaged EEG responses to words and language.—G. Sherrard (Manchester, G.B.).

It is now quite possible to detect, record and measure averaged cortical (V wave) responses to messages recorded on sound-track tape. This could be useful in investigating deaf and language disordered adults and children. Evaluation of this procedure poses several problems:

1) How much of the averaged response has been produced by the message as a series of sounds of varying frequency? (*i.e.*, what is the effect of the meaning of the message, if any?)

2) If, as might be suspected, motivation has a strong bearing on the intensity of response, how can this be studied at the same time?

3) Procedures suitable for adults may be quite unsuitable for young children. How should the messages be modified?

4) What are the best controls?

The problems have been approached as follows:

1) A 64-word message, each word being approximately 250 msec long and separated by 2 sec from its fellow, is used to produce a V potential complex, and compared with the same tape wherein each word is reversed.

2) Students are used, and the message in (1) is the standard instruction for a CNV experiment. The CNV is used to monitor alertness, concentration, and motivation between forward and reverse messages.

3) The above procedure is tried with young, normally hearing children aged between 7 and 12 years, and compared with messages involving only the serial counting of numbers (*e.g.*, the spoken words "one" to "eight" repeated in eight groups, making 64 words).

4) Controls are produced by alternating words and their reversed equivalents in the message, and by randomizing this method of alternating. These two "message-stimuli" are compared with the straight-forward word-reversal described in (1).

The amplitudes and latencies of the responses in all these studies are compared and correlated.

38. EEG changes produced by heroin and methadone.—J. Roubicek, A. Zaks, and A. M. Freedman (New York, N.Y., U.S.A.).

Studies of the effects of narcotics on the EEG have been reported sporadically. The recent interest in methadone and its use in the treatment of heroin addiction provided an opportunity to examine the chronic effect of methadone and its interaction with acute intravenous heroin.

Intravenous heroin yields increased alpha abundance, slowing of alpha frequency, theta activity (occasionally in bursts) and occasional delta bursts. Periods of desynchronization occur.

Chronic methadone yields similar changes to which adaptation occurs after 2-3 months at dosages of 100 mg/day.

The behavioral and EEG effects of intravenous heroin after methadone vary with the dose of heroin (25-75 mg) and the time after last dose of methadone. The EEG changes often appear dissociated from the behavioral changes.

These observations will be related to observations of the percent methadone maintenance treatment of opiate addiction.

39. Semiological relations of the frequency and distribution of six and fourteen per second positive spikes.—Y. Shimoda, Y. Yoshino and K. Tanaka (Yonago, Japan).

Approximately 1200 patients have been registered in our clinics who showed "6 and 14/sec" positive spikes in their EEG. Some demonstrated clinical paroxysmal symptoms such as headache, abdominal pain, heart throbbing, dyspnea, emotional instability, rage, violence and so on. Others showed a wide variety of non-paroxysmal manifestations. There was no demonstrable indication in these patients which would suggest any macroscopic changes in the central nervous system.

The patients were divided into six groups according to the frequency of their spikes: those with spikes at 6/sec, with spikes at 7/sec, or with spikes at 8/sec, in each case with or without 14/sec spikes; those showing only 14/sec spikes, those having spikes of more than two of the 6, 7 or 8/sec frequencies with or without the 14/sec spikes, and those with spikes of other frequencies. The six groups of patients were compared with each other with respect to their symptoms or signs. There appeared to be no close correlation between the semiological features and the frequency of the positive spikes.

The distribution of this EEG pattern over the scalp was also analyzed. In over 30 patients the spikes appeared diffusely over wide areas during the course of clinical paroxysmal manifestations but were only recorded from one or a few areas when the patients were examined in paroxysms-free intervals.

40. Experimental studies on memory during slow sleep stages and REM stages.—K. Jus, A. Kiljan, A. Kubacki, T. Losieczko, H. Wilczak and A. Jus (Warsaw, Poland).

The authors have studied the correlation between the recall of external stimuli applied during different stages of sleep and the polygraphic patterns of reaction to these stimuli. Thirty healthy adults were used as subjects. Acoustic (verbal and non-verbal) stimuli lasting no more than 2 sec and of different intensities were applied during the slow sleep stages (II, III and IV) and during the REM stage with and without eye movements. The subjects were awakened after each series of stimuli in a given sleep stage and asked about the presence or absence of sleep and of dreaming. They were also asked to assess the duration of the period of sleep and the hour at which they awakened. They were also asked about spontaneous recall of the applied stimuli and recognition of stimuli presented in the awakened state.

In the evaluation of results a distinction was made between the reaction during the application of the stimulus itself and the polygraphic patterns after its application. The reaction during application of the stimulus was evaluated in terms of latency, EEG pattern, and interaction of vegetative (EKG, PGR) and EMG reactions. The polygraphic pattern after application of a stimulus was evaluated in terms of its structure and duration in order to test the consolidation hypothesis.

It was found that even with an activation pattern lasting over 1 min with alpha activity and vegetative and EMG patterns after the application of a stimulus does not implicate recall if an "arousal-awakening" pattern was absent during the stimulus itself. The presence of such a pattern does not, however, implicate full recall of the quality and content of the stimulus. The recall of stimuli during the REM stage is often changed with dream content or is even, perhaps, built into the dream itself. The difference in arousal patterns during the REM stage with and without eye movements was not found to correlate with the presence or absence of recall. A correct evaluation of the presence of sleep was observed more frequently after awakening from the REM stage while evaluation of the duration of sleeping and indication of the hour of awakening was correct more frequently after waking from the slow sleep stages.

41. Time interval histogram mode data processing of the alpha rhythm output integration.—S. L. Visser (Amsterdam, The Netherlands).

Use has been made of the method of output integration as originally described by Drohocki. For this investigation special attention has been given to the integration of the output of the alpha rhythm band of broadband frequency analysis.

The number of pulses released by the integrator is a measure of the amount of energy of the alpha rhythm band. The data of this output integration can be processed in two different ways:

a) by counting the number of integrator

pulses per 10-sec period and calculating mean and standard deviations.

b) by determining all time intervals between the integrator pulses and calculating mean and standard deviations.

A randomly selected group of 100 EEGs has been studied. The two parameters studied (coefficient of variation of the number of pulses per 10 sec and that of the time intervals) as a rule varied similarly. The coefficients of variation are either high in both categories or low in both categories (Kendall's rank correlation test, $p < 0.01$). However, this was clearly the case only for normal EEGs with an alpha rhythm of 10 c/sec. In borderline or abnormal EEGs with excess slow or fast activity in the background pattern and with a fast or slow alpha rhythm, this rank correlation was not clearly demonstrable. In all such EEGs, therefore, it is important to determine both parameters because they indicate different information.

42. Evoked responses of different sensory modalities in newborn infants.—A. Hrbek (Goteborg, Sweden).

The presented work is based on the examination of more than 200 premature and mature newborns. Visual, somato-sensory and auditory evoked responses (ER) were studied. Different averaging methods were used.

ERs were present in all the newborns including a premature of 530 g birth-weight (24 weeks fetal age). Visual ERs were most evident in the occipital region, but often present also in the other areas of the scalp. Differentiation between primary and non-specific components was almost impossible. In prematures the development of shape and latency appeared to be dependent on the maturity level.

The somato-sensory ERs consisted of a primary and non-specfic component. They differed from the visual ERs in topography, shape and latency. Primary responses were limited to the sensory projection (Rolandic) area, non-specific components were more widespread with a maximum at the vertex.

Auditory vertex ERs were almost identical to the late components of somato-sensory responses. Primary responses were not demonstrable.

The behavioral states (vigilance level) influenced the shape, amplitude and, to a less extent, also the latency of individual response components. The primary somato-sensory ER was more pronounced in REM sleep and in wakefulness, the late components, on the other hand, were more pronounced in slow wave sleep. Auditory ERs behaved like the late somato-sensory components. Visual ERs did not behave in an uniform way in all infants.

It is suggested that the ER may provide an important tool for studies of the development and the conditions of the nervous system in newborns. Preliminary experiences in infants with nervous system disturbances and also in adult neurologic patients indicate usefulness of ERs in clinical studies.

43. Somato-sensory responses evoked by tendon taps in normal adults and neurologic patients.—M. Hrbkova (Goteborg, Sweden).

Somato-sensory responses evoked by tapping muscle tendons were studied in a group of 6 normal adults and 4 neurologic patients. For response averaging a CAT 400B was used.

The evoked responses (ER) consisted of seven deflections, the first one negative. They were best observed in centro-frontal leads, the short latency deflections being more distinct contralaterally while the late deflections were more widespread. The ERs were similar to responses evoked by electrical stimulation of peripheral nerves described in the literature.

ERs to upper and lower extremity stimulation showed some differences. ERs to leg stimulation were often of simpler shape (fusion of waves 2, 3, and 4) and of longer (about 6 msec) latency. The average peak latency of the first wave was 16.8 msec from the arm and 22.7 from the leg.

Interesting findings in neurologic patients are described. In a case of a transverse spinal cord lesion without any clinical evidence of somato-sensory conduction from the legs, the ER could be determined.

Tumors in the somato-sensory cortical region caused a distinct suppression of the ER from the involved projection area.

In a patient with focal sensory epilepsy the ER in the area of the irritative lesion was markedly enhanced.

Although the group studied was small, the preliminary results are very promising. In accord with other observations, the ER may be very valuable for functional testing of some cortical areas.

44. Fourteen and six per second positive spikes in psychiatric patients and their sibs.—M. Pollack, R. Jaffe, M. G. Woerner and D. F. Klein (New York, N.Y., U.S.A.).

In spite of many studies, the clinical significance of the 14 and 6/sec positive spike EEG pattern in psychiatric patients is still doubtful. If this pattern were associated with psychiatric disorders, one would expect its frequency to be greater in patients than in normals.

The present investigation studied adolescent and young adult hospitalized psychiatric patients and their biological sibs in terms of the prevalence of, and patient-sib concordance for, the "14 and 6" pattern.

Seventy-nine consecutively admitted, primarily middle-class patients, (38 men and 41 women) aged 15-29 (median age 19) were compared with 100 sibs (55 men and 45 women) in the same age range. All subjects were given a psychiatric interview by two examiners prior to the sleep EEG. Twenty-nine patients were diagnosed as schizophrenic, 42 as personality disorders and 8 as neurotic or affective disorders.

On the basis of history and interview the sibs were rated as: normal (57), moderate psychiatric abnormality (31) and severely abnormal (12).

No difference was found between the patient and sib groups in the prevalence of the "14 and 6" pattern (24% for patients, 25% for sibs). There was no relation between the presence of "14 and 6" in sibs, and ratings of their psychiatric abnormality: normal sibs, 28%; moderately abnormal, 35%; and severely abnormal, 16%. The highest frequency was found in the subjects under 17 years old.

For the group as a whole, the presence of the "14 and 6" pattern in patients and their own sibs was not significantly correlated (r=+0.14). Separate analyses by sex indicated significant patient-sib concordance only for male patients and their male sibs (r=+0.60, p.<005).

The findings fail to provide evidence for ascribing clinical importance to the "14 and 6" pattern in psychiatric patients. It appears to be a maturational pattern with the highest frequency in early adolescence.

45. Cerebral impedography in cat, rabbit and cadaver.—S. Tachibana (Stanford, Calif., U.S.A.).

Recently, we have developed a technique of reconstructing the appearance of entire coronal sections of brain using impedance values of brain matter in cat, rabbit, and cadaver. Impedance is monitored constantly from parallel trajectories of probe insertions. The impedance signal from the roving electrode (platinum 0.1 mm diameter) driven at a constant speed is an input of intensity modulation (Z-axis) of oscilloscope, and electrode location (depth) is indicated by the Y-axis by adjusting beam sweep and electrode moving speed. Sequential profiles obtained from paralleled tracts are plotted on the X-axis (lateral) and the resulting image is photographed. The picture of impedography shows three factors, probe location (X and Y) and tissue impedance from all parts, as a function of light intensity. Impedography in living brain and dead brain (cat, rabbit) are basically similar, in the sense that the gray matter with half tone and the white matter with light tone are sharply contrasted, and both the configuration and the location of these tone differences are correlated to those observed in the histological section at the same site even in the brain stem. However, tissue impedance in the living brain is much lower than that obtained in brain postmortem, and occasionally detail changes in the impedography of living brain associated with physiological or pathological factors are appreciable. The multiple probe insertions produce no apparent damage to the animal. The experiments suggest that the method might be applicable to the study of pathological processes in restricted areas of human brain during surgical procedures.

46. Lithium effects on cerebral cortical function in manic depressive patients.—G. R. Heninger (New Haven, Conn., U.S.A.).

Although the lithium ion is known to be effective in treatment of certain psychiatric disorders, the cause for this is not known. A study has been undertaken to quantify cerebral evoked responses (CER) and EEG activity in 18 patients before and after beginning lithium treatment.

Two somatosensory (SER), auditory (AER) and visual (VER) evoked responses and two 17-sec resting EEG samples were obtained on these patients. Also SER recoveries were obtained on 12 patients and AER recoveries on 8 patients. Peak latencies and peak to peak amplitudes were measured for the CERs and 6 quantified intensity measurements obtained from spectral analysis of the EEG samples. Six of the 18 patients had a normal mood and it was possible to record data when the lithium was stopped. Four of the 12 manic and hypomanic patients were cooperative enough to allow numerous recordings and correlation made to objective ratings of behavior.

Therapeutic concentrations of lithium produced 1) increased amplitude and slowing of the EEG, 2) a consistent increase in amplitude of the early primary positive component of the SER, 3) variable increases in amplitude of late components of all CERs with minor latency changes, and 4) little alteration in recoveries of the SER and AER amplitudes. These electrocortical changes occurred 3-5 days after the serum lithium reached a level of 1.0 meq/1 or more, they persisted up to 2-4 days after stopping lithium with serum levels of nearly zero.

The magnitude of changes relate to lithium levels and they generally parallel symptom changes in mania. In the 4 patients studied intensively the changes occurred at the time specific behavioral changes occurred. Similar types of changes have not been observed with other psychotropic drugs and they highlight specific and unusual effects of lithium on cerebral functioning.

47. The EEG in anesthetized juvenile baboons during an experimental investigation of vitamin B_{12} deficiency.—**R. Harris (London, G.B.).**

The EEG has been studied in 39 juvenile baboons during a long term dietary experiment in which a Vitamin B_{12} deficient state is being induced. The weights were between 3.1 and 6.0 Kg. Eighty EEGs were recorded, all the animals had at least one record when they were without any known biochemical abnormality. In some, subsequently the level of B_{12} was beginning to fall but not to a deficiency level.

The records were obtained in the fasting state during anesthesia with Sernylan (phencyclidine hydrochloride: 1.5 mg/Kg i.m.). Needle electrodes were inserted and mainly bipolar recordings carried out.

Considerable fluctuations in the EEG features appeared to be related to the time of recording after the administration of Nembutal. These EEGs appeared to be somewhat different to the paroxysmal EEG activity described by Ellington *et al.* in adult baboons, although the medication was similar. It is possible that this is partly due to differences in recording technique and age.

The relationsip of chronic cyanide toxicity and vitamin B_{12} deficiency is also being examined in these animals following the clinical work of Monekosso and Wilson. No gross EEG changes have been noted after a period of a few months in the groups of animals tested. During acute cynaide tolerance tests the alterations in the simultaneous EEG were no more than could be explained by anesthesia alone.

In baboons, fluctuations of the on-going activity in relation to anesthesia may be important in evaluating results in various experimental situations.

48. Multichannel analysis of electrical fields of averaged evoked potentials.—**D. Lehmann and D. H. Fender (San Francisco and Pasadena, Calif., U.S.A.).**

The human average evoked responses measured on the skull are complex wave forms reflecting the underlying firing of many classes of neurons. A major challenge is the identification of components in the evoked responses, and the linking of these components with specific functions. Latency and amplitude have classically been used as descriptors of the components, although less subjective methods such as factor analysis are now gaining favor. However, much of the wave shape depends on the location of the generators in the brain with respect to the placement on the scalp of both electrodes of a differential pair. There is no proven indifferent electrode on the head. If we expect to find more than one active generator, an analysis of the electrical field on the scalp is necessary in order to determine the location and functional significance of the generators. A small number of electrodes does not allow adequate sampling of the spatial distribution of this field; *e.g.*, a minimum array of 5 by 5 electrodes is required if two generators are to be identified reliably.

We use at least 48 independent amplifying and recording channels. Analysis of the electrical field on the scalp is performed at intervals down to 1 msec. The results of the analysis can be displayed as an animated sequence of three-dimensional maps, or of isopotential plots. The data can also be processed to give the location of the various generators which are active in a specific stimulus condition, or to trace the migration of the generators as a function of time after the evoking stimulus.

49. On the neural mechanism of conditioned lever-pressing in the dog.—**N. Yoshii, K. Miyamoto and S. Hayase (Osaka, Japan).**

To evaluate the change in responsiveness of cortical and subcortical structures and to determine when the changes would occur during continuation of intracerebral stimulation just before lever-pressing in dogs, electrical stimulation (at 7.5-13.5 c/sec) was applied to subcortical structures and the evoked potentials (EP) were recorded from cortical and subcortical areas. Correlations between the control EPs with the animal at rest and those before the lever-pressing were calculated. The algebraic differences between the amplitudes of the control EPs and those of the EPs before lever-pressing were displayed on a map as contour lines. The differences were presumed to indicate that the EP at rest changed into that before lever-pressing by the development of a motor potential (MP), which was necessary to set-up the motor response.

The results showed that the MPs for alimentary lever-pressing and for avoidance lever-pressing appeared over wide areas. The latest large MP was obtained from the sensorimotor cortex, whilst the MP from the hippocampus was the earliest among those recorded from all areas. It was also found that the alimentary MP differed from the avoidance MP in distribution within the sensorimotor cortex. The MPs from other cortical areas were non-specific both to alimentary and avoidance lever-pressing. It appears that the sensorimotor cortex plays a role in alimentary and avoidance lever-pressing which has been specifically initiated, while the hippocampus presumably controls and regulates the MPs of the sensorimotor and other cortical areas.

It has been further found that in the sensorimotor cortex, the change in the late component of the EP was observed several seconds earlier and the early component several hundred milliseconds earlier than the lever-pressing muscle response (EMG). It is suggested that the former change is related to the memory mechanism and the latter to the trigger mechanism of the lever-pressing.

In the paper to be presented the conditioned MP in the sensorimotor cortex during sleep and that before erroneous lever-pressing caused by atropine injection will be discussed.

50. Mechanisms of electroencephalographic and behavioral changes produced by parenteral L-DOPA.—R. N. Harner and R. M. Dorman (Philadelphia, Penn., U.S.A.).

L-dihydroxyphenylalanine (L-DOPA) was administered i.v. to 9 male cats on 14 occasions with prior and subsequent recording of EEG activities from chronically implanted cortical, caudate, hippocampal and lateral geniculate placements. Arterial pressure was monitored on 8 occasions with a catheter placed in the abdominal aorta by the femoral route under brief ether anesthesia.

After the animal recovered from anesthesia and passed into spontaneous slow wave sleep, DOPA was given in doses ranging from 10-15 mg/Kg. There was onset of arousal with cortical desynchronization 20-100 sec later, preceding a small rise of arterial pressure by 15-75 sec. The arterial pressure response was transient, subsiding in 10-20 min, but electrocortical arousal persisted for 2-3 h, associated with darting head movements, arched neck, mydriasis, drooling, piloerection, continuous eye movement, vomiting and defecation. At times the animals looked as if they were hallucinating, as evidenced by following movements of the head and eyes and a peculiar fixity of gaze.

Norepinephrine in doses ranging from 16-32 μg i.v. produced a brief hypertensive effect associated with bradycardia having its onset in 9-10 sec and lasting an average of 125 sec. In an attempt to see if the central effects of L-DOPA were mediated through the formation of norepinephrine, disulfiram was given to block dopamine-beta-hydroxylase. Administration of this drug in doses of 250 mg/Kg i.p., even in the absence of externally administered L-DOPA produced many of the effects seen when L-DOPA itself was administered. In addition, cortical desynchronization was sometimes associated with loss of neck tone, tightly closed eyes and a few rapid eye movements. It appears from these pharmacologic studies that dopamine may be an important neurotransmitter involved in control of sleep and wakefulness.

51. Electroencephalographic evaluation of the anti-epileptic action of Mogadan and other benzodiazopinic derivatives (RO5-4023).—M. Turner, M. D. E. Shugurensky and R. A. Perea (Buenos Aires, Argentina).

Eleven cases of epileptic children with very frequent EEG and/or clinical epileptic discharges resistant to classical anti-epileptic medication were chosen in order to assess the effect of a benzodiazepinic derivate (Mogadan-Roche).

From these 11 cases, 8 were classified as Lennox Syndrome (slow spike-and-wave), 1 as a hypsarrythmia (West Syndrome) and 2 others as typical *absences* (3/sec spike-and-wave).

The drug was given under EEG control, by slow i.v. injection (1 ml of the solution of 10 mg in 15 ml solvent, every 30 sec). Rapid and total disappearance of the epileptic discharges was obtained with doses ranging from 2 to 10 mg (average 4 mg). The lowest dosages occurred with the Lennox Syndrome. The typical *absence* cases needed the highest doses (10 mg) but a stage of clinical and EEG sleep was reached in order to suppress the pathological epileptic discharges. In the hypsarrythmic case disappearance of the slow spike-and-waves was obtained but slow and disorganized background rhythms persisted even after a relatively high dose (3 mg/10 Kg weight).

Of the 6 cases that were submitted to oral treatment with Mogadan, a beneficial effect in the Lennox Syndrome was observed. In the *absence* cases the association with other drugs (Tridione and Luminal) was necessary.

The conclusion is reached that a correlation could be established between the beneficial effects of the drug in the oral and chronic treatment and the antiepileptic effect observed in the EEG control during the i.v. injection.

More cases were submitted to oral treatment using a placebo in comparison to a new benzodiazepinic derivative (RO5-4023) in a double blind test, after the antiepileptic effect was anticipated by the EEG control during the i.v. injection.

52. A continuous monitoring device for cerebral activity.—D. Maynard, P. F. Prior and D. F. Scott (London, G.B.).

Continuous monitoring of cerebral activity over hours or days in both clinical and research situations using conventional EEG equipment presents many problems. This is because of artefacts, the bulk of the recording apparatus and the resulting voluminous paper trace. In addition skilled operation is required. For these reasons a small simple apparatus has been devised the output of which is displayed on a chart recorder running at a paper speed of 5 cm/h. Using this recorder, we have been able to monitor cerebral activity from periods of from several hours to 10 days.

The EEG signal is conveyed from a single pair of biparietal stick-on electrodes with non-microphonic screened leads to the apparatus. After passage through a radio frequency trap the signal reaches a parametric amplifier from which it enters a special wide band filter. This filter has a sharp cut off below 2 c/sec and above 15 c/sec to minimize artefacts. It has a skewed response within the pass-band attenuating the lower frequencies more than the higher ones. The signal, expressed in μV peak to peak forms one of two write-outs on the paper trace. The other comes from a specially devised impedance monitor which indicates not only the state of electrode contact but also blocking or other malfunctioning of the amplifier.

This device has been used in combination with conventional EEGs particularly on a group of 24 patients unconscious following various cerebral insults including cardio-respiratory arrest. It indicates whether cerebral activity remained at a constant level or whether it had increased or decreased and therefore increases the confidence of our predictions about outcome.

It is suggested that this device might be of value for all night sleep recordings possibly with a slightly different filter "shape" and electrode derivation.

53. A method for continuously recording characteristics of EEG topography.–J. C. Shaw (Chichester, G.B.).

A complete analysis of EEG topography requires measurement of cospectral density functions and coherence functions. This analysis is complex and difficult to interpret. The method described in this paper is simpler. It uses a visually observable EEG pattern (*e.g.*, alpha rhythm) recorded from one electrode site as a reference or template signal and examines its distribution at other sites. Only linear associations between activities at different sites are considered.

Three characteristics define the linear association between the activity at an electrode site with that at a reference site. These are:

1. The correlation coefficient corrected for time differences between the two signals.
2. The regression coefficient corrected for time differences.
3. The time difference between the reference signal and that part of the test signal correlated with it.

The correlation coefficient and regression coefficient indicate whether the correlated signals are in phase or out of phase.

A small analogue computer has been programmed to continuously record running estimates of these measures for two channels. Because running estimates are used, changes in these parameters can be monitored and related to other events. The presence of an EEG focus can be detected in the presence of generalized activity provided that the signal is available noise free as a template in at least one channel. Changes of alpha rhythm distribution in relation to mental activity and orienting reflexes have also been studied.

The above technique has the advantage of either graphic or numerical output; it results in data reduction; it gives information about visually observable patterns; and it is theoretically simple. The method is being developed so that simultaneous multichannel on-line topographic analysis will be possible with the aid of a small laboratory digital computer.

54. Intracellular studies of cyclical spike driving in cortical epileptogenic foci.–**D. Prince (Stanford, Calif., U.S.A.).**

Low frequency (1-3/sec) stimulation of afferents may trigger epileptiform events in experimental penicillin foci. During such stimulation cyclical changes in the excitability of the epileptogenic focus may occur so that trains of triggered interictal discharges lasting many seconds alternate with trains of normal evoked responses. Intracellular recordings during such "cyclical spike driving" were obtained to investigate the nature of these long duration changes in excitability. The results of these experiments, which are relevant to the general problem of control mechanism in focal epileptogenesis may be summarized as follows: 1) Neurons generated both normal post synaptic potentials (PSPs) associated with evoked responses, and large depolarization shift (DSs) during surface epileptiform events. 2) During cyclical spike driving, trains of evoked PSP-DS complexes associated with triggered surface epileptiform events alternated with trains of PSPs which were evoked when stimuli failed to trigger surface spikes. 3) Although the latency for PSP generation was constant, the latency for DS triggering varied, being longest at the beginning and the end of the train of triggered epileptiform discharges and shortest in mid-train. 4) The properties of neurons as judged by their membrane potentials, their capacity to generate impulses and the characteristics of evoked PSPs, were the same during periods of the cycle when epileptogenic events could and could not be triggered. 5) The only elements encountered which developed changes in membrane potential that persisted several seconds after an epileptogenic spike and summated with low frequency spike triggering were silent cells which did not generate impulses.

These findings suggest that alterations in the

excitatory drive onto the neurons studied are responsible for limitations in spike triggering. Sequential changes in complex interneuronal cortical organizations or prolonged alterations in non-neuronal (glial) elements may underlie cyclical spike driving and account for changed in excitability of epileptogenic foci which last many seconds.

55. Average EEG responses to sinusoidally modulated light in normal subjects and patient.–H. A. C. Kamphuisen (Utrecht, The Netherlands).

An endeavor was made to relate symmetry or asymmetry of responses to sinusoidally modulated light (SML) to two types of disturbance of cerebral function, *e.g.*, hypofunction and irritation, both from clinical and EEG points of view. Fifty-four normal control subjects and 284 patients suffering from various brain disturbances have been examined.

The patients were grouped in the following ways:

1. On basis of the nature of the cerebral disorder, 3 groups of patients were distinguished, viz., patients in whom either from clinical and/or EEG points of view signs could be discerned indicating (a) hypofunction, (b) irritation, and (c) neither hypofunction nor irritation.
2. According to symmetry and asymmetry of the responses to SML and the nature of the asymmetry 3 other groups were distinguished:

Group I Symmetrical responses (148 patients).

Group II inconsistent asymmetrical responses (34 patients) and

Group III consistent asymmetrical responses (66 patients).

It was found that the two groups of patients with asymmetrical responses to SML have relationships with different forms of cerebral dysfunction. The patients with consistent asymmetrical responses to SML appear highly related to hypofunction, and patients with inconsistent asymmetrical responses to SML seem to be considerably more related to irritation than to hypofunction.

When applying SML at various modulation depths the phenomenon was encountered of "paradoxical diminution" (increase of modulation depth produces decrease of response amplitude). This phenomenon was encountered in all patients with inconsistent and in none of the patients with consistent asymmetrical responses. The phenomenon is related ($p<0.005$) to homolateral irritative function disturbance.

56. Receptive field of striate neurons in waking cats.–H. Sasaki (Boston, Mass., U.S.A.).

The receptive fields of visual-cortical cells in anesthetized animals have been described by several investigators. In the experiments to be described, preparations were immobilized and maintained by galamine triethiodide. Of these, some were dissected upper spinal cord *(encéphale isolé)* and others were only locally anesthetized with lidocaine hydrochloride. Both preparations showed ordinary EEG patterns, *i.e.*, low voltage fast, spindle and/or slow wave activity. Unitary discharges in Area 17 were recorded through tungsten micro-electrodes. A general purpose computer (DEC, PDP-7) was used both for presentation of light stimuli and for data processing.

A feature of the receptive fields of striate neurons in the waking state was that they changed qualitatively as well as quantitatively with lapsed time even under the same stimulus parameters. For instance, the orientation of the axis in the receptive field, reported by Hubel and Wiesel, changes sequentially. In some cases new areas of excitation appear on previously inactive regions on the visual field. These changes occurred predominantly in the waking state. The more reduced the state of wakefulness, the more fixed the pattern of receptive field. Anesthesia by injection of sodium pentobarbital stabilized the configuration of the receptive fields. In contrast to striate neurons, fibers in deep subcortical areas, presumed to be geniculo-cortical, showed simple concentric receptive fields and failed to present any qualitative change in the waking state.

57. Optic evoked potential and behavioral changes induced by the alcohol and acid derivatives of serotonin and tryptamine.–H. C. Sabelli, W. J. Giardian and J. E. P. Toman (Chicago, Ill., U.S.A.).

The intraventricular administration of 140 μg of 5-hydroxytryptophol (5HTOL) and of 5-hydroxyindoleacetic acid (5HIAA) to non-anesthetized rabbits modified averaged photic potentials. The reduction of the slow negative component was similar in magnitude to that observed with the same dose of serotonin (5HT) whereas the effects on fast potentials differed from those of the amine.

In newly hatched chicks not only the i.p. administration of 5HT, tryptamine and their aldehydic derivatives but also of very high doses (60 mg/Kg of 5HTOL) and tryptophol induced sleep. Pargyline (100 mg/Kg/24 h prior) partially prevented the lethargic effect of indoleethylamines and of tryptophol; it also reduced nicotine-induced lethargy.

Mouse exploratory behavior was depressed by tryptophol and enhanced by 5H1AA.

This and other evidence for the pharmacological activity of exogenous deaminated derivatives of indoleethylamines suggest a possible role of the endogenous products of MAO in the modulation of synaptic transmission within the optic pathway, in support of Jouvet's hypothesis that a deaminated metabolite triggers REM sleep.

58. Studies on the cholinergic system of the reticular formation.—W. Baust and H. P. Otter (Dusseldorf, West Germany).

Experiments have been carried out on cats with chronically implanted electrodes as well as on cats with precollicular, intercollicular and C_1 transections. In the *encéphale isolé* preparation two cortical arousals can be observed after injection of acetylcholine into the carotid artery. The first arousal appears immediately after the injection, the second one occurs simultaneoulsy with the increase of blood pressure following acetylcholine-induced hypotension, *i.e.*, with a latency of about 40 sec. In cats with intercollicular section only the late cortical desynchronization can be observed after injection of acetylcholine. After blood pressure is lowered by efferent vagal stimulation, an arousal occurs when blood pressure returns to normal. After cutting the sinuaortic baroceptors the acetylcholine-induced hypotension is markedly prolonged. In this case the second arousal is abolished. These results suggest that the late arousal is only caused by the increase in blood pressure. In cats with precollicular section no arousal can be produced by injections of acetylcholine. Thus, a cholinergic arousal takes place only in preparations in which the connections between reticular formation and cortex are intact.

In cats with chronically implanted electrodes the sleep wakefulness pattern has been studied before and during an i.v. infusion of acetylcholine with a rate of 0.25 μg/kg/min. During the application of acetylcholine, the total duration of wakefulness and of REM sleep is significantly increased, whereas the total duration of nonREM sleep is reduced. The experiments demonstrate that the reticular activating system as well as the structures being responsible for the occurrence of REM sleep are triggered by cholinergic mechanisms.

59. Effects of acetylcholine and atropine upon reticular excitation of cortical neurons.—R. Spehlmann (Chicago, Ill., U.S.A.).

To study neurohumoral mechanisms involved in the reticular activation of cerebral cortex, we applied acetylcholine (ACh) and atropine to single neurons in cat lateral gyrus while their activity was driven by stimulation of the mesencephalic reticular formation (MRF) and the visual path. Drug ions were liberated electrophoretically from micro-pipettes having seven or ten drug barrels which surrounded a protruding central recording barrel. Because general anesthesia alters drug susceptibility, spontaneous firing, and synaptic responses of cortical neurons, *encéphale isolé* preparations were used.

Post-stimulus histograms of several of the neurons that responded to brief tetanic stimulation of the MRF with a prolonged increase in firing rate revealed ACh facilitation and atropine depression of this response. Histograms of nonstimulated firing, computed under otherwise identical conditions, showed less clear-cut drug effects in these neurons. Responses to intermittent retinal illumination and to electrical stimulation of the optic radiation were rarely altered. A few neurons that did show drug effects upon radiation responses also showed, when tested, facilitation of these responses by a conditioning stimulus to the MRF. Atropine suppressed this reticular facilitation of radiation responses. Light responses in these neurons were not altered by either reticular stimulation or drug application.

These results suggest that ACh and atropine acted primarily not upon transmission of specific visual impulses but upon facilitatory input from the MRF. Such a differential drug effect, although not excluding the possibility of pre-synaptic drug action upon the terminals of reticular afferents at cortical neurons, is compatible with the view that endogenous ACh is engaged in the synaptic transmission of excitatory reticular impulses to cortical neurons. This explanation is supported by reports on histo-chemical staining and on ACh liberation from the cortical surface.

60. Spontaneous unit activity in motor and somesthetic cortices during the sleep-wakefulness cycles in the monkey.—Y. Lamarre (Montreal, Canada).

Monkeys had electrodes chronically implanted under a hermetically closed chamber over the perirolandic region, allowing unit recordings from precentral and postcentral neurons during natural waking and sleep. Differentiation between discharges of cortical cells and those recorded from thalamo-cortical radiation fibers was possible following well-known criteria. Several types of neurons were classified as unresponsive or discharging in response to antidromic invasion of the pyramidal tract and to natural, specific thalamic or transcallosal activation. Spontaneous EEG rhythms, potentials of the neck muscles, ocular movements and direct observation of behavior permitted differentiation of wakefulness from different stages of sleep.

About one half of the observed neurons showed marked fluctuations during sleep-wakefulness cycles in both motor and somesthetic areas. The overall amount of spontaneous discharge decreased on arousal from synchronized sleep in 75% of neurons recorded from the precentral gyrus; these neurons were either unresponsive or modulated at short latencies by shocks applied to the appropriate specific (ventro-lateral) thalamic nucleus or by transcallosal stimulation. In some cases, increase of unit discharge preceded by a few seconds and announced appearance of clear-cut behavioral and EEG signs of sleep. Behind the central fissure, equal proportions of neurons increased and decreased their discharges on arousal. All neurons which were found both in the precentral and postcentral gyri to be spontaneously more active during excited wakefulness than during drowsiness or synchronized sleep, could be modulated by gentle passive movements and cutaneous stimulation of the contralateral body half or by shocks to the lemniscal system.

The findings offer the possibility of a classification of various alterations of spontaneous activity in sensori-motor cortex during the sleep-wakefulness cycle related to the neuronal function.

61. Quantitative analysis of the EEG in psychopathological states: human experimental and clinical observations.—G. Marjerrison, R. P. Keogh, and A. E. Krause (Saskatoon and North Battleford, Canada).

The findings of Goldstein *et al.* of a low signal variability in the EEG of chronic schizophrenics using modulus voltage integration has been confirmed. It has been further found that acute schizophrenics, whilst not varying from a non-psychotic population as a group, show low signal variability while hallucinating. Within-patient decreases in rated perceptual psychopathology correlated significantly with increase in the coefficient of variation measure of EEG signal variability.

In a group of chronically hospitalized chronic schizophrenics selected for withdrawn, non-paranoid symptomatology, low signal variability was found to significantly vary with a measure of "state" anxiety—the AACL of Zuckerman *et al.* Chronic schizophrenics with hallucinatory symptomatology induced by MAO inhibition or by experimentally applied stress, showed decreases in signal variability greater than those found under baseline conditions. It has been found that clinical changes in acute schizophrenics during controlled drug treatment were related to changes in EEG variability specifically as predicted on the Perceptual Psychopathology Factor Score—the IMPS of Lorr *et al.* Treatment induced changes in EEG variability also were found to interact with perceptual field dependency as measured by the Rod and Frame Test.

Sensory input attentuation during perceptual deprivation has been examined in acute unmedicated schizophrenics and staff volunteers. Input attentuation produced major changes in the EEG signal variability over time. Again perceptual field dependency interacts with diagnostic status.

Further studies on bilateral integration of the EEG in a series of dominantly right and left-handed patients and normals has shown that correlations between the integrated amplitudes from the two sides were greater in the right-handed. Correlations between right and left-sided signals have been shown to differ with the psychotic-nonpsychotic status and with psychoactive drug treatment.

The findings will be discussed in relation to current theories of perceptual input dysfunction in psychosis.

62. Prediction of the cerebral blood flow from the EEG.—I. A. Sulg and D. H. Ingvar (Lund, Sweden).

Manual analysis of EEG frequency and voltage content offers a cheap simple method to quantitate the EEG. The method used in our studies was developed by one of us. It has been used with advantage in a number of experimental and clinical investigations in which, under normal conditions, statistically significant correlation between the EEG frequency content and the cerebral blood flow was demonstrated.

EEG records from 123 patients with various cerebral disorders were analyzed. The majority were in the subacute stage of their disease. Only analysis outputs from parieto-occipital leads were included in this study. Records which showed focal abnormalities in this region were excluded. Various standard subroutines for statistical processing were used in general purpose computers (IBM 1800 and CDC 3600). The computers were also fed the cerebral blood flow values (rCBF) from the same patients.

By means of stepwise regression analysis it was found that the EEG activity in the alpha and delta bands showed the best correlation to the rCBF. Using only certain few frequencies with the highest correlation to the rCBF, predicted values obtained were closer to the estimated values than in predictions based on the total spectrum analysed (1-20c/sec). The best prediction results were, however, obtained when the statistical predictor was derived from an average measure: the mean period frequency, called by us for the EEG frequency index. When the residuals (*i.e.*, differences between estimated and predicted rCBF values) are plotted in a polynomial regression against the estimated values, it is found that most of the predicted values differ by less than 10 ml/100 g brain weight/min from the measured ones.

Summarizing the results of the prediction trials within the framework of the linear regression equation, it should be pointed out that these trials were a logical part of the project in which the statistical relationship between different parameters of the EEG frequency content were to be correlated to rCBF estimates. The predictor thus tests whether the regression coefficients and "the best linear predictor" derived from this equation really have the functions which in statistical terms support the hypothesis of linear correlation between the EEG and cerebral blood flow within certain conditions. This correlation is probably a consequence of metabolic regulation of the CBF, which implies that the CBF is adapted to the brain activity and that this metabolic regulation is reflected also in the EEG.

63. Changes in visual evoked potentials induced by electrolyte alterations in dogs.—S. I. Lee, D. W. Klass and K. G. Wakim (Rochester, Minn., U.S.A.).

As part of a study of hemodialysis, visual evoked potentials (VEP) summated by CAT have been recorded from 67 curarized dogs. The VEPs obtained by extracranial leads showed prominent surface negative peaks at 43±13 msec and positive peaks at 100±37 msec in controls before dialysis. During 3-6 h of dialysis (standard dialysate) no significant VEP changes occurred from healthy dogs or from animals previously made azotemic by acute i.v. urea loading, bilateral nephrectomy, or ureteral ligation. Overhydration produced no VEP changes until a significant decrease of serum sodium and osmolality occurred. The most significant change of VEPs was observed during dialysis of normal or azotemic dogs, using dialysate with low sodium content (30 mEq/L). This procedure induced significant decrease of serum sodium, chloride, and osmolality levels and frequent paroxysmal (spontaneous or light-induced) EEG changes. There was a consistent gradual increase in latency and amplitude of certain components of the VEPs, most significant ($p<0.01$) in the positive peak at 100 msec, before electrographic seizure discharges. Maintenance or serum osmolality using i.v. urea or mannitol during low sodium dialysis decreased the magnitude of VEP changes and delayed their occurrence, while the incidence of electrographic seizure discharges was not altered.

The present study corresponds well with gross EEG changes reported earlier from this laboratory, suggesting an important role of hyponatremia in producing central nervous system alterations by dialysis.

64. Power spectrum analysis of higher central nervous rhythms in the human EEG.—H. Kuenkel, F. Schweitzer, M. Sternberg and P. Sternberg (Berlin, W. Germany).

The electrical activity of the brain as measured by the amount of delta, alpha and beta percentage during several hundred successive intervals of 1 sec duration shows marked variability. Multichannel simultaneous power spectrum analysis reveals that up to 70% of this variability may depend on the influence of higher central nervous rhythms in the frequency range of respiration, higher-order blood-pressure waves and other far slower ones. Analysis of variance based on orthogonal experimental design gives evidence that the influence of these rhythms is modified by several factors, such as location of the EEG leads, therapy with psychopharmacological agents, time of day and moreover that there are typical interindividual differences.

65. Linear and non-linear properties of evoked potentials and correlates with perception.—F. H. Lopes da Silva, A. van Rotterdam, and A. M. Tielen (Utrecht, The Netherlands).

Methods of analysis of linear and nonlinear systems were used to quantify the "steady-state" potentials evoked by Sinusoidally Modulated Light (SML) recorded from the cortical surface and the lateral geniculate nucleus in unrestrained dogs with implanted electrodes. Harmonic components of the SML evoked potentials were determined by means of discrete Fourier analysis.

In all areas studied essential nonlinearities were revealed particularly by the generation of an important second harmonic component. This characteristic depends upon the rectifying properties of on-off subsystems in visual projection areas.

Furthermore at the marginal gyrus (occipital lobe) a frequency selective system was individualized within the beta frequency range (centered around 28 c/sec). In this cortical area and frequency band the evoked potentials could be described by a linear Transfer Function with the restriction that the modulation depth was lower than 30%. By means of this transfer function it was possible to predict the behavior of the beta frequency selective system to transients; this was checked by means of stimulation with flashes and with Noise Modulated Light (input-output cross-correlation). A close relation was found between the frequency selective system responsible for cortical SML evoked potentials and the dominant mode of spontaneous activity. Outside the linear range nonlinear properties of cortical evoked potentials were revealed by finding saturation and subharmonics of order ½.

Correlates between parameters of the evoked potentials and perception were explored. The flicker fusion sensitivity (De Lange curve) of the dog was determined. A correlate was found at the lateral geniculate nucleus where the attenuation of the second harmonic follows that of the De Lange curve. This correlate indicates that the second harmonic component might reflect stochastic properties of neural aggregates which are also relevant, in the perception domain, for the determination of flicker sensitivity.

66. Slow potential changes recorded from cerebral cortex of dogs.—**A. Kamp, A. J. van Rijn, and J. M. Zwart (Utrecht, The Netherlands).** During an investigation of relations between electrical phenomena of the brain and behavior in dogs, special attention was devoted to slow potential variations. The electrical signals were recorded from chronically implanted electrodes placed on frontal, central, temporal and occipital cortex.

Two types of electrodes were used, silver-silver chloride electrodes were placed on the dura, carbon electrodes were positioned in direct contact with the cortex. The experiments were carried out using multichannel EEG radiotelemetry which permitted recording from freely moving animals. To obtain a controlled and reproducible behavioral situation, the animals were trained to press a pedal on a stimulus presentation in order to obtain a food reward.

Slow potential changes could be observed by averaging the electrical signals in relation to the amount the animal pressed the pedal.

Two negatively increasing potential changes could be distinguished: 1) a rise of potential preceded the pressing of the pedal, 2) a second increase of potential between pedal pressing and the delivery of food. The first potential change is similar to a phenomenon known as "readiness potential" (Kornhuber), preceding voluntary movements. In a certain stage of performance of the animal correct pressings and pressings in between stimuli could be distinguished on the basis of the characteristics of the wave form of this phenomenon.

The second rise of potential preceding the food reward seems to reflect the expectancy of the animal on getting the food. The duration of this phenomenon is related to the time delay between the moment the pedal was pressed and the delivery of food.

Both phenomena have been recorded from the same cortical area, however simultaneously recorded data show different variability. This could indicate that the observed electrical activities reflect different neural processes in the cortical structures underlying the recording electrode.

67. Alterations of evoked neuronal discharges in motor and somesthetic cortices during the sleep-wakefulness cycles in the monkey.—**M. Steriade (Quebec, Canada).** Discharges of single units in precentral and postcentral gyri were evoked by stimulation of specific afferent pathways (at the level of the ventro-lateral and ventralis postero-lateralis thalamic relays or medial lemniscus) and by transcallosal stimulation of homotopic points in monkeys with chronically implanted electrodes during wakefulness and various stages of sleep.

Discharges evoked at 1.5-4 msec latency in the precentral motor cortex by shocks applied to the appropriate (ventro-lateral) thalamic nucleus were reduced or even abolished during arousal in comparison with synchronized sleep. About 20% of the observed neurons in the precentral gyrus were transsynaptically activated by callosal stimulation of the homotopic points with latency values ranging from 3 to 7 msec (especially at 4-5 msec); shock-evoked discharges of all these neurons (some identifiable as pyramidal tract neurons by antidromic responses to stimulation of the medullary pyramid) were also strikingly diminished during natural waking, similarly to those elicited in the same area by thalamic ventro-lateral stimulation. In contrast, discharges of neurons activated by stimulation of the somesthetic afferent pathway, regardless to the site of recording (postcentral or precentral gyri), were obviously facilitated on waking. However, the latter event might be also ascribed to concomitant facilitation, during arousal, of the thalamic specific (ventralis postero-lateralis) relay, considering the increase of the evoked discharges recorded from the thalamo-cortical radiation fibers.

A dissociation between neurons activated by somesthetic afferent messages and those firing to the specific input of the motor cortex, according to fluctuations in responsiveness during sleep-wakefulness cycle is postulated.

68. Behavioral and neurophysiological studies of the sensorimotor rhythm in the cat.—**M. B. Sterman, W. Wyrwicka and R. Howe (Sepulveda and Los Angeles, Calif., U.S.A.).** Automatic food reinforcement of a specific pattern of 12-14 c/sec EEG activity from sensorimotor cortex in the cat (sensorimotor rhythm or SMR) established (a) that this rhythm could function as a conditioned instrumental response, (b) that its direct behavioral correlate was a suppression of movement, (c) that phasic motor activity was never observed in the presence of this rhythm during wakefulness and both the slow-wave and REM patterns of sleep, and (d) that facilitation of the SMR in the waking state resulted in a related enhancement of sensorimotor cortex spindle-burst activity during sleep. Subcortical EEG recordings obtained during conditioned SMR activity disclosed corresponding electrical patterns in the VPL, VPM, and VL nuclei of the thalamus. Late cortical evoked potentials elicited by stimulation of these nuclei were suppressed during both the SMR and slow-wave sleep spindles, the suppression being probably of thalamic origin. These and other neurophysiological findings stress the role of proprioceptive feedback and fusimotor activity in the regulation of phasic motor behavior. Preliminary studies suggest, also, that modification of these mechanisms through manipulation of the SMR can alter susceptibility to drug-induced motor seizures.

69. The advantages of brain signal reconstitution within a resistive analog of the skull.—G. Schuler and E. W. Peterson (Ottawa, Canada).
A variety of EEG signals reconstituted within an electrically resistive volume permits electrical exploration of the volume to provide a sensitive and selective means to study signals arising from discrete areas within the brain.

In theory, EEG signals may arise from such spatially discrete areas as non-propagating epileptic foci, or from temporally discrete areas such as the individual generators of complex brain activity. Such signals travel routes with various conductive properties, but appear almost simultaneously upon all areas of the scalp. If many scalp electrodes pass these signals to low-noise amplifiers connected in a common-average-reference configuration, the resulting amplified signals may be impressed upon corresponding areas of a simple resistive analog of the head. With the scalp voltage pattern reproduced upon the periphery of the resistive analog, the resulting signals within the analog may be profitably studied since parallel averaging provides 'low-noise', and maximal signal areas give spatial information.

In theoretical operation, a low-level epileptic focus could impart submicrovolt spikes to large areas of the scalp, but be undetected by present day EEG techniques. If these submicrovolt spikes were processed by 100 electrode-amplifier units and combined in a resistive analog, the resultant parallel averaging could provide a 10-fold improvement in signal/noise ratio and aid detection. The locus of maximal spike activity within the analog would exactly correspond to the epileptic focus were the animal head electrically homogeneous, but with this not so, the correspondence is imperfect but nevertheless useful.

In practice, a somewhat similar technique has selectively acquired fetal EKG signals and a special 20 channel EEG amplifier and resistive analog of the human skull has been built and tested.

The EEG apparatus, tests and results will be presented.

70. Alterations of micromotoric tonus regulation during paroxysmal EEG activity.—H. D. Weigeldt (Bremen, W. Germany).
During the last seven years, the recording of the "micromotoric tonus" (MMT) in and during traumatic and alcoholic delirious processes has produced more qualified and measurable data about the extent of cerebral functional disorders than the EEG. This has been especially so with the late sequelae of cerebral injuries. The method has also been very useful for controlling the anticonvulsive treatment of epileptics as it can be used as often as necessary without losing its diagnostic validity for the recognition and determination of positive or negative psychotropic drug effects or intoxications. We, therefore, studied the direct influence of spike-wave bursts on the writing pressure records by simultaneous registration of the EEG and the MMT.

Various degrees of curve inhibition (retardation, perseveration, interruption of records) were dependent only to a minor degree on the mode, localization and duration of the paroxysms. No direct simple relation was found between the records, especially if the EEG and MMT were compared for longer periods. Not only the writing speed as an approximate measure of the psychomotor velocity but also various symptoms of the pressure course—also one mode of tonus regulation—permit better recognition of the fluctuations of subcortical regulation and counter-regulation than the conventional EEG. Often from a few up to more than 20 sec before a spike-wave discharge a period of increased lability with pathological symptoms is observed. The writing speed before and after the bursts frequently increases, probably by pre- and postparoxysmal arousal reactions.

It is also noted that simultaneous EEG and MMT recording reveals that similar EEG phenomena may have different clinical meanings, possibly due to brain stem and/or cortical effects. Simultaneous comparisons with the H-reflex, with DC shifts and data on the autonomic system might permit more certain correlation of the phenomena described with subcortical functions.

71. Alterations micromotoric tonus regulation in cerebral disorders.—F. Steinwachs (Aachen, W. Germany).

Since 1950 the method of measuring "micromotoric tonus" regulation (MMTR) has been found to be a diagnostically usable technique after standardizing equipment and methods and objectively evaluating the components of the procedure. Factor analysis studies by Hoffman *et al.*, reliability studies by Hoffman and longitudinal studies throughout the day by Nesswetha *et al.* have confirmed the adequacy of the basic concepts.

The relation of the physiological variables during oxygen deficiency to the parameters of writing pressure were shown to be significantly related in 245 applicants for pilots. Itani and Steinwachs compared 30 patients with brain trauma to a control group and found 24 significant measurements. Herzmann and Steinwachs compared 30 schizophrenics with a control group and found 8 statistically valid symptoms. Nesswetha found significant correlations between cardiovascular reactions and findings in the tonus curve under stress and performance conditions.

After 7 years of comparative analyses of the MMTR and the EEG and clinical symptoms Weigeldt used simultaneous recordings of these procedures for neurophysiological research. He applied these techniques to studies of drug effects, brain disorders and alcohol withdrawal. Von Both has applied the techniques to studies of the effects of Valium and has found 85 statistically valid measurements.

An apparatus has now been built at the Psychological Institute of Rheinisch-Westfalische Technical University of Aachen to read the data continuously for 43 measurements and convert them into digital format. The statistical significance of the measurements can be evaluated by a computer program.

72. Cerebral reactivity in psychiatric and epileptic patients.—V. Floris, C. Morocutti, G. Amabile, G. Bernardi and P. A. Rizzo (Siena, Italy).

The authors have studied the visual evoked potentials (VEP) and the cortical recovery cycle in 45 normal subjects, 15 paranoic schizophrenics, 15 neurotics, 15 endogenous depressed and 15 epileptics. The normals are divided in 3 groups: young, adult and old. For the evaluation of the recovery cycle the ratio R2/R1 of the amplitude of the wave III was first employed. A procedure based on the analysis of covariance for a direct confront of R2 in different groups was then used.

With regards to the VEP to the single flashes in normal subjects, a progressive increase of the amplitude and of the latency can be observed with increase in age. A global decrease of the VEP amplitude can be observed in schizophrenic subjects. In the endogenous depressives the evoked response is of larger amplitude, whilst in neurotic patients it is not possible to discern substantial alterations in comparison with the group of normal subjects. The later waves of the VEP in epileptic patients, especially waves V, are of larger amplitude than in normal subjects.

As far as the recovery cycle amplitudes are concerned, there can be seen in normal subjects a progressive increase in the facilitation period of the primary components of the VEP with increase in age. This super facilitation period is very depressed and almost absent in all the three groups of psychiatric patients, while it is increased in the epileptics.

The comparison of R2 adjusted between different groups showed important differences between epileptics, neurotics, schizophrenics and normal subjects. Such differences were not present in the comparison between psychotically depressed and normals.

The above findings are discussed in the light of the latest physiopathological studies.

73. Cortical intracellular responses to interacting stimuli.—J. B. Veith, U. Kneise and K. Komposch (Erlangen, W. Germany).

Intracellular studies of unitary activity in the anterior sigmoid gyrus (layer V) of the cat were performed to examine the responsiveness to interacting inhibitory single electric shocks. Recently it had been demonstrated that during a depression of the cortical activity due to hyperpolarization of the membrane and induced by stimulation of the caudate nucleus, the introduction of a stimulus to the lateral geniculate body results in a potentiation due to depolarization and thus shortening of the hyperpolarization phase. These results also were in correlation with behavioral experiments. The following observations have important bearing upon the functional organization of cortical networks.

A shock to the lateral geniculate body caused a potentiation not only during a caudate nucleus induced depression, but also during a cortical depression elicited by antidromic (pyramidal tract) or epicortical stimulation. Those stimuli which caused a depressive response if applied as a single shock, had a potentiating effect when introduced while a depression was going on. This effect of the second stimulus, however, appeared only if it was weaker than the conditioning stimulus. This was very obvious especially when epicortical shocks or those to the caudate nucleus were paired using the same stimulation electrodes. The potentiating stimulus was more effective when placed into the second half of the hyperpolarization. If the second shock was of the same strength or even stronger than the first one, then the result was a new depression after a short potentiation. Epicortical or caudate stimulation were more effective in causing a potentiation than the antidromic stimulation.

These findings will be illustrated, and discussed. Relations to behavioral experiments are assumed. It is suggested that the potentiation is a similar nonspecific, cortical effect as the depression.

74. A sixteen channel wave pattern digitizer.—E. Kaiser, R. Magnusson and I. Petersen (Copenhagen, Denmark, and Goteborg, Sweden).

The digitizer is programmed to convert and codify full-wave EEG sections into 14-bit computer words.

The routines comprise conversion of full-wave duration to frequency (five bits), indication whether the ratio of the durations in a half-wave pair is outside a preset interval (one bit), classification of the peak-to-peak amplitude in eight classes (three bits), indication of the number of secondary waves in the full wave (three bits), and indication of the presence and polarity of spikes (two bits).

75. Sleep patterns in malnutrition: a longitudinal study of anorexic patients.—G. W. Fenton and T. M. Elphicke (London, G.B.).

It is a common clinical observation that patients with anorexia nervosa often display sleep disturbance and it has been suggested that this may be related to the malnutrition. The following study was carried out (in collaboration with P. B. C. Fenwick) in order to investigate these observations. Six patients in the Maudsley Hospital metabolic unit suffering from anorexia nervosa were examined longitudinally. All night sleep EEG recordings were performed in the ward on four consecutive nights within ten to fourteen days of admission and the same procedure was repeated when the patients had gained their optimum weight six to eight weeks later. The treatment consisted of refeeding only, no psychotropic drugs being used. Two patients received hypnotics, the doses being maintained unchanged throughout the study. Daily ratings of mood and behavior were recorded throughout their stay in hospital. Five of the patients responded well to treatment, each gaining at least 10Kg; one failed to show an appreciable weight change. All the recordings were performed by a single investigator, who also rated the depth of sleep for each 20-sec period using the Loomis classification. These alphabetic ratings were converted into numerical data to facilitate processing, put on punched tape and analysed by digital computer. The subjects who gained weight displayed changes in their sleep pattern, significantly more time being spent awake and in stage A before treatment while after weight gain the duration of deep sleep (stage D and E) were increased. A significant increase in REM sleep time was also observed on refeeding. The length of time from retiring for the night to first onset of stage C was reduced on retest. The latency of onset of REM appeared to be delayed initially but was significantly less after weight gain. Data concerning changes in sleep pattern throughout each hour of the night were collected and will be presented. No consistent association between change in sleep pattern and alteration in mood could be detected. The patient whose weight remained essentially unchanged did not show any alteration in sleep pattern. These findings confirm the importance of regarding malnutrition and loss of weight as variables which may influence the pattern of an individual's sleep.

76. Contrasting reactions of the evoked auditory response and amplitude histogram to mental arithmetic and eye opening in man.—A. Glass (Birmingham, G.B.).

In earlier studies, the separate and combined effects on the total amplitude histogram (AH) of the EEG of mental arithmetic and eye opening were compared. Visual evoked responses are known to be reduced in amplitude during mental arithmetic, so it was decided to compare the effects of the two main factors, eye opening and calculation, on the overall amplitude of the evoked response to an auditory stimulus (AER).

The EEG was recorded by a Beckman Dynograph in conjunction with an Ampex tape recorder. A trigger pulse was also recorded. Silver disc electrodes were placed at Pz, C3, C4 and P3, P4 positions on the scalp with a reference on the right mastoid. Responses were averaged to a 1000 c/sec tone lasting 150 msec with rise and fall times of 20 msec approximately. The repetition rate of tone was 1/2.7–3 sec. Sixty-four sweeps were averaged by the Biomac 1000 computer both on and off-line. The subject sat in a sound-isolated chamber.

As before with the AHs, the AERs (and AHs) were recorded with eyes closed; eyes closed during mental arithmetic (continuous subtraction of 7's); eyes open; eyes open during mental arithmetic. Any possible order effect was balanced out by the design of the experiment.

With the AER there was little difference in peak-to-peak amplitude whether eyes were open or shut. Continuous subtraction of 7's reduced the peak-to-peak amplitude by up to 50%. This occurred with eyes open or shut, in contrast to the results of AH measures.

It is suggested that this evidence on amplitudes supports the view that the AER is subserved by different cerebral mechanism and pathways than non-evoked electrical activity. The relation of the conscious level to these findings will be discussed.

77. The use of Haar function to automatic EEG analysis.—A. O. Bishop, W. P. Wilson and L. Wilcox (Durham and Clemson, U.S.A.).

The desirability of reducing the cost of medical laboratory examinations, while extending the service to more patients who might benefit from the procedure, predicates a need for new methods of examination and interpretation of results. In EEG, it is clear that computer analysis of data is possible on the digital computer. Unfortunately, current approaches are not clinically applicable. The use of Haar functions is a new approach to analysis of EEG signals. Preliminary work indicates that these functions can be used in the analysis of the EEG. As the approach may allow a screening method to be developed, the computer techniques and use of the functions will be described.

The utility of this mathematical approach is that it allows the computation to be performed on a small high-speed digital computer. All analysis is done in real time. Multiple channels can be analyzed. The clinical and research applications of the technique will be discussed.

78. Extracellular dendritic fields and unit activity of hippocampal neurons during epileptogenesis induced by "abnormal" CSF perfusion.—E. C. Zuckermann and G. H. Glaser (New Haven, Conn., U.S.A.).

Extracellular dendritic fields and unit activity of hippocampal neurons during epileptogenesis were studied by means of bipolar micro-electrodes implanted in the basal and apical dendritic layers, and at the level of somata of dorsal hippocampal pyramidal cells in chronically prepared cats and acute experiments in chronic preparations. Stimulating stainless steel electrodes were located in ipsi- and contralateral hippocampus and cannulae for localized perfusion of the inferior horn were placed above this hippocampal area. Three groups of chronic animals were used (1) normal, and those with a chronic epileptogenic focus produced by (2) cobalt powder and (3) alumina cream. In all the animals seizure activity was triggered by repetitive electrical stimulation of ipsi- or contralateral hippocampal structures and by alteration of normal components of perfused artificial CSF (at rate of 0.05-0.1 ml/min). The changes in CSF were: increase of K^+ to 7-18 μeq/ml; Ca^{++} free fluid, glutamic acid to 20-100 μeq/ml; acetylcholine to 10-100 μg/ml; anticholinesterases neostigmine 2-5 μg/ml and edrophonium 25-100 μg/ml.

Characteristic changes of the extracellular fields were seen to develop during the build-up of epileptogenic activity in both basal and apical dendritic layers along with a progressive recruitment of discharging units in the same period. Some of the changes were common during all types of epileptogenesis, but others characterize the particular conditions of the type of focus or preparation and the epileptogenic agent. An analysis is attempted of spatial and sequential relationships between events occurring at the different levels of the hippocampal pyramidal cell during epileptogenesis. The results are discussed in terms of the roles played by the dendritic expansions and neuronal somata in initiating self-sustained activity.

79. Methohexital activation of "centrencephalic-like" discharge.—B. J. Wilder, L. Musella, G. Van Horn and R. P. Schmidt (Gainsville, Fla., U.S.A.).

The bilaterally synchronous 3/sec spike and wave EEG discharge, which is the electrographic sign of *petit mal* epilepsy, is sensitive to activation by hyperventilation. Much less frequently these "centrencephalic-like" bursts can be triggered by photic-stimulation.

During a study of a new technique to activate temporal lobe foci and to separate primary from dependent secondary temporal lobe foci methohexital (Brevital) was given i.v. to patients with a history of *absence* attacks and EEG evidence of bilateral spike and wave discharge. Twenty-five of 27 patients with previously demonstrated "centrencephalic-like" EEG abnormalities were sensitive to activation with i.v. methohexital. In the majority of these patients, 3/sec spike and wave and polyspike and wave discharge could be provoked by exceedingly small doses of the drug (5-20 mg). These doses, in most instances, did not result in sleep or marked drowsiness. Higher doses of methohexital (40-70 mg), which routinely produced sleep, frequently failed to activate the "centrencephalic-like" discharge. In two patients who were photosensitive, methohexital activated EEG spike and wave and polyspike and wave discharge and at the same time, blocked the response to photic-stimulation.

I.v. methohexital promises to be a useful activation technique in patients with *absence* seizures associated with "centrencephalic-like" discharge patterns. Furthermore, this agent may be a provocative test to assess response to anticonvulsant medication. Possible mechanisms of action are discussed.

80. Paroxysmal activity evoked by painful stimuli in the sleep EEG of epileptics.—J. S. Mendoza (Santo Domingo, Dominican Republic).

It has been found in a group of 74 epileptic children during spontaneously or Nembutal induced sleep that excluding those showing focal or central discharges, 20 produced paroxysmal bursts on light pinprick stimulation of the limbs. There were two main types of bursts: bifrontal discharges at 5-7 c/sec sometimes preceded by a short burst of fast waves and more generalized discharges in the delta range. The stimulus response delay varied between 0.5 and 2.0 sec. In all the recordings auditory and visual stimuli were given but in only 3 records was an auditory stimulus capable of producing a long lasting paroxysmal discharge. Two further cases produced similar discharges from photic stimulation during sleep. The discharges evoked by photic and auditory stimuli did not resemble those produced by the painful stimuli, *i.e.*, frontal theta discharges which were very similar from case to case and appeared to be specific for this type of stimulation.

The occurrence of the bursts is paradoxical since one would expect a painful stimulus to awaken the patient or at least lighten the level of sleep as occurs in non-epileptics. Instead of the expected desynchronization through the ascending alerting system, the evoked theta bursts resemble synchronization of thalamic origin or even 14 and 6/sec positive spikes. This fact is even more evident when the centrencephalic delta waves are evoked. This unusual response from epileptics does not appear to be due to dampening of the reticular system by the narcotic since K complex and other stages of sleep appear normally. These nociceptive bursts have not been found in sleep recordings of non-epileptics.

81. Clinical observations on photosensitive epilepsy.—H. Gerken (Kiel, West Germany).
Follow-up studies were undertaken on 195 photosensitive children. Of these, 168 were suffering from cerebral seizures and the remaining 27 from a variety of other disorders including headache. Only four patients had sporadic photogenic seizures; the remainder had seizures unrelated to photic stimuli.

The clinical picture of photosensitive epilepsy is very varied and includes almost all types of seizure patterns and of illness course. In the group studied febrile and afebrile *grand-mal* seizures were seen the most frequently, with focal seizures and *petit-mal* next in frequency.

Photosensitivity appears dominantly in females. The course is often very unfavorable especially in cases with focal symptoms and onset after the fifth year of life. Two-thirds of the cases studied started their disease before the sixth year of life, *i.e.*, before the age of maximal penetration of a genetically determined photosensitivity. Inquiries into the family histories support the suggestion that there are additional genetic factors, independent from photosensitivity, which are of importance for the manifestation of epilepsy in carriers.

Photosensitivity is regarded as a symptom of a dysfunction of the reticulo-cortical system and this must already exist at a time when the characteristic photoconvulsive response has not yet appeared. It seems that the reticulo-cortical dysfunction is not linked to age but only to its sensitivity to stimulation by the optic path afferents.

82. A mathematical model providing a synthesis between evoked and spontaneous phenomena of the EEG.—P. B. C. Fenwick and J. Dollimore (London, G.B.).
Saunders showed the alpha rhythm to have a Gaussian distribution and to be generated by noise passed through a narrow band filter. McCullough *et al.* have suggested that the CNS is a state determined system. In collaboration with G. W. Fenton these two ideas have been combined by using the auto-regressive model. A model is calculated by fitting it to a length of EEG signal and then various properties of the models are investigated. If random noise is passed through a model, a wave form similar to the original EEG is generated by the model. The model can be transformed into its impulse response and this shows many features which closely approximate to the average evoked potential. It is suggested that evoked phenomena may be better considered by more refined statistical techniques rather than simple measuring of latencies and so on.

83. Strychnine effects on cell membrane properties.—M. R. Klee and W. Heiss (Buffalo, N.Y., U.S.A.).
Decreases in membrane potential, membrane resistance and amplitude of hyperpolarizing afterpotentials are caused in identified neurons of *Aplysia Californica* by adding 0.02-0.2% strychnine sulfate to the bathing solution. Most of those cells showing spontaneous discharges resulting from both endogeneous and synaptically induced activity started with depolarizing afterpotentials which increased in amplitude and caused bursts of spikes which were independent from the synaptic input (persistent after ligature of the axon of these unipolar cells). The nature of the repetitive activity and the sequence of depolarizing waves followed by hyperpolarizations are similar to phenomena seen in cortical and spinal neurons of mammals during strychnine seizure. Reducing the external calcium concentration or addition of cobalt to the strychninized medium caused mem-

brane depolarization of many seconds and a massive increase in conductance, while increases in calcium concentration to 33-88 mM depressed or blocked the bursting activity. Replacement of sodium with tris blocked the long-lasting depolarizations, in contrast to the reported persistance of a depolarization in a sodium-free solution with TEA added. Changes in temperature or in external concentration of potassium and addition of ouabain or copper ions to the bathing medium had no significant influence on the described effects of strychnine. After an increase in spontaneous synaptic activity by 0.2% strychnine solution ortho- and antidromic activation were depressed or even blocked possibly due to an increase in threshold of the presynaptic fibers. Furthermore, the changes in membrane potential and resistance due to iontophoretic application of acetylcholine were altered by strychnine. That is, the depolarizing (D-) response in DINI and DILDA cells, which is blocked in sodium-free solution, was significantly decreased, and the hyperpolarizing (H-) response, which is blocked by copper ions, was increased after strychnine application and reduced during the washing period.

These results suggest that strychnine, in addition to its known interaction with a specific inhibitory transmitter of the mammalian motoneuron, changes properties of the spike generating and subsynaptic membrane and causes repetitive activity even in synaptically isolated neurons.

84. Studies on brain glutamic acid.—V. V. Subbarao (Jaipur, India).

The metabolism of amino acids is of great interest in mental diseases. In this paper some of the changes brought about in cerebral metabolic processes by chemical agents will be presented.

The experiments were performed on albino rats on exposure to cold stress, after treatment with cortisone and reserpine and also on exposure to total darkness. The brain amino acids of the animals were estimated by paper chromatographic techniques. Reserpine and cold stress caused depletion of brain glutamic acid, whereas cortisone and dark exposure increased the brain glutamic acid content.

The significant rise in brain glutamic acid leads to the question whether glutamic acid is directly concerned with seizure processes, although it is not clear what metabolic area is primarily involved.

85. A preliminary study of the evoked response at the time of voluntary movement in normal man.—P. Castaigne, H. Cathala, E. Pierrot-Desseiligny and E. Bussel (Paris, France).

The work to be presented demonstrates the great variability of the large negative wave seen in the averaged EEG when voluntary movement occurs. It has been possible to show this variability by recording 10 to 12 times a series of 100 movements repeated for each subject. The variability affects the amplitude of the wave as well as the latency to the time of maximum negativity which indicates the beginning of muscle movement. The maximum negativity can occur 100 msec before to 100 msec after beginning of the movement but there appears to be no systematic relation in the variations.

The large negative wave is probably the same pattern as that described by Kornhuber *et al.* and Vaughan *et al.* Although this wave might be identified with the Expectancy Wave of Walter, it shows certain differences in amplitude and topography.

86. Cortical steady potential shifts during delayed response performance by monkeys.—S. C. Rosen and J. S. Stamm (Stony Brook, N.Y., U.S.A.).

Monkeys were trained on a two choice delayed response (DR) task which involved 2-sec visual cue presentation, 8-sec delay, and food reinforcement for the correct response. Pairs of non-polarizable Ag-AgCl electrodes were chronically implanted on the surface and in underlying white matter of several cortical areas. Bipolar ECoG recordings with DC amplifiers were obtained throughout testing and were computer averaged. Recordings from cortex contralateral to the responding (preferred) hand revealed surface negative steady potential (SP) shifts of 25 to 100 μV from: (1) occipital cortex during presentation of the cue and reinforcement lights, (2) premotor cortex in relation to the instrumental response, and (3) prefrontal cortex prior to and after the start of the delay period and again following the instrumental response. SP shifts from posterior parietal cortex were not clearly associated with events of the DR trial. When the monkeys were then tested with cues of 4, 6, and 8 sec duration, it was found that the prefrontal SP shifts reached maximum negativity at the start of the delay period, regardless of cue duration, and returned to baseline level during the last 5 sec of the delay. The magnitude of the prefrontal shift was also a function of the level of correct responses, with higher correct scores correlated with greater shifts. SP shifts from prefrontal cortex ipsilateral to the responding hand were less than those from contralateral cortex. During transfer tests with the nonpreferred hand the magnitude of prefrontal SP shifts increased in both hemispheres. The surface negative SP shifts are interpreted as reflecting increased excitation, and hence greater involvement of the underlying neuronal structures at critical times during the DR trial. The prefrontal SP shifts would, therefore, implicate this cortical area in the DR task during the brief period at the beginning, but not during the later portions, of the delay period. The present findings also indicate interhemispheric differences and possible cerebral dominance in monkeys.

87. Effects of 24 hour REM deprivation on serum growth hormone levels in humans.—E. Othmer, V. Daughaday, and S. Guze (St. Louis, Mo., U.S.A.).

The study was designed to explore the relationship of rapid eye movement sleep (REM) measured by the EEG and the level of somatotrophic (growth) hormone (GH) in blood serum measured by a radioimmunoassay method. Previous studies suggest a possible relationship of the onset of slow sleep to GH, consisting of an early GH peak that levels off as the night progresses.

Our method was to record the EEG, electro-oculogram and EMG of male subjects during: (a) 24 h of baseline, (b) 24 h of REM deprivation by awakening, and (c) 24 h of recovery following REM deprivation. GH serum concentrations were determined from blood samples taken every 20 min from an indwelling catheter. We elected to use 24-h time units because a somewhat periodic appearance of REM activity has been demonstrated under special resting conditions throughout the night and day previously. Twenty-four hour curves of GH concentration during the baseline period were compared with those measured during 24 h of REM deprivation and 24 h of REM recovery. The results show that GH levels are significantly increased during REM deprivation in comparison to the baseline and that elevated GH concentration of a somewhat higher degree can be observed also during REM recovery.

These results indicate that REM deprivation methods activate REM production (as expressed by an increase of REM onsets during deprivation and REM percentage during recovery) as well as GH release (as expressed by elevated levels over 24 h during REM deprivation and recovery). This finding suggests a functional relationship between those pontile areas responsible for REM regulation and those areas of the hypothalamus that control GH release, and thus seem to lend evidence to former speculations that REM has a metabolic function.

88. Sleep-onset REM in normals.—M. P. Hayden (St. Louis, Mo., U.S.A.).

Episodes of fast-frequency, low-voltage EEG activity accompanied by rapid eye movements (REM), appear periodically during night sleep but normally not at sleep-onset. Our experiments were designed to test the conditions which need to be fulfilled in order for normal subjects to have sleep-onset REM.

Three male subjects were kept in bed for 24 h. The light was out from 10 p.m. to 7:30 a.m. EEG, EMG, EOG were recorded during baseline and awake conditions. During baseline condition, undisturbed night sleep from 10 p.m. until 7:30 a.m. was allowed prior to the awakening procedure. During awake condition, subjects were awakened by sound and interview whenever they entered stage 2 for more than 3 min or entered a deeper stage of sleep. The onset of REM under this condition was considered to be a sleep-onset REM.

During baseline condition, our three subjects had 10 REM periods all together during the daytime. Seven out of these 10 periods met the criteria for sleep-onset REM. Four of these did not even show spindle sleep before the onset of REM. Inspite of the scheduled awake conditions, one subject could not be kept awake. His eleven REM periods did not meet sleep-onset REM criteria. A second subject was kept awake successfully for most of the 24 h of recording, but he showed only one REM period which failed to meet REM-onset requirements. A third subject had 6 REM periods. Only the last 2 were sleep-onset REM.

Our results show that sleep-onset REM can be demonstrated in normals when the subject is well rested. The occurrence of sleep spindles prior to REM seems not to be a necessary requirement for the appearance of a REM period.

89. The electroencephalogram in speech disorders of children.—M. Dawson and F. C. Rose (London, G.B.).

EEGs were performed on 85 children, all of whom had severe speech disorders. The severity of the speech disorders in these children was such that it merited admission to the only two schools solely for speech disorders in Great Britain; these are Moor House School, Oxted, Surrey, where there are 61 pupils between the ages of 9 and 16, and John Horniman School, Worthing, Sussex, where there are 24 pupils between the ages of 5 and 9.

The disorders may be broadly divided into those of language—dysphasia and those of speech—dysarthria. The language disorders are either predominantly expressive or predominantly receptive. The latter group form the most incapacitated children from the point of view of failure to communicate. This group of receptive aphasics can be divided on their history into acquired and developmental. The acquired group invariably has an abnormal EEG initially which usually improves. The developmental group of receptive aphasia often, but not invariably has an abnormal EEG.

In the dysarthric group there is a close

correlation between the severity of the speech disorder and the EEG abnormality.

The implications of these EEG findings are discussed in relationship to the aetiology of the many types of speech disorders in children.

90. Effect of hippocampal stimulation on unit activity of hypothalamic, preoptic and basal forebrain areas.–C. E. Poletti, M. A. Kinnard and P. D. Maclean (Bethesda, Md., U.S.A.).

The effects of hippocampal volleys and after-discharges on unit activity in hypothalamic, preoptic, and basal forebrain areas are being studied in awake sitting squirrel monkeys. Most of the present sample of 490 units have shown a slow spontaneous firing rate (0.1-5/sec). With single or paired shocks to the anterior and posterior hippocampus evoked responses and changes in firing pattern have been observed in 12% (33/268) of units in the hypothalamus; 36% (25/70) in preoptic areas; and 30% (45/152) in basal forebrain structures (n. of diagonal band, n. accumbens, gyrus rectus, and olfactory tubercle). The three structures with the highest percentage of responses are nucleus of the diagonal band (47%), medial preoptic area (41%), and lateral septum (31%). Of 102 responding units, 95 were predominantly excited and 7 inhibited. Average latencies for units ranged from 15-80 msec, with latencies of 10 msec or less being found in lateral hypothalamus, medial and lateral preoptic areas, lateral septum, n. accumbens, and n. of the diagonal band. Stimulation of anterior and posterior parts of the hippocampus were equally effective in evoking unit responses in the three explored regions. One-fifth of the units responded to ipsilateral anterior and posterior stimulation, whereas 8% were affected by contralateral volleys. Observations were made on the effect of hippocampal after-discharges on 27 units in the three different regions. During an after-discharge excitation was twice as frequent as inhibition. When changes in the firing rate occurred following the after-discharge the direction of change was invariably opposite to that during the after-discharge and lasted 1-11 min.

91. Sleep EEG patterns in a case of Down's syndrome–before and after 5-HTP.–J. C. M. Lee, E. M. Ornitz, P. E. Tanguay and E. R. Ritvo (Los Angeles, Calif., U.S.A.).

Down's syndrome sleep EEG patterns have been studied in different age groups. Particular attention has been given to REM sleep time. The results of these studies have varied in different investigations.

REM sleep time has been shown to correlate with age and the degree of mental retardation. EEG studies of adolescent Down's syndrome have shown reduction of REM sleep time in severely retarded patients, but not in moderately retarded patients. A study of newborn mongol babies also showed reduced REM sleep time. Recently, a case of Down's syndrome treated with 5 Hydroxytryptophan (5-HTP) from 3 days of age was reported. Throughout the first year the child had a normal percentage of REM sleep time, but it was impossible to state whether or not the medication itself had had an effect in normalizing the sleep cycle. To clarify this question, we present a case of a 6-month old baby with Down's syndrome in which sleep EEG data have been collected before and after 5-HTP treatment. We also studied four normal 6-month old babies. In the Down's syndrome baby, there were no sleep pattern changes after medication. There was no reduction of REM sleep time in the Down's syndrome baby when sleep patterns were compared to the normals.

Data on averaged auditory evoked responses to clicks and development testing of the patient will also be presented.

92. Relations between EEG activity and post-synaptic potentials of spinal motoneurones during seizure discharges.–E. J. Speckman and H. Caspers (Munster, W. Germany).

In anesthetized rats i.v. injections of 20-50 mg/Kg of Metrazol evoke cortical seizure discharges which do not affect the spinal motoneurones if the cord has been transected. However, with intact motor pathways the membrane potentials of the motoneurones show considerable fluctuations which coincide with the seizure discharges. During experiments the following observations have been made:

1. The first administration of the drug is followed by a prolonged neuronal depolarization whose time course corresponds to the initial negative DC shift at the cerebral cortex.
2. Each single EEG spike is associated with a sequence of motoneurone postsynaptic potentials which can be divided into a fast and a delayed response. The fast components arise after a latency of some msec and represent either EPSPs or IPSPs with a duration up to 100 msec. The delayed responses consist of polysynaptic EPSPs accompanied by a series of propagated discharges. Both voltage and time course depend on the steepness of the EEG spikes.
3. With increasing frequency of cortical seizure discharges the polysynaptic EPSPs sum up to a sustained depolarization. In this condition the firing pattern of the motoneurones turns from the clonic to the tonic form. Occasionally, excessive depolarization occurs, upon which spike generation fails.

4. Extinction of EEG seizure discharges by an increase of pCO_2 is associated with a moderate hyperpolarization of the motoneurones. Simultaneously the evoked postsynaptic potentials disappear.

The induced response patterns of spinal motoneurones during cerebral convulsive discharges resemble those observed in the immediate area of active foci.

93. Correlations between different EEG patterns and serum concentrations during Phenothiazine therapy.—H. Helmchen, and S. Kanowski (Berlin, W. Germany).

Changes in background activity and appearances of paroxysmal rhythmic and dysrhythmic discharges during therapy with neuroleptic drugs are well known. These changes have been followed in 282 EEGs taken from 50 patients over a 30-day period while on a constant dose of Perazine. The frequencies of the alpha dominant type EEG, the small amplitude EEG, regular 7 to 8 c/s activity and irregular activity increased significantly during the course of Perazine therapy. The same was true for continuous and paroxysmal dysrhythmias and even focal disturbances appeared more often under this therapy. Left-sided foci were more common than those appearing on the right. Continuous and grouped abnormal monorhythmic activity appeared mainly under therapy. Generalized slowed and irregular activity of pathological amounts was not seen. Hypersynchronous high voltage discharges developed in only two patients while under therapy. The serum concentration of Perazine was determined prior to the EEG being taken. Correlations have been made using a special computer program between the EEG changes under Perazine therapy and the averaged and special serum concentrations of the Perazine.

94. Memory and vigilance: spectral EEG analysis during learning in humans.—M. Koukkou, J. M. Madey and C. L. Yeager (San Francisco, Calif., U.S.A.).

Behavioral experiments indicate that learning is facilitated with increased vigilance. The level of vigilance can be assessed using the spectral distribution of wave frequencies in the EEG. We tested the hypothesis that the degree of vigilance after presentation of memory material determines the quality of memory storage in normal humans. Short, meaningful sentences were presented to sleeping subjects via a loudspeaker. These presentations resulted in brief periods of increased vigilance. Retention of the sentences was tested after the experiment; the results were classified as spontaneous recall, or possibility to recognize, or "no memory".

The parieto-occipital EEGs recorded during 90 sec after the presentations were subjected to a spectral analysis (period analysis) in 5-sec intervals. The spectra of corresponding intervals for the same class of recall were averaged over all subjects. The average EEG spectra during 5 to 15 sec after the presentation showed a wakefulness-type frequency distribution for the cases of spontaneous recall and recognition, and a sleep-type distribution for the cases of "no memory". The EEG spectrum for the cases of recognition showed an increase of slower frequencies and a reduction of higher frequencies at 25 to 35 sec after the presentation. With further increase in time after the presentation, the spectrum for the cases of recognition, and later the spectrum for the cases of spontaneous recall approached the sleep distribution.

In addition, EEG spectra obtained during learning of new sentences were compared with spectra during relearning of sentences which were familiar to the subjects. Within the same class of recall, distinctly higher levels of vigilance were associated with learning of unfamiliar material than with relearning of familiar material.

Our results demonstrate a systematic relation between the level of vigilance (objectively assessed by computer analysis of the EEG) during learning and the quality of the memory storage.

95. Bizarre EEG of striate cortex in blind squirrel monkeys.—H. Sakakura and R. H. Doty (Osaka, Japan and Rochester, N.Y., U.S.A.).

In normal, unanesthetized squirrel monkeys oscilloscopic recordings from electrodes with 1 mm tip separation in the striate cortex often show 40-60/sec oscillations at 100-300 μV, for several seconds when room lights are turned on; and similar oscillations may occur for a briefer period with onset of darkness. Such oscillations, however, are often absent or may be suddenly curtailed by eye movements or change of attention. There is no prominent alpha rhythm. Responses of striate cortex to electrical pulses to optic radiation are strongly influenced by light versus darkness or by state of alertness (*e.g.*, wakefulness versus slow wave sleep). After bilateral enucleation of the eyes, the EEG of striate cortex becomes flat, punctuated by sporadic spikes, at 200-300 μV, lasting 100 msec. Many but not all of these spikes are correlated with eye movements (as indicated by the EMG of the eye muscles after enucleation). These spikes are sometimes followed by a burst of large amplitude slow waves. After several weeks the slow waves occur more often, occupy more of the record and sometimes have faster activity superimposed on them, but continue to be interrupted by flat periods lasting about 1 sec. The response evoked by stimulation of the optic radiation gradually increases. From the fifth day on it exceeds any recorded in the intact monkey during wakefulness. The percentage of time spent in slow wave and REM sleep did not change in the one monkey studied so far, although there seemed to be a change in distribution of sleep throughout a 24-h period. In addition, there is a permanent increase of 12/sec spindle bursts in the sensorimotor areas. Thus, some aspect of normal retinal activity must exert continual control over electrical patterns of the brain as well as excitability of the striate cortex.

96. Temporal and spatial summation in generation of somatosensory evoked potential.—T. S. Prevec (Ljubljana, Yugoslavia).

The somatosensory cerebral evoked potential (CEP) has failed to reveal many of the functional properties of the afferent system which have been demonstrated in psychophysical studies and by experimental work on animals. The aim of this investigation was to study interaction between somatosensory stimuli simultaneously applied to several sites or temporally dispersed. The stimuli were electrical pulses, threshold or subthreshold for the CEP, which was recorded from the scalp over the primary somatosensory region (120 responses were summated, analysis time being 100 msec). Spatial interaction of stimulation was studied by applying electrically identical stimuli to several fingers of the hand. To study temporal interaction, one, two, three, five or eight successive stimuli were added to a single subthreshold stimulus at intervals of 2 msec.

The results show a summation of responses to spatially separated stimuli, however, the amplitudes of individual deflections of the CEP never reached those obtained with a stimulus supramaximal for CEP, such as a tap to the thenar eminence.

Successively added stimuli also increased the amplitude of the CEP. The larger the amplitude of the first positive deflection of the CEP when evoked by a single stimulus, the shorter was the train of successive stimuli needed to give the maximum amplitude obtainable with such stimulation. Similarly as with spatially separated stimuli, trains of threshold stimuli did not usually elicit CEP of the maximum amplitude.

The effects of both temporal and spatial summation were most clearly manifested in the peak-to-peak amplitude of the second positive and the following negative wave (with the respective peak latencies between 38 and 47 msec and between 50 and 90 msec).

97. Feedback method: a new look at functional EEG.—T. B. Mulholland (Bedford, Mass., U.S.A.).

Feedback EEG is an example of applied cybernetics in clinical and experimental neurophysiology. The response of the occipital alpha rhythm is connected to a visual display by an external path. By viewing the display, the person makes a closed loop. The alpha feedback system, first reported by Adrian, has many applications which are extensions of the concept of "functional EEG" introduced twenty years ago by Liberson and Gastaut. Other applications of feedback EEG are unprecedented and lead to an entirely new direction in EEG research.

Application of feedback EEG is developed from basic research which has shown that (1) feedback from EEG to the display constrains the EEG alpha-activation cycle, reducing unpredictable or uninformative variation; (2) the constrained system can be disturbed, showing an initial response followed by a recovery to near baseline conditions; (3) the disturbance and recovery of the feedback system is an index of stimulus parameters and complex variables of visual control; (4) EEG processes which are not consciously known can be brought into awareness by informational feedback. Combined with training, voluntary control of these processes can be learned; (5) by means of the feedback path information displays and appliances can be automatically regulated by the EEG processes to which they are connected. Combined with training, voluntary control of the display or appliance can be learned; (6) by controlling the parameters of the feedback path the EEG response can be controlled. If these determine a behavioral response, then it can be controlled.

98. Intra and inter individual variability of the averaged evoked potential in normal and chronic schizophrenic subjects.—K. Lifshitz (Orangeburg, N.Y., U.S.A.).

The spatio-temporal configuration of electrical activity in the brain has been considered as the representation of information processing. The average evoked cortical potential (AEP) is considered as a sample of this processing. We have hypothesized that the difficulties encountered by some schizophrenics are due to an inability to precisely replicate these spatio-temporal electrical patterns.

In a group of chronic schizophrenics (N=16) and "normal" individuals (N=16), we have investigated the intra-individual and inter-individual replicability of the AEP under various stimuli conditions. In addition to investigating this question by the repeated presentations of the same stimuli, we have also studied the relationship between the separate presentation of an auditory stimulus and a visual stimulus, and the simultaneous presentation of these two different stimuli. The two-modality stimulus case has been investigated by utilizing a constrained, weighted, linear summation technique to produce a synthesized two-modality AEP from the AEPs to individual stimuli. Inter individual variability has been evaluated by comparing individual AEPs to a group mean AEP. Replicability of the AEP has been judged by utilization of correlation coefficients and by treating the AEPs as unknowns in identification paradigms.

Our initial results indicate that the intra-individual replicability of an AEP as judged by correlation coefficients was significantly ($P<0.01$) poorer in the schizophrenics. In our intra-individual identification paradigm, for the single modality case, our identification was very significantly better than chance in the normals ($P<10^{-8}$); while for the schizophrenics it was not significantly better than chance. For the two-modality case, identification was significantly better than chance ($P<0.01$) in the normals but not in the schizophrenics. In our inter individual identification paradigm, a commonality of AEP information representation "code" was indicated at a significant level in the normals ($P<0.0001$), but not in the schizophrenics.

99. Encephalophonography.—I. Sherwin and H. T. Castillo (Boston, Mass. and West Haven, Conn., U.S.A.).

Common in the experience of electrophysiologists when recording unit activity from a variety of sources is the fact that an auditory monitor frequently provides much more information about the activity under investigation than may be obtained from visual display (ink writer or oscilloscope). With this in mind it seemed reasonable that complimentary visual and auditory analysis of cerebral bioelectric potentials (EEG) might provide more information than visual inspection alone. The ensemble of electronic components used to produce the audible EEG consists of standard "off-the-shelf" instruments found in most neurophysiology laboratories and may collectively be referred to as an encephalophone. In practice the "brain waves", led from the scalp via needle electrodes, are amplified and passed to a voltage controlled oscillator. The resulting FM electrical signal is fed to a commercial home tape recorder for storage and conversion to an acoustical signal. The final sound heard by an observer has both frequency and amplitude modulation; the FM characteristic is a result of the electrical design and the AM is due to the phenomenon of equal loudness contours.

The normal alpha rhythm is easily recognized as a distinct chirping sound. Destructive and irritative brain lesions on the other hand produce sounds that are identifiable as being distinctly different from those of normal brains.

Preliminary clinical trials suggest that this method may provide a convenient and rapid means of detecting normal and abnormal electrical activity of the brain.

A miniaturized version of the encephalophone might find utility as a bedside "stethoscope" for the brain, as well as providing the design basis for a patient-worn seizure detection and warning device.

100. EEG and clinical arousal induced by bilateral long-term stimulation of pallidal systems in traumatic vigil coma.—R. Hassler, G. Dalle Ore, A. Bricolo, G. Dieckmann and G. Dolce (Frankfurt am Main, Germany, Verona, Italy, Homburg/Saar, Germany, Darmstadt, Germany).

The growing number of patients suffering from traumatic apallic syndrome, who survive for months and even years, requires new more active therapeutic approaches. Assuming that the vigil coma is due to a blockage of the unspecific projection system to the forebrain rather than of the specific system, we have stimulated in 2 patients the right *lamella pallidi interna* and the base of the left VA simultaneously with stereotaxically implanted flexible bipolar electrodes three times daily for 30 min over a period of three weeks. At the same time, while in the state of vigil coma (5 and 3 months after head trauma) we have made polygraphic recordings in these patients.

On bilateral stimulation (25/sec) in the above-mentioned regions an immediate desynchronization appears in all EEG recordings on both sides accompanied by a disappearance of a unilateral delta focus, whereas on unilateral stimulation (VA 25/sec) the previous asymmetry is replaced by alpha activity. Clinically, stimulation of VA brought about opening of the eyelids and contralateral conjugate gaze movements and, after some days, even spontaneous hand movements. Bilateral simultaneous stimulation produced a stronger behavioral arousal combined with apparently spontaneous arm movements. After 20 days of stimulation the level of consciousness was definitely improved, the patients exhibited an emotional interest in their surroundings with appropriate associated movements and could vocalize. In addition, their relatives were convinced that they were recognized by them for the first time.

After the end of stimulation the level of consciousness obtained was preserved but no further progress in conscious state occurred. In a third case studied in Homburg/Saar further improvement appeared in the six months subsequent to removal of their stimulation electrodes. Despite the recovery of spontaneous respiration, however, the other two patients died from infection some months later.

101. Evoked potentials and background activity—extent of linear interaction.—M. S. Weiss (Pullman, Wash., U.S.A).

The extent of a linear relationship between some of the properties of evoked potential (EP) amplitude and background neuroelectric activity was evaluated using data obtained from cats with electrodes chronically implanted in both sensory specific (auditory) regions and non-specific subcortical and cortical regions of the brain. The average and standard deviation of the EP amplitude was measured as was the root-mean-square (RMS) level of the prestimulus activity. The data for these measurements were obtained during a sequence of conditioned changes in behavior. Under conditions of controlled motor activity and stimulus intensity, one burst of tone became a positively reinforced conditioned stimulus (CS) and a second different tone, a negatively reinforced CS. The effects of the establishment and extinction of this differentially conditioned approach response on the relationship between the RMS level of prestimulus activity and the average magnitude and standard deviation of the EP were analyzed.

The results indicated that the prestimulus RMS level of activity and the EP standard deviation were strongly correlated (overall correlation of 0.97), and essentially equal in value. This relationship was independent of the stage of conditioned behavior, but was dependent on the anatomical region from which the data were obtained. There was a weaker correlation between the prestimulus RMS level and the EP magnitude (overall correlation 0.73) which was also independent of stage of conditioning and dependent on the anatomical region analyzed. There was also a trend with structures having low correlations between prestimulus RMS level and EP standard deviation tending to have low correlations between prestimulus RMS level and EP standard deviation tending to have low correlations between prestimulus RMS level and EP magnitude.

Thus, both magnitude and variability of the EP depends on the level of background activity though the detailed nature of this dependence remains to be elucidated and may vary according to the region of the brain which is examined.

102. Visual evoked responses in normal, acallosal and "spilt brain" patients.—G. C. Galbraith, R. E. Saul, J. B. Gliddon (Los Angeles, Calif., U.S.A.).

The visual evoked response (VER) was recorded in ten normal subjects (age range 9-32 years); in one patient with confirmed agenesis of the corpus callosum (age 21 years); and one patient with surgically sectioned corpus callosum and anterior commissure (age 35 years). In all subjects clinical scalp tracings were considered normal.

VERs were recorded from scalp electrodes placed over left and right hemispheres, as well as along the midline. Visual stimuli consisted of 2.2° black triangles centered within 3.8° circular light fields displayed for a duration of 100 msec. Stimuli were flashed in a predetermined random order into the left (L) or right (R) lateral visual field (7° lateral to a point of fixation), or simultaneously into both (B) fields. A Honeywell 1200 computer was used to unscramble the random order and graph the averaged VERs.

VER amplitudes for six electrode sites were compared by means of the following ratio: B/(L+R)½. Results from the normal subjects showed ratios clustering about a mean value of 1.20. That is, amplitudes during the B condition were 20% larger than the average of L and R amplitudes. Ratios from the split brain patient did not differ from normal, (mean ratio = 1.21). The acallosal patient, however, showed ratios ranging from 1.78 to 2.10 (mean ratio = 1.96) with the smallest ratio (1.78) being greater than the largest ratio seen in any of the normal subjects (1.67). However, both patients showed patterns of left-right VER asymmetry not seen in the normals.

Independent behavioral testing showed that the acallosal patient could detect dissimilar patterns in the left and right visual fields whereas the split-brain patient could not.

These results will be discussed in terms of the role played by the corpus callosum in the VER and in processing visual information projected to different hemispheres. Possible developmental differences in the visual system of the acallosal patient will also be discussed.

103. EEG power spectral analysis of newborn infants' sleep states.—A. H. Parmelee (Los Angeles, Calif., U.S.A.).

Infants' EEG patterns change rapidly with maturation, therefore, we chose to define sleep states by physiological parameters other than EEG. The criteria for the two major sleep states are: Quiet Sleep—eye and body movements absent and regular respirations; Active sleep—eye movements and body movements present and irregular respirations.

A coding system for EEG patterns was established without reference to other parameters.

In full term neonates four visually recognizable patterns were identified, similar to those described by Dreyfus-Brisac. These are the *trace alternant* with bursts of large amplitude slow waves, alternating with small amplitude fast activity (Code 407), continuous large amplitude slow waves (Code 405), large amplitude slow waves with periods of rhythmic faster activity intermixed (Code 403), and irregular continuous small amplitude mixed activity with frequent periods of rhythmic activity (Code 402).

Eye movements, body movements, respiration and EEG were visually coded for each 20-sec epoch of 3 h interfeeding polygraphic recordings done on 10 full-term newborns. Using the stated criteria for Quiet and Active Sleep, the frequency of occurrence of each of the four EEG patterns in these two states was determined. Pattern 407 was predominantly associated with Quiet Sleep and 402 with Active Sleep. While 405 and 403 were found in both states, 405 occurred more commonly with Quiet and 403 with Active Sleep.

Power spectral analysis was done on 3-4 min artifact-free samples of each EEG pattern taken from records of 5 full-term newborns recorded on magnetic tape. The percentage of power in four frequency bands was calculated.

The ratios of power found in various frequency bands also differentiated the two sleep states. The Delta/Theta ratio in Active Sleep was 5.4 and in Quiet Sleep 7.9, while the Delta/Sigma ratio was 1.9 in Active Sleep and 2.8 in Quiet Sleep.

104. Statistical characteristics of spontaneous seizure discharges recorded by radiotelemetry over 24 hour periods in man.—J. R. Stevens, B. Lonsbury, H. Kodama and L. Mills (Portland, Ore., U.S.A.).

Continuous 24-h recordings of EEG by radio telemetry from freely moving subjects with seizure disorders have been subjected to statistical analysis in which quantitative relationships between seizure duration and interictal interval were examined. Statistical techniques which have been applied to analysis of single spike trains were employed in the analysis of seizure dicharges and intervening intervals. The spectrum of seizure durations and intervals is presented graphically, and analyzed with respect to internal variance and cross correlation. The relationship of ictal discharge to the circadian cycle of physiologic events and to changes in mood and behavior was also examined.

Results from patients with *petit mal* epilepsy indicate distinct patterns of diurnal and nocturnal ictal events. Automatic numeration of ictal and interictal EEG spikes per unit of time indicates a relatively steady rate of spike discharge interrupted by periods of REM sleep and behavioral arousal. In the subjects studied, nocturnal seizures show less variance in duration and are exponentially distributed as are intervals between onsets. Interictal single spikes are also distributed exponentially. In contrast, daytime seizures are fewer in number, longer, show greater variability in duration and interval, and have either a multimodal or symmetric single mode distribution with respect to both duration and interictal interval (*i.e.,* do not fit an exponential function). A positive relationship between seizure duration and length of ensuing seizure-free interval is evident in several studies. Treated in this way, seizure discharges and intervening intervals are analyzed as stochastic processes, the mathematical formulation of which may permit inferences with respect to underlying physiological determinants of seizure onset and termination.

105. Visceral modulation of somatic brain stem reflexes: vagal neurogram correlates.—M. H. Chase, S. Torii, and Y. Nakamura (Sepulveda and Los Angeles, Calif., U.S.A.).

We recently reported that stimulation of the cut central end of the cervical vagus nerve was capable of modifying the amplitude of brain stem somatic reflexes in immobilized *encéphale isolé* cats. Following excitation of the vagus nerve with a single pulse the monosynaptic masseteric reflex (Mass. R.) was initially suppressed (5 to 35 msec) and then facilitated (35 to 100 msec), whereas the polysnaptic digastric reflex (Dig. R.) was continually suppressed (5 to 100 msec). Repetitive vagal stimulation (100 c/sec) for periods of 10 sec led to Mass. R. facilitation and Dig. R. suppression. We now report an analysis of the vagal fiber systems responsible for these reflex responses. The excitation of specific fiber groups was correlated with changes in reflex amplitude by simultaneously monitoring the induced vagal neurographic activity and the reflex responses. Excitation of rapidly-conducting fiber systems (>20m/sec) had no effect on either the Mass. R. or Dig. R., whereas, excitation of a slower-conducting fiber group (approximately 10 to 20 m/sec) affected the Mass R. and Dig. R., as described above. This slow-conducting vagal system is primarily of thoracic origin, and, thus, we conclude that activity from visceral receptors within the thoracic cavity can profoundly influence somatic reflexes, and, as we have shown previously, initiate correlated patterns of EEG activity.

106. Self photo-desensitization in man and baboon.—J. A. Wada, A. Teraro and H. E. Booker (Vancouver, Canada, and Madison, Wis., U.S.A.).

Self-induced photo-sensitive seizures have been shown to possess certain common features, such as female predominance in the younger age group, light sensitivity and prevalence of mental retardation, regardless of exact clinical or electrographic manifestations involved. In spite of increasing attention paid to these problems, the mechanism underlying self-seizure induction remains obscure.

It is the intention of this presentation to describe results of some of our preliminary exploration in this area in photo- sensitive patients, with a tendency to self-stimulation, who have been given complete control of a photic stimulator in a laboratory setting. It was found that these patients were capable of desensitizing themselves from flicker-induced electrographic and clinical seizures when they were given control of a photic stimulator which was preset at a given parameter.

This finding will be contrasted with the results of our study in a group of photogenic Senegalese baboons which have similarly self-photo-desensitized themselves for a maximum period of up to three months in a comparable laboratory situation.

107. Maturation of visual cortical and subcortical evoked responses and EEG after discharge in unanesthetized kittens.–G. H. Rose and S. P. Gruenau (Omaha, Neb., U.S.A.).

Algebraically summated cortical responses evoked by light flash obtained in 60 cross-sectional and longitudinal age samples from 35 unanesthetized kittens with implanted electrodes and 25 preparations under Flaxedil are compared with similar recordings previously obtained by Rose and Lindsley from lightly anesthetized kittens. Pilot data on subcortical responses were also obtained.

These results show that the maturational changes in the wave form of the visual electrocortical responses in the first two weeks of life are highly similar in the anesthetized and unanesthetized kitten. The responses begin with a long latency negative wave at 0-4 days which is preceded, between 8-10 days, by a shorter latency positive-negative complex resulting in a clearly differentiated positive-negative-negative wave form at 14 days of age. Such a sequence, present in both unanesthetized conditions, is best obtained in the preparations under Flaxedil which permit maximal conditions of controlled focused stimulation identical to that utilized in the original studies on anesthetized kittens.

Beyond two weeks of age, differences occur in the wave form of the visual evoked potentials as a function of anesthesia. Whereas in the anesthetized preparations the adult-like wave form at 30 days consists of a single diphasic positive-negative response, the evolvement of the adult-like wave form in unanesthetized kittens is more complex, usually consisting of an initial double positive deflection.

In addition to maturational changes in cortical evoked activity, there exists in the unanesthetized kittens, parallel changes in the cortical after-discharge to flash characterized by large amplitude spindling in the youngest animals to be gradually replaced, between 10-14 days, by low voltage desynchronized activity typical of adult electrocortical arousal.

108. Prospective study of EEGs in children of low birth weight.–N. L. Auckland, M. Cox, J. U. Crichton, and H. G. Dunn (Vancouver, Canada).

In a prospective study of 500 children with a birth weight of 2041 g or less, 278 had EEGs recorded in the nursery, 249 at about 1½ years, and so far 127 at 6½ years. Among the neonatal records 30% were considered borderline or abnormal. At 1½ years, 22% were interpreted as borderline or abnormal, in contrast to only 2% of the tracings recorded from 98 control children of full birth weight (above 2500 g) at the same age. The correlation between EEG abnormalities in individual children of low birth weight in the neonatal period and at 1½ years is poor, and most of the neonatal abnormalities appear to resolve.

At 6½ years, no fewer than 63 (50%) of the 127 children of low birth weight examined to date have borderline (18) or abnormal (45) records. The commonest EEG abnormalities (sometimes combined) in these cases are spike-wave or sharp-and-slow wave discharges in 21, bilateral spikes or sharp waves in 11, slow dysrhythmia in 11, persistent asymmetry in 10, mixed dysrhythmia in 8, and focal spikes or sharp waves in 7. Only 6 of the 39 children with discharges have ever had seizures. Positive spikes at 14 and 6/sec were found in 5 cases. Thrity-five of the 63 children with abnormal or borderline records previously had an EEG performed at a mean age of 17 months, and only about 1/3 (13) of these previous tracings were interpreted as abnormal. It is concluded that EEG abnormalities occur in nearly ½ of school entrants with a birth weight of 2000 g or less and that about 2/3 of these abnormalities only became evident after the age of 1½ years.

109. Phase of alpha wave, habituation and contingent blocking.–V. Milstein (Portland, Ore., U.S.A.).

This research tested the hypothesis that habituation of the alpha attenuation response (AAR) will be more rapid when the stimulus is presented on the surface negative phase of the alpha wave than when it is presented at other points on the wave.

Conversely, contingent alpha blocking to click-flash procedure will occur more rapidly when the click is presented on the positive phase of the alpha wave.

Subjects with persistent, moderately large amplitude alpha activity were randomly assigned to a group stimulated at one of the following points and 180° from it: peak, trough, midpoints of the up-and-down-going alpha wave. The activity from vertex to left and to right occipital regions was differentially amplified and processed separately by two "Alpha Triggers" which continuously monitored the EEG, recorded when alpha activity was present, and presented the stimuli at the preselected points on the wave.

With a continuous background of white noise, 40 single flashes of light were presented irregularly during runs of alpha activity, with at least 5 sec and one unstimulated train of alpha waves occurring between stimuli. The subject then received 40 click stimuli in the same manner over the white noise background. After a brief delay, the clicks were paired with and preceded the flashes of light by 0.5 sec. After a rest period, the Alpha Trigger was set 180°, + 90° or - 90° from where it was originally.

The results indicated that these subjects demonstrate more rapid and more regular habituation of AAR than did subjects who were presented with stimuli not locked-into a particular point on the alpha wave. Presenting stimuli at the midpoint of the surface negative wave resulted in more rapid habituation for flash but not for click stimuli. Whereas the results of the contingent blocking procedure did not reveal reliable differences between phases, there was a tendency for those subjects stimulated at the trough of the wave to demonstrate contingent attenuation most often.

110. The significance of low voltage fast activity in interictal records of temporal lobe epilepsy. —F. Rotondi Serra (Palermo, Italy).

Approximately 3000 cases of temporal lobe epilepsy seen over the last twelve years were subdivided into various groups on the basis of the dominant or exclusive symptoms of the psychomotor syndrome.

In all the groups the interictal tracings have been frequently characterized by low voltage fast activity (30 to 45% varying with symptomatology). In analyzing this observation either a neurochemical or a neuronal approach could be made. From a neurochemical standpoint consideration must be given to the severe metabolic changes found by Tower in epileptogenic foci as well as the turnover of ATP described by Dosseva. Furthermore, particular attention could be paid to the turnover of free and polymerized nucleotides in both the pre and postictal stages as suggested by Bonavita. The relatively high postictal increase in uridine monophosphate content could be considered as an imporant mechanism of cell membrane permeability.

It is possible that the low voltage fast activity could be interpreted, as indicated by Walter, as the result of metabolic and neuronal changes which characterize the physiopathology of convulsions also in the interictal stage. From a neuronal point of view the findings could be interpreted as the result of an initial participation of the neocortex to an ictal discharge in the subcortex. By means of evoked potential techniques the postictal silence could be interpreted not as a complete neuronal extinction but as a selective inhibition of the highest cortical layers which Eccles suggests might be responsible for afferent collateral circuits. A further suggestion is that the postictal record could be a deficit phenomenon related to the exhaustion of the perilesional neurons immediately after discharging.

The results of automatic frequency analysis of low voltage fast records might give further insight into and explanations for the different approaches.

111. Analysis of the interrelations between frequency bands of the EEG by means of the bispectrum.—B. Kleiner, P. J. Huber and G. Dumermuth (Zurich, Switzerland).

The more or less random character of the spontaneous EEG activity justifies the application of mathematical models developed in time series analysis. Among these methods numerical spectrum analysis has proved to be a powerful tool for analyzing and quantifying EEG data, especially background activity. A first step is the spectral decomposition of a given EEG sample into its frequency components, giving (after appropriate smoothing) the well-known variance or power spectrum. However, the power spectrum gives complete information about the statistical properties of an EEG sample only under the assumption that the underlying process is Gaussian. Recent investigations carried out in our EEG laboratory show that the amplitude distribution already deviates from normality in a major part of resting EEGs from healthy subjects. This implies that in these cases the power spectrum gives only partial information and higher order moments should be investigated. Analogous to the power spectrum S(w), which is the Fourier transform of the autocovariance R_j=Ave($X_t S_{t+j}$), the bispectrum B(w_1,w_2) represents the spectral counterpart of the second order autocovariance $R_{j,k}$=Ave($X_t X_{t+J} X_{t+k}$). Therefore, the bispectrum may be considered as the spectral decomposition of the third central moment (which determines the skewness of the amplitude distribution). As skewness may arise either from interrelations between frequency components (due to nonlinearities) or from non-stationarity, the bispectrum may display important additional information about the properties of a stochastic signal such as the EEG. Obviously this information may prove to be of great value in the investigation of harmonic relationships between different frequency bands, *e.g.*, between α and β activity, or between α activity and slow posterior rhythms. In addition some new insights into the non-linear aspects of the EEG generating process might be expected.

Because of the lengthy calculations, the computation of a bispectrum is a tedious and very time consuming task and until today only a few bispectra of geophysical data have been calculated. The introduction of the Fast Fourier Transform and our previous experience with this alogrithm in EEG analysis form the basis of a program which computes the bispectrum of an EEG sample within reasonable time.

Bispectra of artificial signals will be shown in order to explain the basic aspects of the extension of conventional spectrum analysis, and selected examples of bispectra of actual EEG data will demonstrate the interesting possibilities which this method offers for EEG analysis.

112. EEG changes during arch aortography.–S. Satran, E. O. Lipchik, C. O. Barley and K. Coast (Rochester, N.Y., U.S.A.).

EEG studies were performed on 19 patients (mean age 66 years) during four vessel arch aortography. All patients had signs and symptoms of occlusive vascular disease. In 10 patients X-ray studies revealed surgically significant extracranial stenoses of the internal carotid arteries. During angiography no changes were noted in the overall background activity of the EEG. Minor EEG abnormalities in the pre-angiographic records were not more manifest during or after arteriography. No untoward responses were noted during the angiographic procedures.

Eight patients had carotid endarterectomy and follow-up EEGs 3-4 days after surgery. Six patients had accentuation of minor weight EEG abnormalities present before surgery. The most frequent change was the occurrence of high voltage polyrhythmic mid-temporal delta activity.

Arch aortography performed for the diagnosis of occlusive cerebrovascular disease is a procedure of low risk which does not alter the EEG.

113. Frequency analysis of the EEG under different behavioral states.–D. Giannitrapani (Chicago, Ill., U.S.A.).

Current methods of computer EEG analysis permit exploration of electrocortical activity changes under different behavioral states with a degree of precision not previously available. The current experiment was designed to study these changes during activities involving different kinds of auditory, visual and conceptual functions. Thirty-two right-handed males had EEGs recorded from 16 areas onto digital tape. The results of a spectral analysis in 17 frequency bands from 1 to 33 c/sec were analyzed.

To study auditory involvement the subject listened with eyes closed to white noise, music and verbal stimulation. Differences among the conditions, between each condition and the two control periods (awake, resting, with eyes closed at the beginning and end of the experiment) were analyzed to determine the location and frequency component involved.

To study the correlates of patterned and unpatterned vision the subject looked at a poster for the first condition and through diffusing goggles for the second. The EEG during mental arithmetic was also compared with the resting conditions.

Arithmetic showed increase in fast activity (21 to 33 c/sec) bilaterally, anteriorly more in prefrontal areas; for Noise, an increase in fast activity (23 to 31 c/sec) in prefrontal and temporal areas bilaterally. Music simulated Noise but more weakly, with decrease at 19 c/sec and increase at 33 c/sec in the left occipital area. Voice simulated Noise, but in slightly higher frequency bands (27-33 c/sec). Voice also showed a decrease in alpha activity in the R. post temporal and R. occipital areas, and decrease in 19 and 33 c/sec in the L. occipital area.

The two visual conditions showed overall changes in the prefrontal, temporal, post temporal, parietal and occipital areas, as well as selected changes in other areas. The relevance of these findings in light of current neuroanatomical knowledge is discussed.

114. Correlation between prostaglandin release from cerebral cortex and electrocorticogram in unanesthetized cats.–P. B. Bradley and G. M. R. Samuels (Birmingham, G.B.).

A prostaglandin-like material has been found in superfusates of cerebral cortex in unanesthetized *encéphale isolé* cat preparations. The material was assayed on the rat uterus and identified by thin-layer chromatography. The level of spontaneous release of the prostaglandin-like material was higher than that which had been found previously in anesthetized preparations and it increased still further with electrical stimulation of the reticular formation at levels which induced electrocortical arousal. Administration of chlorpromazine (1.0-8.0 mg/kg) not only depressed the spontaneous release of prostaglandins, but blocked the increase evoked by stimulation, concomitantly with blocking electrocortical arousal. Increasing the stimulating voltage to restore the arousal response also restored the evoked release of prostaglandins. Most of the prostaglandin-like material released spontaneously was represented by 'E' type compounds, whereas the increase with stimulation was mainly of the 'F' compounds. It is thought that, whilst the prostaglandins are unlikely to be synaptic transmitters in the central nervous system, they must have some function connected with neuronal mechanisms.

115. The EEG in acute barbiturate intoxication, with particular reference to isoelectric EEGs. —S. Sament and A. D. Huott (Boston, Mass., U.S.A.).

The EEGs in 26 cases of acute barbiturate intoxication have been classified as follows:

Stage I Normal EEG with small amplitude fast activity (1 case)
Stage II Predominantly alpha with some theta activity (9 cases)
Stage III Predominantly theta activity (5 cases)
Stage IV Predominantly delta activity (3 cases)
Stage V Isoelectric with bursts of sharp activity (2 cases)
Stage VI Completely isoelectric (6 cases)

Stages I-III were associated with drowsiness or confusion.

Stages IV-VI were associated with coma, and these three stages could not be distinguished clinically, or by barbiturate levels.

In Stage IV, all patients survived. In Stage V, one patient survived. In Stage VI, all patients died. Causes of death were cardio-respiratory failure and anoxia, pneumonia, and renal failure. If these complications can be prevented, all cases of barbiturate intoxication are potentially reversible. The blood barbiturate correlated poorly with the state of consciousness, or the EEG. Other investigators have shown that the EEG is the best single measure of the depth of barbiturate narcosis and that it was superior, in this respect, to clinical or biochemical testing: these studies were performed experimentally on cats and also during thiopentone anesthesia in man. The present study shows the same conclusions for barbiturate intoxication in man. There is a direct correlation between the EEG changes, described above, and the complications that might be anticipated. Thus cardiac arrest has occurred only during Stage VI, whereas respiratory failure occurred during Stage III-VI. The present study also shows that depression of tendon jerks, absent pupillary and corneal reflexes, and immobility of the eyes do not, in themselves, indicate a poor prognosis.

116. Rhythmic afterwaves to flashes in relation to amplitude and phase of foregoing and subsequent alpha activity.—J. S. Barlow and R. W. Lansing (Boston, Mass., U.S.A.).

Although a number of aspects have been previously described concerning the relationship between intrinsic or background alpha activity and the rhythmic waves of alpha frequency which are induced by slowly repeated flashes, the exact nature of their interaction has remained unclear. In the present study, we have explored this question further in a series of recordings of EEGs from normal subjects presented with slowly repeated flashes at randomized intervals. Amplitude of background alpha was obtained by full-wave rectification and smoothing (*i.e.*, envelope detection) of the 7-14 c/sec filtered EEG. Averages of both the envelope (*i.e.*, of alpha spindles) and the raw EEG were computed with respect both to the stimuli and with respect to the phase of the foregoing (as well as the subsequent) background alpha activity. Averages were further apportioned according to the instantaneous amplitude of the immediately foregoing alpha activity, by means of an electronic kick-sorter operated in conjunction with a level detector whose input was the alpha envelope.

Preliminary results from the study suggest the following: (1) The average amplitude of rhythmic afterwaves is not dependent on the amplitude of the immediately foregoing alpha activity. (2) In contrast, the trend of amplitude of the envelope of the EEG following each stimulus is dependent on the amplitude of the immediately foregoing alpha rhythm, such that larger amplitudes tend to diminish, and smaller amplitudes to increase, on the average, immediately following a flash, waves of a foregoing alpha spindle, irrespective of their amplitude, can remain in phase with themselves for a relatively long period (*e.g.*, through two successive flash-intervals). (4) In contrast, flash-induced rhythmic afterwaves tend to be disrupted, or reset in phase, by successive flashes. (5) Alpha waves that reappear following alpha-blocking to flash are largely independent, with respect to phase, of the foregoing alpha activity, *i.e.*, the alpha rhythm does not reappear "in phase" with itself.

These findings will be discussed in relation to the general problem of the origin of alpha activity.

117. An EEG interval spectrum analyser.—J. F. Toennies (Freiburg, W. Germany).

The new analysing system has the following properties:

a) it does not classify into specific frequency bands,

b) it measures each individual EEG wave as a time interval between a given point on one wave to the corresponding point on the next wave,

c) the interval is determined as a strictly aperiodic process independent of proceding or following waves,

d) the interval durations are electronically transformed into ordinate values lying between 1 sec and 33 msec (1 to 33 c/sec) with the smallest interval differences exactly marked,

e) each ordinate value is represented by a single black point up or down on the scale depending on interval duration. A frequency range of 1 to 30 c/sec requires a scale height of 80 mm,

f) the time axis is at 5 or 10 mm/min or 20 times slower than a conventional EEG recording. This permits a long term analysis period without missing any details. A full night sleep record is concentrated onto 2 m of paper and a 3-h narcosis trial onto 1 m,

g) the recording is performed 'on-line' for a single channel and for multi-channel records may be stored on magnetic tape,

h) as the interval measuring technique is amplitude insensitive an equally time condensed record of the actual EEG is taken simultaneously with the interval analysis.

118. Correlation of electroencephalographic, reaction time and auditory thresholds on 24 hour recording.—J. C. Corvalan (St. Louis, Mo., U.S.A.).

The first curve of depth of sleep was published by Kohlschutter (1862) who saw after an initial increase, a negative correlation between duration of sleeping time and intensities of sound required to awaken the sleeper. Lambranzi (1900) stimulated the auditory, visual and olfactory system with the purpose of developing a complete curve of sleep. Davis (1939) used auditory stimulus of constant intensity during different EEG stages and measured the reaction time. It was interpreted that the length of stimulation time correlated with depth of sleep. Williams (1964) considered the intensity of sound required to produce arousal (auditory threshold) as the variable that would reflect depth of EEG-sleep. The general opinion was that there is a direct, positive correlation between the EEG (stage W,1,2,3,4, and REM) and both reaction time and auditory thresholds. It was assumed that each EEG stage would require the same stimulus for arousal and that was an expression of other variables that were present consistently.

The present study was designed to test that hypothesis. Our method was to stimulate two groups of subjects: in Group 1, reaction time to an auditory stimulus of constant intensity was measured; in Group II for auditory thresholds, a response to a step-like increase in the intensity of the stimulus was recorded. Within a 24-h period, commencing at 10 pm, this sound stimulation in both groups I and II, was used during different stages of EEG sleep, until a specific motor response (three eye movements) was obtained.

The results for Group I showed that the reaction time of the REM stage of sleep decreased with progress of absolute time during the 24-h period. The other stages of EEG sleep did not reveal such a time correlation. There was also no observable consistency of reaction time for any other EEG stage. The results for Group II, in stage 4 and stage REM, showed an initial increase in threshold, followed by a decrease in the remainder of the 24-h period.

Our conclusion was that stages of sleep did not present a constant auditory threshold and reaction time, but a dependency upon absolute time.

119. Organization of interneurons in a thalamic relay nucleus.—T. Desiraju and D. P. Purpura (New York, N.Y., U.S.A.).

Intracellular studies of neurons in nucleus ventralis lateralis (VL) have disclosed a wide spectrum of interneuronal responses to stimulation of the brachium conjunctivum (BC), ansa lenticularis (AL) and thalamic internuclear pathways linking VL with medial nonspecific thalamic nuclei (MTh). Monosynaptic convergence of BC and AL projections onto VL neurons is established in the present study. The proportion of such elements exhibiting monosynaptic EPSPs to AL stimulation is small compared to BC stimulation. VL neurons exhibiting monosynaptic convergence develop prolonged IPSPs following BC-evoked EPSPs but such IPSPs do not succeed monosynaptic EPSPs elicited by AL stimulation. These observations are not consistent with a recurrent inhibition hypothesis but suggest rather a differential distribution of BC afferents to a parallel inhibitory interneuron pool. Disynaptic and polysnaptic responses of VL neurons to BC and AL stimulation may consist of similar or reciprocal PSP patterns. This holds chiefly for interneuronal organizations activated 2-6 msec after the time neurons exhibit monosynaptic EPSPs. Very long latency PSPs to AL stimulation are observed in a large proportion of VL neurons but these PSPs are rarely elicited by BC stimulation. MTh-stimulation generally evokes EPSP-IPSP sequences in VL elements that are similar to the long latency PSP patterns initiated by AL stimulation. Interactions between AL and BC evoked PSPs with long latency MTh-evoked EPSP-IPSP sequences are observed which indicate some separation of the interneuronal pools generating these different activities. Stimulation of VL neurons activates, via short-latency pathways, MTh-neuronal organizations involved in generating the prolonged PSP sequences characteristic of diffuse thalamic spindle activity. The data indicate both convergence and differentiation of AL and BC inputs to VL neurons and widespread engagement of nonspecific interneuronal organizations by lenticulofugal projections.

120. Nonfocal grand mal seizures as seen through high frequency recordings.—E. Rodin, T. Onuma, S. Wasson, J. Porzak and M. Rodin (Detroit, Mich., U.S.A.).

In an effort to determine the mode of onset of clinically nonfocal *grand mal* seizures in cats subjected to systemic administration of Megimide of Metrazol, conventional EEG techniques were found to be unsatisfactory. Since it is felt that high frequency activity might be a better indicator, the use of a 6 channel Mnemotron Tape Recorder and a Grass Model 78 Electroencephalograph with additional filters which eliminate most activity below 1,000c/sec allowed identification of the presence of frequency components in the Kc/sec range through conventional stainless steel depth electrodes. By recording at a tape speed of 30 in./sec and playing it back at a tape speed of 1 7/8 in./sec, it was possible to display the information on the inkwriter of the Grass Model 78. High frequency activity could be recorded from all cerebral structures that have been sampled, but it was most intense in the brain stem reticular formation. During the myoclonic jerking leading up to the generalized seizure, there was paroxysmal increase in the amount of reticular as well as cortical firing. The animal fell over on its side and entered the behavioral *grand mal* seizure when the brain stem structures began to show continuous rather than intermittent firing. The transition of the tonic to the clonic phase was accompanied by a gradual decline in firing intensity. The clonic phase appeared to be a composite of brain stem, limbic system, and cortical events with different structures initiating intermittent discharges at different times. What appeared to be one *grand mal* seizure consisted usually of two or three different attacks which could originate in separate areas.

Recordings in this high frequency band significantly expand the view of electrophysiological cerebral events and will have to be incorporated in all future work dealing with electroclinical relationships.

121. Role of biochemical systems in mechanisms of pathological responses in Parkinsonian patients.—A. D. Anitchkov, D. K. Kambarova, A. N. Shandurina and Y. V. Shmatkov (Leningrad, U.S.S.R.).

The factors causing the symptoms of Parkinsonism were studied with stereotaxic, neuropharmacological and electrophysiological techniques. Adrenergic, cholinergic and serotoninergic systems were modified by drugs having selective and mainly central effects. Electrosubcorticograms (ESCoG), evoked responses (ER), muscle tone, velocity of movements, tremor, hemodynamic indices and the results of psychological tests were studied.

It was found that the factors mediating the main symptoms of the disease (rigidity, tremor and akinesis) showed a polybiochemical basis with varying degrees of significance of each biochemical system. This was clearly revealed in cases with disturbed function.

Adrenergic and serotoninergic systems are of the greatest significance in normalizing the extrapyramidal dysfunctions. From work to date it appears that disturbance of adrenergic structures is characteristic of Parkinsonian symptoms, while the role of sereotoninergic and cholinergic structures is anomalous. The serotoninergic structures affected produce bimodal changes in the ESCoG when recording from the ventro-lateral (VL) and central thalamic nuclei, the pallidum (gl. pal.) and the caudate nucleus. The drug Dezeril produces reduction in akinesis as well as hemodynamic changes which appear also with stimulation of the VL and gl. pal. In some areas of the brain (gl. pal., VL and g. precentralis) changes in the electrical activity appeared after giving cholinolytics and correlated with changes in muscle tone. In other areas (n. centralis) there was no related change. The influence of cholinolytics depends on whether the patient is taking antiparkinsonian drugs.

It is apparent that the areas studied partake in motor functions although the serotoninotropic drugs are not limited to these areas. It is possible that the Parkinsonian symptoms are carried through cholinergic systems controlling motor functions and that the adrenergic and serotoninergic systems are depressed.

122. The human EEG during 'in extremis' conditions.—E. P. Petushkov (Leningrad, U.S.S.R.).

Clinico-physiological studies of criteria of brain function during 'in extremis' states is one of the aspects of contemporary clinical neurophysiology.

Perfection and knowledge of the reliability of these criteria is now very necessary because of the newly arisen problem in medicine–that of transplanting vital organs in man. It would obviously be expedient to use data from purposely altered functional states–such as hypothermia–to study these criteria.

From data obtained during deep hypothermia with an intra-esophogeal temperature of 23°C, it has been found that the brain tolerates quite well complete cessation of circulation for periods of 15 to 17 min. During this period there is a bioelectrical silence of the cortex with bursts of synchronized slow waves every 8 to 10 sec. An increase in this interval up to 12 sec with decrease in amplitude of the bursts indicates deterioration of the state of the brain. Under these conditions the EEG data have proved to be the main criterion for expediency in efforts to sustain normal functioning of the organs of the patient.

123. Characteristics of bioelectrical events in subcortical structures during different phases of sleep in man.–N. I. Moiseeva, S. A. Movsisiants and A. I. Trohatchev (Leningrad, U.S.S.R.).

In 11 patients with implanted electrodes, bioelectrical potentials of ventro-lateral and posterior thalamic nuclei, hypothalamus, n. subthalamicus, pallidum, putamen, caudate nucleus, substantia nigra, amygdala, hippocampus and white matter were studied during different phases of sleep as determined by the EEG.

The electrical patterns corresponding to the various stages of sleep develop in different ways in different structures. One common feature is that the sleep spindles of the C phase of Loomis occur everywhere except in the caudate nucleus. The spindles are less obvious than in the EEG. During the B_2 phase slow waves either appear or are enhanced. During drowsiness and sleep, dynamic interrelated activity changes are observed in the various deep structures as well as varying interrelations between the changes in depth and the EEG.

During dreaming electrical patterns of the subcortical structures become similar to those of the EEG–amplitudes decrease while sharp and fast waves are enhanced. After electrical lesions in a few subcortical structures dreaming ceased to be accompanied by the paradoxical phase of sleep.

During drowsiness and sleep, nerve impulse activity was studied in the n. subthalamicus, ventral thalamic area and the hippocampus. Continual gradual decrease in firing rate was everywhere observed during the development of sleep. On awakening the firing rate increased.

Mathematical processing of the data derived from depth electrography disclosed regular changes in some structures occurring with the development of sleep and peculiarities of certain types of activity related to other activities in the same structures. The data suggest that for sleep patterns in man the ventro-lateral thalamic nucleus and the putamen-pallidum-substantia nigra system play an essential role.

124. Oxygen availability in the human brain during forms of mental activity.–V. B. Gretchin (Leningrad, U.S.S.R.).

Studies of the available Oxygen (O_2a) in various structures of the brain with implanted electrodes has proved to be a useful method for investigating some forms of mental activity. It has been found that a distinct relation exists between the alerting factor and O_2a levels–the greatest changes in O_2a occurred at the beginning of psychological testing. Changes during specially designed 'talking' tests also confirmed this. It has been demonstrated that in alerting there is a non-reproducibility of results on consecutive testing and that this is dependent on the background. However, some subcortical structures show reproducible changes of O_2a levels during mental activity of the operative memory type. The character of the changes varied in different structures and in some depended on whether the performances of the tests were done correctly or incorrectly or whether the correctness was evaluated by the subject himself. In some structures this suggests the features of an error detector. Experiments have also shown changes of O_2a levels with emotional responses but the character and structural distribution were different from those during operative memory tests.

125. The role of electrical conductivity in the spread of epileptiform activity in the cortex. –N. Y. Belenkov and V. D. Chirkov (Gorky, U.S.S.R.).

Evidence has been presented at previous meetings to suggest that transmission and synchronization of epileptiform (strychnine-induced) electrical activity might occur through ephaptic mechanisms. Further evidence is presented from experiments on 13 nonanesthetized cats in which the electrical conductivity between the site of epileptiform activity and isolated cortex is artificially increased or decreased.

The animals, under light anesthesia, had wide removal of the cranium and dura and a small island of isolated cortex prepared by sub-pial resection. Ag-AgCl electrodes recorded cortical activity and tungsten micro-electrodes recorded both extracellular neuronal activity and slow (EEG) potentials from the slab. Epileptiform activity was induced by a strychnine crystal applied to the suprasylvian gyrus. Increase in conductivity was made by placing a small strip of silver between the focus and the slab (4-5 mm away from the epileptogenic focus), decrease by placing a grounded silver strip between the two. It was found that an increase in conductivity raised the amplitude of potentials in the slab from 68 μV to 143 μV. Decrease in conductivity reduced the amplitude to 45 μV.

Activity from 430 neurons was recorded in the slab. With an increase in conductivity the number of excited neurons increased by 10% and no changes were demonstrated on the inhibited cells. With decrease in conductivity the number of excited neurons decreased by 14% and the inhibited cells by 4.5%.

The findings indicate that the ephaptic factor is more effective when the resistance to current spread decreases and demonstrate the effects of passive conductivity of biocurrents. They also confirm our suggestion of the part played by electrical fields in the synchronization or neuronal activity.

126. The visual evoked response dispersion curve: its relation to cerebral stochastic and deterministic mechanisms.—V. Constantinescu and E. Crighel (Bucharest, Rumania).

Some of the mechanisms involved in the process of information transmission are stochastic in character. Such mechanisms, generally, do not start from an always identical initial state, but from the random state existing at the moment of appearance of the signal. They subsequently develop in a stochastic way.

On these grounds the authors consider that averaging techniques and those derived from it have the disadvantage of eliminating precisely the stochastic components considered as noise and retaining the deterministic ones which carry much less information.

Therefore, as a further investigative method, the following was devised and tested. By statistical processing of evoked responses (ER) groups in man and cat, under different physiological conditions, the variation of dispersion with time was computed and plotted as a curve D = f(t) with three distinct periods. In man the first period following the signal was characterized by a very large dispersion with a latency of 35 to 40 msec and lasting for 130 msec, the second lasted 100 to 170 msec with a small dispersion and the third exhibited again a high dispersion. In cat the same dispersion curves were found but with shorter latencies.

Taking into account the constant character of the flash and the equiprobability of the stochastic external disturbances, the authors consider that the dispersion curves of the ER indicate that the biologic system involves some mechanisms answering in a deterministic way and some answering in a stochastic way to external signals, and that in each of the three periods one or the other type of mechanism is prevalent. These results are in agreement with physiological data and could form the basis for a mathematical model.

It is also possible to consider that the dispersion D at a given moment is the resultant of three components: the variation of (i) latencies, (ii) amplitudes and (iii) patterns of the analyzed group of ERs. The global curve D = f(t) seems, however, to be more useful for interpretation and closer to the biologic phenomenon than the splitting in these three components.

127. The amplitude of slow evoked cortical responses in relation to temporal features of stimulation.—H. H. Rothman and H. Davis (St. Louis, Mo., U.S.A.).

A series of experiments were run to determine how slow evoked cortical responses were affected by temporal features of auditory and shock stimulation, in human subjects. The response was recorded extracranially between vertex and right mastoid. Amplitude was measured from the 100 msec negative peak (N_1) to the 200 msec positive peak (P_2).

One experiment explored how irregular interstimulus intervals affected responses, compared to strictly regular intervals. Irregularity generally enhanced response amplitude though its specific effect depended on the particular subject and modality, and certain subjects did not consistently produce the effect at each session. A slightly modified experiment with shocks alone showed a more consistent effect.

Also, in the modified experiment, response recovery was recorded as a function of the interval between the successive shocks. Both regular and irregular schedules of stimulation were used. The shapes of the recovery curves were quite similar for both schedules, but the absolute amplitudes were slightly larger for irregular presentation, in accord with the findings above.

The modified experiment also furnished data regarding the effects of the immediate preceding interval on response amplitude, compared to the next-earlier preceding interval. The next-earlier preceding intervals were found to have no discernible effect for the subject group as a whole (n=4). In addition, if the immediate preceding interval was short (about 0.5 sec) then an increase in background stimulation rate caused a profound decrease in response amplitude.

The findings suggest that the slow evoked response is influenced by the most recent preceding event, and by a summation of events earlier than the most recent, but not by individual events earlier than the most recent.

128. Classification of deviant average evoked responses.—K. A. Kooi and A. G. Clague (Ann Arbor, Mich., U.S.A.).

Experience with the localization of 36 supratentorial tumors through multiareal recording of average visually evoked responses has shown that the alterations of compound evoked potentials may be classified descriptively according to 1) segment of the response affected, 2) type of change, and 3) area of maximal deviation. The effects of discrete lesions are typically selective, involving only a portion of the response, and variously manifested by augmentation or diminution of voltage, advanced or delayed peak culmination, rounding, atypical distribution, spatial stereotypy, or fusion of components. Anomolous waves, not corresponding to any known event, may be observed.

Each of the 3 normally occurring surface-negative waves (peak latencies of approximately 40, 90 and 150 msec respectively) may be differentially affected in respect to the others. Local augmentation of voltage is largely limited to the initial surface negativity (I) or subsequent positivity (II) or both. The second surface negativity (III) is rarely augmented but is commonly depressed, without constant relation to alterations of preceding waves. Of all components, the third surface negativity (V) is most likely to evidence depression, often in conjunction with the preceding positivity.

Recognition of the presence of deviant activity generally requires the existence of a substantial asymmetry between responses recorded from homologous cerebral regions. Detection of the side and area of involvement rests upon the establishment of 1) lack of correspondence of the observed pattern with the expected normal pattern for the region in question and 2) lack of correspondence of the pattern with that evident in the remainder of the areal samples, both ipsi- and contralateral to the site under study.

Satisfactory localization of most supratentorial tumors can be achieved on the basis of the foregoing considerations.

Twenty-four-point spatiotemporal arrays of responses recorded from representative patients will be utilized to illustrate various aspects of the classification procedure.

129. EEG spectral analysis in coma.—F. Ferillo, C. Rivano, G. Rosadini, G. F. Rossi and C. Turella (Genova, Italy).

A spectral analysis of the EEG activity of patients in comatose states of variable degree due to organic brain lesions has been made.

(1.) Oscillatory periodic potentials ("rhythmic" activity) are recorded in all degrees of coma except in the terminal stage of vegetative coma or coma *"dépassé"*. A certain organization of the cerebral electrical activity is therefore compatible with a severe disorganization of cerebral functioning.

(2.) The dominant rhythmic activity belongs to the delta band. Theta as well as alpha rhythms can be recorded. No clear-cut relation between depth of coma and type of rhythmic activity is apparent.

130. On the diagnosis of cerebral death—a prospective study.—J. Korein and M. Maccario (New York, N.Y., U.S.A.).

The initial criteria used for admission to the study included coma, fixed dilated unreactive pupils, absent corneal reflexes, absent deep tendon reflexes, and absent clinical response to any painful stimuli. Clinical data that were pertinent to the evaluation such as drug toxicity, hypothermia, metabolic disorders and encephalitis were carefully documented. Later some patients were also included in whom these criteria were not completely present, but in whom the progressive course suggested that they might soon be in the previously described state.

The following provocative procedures were carried out during the EEG recording: delivery of painful stimuli, ice water caloric stimulation, photic stimulation, and Methylphenidate hydrochloride (Ritalin), 50-100 mgs i.v. The data were recorded using an 8-channel Grass EEG Model 6A, and a 4-channel magnetic tape recorder for subsequent analysis of evoked responses.

No patient was pronounced dead by the use of these criteria during the course of the study, and full supportive therapy was continued to the time of final cardiovascular collapse. Serial EEGs from 4 to 48 h apart were taken in patients who survived for that period of time. Thus far, a total of 28 patients were studied with 58 EEGs. Of the 28 studied, 25 had isoelectric EEGs prior to their death. Six of these isoelectric records had some muscle artifact in the EEG tracing indicating that peripheral activity was still present. All patients in this study died. Caloric stimulation, photic stimulation, and Methylphenidate hydrochloride injection occasionally produced phenomena such as shivering, decerebrate movements and muscle artifacts which will be described. In four patients, a phase of the EEG prior to death was observed which was characterized by a sequence of cyclic activity of sharp spikes, slowing, triphasic waves and suppression bursts, with a periodicity ranging from 30 sec to 3 min.

131. A comparison of electroencephalography, rheoencephalography and tests of dyslipidemia in affective syndromes of late onset. —V. Predescu and I. Roman (Bucharest, Rumania).

One hundred patients with affective syndromes diagnosed as due to cerebral arteriosclerosis and 100 patients with presenile affective syndromes were studied. All were males and in the age range of 50 to 65 years. In the patients with cerebral arteriosclerosis the following were recorded: altered eyegrounds 82%, dyslipidemia 62%, EEG changes 75%, RheoEG abnormalities 76%. In the patients with presenile affective syndromes the following were found: dyslipidemia 35%, EEG changes 54%, and RheoEG abnormalities 51%. These latter findings showed similar patterns to those seen in incipient cerebral arteriosclerosis. The RheoEG correlates best with the EEG, dyslipidemia and eye ground changes in cerebral arteriosclerosis and less in the presenile affective syndromes.

From study it has been found that: a) the presence of biochemical, EEG and RheoEG abnormalities suggest the presence of cerebral arteriosclerosis even in its early and treatable stage, b) changes in the RheoEG suggest the possibility of the presence of cerebral arteriosclerosis in patients with the affective presenile psychoses, c) the EEG changes in cerebral arteriosclerosis are more commonly of a lesional than functional type while the reverse is true in the case of affective presenile psychoses; and d) the correlation of these various tests might help in differentiating organic from functional EEG change, and is useful in the classification of the psychotic syndrome, in determining its cause and, consequently, in selecting a more appropriate therapy.

132. Inter-relationships of EEG activity and information processing on paced and unpaced tasks in epileptic children.—H. Fairweather and S. J. Hutt (Oxford, G.B.).

Studies of the effects upon cognitive and perceptual motor skills of generalized spike-wave paroxysms in the EEG have shown effects varying from little or none to massive impairment. This kind of inconsistency has led some writers to the conclusion that the spike-wave paroxysm is a bioelectrical epiphenomenon with no reliable behavioral correlates. This may be due to lack of consideration of relevant variables in such psychological tests, some of which may be usefully specified in terms of the mathematical theory of communication. These include the nature and amount of information involved, the rate at which it has to be processed, and the age and level of practice of subjects. If a possible general theory were that bioelectric interference impaired performance most noticeably at or near optimum rates of information processing, this rate might be determined not only by considerable extension along a single parameter, but also by combinations of two or more of these; and perhaps more pertinently, some causal factors might be isolated only by use of both approaches.

Accordingly, in the present study 6 - 12 year old epileptics were investigated under EEG control on a choice reaction task with three different information loadings, and under conditions of either self-pacing or pacing at the same mean rate resulting from this.

Results suggests that the primary effect of spike-wave paroxysms is to slow reaction times with the consequence that, in temporally-limited (*i.e.*, paced) tasks, information transmission is reduced. It is theorized that this may be regarded as a specific case of the more general effects of the neural "noise" in developing organisms, as both this and the informational analogue of response equivocation show a declining function with age.

133. EEG activity in newborns delivered from mothers with and without full anesthesia.—G. Modena, M. Angiolillo, R. Bertelli and M. Bini (Mantova, Italy).

EEG recordings have been made on 30 children within half an hour of controlled delivery with the mother under full anesthesia. These records have been compared with those taken from newborns under the same conditions except that the mothers delivered without anesthesia.

The results obtained in the two groups are identical.

134. Operant conditioning of EEG in the unrestrained chimpanzee.—J. M. R. Delgado, V. S. Johnston, J. D. Wallace, and R. J. Bradley (New Haven, Conn., Holloman A. F. B., and Albuquerque, N.M., U.S.A.).

This report deals with the successful application of operant conditioning principles to the manipulation of amygdala spindling in the chimpanzee.

EEG activity in the amygdala was recorded via telemetry from the unrestrained animal and 28 c/sec spindle bursts were recognized by on-line computer. Radio stimulation in aversive areas of the mesencephalic reticular formation was made conditional upon spindle occurrence.

It was possible to achieve either unilateral or bilateral suppression of 28 c/sec activity by appropriate manipulation of the reinforcement contingencies.

The relationship between the amygdala spindle and olfactory input was investigated and the behavioral effects of spindle suppression were tested using an olfactory discrimination task. Results suggest that spindling is not directly related to the central processing of olfactory information *per se*. The significance of nasal air-flow and arousal factors in the control of amygdala activity will be discussed.

135. Slow changes in the membrane potentials of glial cells and neurons following nerve impulses.—**J. G. Nicholls (Boston, Mass., U.S.A.).**

Neurons in the central and peripheral nervous system are closely in contact with glial or Schwann cells. Potassium (K) can collect in this intercellular space. This paper discusses the effect of K accumulation from action potentials and of a slow neuronal hyperpolarization. Since the membrane potential of a glial cell behaves like a K electrode, this potential follows changes in external K and an intra-glial cell electrode follows the K levels in the space between nerve and glial cell. Leech ganglia have been used since they permit simultaneous recording of glial cells and neurons. Due to the high propagation safety factor in the fiber, removal of glial cells and change in surrounding K concentration are unlikely to produce demonstrable change. However, at synapses, variation of surrounding K concentrations might produce effects on release of transmitter substances, postsynaptic potentials and the initiation of impulses. It has been found that small increases in K (around 3 mM) can cause changes in the frequency of spontaneously active cells and in the frequency of synaptic potentials. It is possible that the activity of one neuron could influence the activity of some adjacent ones and shield others. Furthermore, since prolonged trains of impulses can produce hyperpolarization of up to 20 mV which declines over 15 min and since evidence suggests this is related to some electrogenic pump, a glial depolarization with a neuronal hyperpolarization might interact to produce some of the recorded extracellular potentials.

136. Strychnine effect on cord dorsum potentials. —**A. Wagner (Frankfurt am Main, W. Germany).**

The experiments were performed on 40 cats, anesthetized with Nembutal, using conventional methods for recording from motoneurons and the dorsal surface of the spinal cord. Either muscle nerve or the cut end of dorsal root L 6 were stimulated. Activity was displayed on an oscilloscope and filmed and also fed directly into a CAT computer.

Before strychnine, with 10 msec stimulus intervals, refractory phase of the N 1 wave did not exist. With 0.5 - 1.5 msec intervals a distinct augmentation was found. Following strychnine injection, however (0.2 mg/kg i.v.), even with 50-100 msec intervals, amplitude of the N1 wave was greatly reduced and the P component completely abolished. Further increasing the intervals up to 175-300 msec the P wave clearly emerged again. The described behavior of the cord dorsum potentials corresponded in phase to those induced by strychnine on the cerebral cortex but with opposite polarity. Intracellular recording during strychnine injection revealed increased amplitude and duration of the polysynaptic EPSPs. At the same time, the negative N1 wave was followed by a positive P wave which was fully synchronous with secondary EPSPs in intracellular records. Following strychninisation, 50-100 mg/kg of guaiacol-glycerinether (MY-301) was administered and change of the polysnyaptic EPSPs in the opposite direction from that induced by strychnine was seen, *i.e.*, there was a reduction of their amplitude and also a normalization of the cord dorsum potentials with a decrease and abolishment of the P component.

137. Variability of visual evoked responses in epileptic patients.—**C. H. Lucking (Munich, W. Germany).**

Visual evoked potentials (VEP) were studied in 45 epileptic patients and compared with those from 30 normal persons. The purpose of this investigation was to look for typical alterations and a diagnostic value of the VEP in epilepsy. In contrast to the relatively high inter-individual stability of the VEP in normal persons, epileptic patients showed a great variability of amplitude, shape and latency of the VEP. Patients with epileptiform patterns in the EEG showed a larger alteration of the evoked responses than those without such patterns. But no typical alteration could be shown which may be related to the different types and etiologies of epilepsy except in patients with spike-wave patterns who often had a pronounced negativity corresponding to wave V of Cigánek, and the photosensitive epileptics, who showed a high voltage VEP of up to 80 μV. No significant differences of the VEPs of both sides were found in patients with a unilateral temporal focus. The majority of the VEPs from epileptic patients showed a slightly longer latency of waves IV - VI than normals. This has no diagnostic significance but may be interesting for pathophysiological considerations. The correlation between the amplitude of EEG and VEP was close no matter whether the person was epileptic or not.

138. Wave length analysis of the EEG—the alpha profile.—**J. D. Frost (Houston, Tex., U.S.A.).**

Clinical EEG reports usually include some statement regarding alpha frequency and often a comment about its constancy or stability. An on-line computer method is described which automatically quantifies these aspects. The scheme treats EEG frequency in a manner independent of amplitude, and is somewhat similar to Tecce and Mirsky's technique but differs in that a precise wave length measurement is made and activity outside the alpha range is excluded.

Filtered occipital activity (6-14 c/sec) enters an electronic circuit which determines wave lengths by measuring the time interval between successive positive-going baseline crosses. Each measurement is checked to determine if it falls within the "alpha range" of 56-174 msec (6-17 c/sec), and, if not, this value is discarded. If the measurement meets this requirement, a count of one is added at a particular computer-memory location which corresponds to the measured wave length. Sixty memory locations are used, each representing one of the possible wave length values between 56 and 174 msec (2 msec resolution). These locations are thus used to keep score of the number of waves which fall into different wave length categories. Analysis continues until a total of 1000 counts are contained in memory, indicating consideration of 1000 alpha waves. Total time required to complete the analysis is recorded, since it depends upon the average frequency of the alpha activity and the percentage of time it is present, and consequently provides a measure of the alpha index.

Memory contents are plotted in the form of a histogram, or alpha profile, providing a quantitative measure of the range of alpha activity, with the abscissa corresponding to wave length and the ordinate to the number of waves in each category. The mode correlates with the electroencephalographer's alpha frequency determination, while the spread of the distribution can be quantitative measure of alpha variability.

139. The Modal alpha wavelength.—J. R. G. Carrie (Houston, Tex., U.S.A.).

Occipital EEG signals were detected in 67 subjects under standardized experimental conditions. Histograms (profiles) showing the frequency of occurrence of waves of different duration in a sample of 1000 consecutive waves in a pass-band which included the alpha range were derived using the technique developed by Frost.

No correlation was found between modal height and the wave length at which the mode was located. These was significant positive correlation (+0.80) between the location of the mode and the alpha frequency as assessed by visual inspection and manual measurement of the ink-written EEG record. With a technique having this degree of temporal resolution (2-msec separation of the histogram ordinates), the maximum representation of the modal alpha component in the 67 subjects was 16.6% of the sample of 1000 oscillations; the minimum modal representation was 2.5%; the average modal representation was 5.7%.

Since the height of the profile mode is one indicator of the stability or monorhythmicity of the most prominent alpha component, it was predicted that there would be a correspondence between this profile characteristic and the relevant elements in the verbal reports based on visual assessment. An experienced electroencephalographer wrote verbal reports on each EEG recording without knowledge of the type of analysis to which his assessments would be subjected. It was found that the verbal reports could be divided into four categories with regard to content describing the alpha-activity stability. The average magnitudes of the modes in the corresponding four groups of EEG histogram profiles differed from one another. These differences were highly significant when the groups categorized as showing poorly sustained or uncountable alpha rhythms on visual assessment were compared statistically with the group whose alpha frequency was stated without any comment on the alpha-wave form stability.

140. The physiological interpretation of amplitude histograms of the EEG.—R. Elul (Los Angeles, Calif., U.S.A.).

The amplitude probability distribution of the EEG is closely correlated with behavior. In the idle adult, fronto-occipital EEG activity is Gaussian 60-80% of the time, falling to 30-50%, during performance of mental tasks. There are several possible interpretations of the observed decrease in Gaussian EEG.

a) Data will be presented which indicate that cortical neurons may be identified with the unitary generators of the EEG. Any gross electrode reflects the summed activities of many thousands of neurons. However, the Central Limit Theorem of statistics indicates that the probability distribution of the sum is unaffected by changes in the behavior of individual generators. With regard to the EEG it is therefore clear that this does not provide an explanation for the experimental observations.

b) The sum of 2 Gaussian distributions of unequal mean and variance is not Gaussian. Hence, it is possible that during mental task performance that there is a decrease in duration of stationary EEG periods. Long epochs of EEG could appear non-Gaussian, but be the sum of shorter Gaussian periods with different means and variances. If this is correct, decrease in Gaussian activity should be

correlated with increased variation of the mean and variance of short EEG periods. Although in general the EEG cannot be considered stationary for periods longer than 2-5 sec, the fall in Gaussian behavior is not correlated with increased fluctuations of the mean and variance.
c) As transition from Gaussian to non-Gaussian reflects an increase in mutual interaction between individual generators, it is the only possibility presented here which is compatible with, and supported by, classical probability theory. In fact, it follows as a direct corollary from the Central Limit Theorem of statistics.

Analysis of the data presented here thus indicates that amplitude histograms of the EEG provide a criterion for evaluation of inter-neuronal interactions in different behavioral states.

141. On automatic methods of sleep staging by spectra of electroencephalograms—L. E. Larsen and D. O. Walter (Los Angeles, Calif., U.S.A.).
This research grew out of a comparison of the multiple regression (MR) technique for sleep stages classification and the technique of multiple discriminant analysis as previously used by this laboratory. Using spectral data kindly provided by Dr. L. C. Johnson, a simple, routine application of the latter method showed a marked improvement in the identification of Stage 3 sleep (from 0% to 77% agreement on equivilent samples) and a less impressive improvement on the identification of REM (from 70% to 75%) with a somewhat variable loss in the other stages the worst being a drop from 91% rate for Stage 4 with MR to 69% for multiple discriminant analysis.

A prominent source of error in both techniques resided in the difficulty of identifying low-alpha subjects in Stage 1 sleep and high-alpha subjects in REM. These findings prompted a systematic study of whether high and low-alpha subjects (as identified by the waking records) differ in other stages of consciousness. We found that high and low-alpha subjects were easily discriminated in all stages studied except REM where only one record was misclassified from each group.

Subsequently, many techniques were investigated for their ability to improve the operation of the multiple discriminant method. The combination of a layered decision process (based on the identification of "clumps" in the test space) and the use of smoothly curved decision boundaries (*i.e.*, quadratic discriminant functions) raised the level of performance on the so-called testing data sample to the following levels of percent agreement with clinical classification: Waking, 91%; Stage 1, 64%, REM, 66%; Stage 2, 85%; Stage 3, 85%; and Stage 4, 85%. We conclude that spectra are adequate measurement parameters for all sleep stages with the possible exception of Stage 1 and REM where the level of performance is marginally acceptable.

142. Drive and performance related aspects of the CNV in Rhesus monkeys.—R. P. Borda (Houston, Tex., U.S.A.).
The "contingent negative variation" (CNV) was studied in rhesus monkeys using epidural and subcortical electrodes and long time-constant amplifiers. The CNV has been linked in the literature with psychological concepts such as motivation, expectancy, attention, and conation.

This study sought to determine the effects of two levels of drive, as determined by normal diet or total deprivation of food, on the amplitude of the CNV in subjects trained to respond for a food reward. Recordings made over a period of several months from four subjects led to the following conclusions:

1) At least two independent negative slow potentials are present during the course of conditioning with a paradigm of this type. One is frontal dominant and the other maximal near the central sulcus, and the two may summate to produce the CNV typically recorded from the scalp.

2) The central-dominant potential decreases in amplitude and overtraining, reappearing only briefly following periods of food deprivation.

3) The frontal-dominant potential reaches its maximum amplitude early in training and continues to be present as long as the subject maintains a high level of performance.

4) Food deprivation is associated with a larger amplitude frontal-dominant potential than that recorded during periods of normal diet, but the subject's performance is also a factor. It is suggested that food deprivation acts to increase the probability of the subject's detecting the stimuli and making a correct response, and that the CNV may, therefore, be the electrical sign of activation of a basic mechanism of selective attention subserved by nonspecific thalamocortical pathways.

5) It is suggested that the term "contingent negative variation" be reserved for the frontal-dominant component which is uniquely associated with the type of stimulus-response paradigm used in this study.

143. Differential effects of repetitive visual stimulation on alpha rhythm and average visual evoked potentials.—G. F. Wilson, and D. B. Lindsley (Los Angeles, Calif., U.S.A.).
The purpose of this study was to contrast the effect of visual stimulation upon a diffuse alpha

generator mechanism and that of locally generated rhythmic potentials.

Average evoked potentials (AEPs) and alpha rhythms were recorded from electrodes placed bilaterally over occipital and parietal areas referenced to the ear lobes. Flashes were presented to the right and/or left visual fields of one or both eyes and could be delivered either in or out of phase.

Evoked potentials were obtained by averaging from the onset of flashes; alpha rhythms were studied by averaging unfiltered EEG activity for 250-1000 msec epochs before and during repetitive stimulation. Alpha averaging was triggered by an amplitude criterion individually determined for each subject.

The alpha averages and the AEPs to repetitive stimulation produced relatively simple sinusoidal wave forms whose amplitude was largest when stimuli were presented at 10 c/sec and decreased when the stimulus frequency was varied either above or below 10 c/sec. The amplitude of alpha averages was considerably greater than that of the rhythmic AEPs recorded from the same electrode . Alpha amplitude was smallest at the inion and largest over more anterior occipital and parietal areas. The amplitude of AEPs was maximal at the inion and was reduced at more anterior recording sites.

As frequency of photic stimulation varied, frequency of alpha remained constant while frequency of AEPs followed the rate of stimulation. Out of phase flashes presented to the two eyes or to the two visual fields produced amplitude reductions and wave form changes in the AEPs at all stimulus frequencies, but produced only amplitude reductions in the alpha averages when the repetitive stimulation was in the neighborhood of 10 c/sec.

These results provide a basis for the differentiation of diffusely distributed alpha activity, presumably controlled by a nonspecific thalamic generator, and regionally confined rhythmic potentials which closely follow the frequency of the repetitive stimulation and apparently reflect the influence of local generators associated with specific thalamic control centers.

144. Inter- and intra-hemispheric interactions of average visual evoked potentials.—J. D. Wicke (Los Angeles, Calif., U.S.A.).

Repetitive flashes of 5-20 c/sec were presented binocularly to the left and/or right visual fields to investigate inter-hemispheric relationships, and monocularly to one visual field of each eye to investigate intra-hemispheric relationships. Flashes were either in phase or 180° out of phase with respect to the left and right visual fields, or with respect to the two eyes. In order to insure that each cerebral hemisphere received information from only one visual field, the flashes to each of the visual fields were separated by a continuously illuminated central adapting field. Average evoked potentials (AEPs) were obtained from scalp electrodes placed bilaterally over the occipitals (AEPs) were obtained from scalp electrodes placed bilaterally over the occipital and parietal areas and were referenced to the ear lobes. The AEPs were relatively simple sinusoids which followed the frequency of the flash trains.

With respect to inter-hemispheral comparisons the following results were obtained. 1. Simultaneous stimulation of the right and left visual fields of both eyes produced larger AEPs than when only homonymous half fields of both eyes were stimulated. 2. AEPs recorded bilaterally were similar whether flashes were presented to the right or left half of the visual fields. 3. Stimulation of the same visual fields of the two eyes 180° out of phase caused a marked reduction in the amplitude and a modification of the wave form of the AEPs.

Intra-hemispheral comparisons provided the following results. 1. Bilateral stimulation of homonymous half fields produced larger AEPs than unilateral stimulation. 2. Stimulation of the same visual half field of either eye separately produced similar AEPs bilaterally. 3. Stimulation of the same visual half field of both eyes with flashes 180° out of phase caused interaction and cancellation of AEPs.

145. Human evoked potentials as a function of stimulus information content in an expectancy—reaction time situation.—M. D. Buck (Los Angeles, Calif., U.S.A.).

The purpose of this study was to devise a stimulus-response situation which would allow three stimuli presented 1 sec apart and preceding the response to define the limits of the periods during which anticipation or expectancy could be established, and endow the second stimulus with more or less information content. Given these conditions, the goal was to determine the effect of them upon the average evoked potentials. The response itself was a simple finger press upon a right or left key, depending upon the nature of the information contained in the third stimulus.

The first stimulus, a tone-pip of medium pitch, was always a Warning Stimulus (S_w); the second stimulus, a tone-pip of either high or low pitch, served as an information carrying stimulus, and is referred to as a Discriminative Stimulus (S_d); the third stimulus, which consisted of a change in a visual fixation figure, indicated which of two keys to press and is called the Imperative Stimulus (S_i). The fixation figure, presented in a three-field tachistoscope was observed throughout with fixation maintained upon the center of a cross inscribed in a circle. The change in the figure, which constituted the S_i, was effected by having an open sector pointing right or left. In the information situation the S_d of high or low pitch carried information agreeing with that in the S_i and thus allowed the subject to prepare for the correct response following S_i. In the no-information situation the S_d was always of high pitch and simply marked time until the S_i. Instructions to the subject determined whether S_d would be informational or not.

Cortical evoked potentials were recorded from somatosensory and vertex scalp electrodes, using long time-constant amplifiers. Averages were obtained by means of a CAT computer. Reaction times were measured from the S_i.

Results show that there are significant differences in the nature of the CNV under the different conditions.

146. Relationships between motor potentials and CNV.–K. Syndulko (Los Angeles, Calif., U.S.A.).

The purpose of this experiment was to determine what relationships exist between the motor potential (MP) and the contingent negative variation (CNV). Each human subject was studied under three different conditions. Condition I was a choice reaction time task in which the subject was instructed to make a right or left hand movement, after presentation of one of two visual patterns. Condition II involved the same stimuli and responses, but included a tone stimulus preceding both visual stimuli by 1 sec. In Condition III the tone was high or low indicating which of the two visual patterns was to follow and allowing the subject to anticipate the specific responses he was to make.

The visual stimuli were presented via 2 channels of a 3-channel tachistoscope. The third channel was used to display a continuously present fixation point. Subjects were given practice trials before each of the three conditions.

Steady potential changes were recorded at sites presumed to overlie the motor hand area of each hemisphere as well as from points anterior and posterior to the motor sites, from the vertex and from a site on the forehead to monitor eye movements. EMG activity was recorded from forearm muscles involved in the response. Both MPs and CNVs were averaged either backward from the response or foreward from the warning stimulus.

The plan of the experiment permitted comparison of motor potentials which are assumed to arise from a specific locus, and CNVs, which are assumed to have a different distribution. Condition I provides an imperative stimulus to a motor response but without warning and anticipation, Condition II provides only general expectancy and a pre-imperative stimulus period favoring CNV, and Condition III provides a specific and directed motor expectancy favoring the MP.

147. Behavioral and electrophysiological responses in a two flash discrimination task in the cat.–C. K. Peck (Los Angeles, Calif., U.S.A.).

The purpose of this study was to train cats to discriminate two brief flashes presented as a pair from a single flash and then to reduce the temporal interval between the paired flashes until discrimination of two from one was no longer possible. Electrodes implanted in the optic tract, lateral geniculate body and the visual cortex permitted concurrent recording of responses to the visual stimuli.

The behavioral task associated with this visual temporal discrimination involved a "go/no-go" procedure. On each trial the stimulus was either a single flash or a pair of flashes separated by a variable interval. During initial training the inter-flash interval was 250 msec but was subsequently reduced to a value as low as 20 msec which was well below the behavioral threshold at approximately 75 msec. Stimuli were presented only when the cat faced a transparent plastic panel upon which the flashes appeared. On any one trial the stimulus was repeated at 1.5 sec intervals until 5 stimuli had been presented or until the cat pressed the panel. A press following a paired flash provided a milk reward; a press following a single flash delayed the start of the next trial 15 sec.

Fairly stable behavioral thresholds have been obtained and data will be presented concerning these and associated electrical responses to the flashes at each of the levels of the visual system sampled. Of particular interest is the question whether separation of the responses to the two flashes occurs when the behavioral discrimination is just possible as opposed to when it is not.

148. Polygraphy and its applications in the study of stabilized medullary lesions.–A. Heilporn (Brussels, Belgium).

The author presents findings from 500 cases of medullary lesions all with chronic and severe sequelae. Special emphasis is laid on changes in the vasomotor and thermoregulatory functions, in blood pressure and cardiac rhythm, in their relation to type and level of the lesion.

Polygraphic recordings were made simultaneously from regions above and below the level of the lesion under conditions of rest and of varying body positions and body temperature. Emphasis is placed on the necessity of understanding and knowing the reactions since widespread effects appear throughout the body or else appear in areas very distal to the site of the lesion.

149. Paradoxical activating EEG responses to the intracarotid Amytal test in focal and multifocal bilateral epilepsies.—G. B. Ricci, P. Silipo and F. Gagliardi (Rome, Italy).

The test was performed in a total of 64 patients. Of these, 26 had unilateral and 37 bilateral epileptogenic foci, in 18 the injection was followed by an increase in epileptiform EEG activity and in two also by seizures.

Two principal types of responses were found: 1) a paradoxical response with injection on both sides—this occurred with 5 cases of unilateral and 5 cases of bilateral foci; 2) a response observed with injection on one side only—this occurred with 3 cases with injection on the opposite side, in 4 cases on the same side and in 1 case with bilateral independent foci.

It is suggested that these phenomena depend on the abolition by the Amytal of defenses against epileptic activity that normally exist on the same and/or opposite side to the foci. This concept is supported by the clinical improvement that occurs in these cases with use of non-barbiturate therapy and also, in cases of independent bilateral foci, by the shifts that occur in relation to the drugs used. Further proof seems to lie in the results of surgery which aims to save the defense system particularly after exploration with the use of topical KCl (25%) to produce spreading depression. Further recent work by the authors also stress this idea since it has been found that excellent post-operative results occur in patients showing paradoxical responses to contralateral Amytal injections.

The experiments underline the fact that the epileptic disturbance should be considered as a dynamic process which such mechanisms as defense systems, although improperly understood, coming into effect.

150. The electroencephalogram in endemic juvenile goiter and in acute goiter.—L. Pacini, M. Mortara and R. Rubino (Milan and Alessandria, Italy).

EEG studies were carried out in 27 cases of endemic juvenile goiter and in 5 cases of acute goiter from endemic areas. In the patients with endemic goiter the EEG was abnormal in 26 cases (96.3%) and within normal limits in 1 case. The most common changes were in the appearance of theta rhythms at 4 to 5 c/sec in 14 and at 5 to 7 c/sec in another 9 cases. This activity was of regular form, sometimes paroxysmal and of medium to high voltage. In 3 records the theta rhythms were associated with fairly frequent delta activity of moderate to distinctly high voltage and often rhythmic. In 24 cases, in addition to the above anomalies there were sharp, spike and spike slow wave complexes. The theta and delta rhythms were accentuated by hyperpnea although they were already fairly marked in the resting state. The epileptiform patterns were present before hyperpnea in 11 cases and appeared during overbreathing in 13 other cases.

In the 5 patients with acute goiter the EEGs showed theta rhythms of 4 to 5 c/sec in 1 case, of 5 to 7 c/sec in 2 cases and intermixed theta and delta activity in the other 2 cases. The patterns and voltages were similar to those for the juvenile endemic goiter. Hyperpnea again made the changes more marked and in 4 of these 5 cases high voltage sharp waves appeared only during this test.

These EEG findings are unlike those of other workers in so-called primary hyper and hypothyroidism but are like those reported in the secondary condition. The changes described above would suggest diencephalic-hypophyseal disturbance.

151. EEG and the measurement of visual performance.—W. Clusin (Chicago, Ill., U.S.A.).

Investigators concerned with the relationship between EEG and higher cortical organization have long suspected that features of the alpha rhythm might correlate with intelligence. Although measurements of the IQ and alpha amplitude have been unproductive, relating studies of alpha index have produced controversial results.

The dubious reliability of such correlations is not surprising since the alpha rhythm is rather specifically associated with the neural activity of the visual system. Whereas most IQ tests take account of perceptual and occular-motor performance, there is little to suggest that intelligence is primarily a property of the visual apparatus.

The present experiment was performed to determine whether alpha activity would be related to a subject's performance on a more specifically visual task. For this purpose, we employed the scaled score of Wechsler's Coding subtest, which measures the speed and accuracy of transcribing digits into corresponding abstract symbols.

Digitized EEG signals were recorded on magnetic tape from 16 monopolar electrodes from a sample of 32, 11 to 13 year old right-handed males. The power-density of the activity in each of several frequency bands was calculated by a computer. The alpha score obtained for each electrode was a combined measurement of alpha amplitude and alpha index.

We found that Spearman correlations between alpha activity and Coding were positive at all electrode loci, and significant (p=0.005, one-tailed) in 12 of the 16 areas. Our correlations were no less significant in anterior electrodes. The highest correlation, 0.70, reached a significance of $p<0.00005$.

The hypothesis that these correlations reflect an association between alpha activity and visual performance is supported by the fact that the power density of activity outside the alpha range was not significantly correlated with Coding and that the alpha scores were not related to Full IQ, or other such non-visual measurements as Information, Comprehension, and Vocabulary.

152. Inertia of the nervous processes of the brain. –J. G. Kratin (Leningrad, U.S.S.R.).

When positive and negative conditioned reflexes have been formed, the electrical reactions of the brain can be recorded as a switch from resting EEG activity to various activated rhythms. The duration and intensity of the EEG response depends on stimulus quality. A positive signal evokes a long lasting and prominent reaction. A fine negative differential stimulus also activates the EEG and the finer the differentiation the longer the EEG reaction. Only a gross differentiation induces little or no change. Repetitive presentation of gross differential stimuli restores the resting EEG pattern after cessation of the positive or fine negative stimuli. The length of time required for this restoration reflects the degree of inertia of the brain function.

The inertia of inhibition, which is manifested as negative after-activity, is of special interest. This problem was explored in experiments on cats. Negative after-activity results from repetition of differential stimuli and consists of a blocking of the subsequent action of positive signals. For gross differentiation this effect appears after many negative stimuli and for fine differentiation after only several stimuli. In both cases effector blocking persists during desynchronization of the EEG, a change which reflects acceptance of the signal by the system and its excitation.

These findings suggest a duality of CNS inhibition: while the analyser system is in a state of excitation the effector mechanism is blocked. A more intense state of after-inhibition develops with a diffuse inhibitory state and is reflected in the slow wave EEG patterns. It can be eliminated by gradual activation of the EEG from repetitive positive signals.

It is suggested that EEG recordings of the inertia of processes of the brain show the same external manifestations as behavior (rest and inaction) and underlying these, there exist many interactions of different nervous processes.

153. The role of some subcortical structures of the brain in the forming of internal conditioned inhibition.–N. F. Suvorov (Leningrad, U.S.S.R.).

Studies of behavioral reactions suggest there are structures and inhibitory mechanisms in the CNS which modulate the parameters of the excitatory process or block output. Both innate and acquired forms of inhibition exist and can be investigated by the method of conditioned reflexes. The behavioral studies of inhibition are now complemented by neurophysiological techniques. In this paper the dynamics of bioelectrical activity (EEG, primary and evoked responses and neuronal activity) has been studied in different regions of the brain, (thalamus, basal ganglia, amygdala, hypothalamus and midbrain reticular formation) during acute interrupted extinction of the orientating reaction and during differential, extinctive and other forms internal conditioned inhibition.

It has been shown that the inhibitory systems of the brain (head of caudate nucleus, n. basolateralis of amygdala, n. medialis of thalamus) partake in forming conditioned inhibition. Destruction of these structures causes delay in forming conditioned inhibition. Low frequency stimulation of some of these structures hastens formation of inhibition, but the genesis of formation of conditioned inhibition is not identical in all of them.

Some structures take part in forming inhibitory responses directly (n. caudate and septum) others only are involved indirectly; that is, they do not belong functionally to systems involved in the formation of the act which is inhibited. It is suggested that the principle of vertical organization of nervous processes in the brain during formation of acquired forms of inhibition is important.

154. Microphysiology of cortical single neurons in Papio Papio.–F. Morrell, R. Naquet and C. Menini (Stanford, Calif., U.S.A. and Marseille, France).

The baboon, Papio Papio, may display epileptic seizures when exposed to stroboscopic illumination; previous investigations have indicated that the seizures originate in the pre-frontal cortex of both hemispheres. In the present study, single unit analysis of area 6 and occipital neurons was carried out by means of extracellular micro-electrodes. The sensitivity of these cells to various stimulus modalities was explored. (a) In area 6, striking correlations were observed between single unit activity and both surface and depth epileptiform or paroxysmal discharge as viewed with gross electrodes; (b) neither spontaneous or photically elicited unit abnormality was observed in occipital cortical units; (c) cellular discharge patterns in frontal cortex were similar to those observed in focal epileptogenic lesions in man and experimental animals; (d) the cellular discharge could not be attributable to spread in a volume conductor and hence was assumed to have arisen locally; and (e) paroxysmal discharges were more easily elicited by visual stimuli than by other stimulus modalities tested.

155. Cell firing related to active inhibition in visual cortex of cats.—M. Demetrescu (Irvine, Calif., U.S.A.).

Previous findings concerning the recovery cycle of cat's visual cortex to thalamocortical evoked potentials (EP) and corresponding time-locked cell firing demonstrated that pairing intervals of thalamic pulses as low as 5 msec can still elicit full size cortical responses (preparations with subcortical lesions of lower reticular formation and/or caudate nuclei). Exhaustion being thus ruled out, active inhibition triggered by the first lateral geniculate (LG) pulse remains the only explanation of refractoriness extending from less than 5 to over 60 msec in the normal brain, either activated or under barbiturate anesthesia.

In intact brain Nembutal preparations, the first pulse starting the recovery cycle does not need, however, to reach the threshold at which the EP or short-latency firing of most cells is elicited in order to trigger inhibition of responses to a second suprathreshold pulse following at 5-60 msec. Metal micro-electrode (2-6 u tip diameter, platinum-black coated) recording of multiple cell firing showed, in certain specific positions at the depth of reversal of polarity of phases 2-5 of the EP, relatively small spikes following at 3-15 msec the first subthreshold LG pulse. This type of firing only occurred in connection with inhibition of the second response. These hard to find and probably small neurons displayed repetitive firing over 5-12 msec (3-5 spikes), usually masked by firing of other cells at higher intensities from the first LG stimulus. The latency of the first such spike decreased from 15 to 3 msec by increasing the LG stimulus triggering it, which also increased the efficiency of inhibiting the responses to the second LG stimulus (kept constant). It is believed that these small spike cells are intimately connected with the inhibitory mechanism, most of it being located intra-cortically.

156. Somatic representation in the human thalamus.—N. de M. Rudolf (London, G.B.).

Recordings of cellular activity along one or more linear trajectories of up to 25 mm in length have been made in more than 50 stereotaxic operations in order to locate functional thalamic regions as a guide to the placing of lesions for relief of involuntary movements.

Entry was through a frontal burr hole and all trajectories inclined downwards posteriorly and medially at various angles and positions. The sites on a three-dimensional co-ordinate system of findings such as the presence or absence of spontaneous discharges, modifications of spontaneous activity by peripheral somatic stimuli and in the case of Parkinsonism, rhythmic bursts of discharges at or near the tremor frequency, have been collated. Interpretative generalizations concerning the spatial arrangement of somatic representation in the thalamus are presented.

157. Evolution of reactivity to auditory stimuli. —S. Dongier and M. Degossely (Liege, Belgium).

In previous work on auditory stimulation and startle reaction we have shown the clinical interest of such studies in psychiatry especially in hysteria, in autogenic training and industrial psychology (sensitivity to noise.)

However, the influence of habituation on these patterns has not been sufficiently evaluated and the present study tries to tackle this problem.

Two series of auditory stimuli are given at irregular intervals at the beginning and at the end of a routine EEG, in order to compare their effect and to establish if possible, correlations with reactivity to other stimuli and with clinical data.

Three-hundred subjects (ambulatory psychiatric patients of both sexes) have been studied. In 50 of them the tones were different in each of the series (512 and 1024 c/sec).

In 31% there was no effect on the primary record. In 27%, a decrease in amplitude and/or persistence of evoked potentials is observed. In 24%, the results in both series are comparable, in 11% there is an increase in the second series and 7% of the results are not homogeneous enough for a reliable conclusion.

The group with no visible reaction is also less reactive to other forms of stimulation. The group with more habituation is less photo-sensitive. The groups with no change or increased reactivity is more sensitive to both hyperventilation and photic stimulation. More hysterical patients are found in these latter groups.

158. On the physiological role of a 55 c/sec rhythm produced by the olfactory bulb.—D. M. Gedevani (Tbilisi, U.S.S.R.).

A spontaneous rhythmic activity at 55 c/sec (range 50-60 c/sec) and a related rhythm of 2-5 c/sec was described by the author in olfactory bulb of rabbits, cats, dogs and humans and has also been described by Adrian and other neurophysiologists. The work of the author indicates that these activities are an expression of orienting and emotional responses and may be caused by any external or internal stimuli as well as by olfactory stimuli. The 55 c/sec rhythm appears to be as important as the alpha rhythm of Berger.

Oscillographic studies of unilateral salivary and motor conditioned reflexes have shown that during their formation the behavior of the 55c/sec activity is modified in a specific way, thus suggesting that this rhythm partakes in the formation of the reflex processes. The 2-5 c/sec activity does not necessarily accompany the appearance of the 55 c/sec rhythm.

A bionic model of the 55 c/sec rhythm–the "orienting reflex model" (Gedevani and Eidelman)–together with a physical and mathematical analysis of it have indicated that the smooth rhythmicity of the waves is due to an ordered but not completely synchronized neuron activity in the bulb. This occurs if each discharge of the recruited neuron follows the other by not more than 0.1 msec. The amplitude of the waves and their duration depends on the number of discharges making up each wave.

It appears that the EEG pattern of the orienting response represents the form of each wave, (*i.e.*, the number of discharges), the number of waves in each burst, and the interval between each of the bursts or spindles. These characteristics obviously are information bearing and stimulate other parts of the brain appropriately. The 55 c/sec rhythm appears also in the frontal poles of the brain which further suggests paleobiological relationships.

159. EEG patterns as an index of clinical activity of psychoactive drugs.–M. Fink and D. M. Shapiro (New York, N.Y., U.S.A.).
The human scalp record of cerebral electrical activity is easily recorded, sensitive to drug effects and related to clinical behavior. Frequency analysis, amplitude integration, averaged evoked response, activated EEG to barbiturates and chloralose, and changes during all night sleep recording are among the many methods of analysis that have been investigated.

In a review of the effects of psychoactive drugs in man a classification of drugs emerges which is related to the clinical efficacy of the compounds. This classification is being applied to the identification of the clinical effects of new, potentially psychoactive compounds.

1. The EEG pattern of cyclazocine is similar to that of imipramine, and in clinical trials it was found to be an active antidepressant.

2. The EEG patterns of thiothixene and trifluperidol are similar to chlorpromazine. The psychoactive range is in the same class.

3. The EEG patterns of fenfluramine, an anorexigenic compound, are most like 50 mg amobarbital and differ from dextroamphetamine. In clinical trials, the principal secondary effects have been sedation and drowsiness.

4. Time-dose studies of 50 mg and 100 mg amobarbital and 300 mg sustained release amobarbital showed different patterns for the different drug forms.

5. The separation of sympathomimetic and anticholinergic hallucinogens by EEG criteria provides a basis for the selection of appropriate antagonists.

Quantitative EEG provides a useful means of identifying and classifying psychoactive drugs in man for therapeutic purposes.

160. Effects of cigarette withdrawal on sleep and dream patterns.–J. D. Kales, T. A. Preston, and T. L. Tan (Los Angeles, Calif., U.S.A.).
A. Kales, in our laboratory, has noted that psychiatric patients frequently reported more dreams in association with the cessation of chronic cigarette usage. Three subjects were studied for nine consecutive laboratory nights. They were continuously monitored with EEG, EKG, and EOG. The first four nights followed days during which subjects continued to smoke as usual (2-3 packs/day). Starting on the fifth day, subjects completely abstained from smoking so that nights 5 - 9 represented withdrawal nights.

The results are not conclusive as to whether subjects had a slight decrease in REM sleep while smoking. The most striking finding was a moderate increase in the percentage of REM sleep and the absolute amount of REM time on withdrawal nights as compared to "cigarette" nights. The results also suggested a decrease in the onset of the first REM period of the night on "non-cigarette" (5-9) as compared to cigarette (1-4) nights. In addition, upon final awakening in the morning, subjects' estimates of how much they had dreamed during the night showed a slight increase on non-cigarette nights.

161. Effectiveness of sleep medications: all night studies of hypnotic drugs.–A. Kales, M. B. Scharf and C. Allen (Los Angeles, Calif., U.S.A.).
This report summarized work to date regarding the effects of sleep medications in inducing and in maintaining sleep.

Drugs evaluated include chloral hydrate 1000 mg, glutethimide 500 mg, flurazepam 30 mg and Sominex (which contains 25 mg of methapyrilene hydrochloride and 0.25 mg of scopolamine aminoxide hydrobromide). In the studies, insomniac subjects were continuously monitored in the laboratory with EEG, EMG, and EOG. The first three drugs were evaluated over 22 consecutive nights; the first 7 were in the laboratory (nights 1-4: placebo-baseline and nights 5-7: active drug). On nights 8-15, subjects slept at home and took the active drug each night at h.s. The last 7 nights (16-22) the subjects slept in the laboratory (nights 16-18: active drug and nights 19-22: placebo-withdrawal).

The results were as follows: flurazepam significantly decreased sleep latency and total wake time after sleep onset for both sets of drug nights in the laboratory. While at home on the drug, the subjects reported that they slept well. Chloral hydrate and glutethimide significantly decreased sleep latency on nights 5-7 whereas by nights 16-18 sleep latency had returned to baseline levels. While sleeping at home on the drug, the subjective reports tended to be unfavorable. The results indicate that flurazepam significantly induced and maintained sleep over the entire two week drug period. Chloral hydrate and glutethimide significantly induced sleep on the first three drug nights. However, on nights 8-15 it appeared that the effectiveness of these drugs had decreased considerably, and by the last three drug nights they were ineffective.

In a study of insomniac subjects, the effectiveness of two tablets of Sominex was evaluated with the following schedule: nights 1-3, baseline-placebo; nights 4-6, active drug; and nights 7 and 8, placebo-withdrawal. Sleep latency and total wake time after sleep onset did not change on drug nights, indicating that the drug was ineffective in inducing or maintaining sleep.

FREE COMMUNICATIONS IN ELECTROMYOGRAPHY

1. **Anal sphincter electromyography: description of urethro-anal reflex.–A. P. Ruskin and J. E. Davis (New York, N. Y., U.S.A.).**

A study was undertaken to observe the electromyographic response of the anal sphincter to several urogenital procedures including bulbocavernosus reflex and intraurethral stimulation. The patients were placed in a modified lithotomy position and coaxial needle electrode insertion was made in the anal sphincter. The electromyographic output was observed in the resting condition and also with a voluntarily increased intraabdominal pressure. A bulbocavernosus reflex was elicited first by compression of the glans penis. Then passage of various sized sounds or catheters was carried out with observations being made at progressive depths of penetration and withdrawal.

A technique for localizing the anal sphincter and establishing a base line was established. Passing a sound or catheter, which causes distention of the urethra, likewise produces a reflex contraction of the anal sphincter, demonstrated by an increase in electrical output. Furthermore, this burst of activity appears to occur specifically with dilatation of the posterior part of the urethra in the region of the bladder neck. This response is much more pronounced than that produced by the sound in other portions of the urethra. It is independent of local anesthesia and therefore not of sensory origin. The authors postulate the presence of a previously unrecorded urethro-anal reflex dependent on dilatation of a reflexogenic zone just anterior to the bladder neck.

2. **EMG and muscle tension studies of myotonia induced by 25-azacholesterol.– A. Eberstein and J. Goodgold (New York, N.Y., U.S.A.).**

Myotonia was induced in white, Wistar rats with daily subcutaneous injections of 25-azacholesterol. After seven weeks of injections, the rats developed obvious clinical symptoms of myotonia. Electromyographic examination demonstrated (1) that the fast-twitch muscles (*e.g.*, anterior tibial) develop myotonia earlier than the slow-twitch muscles (soleus), (2) that with prolonged drug administration the soleus muscle becomes as much involved as the anterior tibial, and (3) female rats follow the same delayed time course in development of myotonia as occurs in the soleus of male rats.

In vivo, isotonic tension measurements were performed with myotonic muscle. The response of the muscle to trains of tetanic stimuli was characteristic of myotonic muscle: an increase in tension after cessation of stimulus or after spasm and an increased relaxation time. Occlusion of the arterial blood supply to the muscle resulted in almost immediate disappearance of the prolonged relaxation. Venous occlusion did not alter the response in any way.

3. **Myasthenic-like response in patients with neuropathy.–O. Miglietta (Welfare Island, N.Y., U.S.A.).**

The electrical response of the abductor pollicis brevis evoked by a brief train of stimuli was studied in 10 normal subjects and in 18 patients with diabetic neuropathy. The median nerve was stimulated at the wrist with trains of 25 pulses at pulse rates of 10, 20, 50, 100, 200, and 500/sec.

The response in general increased in amplitude and decreased in duration in all normal subjects with stimulating rates of 10, 20, 50, and 100/sec. An average maximal increase in amplitude of 29% occurred with a rate of 20/sec. The response rapidly decreased to an average of 59%, with a rate of 200/sec. At 500/sec generally no response could be recognized after the first one.

In the patient group a common finding was a rapid and earlier decrement of the evoked action potentials. At 10/sec stimulation, 3 patients already showed a decrease of 13%. At 50/sec the response decreased an average of 24% in 8 patients; and at 100/sec it dropped by an average of 28% in 16 of the 18 patients. The myasthenic-like response occurred at frequencies that facilitated a normal muscle or left it unchanged. The rate of decrement was faster and more severe, the more rapid the stimulation. Usually no changes were seen in patients or in normal persons with a rate of stimulation below 5-10/sec.

4. **The control of muscle tone in man.–J. W. Lance (Kensington, Australia).**

Reflex spread or irradiation depends upon propagation of a vibration wave from the point percussed to the spindle receptors of muscles participating in the reflex contraction. This accounts for clinical phenomena such as the "inverted supinator reflex". Continuous vibration of muscle belly or tendon in man produces a tonic contraction of the muscle vibrated by repetitively exciting group Ia fibers arising from muscle spindles. Vibration-induced tonic contraction therefore stimulates the natural reflex response to muscle stretch, and serves as a model for study of tonic mechanisms in man. The augmenting quality of normal tonic contraction depends upon supraspinal reinforcement, and is absent in spinal man or cat.

Vibration of muscle suppresses tendon jerks

and H reflexes by a process of presynaptic inhibition. The latter has been demonstrated by neurophysiologic studies in the cat. The fact that the monosynaptic reflex is inhibited by peripheral vibration while a tonic contraction is in progress suggests that the tonic reflex depends at least in part upon a polysynaptic pathway.

Vibration-induced tonic contraction is normal in Parkinson's disease but is diminished or altered in character in upper motor neurone lesions. In spastic patients, the normal augmenting tonic contraction may be replaced by an extensor thrust in response to vibration. This implies that the tonic stretch reflexes of spasticity are not simply exaggerated normal responses, but employ only part of the normal pathway, being deprived of the supraspinal connexions required for the normal graded reflex contraction.

The fact that tonic mechanisms in the intact subject depend upon bulbospinal connexions which are in turn influenced by the motor cortex and cerebellum, accounts for the ways in which muscle tone may be altered independently of tendon jerks, which rely solely upon the excitability of the monosynaptic arc.

5. Clinical application of sensory nerve action potentials.—K. Sato and H. Ishijima (Tokyo, Japan).

Sensory loss is one of the most important signs of a nerve lesion. However, it is difficult to measure a disturbance of sensory function objectively without interrogating the patient. Recently, many investigators have contributed information by measuring the sensory nerve action potential, a relatively new field of electrodiagnosis. Our own recent reports have dealt with sensory nerve action potentials in normal persons and in patients with peripheral neuropathies. This report deals with sensory nerve action potential examination of upper and lower extremities in normal and pathological states.

Two hundred and thirteen normal subjects were examined and the action potentials analysed for wave-form, amplitude, latency and conduction velocity, in relation to sex and age. In addition, the motor nerve conduction velocity was compared with sensory nerve conduction velocity.

Two hundred cases of various kinds of nervous disorder were examined, and all of them showed abnormalities, such as lack of action potentials, low amplitude or long latency (low conduction velocity). Several cases showed these abnormalities even without demonstrable sensory loss, indicating that this test was very sensitive. Serial observations were made in several cases and the action potentials became normal after symptoms had completely disappeared.

It is concluded that this examination can be of practical value in the investigation of sensory disorders, especially in cases of minor peripheral nerve damage.

6. Conduction velocity, electromyography and H-reflex studies after phenol nerve block for the management of spasticity.—A. A. Khalili and H. B. Betts (Chicago, Ill., U.S.A.).

Two hundred ninety-three nerve blocks with 2 and 3% phenol solutions in distilled water have been performed in 120 patients with spasticity of various etiology. Clinically, spasticity was diminished or relieved without gross sensory loss. The average duration of relief of spasticity in 72 nerve blocks with completed follow-up was 298 days ranging from 10 to 754 days. In 10.5% slight to moderate paresthesia developed following the block. Diminution or emergence of voluntary movement was noticed in some patients.

Following the block, motor and sensory conduction velocity in some patients was unchanged, in others they were increased or diminished. Electromyography showed partial denervation in the related muscles. Amplitude ratio study of M-response and H-reflex distal and proximal to the area of block, and Achilles tendon reflex showed abolition of tendon jerk, depression of proximal M-response, proximal H-reflex and distal H-reflex immediately after the block. In some patients distal M-response, following the block, was increased.

It can be concluded that 2 and 3% phenol solutions in distilled water have a rather selective blocking effect and primarily affect gamma motor, small alpha motor and group I-a afferent fibers. The reason for rise in distal M-response is under investigation.

7. Studies concerning the role of the safety factor in injured nerve.—F. A. Davis (Chicago, Ill., U.S.A.).

The ratio of the action current of a nerve fiber to the minimum current necessary to maintain impulse conduction is known as the safety factor. Tasaki found a value of 5-7 in amphibian myelinated nerve. Theoretically if the safety factor is decreased by axonal injury or disease, the conduction mechanisms should become more labile and might fail with adverse alterations in pH, electrolytes, temperature, etc., even though similar changes do not block normal nerve. On the other hand, conditions that increase the safety factor might improve function in injured nerve.

It has been found that excised frog sciatic nerves that are injured by pressure but are still capable of conducting impulses have an altered response to temperature. Conduction block begins around 26τC and is marked (30-40%) by 28°C. Normal nerves do not begin to block until 32-33°C and not until 33-35°C is it comparable to injured nerve. Conduction markedly improves in the experimental nerves when the localized lesion is bathed in low calcium Ringer's solution. This had been predicted on the basis that calcium ion depletion lowers the threshold for excitation and therefore might increase the safety factor.

Direct current injuries were also made in the region of one sciatic nerve in intact frogs. Animals that demonstrated little or no significant impairment developed a severe, transient paralysis of the affected limb after both legs were immersed in warm water for several minutes (a brief film will be shown). When studied *in vitro*, the sciatic nerve injured by direct current showed the same type of temperature response seen after the pressure lesions.

These findings support the safety factor thesis discussed above. The possible clinical significance of this concept is currently being explored.

8. Maximum conduction velocity and range of conduction velocity in motor fibers of the deep peroneal nerve in patients with chronic renal insufficiency.—D. van der Most van Spijk, S. Dijkstra and F. G. I. Jennekens (Utrecht, Netherlands).

It is well known that motor nerve conduction velocity may be low in patients with chronic renal insufficiency. The aim of the present study was to investigate: (1) the relation between the amount of slowing and the degree of renal failure, and (2) the relation between the amount of slowing and the extent of the clinical signs of neuropathy. Motor nerve conduction velocity was determined in the deep peroneal nerve of 61 patients, not treated with hemodialysis.

In order to obtain information about the conduction velocity in rapidly and slowly conducting fibers, we used a modification of Hopf's method. In our modification the area of the response was measured. It is our opinion that the end of the nerve fiber blockade may not be accurately determined. Therefore, we did not turn our attention especially to the time difference between the last maximal and last minimal second response, but we measured the whole range of time differences between these two extreme values.

The results were as follows: (1) The mean conduction velocity of 46 patients with serum creatinine level above 100 mg/1 appeared to be significantly lower than the mean conduction velocity of 15 patients with serum creatinine content between 20 and 100 mg/1. (2) The mean conduction velocity in patients with or without clinical signs of neuropathy was lower than that in a control group of 21 healthy normal subjects. (3) The slowing of conduction appeared to be more pronounced in the patients with a more severe neuropathy. (4) Conduction velocities more than 50% below normal have been recorded. (5) In cases of uremia with low motor conduction velocity a slowing of conduction in all alpha motor fibres of the N. peroneus profundus was observed.

9. The silent period during control of skilled motor performance.—R. Herman (Bronx, N.Y., U.S.A.).

When isometrically contracting triceps surae muscle is suddenly "unloaded", a period of electrical silence (silent period) appears in the electromyogram (EMG) of the agonist muscle and a reflex discharge is observed in EMG of the antagonist tibialis antericus muscle at a time consistent with spinal cord transmission. Complete narcotization of the common peroneal nerve does not influence the duration of the silent period. This suggests the silent period is due to reflex withdrawal of motoneuron support due to a decrease in muscle afferent discharge. The rate of change of load (*i.e.*, rapid or slow decrement of load) influences both the duration of the silent period and the amplitude and duration of the EMG burst following the silent period. Such alterations in EMG activity imply that the velocity of unloading and/or the resultant isotonic movement of the limb enhance muscle spindle discharges. The silent period and the associated motor burst are also altered during repetition of a task utilizing a particular decrement of load during visual tracking of angular position of the ankle. Reduction in errors during repeated trials apparently is due to adjustment in local feedback circuits as well as adjustment in the magnitude of response to somatic stimuli. The silent period increases in duration and terminates in a motor burst which is reduced in amplitude and duration. When visual information is not utilized, the silent period and EMG bursts during the initial trial are similar to the silent period and EMG bursts during the performance of a learned task. It appears that such modifications during visual tracking are due to alterations in fusimotor activity and that sensory information derived from visual stimuli provide high gain on the muscle servo system; this is eventually altered when vision no longer plays a dominant role in the acquisition of a task.

10. The peripheral neuropathy of Krabbe's (globoid) leucodystrophy.—L. Gutmann, G. Hogan and S. M. Chou (Morgantown, W. Va., U.S.A.).

Krabbe's disease (globoid leucodystrophy) has

been thought of as a disorder limited to the central nervous system. Involvement of peripheral nerves has not been appreciated until the past few years. Twelve such cases have now been reported.

This presentation emphasizes the peripheral neuropathy of this disease as studied clinically, electrophysiologically and pathologically in a young girl. The diagnosis of a severe peripheral neuropathy was made at age 22 months on the basis of electromyographic studies and histological examination of the sural nerve. Additional histological studies on brain and peripheral nerves were performed 6 months later at the time of autopsy.

At a time when a peripheral neuropathy was not clinically apparent because of the presence of hyperreflexia related to central nervous demyelination, motor conduction velocities in four nerves studied were slow, ranging from 18.5 to 24.4 m/sec. Distal sensory latencies were also very prolonged. Despite these marked abnormalities the amplitudes of the evoked muscle and nerve action potentials were relatively normal suggesting that segmental demyelination was the predominating defect in the nerves. This was substantiated by pathological studies.

Pathologically, the peripheral nerve changes in Krabbe's disease differ from those of metachromatic leucodystrophy. The nerves in Krabbe's disease are abnormal in size, color and consistency while they appear grossly normal in metachromatic leucodystrophy. Histologically endoneurial fibrosis occurs in Krabbe's disease whereas brown metachromasia is present in metachromatic leucodystrophy.

The failure to fully appreciate the peripheral neuropathy of Krabbe's disease is most likely related to the overwhelming central nervous system involvement and its clinical manifestations. Conduction studies and biopsy of peripheral nerves are helpful in recognizing this neuropathy. It is proposed that the peripheral neuropathy is a consistent component of this disease.

11. Anal sphincter electromyography in adults. —G. W. Waylonis (Columbus, Ohio, U.S.A.).
Electromyography of the external anal sphincter was first described in 1930 by Beck, with Newman (1949), Kawakaimi (1954), Traverner (1959), and Covine (1959) also describing their interest in this muscle. Ingberg and Johnson (1962) and Chantraine, Lloyd and Swinyard (1966) described clinical application of the technique in spina bifida associated with myelomeningocele. Archibald and Goldsmith (1967) described some other clinical applications of the technique. Bailey, Powers and Waylonis (1968) reported a series of 184 children with genitourinary tract problems in which the electromyogram played a major role in assisting the urologist to diagnose a neurogenic state of the bladder. At that time it was proposed that the technique might have useful applications in the adult age group as well.

The present report concerns our further observations in the technique of anal sphincter electromyography and presents the results of our observations in a series of 39 adult patients. Conditions in which the EMG has proved helpful include: chronic enuresis, acute enuresis, acute urinary retention, acute and chronic groin and rectal pain syndromes, acute and chronic bowel problems. These symptoms have been observed in patients with lower lumbar and sacral anomalies, acute herniated disc syndromes, chronic degenerative disc syndromes, arachnoiditis, and diabetic neuropathy. Case reports will be presented.

12. Cutaneous nociceptive reflexes in humans. —M. M. Gassel and K. H. Ott (San Francisco, Calif., U.S.A.).
The excitability changes in a population of triceps surae motoneurones was investigated after cutaneous stimulation of the foot and leg in humans. A regulated system was evolved for eliciting the monosynaptic reflex and delivering an unvarying single-shock stimulus. The excitability changes were evaluated by the classical recovery curve. A new accelerated method for recording mononeurone excitability was also utilized. The technique is based upon the observation that during voluntary activity motor unit discharge increased with periods of reflex facilitation and decreased with inhibition of the reflex. This relationship was established in a population of triceps surae motoneurons in which the recovery curve of monosynaptic excitability had earlier been elicited by the same conditioning stimulus. A graph representing the amount of muscle activity was fashioned by passing the electromyogram through an absolute value rectifier circuit to sum both the positive and negative phases of the motor unit potential and then averaging 250-500 traces by computer. The computer sweeps are triggered by the conditioning stimulus and the recording made from tonically active triceps surae motoneurones.

There are early excitability changes with local sign mediated by group II cutaneous fibers. There is facilitation on stimulation of the dorsum of the foot and of the leg and inhibition on plantar stimulation of the distal foot. A prominent late increase in excitability occurs without local sign, mediated by group III fibers and by long-loop spinobulbo-spinal reflexes. Reliable changes in motoneurone excitability with serial alterations in electrode placement support the concept of an intricate organization of the receptor fields of flexion and extension reflexes with considerable overlapping and interaction.

13. Conduction velocity in the posterior tibial nerve of juvenile male baboons.—R. Harris (London, G.B.).

Nerve conduction studies have been carried out in 36 juvenile male baboons weighing 3.1 to 6.0 kg. These animals are involved in a dietary experiment to study the effects of vitamin B_{12} deficiency and chronic cyanide toxicity. Measurements have been made on two or more occasions in each animal and at least one of these was at a time when there were no biochemical abnormalities. The examinations were carried out under anaesthesia with phencyclidine hydrochloride and pento-barbitone. The body and limb temperatures were monitored during the procedure.

Motor conduction velocity in the posterior tibial nerve to the flexor hallucis brevis muscle was determined and conduction in the afferent fibers was measured by recording action potentials from the nerve at the knee following stimulation at the ankle. Supra-maximal stimulation, and stimulation below the motor threshold were carried out. Sensory action potentials were recorded over the nerve at the ankle after stimulating the digital nerves of the first digit.

The results show uniformly slower velocities than those reported in the forearm nerves of adult baboons. There have been no changes in velocities or other measurements during the first few months of the experiment which might be due to a peripheral neuropathy but there does appear to be some relationship between the body weight (*i.e.*, age) and velocity.

14. Neuronal mechanisms of the Achilles tendon jerk and of the ischemic hind-limb rigidity. —B. Fujimori, M. Kato, T. Yamauchi and Y. Hirata (Sapporo and Niigata, Japan).

First, neuronal mechanisms of the Achilles tendon jerk were analysed in normal cats, by recording reflex responses in the ventral root, afferent volleys in the dorsal root, and the respective unit discharges. Comparison was made between the reflex responses and afferent volleys produced by the tendon tap and those elicited by electrical stimulation of the gastrocnemius nerve.

Secondly, as an extension of our previous experiment, synapses of the intracellularly stained motoneurons were observed under the electron microscope in order to investigate the mechanisms of the ischemic hind-limb rigidity.

(1) The majority of reflex discharges (72.2% of 97) of single motoneurons following a single tendon tap were considered to be monosynaptically evoked. However, other similarly elicited ventral root unit reflex discharges (27.8%) were polysynaptic as judged by their latencies. (2) Reflex responses in the ventral root elicited by the tendon tap were more susceptible to variations of stimulus or experimental conditions than those set up by electrical stimulation of the muscle nerve. This may be attributed mainly to the processes of temporal and spatial summation of synaptic transmission, in view of the marked asynchrony of group Ia afferent discharges elicited by tendon tap in contrast to their synchrony following electrical stimulation observed in the present experiment. These results may be useful for the evaluation of the tendon jerk in contrast to the H-reflex. (3) Electron microscopic study revealed certain specific features in preparations with chronic ischemic hind-limb rigidity. However, in the few cases examined no significant change in ratio of synaptic knobs containing two types of vesicles could be seen that would explain the enhanced level of activity of the motoneurons.

15. Electromyography and nerve conduction in bronchial carcinoma.—A. M. M. Fleming, J. A. R. Lenman, M. A. H. Robertson and H. H. R. Samarasinghe (Dundee, G. B.).

An unselected series of patients affected by bronchial carcinoma has been studied in association with matched controls in order to investigate the relationship between bronchial carcinoma and associated forms of neuropathy and myopathy. In each patient electromyographic studies were carried out and nerve conduction velocity was measured in the upper and lower limbs. The latency of the H reflex in the posterior tibial nerve was determined. Each patient submitted to neurological examination according to a standard protocol and to haematological and biochemical study. The controls were matched for sex and age within five years and had no clinical evidence of carcinoma, neurological disorder or diabetes. The conduction velocity studies were carried out in both patient and control populations and electroencephalograms were also recorded in each patient and control.

In the present report the electrophysiological findings in peripheral nerve and muscle are considered and correlated with clinical and biochemical observations. In a small proportion of cases there was clinical evidence of neurological disorder and the electrophysiological findings in these cases are considered in relation to those in which electromyography or nerve conduction measurement showed abnormality in the absence of clinical disability. The distribution and range of nerve conduction velocity in the series of patients with bronchial carcinoma is compared with that in the control population and the possible significance of minor abnormalities in terms of underlying pathology is discussed.

16. Motor unit frequency control in facial neuropathy.–J. H. Petajan (College, Alaska, U.S.A.).

Using audiovisual feedback of motor unit action potentials, the ability of 11 patients with facial neuropathy to control firing rate was examined. The following mean interspike intervals were determined when firing rate was: (1) at its lowest most stable level, *onset interval* and (2) increased to a level at which recruitment of a second motor unit occurred, *recruitment interval.* Mean onset interval was decreased while mean recruitment interval was unchanged. In 20% of orbicularis oris and 12% of frontalis motor units studied a second motor unit was not recruited despite high firing rates while in normal subjects recruitment always occurs. The findings can be explained by a loss of larger motor units as would be produced by ischemia or pressure block. Regardless of the number of motor units lost in any territory, if recruitment can occur, then it occurs when the primary unit reaches a critical firing rate, the normal recruitment interval.

17. Threshold and conduction velocity in human median nerve sensory fibers.–W. C. Wiederholt (Columbus, Ohio, U.S.A.).

Fast conducting nerve fibers have a lower threshold than slow conducting fibers. Contrary to this generally accepted fact, Hodes *et al.* concluded from study of human motor nerves that fibers of low threshold conduct more slowly than those of high threshold. Recently, Wiederholt demonstrated in isolated mixed mammalian nerves that increasing stimulus intensities produce progressive shortening of latency, no change of conduction velocity, but movement of the effective point of excitation away from the stimulating cathode.

Conduction velocity in median nerve sensory fibers and its relation to stimulus intensity was studied in 30 normal subjects. Sensory fibers were stimulated with square pulses (0.1 msec, 30 to 110V) at the base of the third digit. Evoked nerve action potentials were recorded simultaneously from electrodes distal and proximal to the carpal tunnel. The distance from the distal electrode to the first electrode proximal to the carpal tunnel averaged 3.8 cm and between electrodes proximal to the carpal tunnel 1.94 cm. Conduction times between electrodes were used to calculate conduction velocities.

With just supramaximal stimulation conduction velocity across the carpal tunnel was 54.4±10.3 (S.D.) m/sec and proximal to the carpal tunnel 64.3±9.3 m/sec. When stimulation was increased from minimal (30 to 40 V) to just supramaximal (80 to 110 V), latency from shock artifact to beginning of the evoked potential (proximal to carpal tunnel), decreased from 2.24±0.24 msec to 2.08±0.23 msec but conduction velocity remained the same. This could result from movement of the effective point of excitation 1.04±0.32 cm away from the stimulating cathode.

The results suggest that (1) the fastest conducting sensory fibers in the human median nerve have a lower threshold than slower conducting fibers, and (2) the effective point of excitation moves away from the stimulating cathode as intensity of stimulation is increased.

18. Effect of local temperature on resting membrane potential in rat muscle.–T. Nakanishi and F. H. Norris, Jr. (San Francisco, Calif., U.S.A.).

The resting membrane potential (RMP) of human muscle has been measured as a diagnostic tool, but large variations have made determination of the normal range difficult. As one of the technical causes of such variation, the effect of local temperature on the RMP was investigated in rat muscle *in vivo*. The longissimus dorsi medialis muscle was irrigated with Liley's solution at various temperatures and RMPs measured within a depth of 1 mm from the surface using 3 M KCl-filled micropipette electrodes. The muscle RMP increased and decreased as the local temperature was raised and lowered between 25 and 44°C. Two experiments were performed. In one, fibers were studied for long periods of time while serial RMP measurements were made. The coefficient of the RMP was 1.3±0.6 (S.D.)μV per degree with a Q_{10} of 1.21±0.03 for increasing temperatures; the coefficient was 1.4±0.7 μV per degree with a Q_{10} of 1.25±0.05 for decreasing temperatures. In the second experiment, 20 different fibers were impaled successfully at each of several temperatures. The coefficient of the RMP was 1.0±0.4 μV per degree with a Q_{10} of 1.15±0.08 for increasing temperatures; the coefficient was 1.1±0.3 μV per degree with a Q_{10} of 1.16±0.07 for decreasing temperatures. These linear relationships of RMP and temperature might account for some of the reported variations of the normal RMP.

19. Subclinical lead neuropathy in man.–P. M. Fullerton and M. J. G. Harrison (London, G.B.).

Guinea pigs given lead acetate orally for several months often develop peripheral neuropathy, associated in some instances with considerable slowing of conduction. Pathological changes of segmental demyelination have been demonstrated in such animals.

Although lead poisoning is still a common industrial problem, paralysis is rare. Nevertheless, it is possible that subclinical damage might be reflected in abnormalities of nerve conduction. Nineteen men who had worked in a lead battery factory for between 5 months and 13 years were therefore examined. All had raised blood lead levels and some were anemic, but none had any abnormal neurological symptoms or signs. Twelve age matched control subjects were studied for comparison.

The lateral popliteal nerve was stimulated at knee and ankle and the muscle action potential recorded through surface electrodes over extensor digitorum brevis. The afferent volley was recorded from the lateral popliteal nerve at the head of the fibula following stimulation at the ankle. There was no statistical difference between the two groups for maximal motor conduction velocity, nor for the velocity or amplitude of the afferent volley. If slowing of conduction occurred in only a proportion of the nerve fibers, then maximal velocity might remain normal, but the muscle action potential would become increasingly dispersed the longer the conduction distance. As an indication of dispersion, the amplitude of the muscle response following stimulation at the knee was expressed as a percentage of that following stimulation at the ankle. The value for the lead workers was 84.8% (S.D. 12.7) and for the control group was 95.4% (S.D. 6.9). These differences are statistically significant and suggest that some fibers in the lead workers were conducting at a reduced velocity.

20. Stretch reflex and shortening reaction. A quantitative analysis of phasic and tonic stretch reflex in clinical states of spasticity and rigidity.—E. Esslen (Zürich, Switzerland).

A method (Electro-Tono-Myography) is described, to perform strictly defined active and passive extension and flexion movements and to record and analyse quantitatively phasic and tonic stretch reflexes in patients suffering from central motor disorders. In the course of these investigations a new phenomenon has been observed, called shortening reaction. It is mainly manifest in extrapyramidal diseases. Stretch reflex and shortening reaction are based on normal neurophysiological mechanisms, controlled by higher brain centers. In central motor disorders they are more or less released from central control. Comparisons of stretch reflex and shortening reaction before and after stereotactic operations on the thalamus reveal a differential effect on both.

21. A study of the diseased nerve in carpal tunnel syndrome.—K. Mechelse and B. Matricali (Leyden, The Netherlands).

In patients with a carpal tunnel syndrome, the conduction velocity of the exposed median nerve was measured during operation. After section of the ligamentum carpi transversum, a number of electrodes with fixed distances of one centimetre were placed on the nerve. The nerve was then stimulated successively through the various electrodes and the muscle response recorded from the m.abductor pollicis brevis. Voltage of the threshold stimulus and the latency of the muscle response were measured. Then the nerve response was recorded from various points of the nerve which was stimulated either distally or proximally at different distances from the recording point.

The result was that in most cases the threshold voltage of the muscle response was significantly higher in a certain part of the nerve. Sometimes the muscle response obtained by stimulating this part was either absent or of lower amplitude. Conduction velocity as derived from the latency and distance measurements increased clearly distal to this point. Further studies of the nerve response seem to confirm that nerve conduction is slowed and refractory period is longer particularly in this part of the nerve. Anatomical changes, when present, were observed in this part of the nerve.

In all operations performed, the m.opponens pollicis originated across the median nerve on the ligamentum carpi transversum. In a number of hands studied on the dissecting table, this origin never crossed the median nerve except in one case with a clear cut partial thenar atrophy. It is concluded that these carpal tunnel syndromes are related to the action of an aberrantly originating muscle on the nerve.

22. Motosensory afferents in human peripheral nerve to mechanical stimulation of muscle receptors.—H. M. Krott and H. M. Jacobi (Dietenbronn, Germany).

There have been many unsuccessful attempts to record the afferent discharge in the human peripheral nerve preceding the ankle jerk to mechanical stimuli. In the positive report of Hagbarth and Vallboit is difficult to distinguish between afferents from muscle, joint and skin.

Methods: In order to get exclusively muscle afferents with the T-reflex, records were taken from the femoral nerve and from the ramus muscularis of the tibial nerve by means of semimicroelectrodes. The criterion for a correct position of the electrode tip in the nerve was an optimal H-reflex following threshold stimulus, with M-response and without any sensation. The contact of the hammer-stimulator with the Achilles or patellar tendon, respectively, was used to trigger the Mnemotron Computer of Average Transients.

Results: In normal subjects and in patients with spasticity it was regularly possible to record the T-reflex afferents in both nerves, the latency being 8-10 msec. The T-discharge is less synchronized than the H-discharge. By contrast there was no T-discharge in 7 patients with polyneuritis.

The following control experiments were done: (1.) Electrical artifacts due to movement were excluded by simultaneous paraneural recording near the electrode in the nerve under identical recording conditions. (2.) Stimulation of skin and deep receptors in the sensory innervation area of the nerve did not give any afferent discharge. (3.) Complete Procaine block of distal parts of the femoral and tibial nerves, respectively, did not change the recorded afferent muscle response.

23. Peripheral nerve regeneration and muscle receptor reconstruction.—S. Homma (Chiba, Japan).

Tibial nerve of adult cats was cut at the level of the popliteal fossa and the perineurium of the cut ends was carefully sutured immediately after the cutting with the aid of special platinum rings. Daily injection of vitamin B_1, B_6 and B_{12} complex was continued for 20 to 60 days.

Alpha efferents and group I afferents were known to regenerate at 15 days after operation, gamma efferents and group II afferents at 25 days. Two tension receptors were found about 30 days and several stretch receptors after 50 days following the operation. The slope obtained from the relation between frequency of the group Ia discharge and muscle extension was in these "regenerated stretch receptors" less steep than in the normal muscle spindle. Whether the tension receptors which appear in the very early stage of recovery belong to Golgi tendon organ or develop into muscle spindles, is still not known. Several histological preparations of "regenerated" muscle spindle and Golgi tendon organs will be shown.

In cats having such "raw" stretch receptors, the size of muscle contraction produced by the stimulation of regenerated alpha efferent nerves was approximately 50% of the intact side. It is proposed that the animal at this stage be called an "alpha animal".

24. Vibratory stimulation of muscles and optimal frequency as tested by fixed rate of motoneuronal discharge.—H. Kobayashi and S. Watanabe (Chiba, Japan).

Cats were anesthetized and forced vibration was applied to the isolated tendon of the gastrocnemius or soleus muscles by the use of function generator, power amplifier and electromagnetic vibrator. The excursion of vibration was monitored by a photoelectric device. The frequency and intensity of gated vibratory stimuli were varied to evoke a certain fixed rate of ventral root discharge at L_7-S_1 segments. A "response area" curve was plotted for each unit from the varied values of the above two parameters. Most of the gastrocnemius motoneurons were known to have an optimal (minimal) threshold of vibratory amplitude around 100-120 c/sec. It is proposed that this be designated an "optimal frequency" in muscle vibration.

Further experiments were done to determine whether or not there is shift in the optimal frequency during post-tetanic potentiation which was effected by repetitive electric stimulation of the afferent side of monosynaptic reflex arc. In most of these experiments it was observed that optimal frequency shifted to a slightly higher range after post-tetanic stimulation. Shifts of the optimal frequency were also observed in soleus muscle experiments when the synergist (gastrocnemius) muscle was tonically stretched.

25. Further contributions to electromyography in internal medicine.—C. Serra (Naples, Italy).

In previous papers the spontaneous EMG of different chronic occlusive arterial diseases (Buerger's disease, arteriosclerotic arteropathy) has been systematically explored. Furthermore, the spontaneous and evoked EMG of diabetic arterial disease has been explored.

(1) More recently a comparative evaluation of nerve functional status in different chronic occlusive arterial diseases has been performed. Motor and sensory nerve conduction velocities (NCV) of 40 patients with chronic arterosclerotic occlusive disease have appeared to be borderline. A significant shift from normal values in both motor and sensory nerve has been observed frequently in 30 patients with diabetic arterial disease, with low conduction velocity values in most cases.

(2) Spontaneous and evoked EMG of a series of 40 hypersplenism patients has revealed frequent impairment of myoelectric patterns before splenectomy and a trend to normal values for the same muscles after surgery. The hypothesis of a direct peripheral influence of hypersplenism on motor unit action potentials, through the release of a toxic factor (DE FRANCISCIS' hyperoxylienine) could be advanced.

(3) EMG and electrodiagnostic investigations on a series of 40 patients with malignant blood diseases (lympogranuloma, chronic myeloid leukemia, lymphosarcoma, histioleukemia, multiple myeloma, acute myelosis). In lymphosarcoma, EMG traces of mixed patterns without significant

NCV abnormalities have been observed; in myeloma multiple, constant neurogenic patterns with reduction of motor NCV; in histioleukemia, frequent neurogenic patterns with reduced motor NCV; and in acute myelosis, slight neurogenic impairment with constant reduction of NCV of motor nerves have been observed. Mixed patterns with reduced motor NCV values occurred in malignant lymphogranuloma patients, whereas slight changes in spontaneous and evoked EMG occurred in chronic myeloid leukemia.

Sensory nerve conduction determinations have been of no diagnostic importance in differentiation of various neuromuscular disorders of blood diseases.

26. Sensory finger innervation as evidenced by nerve action potentials.—H. R. Muller, V. Skorpil and G. Muheim (Basal, Switzerland). Registration of sensory nerve action potentials from individual finger nerves has not been possible until now, since methods used were either simultaneous stimulation of the finger nerves, or antidromic registration of the sensory nerve action potentials from the radial and ulnar collateral nerve after stimulation at the wrist.

Therefore, a special needle electrode was used for bipolar antidromic registration of the sensory nerve action potential of single finger nerves. Two platinum needles were incorporated 10 mm apart in a plastic plate, the exposed length of the needle being 2.5 mm. The two points were stuck into the skin of the middle phalanx over the course of the volar nerve, and the two electrodes were fixed with adhesive tape to the finger. Spread of the sensory nerve action potential from the contralateral nerve by volume conduction was excluded by the fact that in two cases of recent finger nerve transsection, no potential could be recorded from the severed finger nerve, although the contralateral nerve was intact.

The innervation of the fingers was studied in 40 hands of 40 healthy subjects by antidromic stimulation of the median and ulnar nerves at the wrist. The following types of innervation could be recorded:

In 37 cases both sides of the fourth finger showed a double innervation by ulnar as well as by median nerve. In 3 of these cases this double innervation concerned both the fourth and fifth finger, and in 2 the third and the fourth finger. In these fingers, the amplitude of the potential was higher on the radial side when the median nerve was stimulated, and higher on the ulnar side when the ulnar nerve was stimulated. In only 3 cases, the fourth finger was innervated entirely by the median and the fifth by the ulnar nerve.

27. Thiamine deficiency neuropathy in rats.—K. Kunze and E. Muskat (Giessen, Germany). Affections of central and peripheral nervous system during thiamine deficiency are well known. Concerning affection of the peripheral nervous system, it is not clear to what extent this could be caused by starvation, or if it is due primarily to thiamine deficiency.

One hundred male Wistar rats divided into three feeding groups have been investigated over a time of about six months. Group I got full food, with all vitamins. Group II got 30% of necessary thiamine. Group III got full vitamin requirement, but only as much food as group II (pair fed to group II). Besides continuous weight control, rats of all groups have been investigated electromyographically, with special attention to evoked potentials, motor conduction and neuromuscular transmission (N. ischiadicus).

During the trial, weight increase of rats in group I continued, whereas weight increase of group II and III stopped. Rats of group II showed increasing muscular atrophy and paresis and severe disturbances of trophic function. In group II denervation potentials appeared 8-10 weeks after starting the trial. In addition a decrease of motor conduction velocity to nearly half the normal value and a drop of the amplitude of evoked potentials (measured under standard conditions) was found. Addition of SO_2 (400 mg/kg/day) to the thiamine deficient diet led to earlier detection of the neuropathy. No signs of neuropathy could be found in animals of group I and III. With thiamine administration to group II animals, neuropathy diminished with an increase of motor conduction velocity.

These findings suggest an affection of peripheral nerve, probably the myelin sheath, in thiamine deficiency. Thiamine deficiency as an important additional pathogenetic factor in some kinds of human polyneuropathies will be discussed.

28. Changes in the flexion reflex with repetitive cutaneous stimulation in spinal man.—M. R. Dimitrijevic and P. W. Nathan (Ljubljana, Yugoslavia and London, G.B.). A study was made of the changes that occur in the flexion reflex with repeated cutaneous stimulation. It was carried out on 10 patients with complete division of the spinal cord, and on 5 normal subjects. The flexion reflex was induced by electric and other stimuli applied to the plantar surface.

How frequently a minimal noxious stimulus has to be applied to be responded to by the spinal cord as one of a series or as a single stimulus was determined. The response to a noxious stimulus well above threshold applied repetitively passes through the following phases: build-up, constancy, fluctuation, diminution, and absence of response. The faster the stimulation rate and the stronger the stimulus, the sooner each phase is reached. These phases do not occur simultaneously in all muscles. When repeated stimulation at one site has brought the responding motor units to the phase of absence of response, their response can be restored by stimuli of the same or of other kinds applied anywhere else in the limb. The site from which their activity can be restored can be as near as 4 cm from the first site. Stimulation of the same or different kinds applied to the contralateral limb also restores the response of these motor units. But in all cases the restoration of activity is evanescent. Repetitive stimulation at the second site soon evokes no response from these motor units; this phase is reached much sooner than it would have been had the first site not already been brought to this phase before.

29. Anomalous peroneal nerve distribution detected by electromyography.—E. Infante and W. R. Kennedy (Minneapolis, Minn., U.S.A.).

During the determination of peroneal nerve conduction velocities in some patients, the amplitude of the evoked response, recorded by surface electrodes over the extensor digitorum brevis muscle, is considerably larger when this nerve is stimulated at the level of the knee than when it is stimulated at the ankle. In these patients stimulation behind the lateral malleolus elicited an additional response. This suggested the existence of an anomalous branch of the nerve to this muscle. Because we could not find a description of the electrical phenomenon in the literature, we studied its incidence.

The peroneal nerve was stimulated supramaximally at the knee, ankle and behind the lateral malleolus in 148 patients with diverse neurological disorders and 56 healthy controls. Bilateral testing was done in 122 persons. Of a total of 326 nerves tested, 61 (19%) gave positive response. Four of these 1.2% were bilateral. There was no significant difference between patients and controls. In 13 of 61 positive responses, or 3.9% of all nerves tested, the amplitude of the evoked response was higher after stimulation at the knee than after simulation at the ankle. In these cases the average response to stimulation at the lateral malleolus was 1.5 millivolts. These cases (3.9%) are of clinical importance in evaluation of nerve conduction studies. The remainder of the cases gave responses averaging 0.16 millivolts. They are likely to be overlooked in clinical testing.

It is concluded that in 19% of peroneal nerves there is an anomalous muscular branch coursing around the lateral malleolus and innervating a portion of the extensor digitorum brevis muscle. This branch corresponds to the "accessory peroneal nerve", first described in man by T. H. Bryce (1897). In 3.9% of nerves it is of sufficient size to lead to confusion of the electromyographer who is unaware of its existence.

30. Multiple distal neuritis of the shoulder girdle: an electromyographic clarification of "paralytic brachial neuritis".—G. H. Kraft (Seattle, Wash., U.S.A.).

Fifteen patients with acute shoulder pain followed by weakness of muscles of the upper extremity were evaluated electrodiagnostically. This disease is commonly known as "paralytic brachial neuritis", and is generally considered to be a disorder of the brancial plexus. In order to determine the site of nerve dysfunction and the natural course of the disease, serial electromyographic and nerve conduction studies were performed. In addition to standard nerve conduction velocities, nerve conduction through the brachial plexus, and latencies from Erb's point to the trapezius, biceps, deltoid, supraspinatus and infraspinatus muscles were measured. Normal values for these latencies were also established.

Nerve conduction velocities and conduction through the brachial plexus showed no abnormalities. However, latencies to affected muscles showed prolongation, while unaffected muscles innervated by the same peripheral nerves had normal latency values. This, and the pattern of denervation, could best be explained by the involvement of distal portions of peripheral nerves.

Bilateral disease was present in one-third of the patients. The most commonly affected nerve was the branch of the suprascapular to the supraspinatus muscle. Next most frequently involved nerves were the branch to the infraspinatus and the axillary. The 11th cranial nerve was affected in four patients. Branches of other peripheral nerves were occasionally affected. The course of the disease was variable. Maximum involvement usually occurred at the onset of symptoms, but occasionally other nerves became affected during the first several weeks. Recovery was complete after several months in mildly paretic muscles, but never complete in paralyzed muscles.

Since nerve latency determinations suggest that the site of nerve dysfunction in "paralytic brachial neuritis" is the distal portion of nerves innervating the shoulder, a more appropriate name would be "multiple distal neuritis of the shoulder girdle".

31. Electromyography in surgery of the hand.—J. E. Stern and M. H. Leonard (El Paso, Texas, U.S.A.).

The value of EMG in surgery of the hand is predicated on: (1.) a knowledge of peripheral neuroanatomy: cells, roots, trunks, cords, nerves, junctions, muscles; (2.) a knowledge of peripheral neuropathology (and psychopathology): neurotmesis, axonotmesis, neurapraxia, ischemic-hypoxic and metabolic neuropathy, conversion reaction; and (3.) a knowledge of electromyography and electromyophony: artefacts; standardization; time relationships; positive sharp waves; fibrillation; nascent, polyphasic, and giant units; dystrophic and myotonic potentials.

The EMG is useful in identifying: (1.) the true *nature* of a lesion; (2.) the true *level* or levels of a lesion (as opposed to the level of muscular, tendinous or osseous trauma); (3.) the presence of *multiple* peripheral nerve lesions; (4.) the presence or absence of *regeneration*; and (5.) *compression syndromes,* if the motor fibers are sufficiently involved.

In 41 patients, 47 nerves were studied by surgical and clinical methods. The overall percentage of electrographic accuracy was 79, including false positives and false negatives. No matter how obvious the case, the initial study of a patient should involve a complete survey of the affected part. Most of these points will be documented with slides; some with brief case reports.

32. Latency variation of single human motoneurones in the H-reflex.—J. Trontelj (ljubljana, Yugoslavia).

Using Ekstedt's criteria for single muscle fiber action potentials, it is possible to isolate responses of single muscle fibers in the H-reflex of human calf muscles. The H-reflex of individual motoneurones shows considerable variation of latency ranging between 400 and 2500 μsec, with most between 500 and 1500 μsec. That a large proportion of this variation is due to fluctuation of excitability of spinal motoneurones has been concluded from the fact that (1) the latencies of direct (M) responses of single muscle fibers recorded in the same experimental conditions varied much less, *i.e.,* less than 120 μsec in over 90% and (2) the Jendrassik manoeuvre not only tends to increase the proportion of effective stimuli, but also to shorten the latency of the responses. In a minority of instances, the opposite effect was observed; the latencies of some motoneurones lengthened with higher stimulus amplitudes. The latencies could also be shortened by increments of 5-10% in the stimulus amplitude (presumably depolarizing more Ia fibers). Subthreshold conditioning stimuli applied through the same electrodes produced prolongation of latencies and blocking of responses at intervals between 1 msec and 1 sec and shortening at intervals below 0.75 msec. Shortening of the latencies was more readily obtained at lower amplitudes of the conditioning stimulus, while at higher amplitudes the latencies could occasionally be lengthened.

These effects can be explained in part by spatial and temporal summation of EPSP's and IPSP's at synapses on motoneurones. This process can either shorten or lengthen rise time of the excitatory membrane potential of the spinal motoneurone and enhance or delay the propagation of action potentials. Latency of the reflex response can thus reflect fine changes in excitability of individual motoneurones resulting from variation of the afferent inflow or other factors influencing their threshold.

33. Electrophysiological and histological studies in patients with Friedreich's ataxia.—J. G. McLeod (Sydney, Australia).

Nerve conduction studies have been performed on 9 patients with Friedreich's ataxia, whose ages ranged from 11 to 69 years, and in 20 control subjects. Motor conduction velocities in the median, ulnar and lateral popliteal nerves of the patients with Friedreich's ataxia were 46.0±4.9 m/sec, 44.6±3.3 m/sec and 36.3±3.1 m/sec, respectively, and were significantly less than those of the control subjects. Sensory action potentials were absent from the median and ulnar nerves at the wrist in seven of the patients and were reduced in amplitude in the other two patients. Lateral popliteal nerve action potentials were absent in all nine patients.

Sural nerve biopsies were performed in four patients. There was a marked reduction in the number of large diameter (9-14μ) fibers in all the nerves. Single fibers teased from the nerves were poorly myelinated and their internodal lengths were reduced. It is concluded that in patients with Friedreich's ataxia there is impairment of motor and sensory conduction which is related to the histological abnormalities present in the peripheral nerves.

34. A study of excitability of spinal motoneurones in hemiplegia.—F. Gracanin (Ljubljana, Yugoslavia).

One of the features of spasticity in hemiplegia is fluctuation of excitability of spinal motoneurones, which is shown by a variation of the amplitude of the tendon jerks and the H-reflex.

The purpose of this study was to find an index of excitability of the spinal motoneurone pool which would be more reliable than the amplitude of the tendon and H-reflex. The absolute refractory period for the H-reflex conditioned by a preceding H-reflex was not always found to be proportional to the excitatory state of the tested motoneurone pool, as it frequently did not differ significantly on the affected and healthy side. The attempts to use a tendon jerk (the amplitude of which was always higher on the affected side) as a conditioning stimulus instead of an H-reflex also failed to demonstrate any major differences between the two sides. These, however, did appear when a muscle stretch was introduced as a conditioning stimulus to test the refractory period of two H-reflexes. A stretch caused an increase in the amplitude of the second H-reflex on the affected side. This was constant with the interval between the conditioning stretch and the first H-reflex between 20 and 100 msec. The effect was not obtained on the healthy side and in normal subjects.

It is believed that normal supraspinal control limits or prevents the conditioning effect of a tendon jerk on the refractory period of the H-reflex induced by a preceding H-reflex.

35. Electrodiagnostic indices in patients with renal dialysis.—W. T. Liberson, M. Gratzer and A. W. Zalis (Hines, Ill., U.S.A.).

Electrodiagnostic procedures were applied to 21 patients with renal neuropathy, undergoing dialysis. The presence of fibrillation, decreased motor conduction velocities and/or increased chronaxies were investigated. Only one patient showed none of the above abnormalities. Nineteen patients showed slowing of motor conduction (below 35 m/sec in the lower extremities and/or below 40 m/sec in the upper). Only ten patients showed fibrillation (5 in only one muscle, 5 in more than one). Twelve patients had increased chronaxies in some muscles (only in 3 patients were the chronaxies increased above 5 msec; in the others they were above 1 msec). The lower extremities were more involved than the upper ones; 23% had normal conduction velocities for the former (average, 30 m/sec) and 40% had normal conduction velocities for the latter (average, 39 m/sec).

Although each electrodiagnostic abnormality could be seen independently, there was some association between them. Average conduction velocity (lower extremities) was 27 m/sec in patients with fibrillation in more than one muscle and chronaxies above 1 msec appeared in 44% of all data collected in these patients. The corresponding figures were 27 m/sec and 40% for the patients with only one fibrillating muscle and 30 m/sec and 22% for those with no fibrillation. Eight patients died. The average conduction velocities in these patients were 4 to 5 m/sec below those for the whole group.

The decrease in conduction velocity, undoubtedly related to demyelination, may be associated with axonic involvement witnessed by the moderately increased muscle chronaxies and, particularly, fibrillation. Moderately increased chronaxies were found in experimental diphtheric neuropathy which is characterized mainly by demyelinization. The advisability of applying combined electrodiagnostic procedures to patients with neuropathies is stressed.

36. Voluntary control of motor unit activity by visual and aural feedback.—R. G. Baginsky (Bedford, Mass., U.S.A.).

Most clinical electromyographers have been employing audiovisual feedback empirically. Only very recently a few investigators have been conducting research using such a feedback mechanism on an experimental basis. Our investigation involved 20 righthanded informed volunteers of both sexes, 21-25 years of age, students or graduates of paramedical professions. A dual-channel electromyograph, providing visual and audio monitoring of muscle signals, and bipolar coaxial needle electrodes were employed as follows.

(1.) Needle electrodes were inserted in the right abductor pollicis brevis and the right opponens pollicis. Signals from the right abductor pollicis brevis were displayed on channel A. Signals from the right opponens pollicis were displayed on channel B.

(2.) Channel A was used alone. Within a few minutes the subject learned to relax completely displaying electrical silence. On minimal volition he was able to recruit one single motor unit upon command. He then was taught to abduct his right thumb moderately displaying three different motor units. He now was pointed out the motor unit with the highest voltage and asked to reproduce it at will. As a rule after a few minutes the subject was able to repress all other units and to display the desired one.

(3.) The same experiment was repeated on channel B with motor units of right opponens pollicis.

(4.) Both channels were used simultaneously and patient was asked to contract first the right abductor pollicis and then the right opponens pollicis. Initially there was an interference pattern on both channels. Within a few minutes the interference pattern on channel A could be repressed at will on contraction of the opponens and the interference pattern on channel B could be repressed during contraction of the abductor. Again the individual was trained to recruit only the motor unit with the highest voltage. Audiovisual feedback or visual feedback and aural feedback, alone, were employed. Fastest results were obtained with audiovisual feedback. The mechanism of individual motor unit control will be discussed.

37. Normal human flexor reflexes.—B. Shahani and R. R. Young (Oxford, G.B. and Boston, Mass., U.S.A.).

Human flexor reflexes were evoked by trains of electrical stimuli administered through intradermal needles in the sole of the foot and recordings were routinely made over tibialis anticus and gastrocnemius. The subjects were awake, unsedated and lay supine with hips and knees fully extended and ankles at 90°. Five normal subjects were studied repeatedly and more than thirty patients with classical neurological lesions were studied subsequently.

The normal flexor reflex response consists of two discrete components in tibialis anticus—a brief, synchronous response at latency 60 to 80 msec and a prolonged asynchronous response with latency 120 to 400+ msec. With gradually increasing stimulus current, the latency of the initial component shortens relatively little, but that of the second component shortens over a wide range. Both components increase in duration as well and eventually fuse. Whereas single stimuli were capable of producing both components in *some* normal subjects, trains of stimuli were adequate for the production of both components and were supramaximal in *all* subjects.

Excitability curves were plotted using two equal stimuli, or trains of stimuli, through the same electrodes at various intervals. An initial phase of facilitation is present, lasting 2 to 4 sec after the first stimulus. During this phase, the reflex response to the second stimulus train is of much larger amplitude and duration. This is followed by a period of subnormality lasting 5 to 10 sec during which the response to the second stimulus train is much smaller in both dimensions and often absent. The latency of the second component varies inversely to the size of the reflex during these two phases. It is necessary to separate equal stimuli by at least 60 sec if identical responses are to be achieved consistently. Findings in patients with different pathological conditions aid in identification of human flexor reflex afferents.

38. Electromyographic studies of facial muscle activity in speech.—A. Persson, R. Leanderson and S. Ohman (Stockholm, Sweden).

Fine concentric needle electrodes were used to record the EMG from different muscles of the face while subjects read aloud a list of nonsensical utterances of Swedish vowels and consonants embedded in a fixed linguistic context. The object was to study the manner in which facial muscles are employed in speech.

Two different types of activity were observed. Tonic EMG activity occurred in levators and depressors of the upper and lower lips both between and during the utterances. This activity, evidently associated with basic speech posture, precedes by several hundred milliseconds the activity due to the articulatory movements of the utterances.

Articulatory modulation may be either excitatory or inhibitory. About 100 msec before utterance of the consonants [p] and [b], bursts of activity appear in M. orbicularis sup. and inf., M. mentalis and M. depressor anguli oris. Signs of inhibition, *i.e.,* disappearance or strong reduction of activity in muscles that contract tonically between utterances, are always visible in traces from M. labii sup. during utterance of the vowel [u] and M. depressor labii inf. during utterance of both [y] and [u]. Inhibition was always well synchronized with increased activity in antagonistic muscles. Functional differences between muscle groups associated with basic posture and those associated with articulatory modulation suggest that facial muscles are divided into tonic and phasic units.

In general the EMG pattern associated with a given sound varies considerably with the linguistic context, *e.g.,* a bilabial gesture ([p], [b]) is weaker in a [u-u] context than in an [i-i] context. Data suggest that articulatory control is mediated by sensory feedback from receptors in the facial region.

Patients with dysarthria (Parkinson's disease) have a greatly increased basic posture activity. Modulatory activity is thereby less prominent and appears to be independent of context. Coordination between muscle groups is impaired and inhibition is often replaced by increased activity.

39. Median nerve conduction variant.—J. J. Powers and J. L. Melvin (Columbus, Ohio, U.S.A.).

Prolonged distal latencies combined with normal proximal latencies are occasionally found by some electromyographers in doing nerve conduction studies. If a conduction velocity were to be calculated, it would appear to be unphysiologically fast. The reason for this discrepancy is often unclear.

We are presenting a case history of a patient with complaints of night pain, numbness of both thumbs and weakness of the thenar muscles of both hands which has been progressive over the past nine months. Median and ulnar latencies were done. Slow distal median motor latencies were present bilaterally. Sensory latencies were not obtainable. The right distal median motor latency to the thenar eminence was 7.8 msec. The left distal median motor latency was 6.2 msec. On stimulation of the right median nerve at the elbow, two latencies, at 7.0 and 12.0 msec, were obtained. Median latencies of 7.0 and 10.0 msec from the elbow to the thenar eminence were obtained on the left. This discrepancy was resolved by blocking the ulnar nerve. It is postulated that the patient has bilateral crossed innervation between the median and ulnar nerves, as well as bilateral carpal tunnel syndrome.

The case is presented to point out the need for carefully observing the configuration of the response obtained with surface electrodes in order to differentiate the response of a single nerve latency from one obtained in a muscle which has been cross innervated. Post-operative followup is included.

40. Sensory conduction in peroneal, posterior tibial, and sural nerves using averaging techniques.—R. E. Lovelace, S. J. Myers, and L. Zablow (New York, N.Y., U.S.A.).

Conduction in sensory fibers of the peroneal and posterior tibial nerves following digital stimulation was measured with new techniques. Utilizing an Analog Averager (TECA Corp), nerve action potentials as low in amplitude as 0.1 μV have been recorded with surface electrodes. Accurate location of surface markings of these nerves between toe and knee is essential, since some locations required the averaging of up to 400 sweeps over the nerve in order to obtain readable potentials.

In the normal series (ages 23 to 42) consistent responses were obtained at every attempt. Conduction in the sensory fibers of the peroneal nerve from the interdigital nerves of the big toe computed from recordings at ankle and knee, had a mean peak velocity of 50.3 m/sec (range 41.4 to 55.6). Posterior tibial sensory fibers had a mean peak velocity of 50.6 m/sec (range 45.3 to 56.8) from ankle to knee, with both nerves showing the same mean amplitude of 0.4 μV at the knee.

In 15 patients (ages 16 to 65) with various forms of peripheral neuropathy, those with severe neuropathy often had no responses. Those with mild and moderate neuropathy showed variable responses, generally with amplitudes of nerve action potentials at the knee of 0.1-0.4 μV. The peak velocity means were 38.0 m/sec (range 25.5 to 48.6) for the peroneal and 33.4 m/sec (range 26.5 to 37.5) for posterior tibial.

Sural nerve potentials were of somewhat higher amplitude, but a significant technical difficulty was the variation in the anatomical course of the nerve. Good correlation of *in vivo* sural conduction velocity with the velocity of the excised nerve in a constant temperature chamber was obtained.

This technique could be of considerable diagnostic value in mild and moderate sensory neuropathy.

41. Are all motor end-plates equally affected in a myasthenic muscle? A single fiber electromyography study.—J. Ekstedt, E. Stålberg and A. Broman (Uppsala, Sweden).

When recording from *two* muscle fibers belonging to one and the same motor unit, there is a variability in the interpotential intervals of consecutive discharges. This variability, *the jitter,* is normally of the order of 20 μsec (expressed as S.D.). This is mainly due to a variablity in the synaptic delay.

In patients with myasthenia gravis the following observations were made.

a) Some jitter recordings in a muscle could be normal, others increased up to tenfold, often with frequent blocking.

b) Pairs of action potentials from two muscle fibers from the same motor units were chosen, where only one of the action potentials was subject to occasional blocking. At low innervation rate both action potentials usually occurred together without any blocking. When increasing the stimulation rate, one action potential now and then dropped. This could have the effect of a considerable decrease of the rate of the blocking potentials.

c) With electrical stimulation of intramuscular nerve-twigs, it was possible to record up to six muscle fibers from the recording electrode, when stimulation rate was low (0.5/sec). The jitter between the stimulation artefact and the potentials could be normal or increased. When increasing the stimulation rate, one after the other of the single action potentials dropped. The order of dropping was correlated to the initial size of the jitter. At a stimulation rate above 10/sec only those single fiber potentials remained which originally had a normal jitter. These action potentials could withstand a stimulation rate of 15/sec for several minutes without any increase of jitter or blocking.

Thus, in a myasthenic muscle the different motor end-plates are affected to a different degree. Some are even entirely normal.

42. Experimental studies on the pathophysiology of spasticity.—P. J. Delwaide and C. A. Penders (Liege, Belgium).

Current theories hold that hyperreflexia in pyramidal tract disease is best understood by postulating a hyperactive gamma system. This conception is based on analogies with decerebrate rigidity in the cat and on Procaine experimentation in man. However, neurophysiological contributions suggest other hypotheses and a need for further investigation in man.

The study consisted of finding an electrophysiological test which would show significant modification in all cases of spasticity and analyzing its physiological mechanisms.

The Hoffman (H) reflex and the Achilles tendon reflex in normal and spastic subjects were systematically compared under a variety of experimental conditions. The most pronounced electrophysiological anomalies appeared when spinal regulatory mechanisms were activated maximally by a continuous discharge of muscle afferents achieved with a vibrator (100-150 c/sec) applied to the Achilles tendon. Under these conditions, the Hoffman and tendon reflexes were strongly inhibited in normal subjects. The magnitude of inhibition was expressed by H reflex recruitment curves. Provided rigorous controls are applied, such inhibition may be measured quantitatively. In spastic patients, inhibition was markedly reduced in every case, indicating that this response may be used as a supplemental test for diagnosis of spasticity.

The mechanism of inhibition during vibration of the Achilles tendon was studied by (1) analyzing the mechanisms activated during the test (repeated stretching of soleus muscle via passive sinusoidal ankle movements; controlled and selective stretching of the soleus) and (2) testing the excitability of the soleus motor nucleus simultaneously via mono- and polysynaptic pathways. The results strongly suggest that the inhibition depends on a presynaptic inhibitory mechanism acting on IA afferent fibers. In the presence of spasticity, this mechanism becomes inefficient. Consequently, the hyperreflexia of spasticity should be interpreted not exclusively as a hyperactivity of the fusimotor gamma system, but as an absence of physiological control over the afferents arising from muscle spindles.

43. Familial chronic polyneuropathy with crampiform manifestations.—G. Avanzini, M. Caccia and S. Negri (Milano, Italia).

The authors report two cases, father and daughter, affected by a chronic polyneuropathy associated with crampiform contractions. The clinical examination demonstrated that the deep reflexes were absent in the father and decreased in the daughter; only later the father developed cutaneous sensory loss in feet and hands in a glove and stocking distribution.

The EMG study showed in both cases a serious and distally predominant neurogenic damage, with slowing of the motor conduction velocity in all the nerves examined (ulnar, median, sciatic—external popliteal of both sides). Signs of denervation (fibrillation) and signs of collateral regeneration (enlargement of the motor units and fasciculation) were present.

The EMG pattern of the crampiform contraction revealed a discontinuous recruiting of polyphasic action potentials, with increased duration, probably constituted by biphasic or triphasic regrouping potentials. These groups may have repetitive characteristics.

The observations are discussed in relation with the nosographic classification of the syndrome and the pathogenesis of the crampiform manifestations and their possible connection with a lesion of the intramuscular nerve branches.

44. Logarithmic amplification: a new method of electromyographic presentation.—J. B. Rogoff (New York, N.Y., U.S.A.).

In a paper published in 1964, Simpson noted "a small negative wave which is sometimes recorded immediately before the main muscle complex. It may be a nerve action potential in the terminal fibers...and may only be seen with high amplification."

The conventional linear amplitude display of electromyographic information permits the observation of signals differing in amplitude by no more than 10 or 20 to 1 at a given amplifier gain setting. Signals beyond this range in amplitude either appear too small or fall beyond the screen. It is possible to construct a logarithmic amplifier whose output is proportional to the input multiplied by a gain factor that is not a constant, but changes as the logarithm of the input voltage.

A linear amplifier set at 16 mv amplitude for total vertical deflection shows no evidence of any displacement of the base line before the motor response. However, if the sensitivity of this amplifier is increased to 80 μV, a very clear small displacement is noted. The motor response is now completely off the screen.

Using a logarithmic amplifier, the motor action potential is clearly visible, as is the response which precedes the motor response. Graphs of responses will be presented, together with description of the amplifier.

DEMONSTRATIONS AND EXHIBITS

1. A new on line spectral analyser of EEG signals (ATREEG).–E. J. Caille, J. Bertheas and J. Mounier (Toulon, France).

A need exists for spectral analysis of both the physiologic (vigilance measure) and pathologic (head injury) EEG.

With assistance from DGRST we have built a compact analyser of small size (100 cubic inches) which is adaptable to any EEG polygraph and able to deliver "on line" the spectrum of each EEG derivation.

The signals are sampled 100 times per second from the output of a single lowpass filter (0 to 25 cps) at 256 levels. Every 10 ms, the impulses are registered on a recirculating delay line, producing a time compression of about 500.

The spectrum of the EEG signal is averaged for a variable epoch of 20 to 120 sec. This epoch satisfies all the possible EEG synchronization states, from the basic α rhythms to $\beta 2$ desynchronization rhythms, in association with all stages of hypervigilance.

The three spectrograms can be registered simultaneously, without depriving the clinician or experimenter of the conventional EEG write-out.

Regeneration of the spectral analysis every 8 seconds allows testing of the viability of the analysis, built continuously with commutable integration epochs. Such a control is expensive and takes much time, even with UNIVAC 1108 and IBM 360/44 computers that we used during the previous investigations.

The sharpness of such a resolution, achieved with the ATREEG instrument, explains more objectively the different sleep phases and wakefulness cycles; for example, to point out the "rectangular" spectrum of the paradoxical sleep phase which can no longer be mistaken for the "Gaussian" spectrum of the drowsy phase.

This design has considerable advantages as compared with filter-set analysers. It introduces little phase distortion between the investigated frequency bands. The addition of a correlator will allow a study of coherence relations between different areas of the scalp.

2. Pioneers in the electrophysiology of the nervous system 1875-1929.–M. A. B. Brazier (Los Angeles, Calif., U.S.A.).

The exhibit consists of several panels, each depicting the first public description and, where possible, the first published photograph of a classical discovery in the electrical activity of the nervous system. Each panel will display a portrait of the discoverer, a reproduction of his own description and in the great majority of cases the first published photograph of the results.

The panels will include:

The first descriptions of the EEG (1875) (1890).

The first DC studies of brain potentials (1875) (1883) (1890).

The first reports of the effect of flicker on brain potentials (1887).

The discovery of alpha-blocking after sensory stimulation (1890).

The first descriptions of evoked responses (acoustic and visual) recorded at the cortex (1890) (1903).

The first recorded response of a nerve to a single stimulus (1898) and the first demonstration of the refractory period (1899).

The first recordings from the cerebellum (1911).

The first published photographs of the EEG (1913, 1914).

The first photographs of responses (recorded from the cortex) and evoked by sciatic stimulation (1913).

The first studies of experimental epilepsy (1912) (1914).

The first recorded responses in a sensory nerve trunk initiated by a natural excitation excluding artificial electrical stimuli (1915 and 1924).

The first potentials from a single sensory nerve fiber (1926).

The first unit potentials from a single motor nerve fiber (1928).

The first unit potentials recorded from single muscle fibers (1929).

The first EEG to be recorded from man (1929).

3. Computer calculation of two targets trajectory and position of electrode point during penetration in human brain.–F. Peluso and J. Gybels (Leuven, Belgium).

For obvious reasons it may be important 1) to reach two different targets in the human brain through one electrode trajectory and 2) to know exactly for each distance from target where the electrode point is situated with respect to a chosen coordinate system. The exhibit presents a method to do this easily. All information needed is available on lateral and AP X-Ray pictures. The necessary mathematics, which are actually calculated by computer fed with a program written in Fortran IV, are developed.

4. Computer calculation of two targets trajectory and position of electrode point during penetration in human brain.—F. Peluso and J. Gybels (Leuven, Belgium).

For obvious reasons it may be important 1) to reach two different targets in the human brain through one electrode trajectory and 2) to know exactly for each distance from target where the electrode point is situated with respect to a chosen coordinate system. The demonstration shows calculation of any trajectory requested by a computer fed with a program written in Fortran IV. The information needed is available on the lateral and AP X-Ray pictures.

5. Routine transmission of EEG by telephone from a distant community.—D. R. Bennett (Salt Lake City, Utah, U.S.A.).

The availability of medical care and health facilities in the Inter-mountain Region of the United States of America for optimal care of patients with neurological disease is limited. Major factors are a sparse population spread over a vast area and the concentration of physicians knowledgeable in these fields in the Salt Lake Valley region. Consequently patients must often travel long distances for diagnostic procedures such as an electroencephalogram. The problems of distance, increased expenses secondary to travel, and delays in obtaining reports frequently influence the physician not to obtain an EEG in patients. The major drawback in the establishment of independent laboratories in outlying communities is the lack of professional personnel experienced in EEG interpretation. One such region is the Magic Valley area of Idaho with a population of approximately 80,000 and Twin Falls, the major city. This town is approximately 240 miles from Salt Lake City.

Since November 1968 six channels of EEG have been routinely transmitted by telephone from the Magic Valley Memorial Hospital in Twin Falls, Idaho to the University of Utah Hospital in Salt Lake City.

This panel exhibit illustrates the technique, the results, interesting records that were transmitted, as well as a cost analysis of the transmission project.

At specified times during the Congress, EEG's will be transmitted by telephone from Twin Falls, Idaho, to the exhibit area.

6. Correlates of depth spiking in EEG scalp activity.—B. Saltzberg (New Orleans, La., U.S.A.).

The application of digital matched filters to the problem of detecting in scalp EEG specific patterns which correlate with spiking at depth will be demonstrated using EEG data collected from primates. Scalp recordings from implanted primates that exhibit depth spiking activity will be analyzed on the Time/Data 100 computer. The T/D 100 will convolve the scalp EEG signal with a noise-corrected reference pattern (matched digital filter). This reference pattern is determined by carrying out the following operations on the T/D 100:

a) synchronous averaging triggered on depth spikes,
b) complex Fourier analysis of the snychronous average a),
c) power spectral density analysis of the background activity,
d) multiplication of b) by the reciprocal noise spectrum, and
e) Fourier series inversion of d).

The pattern obtained in e) is continuously compared with the incoming scalp EEG signal and the degree of matching is presented at the output of the so-called "matched filter."

7. UCLA Brain Information Service. (Los Angeles, Calif., U.S.A.).

The Brain Information Service will demonstrate its retrieval system. Retrieval will be via typewriter terminal, which can be operated by a librarian or by a scientist. The terminal will connect to the Health Sciences Computing Facility 360/91 at UCLA. The programs and terminal are the same as a system now operating in the BIS office at UCLA and connected to the HSCF computer. The file is 100,000 citations to articles in basic neurology, published since 1960. An indexing term vocabulary of 17,000 terms in an alphabetical and hierarchical listing will be used in phrasing search requests.

8. Three programs for assisted interpretation and analysis of electroencephalograms.—S. L. Sherwood (Palo Alto, Calif., U.S.A.).

The first program requires "eyeball" reading of the conventional EEG, but is automated from that point on. The instrument uses a Varian Data 620i and its teletype interface. A list has been devised of descriptors falling into three categories: (1.) clinical condition of patient, (2.) wave forms found, and (3.) sites where such wave forms occur. This list is derived and abbreviated from personal communications with A. Remond and the Standard Glossary proposed by FISEEG. The appropriate descriptors are "ticked off" manually on a sheet; by means of sine mnemonics they are entered into the data processor. The data processor then gives an account of the EEG in English and derives its conclusions in terms of NORMAL,

MODERATELY ABNORMAL, AND HIGHLY ABNORMAL automatically, also indicating site or ddiffuse abnormality. The English print-out lacks verbs and negative statements. The latter, unexpectedly, has caused some trouble with users of EEG reports; but using a minimal number of hand-written comments, this program becomes acceptable.

The first program has now been in daily use for six months. A second program is the natural extension of the first. By means of a magnetic tape recorder, the original data will be transformed from analogue to digital form and analyzed by the machine in terms of distributions of fast Fourier transforms. This method somewhat resembles methods used by Adey at UCLA. Reviewing the article by E. D. Brigham and R. E. Morrow, it can be seen that such an analysis approximates pattern recognition. To quote Marshall McLuhan: "Information overload equals pattern recognition."

Like the previous program, making use of analogue to digital and digital to analogue conversion, the last two programs attempt (1.) the ratio of amplitude over time (Abandonment of the Absolute), and (2.) true pattern recognition, such as a spike, will be recognized as such only when it is followed by a slow wave, thus distinguishing it from muscle and other non-cerebral potentials. For instance, the detection of electrocerebral seizures obtained by a method described in 1968 can be fully automated and save personnel time and expense, especially when employing for the patient's comfort, a telemetering system. Appropriate lists and block and flow–diagrams will be demonstrated.

9. A small computer or data processor for assistance in EEG analysis and interpretation.–S. L. Sherwood (Palo Alto, Calif., U.S.A.).

1. A data processor of relatively small capacity (4096 words at 16 bits per word, Varian Data 620i), is used to assist the electroencephalographer, after perusal of an EEG tracing, in describing the record, printing-out a summary report derived from a list of descriptors and, through a simple logic, producing a conclusion.

2. The extension of this, namely, a fully automated EEG report, can be based on imitating what the EEG-er does: recognize "frequencies," their predominance and anatomical distributions. Algorithms to accomplish this are now available in the form of Fast Fourier Transforms.

3. Criteria other than the usual voltage–over–time records may contain more information; impedance and frequency changes, related to behavior, may well yield such information more quickly and clearly than the familiar EEG reports.

4. Pattern recognition, such as a tell-tale spike and wave, is well within the capabilities of a modern small data-processor, and appropriate methods are proposed.

10. Minimal electroencephalographic recording techniques in suspected cerebral death.–D. Silverman, R. L. Masland, M. G. Saunders and R. S. Schwab (Philadelphia, Penn., U.S.A.; New York, N.Y., U.S.A.; Winnipeg, Canada; and Boston, Mass., U.S.A.).

Because of frequent lack of appreciation of the characteristics of the "isoelectric" EEG, the Committee has redefined this state as "electrocerebral silence" and recommended the following minimal techniques, listed in the order in which the test would be performed, together with the rationale for each recommendation.

1. Ten scalp and ear-lobe reference electrodes, to be sure absence of activity is not a focal phenomenon.

2. Interelectrode resistances under 10,000 ohms. High resistances attenuate signals or single high resistance electrodes predispose to artifact.

3. Deliberate creation of single electrode artifact by manipulation on patient-input recording to prove channels are recording and that input switch settings match electrode placements.

4. Long interelectrode linkages (10 cm). Amplitude diminishes as interelectrode distance lessens.

5. Sensitivity increased to 3.5 and to 2.5 μV/mm or better. Since pen line is ¼ mm wide, 2 μV activity cannot be seen at sensitivity of 7.5 μV/mm and is barely visible at 3.5 μV.

6. During part of recording, longest time constant used, with high frequency filters off. Filters attenuate signals in specific frequency bands; the slower frequencies are more critical.

7. Monitoring devices: ECG recommended in one channel; others as needed in a second channel. EEG is composite of brain potentials, physiologic signals, machine and environmental noise; monitors enable one to subtract the latter three to indicate the underlying true brain waves.

8. Sensory stimulation with sound, light and pain. Absence of cortical responses is necessary for electrocerebral silence.

9. Thirty-minute recording time. Runs of low voltage activity separated by minutes of electrical silence may occur and would be missed in brief recording.

10. Repeat record in 24 hours (International Committee recommends 12 hours). Revival time after electrocerebral silence is unknown in the human. Systematic research is needed; until then we recommend a conservative course. Only exceptions noted are cases of massive overdoses of CNS depressants.

11. Remote spectral and discriminant analysis of EEGs.—D. O. Walter, J. Hanley, J. Berkhout, L. Rovner, J. R. Zweizig, H. Okada and W. R. Adey (Los Angeles, Calif., U.S.A.).

We have used packaged solid-state amplifiers and audio-band FM modulators to transmit EEGs over standard telephone circuits to a central computer system and to retransmit analytic results back to the source, if desired.

If the computer system is that of the Space Biology Laboratory, a small, time-shared general-purpose computer (Scientific Data Systems 930) will acquire the data, and transmit it to a special-purpose frequency-domain computer (Time/Data 100) for Fourier transformation; the transformed data is converted to spectra, and cross-spectral derivatives such as coherence. Spectra and coherence will be collected by the 930 for several adjacent epochs. When collection is complete, the 930 will calculate contours of spectral intensity or of coherence and transmit these maps back to the point of acquisition, for presentation on a storage oscilloscope; the maps can also be plotted on paper for later reference.

If the computer system is that of the Data Processing Laboratory, a medium-sized time-shared general-purpose computer (SDS 9300) will acquire the data and transmit it to a large time-shared general-purpose machine (IBM 360/91) in the Health Sciences Computing Facility, where it will be spectrally analysed as above. This system can also retransmit contour maps, or the results of other forms of analysis. We plan to demonstrate step-wise discriminant analysis and have the computer system transmit to the Congress the plots of discrimination achieved either from live data or from previously recorded sleep EEGs.

12. Visual potentials evoked by pattern reversal. —H. B. Morton and W. A. Cobb (London, G.B.).

The abrupt displacement of a regularly alternating black and white pattern by one unit is an effective stimulus for evoking cortical potentials in human subjects.

The use of such a stimulus will be demonstrated. It is produced here by using a mirror mounted on a standard ECG pen motor to deflect (by one square) a checker board pattern which is projected onto a screen. Fixation lamps, viewed in the plane of the projected image, allow the subjects gaze to be fixed to provide full field, half field, or quadrant stimulation.

A Digitimer pulse generator is used to drive the mirror motor and thus abrupt movements (or other, *e.g.*, ramp, exponential) at varying repetition rates can be produced. The cortical evoked potentials recorded from a transverse line of electrodes placed 3 cm above the inion will be averaged in a Biomac 1000 averaging computer.

The potentials evoked by this stimulus exhibit properties which differ from those evoked by flash stimulation. In particular, the response is derived almost entirely from foveal stimulation, it is relatively simple and notably free from rhythmic late components (after-discharge). It is more constant than the flash-evoked responses from time to time and subject to subject, and results suggest that it is possible to stimulate selectively the left or right cerebral hemispheres by half visual field stimulation.

13. Automatic conversion of ink-tracings to analog electrical form.—J. S. Barlow, Boston, Mass., U.S.A.).

This exhibit will describe and demonstrate a continuous multichannel automatic curve reader, designed and constructed in this laboratory, for reconversion of ink-tracings and similar data to their electrical form. Specially designed electronic units and self-contained photoelectric scanning pens are operated in conjunction with standard EEG's or polygraphs, through which the original tracings are rerun for transcription. The number of channels is optional and easily expandable, and the special components are compact and readily portable, a minimum of time being required to prepare a standard ink-writing instrument for transcribing purposes.

The system has two modes of operation (determined by a selector switch), scanning and line-following. In the former, appropriate for tracings of high slopes such as EEG's, the scanning pens scan the tracing at a fixed amplitude. In the latter, which is more appropriate for small-slope tracings (*e.g.*, GSR's), the scanning pen, employing a very much lower amplitude together with a feedback loop, actually traces over the original curve. In either case, the output of the system is a time-varying analog voltage, *i.e.*, the form in which the original data were recorded (high contrast should be used, *i.e.*, black ink on red-grid paper), which can then be fed to another ink-writing machine for copying purposes, or into a computer (either directly or via a communications linkfor analyses. Within the limits of the frequency response of the original recording and that of the curve-reader system itself, the resulting output is the equivalent of having available a magnetic-tape recording of the original data. The system has the advantage over the latter, however, in that editing of the recordings can be done under direct visual control.

The exhibit will indicate the principles of operation of the system and will illustrate and demonstrate its capabilities in a number of different applications.

14. Recent brain research in China.—J. S. Barlow (Boston, Mass., U.S.A.).

The great majority of papers on brain research in China in recent years have been published in Chinese-language journals and hence have remained largely inaccessible to other workers since there have been no translation programs of the types that have existed for Russian-language materials. Accordingly, most investigators are unaware of details of the work of their Chinese colleagues. Yet, at least until quite recently (mid 1966), the field has been an active if small one in China, and has covered a variety of topics including electrophysiology, neurochemistry, neuropharmacology, neuropsychology, and instrumentation. Standard techniques and instruments, a number of Chinese manufactures, have been employed, and close familiarity of Chinese scientists with the work of other investigators is indicated by the bibliographies in the papers.

This exhibit draws attention to this largely unknown work of our Chinese colleagues by listing of a number of papers published in the Chinese-language *Acta Physiologica Sinica* and the *Acta Psychologica Sinica* from 1962 to 1966. Portions of some of the original papers and their translations (a number of which have been completed by this investigator as a part of a continuing program) will be included, as well as examples of renditions in Chinese of difficult technical terms. The exhibit will also include a map of China indicating the institutions of origin of these papers, and a list of non-Chinese investigators whose published work has been cited in Chinese papers.

15. Selection of patients for surgical treatment of temporal lobe epilepsy by use of chronically implanted depth electrodes.—R. D. Walter and P. A. Crandall (Los Angeles, Calif., U.S.A.).

This demonstration consists of a film depicting the stereotactic technique of depth electrode implantation into the amygdala, pes hippocampus, and hippocampal gyrus. Depth recordings from these areas will be illustrated showing "resting" abnormalities. During electrical stimulation at electrode sites, a split screen simultaneously presents depth electrode recordings and the patient's reaction during an aura and in a confusional state. The criteria for selection for surgery will then be presented, which includes:

1.) Assessment of the resting recordings for the area of maximal abnormality.

2.) The site of origin of electrical changes during a clinical seizure.

3.) Results obtained by depth electrode electrical stimulation.

4.) Results from pharmacological studies.

A technique for surgical resection will also be illustrated.

16. Transdermal stimulation of the brain in free primates.—J. M. R. Delgado (New Haven, Conn., U.S.A.).

A system has been developed for transdermal electrical stimulation of the brain with radio control of pulse duration, frequency and intensity. The system is based on implantation underneath the skin of an encapsulated, batteryless, solid state 3 channel instrument measuring 28 mm in diameter by 10 mm thick, with common lead plus three different electrodes introduced stereotaxically in the depth of the brain. Power and coded information are provided by transdermal coupling between the emitting and receiving coils. Depending on frequency the signal either charges a storage capacitor or activates one of the three stimulation channels. A pulse width modulation technique is used to control constant current intensity of stimulation, thus insuring reliability with a wide range of tolerance of possible changes in the received signals or in brain impedance.

Transdermal stimulation of motor pathways, tested for months in several monkeys and in one chimpanzee, has demonstrated good electronic performance, biological tolerance of instrumentation, reliability of evoked motor responses, stability of local excitability, and the possibility of efficient transdermal long-term electrical stimulation of the brain in unrestrained animals.

These experiments provide the technical possibility of long-term electrical stimulation of the brain for therapeutic purposes in man. Intractable pain, involuntary movements, and certain behavioral disturbances could be treated by programmed electrical stimulation of inhibitory areas of the brain. Instrumentation and live animal demonstrations will be presented.

17. Effects of impoverished environments upon time series functions of the developing brain. —J. W. Prescott, B. Saltzberg and L. Lustick (New Orleans, La., U.S.A.).

Interest and concern by the scientific and social communities have recently focused upon the possible consequences of early deprivations—nutritional, sensory, cognitive—upon the developing brain and behavior. Preliminary evidence suggests marked impairments of brain function associated with malnutrition and sensory-cognitive deprivations experienced during the early formative periods of development. These findings have raised questions concerning the permanence or reversibility of such brain impairments and the necessity to provide objective and quantitative descriptions of these effects in human populations.

This demonstration program proposes to illustrate a variety of analytic procedures derived with the TIME/DATA 100 computer and FABRI-TEK hybrid computer which appear to be sensitive to early deprivational insults upon developing brain function. A variety of experimental-clinical case studies have been obtained from human and nonhuman primates that illustrate the effects of early malnutrition, neonatal anoxia, and sensory deprivations upon brain electrical activity and, in some instances, upon learning performance deficits. The above data has been collected on magnetic tape and will be processed with large video output display monitors as a "live demonstration" progress report.

18. On-line full text retrievel of *Epilepsy Abstracts*.—J. K. Penry and J. F. Caponio (Bethesda, Maryland, U.S.A.).

This exhibit provides an opportunity for the investigator to communicate directly with published literature on epilepsy without the interposition of a computer programmer or the use of extensive codes. The investigator will be able to use the actual language of the literature to search not only citations and index terms, but also the full text of each abstract. For example, one may request titles of all abstracts in which both terms "spike-wave" and "genetics" appear.

The Epilepsy Information Program of the NINDS, established as a consequence of recommendations of the Public Health Service Advisory Committee on the Epilepsies, launched its first issue of *Epilepsy Abstracts* in November 1967. The program, which employs existing biomedical literature resources and facilities, has been designed whenever practical to serve as the national focal point for the collection, storage, retrieval, and dissemination of information relating to the epilepsies. Its main objectives are to stimulate research activity in the epilepsies and to provide a service for investigators and clinicians conducting research in this area.

In addition to the major product, *Epilepsy Abstracts,* distributed internationally to more than 3000 researchers and clinicians, the Epilepsy Information Program has made notable progress toward its goal of a computer-based secondary information system for epilepsy. The introduction in May 1969 of Data Central, an on-line interactive computer-controlled information storage and retrieval system, made possible for the first time a complete text search by computer across the full range of the world's current epilepsy information. NINDS Epilepsy Information retrieval is accomplished through direct communication using a terminal (teletypewriter or CRT display) and a remote computer located at Data Corporation, Washington, D.C. The "EPIL" file stored in the computer responds to the queries, instructs in the sequence of operation, conducts searches as requested and prints out or displays part or all of epilepsy abstracts pertinent to the queries. Several options are available.

The retrievable elements are subject category, abstract number, author(s), English title, foreign title, language of original document, publication volume, indexing terms (primary and secondary), and complete informative abstract.

The retriever can choose a standard format for output or specify the particular items of bibliographic information needed.

Members of the Congress will be able to interact personally with the "EPIL" data file and search for technical information pertinent to their interests.

19. Bizarre EEG of striate cortex in blind squirrel monkeys.—H. Sakakura and R. W. Doty (Osaka, Japan and Rochester, N.Y., U.S.A.).

In normal, unanesthetized squirrel monkeys oscilloscopic recordings from electrodes with 1 mm tip separation in the striate cortex often show 40-60/sec oscillations, 100-300 μV, for several seconds when room lights are turned on; and similar oscillations may occur for a briefer period with onset of darkness. Such oscillations, however, are often absent or may be suddenly curtailed by eye movements or change of attention. There is no prominent alpha-rhythm. Responses of striate cortex to electrical pulses to optic radiation are strongly influenced by light versus darkness or by state of alertness (*e.g.,* wakefulness versus slow wave sleep). After bilateral enucleation, the EEG of striate cortex becomes flat (!), punctuated by sporadic spikes, 200-300 μV, lasting 100 msec. Many, but not all, of these spikes correlate with eye movements (as indicated by EMG of eye muscles after enucleation). These spikes are sometimes followed by a burst of high-amplitude slow waves. After several weeks the slow waves occur more often, occupy more of the record and sometimes have faster activity superimposed on them, but continue to be interrupted by flat periods lasting about 1 sec. The response evoked by stimulation of the optic radiation gradually increases. From the fifth day on it exceeds any recorded in the intact monkey during wakefulness. Percentage of time spent in slow wave and REM sleep did not change in the one monkey studied so far, although there seems to be a change in distribution of sleep throughout a 24-hour period. In addition, a permanent increase of 12/sec spindle bursts occurs in sensorimotor areas. Thus, some aspect of normal retinal activity must exert continual control over electrical patterns of the brain as well as excitability of the striate cortex.

20. Techniques in EMG examination.—**E. W. Johnson, J. L. Melvin and R. Potts (Columbus, Ohio, U.S.A.).**

This exhibit presents on videotape the various steps used in the electromyographic examination. Five steps illustrate on videotape the audio and visual techniques of the examination. The demonstration will include nerve conduction studies of both motor and sensory fibers of the median, ulnar nerve and radial nerves; motor conduction studies of the tibial, peroneal and femoral nerves. In addition, the demonstration will display elicitation of the "H" reflex.

21. An experimental model of petit mal epilepsy: electrical and behavioral correlates of acute bilateral epileptogenic foci in monkey cerebral cortex.—**E. M. Marcus and S. Jacobson (Boston, Mass., U.S.A.).**

We have reported that acute bilateral epileptogenic foci, initiated by application of estrogen to the cortical surfaces, interact to produce synchronous and symmetric spike and slow wave discharges similar to those of *petit mal.* This model will be demonstrated as an acute experiment in the monkey under ether anesthesia, Flaxedil and controlled respiration. The characteristic effects of hyperventilation will also be demonstrated.

Behavioral correlates of acute symmetrical foci in the monkey will be seen related to the simultaneously displayed EEG on video tape. These studies demonstrate the relative correlation of bilateral synchronous bursts of 3 cps spike-slow wave complexes produced by bilateral superior-anterior premotor foci with short staring spells resembling *absence* seizures. There is interruption of motor activity and apparent impairment of awareness during the discharges. Bilateral foci more posterior in premotor cortex produced *absence* seizures with greater myoclonic components and bilateral bursts of polyspikes-slow waves in the EEG. Bilateral foci in premotor areas produce repetitive spike discharges associated with myoclonic jerks with no definite *absence* seizures. Parietal foci produce occasional bilateral jerks without *absence* seizures. In contrast bilateral foci in anterior prefrontal areas produced bilateral non-propagated polyspike discharges of 6-12 second duration with no myoclonus and little if any impairment of awareness or activity.

More recent studies of bilateral foci in other cortical locations suggest that a certain dissociation of the 3 cps spike-slow wave complex and of *absence* seizure may result.

22. EEG tutorial environment—an exhibit of self-instructional programs.—**R. G. Bickford, R. A. Nichols, R. Marchand and R. Livingston (San Diego, Calif., U.S.A.).**

As part of the neurosciences study plan at UCSD, the Office of Learning Resources and Neurosciences Department have developed an integrated self-instructional system. This has been tested and validated in the Charter Class of medical students.

The present exhibit extends this concept into EEG and related fields. The exhibit centers around the topic of photic stimulation and photo-epilepsy. Thus, it has self-instructional aspects dealing with the normal EEG response of the visual system to photic stimulation, the general subject of photo-epilepsy illustrated by sound and simultaneous EEG movies of relevant clinical cases, and the interpretation of the photic stimulation tests in clinical electroencephalography.

INDEX OF AUTHORS

VOLUME 27, 1969

(The numbers followed by P refer to abstracts from Society Proceedings)

ABABEI, L., 637P
ABBINK, F., 627P
ADAMS, A. E., 627P
ADELMAN, W. J., see COLE, K. S., 556
ADEY, W. R., 732P
ADEY, W. R. and TOKIZANE, T. (Eds.). Structure and function of the limbic system. A book review by O. J. ANDY, 110
ADEY, W. R., see BERKHOUT, J., 457
AHMED, M., see THACORE, V. R., 605
AKHUNDI, M. N., 323P
ALAJMO, Y., 624P
ALEXANDROVA, ZH. G., 447P
ALLEN, C., 710P
AMABILE, G., 99P, 680P
AMATI, A., 101P
ANDERSEN, P. and ANDERSSON, S. A. Physiological basis of the alpha rhythm. A book review by D. P. PURPURA, 222
ANDERSSON, S. A., see ANDERSEN, P., 222
ANDY, O. J., 551P
ANDY, O. J., see ADEY, W. R., 110
ANGEL, A. An analysis of the effect of 1,2-dihydroxybenzene on transmission through the dorsal column sensory pathway, 392
ANGELERI, F., 101P
ANGIOLILLO, M., 701P
ANITCHKOV, A. D., 697P
ANOKHIN, P. K., 322P
ANTOGNETTI, P., 100P
ARFEL, G., 108P
ARFEL, G., CASANOVA, C. et COULMANCE, M. Aspects dynamiques de l'électroencéphalogramme humain. Premiers résultats d'une étude radio-télémétrique, 225
ARNAL, D. et GERIN, P. Étude du bruit résiduel des potentiels évoqués moyens, 315
ARSENI, C., 631P, 632P
ASAO, H. and OJI, K. Hepatocerebral degeneration. A book review by J. REIHER, 456
ASGIAN, B., 656P
ASSAEL, M. I., 218P, 220P
ATA-MURADOVA, F. A., 322P
ATSEV, E., 444P
AUCKLAND, N. L., 692P
AUERBACH, E., 217P
AVANZINI, G., 727P
AVANZINI, G. L., 97P
AVIRAM, A., 217P
BAGINSKY, R. G., 724P
BAKLAVADJAN, O. G., 323P
BALDY-MOULINIER, M., 105P
BALL, G. G., 663P
BALTIEV, A., 636P
BARENSTEN, R. I. and LOCKARD, J. S. Behavioral experimental epilepsy in monkeys. II. Video-tape control gate for the detection and recording of motor seizures, 89
BARJAKTAREVÍC-NIKOLIĆ, K., 553P
BARLEY, C. O., 694P
BARLOW, J. S., 545P, 695P, 732P, 733P
BARNHART, D. A., 549P
BAROLIN, G. S., 211P
BARTOLUCCI, G., 662P
BAUST, W., 626P, 675P
BEAUMANOIR, A., 106P
BECHTEREVA, N. P., 323P
BECK, E. C., see RHODES, L. E., 364
BEDDOW, R., 551P
BEHROOZI, K., 220P
BELENKOV, N. Y., 698P
BENEDETTI, A., 99P
BENNETT, D. R., 730P
BENTAL, E., 216P
BENTE, D., 628P
BERGMANN, F., 220P, 221P
BERGSTRÖM, R. M., see FRUHSTORFER, H., 346
BERKHOUT, J., 732P
BERKHOUT, J., WALTER, D. O. and ADEY, W. R. Alterations of the human electroencephalogram induced by stressful verbal activity, 457
BERMAN, A. L. The brain stem of the cat. A book review by W. J. S. KRIEG, 111
BERMOND, F. et BERT, J. Étude des effets électrophysiologiques de la psilocybine chez un cercopithecinae, *Papio papio*, 48
BERNARDI, G., 99P, 680P
BERT, J., see BERMOND, F., 48
BERTAMINO, F., 97P
BERTELLI, R., 701P
BERTHEAS, J., 729P
BERTI CERONI, G., 99P
BETTINGER, L. A., see THOMPSON, R. F., 146
BETTS, H. B., 714P
BETZ, E., 621P
BICKEL, H., 625P
BICKFORD, R. G., 546P, 735P
BIGOT, B., 107P
BIMAR, J., 451P
BINI, M., 701P
BINNIE, C. D., 334P, 335P
BINNIE, C. D., COLES, P. A. and MARGERISON, J. H. The influence of end-tidal carbon dioxide tension on EEG changes during routine hyperventilation in different age groups, 304
BIRCH, H., see THOMPSON, F. R., 146
BISHOP, A. O., 682P
BLOKZIJL, E. J., 215P
BODNAR, V., 636P
BOGDAN, F., 631P, 633P
BOGEN, J. E., 660P
BOHNERT, B., 626P
BOMSHTEIN, O. Z., 329P
BONDARCHUK, A. N., 323P
BOOKER, H. E., 691P
BOONSTRA, S., 215P
BOONSTRA, S., see NOTERMANS, S. L. H., 337
BORDA, R. P., 704P
BORNSTEIN, B., see ELIAN, M., 601
BOSTEM, F., 451P
BOSTEM, F. H., 647P
BOZSODI, I., 631P
BRADLEY, P. B., 694P
BRADLEY, R. J., 701P
BRADLEY, W., see TEAGUE, C., 92

BRADLEY, W. E., see CONWAY, C. J., 199
BRAHAM, J., 217P
BRAM, S., 100P
BRAUN, M., see FEINBERG, I., 128
BRAUNER, E., 636P
BRAVACCIO, F., 96P
BRAZIER, M. A. B., 549P, 659P, 729P
BRICOLO, A., 689P
BRICOLO, A., see HASSLER, R., 306
BRIGNOLIO, F., 98P
BRITAIN, R. P., 335P
BROMAN, A., 726P
BROȘTEANU, E., 631P, 635P
BROȘTEANU, R., 632P
BROUGHTON, R., MEIER-EWERT, K.-H., and EBE, M. Evoked visual, somato-sensory and retinal potentials in photosensitive epilepsy, 373
BROUGHTON, R., see EBE, M., 429
BROUGHTON, R. J., 548P
BROVERMAN, D. M., see VOGEL, W., 186
BROWN, B. B. Effect of LSD on visually evoked responses to color in visualizer and non-visualizer subjects, 356
BUCK, M. D., 705P
BUCY, P. C., see DI CHIRO, G., 223
BURAKOVA, N. S., 331P
BURIAN, K., 213P
BUSHART, W., 622P
BUSSEL, E., 684P
BYFORD, G. H., 665P
CABRAS, P., 662P
CACCIA, M., 727P
CAILLE, E. J., 729P
CĂLCĂIANU, G., 630P
CÂMPEANU, E., 632P
CAPONIO, J. F., 734P
CARRIE, J. R. G., 703P
CARRINGTON, J. H., 653P
CARTA, F., 97P
CASANOVA, C., 108P
CASANOVA, C., see ARFEL, G., 225
CASATI, C., DAGNINO, N., FAVALE, E., MANFREDI, M., SEITUN, A. and TARTAGLIONE, A. Functional changes of somato-sensory system during deep sleep, 289
CASPERS, H., 686P
CASTAIGNE, P., 684P
CASTILLO, H. T., 689P
CATHALA, H., 684P
CATIER, J., 105P
CERCEL, I., 636P
CHASE, M. H., 691P
CHAUMONT, P., 107P
CHIRKOV, V. D., 698P
CHOU, S. M., 715P
CHRISTIAN, W. Klinische Elektroenzephalographie. Lehrbuch und Atlas. A book review by H. PETSCHE, 453
CIGÁNEK, L., 663P
CIGÁNEK, L. Variability of the human visual evoked potential: normative data, 35
CIGÁNEK, L., see KRATIN, J. G., 453
CINCĂ, I., 639P
CLAGUE, A. G., 700P
CLUSIN, W., 707P
COAST, K., 694P
COBB, W. A., 648P, 732P
COCCAGNA, G., 99P
COCCHI, A., 100P
COCULESCU, M., 638P
COHEN, B., 547P
COHN, R., 545P
COLE, K. S. Membranes, ions and impulses. A book review by W. J. ADELMAN, 556
COLES, P. A., see BINNIE, C. D., 304
COLLARD, M., 109P
CONRAUX, C., 109P
CONSTANTINESCU, V., 699P
CONWAY, C. J. and BRADLEY, W. E. Z-axis modulation in neural spike display, 199
COOPER, R. and HULME, A. Changes of the EEG, intracranial pressure and other variables during sleep in patients with intracranial lesions, 12
CORBAT, F., 108P
CORDONE, A., 98P
CORVALAN, J. C., 696P
COSI, V., 100P
COSTA, E., 636P
COSTAN, C., 637P
COSYNS, P., 657P
COULMANCE, M., 108P
COULMANCE, M., see ARFEL, G., 225
COWEY, A., see SCHWARTZKROIN, P. A., 594
COX, M., 692P
CRANDALL, P. A., 733P
CRAWLEY, J. W., 549P
CREUTZFELDT, O., 627P
CREUTZFELDT, O., see HESS, W. R., 224
CREUTZFELDT, O. D., see LEGEWIE, H., 470
CRICHTON, J. U., 692P
CRIGHEL, E., 632P, 638P, 699P
CRISTESCU, C., 629P, 630P, 638P
CRISTIAN, C., 632P, 635P
CROW, H. J., 332P, 665P
CROWELL, D. H., see JONES, R. H., 436
CZEKAJEWSKI, J., EKSTEDT, J. and STÅLBERG, E. Oscilloscopic recording of muscle fiber action potentials. The window trigger and the delay unit, 536
DAFNY, N., 218P, 219P
DAGAN, D., 221P
DAGNINO, N., see CASATI, C., 289
DALLE ORE, G., 689P
DALLE ORE, G., see HASSLER, R., 306
DALY, D. D., 551P
D'ANNA, R., 99P
DAPRES, G., 105P
DASCALOV, D., 447P
DAUGHADAY, V., 685P
DAVIES, A. C., 334P
DAVIS, F. A., 714P
DAVIS, H., 699P
DAVIS, J. E., 713P
DAWSON, M., 685P
DEACON, P. A., see PRIOR, P. F., 422
DE BIOLLEY, M. D., 452P
DEGOSSELY, M., 709P
DELGADO, J. M. R., 701P, 733P
DELLO IOIO, G., 97P, 101P
DELSEDIME, M., 98P
DELWAIDE, P. J., 727P
DEMETER, A., 638P
DEMETRESCU, M., 709P
DE NEGRI, M., 97P
DENISCHI, A., 636P
DENOTH, F., 98P, 100P, 101P, 102P
DERBYSHIRE, A. J., 547P
DE SEZE, S., 107P
DESIRAJU, T., 696P
DIAMOND, S., 547P
DI BERNARDO, C., 102P

DI CHIRO, G., SCHECTER, M. M. and WICKBOM, I. An atlas of pathological pneumoencephalographic anatomy. A book review by E. D. GEORGE and P. C. BUCY, 223
DIECKMANN, G., 619P, 663P, 689P
DIECKMANN, G., see HASSLER, R., 306
DIMITRIJEVIĆ, M., 553P
DIMITRIJEVIĆ, M. R., 721P
DIMITRIU, S., 636P
DI PERRI, R., 97P
DIXON, K., 104P
DODDS, S., 544P
DODGE, F. A., 219P
DOENICKE, A., 212P
DOLCE, G., 689P
DOLCE, G., see HASSLER, R., 306
DOLLIMORE, J., 683P
DONCHIN, E. Discriminant analysis in average evoked response studies: the study of single trial data, 311
DONGIER, M., 108P
DONGIER, S., 709P
DOOSE, H., 625P
DORAZCO-VALDES, J., 659P
DORMAN, R. M., 672P
DOTY, R. H., 687P
DOTY, R. W., 734P
DRACHMAN, D. A., see ELIA, J. C., 640
DRAGOMIRESCU, V., 630P
DRAVET, C., 105P
DREYFUS, P., 107P
DREYFUS-BRISAC, C., 106P
DRIVER, M., 664P
DRIVER, M. V., 332P
DUBIKAITIS, V. V., 449P
DUCAS, P., 107P
DUFFY, F. H., see LOMBROSO, C. T., 238
DUMERMUTH, G., 693P
DUMITRU, E., 632P
DUMON-RADERMECKER, M., 452P
DUNLOP, C. W. A stereotaxic frame assembly for investigating the cat auditory system, 614
DUNN, H. G., 692P
DÜRRIGL, V., 552P, 553P
DUSTMAN, R. E., see RHODES, L. E., 364
DIJKSTRA, S., 715P
EBE, M., 657P
EBE, M., MEIER-EWERT, K.-H. and BROUGHTON, R. Effects of intravenous diazepam (Valium) upon evoked potentials of photosensitive epileptic and normal subjects, 429
EBE, M., see BROUGHTON, R., 373
EBERSTEIN, A., 713P
EDELSON, A., and HOLDSTOCK, T. L. A printed circuit swivel for recording from freely moving animals, 209
EDERY, H., 219P
EKSTEDT, J., 726P
EKSTEDT, J., HÄGGQVIST, P. and STÅLBERG, E. The construction of needle multi-electrodes for single fiber electromyography, 540
EKSTEDT, J. and STÅLBERG, E. The effect of non-paralytic doses of D-tubocurarine on individual motor endplates in man, studied with a new electrophysiological method, 557
EKSTEDT, J. and STÅLBERG, E. Abnormal connections between skeletal muscle fibers, 607
EKSTEDT, J., see CZEKAJEWSKI, J., 536
ELFERT, J., see TEAGUE, C., 92
ELIA, J. C. The dizzy patient. A book review by D. A. DRACHMAN, 640
ELIAN, M., 216P
ELIAN, M. and BORNSTEIN, B. The Kleine-Levin syndrome with intermittent abnormality in the EEG, 601
ELLINGSON, R. J. and SCHAIN, R. J. EEG patterns in juvenile cerebral lipidosis, 191
ELLIS, R. R., 664P
ELPHICKE, T. M., 681P
ELUL, R., 703P
EMBRY, T. E., 551P
ENCINOZA, O., 624P
ENGE, S., 211P
ENGEL, R., 662P
ENGELMAN, K., see WYATT, R. J., 529
ERMIRIO, R., 97P
ESSLEN, E., 719P
ESTRIN, T., 658P
ETTLINGER, G., 664P
FAGANEL, J., 553P
FAIBIȘ, A., 639P
FAIRCHILD, M. D., JENDEN, D. J. and MICKEY, M. R. Discrimination of behavioral state in the cat utilizing long-term EEG frequency analysis, 503
FAIRWEATHER, H., 701P
FANAGORSKAYA, T. P., 450P
FAVALE, E., see CASATI, C., 289
FEINBERG, I., BRAUN, M. and SHULMAN, E. EEG sleep patterns in mental retardation, 128
FEINSOD, M., 217P
FELDMAN, M., 547P
FELDMAN, S., 218P, 219P
FENDER, D. H., 671P
FENDER, D. H., see LEHMANN, D., 142
FENTON, G. W., 681P
FENWICK, P. B. C., 683P
FERLINZ, R., 622P
FERNER, U., 628P
FERRILLO, F., 101P, 700P
FERRO, F. M., 100P
FERRO-MILONE, F., 98P, 100P, 101P
FICHSEL, H., 660P
FILCESCU, V., 629P, 630P, 638P
FILDIŠEVSKI, P., 553P
FINK, M., 710P
FINK, M., see ITIL, T. M., 76
FLEMING, A. M. M., 717P
FLEMING, D. E. Modified pupillary diameter and evoked potential component variation in waking cats, 84
FLOREA-CIOCOIU, V., 639P, 656P
FLOREA-CIOCOIU, V., see ROGOZEA, R., 162
FLORESCU, D., 637P
FLORIS, V., 680P
FLUGEL, K. A., 624P
FORNER, P., 622P
FÖRSTER, C., 211P
FRA, L., 98P
FREEDMAN, A. M., 667P
FRIGYESI, T. L., 546P
FROST, J. D., 550P, 702P
FRUHSTORFER, H. and BERGSTRÖM, R. M. Human vigilance and auditory evoked responses, 346
FUJIMORI, B., 717P
FULLERTON, P. M., 718P
FUNFGELD, E. W., 622P
GABERSEK, V., 109P
GAGLIARDI, F., 707P
GALBRAITH, G. C., 690P
GAMBI, D., 97P, 101P
GANDIGLIO, G., 97P
GANDINI, S., 102P

GANDINI-COLLODEL, E., 102P
GANGLBERGER, J. A., 213P, 214P
GASSEL, M. M., 716P
GASTAUT, H., 105P, 643P
GEDEVANI, D. M., 709P
GEIER, S., 108P
GENTILOMO, A., 98P
GEORGE, E. D., see DI CHIRO, G., 223
GERHARD, L. Atlas des Mittel- und Zwischenhirns des Kaninchens. A book review by H. PETSCHE, 555
GERIN, P., see ARNAL, D., 315
GERKEN, H., 625P, 683P
GESTRING, G. F., 213P, 214P
GIAMMANCO, S., 99P, 102P
GIANNITRAPANI, D., 694P
GIANNITRAPANI, D. EEG average frequency and intelligence, 480
GIARDIAN, W. J., 674P
GIRETTI, M. L., RUCCI, F. S. and LA ROCCA, M. Effects of lowered body temperature on hyperoxic seizures, 581
GIUNTA, F., 97P
GLASER, G. H., 547P, 682P
GLASS, A., 681P
GLIDDON, J. B., 690P
GLOOR, P., 649P
GOGOLÁK, G., LIEBESWAR, G. and STUMPF, CH. Action of drugs on the electrical activity of the red nucleus, 296
GOLDHAMMER, Y., 217P
GOODGOLD, J., 713P
GOZARIU, L., 636P
GRACANIN, F., 723P
GRANDSTAFF, N. W. Frequency analysis of EEG during milk drinking, 57
GRATZER, M., 724P
GRAY, J. A., 663P
GREEN, J. B., 666P
GRETCHIN, V. B., 448P, 698P
GROLL-KNAPP, E., 213P, 214P
GROSS, C. G., see SCHWARTZKROIN, P. A., 594
GROSS, H. P., 625P
GROVES, P. M., see THOMPSON, R. F., 146
GRUENAU, S. P., 692P
GRUNFELD, Y., 219P
GRUSON, R., 625P
GULIAN, E., 637P
GUMNIT, R. J., see YAHR, M. D., 336
GUSSELNIKOV, V. I., 325P
GUSSELNIKOVA, K. G., 325P
GUTMANN, L., 715P
GUTTMANN, G., 213P, 214P
GUZE, S., 685P
GYBELS, J., 657P, 729P, 730P
HÄGGQVIST, P., see EKSTEDT, J., 540
HAIDER, M., 213P, 214P
HAJNŠEK, F., 552P, 554P
HALER, C., 637P
HAMILTON, L. R., 547P
HAMMA, I., 657P
HAMONET, C., 107P
HANLEY, J., 732P
HANSOTIA, P., 335P
HANSOTIA, P., HARRIS, R. and KENNEDY, J. EEG changes in Wilson's disease, 523
HARDEN, A., 333P
HAREL, D., 219P
HARIZANOV, R., 446P
HARNER, R. N., 672P
HARRIS, J. A., 546P
HARRIS, R., 333P, 335P, 671P, 717P
HARRIS, R., see HANSOTIA, P., 523
HARRISON, M. J. G., 718P
HASSLER, R., 689P
HASSLER, R., DALLE ORE, G., DIECKMANN, G., BRICOLO, A. and DOLCE, G. Behavioural and EEG arousal induced by stimulation of unspecific projection systems in a patient with post-traumatic apallic syndrome, 306
HĂULICĂ, I., 637P
HAYASE, S., 671P
HAYDEN, M. P., 685P
HEILPORN, A., 706P
HEINEMANN, U., 626P
HEISS, W., 683P
HELLER, H., 620P
HELMCHEN, H., 624P, 687P
HENDRIX, D. E., 661P
HENINGER, G. R., 670P
HENRY, C. E., 551P
HERMAN, R., 715P
HESS, W. R. Hypothalamus und Thalamus. Experimental-Dokumente. A book review by O. CREUTZFELDT, 224
HIRATA, Y., 717P
HIRSCH, H., 629P
HOFFMANN, I., 624P
HOGAN, G., 715P
HOHLWECK, H., 621P
HOLDSTOCK, T. L., see EDELSON, A., 209
HOMMA, S., 720P
HOOSHMAND, H., 550P
HOPF, G., 620P
HOSSMANN, K. A., 619P
HOWE, R., 678P
HRBEK, A., 669P
HRBKOVA, M., 669P
HRUBY, S., 213P
HUBER, P. J., 693P
HUEY, T. E., 551P
HUGHES, J. R., 661P
HUGHES, J. R., see LIPMAN, I. J., 43
HUGON, M., 646P, 652P
HULME, A., see COOPER, R., 12
HUMMEL, P., 105P
HUOTT, A. D., 695P
HUTT, S. J., 701P
HUTT, S. J., see LENARD, H. G., 121
ILYANOK, V. A., 325P
INANAGA, K., 665P
INFANTE, E., 722P
INGVAR, D. H., 621P, 676P
INVERNIZZI, G., 100P
IRWIN, D. A., see REBERT, C. S., 152
ISHIJIMA, H., 714P
ISHIYAMA, Y., 657P
ITIL, T., 658P
ITIL, T. M., SHAPIRO, D. M., FINK, M. and KASSEBAUM, D. Digital computer classifications of EEG sleep stages, 76
ITTU, C., 629P
ITTU, E., 629P
IVANOVA, M. P., 325P
IVRIANI, I., 220P
IWATA, Y., see JINNAI, D., 404
JACOBI, H. M., 719P
JACOBSON, A., see NAITOH, P., 2
JACOBSON, S., 735P
JAFFE, R., 669P
JANKO, M., 553P

JANTSCH, H., 213P
JENDEN, D. J., see FAIRCHILD, M. D., 503
JENNEKENS, F. G. I., 715P
JENSEN, D. R., 662P
JINNAI, D., MOGAMI, H., MUKAWA, J., IWATA, Y. and KOBAYASHI, K. Effect of brain-stem lesions on Metrazol-induced seizures in cats, 404
JÖBSIS, F. F., see O'CONNOR, M. J., 280
JOHN, E. R. and MORGADES, P. P. A technique for the chronic implantation of multiple movable microelectrodes, 205
JOHN-LOE, P. ST., 664P
JOHNSON, E. W., 735P
JOHNSON, G., 656P
JOHNSTON, V. S., 701P
JONES, R. H., CROWELL, D. H. and KAPUNIAI, L. E. A method for detecting change in a time series applied to newborn EEG, 436
JONKMAN, E. J., 215P
JONKMAN, E. J., see OOSTERHUIS, H. J. G. H., 23
JOPPICH, G. und SCHULTE, F. J. Neurologie des Neugeborenen. A book review by H. F. R. PRECHTL, 112
JOSEPH, M. E., 547P
JOVANOVIC, U. J., 626P
JURKO, M. F., 551P
JUS, A., 668P
JUS, K., 668P
KADYROV, G. K., 322P
KAESER, H. E., 106P, 108P
KAISER, E., 681P
KALES, A., 710P
KALES, A., see NAITOH, P., 2
KALES, J. D., 710P
KALYUZHNY, L. V., 325P
KAMBAROVA, D. K., 697P
KAMP, A., 678P
KAMPHUISEN, H. A. C., 674P
KANOWSKI, S., 624P, 687P
KAPUNIAI, L. E., see JONES, R. H., 436
KARADŽIĆ, V., 552P, 554P
KASSEBAUM, D., see ITIL, T. M., 76
KATO, M., 717P
KATO, M., see LÜDERS, H., 425
KEESEY, U. T. and NICHOLS, D. J. Changes induced in stabilized image visibility by experimental alteration of the ongoing EEG, 248
KENNARD, M. A., 544P
KENNEDY, J., 335P
KENNEDY, J., see HANSOTIA, P., 523
KENNEDY, W. R., 722P
KEOGH, R. P., 676P
KEREM, J., 219P
KHALILI, A. A., 714P
KHANANASHVILI, M. M., 330P, 331P
KHOSABOV, G. A., 331P
KHRIZMAN, T. P., 450P
KILJAN, A., 668P
KINNARD, M. A., 686P
KIPRYAN, T. K., 323P
KLAIBER, E. L., see VOGEL, W., 186
KLASS, D. W., 677P
KLEE, M. R., 617P, 618P, 683P
KLEIN, D. F., 669P
KLEINER, B., 693P
KNEISE, U., 680P
KNOTT, J., 551P
KOBAYASHI, H., 720P
KOBAYASHI, K., see JINNAI, D., 404
KODAMA, H., 691P
KOENIG, M. P., 107P
KOFES, A., 628P
KOGAN, A. B., 326P
KOHLER, M., 622P
KOLLAR, E. J., see NAITOH, P., 2
KOMPOSCH, K., 680P
KONOVALOV, V. F., 326P
KOOI, K. A., 700P
KOPPEN, G., 619P
KOPYLOVA, T. V., 449P
KOREIN, J., 700P
KOTTLER, A. H., 624P
KOUKKOU, M., 687P
KRAFT, G. H., 722P
KRATIN, J. G., 708P
KRATIN, J. G., Electrical reactions of the brain to inhibitory signals. A book review by L. CIGÁNEK, 453
KRAUSE, A. E., 676P
KREINDLER, A., 637P, 655P
KRIEG, W. J. S., see BERMAN, A. L., 111
KROTT, H. M., 719P
KRUSE, R., 625P
KUBACKI, A., 668P
KUBICKI, ST., 623P
KUENKEL, H., 677P
KUGLER, J., 211P, 212P
KUHN, R., 106P
KUN, K. J., see VOGEL, W., 186
KUNZE, K., 721P
KUPFER, D. J., see WYATT, R. J., 529
KURMUKOV, A. G., 326P
KUROIWA, Y., see LÜDERS, H., 425
KUZMINSKY, T., 216P
LA GRUTTA, V., 99P, 102P
LAMARRE, Y., 675P
LAMY, M. L., 647P
LANCE, J. W., 713P
LANGE, G. W., see MARSDEN, C. D., 169, 179
LANSING, R. W., 695P
LA ROCCA, M., see GIRETTI, M. L., 581
LARSEN, L. E., 704P
LAUB, M., 212P
LAVARELLO, P., 101P
LAVY, S., 217P, 218P, 219P
LEANDERSON, R., 725P
LEE, B. B., MANDL, G. and STEAN, J. P. B. Micro-electrode tip position marking in nervous tissue: a new dye method, 610
LEE, J. C. M., 686P
LEE, R. G., 546P
LEE, S. I., 677P
LEE, Y. H., see ORNITZ, E. M., 195
LEENSTRA-BORSJE, H., 215P
LEFEBVRE, J., 107P
LEGEWIE, H., 627P
LEGEWIE, H. and PROBST, W. On-line analysis of EEG with a small computer (period-amplitude analysis), 533
LEGEWIE, H. SIMONOVA, O. and CREUTZFELDT, O. D. EEG changes during performance of various tasks under open- and closed-eyed conditions, 470
LEHMANN, D., 671P
LEHMANN, D. and FENDER, D. H. Averaged visual evoked potentials in humans: mechanism of dichoptic interaction studied in a subject with split chiasma, 142
LEHTINEN, I. and VALLEALA, P. Thalamo-cortical recruiting responses during sleep characterized by a low voltage fast EEG, 412

LELORD, G. et MAHO, C. Modifications des activités évoquées corticales et thalamiques au cours d'un conditionnement sensoriel. I. Localisation des réponses et variations avec la vigilance, 258
LELORD, G. et MAHO, C. Modifications des activités évoquées corticales et thalamiques au cours d'un conditionnement sensoriel. II. Évolution des réponses avec les stades du conditionnement, 270
LEMMI, H., 550P
LENARD, H. G., VON BERNUTH, H. and HUTT, S. J. Acoustic evoked responses in newborn infants: the influence of pitch and complexity of the stimulus, 121
LENMAN, J. A. R., 717P
LEONARD, M. H., 723P
LERIQUE, J. L., 107P
LERMAN, P., 216P
LESÈVRE, N., 445P
LETALLE, A., 105P
LEVY, P. A., 335P
LEWIS, A. S., 333P
LEWIS, M. J., 335P
LEWIS, S. A., 335P
LIBERSON, W. T., 665P, 724P
LIEBESWAR, G., see GOGOLÁK, G., 296
LIFSHITZ, K., 688P
LINDSLEY, D. B., 704P
LIPCHIK, E. O., 694P
LIPMAN, I. J. and HUGHES, J. R., Rhythmic mid-temporal discharges. An electro-clinical study, 43
LITTLE, S. C., 551P
LIVINGSTON, R., 735P
LLOYD, D. S. L., 334P, 335P
LOCKARD, J. S., see BARENSTEN, R. I., 89
LOMBROSO, C. T., DUFFY, F. H. and ROBB, R. B. Selective suppression of cerebral evoked potentials to patterned light in amblyopia ex anopsia, 238
LONSBURY, B., 691P
LOPES DA SILVA, F. H., 677P
LORENZONI, E., 212P
LORIZIO, A., 98P
LOSIECZKO, T., 668P
LOVELACE, R. E., 726P
LUCIANO, L., 97P
LUCKING, C. H., 628P, 702P
LÜDERS, H., KATO, M. and KUROIWA, Y. Cortical evoked potentials in hepatolenticular degeneration, 425
LUDIN, H. P., 107P
LUGARESI, E., 99P
LUPU, I. M., 629P, 633P
LUSTICK, L., 733P
LUTCKE, A., 625P
LUX, H. D., 618P
LUYENDIJK, W. (Editor). Progress in brain research. Vol. 30. Cerebral circulation. A book review by L. MOLNÁR, 454
LYNNE, S. H., 551P
MCADAM, D. W. and SEALES, D. M. Bereitschafspotential enhancement with increased level of motivation, 73
MACCARIO, M., 700P
MCDONALD, R. T., 551P
MCGEE, F. E., 546P
MACHEK, J., 546P
MACLEAN, P. D., 686P
MCLEOD, J. G., 723P
MADEY, J. M., 687P
MADJAREVIĆ, N., 553P
MAGGINI, C., 99P
MAGNUS, O., see OOSTERHUIS, H. J. G. H., 23
MAGNUSSON, R., 681P
MAHO, C., see LELORD, G., 258, 270
MAÎTRE, L., 104P
MAJEAU, D. A. and PLEASONTON, A. K. An electrode for the study of lingual sensitivity, 440
MAJKOWSKI, J. and MORGADES, P. P. Primary auditory evoked potentials after section of brachium of the inferior colliculus, 587
MANCIA, M. Electrophysiological and behavioural changes owing to splitting of the brain-stem in cats, 487
MANDELL, A. J., see WALLACH, M. B., 563, 574
MANDL, G., see LEE, B. B., 610
MANFREDI, M., see CASATI, C., 289
MANN, L. B., 660P
MANTOVANI, M., 99P
MARCHAND, R., 735P
MARCUS, E. M., 735P
MARCUS, R. J., see WINTERS, W. D., 514
MAREŞ, V., 636P
MARGERISON, J. H., 335P
MARGERISON, J. H., see BINNIE, C. D., 304
MARJERRISON, G., 676P
MARSDEN, C. D., MEADOWS, J. C., LANGE, G. W. and WATSON, R. S. Variations in human physiological finger tremor, with particular reference to changes with age, 169
MARSDEN, C. D., MEADOWS, J. C., LANGE, G. W. and WATSON, R. S. The relation between physiological tremor of the two hands in healthy subjects, 179
MARTIN, F., 106P
MARTIN, R., 653P
MARULLO-REEDTZ, G., 100P
MASHKOVSKY, M. D., 326P
MASLAND, R. L., 549P, 731P
MASON, A., see ORNITZ, E. M., 195
MATOUSEK, M., 667P
MATRICALI, B., 719P
MAYNARD, D., 672P
MAZZELLA, G. L., 100P
MEADOWS, J. C., see MARSDEN, C. D., 169, 179
MECHELSE, K., 719P
MEIER-EWERT, K.-H., see BROUGHTON, R., 373
MEIER-EWERT, K.-H., see EBE, M., 429
MELBY, G., 546P
MELVIN, J. L., 725P, 735P
MENDELS, J., 659P
MENINI, C., 708P
MERA, A., 218P
MERDJANOV, C., 446P
MERREM, G. (Editor). Chemische, physikalische und radiologische Probleme in der Neurochirurgie. A book review by A. ROSS, 555
MESSINA, C., 98P
MEZAN, I., 445P
MIČIĆ, D., 554P
MICKEY, M. R., see FAIRCHILD, M. D., 503
MIGLIETTA, O., 713P
MIHUL, V., 636P
MILLS, L., 691P
MILSTEIN, V., 544P, 692P
MILSTEIN, V. Implantation of sterile electrodes in chronic animals, 442
MINGRINO, S., 99P
MITSCHKE, H., 660P
MIYAMOTO, K., 671P
MNUKHINA, R. S., 327P
MODENA, G., 701P
MOFFETT, A. M., 664P
MOGAMI, H., see JINNAI, D., 404

Moiseeva, N. I., 698P
Moisiu, M., 637P
Molnár, L., see Luyendijk, W., 454
Monnier, M., 107P
Monod, N., 107P
Mora, E., 98P
Morariu, M., 636P
Morgades, P. P., see John, E. R., 205
Morgades, P. P., see Majkowski, J., 587
Mori, K., see Winters, W. D., 514
Morocutti, C., 99P, 103P, 680P
Morrell, F., 708P
Mortara, M., 707P
Mortillaro, M., 622P
Morton, H. B., 732P
Mounier, J., 729P
Movsisiants, S. A., 449P, 698P
Mršulja, B., 552P
Muheim, G., 108P, 721P
Mukawa, J., see Jinnai, D., 404
Mulholland, T., 548P, 688P
Müller, H. R., 106P, 108P, 721P
Muller, J., 628P
Muratorio, A., 99P
Musella, L., 682P
Muskat, E., 721P
Musolino, G., 100P
Myers, S. J., 726P
Naghiu, A., 633P
Nagy, J., 638P
Naitoh, P., Kales, A., Kollar, E. J., Smith, J. C. and Jacobson, A. Electroencephalographic activity after prolonged sleep loss, 2
Nakamura, Y., 691P
Nakanishi, T., 718P
Naquet, R., 451P, 708P
Nashold, B. S., 550P
Nathan, P. W., 721P
Naumova, T. S., 327P
Negri, S., 727P
Nekrasova, L. I., 325P
Neştianu, V., 638P, 639P, 656P
Newsom, T. D., 549P
Nicholls, J. G., 702P
Nichols, D. J., see Keesey, U. T., 248
Nichols, R. A., 735P
Nicolescu-Catargi, A., 633P, 638P
Niedermeyer, E., 544P, 661P
Nir, I., 220P
Nolte, R., 625P
Norris, F. H., 718P
Notermans, S. L. H., 215P
Notermans, S. L. H. and Boonstra, S. Electroencephalographic findings in experimentally induced intracranial hypertension, 337
Obrist, W. D., see Waszak, M., 113
O'Connor, M. J., Rosenthal, M. and Jöbsis, F. F. Long-term EEG changes during direct cortical stimulation, 280
Oehlschlägel, H. K., 618P
Ohman, S., 725P
Oji, K., see Asao, H., 456
Okada, H., 732P
Oniani, T. N., 328P
Onuma, T., 545P, 697P
Oosterhuis, H. J. G. H., Ponsen, L., Jonkman, E. J. and Magnus, O. The average visual response in patients with cerebrovascular disease, 23
Ornitz, E. M., 686P
Ornitz, E. M., Ritvo, E. R., Lee, Y. H., Panman, L. M., Walter, R. D. and Mason, A. The auditory evoked response in babies during REM sleep, 195
Ornitz, E. M., Ritvo, E. R., Tanguay, P. E., and Walter, R. D. EEG spikes and the averaged evoked response to clicks and flashes, 387
Osenar, S. B., 547P
Oswald, I., see Thacore, V. R., 605
Othmer, E., 685P
Ott, K. H., 716P
Otter, H. P., 675P
Overton, D. A., 546P, 662P
Paal, G., 624P
Pacini, L., 707P
Paddison, R. M., 551P
Pallestrini, E. A., 97P
Palley, N., 653P
Panait, G., 636P
Panman, L. M., see Ornitz, E. M., 195
Papajewski, W., 617P, 618P
Papini, M., 662P
Parmelee, A. H., 690P
Parnas, I., 220P, 221P
Pascu, I., 656P
Passerini, D., 98P
Passouant, P., 105P
Pateisky, K., 211P
Paul, R., 333P
Pavlygina, R. A., 327P
Pazzaglia, P., 99P
Peck, C. K., 706P
Peluso, F., 657P, 729P, 730P
Penders, C. A., 727P
Peneva, L., 446P
Penry, J. K., 734P
Perea, R. A., 672P
Perfetti, C. C., 101P
Perl, E. R., 650P
Persson, A., 725P
Petajan, J. H., 718P
Petajan, J. H. and Philip, B. A. Frequency control of motor unit action potentials, 66
Petersen, I., 681P
Peterson, E., 653P
Peterson, E. W., 679P
Peterson, H. W., 551P
Petrescu, M., 638P
Petrescu, S., 638P
Petrov, P., 446P
Petrovanu, I., 636P
Petsche, H., see Christian, W., 453
Petsche, H., see Gerhard, L., 555
Petushkov, E. P., 697P
Philip, B. A., see Petajan, J. H., 66
Pierrot-Desseiligny, E., 684P
Pintilie, I., 630P, 638P
Pleasonton, A. K., see Majeau, D. A., 440
Poenaru, S., 635P, 636P
Poilici, I., 632P, 638P
Poiré, R., 106P
Poletti, C. E., 686P
Polikanina, R. I., 327P
Pollack, M., 669P
Ponsen, L., see Oosterhuis, H. J. G. H., 23
Poole, E. W., 332P, 666P
Popescu-Tismana, G., 637P, 655P
Popova, N. S., 327P
Popoviciu, I., 656P
Popoviciu, L., 633P, 635P

Porzak, J., 545P, 697P
Potts, R., 735P
Powers, J. J., 725P
Prechtl, H. F. R., see Joppich, G., 112
Predescu, V., 633P, 634P, 701P
Prescott, J. W., 733P
Preston, T. A., 710P
Prevec, T. S., 688P
Prince, D., 673P
Prior, P. F., 333P, 672P
Prior, P. F. and Deacon, P. A. Spontaneous sleep in healthy subjects in long-term serial electroencephalographic recordings, 422
Probst, W., 627P, 628P
Probst, W., see Legewie, H., 533
Prull, G., 622P
Puca, F. M., 96P
Purpura, D. P., 545P, 645P, 696P
Purpura, D. P., see Andersen, P., 222
Purpura, D. P., see Yahr, M. D., 336
Puskás, G., 630P
Quai, I., 630P
Quattrini, A., 101P
Rabinovitch, M. Ya., 328P
Racotta, R., 639P
Radvanyi, M. F., 106P
Rahamimoff, R., 219P
Rakić, L., 554P
Ravenna, C., 99P
Rebert, C. S. and Irwin, D. A. Slow potential changes in cat brain during classical appetitive and aversive conditioning of jaw movement, 152
Redding, F. K., 547P
Reichenmiller, H. E., 623P, 626P
Reiher, J., see Asao, H., 456
Reilly, E. L., 549P
Rémond, A., 334P, 445P
Rhodes, L. E., Dustman, R. E. and Beck, E. C. The visual evoked response: a comparison of bright and dull children, 364
Ricci, G. B., 707P
Riemann, O., 626P
Rinaldi, F., 96P
Rischmaui, R., 628P
Rittmeyer, P., 622P
Ritvo, E. R., 686P
Ritvo, E. R., see Ornitz, E. M., 195, 387
Rivano, C., 96P, 98P, 101P, 700P
Rizzo, P. A., 99P, 680P
Robb, R. M., see Lombroso, C. T., 238
Roberton, N. R. C., 333P
Robertson, M. A. H., 717P
Rodin, E., 545P, 697P
Rodin, M., 697P
Roger, J., 105P
Rogina, V., 553P
Rogoff, J. B., 727P
Rogozea, R., 655P
Rogozea, R., Ungher, J. and Florea-Ciocoiu, V. The influence of intra-hippocampal gamma-aminobutyric acid on the orienting reflex, 162
Roitbak, A. I., 328P
Roman, I., 632P, 633P, 634P, 635P, 701P
Rosadini, G., 96P, 101P, 700P
Rosadini, I., 96P
Roșca, V., 637P
Roschina, L. F., 326P
Rose, F. C., 685P
Rose, G. H., 692P
Rosen, M. G., 661P
Rosen, S. C., 684P
Rosenfalck, A., 654P
Rosenthal, M., see O'Connor, M. J., 280
Ross, A., 211P
Ross, A., see Merrem, G., 555
Rossi, G. F., 96P, 700P
Rothman, H. H., 699P
Rotondi Serra, F., 693P
Roubicek, J., 667P
Rougeul, A., 105P
Rovner, L., 732P
Royer, J., 106P
Rubino, R., 707P
Rucci, F. S., see Giretti, M. L., 581
Rudolf, N. de M., 709P
Ruskin, A. P., 713P
Rusnac, C., 630P
Sabelli, H. C., 674P
Sager, O., 639P, 656P
Sakakura, H., 687P, 734P
Sala, E., 98P
Saltzberg, B., 730P, 733P
Samarasinghe, H. H. R., 717P
Sament, S., 695P
Samuels, G. M. R., 694P
Santini, M., 545P
Santoni Mendoza, J., 682P
Sasaki, H., 674P
Sasaki, K., 663P
Sato, K., 714P
Satran, S., 694P
Sauer, R., 107P
Saul, R., 660P
Saul, R. E., 690P
Saunders, M. G., 549P, 731P
Sayed, Z. A., 335P
Sayers, A. and Stille, G. A novel method for preparing and implanting brain electrode assemblies in rats, 87
Schaefer, K. P., 619P, 620P
Schain, R. J., see Ellingson, R. J., 191
Scharf, M. B., 710P
Schecter, M. M., see Di Chiro, G., 223
Scheich, H., 626P
Scherzer, E., 212P
Schmalbach, K., 623P, 624P
Schmidt, R. F., 617P
Schmidt, R. P., 649P, 682P
Schmitz, H., 627P
Schneider, F., 630P
Schott, D., 619P
Schuler, G., 548P, 679P
Schulte, F. J., 625P
Schulte, F. J., see Joppich, G., 112
Schwab, R. S., 549P, 731P
Schwartzkroin, P. A., Cowey, A. and Gross, C. G. A test of an "efferent model" of the function of inferotemporal cortex in visual discrimination, 594
Schweitzer, F., 677P
Scibetta, J., 661P
Scott, D. F., 672P
Scott, J., see Wyatt, R. J., 529
Seales, D. M., see McAdam, D. W., 73
Seitun, A., see Casati, C., 289
Semerano, A., 99P
Serbănescu, A., 639P
Sergeeva, L. N., 327P
Serra, C., 720P
Shagass, C., 546P, 662P

SHAHANI, B., 725P
SHANDURINA, A. N., 450P, 697P
SHAPIRO, D. M., 710P
SHAPIRO, D. M., see ITIL, T. M., 76
SHARF, B., 216P
SHARF, M., 216P
SHARP, S., 551P
SHAW, J. C., 673P
SHEPOVALNIKOV, A. N., 451P
SHERRARD, G., 667P
SHERWIN, I., 689P
SHERWOOD, S. L., 730P, 731P
SHIMODA, Y., 668P
SHMATKOV, Y. V., 697P
SHNEIDOROV, V. S., 451P
SHUBIN, H., 653P
SHUGURENSKY, M. D. E., 672P
SHULMAN, E., see FEINBERG, I., 128
SIANI, C., 97P
SIEPRATH, H., 622P
SILIPO, P., 707P
SILVEANU, R. A., 638P
SILVERMAN, D., 549P, 731P
SIMONE, F., 100P
SIMONOVA, O., 627P
SIMONOVA, O., see LEGEWIE, H., 470
SIPOS, C., 656P
SIRIAN, S., 655P
SJOERDSMA, A., see WYATT, R. J., 529
SKORPIL, V., 721P
SKREBITSKY, V. G., 324P, 329P
SLAVOVA, R., 446P
SMIRNOV, V. M., 323P
SMITH, J. C., see NAITOH, P., 2
SNYDER, F., see WYATT, R. J., 529
SOKOLOV, E. N., 644P
SOLOGUB, E. B., 450P
SOMMER-SMITH, J., 103P
SOREL, L., 452P, 655P
SOREL, M. L., 452P
SPECKMAN, E. J., 686P
SPEHLMANN, R., 675P
SPEHLMANN, R. Multi-barreled coaxial micro-pipettes with independent control of the central recording barrel, 201
SPIESS, J., 107P
SPIRA, M., 220P, 221P
SPÎRCHEZ, T., 635P
SPOONER, C. E., see WALLACH, M. B., 563, 574
SPOONER, C. E., see WINTERS, W. D., 514
SPUNDA, C., 212P
STÅLBERG, E., 726P
STÅLBERG, E., see CZEKAJEWSKI, J., 536
STÅLBERG, E., see EKSTEDT, J., 540, 557, 607
STAMM, J. S., 684P
STANCIU, E., 631P
STĂNESCU, B., 635P
STĂNESCU, V., 635P
STANEVA, M., 446P
STARITA, A., 101P
STAROBINETS, M. KH., 329P
STEAN, J. P. B., see LEE, B. B., 610
STEFĂNICĂ-MOTOC, L., 635P, 636P
STEIN, H., 217P
STEINER, F. A., 105P
STEINER, J. E., 220P
STEINMANN, H. W., 626P
STEINWACHS, F., 620P, 679P
STERIADE, M., 678P
STERMAN, M. B., 678P
STERMAN-MARINCHESCU, C., 655P
STERN, J. E., 723P
STERNBERG, M., 677P
STERNBERG, P., 677P
STEVENS, J. R., 544P, 691P
STILLE, G., see SAYERS, A., 87
STOIAN, D., 635P, 636P
STORM VAN LEEUWEN, W., 214P
STRAUMANIS, J. J., 662P
STUMPF, CH., see GOGOLÁK, G., 296
SUBBARAO, V. V., 684P
SUKHOV, A. G., 330P
SULG, I. A., 621P, 676P
SULMAN, F. G., 220P
SUPIN, A. Y., 330P
SUPINO, V., 97P
SUVOROV, N. F., 708P
SUWELACK, K., 627P
SYNDULKO, K., 706P
SZABÓ, L., 633P, 635P
SZÜCS, K., 631P
TACHIBANI, S., 670P
TAESCHLER, M., 104P
TAN, T. L., 710P
TANAKA, K., 668P
TANGUAY, P. E., 686P
TANGUAY, P. E., see ORNITZ, E. M., 387
TARTAGLIONE, A., see CASATI, C., 289
TCHAVDAROV, D., 444P, 445P
TEAGUE, C., ELFERT, J., TIMM, G. and BRADLEY, W. Specular reflectance photometric detection of cortical displacement, 92
TEODORESCU, C., 637P
TERARO, A., 691P
TERBANCEA, M., 630P
TERZI, A., 632P, 635P
TESSITORE, V., 102P
THACORE, V. R., AHMED, M. and OSWALD, I. The EEG in a case of periodic hypersomnia, 605
THIEBAUT, M. S., 109P
THIEFFRY, S., 651P
THOMPSON, R. F., BETTINGER, L. A., BIRCH, H. and GROVES, P. M. Comparison of evoked gross and unit responses in association cortex of waking cat, 146
TIELEN, A. M., 677P
TIMM, G., see TEAGUE, C., 92
TIZARD, J. P. M., 333P
TOENNIES, J. F., 696P
TOKIZANE, T., see ADEY, W. R., 110
TOMAN, J. E. P., 674P
TONALI, P., 101P
TORII, S., 691P
TROHATCHEV, A. I., 698P
TROKHACHEV, A. T., 323P
TRONTELJ, J., 723P
TRUBATCHEV, V. V., 447P
TUDOR, I., 631P
TURCU, T., 636P
TURELLA, C., 700P
TURNER, M., 672P
TZENOV, A., 446P
TZICALOVA, R., 445P
ULETT, G. A., 658P
UNGHER, J., 655P
UNGHER, J., see ROGOZEA, R., 162
URMANCHEEVA, T. G., 331P
URSONIU, C., 630P
USUNOFF, G., 444P

UZGALIS, R., 658P
VACCA, L., 96P
VALLEALA, P., see LEHTINEN, I., 412
VALLI, G., 98P
VAN DER MOST VAN SPIJK, D., 715P
VAN HORN, G., 682P
VAN ROTTERDAM, A., 677P
VAN RIJN, A. J., 678P
VARTANIAN, G. A., 447P
VASILESCU, C., 637P
VASILEVSKY, N. N., 331P
VASSILEVA, B., 446P
VASSILEVSKY, N. N., 447P
VÂTĂ, A., 636P
VATTER, O., 628P
VEITH, J. B., 680P
VEKSHINA, N. L., 324P
VELJKOVIĆ, J., 553P
VERDEAUX, G., 104P
VERDEAUX, J., 105P
VESKOV, R., 554P
VIDART, L., 108P
VISSER, S. L., 215P, 668P
VIVIANI, P., 98P
VLADIMIROVA, G., 446P
VOGEL, P. J., 660P
VOGEL, W., BROVERMAN, D. M., KLAIBER, E. L. and KUN, K. J. EEG response to photic stimulation as a function of cognitive style, 186
VOLANSCHI, D., 637P
VOLAVKA, J., 667P
VOLZ, CH., 625P
VOLZKE, E., 625P
VON BERNUTH, H., see LENARD, H. G., 121
VON WESTERNHAGEN, B., 618P
VORONIN, L. L., 324P, 448P
VORONKOV, G. S., 325P
VUILLON-CACCIUTTOLO, C., 451P
WADA, J. A., 691P
WAGNER, A., 617P, 618P, 702P
WAKIM, K. G., 677P
WALKER, A. E., 643P
WALLACE, J. D., 701P
WALLACH, M. B., WINTERS, W. D., MANDELL, A. J. and SPOONER, C. E. A correlation of EEG, reticular multiple unit activity and gross behavior following various antidepressant agents in the cat. IV, 563
WALLACH, M. B., WINTERS, W. D., MANDELL, A. J. and SPOONER, C. E. Effects of antidepressant drugs on wakefulness and sleep in the cat, 574
WALLACH, M. B., see WINTERS, W. D., 514
WALTER, D. O., 704P, 732P
WALTER, D. O., see BERKHOUT, J., 457
WALTER, R. D., 733P
WALTER, R. D., see ORNITZ, E. M., 195, 387
WALTER, W. G., 645P, 665P
WASSON, S., 545P, 697P
WASZAK, M. and OBRIST, W. D. Relationship of slow potential changes to response speed and motivation in man, 113
WATANABE, S., 720P
WATSON, R. S., see MARSDEN, C. D., 169, 179
WAWERNIA, E., 635P, 639P
WAYLONIS, G. W., 716P
WEIGELDT, H. D., 620P, 679P
WEIL, M. H., 653P
WEINBERG, H., 665P
WEISS, M. S., 690P
WEISSE, Y., 625P
WERMAN, R., 221P
WETZEL, N., 661P
WICKBOM, I., see DI CHIRO, G., 223
WICKE, J. D., 705P
WIEDERHOLT, W. C., 718P
WILCOX, L., 682P
WILCZAK, H., 668P
WILDER, B. J., 682P
WILSON, G. F., 704P
WILSON, W. P., 549P, 550P, 551P, 682P
WINTER, A., 332P
WINTERS, W. D., MORI, K., WALLACH, M. B., MARCUS, R. J. and SPOONER, C. E. Reticular multiple unit activity during a progression of states during a progression of states induced by CNS excitants. III, 514
WINTERS, W. D., see WALLACH, M. B., 563, 574
WOERNER, M. G., 669P
WOODS, J., 548P
WYATT, R. J., ENGELMAN, K., KUPFER, D. J., SCOTT, J., SJOERDSMA, A. and SNYDER, F. Effects of *para*-chlorophenylalanine on sleep in man, 529
WYRWICKA, W., 678P
YAHR, M. D. and PURPURA, D. P. (Editors). Neurophysiological basis of normal and abnormal motor activities. A book review by R. J. GUMNIT, 336
YAKOVLEV, N. M., 447P
YAMAGUCHI, E., 665P
YAMAUCHI, T., 717P
YEAGER, C. L., 687P
YOSHII, N., 671P
YOSHINO, Y., 668P
YOSIPHOV, T., 444P
YOUNG, R. R., 725P
ŻABLOW, L., 726P
ŻAGAMI, M. T., 99P
ŻAKHAROVA, I. N., 325P
ZAKHER, YU. YA., 447P
ZAKS, A., 667P
ŻALIS, A. W., 724P
ŻAPPOLI, R., 96P, 102P, 636P
ŻAREA, L., 636P
ZATTONI, J., 97P, 103P
ŽEŠKOV, P., 553P
ZION, T. E., 549P
ZUCCONI, G., 101P
ZUCKERMANN, E. C., 547P, 682P
ZWART, J. M., 678P
ZWEIZIG, J. R., 732P
ZYSNO, E. A., 623P, 626P

INDEX OF SUBJECTS

VOLUME 27, 1969

(The numbers followed by P refer to abstracts from Society Proceedings)

ALPHA RHYTHM, amplitude and phase, related to rhythmic after-waves to flashes, 695P
— and drugs, 626P
— and expectancy waves, 626P
— and motor activity, 626P
— in eye movements, 548P
— time interval histogram, mode data processing, 668P
ALPHA WAVE, habituation and contingent blocking, 692P
AMBLYOPIA EX ANOPSIA, visual evoked response, 238
AMNESIA, retrograde, experimental, EEG, 212P
ANALYSIS, alpha wave-length, modal, 703P
— beta activity, 212P
— bispectrum, of EEG frequency bands, 693P
— computer, cortical responses, thalamus stimulation, 213P
— computer, on-line, of period–amplitude, 533
— discriminant, in average evoked response studies, 311
— EEG, 730P
— EEG, amplitude histograms, 703P
— EEG, and signal comparator procedure, 628P
— EEG, and simple arithmetic, 665P
— EEG, automatic, and use of Haar function, 682P
— EEG, averaged responses to words and language, 667P
— EEG, computer, 731P
— EEG, determination of sensitivity, 213P
— EEG, digital amplitude and interval, 628P
— EEG, electronic, 621P
— EEG, fields of average velocities-of-change method, 449P
— EEG frequency, 694P
— EEG, in schizophrenia, quantitative, 676P
— EEG, mathematical model of evoked and spontaneous activity, 683P
— EEG, on-line spectral analyser, 729P
— EEG, power spectral, of sleep states in newborns, 690P
— EEG, power spectrum, of higher CNS rhythms, 677P
— EEG, remote spectral and discriminant, 732P
— EEG, spectral, in anoxia, 451P
— EEG, spectral, in coma, 700P
— EEG, spectral, during learning, human, 687P
— EEG, wave length, 702P
— Fourier and aperiodic interval, 627P
— interval, of cerebral vascular processes, in serial studies, 622P
— potentials, by cross correlating EEG and prescribed template, 547P
— sleep stages, by EEG spectra, 704P
— statistical, EEG responses and maturation, 662P
— statistical, spontaneous seizure discharges recorded by radiotelemetry, 691P
ANNOUNCEMENTS, American Board of Qualification in Electroencephalography, 435
— Society for Neuroscience, 421
— Society of Biological Psychiatry, 421
— Third European Symposium on Epilepsy, 224
APNEA, in hypersomnia, classification, 99P
AROUSAL, induced, and post-traumatic coma, 306
AUDITORY evoked potentials after section of brachium, inferior colliculus, 587
— evoked potentials, in children, 195
— evoked potentials, in newborns, 121
— evoked responses, in normal subject, 98P
— responses, and human vigilance, 346
— responses, and partial bilateral fornicotomy, 655P
— responses to mental arithmetic and eye opening, 681P
— stimulation, transmission pathways to anterior sigmoid gyrus, 639P, 656P
— stimuli, reactivity to, 709P
— threshold, and EEG reaction time, 696P
BASAL GANGLIA, caudate nucleus, effects on posterior hypothalamus, 218P
— caudate nucleus, somato-motor effects of stimulation, 99P
— caudate nucleus stimulation, 545P
BEHAVIOR, and L-DOPA, 672P
— disturbances and EEG, 106P
— EEG frequency analysis, in cat, 503
— EEG, in conditioning, in cat, 152
— effects of psychodysleptic drugs, 105P
BEREITSCHAFTSPOTENTIAL, and motivation, 73
BERGER, HANS, work of, 649P
BLOOD FLOW, and EEG, prediction, 676P
BOOK REVIEWS, see *Table of Contents*
BRAIN, developing, time series functions; effects of impoverishment, 733P
— glutamic acid studies, 684P
— nervous processes inertia, 708P
— research in China, 733P
— signal reconstitution, and EEG, 679P
BRAIN-STEM reflexes, visceral modulation, 691P
— reticular excitation, cortical neurons, effects of acetylcholine and atropine, 675P
— reticular formation, cholinergic system, 675P
— splitting, EEG and behavioral changes, in cats, 487
— stimulation, and lateral geniculate body transmission, 547P
CAUDATE NUCLEUS, see BASAL GANGLIA
CEREBRAL ischaemia, and hyperbaric oxygenation, in rabbit, 622P
— responses, in epilepsy, 666P
— responses, vasomotor, to posterior hypothalamus and mesencephalic reticular formation, 655P
— vascular resistance, and EEG, in hyperventilation, 445P
CEREBRAL CORTEX, activity higher than 14 c/sec, 96P
— epileptiform activity and electrical conductivity, 698P
— epileptiform activity, experimental, 331P
— evoked potentials, protracted, and slow auditory stimuli, 665P
— focal epileptiform activity, in rats, 330P
— isoelectric EEG and death, 214P, 215P
— isolated, characteristics, 330P
— isolated, unit activity, 331P
— lithium, effects in manic depression, 670P
— neurons, and acetylcholine and atropine, 675P
— potential shifts during delayed response performance, 684P

— potentials in hepatolenticular degeneration, 425
— prostaglandin release and ECoG, 694P
— responses, and stimulation of urinary bladder receptors, 322P
— responses, interaction of caudate nucleus in evoking, 638P
— responses to interacting stimuli, 680P
— responses to putamen and pallidum stimulation, 663P
— rhythmicity mechanisms, EEG, 330P
— slow evoked responses, amplitude, and temporal features of stimulation, 699P
— slow potential changes, in dogs, 678P
— striate neurons, receptive fields, in waking cats, 674P
— unit activity during sleep cycle in monkeys, 675P
— unit activity, evoked, during sleep cycle in monkeys, 678P

CHILDREN, EEG, abnormal, in 6-year-olds, 544P
— EEG and behavioral disturbances, 106P
— EEG and low birth weight, 692P
— EEG, brain association areas and voluntary activity, 450P
— EEG in lipidosis, 191
— EEG in measles encephalitis, 211P
— EEG in speech disorders, 685P
— EEG, prognostic value in early years, 107P
— EEG sleep states, newborns, 690P
— epilepsy, petit mal, 625P
— epileptic, EEG and information processing, 701P
— evoked responses in newborns, 669P
— head injuries, electrocerebral findings, 626P
— REM sleep, auditory evoked response, 195
— visual evoked response and intelligence, 364
— visual responses to colored light stimulation, 660P

COMA, post-traumatic, induced arousal, 306

CONDITIONED inhibition, and subcortical structures, 708P
— reflex formation and EEG activity, 328P
— reflexes, cortical derivation, 327P

CONDITIONING, operant, of EEG in chimpanzee, 701P

CONDUCTION VELOCITY, see also ELECTROMYOGRAPHY
— in toxic polyneuritis, 637P

CONTINGENT NEGATIVE VARIATION, and attention, 664P
— and epileptic EEG discharges, 662P
— and motor potentials, 706P
— related to response speed and motivation, 113
— separation of phenomena, 108P

CREUTZFELDT-JAKOB DISEASE, and EEG, 217P

DEATH, and EEG, 332P, 549P
— and isoelectric EEG, 214P, 215P

DENDRITES, properties and activities, 645P

DOMINANCE, trace phenomena, 327P

DREAMS, cigarette withdrawal effects, 710P

DRUGS, acetylcholine and reticular formation, 675P
— Acrisuxine, in epilepsy, 106P
— ACTH, in infantile epilepsy, 97P
— aescine, and EEG in intracranial hypertension, 101P
— alcohol and photic potentials, 674P
— amobarbital (Amytal), 707P
— amphetamine, 514
— and red nucleus activity, 296
— and sleep, effectiveness, 710P
— antidepressants and unit activity, 563
— apzofenum, 326P
— atropine, and reticular excitation of cortical neurons, 675P
— 25-azacholesterol, 713P
— benactyzine, 326P
— benzodiazepine, as anticonvulsant, 105P
— benzodiazepines, EEG, 100P
— Cl 581, and EEG, 100P
— *Cannabis sativa* L. (hashish), psychopharmacological activity, 219P
— catechol, 392
— chloralose and chlordiazepoxide HCl in acute experiments, 220P
— chlordelazine, and EEG, in schizophrenia, 633P
— chlordiazepoxide HCl, and chloralose in acute experiments, 220P
— *p*-chlorophenylalanine, 529
— chlorpromazine, 449P
— D-cycloserine, 446P
— D-tubocurarine, 557
— Depakine, in epilepsy, 452P
— diazepam (Valium), and EEG changes, 544P
— diazepam (Valium), deactivation test in epileptics, 661P
— diazepam (Valium), in epilepsy and normals, 429
— diazepam (Valium), in status epilepticus, 218P
— ethotrimeprazine (Ditran), effects on sleep, 554P
— Fluanxol, and EEG, in schizophrenia, 633P
— GABA, effect on orienting reflex, 162
— gamma-hydroxybutyrate, 521
— heroin, 667P
— 5-HTP (5-hydroxytryptophan), 686P
— L-DOPA, 672P
— lithium, 670P
— lithium, and EEG, 656P
— LSD-25, 514
— LSD, and visually evoked responses, 356
— mescaline, 445P, 514
— methadone, 667P
— methohexital, 682P
— methohexitone, in EEG, 333P
— Metrazol, see pentetrazol
— Mogadon, see nitrazepam
— nitrazepam, 103P, 105P, 672P
— noradrenalin, 446P
— Oxypertin, and EEG, in schizophrenia, 633P
— pentetrazol, 514
— pentetrazol, and brain-stem lesions, 404
— pentobarbital, in pinealectomized rats, 220P
— pentylenetetrazol, see pentetrazol
— phencyclidine, 514
— phenobarbital, 105P
— phenothiazine (Perazine), 106P, 687P
— picrotoxin, and ECoG changes, 444P
— psilocybin, effects in baboons, 48
— psychodysleptic, 105P
— psychotropic, 104P
— RO 5-4023, 672P
— RO 5-4023, anticonvulsant properties, 106P
— sedatives, differentiation, 104P
— serotonin, 446P, 674P
— strychnine, 445P
— strychnine, and cell membrane properties, 683P
— strychnine, and cord dorsum potentials, 702P
— trifluoperazine, 449P
— tryptamine, 674P
— Valium, see diazepam
— vincamine, 326P
— W.Y. 3498, 634P

EEG MISCELLANEA, abnormalities, left temporal region focus, 634P
— abnormal, in first-grade children, 544P
— adult, and pre- and perinatal brain damage, 667P
— after cardiac arrest and resuscitation, in babies,

333P
— after cerebral commissurotomy, 660P
— after glucose infusion, in rabbits, 639P
— after lateral hypothalamus ablation, 325P
— after pinealectomy in rats, 220P
— after sleep loss, 2
— analysis, intersensory interaction, 213P
— and anosognosic syndrome, 450P
— and aphasia, 450P
— and arch aortography, 694P
— and blood flow, prediction 676P
— and brain signal reconstitution, 679P
— and brain-stem splitting, 487
— and cardiac arrest, 332P
— and cell metabolism, 326P
— and cerebral blood flow, after strychnine and mescaline, 445P
— and cerebral circulation, 621P
— and cerebral death, 549P
— and cerebral disaster, 332P
— and cerebral vascular occlusions, 622P
— and cognitive style, 186
— and DC potentials, 545P
— and death, 214P, 215P
— and defensive conditioning, in dogs, 327P
— and differential diagnosis in comatose patients, 626P
— and L-DOPA, parenteral, 672P
— and enuresis, 635P
— and epilepsy, adult, 108P
— and evoked cerebral sensory responses, 666P
— and excitatory picture, single-cell study, 618P
— and Graves disease, 633P
— and hepatolenticular degeneration, 425
— and hyperbaric oxygen convulsions, 219P
— and hyperventilation, 445P, 622P
— and hypochondriasis, 624P
— and hypothyreosis, primary, 446P
— and hypoxia, in newborns, 333P
— and hypsarrhythmia, 216P
— and insane murderers, case studies, 335P
— and Kleine-Levin syndrome, 601
— and law (moot trials), 551P
— and lithium, 656P
— and micromotoric tonus regulation, 679P
— and Mogadon, 672P
— and motor conditioned reflex, 328P
— and oral contraceptives, female, 335P
— and penicillin convulsions, 217P
— and reanimation, 629P
— and resuscitation, 623P
— and RO 5-4023, 672P
— and schizophrenia, 633P
— and sensori-motor rhythm in cat, 678P
— and sensory thresholds, 644P
— and serum concentrations in Perazine therapy, 687P
— and single neuron relationships, statistical analysis, 550P
— and sleep, 552P
— and smoking deprivation, 658P
— and stimuli, real and imaginary, 665P
— and task-performance, open and closed eyes, 470
— and thalamo-cortical responses during sleep, 412
— and timing in nervous system, 545P
— and unit activity, after antidepressives, 574
— and ventral amygdaloid complex, 445P
— and verbal activity, 457
— and visual performance, 707P
— and Wilson's disease, 335P
— beta waves, 624P
— changes in open- and closed-eye conditions, 627P
— comparison with rheoencephalography and dyslipidemia test in affective syndromes, late onset, 701P
— computer classifications in sleep, 76
— conditioned reflexes, 326P
— cortical and thalamic evoked activity, during conditioning, 258, 270
— cortical rhythms and motor reaction, 325P
— cortical stimulation and long-term changes, 280
— development in diffuse cerebral vascular and atrophic processes, 622P
— during conditioning, jaw movement, 152
— Ecatox, in accidental poisoning, 630P
— epilepsy, grand mal, inter-seizure activity, 655P
— excitation, in spinal motoneurons and motor cortex cells, 618P
— frequency analysis in group study, 627P
— frequency spectrum and regional cerebral blood flow, correlation, 621P
— human fetal, during birth, 661P
— hyperventilation and pCO_2, 304
— in acute barbiturate intoxication, 695P
— in acute renal insufficiencies, 106P
— in adults, dying and resuscitated, 333P
— in aircraft crews, 629P
— in Alzheimer's disease, 447P
— in amblyopia ex anopsia, 238
— in anovulatory cycles, 216P
— in anoxia, 451P
— in athletes at 5000 m altitude, 638P
— in behavior of cat, frequency analysis, 503
— in bladder stimulation, 322P
— in cerebral arachnoiditis, and clinical correlations, 449P
— in chemical coke plant workers, 630P
— in children of low birth weight, 692P
— in coma, traumatic vigil, 689P
— in "corpus callosum" cats, 619P
— in craniostenosis, 632P
— in Creutzfeldt-Jakob disease, 217P
— in Devic's disease, 549P
— in Down's syndrome, 686P
— in dyskalemia, 106P
— in epilepsy, 680P
— in goiter, endemic juvenile, and acute, 707P
— in hemiparkinsonism, 101P
— in hepatolenticular degeneration, 218P
— in hypernatremia, 106P
— in hypersomnia, periodic, 605
— in hypertension, 636P
— in hypertension, arterial, 660P
— in hypertension, experimental, 337
— in hyponatremia, 106P
— in hypophyseal dwarfism, 635P
— in industrial medicine, 629P
— in "in extremis" conditions, 697P
— in infants, 323P
— in insomnia caused by affective psychosis, 553P
— in intracranial lesions, 12
— in intracranial metastases, 635P
— in measles encephalitis, 211P
— in medico-legal assessment, 630P
— in meningitis, 636P
— in mental retardation, 128
— in metastatic carcinoma, 659P
— in milk drinking, 57
— in neurosurgery, 643P

— in newborns, delivered from mothers with and without anesthesia, 701P
— in post-convulsive coma, 96P
— in psychiatric forensic evaluation, 631P
— in psychiatric patients, 680P
— in psychopharmacology, 104P
— in retrograde amnesia, experimental, 212P
— in schizophrenia, 676P
— in Schwartz-Bartter syndrome, 106P
— in seizure discharges and synaptic potentials of spinal motoneurons, 686P
— in speech disorders, children, 685P
— in Steinert myotonic dystrophy, 635P
— in stomach operations, 635P
— in subacute sclerosing panencephalitis, 550P
— in uremia, 217P
— in vibration sickness, 446P
— in vit. B_{12} deficiency, in baboons, 671P
— in Wilson's disease, 523
— intelligence and average frequency, 480
— mechanisms of origin, 617P
— mental arithmetic and eye opening, 681P
— minimal techniques in suspected cerebral death, 731P
— of striate cortex in blind squirrel monkeys, 734P
— olfactory bulb studies, 661P
— operant conditioning in chimpanzee, 701P
— peak amplitude restriction, 451P
— petit mal-like discharge, adult, 216P
— potentials, with mixed excitatory and inhibitory components, 617P
— power spectrum analysis, 101P
— premature babies, study, 446P
— prognostic value in young children, 107P
— radiotelemetric study, 108P
— reaction time and auditory thresholds correlation, 24-hour recording, 696P
— reanimation and resuscitation, 647P
— responses, in rabbit, 322P
— responses to auditory stimuli in epileptogenic lesions, 102P
— responses to sinusoidally modulated light, 674P
— self-instructional programs, 735P
— sensitivity determination analysis, 213P
— sleep patterns and diencephalic lesions, 551P
— stabilized image visibility, changes, experimental, 248
— statistical method for automatic analysis, 98P
— stimulation of putamen and pallidum, cats, 619P
— striate cortex, blind squirrel monkeys, 687P
— tectum opticum stimulation in decorticate cats, 620P
— treatment of behavioral disturbances, in children, 106P
— visual responses and maturation, in kittens, 692P

EEG PATTERNS MISCELLANEA, and psychoactive drugs, index of clinical activity, 710P
— and "vertical" montage, 655P
— anomalies during anticonvulsive treatment in epilepsy, 631P
— automatic recognition, 628P
— depth spiking, 730P
— 55 c/sec rhythm in olfactory bulb, 709P
— flat, and frequency analysis, 627P
— flattening, and spinal reflex excitability, 622P
— following hemispherectomy, 99P
— 14 and 6/sec spike frequency in psychiatric patients and sibs, 669P
— in juvenile cerebral lipidosis, 191
— isoelectric, and death, 214P, 215P
— latency changes, and noise in auditory vigilance task, 637P
— reticular multiple unit activity, drug-induced, 514
— rhythmic mid-temporal, 43
— 6 and 14/sec spike frequency, and semiological relations, 668P
— slow potential shifts, in hippocampus stimulation, 547P
— slow potentials during movement in normal and neurotic states, 450P
— spike foci, induced, and learning and memory, in monkey, 664P
— spikes and responses to clicks and flashes, 387
— steady potentials during alertness, anesthesia, and sleep, 329P

ELECTROCORTICAL ACTIVITY, and vegetative afferents, 639P

ELECTROCORTICOGRAM, and cerebral cortex prostaglandin release, 694P

ELECTRODES, see TECHNIQUE

ELECTROMYOGRAPHY, anal sphincter, 713P, 716P
— analysis, motor unit activity, 101P
— and carpal tunnel syndrome, 107P
— conduction velocity, in polyneuropathy, 98P
— conduction velocity, in tibial nerve, 98P
— conduction velocity, in ulnar nerve, 98P
— diagnostic, during renal dialysis, 724P
— examination technique, 735P
— frequency analysis, 100P
— in Achilles tendom jerk and ischemic hind-leg rigidity, 717P
— in bronchial carcinoma, nerve conduction, 717P
— in carpal tunnel syndrome, 719P
— in chronic renal insufficiency, 715P
— in facial neuropathy, motor unit frequency, 718P
— in flexion reflex, in spinal man, 721P
— in flexor reflex, human, 725P
— in Friedreich's ataxia, 723P
— in hand surgery, 723P
— in hyperthyroidism, 107P
— in internal medicine, 720P
— in Krabbe's disease (globoid leucodystrophy), 715P
— in Mouchet's syndrome, 98P
— in muscular dystrophy, oculo-pharyngeal, 100P
— in myasthenia gravis, single muscle fiber study, 726P
— in nerve injury, safety, 714P
— in neuromyotonia, 108P
— in ocular myopathy, 99P
— in paralytic brachial neuritis, 722P
— in paramyotonia, hypertrophy of thymus, 101P
— in peroneal nerve distribution, anomalous, 722P
— in reflexes, cutaneous nociceptive, 716P
— in scoliosis, 636P
— in sensory finger innervation, 721P
— in spasticity, 714P, 727P
— in spasticity and rigidity, 719P
— in stomatology, 636P
— in tetany, 212P, 636P
— in thiamine deficiency neuropathy, in rats, 721P
— in vibratory stimulation of muscles, 720P
— logarithmic amplification, 727P
— median nerve conduction variant, 725P
— motor unit action potential, frequency control, 66
— myasthenic response, in diabetic neuropathy, 713P
— myotonia, induced, 713P
— of facial muscle activity in speech, 725P
— of finger tremor, spectrum analysis, 169
— silent period in control of skilled motor perform-

ance, 715P
Electronystagmography, see nystagmus
Electrophysiology, pioneers in, 729P
Electroretinogram, in optic nerve lesions, 217P
— in rat visual cortex, 657P
Encephalophonography, 689P
Epilepsy, audio-motor, atypical EEG, 97P
— "centrencephalic", 545P
— centrencephalic-like discharge and methohexital, 682P
— cerebral evoked responses in, 666P
— Depakine, clinical results in, 452P
— EEG activity and information processing in children, 701P
— EEG and radiotelemetry, 544P
— EEG anomalies during treatment, 631P
— EEG in sleep under painful stimuli, 682P
— EEG responses to intracarotid Amytal, 707P
— evoked potentials, and diazepam, 429
— experimental, conditioned reflex, 96P
— experimental, cyclical spike driving in epileptogenic foci, 673P
— experimental, in kittens, 623P, 624P
— experimental, in monkeys, 89
— induced by movements, 97P
— infantile, EEG and ACTH, 97P
— mechanism of "triggered" manifestations, 444P
— partialis continua, 633P
— penicillin, in man, 631P
— petit mal, 549P
— petit mal, experimental model, 735P
— photosensitive, 683P
— picrotoxin-induced, 444P
— potentials: visual, somato-sensory, and retinal, 373
— sleep, crises during, 553P
— status, diazepam and EEG, 218P
— status, grand mal, inter-seizure EEG activity, 655P
— status, petit mal, 218P
— status, petit mal, in children, 625P
— status, psychomotor, 211P
— temporal lobe, and chronically implanted depth electrodes, 733P
— temporal lobe, and low voltage fast activity (interictal), 693P
— temporal lobe lesions, and conditioned responses, 102P
— treatment, see drugs
— Unverricht-Lundborg myoclonic, 211P
— visual evoked potentials, 628P
— visual evoked response, variability, 702P
Errata, 754
Evoked potentials, and acute epileptogenic focus, cat, 444P
— and background activity, 548P, 690P
— and trifluoperazine, in psychotics, 449P
— auditory, see auditory
— average, deviant, classification, 700P
— chlorpromazine, in psychotics, 449P
— during conditioning, 103P
— from electrolyte alterations, in dogs, 677P
— function of stimulus information content in expectancy–reaction time situation, 705P
— in newborns, 669P
— linear and non-linear properties, 677P
— variability, intra- and inter-individual, in normal and chronic schizophrenic subjects, 688P
— visual, see visual
Exhibitionism, and temporal lobe seizures, 550P
Eye, movements and eyeblink potentials, scalp distribution, 546P
— movements, EEG, and task performance, 470
Gammaencephalography, in cerebral tumor diagnosis, 632P
Genetics, of photosensitivity, 625P
Graves disease, and EEG, 633P
Head injuries, electrocerebral findings, in children, 626P
Hemispherectomy, EEG, 99P
Hepatolenticular degeneration, and cortical evoked potentials, 425
Hypersomnia, classification, 99P
Hypertension, and EEG, 636P
Hyperventilation, EEG and cerebral vascular resistance, 445P
— pCO_2 and EEG, 304
Hypophyseal dwarsfism, and EEG, 635P
Hypothalamus, blood serotonin titre changes, in rabbits, 324P
— influence on spinal cord potentials, 323P
— lateral, EEG after ablation, 325P
— posterior, caudate n. effects, 218P
— posterior, effects of extrahypothalamic structures on single cell activity, 219P
— somato-motor effects of stimulation, in cats, 99P
Hypothyroidism, CNS effects, 624P
Hypoxia, and EEG in newborns, 333P
Hypsarrhythmia, and EEG, 216P
— in children, 625P
Intoxication, acute barbiturate, and EEG, 695P
— lead, subclinical, EMG study, 718P
Kleine-Levin syndrome, and EEG, 601
Law, and clinical electroencephalography, 551P
Learning, effects of induced spike foci, in monkey, 664P
Leukoencephalitis, van Bogaert's subacute, electroclinical considerations, 633P
Meningitis, and EEG, 636P
Methods, see technique
Micro-electrode study, brain-stem neurons, caloric stimuli and drugs effects, 97P
— cell firing and inhibition, in cat cortex, 709P
— cortical single neurons, in baboon, 708P
— glial cells and neurons, slow changes in membrane potentials after nerve impulses, 702P
— interneurons, in thalamic relay nucleus, 696P
— neuronal mechanisms, temporary connection, 447P
— neuron responses in rabbit cortex, 324P
— neurons, trace effects of stimulation, 448P
— picrotoxin epileptic seizure, 444P
— potentials in spinal motor neurons, correlations, 447P
— red nucleus activity, drugs, 296
Motoneurons, human single, latency variation in H reflex, 723P
— spinal, and CO_2 pressure, 618P
— spinal, and excitation, 618P
— spinal, excitability in hemiplegia, 723P
Mouchet's syndrome, EMG, 98P
Muscle, evoked responses, in nerve lesions, 98P
— resting membrane potential and local temperature, 718P
— skeletal, connections between fibers, 607
— tone control, 713P
Mutism, akinetic, after cerebral contusion, 631P
Nerve, conduction in Friedreich's ataxia, 723P
— conduction velocity and threshold in human median sensory fibers, 718P
— dendritic, effects of Ca^{2+} and Mg^{2+}, 328P
— lesions, and evoked muscular responses, 98P

— mechanism, of conditioned lever-pressing, in dog, 671P
— peripheral nerve regeneration and muscle receptor reconstruction, 720P
— posterior tibial, conduction velocity, 717P
— ventral, giant axons in cockroach, 220P, 221P

NEUROPHYSIOLOGY, clinical, and neurological practice, 649P
— clinical, evolution, 648P
— clinical, future, 645P
— clinical, survey of use of services (in Marseilles, France), 643P
— clinical, discussion of value, 651P

NYSTAGMUS, electronystagmography, binocular and monocular derivations, 109P
— electronystagmography, optokinetic reaction, disturbances, 212P
— optokinetic and vestibular ear, in rabbits, 619P
— vestibular habituation in pendular test, 109P

OLFACTORY BULB, see also RHINENCEPHALON
— ablation, in rats, 102P

ONTOGENESIS, and instinctive inhibition, 327P

OPTIC, cortex, activity modulation by non-visual stimuli, 329P
— optokinetic reaction and nystagmography, 212P

OXYGEN, availability in brain during mental activity, 698P
— availability in human deep cerebral structures, 448P

PARKINSON'S DISEASE, biochemical systems and pathological responses, 697P

PENICILLIN, convulsions, and EEG, 217P

PHENYLKETONURIA, polygraphic recording, 625P

PHOTIC STIMULATION, and EEG in two-flash discrimination task, in cat, 706P
— and orbicularis oculi muscle contractions (photopalpebral reflex), 665P
— EEG and cognitive style, 186
— in hemiparkinsonism, 101P
— Mogadon and responses, 103P
— responses in human subcortex, 550P

PHOTOSENSITIVITY, and genetics, 625P

PSYCHIATRY, EEG, and insane murderers, case studies, 335P

REFLEX, orienting, effect of GABA, 162
— orienting, in newborns, 327P

RESUSCITATION, and EEG, 647P

RHEOENCEPHALOGRAM, in medico-aeronautical expertise, 630P
— in stomach operations, 635P

RHINENCEPHALON, amygdala, ventral, and EEG, 445P
— amygdalo-hippocampal complex activity and induced depression, 637P
— hippocampal neurons, extracellular dendritic fields, and unit activity during induced epileptogenesis, 682P
— hippocampal regional activity, 659P
— hippocampal stimulat on, anatomical substrates, 547P
— hippocampal stimulation and slow potential shifts, 547P
— hippocampal stimulation, effect on unit activity of hypothalamic, preoptic and basal forebrain areas, 686P
— hippocampal theta rhythm, in learning rat, 663P

SEIZURES, hyperoxic, and body temperature, 581
— Metrazol-induced, and brain-stem lesions, 404
— photosensitive, and patient self-desensitization, 691P
— temporal lobe, 550P

SENSORY, focal, attack, 624P
— -motor rhythm and EEG, in cat, 678P
— nerve action potentials, 714P
— somatic, information transfer and processing, peripheral nerve, 654P
— somatic, information transfer and processing, peripheral receptors, 650P
— somatic, information transfer and processing, spinal cord, 646P, 650P
— somatic, recovery functions and television viewing, 662P
— somatic responses, in deep sleep, 289
— somatic responses, in epilepsy, 373
— somatic responses, temporal and spatial summation, 688P
— somatic responses to tendon taps in normal and neurologic adults, 669P

SKIN stimulation and sensation during CNS stimulation, 657P

SLEEP, amino acids in brain of sleep-deprived cats, 554P
— and alertness, steady potentials, 329P
— and auditory response, in children, 195
— and cerebral ammonia metabolism, 637P
— and EEG, in enuresis, 635P
— and EEG, in neonates, 625P
— and EEG, serial, 422
— and erection, periodicity, 626P
— and heart rate, 626P
— and malnutrition, 681P
— and memory in slow and REM stages, 668P
— and spinal reflex activity, 553P
— antidepressives, effects in cat, 574
— cigarette withdrawal, effects on pattern, 710P
— computer classification, effects of tranquilizers, and REM, 658P
— deprivation and glycogenic response, 552P
— EEG activity after deprivation, 2
— EEG activity in epilepsy with painful stimuli, 682P
— EEG analysis in newborns, 690P
— EEG, and peak amplitude restriction, 451
— EEG, and subjective estimates, 333P
— EEG, computer classifications, 76
— EEG in cortex of waking cat, 146
— EEG in infants, 323P
— EEG in intracranial lesions, 12
— EEG in mental retardation, 128
— EEG in 24-hour cycles, 101P
— EEG patterns in Down's syndrome, 686P
— effects of drugs in inducing and maintaining, 710P
— electrogenesis, 553P
— epileptic crises, 553P
— evoked neuronal discharges in monkey cortices, 678P
— in automatism, nocturnal ambulatory, 633P
— in depression, 99P, 659P
— in ischemic cerebrovascular disease, EEG and EMG, 656P
— in schizophrenic patients, 553P
— histamine as waking factor, 107P
— mechanisms, 552P
— narcolepsy, disturbances in rhythm, 553P
— pharmacological changes, 105P
— phases, EEG, 697P
— REM deprivation and serum growth hormone levels, human, 685P
— REM onset, normal, 685P
— responses, thalamo-cortical, and EEG, 412
— somato-sensory system, functional changes, 289

— spectral analysis, in apallic syndrome, 554P
— unit activity, in monkey cortex, 675P
SOCIETY PROCEEDINGS, Austrian, Vienna (November 1967), 211
— Belgian, Brussels (November 1968), 451
— Bulgarian, Sofia (February 1968), 444
— Eastern (U.S.A.), New York (December 1968), 544
— English, London (October 1968), 332
— French-speaking countries, Basel (October 1968), 104
— German, Münster (June 1968), 617
— International, San Diego (September 1969), 641
— Israel, Jerusalem (May 1968), 216
— Italian, Turin (May 1968), 96
— Netherlands, Utrecht (November 1968), 214
— Rumanian, Bucharest (December 1968), 629
— Southern (U.S.A.), Birmingham (October 1968), 549
— Swiss, Basel (October 1968), 104
— U.S.S.R. Moscow–Leningrad (September–March 1968), 447
— U.S.S.R. review of papers (January–June 1967), 322
— Yugoslavia, Zagreb (October 1968), 552
SOVIET PAPERS, see SOCIETY PROCEEDINGS
SPLIT CHIASMA, visual responses, 142
TECHNIQUE, analysis, computer: expectancy, readiness, orienting potentials, 214P
— analysis in average evoked response studies, 311
— analysis, multichannel, of averaged evoked potentials, 671P
— analysis of adaptive autonomic regulation, 102P
— automated, for hemodynamic measurements, 653P
— averaging, in sensory conduction in peroneal, posterior tibial, and sural nerves, 726P
— biopotential analog, 548P
— cerebral impedography, in cat, rabbit, and cadaver, 670P
— computer analysis, neuro-myoelectric data, 100P
— computer calculation, two targets trajectory and electrode point position in brain penetration, 729P, 730P
— computer, digital, classifications of EEG sleep stages, 76
— computer, on-line full text retrieval, Epilepsy Abstracts, 734P
— digitizer, sixteen-channel wave pattern, 681P
— EEG, and micromotor tone recording, 620P
— EEG, computer audiometry, 212P
— EEG, computer interpolation and area display, 546P
— EEG, conversion of ink-tracings to analog electrical form, 732P
— EEG, determination of sensitivity, 213P
— EEG, feedback method, 688P
— EEG, interval spectrum analyzer, 696P
— EEG, moving topological display, 658P
— EEG, newborn, method for detecting change in time series, 436
— EEG, perpendicular referential montages, 452P
— EEG, radiotelemetry, 544P
— EEG, radiotelemetry, dynamic aspects, 225
— EEG, routine long-distance telephone transmission, 730P
— EEG, topography, simultaneous on-line analysis, 673P
— EEG, with micro-electrodes in primary acoustic areas, 639P
— electrode, lingual sensitivity, 440
— electrode assemblies, brain, in rats, 87
— electrodes, sterile, implantation, 442
— EMG audio-visual feedback, and voluntary motor unit control, 724P
— generator, binary sequence, for testing low frequency-wave analysers, 334P
— grand mal seizure, and high frequency recording, 697P
— micro-electrode tip position, marking, dye method, 610
— micro-electrodes, multiple movable, chronic implantation, 205
— micro-pipettes, multi-barreled coaxial, 201
— monitoring device, continuous, for cerebral activity, 672P
— needle multi-electrodes (for single fiber EMG), 540
— neuro- and myostimulator, with impulse memory, 638P
— oscilloscopic recording, muscle fiber action potentials, 536
— photometric detection, cortical displacement, 92
— polygraphy and stabilized medullary lesions, 706P
— radiotelemetry, dynamic aspects, human EEG, 108P
— radiotelemetry, of spontaneous seizure discharges, 691P
— residual noise, average evoked potentials, 315
— stereotaxic frame assembly for cat auditory system investigation, 614
— stimulation, transdermal, 733P
— swivel, printed circuit, for freely moving animals, 209
— synaptic transmission, method for study, 557
— telemetry, of physiological data, 628P
— video-tape control gate for recording motor seizures, 98P
— Z-axis modulation, neural spike display, 199
THALAMUS, computer analysis, cortical responses to stimulation, 213P
— somatic representation, 709P
— stimulation and synaptic effects, 546P
TRANSMISSION, neuro-muscular synapse, regulation, 219P
TREMOR, relation between two hands, 179
— variations, changes with age, 169
UCLA BRAIN INFORMATION SERVICE, 730P
VESTIBULAR stimulation, caloric, polygraphic investigation of reactivity, 638P
— stimulation, motor, EEG, and vegetative reactivity, 632P
VISUAL, amblyopia ex anopsia, cerebral evoked potentials, 238
— average response, in cerebrovascular disease, 23
— cortical responses, Mogadon, 103P
— discrimination, model of inferotemporal cortical function, 594
— evoked potentials, in epilepsy, 628P
— evoked potentials, in rat visual cortex, 657P
— performance, and EEG, 707P
— response, and intelligence, in children, 364
— response dispersion curve, and cerebral stochastic and deterministic mechanisms, 699P
— response, effect of LSD, 356
— response in epilepsy, 373
— response, recorded from scalp, 97P
— responses, and electrolyte alterations, in dogs, 677P
— responses, and pattern reversal, 732P
— responses, binocular addition, with different stimulus intensities, 663P
— responses, dichoptic interaction in split chiasma, 142

— responses, EEG, and maturation, 692P
— responses, harmonics, 352P
— responses in amblyopia ex anopsia, 238
— responses in normal, acallosal, and split-brain patients, 690P
— responses in psychiatric and epileptic patients, 680P
— responses, inter- and intra-hemispheric interactions, 705P
— responses, normative data, 35
— responses, to colored light, in infants and children, 660P
— responses, with modified pupillary diameter, 84

ERRATA

Electroenceph. clin. Neurophysiol., **1969,** *27*: 641–736

p. 659, art. 14: Read "Guadalajara" instead of "Mexico City".
p. 682, art. 80: The author's name should read "J. Santoni Mendoza".